# What People are Saying About the World's Healthiest Foods

*Your book has EXCEEDED my expectations. Healthy recipes, scientific information, colorful charts/pictures, and most importantly, it is written so that everyone can understand what this book has to offer. — Frank*

*Just received my copy of your book and I am blown away with the information. This has to be the most practical, easy to understand manual I have read. Love the quick, easy to make recipes! — MC*

*What a spectacular resource! Thank you for your life-long mission to promote good health and, most importantly, for sharing this information with the world! — Gail*

*What an incredible tour de force! Your book is exactly what I have been looking for—all the healthy ingredients and their amounts listed, the good and bad fish, plus how to best prepare the foods, allergic reactions, and so much more. This is an extraordinary accomplishment, and you are to be highly lauded for such a feat. I stayed up until 3:00 a.m. reading it the other night. Again, this is a fabulous book. You have done a great service to the world with this information all in one book. — Georgia*

*What a gem of a book!! Thank you so much for this comprehensive resource! For a registered dietitian this is a dream to have all of this wonderful information in one place. I so appreciate this informative and inspiring manual. Thank you for your important work. — Suzanne*

*I have been in the book business for 18 years and this is exactly the type of book I am asked about time and time again. George Mateljan's book The World's Healthiest Foods is a must-have read for anyone wanting to eat healthier. It's outstanding. — Kris*

*I received my copy of your new book the other day and I could not believe the quality and the wealth of information that is on all of those pages. This is one book that is definitely going to make great changes, for the better, in people's lives. I have never seen any other book like this one and I don't think I ever will. Thank you so much for your dedication. — Lena*

*Every home, nutritionist and healthcare professional should have this book. This is the best book! — Deebi*

*I love your book. So complete and the information is so reliable, not a bunch of hype. You are really doing a tremendous service. Too bad all the world's people can't know the world's healthiest foods through your book. I am personally indebted to you for all the information I have gotten from your website and now the book. — Tana*

*I purchased your book, and I love it, I love it, I love it. I'm sure you've heard this many times, but George you saved my life. By following your book for almost a month now the digestion difficulties I had were no more. Now, I eat to live, not live to eat, and cherish the importance of healthy foods entering my body. Please continue with your work because it's absolutely fantastic, straight-forward, and realistic. — Hala*

*Congratulations! This was a huge undertaking and it is a great accomplishment to organize so much information into one book. You have truly accomplished the balance between a practical and scientific approach to healthy eating. It contains an unbelievable amount of beneficial information that covers all of the most important aspects of today's Healthiest Way of Eating. This book is one of a kind—an encyclopedia of healthy foods and practical guide for anyone who is trying to improve the way they eat. In one word: BRAVO! Thank you for everything you have done in the past and for how you are inspiring others to not only improve their individual health but to contribute to the health of the whole world. — Zlatko*

*I am in thrilled receipt of your great new book. I have been wanting for years to have something at hand for daily use and now have it to guide me through my daily healthy meal planning. You have provided to knowledge of healing foods. So thanks, George, for being a true philanthropist by helping people to help themselves. There's plenty of "information" on the WEB but you provide information that one can absolutely trust. — Sheila*

*I have been totally engrossed in your new book. From the first time I opened the book I began to learn so many new things. I love the section "The Healthiest Way of Cooking" for each food item. The information on garlic and olives alone was enough to convince me that this essential guide for the healthiest way of eating was worth my investment. This book is beautifully designed, easy to read, and packed full of valuable information. You have my deepest appreciation for working so hard to create this valuable resource. I will use it daily. I will also spread the word to my friends and family about your web site and book. — Jeff*

*Your book is awesome! I am still enjoying reading it; it's like a food Bible, with all the wealth of information it contains. I read a large part of it and must say I really enjoyed the learning experience. So much about oils, organic vegetables, ATP and use of energy... It should be nominated for a book of the decade. — Gasper*

*I just purchased my 6th WHF book (for family & friends). I continue to be very grateful for all your great work. Our country clearly needs to learn to make healthier nutritional choices—either we spend more money on quality food choices (still cheaper than eating out), or we will likely pay in the long run (health care costs). Thanks again—you obviously are really making a difference!! — Lynn*

*I have been reviewing your book and there is so much beneficial information, it's just incredible. What a tremendous amount of effort that will benefit so many people! — Nikki*

*I'm finding it to be an excellent resource for nutritional information, and it is giving me the added benefit of making much better food choices! It's very thorough, containing great recipes and tips from weight loss to food preparation. By having a working knowledge of the beneficial properties that each food has, I find that it's just that much more challenging to put together foods or complete meals that contain the greatest amount of healthy things (vitamins, minerals, etc.). It covers what foods are good for certain medical conditions, what to eat more of to counteract illnesses and so forth. I cannot be without this book now! — Corey*

*I can always count on your unbiased opinions and insights to get me through any doubts or fears. "When in doubt, check with George." You are simply the best out there, period! — Marybeth*

*Thanks so much for giving such important life-supporting information to the world. — Kerry*

*I always thought it was hard to eat right. There was simply too much info out there geared toward all of the ineffective aspects of human nature. People trying to trick the system or do some crazy magic. By reading the World's Healthiest Foods, I have learned so much, and I am much better off now than I ever was. Great info, techniques, recipes, everything here can help anyone who wants to be helped. Fantastic job. — Patrick*

*I am 40+ community college professor. For virtually all of my adult life I've been trying to lose weight, cut down on fatty foods and eat healthily—but without much success. As I worked my way through the stock of information something clicked on in my brain: This is it! This is the grand design in the nutritional cosmos. This is the way I must go. This is the light among the tunnels of information available. Your approach to helping people find and lead a healthy lifestyle through eating WHFoods surpasses all that I've ever purchased and read about. I've been researching and preparing meals based upon WHFoods for the past month. I feel far more alive, alert, enlightened and energized. I now experience greater degrees of balance, equilibrium, sound sleep and no more mood swings. I and my family are forever blessed for discovering this treasure trove of nutritional wisdom. — Michelle*

*Five of my closest friends are eating the World's Healthiest Foods and after 3 days, we really are noticing some big changes, like how much ENERGY we have first thing in the morning!! Your information is very helpful and just makes good basic sense!—Amy*

*Thank you so much for providing this information. In the past few years, I have been doing everything I can to eat healthy and provide healthy meals for my family. With the help of the World's Healthiest Foods, I can know much more about the specific nutrients that are within the whole foods that we are consuming.—Carole*

*I have had high cholesterol levels for years. For a year or so I have been studying the information on your site and adjusting my diet. A few days ago my doctor called me with the lab results—healthier in all areas! And my high cholesterol was down about 50 points. The doctor told me my diet practices have paid off! Your brilliant site is an ever-updated, research-supported, and rewarding resource. Thank you so much.—SM*

*The World's Healthiest Foods are the*
*true expression of vibrant health and energy.*

George Mateljan

# the world's
# healthiest
# foods

## ESSENTIAL GUIDE
## for the Healthiest Way of Eating

# GEORGE MATELJAN

**Winner of the National "Best Books" 2007 Awards**

The World's Healthiest Foods is the winner of the **National "Best Books" 2007 Awards** in the category of Natural Foods and Cooking. One of the largest literary competitions in the United States, the National "Best Book" Awards highlight fantastic books published each year.

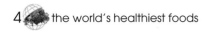
PHOTOGRAPHS BY: *Tenji Cowan*

George Mateljan Foundation
PO Box 25801
Seattle, Washington 98125-1301

book@whfoods.org

This book is for educational purposes only. It is not intended as a substitute for medical advice. Please consult a qualified health care professional for individual health and medical advice. Neither George Mateljan nor the George Mateljan Foundation shall have responsibility for adverse effects arising directly or indirectly as a result of the information provided in this book.

Library of Congress Cataloging-in-Publication Data
ISBN 09-76918544-53995

**The World's Healthiest Foods**
*Essential Guide for The Healthiest Way of Eating*
1st Edition

Science consulting provided by Buck Levin, PhD.

Printed in Canada on acid-free paper.

**How to Order:**  Single copies may be ordered from the whfoods.org website.

# FROM GEORGE MATELJAN

We are entering an exciting new era—an era where the "Healthiest Way of Eating" will be enjoyed by more people, an era in which we will take more personal responsibility for our own health because we realize that this is the way to achieve a lifetime of vibrant health and energy. The emphasis will be placed on enjoying health-promoting foods, which play a major role in keeping your body and mind functioning at their peak. We now know that health, reaching an ideal weight and youthful aging are not just a matter of luck. We can optimize our genetic potential for health every time we eat. We know enough about the messages that specific foods deliver to begin unlocking our genetic health potential right now.

It has long been my strong belief that our future health belongs to selecting and preparing foods that contain the greatest number of health-promoting nutrients. The focus of this book is to answer your questions about what foods are best for the "Healthiest Way of Eating." The World's Healthiest Foods are 100 foods that you can rely on as the foundation of your "Healthiest Way of Eating" because they are known for their nutrient-richness. They are among the best foods to provide you with 100% of all the nutrients—vitamin, minerals, antioxidants and many others—that you need everyday. They are also some of the most flavorful foods in the world.

Scientific evidence is now supporting the fact that only nutrient-rich foods, such as the World's Healthiest Foods, can provide you with all the nutrients you need to promote health. This is because nutrients don't work in isolation but synergistically. The synergy between these nutrients found in the World's Healthiest Foods plays a major role in the expression of our genes, and therefore our appearance, overall health and longevity. I am also now seeing that eating for better health is also the best avenue to achieve an ideal weight.

Since I have experienced firsthand the vibrant health and energy that comes with eating the World's Healthiest Foods, I want to share with you how easily you can incorporate the World's Healthiest Foods as a regular part of your diet by following the "Healthiest Way of Eating Plan."

While writing this book, I also tried to keep in mind how preparing the World's Healthiest Foods could fit into the today's busy lifestyles. Since most of us don't have hours, but usually only minutes, to prepare our food, this book shares with you 500 healthy Mediterranean-flavored recipes in a matter of minutes, many of which you can make in 7 minutes or less—and you can even make a "Dinner for Two in Just 15 Minutes!"

With this book you can easily discover how the nutrient-rich World's Healthiest Foods will solve your quest for the "Healthiest Way of Eating." I wish you the many joys this delicious Mediterranean-style of eating can bring to your life.

Dedicated to help make a healthier world.


George Mateljan

Books by George Mateljan:

Cooking Without Fat

Baking Without Fat

Healthy Living Cuisine

Healthier Eating Guide

Natural Foods Cookbook

## special note to the owner of the world's healthiest foods book:

To thank you for purchasing this book and for your interest in the "Healthiest Way of Eating," I want to present you with three special privileges and services, exclusively for you:

- A free video featuring George Mateljan sharing with you how to make a "5-Course Meal in 15 Minutes" as well as tips on selecting and storing foods, "Healthiest Way of Cooking" techniques and more. The regular price of this video DVD is $15.95.

- Personal answers to any further questions you may have about topics covered in this book, including the World's Healthiest Foods, "Healthiest Way of Eating" and "Healthiest Way of Cooking."

- A free guide, *How To Create a "Healthiest Way of Eating" Group*, which will show you how to create a healthy evening of eating with family and friends.

To access these special privileges, go to www.whfoods.org/privileges and then type in the promotional code **nutrient-rich foods**. Not only will this website offer these three features designed for owners of *The World's Healthiest Foods, Essential Guide for the Healthiest Way of Eating* but it will also be continually updated with special offers, announcements and other information related to the World's Healthiest Foods, "Healthiest Way of Eating" and "Healthiest Way of Cooking."

# contents

**PART 6**    **Biochemical Individuality**                 **717**

This chapter describes how foods affect individuals
differently and helps you determine which foods
are best for you. It addresses such topics as food allergies,
gluten intolerance, lactose intolerance, nightshades,
oxalates, purines and other food constituents that may
be of concern to certain individuals.

**PART 7**    **Health-Promoting Nutrients from the**
**World's Healthiest Foods**                               **733**

Over 30 chapters on nutrients—from antioxidants to zinc,
including information about what foods are the most
concentrated source of each individual nutrient.

**The World's Healthiest Foods'**
**Quality Rating System Methodology**        **805**

**Healing with the World's Healthiest Foods**   **807**

In this section of the book, you'll find an overview of
21 health-related topics—including colds and flu,
fatigue, hair and nail health, skin health, vision health,
memory and others—and what to eat, and what to avoid,
if you are trying to enhance your health in these areas.

**Food Sensitivity Elimination Plan**           **821**

Helps you identify which foods may be problematic
for you and helps you determine if you have
undiagnosed sensitivities to food.

# How to Benefit Most From This Book

The first and most important way to benefit from this book is to familiarize yourself with the World's Healthiest Foods. On page 21, you will find the **Nutrient-Richness Chart**, which presents a list of the foods in order of their nutrient-richness, a reflection of their nutritional value in relation to their caloric content. Nutrient-richness is the primary criteria I used in the selection of the World's Healthiest Foods because their concentration of nutrients is your assurance that the foods you eat will provide you with the foundation of optimal health. (For more on nutrient-richness, see pages 24 and 805.)

Beginning on page 11, you will find a list of over **500 delicious Mediterranean-style recipes** that will help you include the World's Healthiest Foods in your "Healthiest Way of Eating." Rather than one chapter dedicated to recipes, you will find the recipes—including "Flavor Tips" and "Quick Serving Ideas"—featuring specific World's Healthiest Foods in each of the individual food chapters along with color photographs. If you want to learn more about the "Healthiest Way of Cooking" the World's Healthiest Foods, see page 45.

The **"Healthiest Way of Eating" Plan** on page 29 is an easy-to-follow guide that will help you to jumpstart your "Healthiest Way of Eating." It takes the guesswork out of how to begin incorporating the World's Healthiest Foods into your lifestyle by providing you with four weeks' worth of menus. After four weeks on the Plan, you're likely to feel the benefits of enhanced vitality and wellness. It is also a healthy way to lose weight that works, if that is your goal. The Plan and the World's Healthiest Foods are great ways to boost your immune system, fight free radicals, curtail inflammation and support a healthy heart.

If you want information about how to select the safest and most environmentally-sustainable fish and shellfish, see the **Fish & Shellfish Guide** on page 457. It provides information on the sustainability rating, omega-3 fatty acid content and mercury level of many different varieties of seafood.

Because we all have different needs when it comes to health, the section on **Biochemical Individuality**, starting on page 717, will provide you with information on compounds such as oxalates, purines and sulfites, that may be difficult for some individuals to tolerate. Also included in this section is information on food allergies and intolerances.

If you are looking for the foods that are the most concentrated source of specific nutrients (such as calcium, iron and B vitamins) that you need for optimal health, the charts found in each of the individual **Health-Promoting Nutrient** chapters, starting on page 733, will help you determine which foods are the best for you. These chapters also include an extensive review of information relating to each nutrient including how it promotes health, deficiency causes and symptoms, public health recommendations and more. Information about what nutrients we need and why we need them can be found on page 71 in the section on **Eating for Healthier Cells**.

For information about **Healing with the World's Healthiest Foods**, see page 807.

On page 821, you will find information about the **Food Sensitivity Elimination Plan**. I believe every person should read this section because people often do not realize that the food they eat can be the source of many of their everyday health concerns.

To make it even easier for you to select the World's Healthiest Foods, I have included a **Shopping List** on page 879 and 880 that you can copy and use when you go to the market.

You will also find **Q+As** throughout the book. These are answers to questions submitted by readers of the whfoods.org website. I've included them since they may help to answer questions that you have about food, nutrition and healthy cooking. A list of Questions of Interest can be found on page 17.

I have organized this book so that it is very easy to use. My recommendation for the best way to benefit from this book is to start by reading about five or six of your favorite foods. This will familiarize you with how the chapters are organized and what is covered in each of the food chapters. You can use this as a reference book. The World's Healthiest Foods chapters start on page 83. Enjoy!

# Acknowledgments

This book could not have been written without the dedication and hard work of a number of individuals who believe in the benefits of the "Healthiest Way of Eating." It is because of the hard work, extensive knowledge and energy of those researching the World's Healthiest Foods that I could compile and present you with the most accurate and up-to-date information about these foods. Others spent thousands of hours working with me to develop, test and perfect the recipes to ensure that they were not only nutrient-rich and had wonderful flavor, but could be prepared in a minimal amount of time.

I want to acknowledge these people and thank them for their many contributions.

**Tenji Cowan**, who worked with me and contributed in every aspect of the book, including researching, editing, photographing the foods and recipes, and acting as coordinator.

**Stephanie Dara Gailing**, M.S., who worked as a writer and editor and was not only indispensable in providing her background in and knowledge of nutrition education but also her ever-present enthusiasm for this project.

**Joelle Chizmar** (Hartman Group), who designed this book and made it as easy to read as it is attractive.

**Janet Cooper**, for her work on the recipe tips and **Tyua Sereda**, for editing the recipes.

**Rosemary Widener**, has "worked her magic wand" with the typography and the pagination of the book.

**Salugenecists, Inc.,** provided and organized the scientific studies and information about the World's Healthiest Foods and their benefits. Thanks to:

**Dr. Joseph Pizzorno**, President

**Buck Levin**, Ph.D., R.D., Nutrition and Food Expert

**Lara Pizzorno**, M.A.(Lit), L.M.T., M.A.(Div.), Health and Nutrition Specialist, Writer and Editor

**Gary Wehe** and **Terry Taketa**, for their various contributions.

# WORLD'S HEALTHIEST FOODS RECIPE LIST

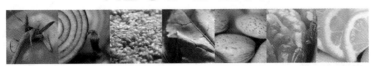

❖Recipes Requiring
No Cooking
* Photo / Recipe Page

## VEGETABLES AND SALADS

### SPINACH
❖Spinach Salad 102
❖Wilted Mediterranean
Spinach Salad 102
❖Citrus Spinach Salad 102
*1-Minute "Quick Boiled" Spinach 103
Creamy Curry Spinach 103

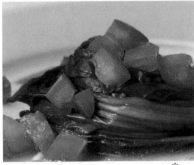
*103

### SWISS CHARD
3-Minute "Quick Boiled"
Swiss Chard 111
Zorba the Greek Swiss Chard 111
Swiss Chard Lasagna 111

### CRIMINI MUSHROOM
5-Minute "Healthy
Sautéed" Crimini Mushrooms 119
Quick Mushroom Stroganoff 119
Crimini Mushroom Sauce 119

### ASPARAGUS
❖Marinated Asparagus Salad 124
5-Minute "Healthy Sautéed"
Asparagus 125
Asparagus with Dijon Caper Sauce 125
*"Healthy Sautéed" Asparagus with
Seafood 125
❖Cold Asparagus Salad 125

### BROCCOLI
❖Chopped Broccoli Salad 132
5-Minute "Healthy
Steamed" Broccoli 133
Asian Flavored Broccoli with Tofu 133
Broccoli with Mustard Tarragon Sauce 133
5-Minute Mediterranean Medley 133

### ROMAINE LETTUCE
❖10-Minute Romaine Salad 139
❖Romaine Turkey Salad 139
❖Spicy Caesar Dressing 139

### SALADS AND SALAD DRESSINGS
❖5-Minute Green Salad with Healthy
Vinaigrette 143
Variations for Healthy Vinaigrette 143
❖Quick and Healthy Caesar Salad 144
❖Greek Salad 144
❖Niçoise Salad 144
❖Waldorf Salad 144
❖Tomato Mozzarella Salad 144
❖Healthy Chef's Salad 144
❖Blue Cheese Dressing and Dip 144
❖French Dressing 144

### COLLARD GREENS
❖Marinated Collard Salad 150
5-Minute "Healthy Steamed"
Collard Greens 151
Thai Flavored Collards 151

### KALE
❖Kale Avocado Salad 158
❖Kale-Apple Smoothie 158
❖Kale Pesto 158
❖Marinated Raw Kale 158
5-Minute "Healthy Steamed"
Kale 159
Spiced Moroccan Kale 159

### MUSTARD GREENS
5-Minute "Healthy Sautéed"
Mustard Greens 163

### TOMATOES
"Quick Broiled" Tomatoes 167
*❖Mediterranean Tomato Salad 168
❖Seafood Tomato Salad 168
❖Quick Salsa 168
❖Tomato Relish 168
❖Fresh Tomato Dip 168
❖No Cook Stuffed Tomato 168
❖5-Minute Tomato Salad Dressing 168
Homemade Tomato Sauce 169

### BRUSSELS SPROUTS
5-Minute "Healthy Steamed"
Brussels Sprouts 177

Brussels Sprouts with Dijon Caper
Sauce 177
Spicy Brussels Sprouts 177
Brussels Sprouts and Apples 177
Nutty Brussels Sprouts 177
Asian Sauce, (for) 177

### GREEN BEANS
5-Minute "Healthy Steamed"
Green Beans 181
Asian Flavored Green Beans 181
Salad Niçoise 181
Marinated Bean Salad 181
Indian Curry Green Beans 181

### SUMMER SQUASH
❖Cool Zucchini Salad 187
❖Zucchini Boat 187
❖Marinated Zucchini 187
3-Minute "Healthy Sautéed"
Summer Squash 189
Mediterranean Summer Squash 189

### BELL PEPPERS
❖Red Pepper Vinaigrette 193
7-Minute "Healthy Sautéed"
Bell Peppers 195
Healthy Fajita 195

### CAULIFLOWER
❖Marinated Cauliflower 198
5-Minute "Healthy Sautéed"
Cauliflower 201
*Curried (Turmeric) Cauliflower 201
Savory Cauliflower 201
Mashed Cauliflower 201
Creamy Cauliflower Soup 201

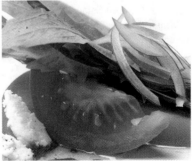
*655

# Recipe List

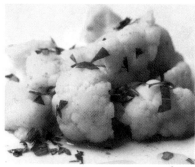

*201

## CELERY
❖Nut Butter Celery Snacks 205
❖Celery Salad 205
❖Refreshing Celery Salad with
 Yogurt 205
❖Celery Relish 205
5-Minute "Healthy Sautéed"
 Celery 207
Sicilian Celery 207
Celery with Shiitake Mushrooms 207
Healthy Sautéed Cod with
 Celery and Olives 208
Homemade Vegetable Broth 209

## FENNEL
❖Beet Fennel Salad 210
❖Apple Fennel Salad 210
7-Minute "Healthy Sautéed"
 Fennel 211
Fennel Mashed Potatoes 211
Fish with Sautéed Fennel and
 Carrots 211

## GREEN PEAS
3-Minute "Healthy Sautéed"
 Snow Peas or Sugar Snap Peas 216
3-Minute "Healthy Sautéed"
 Garden Peas 217
Asian Peas and Shiitakes 217
"Healthy Sautéed" Garden Peas
 and Carrots 217
Peas and Chicken Salad 217
3-Minute Garden Green Pea Soup 217
Honey-Mustard Sauce, (for) 217

## CABBAGE
❖Mayonnaise-Free Coleslaw 224
❖Marinated Cabbage Salad 224
❖Cabbage Spring Roll 224
❖Chinese Cabbage Salad 224
5-Minute "Healthy Sautéed"
 Red Cabbage 225
Carraway Cabbage 225
Easy Spicy Burrito 225

Stuffed Cabbage Leaves 225
5-Minute "Healthy Steamed"
 Cabbage 226
5-Minute "Healthy Sautéed" Red
 Cabbage with Apples 226
4-Minute "Healthy Sautéed"
 Bok Choy 226

## CARROTS
❖Mediterranean Carrot Salad 233
❖Herbed Carrot Salad 233
❖Tahini Carrot Salad 233
❖Pickled Carrot Chips 233
❖Ginger Carrot Zinger 233
5-Minute "Healthy Steamed"
 Carrots 235
Honey Mustard Sauce 235
Orange Carrots 235
Curried Carrot Salad 235
Greek Carrots 235
❖Super Carrot Raisin Salad 235

## WINTER SQUASH
"Slow Baked" Winter Squash 241
7-Minute "Healthy Steamed"
 Butternut Squash 243
Pumpkin with Sea Vegetables 243
Squash and Rice 243
Mashed Butternut Squash 243

## BEETS
15-Minute "Healthy Steamed"
 Beets 247
Creamy Horseradish Beets 247
Orange Spiced Beets 247
Mustard Beets 247
❖Grated Beet Salad 248
❖Mediterranean Beets 248
❖Raw Borscht Soup 248
Marinated Beet Salad 248

## EGGPLANT
7-Minute "Healthy Sautéed"
 Eggplant 257
Quick Eggplant Parmesan 257
Eggplant Dip 257

## GARLIC
❖Spicy Guacamole 262
❖Eggplant Garlic Dip 262
Garlic Dip 263
Bruschetta 263
Garlic Rice 263
Baked Garlic Chicken 263
Garlic Mashed Potatoes 263
Aglio and Olio 266

## ONIONS
❖Onion Spinach Salad 272
❖Marinated Onions 272
5-Minute "Healthy Sautéed" Onions 273
Onions, Potatoes and Olives 273
*Spiced Onion Soup 273
Mediterranean Feast 277

## LEEKS
7-Minute "Healthy Sautéed" Leeks 279
Quick Creamy Leek and Potato Soup 279

## SWEET POTATOES
7-Minute "Healthy Steamed"
 Sweet Potatoes 283
Mashed "Healthy Steamed"
 Sweet Potatoes 283
Sweet Potatoes and Black Beans 283
Sweet Potato Pudding 283
"Slow Baked" Sweet Potatoes 283

## CUCUMBERS
❖Refreshing Pick-Me-Up Drink 288
❖Easy Summer Cooler 288
❖Tangy Gazpacho 288
❖5-Minute Cold Cucumber Salad 289
❖Greek Salad 289
❖Asian Salad 289
❖Yogurt Cucumber Salad 289

## POTATOES
Stuffed Potato 295
10-Minute "Healthy Steamed"
 Potatoes 297
Smashed Potatoes with Garlic 297
Warm Potato Salad #1 297
Warm Potato Salad #2 297

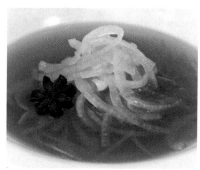

*273

## AVOCADOS
❖3-Minute Avocado Dip 301
❖Avocado Tomato Salad 301
❖Quick Avocado Salad Dressing 301
❖Mexican Avocado Dressing
 or Dip 301
❖Papaya Avocado Salsa 301

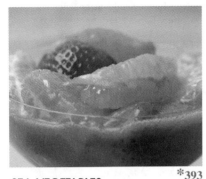

*393

# FRUIT DESSERTS

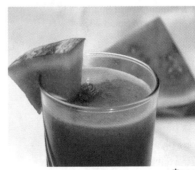

*383

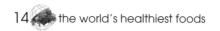

## Recipe List

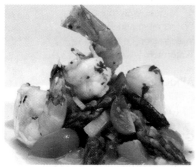

*125

## FISH & SHELLFISH

## NUTS & SEEDS

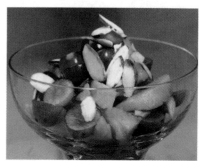

*537

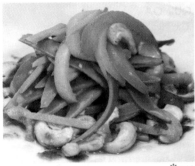

*549

# POULTRY & LEAN MEATS

# BEANS & LEGUMES

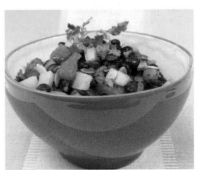

*605

# Recipe List

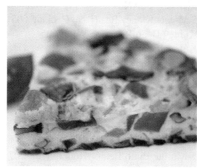

*635

# DAIRY & EGGS

❖Recipes Require No Cooking
* Photo / Recipe Page

# GRAINS

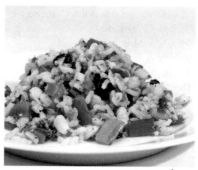

*679

# Questions of Interest

Throughout this book, you can read answers to the most frequently asked questions about the "Healthiest Way of Eating," which may be of special interest to you. Here is a list of the Q&As and their page numbers:

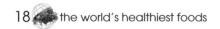

# Questions of Interest

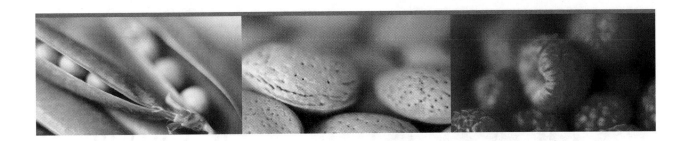

## PART 1

# what are the world's healthiest foods?

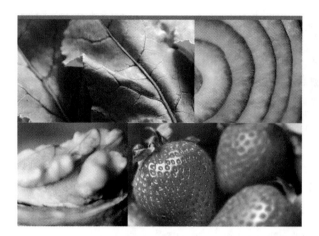

# discovering the world's healthiest foods

My passion for foods that are good for you and my belief that they are the key to vibrant health and energy has been a pivotal part of my life ever since I can remember. It is what inspired me, in 1970, to embark on a journey determined to find the World's Healthiest Foods.

My search to find the World's Healthiest Foods took me to more than 80 countries around the world. I did whatever it took to immerse myself in the native foodways. I went to Florence, Italy, with the desire not only to see the perfection of Michaelangelo's David, but to learn how to cook pasta to perfection. I went to India not only to see the Taj Mahal, but to discover firsthand how locals used spices in their cooking. I went to Paris not only to visit the Eiffel Tower, but to meet French chefs cooking healthy dishes without creams and heavy sauces.

I wanted to discover and experience the foods that are the hallmarks of various regions, especially those from faraway places where people have been known to lead especially long and healthy lives. I found the people of the Greek island of Crete, now believed to be among the healthiest people on earth, enjoying flavorful foods like garbanzo beans, crusty whole grain bread, eggplant, extra virgin olive oil, fish, goat cheese and yogurt. I tasted the sweetest apricots in Turkey and enjoyed the robust flavor of *cavolo nero* (black cabbage) in Italy. In Japan, I learned to enjoy sea vegetables, shiitake mushrooms, sweet potatoes and edamame (soybeans cooked in the pod). I watched the Chinese stir-fry fresh vegetables, and in Alaska, I savored the rich flavor of wild salmon. I joined people savoring spicy black beans in the Caribbean, snacked on pumpkin seeds in Guatemala and ate hearty rye bread in Scandinavian countries.

In Mexico, I also rediscovered the super grain, amaranth, which had been lost for over 300 years, and was honored to share it on ceremonial days with the descendants of the Aztecs. (For more on *Amaranth*, see page 661.)

Delighted by the wonderful tastes and vitality of the healthy, nutrient-rich foods that I discovered were being enjoyed around the world, I began to include them as a regular part of my meals. I started eating whole grain cereal with creamy yogurt and fruit for breakfast. I lunched on salads made with a colorful array of vegetables topped with black beans and an olive oil-based dressing. And for dinner, I would often-times choose seafood such as wild Alaskan salmon seasoned with fresh herbs, Mediterranean-style vegetables drizzled with olive oil and sweet ripe berries for dessert. For snacks, I began to enjoy a variety of nuts, seeds and fruit.

Once I started eating this way, I soon noticed something incredible. At the same time I was enjoying the great flavor of these new foods, my energy was skyrocketing. The foods not only tasted great, but they made me feel great! I realized, from my own experience, what cultures throughout the world have known for millennia—foods that are good for you can make you feel your best while providing you with immense taste enjoyment.

I was so inspired by my newly found vibrant health and energy that I wanted to share my discoveries about these great tasting foods so that others would enjoy and benefit from them as much as I did. So, I created a list of foods I called the World's Healthiest Foods (page 21), which could could serve as the foundation of the "Healthiest Way of Eating," a lifestyle approach that emphasizes whole,

# the world's healthiest foods

## total nutrient-richness chart

### VEGETABLES AND SALADS

| Food | |
|---|---|
| Spinach pg 98 | 65 |
| Swiss Chard pg 106 | 55 |
| Crimini Mushrooms pg 114 | 47 |
| Asparagus pg 120 | 43 |
| Broccoli pg 128 | 40 |
| Romaine Lettuce/Salads pg 136 | 40 |
| Collard Greens pg146 | 38 |
| Kale/Mustard Greens pg154 | 34 |
| Tomatoes pg 164 | 34 |
| Brussels Sprouts pg 172 | 33 |
| Green Beans pg 178 | 33 |
| Squash, Summer (Zucchi.) pg 184 | 32 |
| Bell Peppers pg 190 | 29 |
| Cauliflower pg 196 | 29 |
| Celery/Fennel pg 202 | 25 |
| Green Peas pg 212 | 24 |
| Cabbage pg 220 | 22 |
| Carrots pg 230 | 22 |
| Winter Squash pg 238 | 20 |
| Beets/Beet Greens pg 244 | 15 |
| Eggplant pg 252 | 15 |
| Garlic pg 258 | 15 |
| Onions/Leeks pg 268 | 14 |
| Sweet Potatoes pg 280 | 13 |
| Cucumbers pg 286 | 11 |
| Potatoes pg 292 | 8 |
| Avocados pg 298 | 7 |
| Corn pg 304 | 7 |
| Sea Vegetables pg 310 | 7 |
| Shiitake Mushrooms pg 316 | 5 |
| Olives/Olive Oil pg 322 | 4 |

### FRUITS

| Food | |
|---|---|
| Strawberries pg 344 | 24 |
| Raspberries pg 348 | 18 |
| Cantaloupe pg 352 | 14 |
| Pineapple pg 356 | 12 |
| Kiwi Fruit pg 362 | 11 |
| Oranges pg 368 | 11 |

### FRUITS (cont'd)

| Food | |
|---|---|
| Papaya pg 374 | 11 |
| Watermelon pg 380 | 11 |
| Apricots pg 384 | 9 |
| Grapefruit pg 390 | 8 |
| Grapes/ Raisins pg 396 | 8 |
| Blueberries pg 404 | 7 |
| Cranberries pg 410 | 7 |
| Bananas pg 416 | 6 |
| Plum / Prunes pg 422 | 6 |
| Lemons and Limes pg 428 | 4 |
| Apples pg 434 | 3 |
| Figs pg 442 | 3 |
| Pears pg 448 | 3 |

### FISH AND SHELLFISH

| Food | |
|---|---|
| Tuna pg 464 | 24 |
| Shrimp pg 470 | 23 |
| Salmon pg 476 | 21 |
| Cod pg 484 | 21 |
| Sardines pg 490 | 20 |
| Scallops pg 496 | 14 |

### NUTS AND SEEDS

| Food | |
|---|---|
| Sunflower Seeds pg 506 | 18 |
| Flaxseeds pg 512 | 13 |
| Sesame Seeds pg 516 | 12 |
| Pumpkin Seeds pg 522 | 11 |
| Walnuts pg 528 | 8 |
| Almonds pg 534 | 7 |
| Peanuts pg 540 | 6 |
| Cashews pg 546 | 5 |

### POULTRY AND LEAN MEATS

| Food | |
|---|---|
| Calf's Liver pg 556 | 41 |
| Beef, Grass-Fed pg 560 | 15 |
| Venison pg 566 | 14 |
| Lamb pg 570 | 12 |
| Chicken pg 576 | 11 |
| Turkey pg 582 | 11 |

### BEANS AND LEGUMES

| Food | |
|---|---|
| Lentils pg 592 | 20 |
| Soybeans pg 594 | 20 |
| Kidney B pg 604/Pinto B pg 606 | 19 |
| Lima Beans pg 608 | 18 |
| Black B pg 610 /Navy B pg 626 | 16 |
| Garbanzo Beans (Chickp.) pg 616 | 16 |
| Tofu pg 618 | 16 |
| Dried Peas pg 624 | 14 |

### DAIRY AND EGGS

| Food | |
|---|---|
| Eggs pg 632 | 18 |
| Low-Fat Milk pg 638 | 17 |
| Yogurt pg 644 | 15 |
| Low-Fat Cheese pg 648 | 9 |
| Goat's Milk pg 652 | 8 |

### GRAINS

| Food | |
|---|---|
| Oats pg 664 | 12 |
| Rye pg 668 | 10 |
| Quinoa pg 672 | 7 |
| Brown Rice pg 676 | 7 |
| Whole Wheat pg 682 | 7 |
| Buckwheat pg 686 | 5 |
| Corn (under Vegetables) | |

### HERBS AND SPICES

| Food | |
|---|---|
| Parsley pg 694 | 21 |
| Mustard Seeds pg 696 | 15 |
| Basil pg 698 | 11 |
| Turmeric pg 700 | 11 |
| Cinnamon pg 702 | 10 |
| Cayenne/Rd Chili Pprs pg 704 | 8 |
| Black Pepper pg 706 | 7 |
| Ginger pg 708 | 5 |
| Dill pg 710 | 4 |
| Cilantro pg 712 | 3 |
| Rosemary pg 714 | 3 |

The numbers to the far right of each food indicate their total nutrient-richness. (For more details, see page 805)

nutrient-rich foods prepared with techniques that enhance their flavor and preserve their nutrients.

## modern science supports the world's healthiest foods

I had identified a cornucopia of the healthiest foods through my travels and studies, but I wanted to make sure that the compilation of the World's Healthiest Foods would not be based solely upon my own personal experience. I wanted these foods' inclusion among the World's Healthiest Foods to be supported objectively by modern science.

Therefore, for a food to be included as one of the World's Healthiest, I decided it had to meet strict scientific criteria for nutritional excellence. First, it had to be a food rich in nutrients, such as vitamins, minerals, fiber, protein, essential fatty acids and antioxidants. Additionally, its ability to promote health and vitality had to be supported by the medical literature.

Out of the 23,000 foods for which there is nutritional data available, I found that the World's Healthiest Foods were among those richest in vitamins, minerals, protein, essential fatty acids, fiber and a variety of phytonutrients that act as powerful antioxidants; they were among the most nutritious foods on earth! At the end of each food chapter, you will find a section devoted to the food's Health Benefits, which includes a Nutritional Analysis of its content of over 60 nutrients. To my delight, this analysis demonstrated that the World's Healthiest Foods are a richer source of nutrients than I had ever imagined.

## qualifications to be on the list of the world's healthiest foods

I knew that nutrient-richness and promoting health and vitality couldn't be the only criteria for a food to be included on the World's Healthiest Foods list. These foods had to meet practical criteria as well; they had to be easily accessible and taste good. If you can't easily purchase a food or don't enjoy eating it, you are not going to include it in your "Healthiest Way of Eating."

Therefore, the World's Healthiest Foods had to fulfill the following criteria:

- Be a nutrient-rich food. A World's Healthiest Foods needed to not only be rich in health-promoting nutrients but also be one of the richest sources of nutrients in its food group. The World's Healthiest Foods also have research-demonstrated health benefits, such as preventing chronic disease.
- Be a whole food. The World's Healthiest Foods are

whole foods complete with all their rich, natural endowment of nutrients. They have not been highly processed nor do they contain synthetic, artificial or irradiated ingredients. And whenever possible, they should be organically grown, since organically grown foods not only promote your health but also the health of our planet.

- Be a familiar food. The World's Healthiest Foods are common "everyday" foods. These include the vegetables, fruits, fish/seafood, nuts/seeds, lean meats, legumes, whole grains, and herbs and spices that are familiar to most people.
- Be a readily available food. Although there are many foods that are exceptionally nutritious, many of them are not readily available in different areas of the country. The World's Healthiest Foods are foods that the majority of people can easily find at their local market.
- Be affordable. I selected foods that are not only familiar and available but also affordable, especially if you purchase them locally and in season. When foods are enjoyed in their peak season they are the freshest and of the best quality.
- Taste good. If a food is healthy but doesn't taste good, its health benefits will not be enjoyed. Therefore, these foods had to be rich in flavor and have a pleasing taste. The vibrant taste of many healthy foods is one of the primary reasons they have become increasingly popular.

Since each nutrient-rich food contains a unique nutritional profile that contributes to optimal health, it was also important that the list of the World's Healthiest Foods contain enough variety to meet your personal taste preferences and all your nutritional needs. I cannot tell which of the World's Healthiest Foods you will enjoy the most since I don't know what you like. I leave it up to you to select your favorites and those you feel are the best for you.

Regardless of which you choose, one thing is certain: by eating the World's Healthiest Foods, you will be enjoying those richest in health-promoting nutrients while consuming the lowest number of calories. This is because all these foods are "nutrient-rich," an important concept in nutrition, which I cover in the next chapter, and a key characteristic of all the World's Healthiest Foods.

## are all healthy foods on the list of the world's healthiest foods?

Of course I could not include every healthy food in the world on the list of the World's Healthiest Foods. Pomegranates, for example, are rich in antioxidant phytonutrients, yet they were not included on the World's Healthiest

Foods' list because they are not easily accessible and are relatively expensive. Peaches, cherries, mangoes and other wonderfully healthful fruits are not on the list because they are very seasonal. And hemp seeds, while rich in important nutrients, are not as well-known and versatile as the nuts and seeds chosen for the World's Healthiest Foods. Although every food that offers health-promoting nutrients and benefits could not be included, the list of World's Healthiest Foods provides you with 100 nutrient-rich, familiar foods from which you can choose those that can serve as the foundation for your "Healthiest Way of Eating."

If your favorite nutrient-rich food is not on the list, that doesn't mean that you should not enjoy it or that it is not good for you. I encourage you to include foods such as pomegranates, peaches, cherries, mangoes, hemp seeds and others as part of your "Healthiest Way of Eating." However, selecting from the list of the World's Healthiest Foods is one way to ensure that all the foods you eat are nutrient-rich, easily accessible and affordable.

## why the world's healthiest foods are not all vegetarian

The World's Healthiest Foods contain dairy products, fish, lean meat and poultry. That's because many individuals (because of their unique genetic inheritance and biochemistry) may find animal foods to be beneficial or even necessary to their health. Others—due to their biochemical individuality, personal tastes or philosophy—may choose not to eat these foods. One of the reasons that I included 100, not 10 or 20, foods on the list of the World's Healthiest Foods was to provide you with a selection from which you could choose the ones that best met your individual needs. (For more on *Biochemical Individuality*, see page 717.)

## the benefits of the world's healthiest foods

The benefits of the World's Healthiest Foods are that they are whole, nutrient-rich and unprocessed, characteristics that help keep us connected to nature, the changing of the seasons, the land and the many miraculous aspects of living things. Enjoyment of nutrient-rich foods is an integral part of maintaining optimal health.

In contrast to adulterated, refined or "un-whole" foods, the World's Healthiest Foods are real foods that still retain their natural endowment of nutrients as provided by nature, nutrients essential to the life of the plant or animal. They are not highly processed and contain nothing more than the naturally occurring nutrients intrinsic to the food from which they were derived; none of their nutrients have been removed or altered, and no synthetic, artificial chemicals, whether they be nutrient factors or preservatives, have been added.

Whole foods contain a combination of nutrients that work together synergistically to produce a much more powerful effect on health than any one nutrient alone. Recent research has found that compounds in whole foods differ in molecular size, polarity and solubility; they produce a powerful natural combination that is biologically more available than individual nutrients. The nutrients found in apples are a good example of this. According to Cornell Food Scientist, Rui Hai Liu, one medium apple contains only about 6 mg of vitamin C, however it has enough other antioxidants—such as quercetin, procyanidins, catechins and epicatechins—to produce as much antioxidant activity as 1,500 mg of vitamin C alone. The latest research clearly demonstrates that it is the complex interplay of all the natural components of whole nutrient-rich foods that gives the World's Healthiest Foods their superior nutritional quality as well as their delicious flavors, vibrant colors and rich textures.

### Enjoying the World's Healthiest Foods Will Give You Peace of Mind

- Peace of mind that they are nutrient-rich: Each of the World's Healthiest Foods has been analyzed for its nutrient-richness, and this information can be found in each of the individual food chapters.

- Peace of mind that they promote health: Each individual food chapter contains information on the special health benefits of each food.

- Peace of mind that they are affordable: The World's Healthiest Foods are not exotic foods that can only be found in specialty grocery stores or ethnic food markets. In fact, they are readily available and can be easily found in your local market, most of them year-round. And they are not expensive, especially if you purchase them locally and in season, which is why I included the information about their peak season in each food chapter.

- Peace of mind that they taste great: Whole, nutrient-rich foods are naturally bursting with flavor, and the tips on selecting, storing and cooking each food, plus the delicious and easy-to-prepare recipes included in this book, will help you retain their nutritional value while making them taste their best.

I hope you enjoy discovering the World's Healthiest Foods and the health benefits that they provide as much as I did.

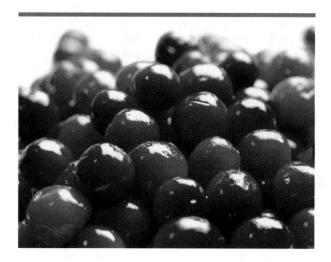

# nutrient-rich foods

## the new paradigm for the healthiest way of eating

**N**utrient-rich foods provide our bodies with the vital nutrients they need for optimal functioning and help us to feel our best. Therefore, one of the most important goals of eating healthy is to eat foods, such as the World's Healthiest Foods, which are the richest in nutrients.

In addition to the importance of considering the nutritional value of all of the foods we eat, we must also consider the number of calories they contain. Taking in too many calories to meet our nutritional needs leads to weight gain, reduced health and diminished energy.

## what is nutrient-richness?

A nutrient-rich food is one that provides the high concentrations of health-promoting nutrients without excess calories— a key feature of all of the World's Healthiest Foods. They are foods that deliver a rich supply of nutrients but a minimal number of calories. They are packed with vitamins, minerals, fiber, powerful antioxidants and phytonutrients that science believes are at the foundation of health promotion, disease prevention and longevity. Studies have shown that animals eating nutrient-rich foods without excess calories live 50% longer than normal.

The new paradigm in healthy eating is the following:

World's Healthiest Foods = $\frac{\text{Maximum Nutrients}}{\text{Minimal Calories}}$

This concept is important for everyone who wants to feel his or her best and/or is trying to lose weight. I use the term "nutrient-rich" to describe this important characteristic of the World's Healthiest Foods; scientists often refer to this quality as "nutrient-dense."

Nutrient-richness compares the absolute nutritional content of a food to its caloric content to discern whether the food has significant nutritional value. If a food is very high in one or more nutrients, but very low in calories, it can be described as "nutrient-rich" because it uses up very little of your day's calories but is a rich source of nutrients. Conversely, if a food is low in nutrients but high in calories, it is the opposite of nutrient-rich—it is "nutrient-poor," giving you very little in terms of nutrition, but using up a lot of your day's calories. Each of us has a budget of calories to take in each day to maintain our optimal weight and look and feel our best. Therefore, nutrient-rich foods, like the World's Healthiest Foods, are those that give you the most health-promoting nutrients for the number of calories you consume.

## how to calculate nutrient-richness

When nutritionists calculate nutrient-richness, they take nutrients and divide by calories. For example, there are 123 mg of vitamin C and 44 calories in a cup of cooked broccoli. If you take 123 and divide it by 44, you get 2.8 or

$\frac{\text{Broccoli with 123 mg vitamin C}}{44 \text{ calories}} = 2.8$

Translated into nutrition language, this result means that you get 2.8 mg of vitamin C for every calorie of broccoli you eat. In other words, broccoli is a food in which vitamin C comes pretty cheap in terms of its caloric "cost." When you get your vitamin C from broccoli, it doesn't cost you very much. To get 60 mg of vitamin C, the current Daily Value, you would only need to eat 18 calories' worth of broccoli, or less than a cup. Nutritionists therefore call broccoli a "nutrient-rich" food when it comes to vitamin C.

When it comes to vitamin C, one example of a nutrient-poor food is fried onion rings. A cup contains about 200 calories and less than 1 milligram of vitamin C. It would take over 17,000 calories' worth of fried onion rings to give you the Daily Value for vitamin C! In other words, fried onion rings are anything but a bargain when it comes to vitamin C.

Another example is the difference between the nutrient-richness of white bread and whole wheat bread. You would have to eat between $2^{1}/_{2}$ and 5 slices of white bread in order to get the same amount of vitamin E as is found in one slice of 100% whole wheat bread. Those extra slices will cost you as much as 320 extra calories!

## unique charts highlight the nutrient-richness of the world's healthiest foods

To fully illustrate the exceptional nutrient-richness of the World's Healthiest Foods and to give you a fast, simple, yet highly reliable way to meet your personal nutrition needs, a team of top nutritionists and I designed an original nutrient-richness rating system. The system took nutrient-richness as well as absolute nutrient contribution into consideration, applying standards that allowed us to qualify foods as sources of nutrients. To learn more about the details of how the World's Healthiest Foods Quality Rating System was devised, please refer to page 805.

One feature of this nutrient-richness ranking system is that it qualitatively rates foods as excellent, very good or good sources of individual nutrients based upon their nutrient-richness and nutrient contribution. This qualitative rating system is featured in three different types of charts found in this book:

- **THE NUTRIENT-RICHNESS CHART** can be found at the beginning of each food chapter and identifies which nutrients are concentrated in that food. For example, in the Nutrient-Richness Chart for Oranges (page 368) you'll see that they are an excellent source of vitamin C, a very good source of dietary fiber and a good source of folate, vitamin B1, potassium, vitamin A and calcium. The chart for each food will give you insight into its special nutrient endowment.

- **THE TOTAL NUTRIENT-RICHNESS CHART** is like a snapshot of the overall nutrient-richness for each of the World's Healthiest Foods. Each food has a unique overall nutritional profile, featuring different nutrients in different quantities. While all the World's Healthiest Foods are naturally nutrient-rich, some are more "rich" than others. For example, how do two incredibly nutrient-rich vegetables—spinach and broccoli—compare to one another? A glance at the Total Nutrient-Richness Chart (page 21) will show you that spinach is actually a bit more nutrient-rich than broccoli, having an overall rating of 65 while broccoli has a rating of 40 (the total nutrient-richness rating for each food is located at the top of its individual Nutrient-Richness Chart). This is not to say that spinach is necessarily better than broccoli, but it does give you an easy way to compare the total nutrient-richness of different foods.

- **THE HEALTH-PROMOTING NUTRIENT CHART** can be found in the individual nutrient chapters and identifies the foods that are the best sources of a particular nutrient. For example, in the chart for Calcium (page 738), you'll see that spinach and collard greens are excellent sources of this mineral (while numerous other foods are either very good or good sources). The Health-Promoting Nutrient Charts can serve as valuable tools for helping you to make decisions as to which foods can help you to meet your personal health and nutrition needs. You can use the Health-Promoting Nutrient Charts to see which foods are excellent, very good and good sources of the nutrients in which you are interested.

## every day with the world's healthiest foods

Over the course of each day, we need a wide variety of nutrients. This list of nutrients includes vitamins, minerals, protein, carbohydrates, fats, fiber, antioxidants and others. No matter what your health goals are (e.g., trying to lose weight, trying to get more energy or any other goal), it's always best to get the widest variety of nutrients you can for the least amount of calories. If you have to consume too many calories to get the optimal amount of nutrients, you'll inevitably gain excess weight.

That's where the World's Healthiest Foods come in. As a group of 100 foods, they give you the fullest variety of nutrients for the least amount of calories. Their nutrient-richness is one of their most important features, a quality that makes them an integral component of a "Healthiest Way of Eating" that promotes vibrant health and energy and optimal weight management.

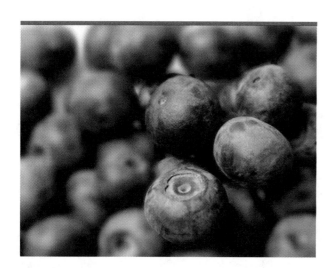

# how the world's
# healthiest
# foods
# keep you
# healthy

Study after study shows that nutrient-rich foods, such as the World's Healthiest Foods, are essential for optimal health. Researchers have found that nutrient-rich foods are the most effective for the prevention of disease because they contain a synergistic blend of nutrients including vitamins, minerals, fiber, fatty acids and other important compounds; in addition, fruits, vegetables, whole grains, legumes, nuts/seeds and herbs/spices contain over 800 identified phytonutrients (plant-based nutrients), such as carotenoids and flavonoids.

Recognizing the nutrient synergy provided by the World's Healthiest Foods is very important since research clearly shows that nutrients do not work in isolation; they can only fully do their work when their activity is complemented by the actions of many other nutrients. All are interrelated in a complex system supportive of the life of the plant or animal from which the food was derived. The more research is done, the more complex this life-giving nutrient web is revealing itself to be. Whole foods contain a wide variety of nutrients to ensure that the right combination is available for each individual nutrient to function optimally. For example, many foods that contain calcium also contain magnesium, which aids in calcium's absorption.

Yet we have just scratched the surface of understanding the role of different nutrients in our food as it is estimated that there are over 40,000 phytonutrients that have the potential of working synergistically to promote health! (For more on *Phytonutrients*, see page 743). While we may not yet know their specific functions (100 years ago, we did not even know the functions of vitamins because they had not yet been discovered), we do know that including the World's Healthiest Foods into your "Healthiest Way of Eating" can vastly increase your probability of enjoying the many benefits that phytonutrients provide. Perhaps the secret to vibrant health and energy, longevity and the fountain of youth rests right in front of us—in the synergistic activity of nutrients, many of which are yet unknown, but are found in nutrient-rich foods such as the World's Healthiest Foods.

## nutrient synergy: an example

Hundreds of epidemiological studies have looked at the relationship between whole, nutrient-rich foods, such as the World's Healthiest Foods, and chronic diseases such as cardiovascular disease, diabetes and cancer. What they have consistently found is that nutrients working together provide greater benefit than ones working alone. Recent research conducted on the health benefits of almonds provides a great example:

Researchers found that the flavonoid phytontutrients found in almond skins team up with the vitamin E present in their meat to more than double the antioxidant power delivered by either one of these nutrients separately. They identified twenty potent antioxidant flavonoids in almonds, some of which are well-known as major contributors to the health benefits derived from other foods.

The effects of almond flavonoids alone on LDL cholesterol levels was dramatically different when compared to the effects of these flavonoids working in combination with the vitamin E also found in almonds. While almond skin flavonoids alone enhanced LDL's resistance to oxidation by 18%, when almond meat's vitamin E was added, LDL's resistance to oxidation was extended by 52.5%! This study demonstrates the dramatic increase in health benefits that comes from nutrients working synergistically.

If the nutrients in just one of the World's Healthiest Foods, such as almonds, can work together so dramatically to increase their health-promoting benefits, think of the increased number of benefits that can be derived by enjoying a diversity of whole, nutrient-rich foods.

Eating more whole, nutrient-rich foods has consistently been shown to result in decreased incidence of disease. Individuals eating diets that contain the most fresh vegetables, fruits, legumes, nuts, seeds, and whole grains are always found to have the lowest disease risk.

## whole, nutrient-rich foods protect against cardiovascular disease

In two of the largest, most significant studies that have looked at the relationship between diet and cardiovascular disease—the DART study and the Lyon Heart Study— a whole foods diet consistently and significantly reduced cardiovascular disease (CVD) risk and mortality.

According to a recent news roundup in the British Medical Journal, the combined evidence of a number of large population-based surveys suggests that for every additional portion of fruit or vegetables eaten, the risk of heart disease is reduced by 4%. In one population study, postmenopausal women who ate 10 daily servings of fruit and vegetables lowered their risk of heart attack by 40%!

In the Lyon Heart Study, those following simple guidelines —increasing their consumption of vegetables, fruit, whole grains and legumes; eating healthy fats such as those found in olive oil, nuts and seeds; and decreasing their consumption of saturated fat—were found to have reduced their risk of death from cardiovascular disease by an amazing 70% after 27 months.

The DASH (Dietary Approach to Stop Hypertension) study demonstrated that a higher intake of whole grains, fruits and vegetables can lower blood pressure. In this trial, a whole foods diet produced an average drop of systolic/diastolic blood pressure of 12mm/6mm in a group of individuals with moderately elevated blood pressure.

Why are all these studies producing such consistently positive results? Here are just a few of the reasons:

- Foods rich in soluble fiber, such as oats, beans and nuts, have been shown to lower LDL ("bad") cholesterol significantly, not only in persons with high cholesterol but even in healthy subjects.

- The fiber in a whole foods diet also lowers serum triglycerides, its potassium and magnesium drop blood pressure, and its rich supply of antioxidants—such as vitamin E—protect cholesterol from free-radical damage.

- Diets rich in plant foods are also high in arginine, an essential amino acid that our bodies use to produce nitric oxide (NO). A vasodilator, NO relaxes blood vessels, improving blood flow.

With all these beneficial actions, it's not surprising that epidemiological studies indicate that a whole foods diet protects against CVD. Penny Kris-Etherton, a well-known researcher from Penn State University, and colleagues have noted that this is most likely due to the fact that a fruit and vegetable-rich diet naturally contains not only antioxidants but also a wide array of active compounds that act synergistically to prevent disease and promote health.

## whole, nutrient-rich foods protect against cancer

Bruce N. Ames, Ph.D., the renowned University of California-Berkeley biochemist whose work focuses on the relationship between diet and maintaining health, has noted that more than 200 epidemiological studies indicate that a diet high in fruits and vegetables can reduce cancer risk. A whole foods diet is richly endowed with all the well-known vitamins and minerals, as well as thousands of phytonutrients whose benefits researchers are just beginning to uncover.

The following provide just a few examples:

- Substantial evidence suggests that folic acid—abundant in vegetables, especially leafy greens—reduces the risk of colon cancer as well as cardiovascular disease.

- Broccoli and other members of the cruciferous vegetable family contain glucosinolates that switch on and turn up enzymes that detoxify carcinogenic substances.

- Powerful anthocyanins found in blueberries, which have a dramatic ability to penetrate cell membranes and provide cells with antioxidant protection, can decrease levels of inflammation and help prevent DNA damage throughout the body.

- Regular consumption of tomatoes, which are rich in a phytonutrient called lycopene, is highly correlated with a lower risk of developing prostate cancer.

## whole, nutrient-rich foods team up to provide greater cancer protection

A study presented on July 15, 2004, at the two-day WCRF/AICR International Research Conference on Food, Nutrition and Cancer in Washington, D.C., examined the effect of eating whole foods in combination instead of isolated nutrients. Not surprisingly, it showed that the benefits of consuming a variety of healthful foods beat consuming single nutrients by many a mile.

According to this research, eating broccoli along with tomatoes maximizes the cancer protection both foods provide. In the study, laboratory animals fed a tomato-and-broccoli combo had much less prostate tumor growth than animals given diets containing either food alone or normal animal chow diets supplemented with lycopene or finasteride (the drug commonly prescribed to men with benign prostatic hyperplasia, or BPH).

At a press conference, lead researcher John W. Erdman, Ph.D., Professor of Food Science and Human Nutrition at the University of Illinois at Urbana, explained the rationale behind this new approach to nutrition research:

"We decided to look at these foods in combination because we believed it was a way to learn more about real diets eaten by real people. People don't eat nutrients; they eat food. And they don't eat one food; they eat many foods in combination."

Erdman also noted, "Studies that examine individual substances in isolation are simply not designed to tell us anything about the interactions that occur among those substances, much less among foods that each contains its own anti-cancer arsenal."

Erdman and his colleagues reported their results on research testing the interaction of substances and their effect on cancer in the November 2003 issue of the *Journal of the National Cancer Institute*. In this study, lycopene alone offered laboratory animals little protection from prostate cancer, while diets containing freeze-dried tomato powder greatly improved their prostate cancer survival.

The conclusion these and other scientists have drawn from hundreds of studies is that cancer protection must come from a combination of phytonutrients, not isolated nutrients. In an article in the December 2004 issue of the *Journal of Nutrition*, Dr. Rui Lui of Cornell University summed up current thinking when he wrote:

"The additive and synergistic effects of phytonutrients in fruits and vegetables are responsible for these potent antioxidant and anticancer activities, and the benefit of a diet rich in fruits and vegetables is attributed to the complex mixture of phytonutrients present in whole foods. This explains why no single antioxidant can replace the combination of natural phytonutrients in fruits and vegetables to achieve the health benefits. The evidence suggests that antioxidants or bioactive compounds are best acquired through whole-food consumption. We believe that a recommendation that consumers eat 5 to 10 servings of a wide variety of fruits and vegetables daily is an appropriate strategy for significantly reducing the risk of chronic diseases and to meet their nutrient requirements for optimal health."

## whole, nutrient-rich foods protect against diabetes

A nutrient-rich foods diet also provides well-established benefits for persons with diabetes. In fact, data collected in the Nurses' Health Study suggest a whole foods diet may be the most successful treatment available for managing onset of the insulin resistance that characterizes early stage type 2 diabetes. A whole, nutrient-rich foods diet provides not only high levels of anti-inflammatory antioxidants and phytonutrients, which lessen the damage that high blood levels of glucose would otherwise cause, but an excellent supply of fiber, which slows digestion, lowers insulin requirements, provides better control of blood glucose and reduces blood cholesterol levels. The importance of whole foods is reflected in the U.S. Department of Agriculture's new food pyramid, which specifically calls for including whole grains in your diet.

## practical tip for optimal health

Take the advice of numerous researchers and health organizations. Eat a diet abundant in fruits, vegetables and other nutrient-rich foods, restrict your intake of foods that are high in saturated fats and sugars and combine it with an active lifestyle to prevent or fight chronic diseases including obesity, cancer, cardiovascular diseases and diabetes. The following chapters will help you discover more about this "Healthiest Way of Eating."

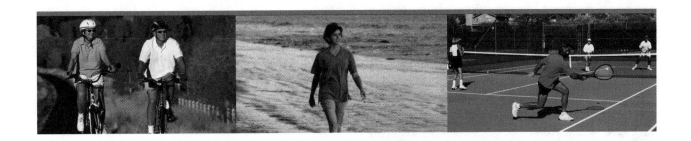

## PART 2

# the healthiest way of eating plan

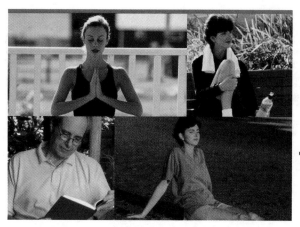

# HOW TO EASILY INCORPORATE
# the world's healthiest foods into your lifestyle

## The Self-Care Revolution

We are at a cultural turning point. This shift towards self-care is reflected in the growing interest in lifestyle activities such as a healthy way of eating, daily exercise, meditation, and the use of herbal teas and botanical medicine, all of which honor the whole self and don't view the body as if it were separate from the whole person. Our growing awareness of how to best support our unique individuality is a journey that will lead to better health and greater energy. Self-care activities enable you to respect your uniqueness and take charge of your own well-being.

## The World's Healthiest Foods: an Integral Part of Self-Care

I believe that the most important part of this growing self-care movement is the understanding of how nutrient-rich foods are vital to our health and well-being. As modern scientific research continues to uncover why nutrient-rich foods promote health and longevity, it becomes increasingly clear why the World's Healthiest Foods are at the core of self-care. They are nutrient-rich foods that will supply your body with all of the health-promoting nutrients you require for vibrant health, including vitamins, minerals and powerful antioxidants. Nothing is more valuable than optimal health, and eating nutrient-rich foods, such as the World's Healthiest Foods, is the best way to achieve it.

## Eating Healthy is Easy with the "Healthiest Way of Eating" Plan

The "Healthiest Way of Eating" Plan is a simple guide that you can follow to achieve your healthy eating goals. By following the Plan, you'll see how easy it is to incorporate nutrient-rich foods, like the World's Healthiest Foods, into your healthier lifestyle and turning them into flavorful meals is actually simple and takes a minimal amount of time. You'll begin to savor nutrient-rich foods so much that you'll lose your desire for nutrient-poor foods, processed foods that do little but provide empty calories. To best help you achieve your healthy eating goals, I designed the Plan so that it was in two phases, each with a specific aim that could best assist you in the ongoing quest towards your "Healthiest Way of Eating." The Plan is composed of two phases—Phase One and Phase Two—that are described in detail in the following pages.

You will notice that when you follow the "Healthiest Way of Eating" Plan, you will not only gain more enjoyment from the food you eat, but a new appreciation of all that food can do for you. By selecting whole, natural foods as opposed to foods that are manufactured and highly processed, and learning about the history, origin and health benefits of these foods you will be better able to attune yourself to those that are best suited to promoting your optimal health.

## Preparation is Minimal with the "Healthiest Way of Eating" Plan

Eating healthy doesn't need to take more time. With the "Healthiest Way of Eating" Plan, you'll see how easy it is to prepare meals that are not only rich in flavor but take only minutes to make. The Plan highlights many recipes featured in the book: more than 95% actually take less than 7 minutes to prepare!

## It Doesn't Cost More to Eat Healthier

The World's Healthiest Foods, which are whole, unprocessed foods, are the cornerstone of the "Healthiest Way of Eating" Plan. Processing and packaging add greatly to the cost of food; you pay more and get less. Preparing meals with the World's Healthiest Foods will probably turn out to be less expensive than purchasing foods that have been processed and packaged. Because the World's Healthiest Foods are among those richest in nutrients for the amount of calories they deliver, they are a nutritional bargain!

## The Key Features of the "Healthiest Way of Eating" Plan

The key features of the "Healthiest Way of Eating" Plan are incorporated into each day of the Plan. They include:

- **Healthier Lifestyle Tea (hot green tea with lemon)**
  Green tea (see page 716) is not only delicious but is renowned for its health-promoting properties. These have been linked to its high concentration of catechin phytonutrients, which have a wide variety of protective benefits, many related to their potent ability to fight free radicals. Adding 1 tsp lemon juice per cup of green tea not only gives it a refreshing taste but additional benefits. Lemon juice is a concentrated source of vitamin C, and hot water and lemon is a very cleansing and energizing beverage. (In Phase One, I recommend drinking one cup of Healthier Lifestyle Tea 15 minutes before each meal.) If you're sensitive to caffeine, you can drink decaffeinated green tea.

- **Fresh fruits with every meal and/or as snacks**
  Not only are fruits delicious and filled with vitamins, minerals, fiber and phytonutrients, which act as powerful antioxidants, but they contain enzymes that help the digestive process; this is why many traditional cultures always include fruit as part of a meal. Many fruits also have a low or medium glycemic index.

- **Large salad for lunch**
  Four cups of salads (made from romaine, red or green leaf, butterhead or bibb lettuce, spring or herb salad mixes or baby spinach) provide a delicious way to increase your intake of nutrient-rich vegetables. They fill you up and provide you with the nutrition that manifests in a vibrantly healthy appearance and the energy to be at your best throughout your day.

- **Two vegetable side dishes for dinner**
  Eating lightly cooked vegetables as a side dish with dinner is a great way to enjoy vegetables. The reason I suggest two different types of vegetables is because not only do they contain a wide range of health-promoting nutrients not often available in other foods, but vegetables are low in calories and rich in fiber. They'll easily satisfy your appetite, helping you to reach and maintain your optimal weight.

## Why the "Healthiest Way of Eating" Plan Can Change Your Life

The nutritional profiles of the World's Healthiest Foods show that they are nutrient-rich foods that can provide all of the nutrients your body needs. The exciting news in nutritional science is increased understanding of how the interaction of eating healthy, nutrient-rich foods can affect gene expression. In other words, a genetic predisposition to heart disease, diabetes or inflammation may be altered by dietary modifications and eating foods that are more beneficial for you. Therefore, enjoying the World's Healthiest Foods, which are the foundation of the "Healthiest Way of Eating" Plan, can influence how healthy you will be, and following the Plan can change your life!

I have included 100 foods on the list of World's Healthiest Foods because I don't believe that optimal overall health can rely on just one or two foods. Superfoods or power foods (those foods very rich in specific nutrients) such as tomatoes, blueberries or flaxseeds have wonderful health-promoting benefits on their own. But, it is the wide combination of nutrient-rich foods, such as the range of the World's Healthiest Foods, that can supply thousands of nutrients, which protect against disease and work together synergistically to achieve vibrant health and energy. The list of 100 foods also allows you to select the ones you like the best.

The "Healthiest Way of Eating" Plan will show you how easy it is to incorporate the World's Healthiest Foods into your lifestyle. It will also show you how easy it is to prepare them using the 'Healthiest Way of Cooking" methods and how these methods not only preserve nutritional value but enhance the flavor and texture of food as well. Since the Plan includes 2 month's worth of ideas for healthy eating, it takes the guesswork out of it. It allows you to enjoy the foods, and enjoy the way you will feel as you embark on the "Healthiest Way of Eating." I have seen with my own eyes how people I know start to have more energy, look more youthful and have glowing skin when they eat healthier as with the "Healthiest Way of Eating" Plan.

## What are the Nutritional Benefits of the Plan?

On page 42 you will find the Nutritional Analysis of Week 1, Day 1, a representative example of the wealth of health-promoting nutrients you can derive from following the Plan and enjoying the World's Healthiest Foods. Each day of the "Healthiest Way of Eating" Plan can provide you with more than 100% of most of the nutrients essential for vibrant health and energy!

# PHASE ONE
# 4 weeks to the healthiest way of eating

In each of the four weeks of Phase One, emphasis is placed on one group of the nutrient-rich World's Healthiest Foods. Studies have shown that it takes at least four weeks to begin changing eating habits, so the initial phase of the "Healthiest Way of Eating" Plan will help you to start eating healthier by learning how easy it is to include more of the foods so often neglected in our diets—fruits, vegetables, fish, nuts, seeds and beans—which have been proven to be essential for vibrant health and energy.

These foods provide the vitamins, minerals, antioxidants, fiber and essential fatty acids necessary to build and maintain a healthy body. They fight free radicals responsible for premature aging, curtail inflammation and promote a lean, energized body, a healthy heart and strong immune system. A diet deprived of these foods not only cannot deliver the many nutrients essential for vibrant health, but leads to nutrient deficiencies that promote physical degeneration and disease.

These initial weeks lay the foundation for Phase Two of the "Healthiest Way of Eating" Plan, which is designed to last you a lifetime. You are never too young or too old to benefit from the "Healthiest Way of Eating" Plan; I know it will prove to be the best possible investment of your time.

### An Easy Way to Follow the "Healthiest Way of Eating" Plan: Phase One

The purpose of the "Healthiest Way of Eating" Plan is to help you enjoy meals and snacks centered around flavorful foods that will optimize your health. Phase One will take you through the steps that are helpful in achieving this goal:

1. **IN WEEK 1**, you will add more antioxidant-rich fruits to your "Healthiest Way of Eating."

2. **IN WEEK 2**, you will add more immune-enhancing salads and vegetables to your "Healthiest Way of Eating."

3. **IN WEEK 3**, you will add more natural anti-inflammatory cold-water fish, shellfish, flaxseeds and walnuts to your "Healthiest Way of Eating."

4. **IN WEEK 4**, you will add heart-healthy nuts and seeds and cholesterol-lowering beans to your "Healthiest Way of Eating."

After 4 weeks on the "Healthiest Way of Eating" Plan, you will start to see the benefits of eating healthier. You'll probably feel more energetic, revitalized, and you may also lose weight if that is your goal. You will begin to relish the taste of nutrient-rich World's Healthiest Foods and lose your desire for nutrient-poor foods.

### How to Follow Phase One

You begin Phase One by selecting one meal daily from the options provided for breakfast, lunch, dinner and snacks; these can be enjoyed interchangeably. Try something new each day and add extra taste and nutrition to your meals.

You will notice that there is no week that focuses on grains, dairy, poultry or lean meats. This is because most people do not have any difficulty including these foods in their diet. I want to help you include more vegetables, fruits, fish, nuts, seeds and beans into your "Healthiest Way of Eating" because these foods are those that are more challenging for people to integrate into their lifestyle. I highly recommend regular exercise with this Plan.

Phase One provides you with ideas of how to easily incorporate fruits, vegetables and nuts, seeds and beans into your meals in an enjoyable way. By including just one meal per day from Phase One (lunch or dinner), you will begin to experience how nutrient-rich foods can contribute to a true state of vibrant health and energy that makes life such a joy.

While I provide suggestions for 3 meals and snacks, portions are not identified in Phase One. Please use my suggestions as a guideline and feel free to adjust the portion size and the foods you eat to meet your personal "Healthiest Way of Eating" goals.

# week 1

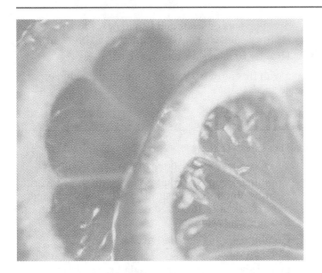

Welcome. In Week 1, you will be adding more fresh, antioxidant-rich fruits to the "Healthiest Way of Eating" Plan. Fruits are a highly concentrated source of hundreds of potent antioxidants, which provide their own unique forms of protection against the cellular damage caused by free radicals. If you have concern about increased blood sugar levels due to the sweetness of some fruits, select those with a lower glycemic index (see page 342). I always recom-mend eating the whole fruit over drinking juice.

Eating fruits is an excellent way to increase your intake of raw foods. They are especially good enjoyed after a meal since they help aid digestion. Enjoying fruit for dessert is a practice that has been followed for generations in healthy traditional diets.

This week you will also discover how to enjoy fresh fruits as a dessert without baking.

There are 19 different fruits (page 335) from which to choose on the list of World's Healthiest Foods. Four servings of fruits per day is a great goal to work towards (one serving equals 1/2 cup fresh fruit or 3/4 cup fresh squeezed juice with pulp).

## Breakfast:

Healthier Lifestyle Tea

Fruits provide an energizing addition to your breakfast. Choose from the following:

- Fruit bowl with banana, berries, walnuts, and ground flaxseeds, topped with vanilla yogurt
- Breakfast Power Smoothie (page 419)
- High-fiber cereal topped with fresh fruits (such as apples, pears, apricots), nuts, and soymilk
- Orange French Toast (page 371) spread with almond butter and sprinkled with sliced strawberries

## Lunch:

Healthier Lifestyle Tea

Here are some meal suggestions from which to choose:

- Combine 4 cups of salad greens with your favorite Healthy Vinaigrette (page 143). Top with 4 oz shrimp or fish, orange sections and pumpkin seeds
- Citrus Spinach Salad (page 102) with 4 oz cooked chicken or salmon
- Chinese Cabbage Salad with 4 oz chicken (page 224)
- Fresh fruit salad with apples, bananas, papaya and pineapple, topped with plain yogurt, and walnuts and cashews

Dessert: Fresh fruit such as an apple, 2 plums or 1 kiwifruit

## Dinner:

Healthier Lifestyle Tea

Start your dinner with 2 cups of mixed green salad with Healthy Vinaigrette Dressing of your choice (page 143). Top with 1/2 cup of sliced pear or apples, toasted nuts or goat cheese.

Here are 5 entrées to choose from:

- "Quick Broiled" Chicken (page 579) with Orange and Avocado Salad (page 371)
- "Quick Broiled" Salmon (page 481) with Ginger Papaya Salsa (page 377)
- Pineapple Chicken Salad (page 359)
- Spicy Shrimp Asian (page 475) (optional: add 1 cup diced pineapple)
- Black Beans and Butternut Squash (page 613)

Entrées should be served with 2 vegetable side dishes, such as:

- Broccoli (page 133) with Red Onions sprinkled with tamari (soy sauce) and sesame seeds
- Creamy Curry Spinach (page 103) and Crimini Mushrooms (page 119)
- Brussels Sprouts and Apples (page 177) with Garden Peas (page 217) or Mediterranean Feast (see page 276)

Dessert: 5-Minute Apricot Fruit Cup (page 387)
Pineapple Fruit Salad (page 359)
5-Minute Raspberry Almond Parfait (page 351)

## Snacks:

- Fresh fruit, such as grapes, pears or tangerines with your favorite nuts
- Fig and Almond Treat (page 445)
- 10-Minute Apricot Bars (page 387)

# week 2

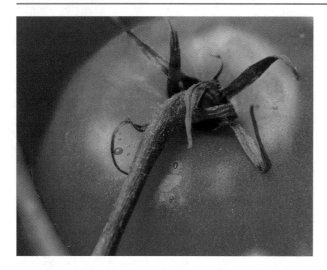

In Week 2, you will be including more immune-supporting vegetables and salads into the "Healthiest Way of Eating" Plan. You will find that adding more vegetables and refreshing salads to your diet is easy, fun and quick (most cooked vegetables can be prepared in 7 minutes or less).

Salads are an especially easy addition to any meal as they require no cooking time; you can now even find prewashed organic varieties of lettuce that are readily available. There are 34 vegetables in the Vegetable section (page 85) from which to choose. For optimal health, it is recommended to eat at least 5 servings of vegetables per day with one serving equaling 1/2 cup cooked vegetables, 1 cup raw vegetables, or 3/4 cup vegetable juice.

This week you will eat healthier and boost your immune system by selecting at least one of the meal or snack options each day. You will find that you can even enjoy vegetables for breakfast! In countries that are renowned for health and longevity such as Japan, China or those along the Mediterranean, vegetables are a traditional part of breakfast.

## Breakfast:

Healthier Lifestyle Tea

Start your day with an energizing breakfast.

Choose from the following:
- Whole grain bagel with sliced low-fat cheese, tomato, and avocado
- Poached Omega-3 rich Eggs (page 634) with 5-Minute Collard Greens (page 151) or 1-Minute Spinach (page 103) and shiitake mushrooms
- Sprinkle nuts or seeds and tamari (soy sauce) on steamed spinach, kale or asparagus and brown rice
- Healthy Breakfast Frittata (page 635)

Serve with fresh fruit such as 1/2 grapefruit, melon or orange slices.

## Lunch:

Healthier Lifestyle Tea

Here are some meal suggestions from which to choose:
- Combine 4 cups of salad greens with your favorite Healthy Vinaigrette (page 143). Top with canned tuna, chicken or turkey slices, as well as tomatoes, avocado and walnuts
- Combine 4 cups of salad greens with Curry Chicken Salad (page 579)
- Quick and Healthy Caesar Salad (page 144), topped with 4 oz cooked salmon, Parmesan cheese and walnuts
- Spinach Salad (page 102), topped with crumbled goat or feta cheese, red bell pepper slices and sautéed shiitake mushrooms (page 319)

Dessert: Fresh fruit such as grapes or pears

## Dinner:

Healthier Lifestyle Tea

Start your dinner with 2 cups mixed green salad with dressing of your choice (pages 143–144) and top with Marinated Onions (page 272), cucumber slices, red bell pepper or shredded beets.

Here are 5 delicious entrées to choose from:
- "Quick Broiled" Salmon with Ginger Mint Salsa (page 481)
- "Quick Broiled" Chicken with mustard (page 579)
- Quick Eggplant Parmesan (page 257)
- "Quick Broiled" Tuna Steak (page 469) with sautéed shiitake mushrooms (page 319) and garlic
- Sweet and Sour Tofu (page 319) with brown rice

Entrées should be served with 2 vegetable side dishes such as:
- Greek Carrots (page 235) with Green Beans (page 181)
- Summer Squash (page 189) and Asparagus (page 125) with grated Parmesan cheese or Mediterranean Feast (see page 276)
- Shiitake Mushrooms (page 319) with Red Onions (page 273). Sprinkle with lime juice and green onions

Dessert: Blueberries with Cashew Almond Sauce (page 407) kiwifruit with Lemon Sauce (page 365)

## Snacks:
- Hummus (page 617) served with crisp vegetables such as celery or bell peppers
- Super Carrot Raisin Salad (page 235)
- 3-Minute Avocado Dip (page 301) with crudités (carrot sticks, cucumber and broccoli)

# week 3

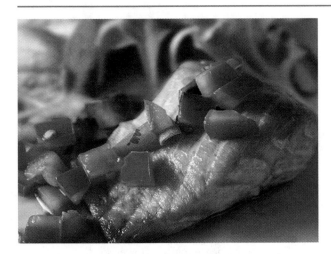

In Week 3, you will add more natural anti-inflammatory cold-water fish and shellfish into the "Healthiest Way of Eating" Plan. These foods provide special anti-inflammatory protection because of their concentration of omega-3 fatty acids, nutrients at the foundation of anti-inflammatory diets. The latest scientific research reports that omega-3 fatty acids should be part of one meal every day, and fish and shellfish are a great source of these hard-to-find healthy fats.

For optimal health, we need 2.5–4 grams of omega-3 fatty acids per day. There are 6 varieties of fish and shellfish rich in omega-3 fatty acids to choose from on the list of World's Healthiest Foods. (Flaxseeds and walnuts are also an excellent source of omega-3s for vegetarians and other individuals who do not eat fish.) Read more about fish and shellfish on page 457 and use the Fish & Shellfish Guide to find which fish and shellfish are safe to eat and the most sustain-able (page 453). It's easy to add more fish to your diet since canned salmon, tuna and sardines are readily available, inexpensive, and convenient.

## Breakfast:

Healthier Lifestyle Tea

Start your morning with healthy omega-3s. Choose from the following:

- 10-Minute Energizing Oatmeal (page 667) with fresh fruit and ground flaxseeds

- High Energy Breakfast Shake (page 347) with 2 TBS ground flaxseeds
- Canned salmon with Poached Eggs (page 634) sprinkled with turmeric and whole grain toast
- Poached Eggs over Greens (page 635) made with omega-3 rich eggs, mushrooms and turmeric

Serve with orange slices or 1/2 cantaloupe with mint

## Lunch:

Healthier Lifestyle Tea

Here are some meal suggestions from which to choose:

- Spinach Salad (page 102) topped with canned sardines or salmon, tomatoes, red onions and walnuts

Combine 4 cups of salad greens with:

- Shrimp Salad (page 475) and Ginger Healthy Vinaigrette (page 143)
- Niçoise Salad (page 144) with Healthy Vinaigrette (page 143) and ground flaxseeds
- "Quick Broiled" Tuna Salad (page 469) with cucumbers, red onions and your favorite Healthy Vinaigrette (page 143)

Dessert: Fresh fruit such as Papaya with Lime (page 337) Grapes in Honey-Lemon Sauce (page 399)

## Dinner:

Healthier Lifestyle Tea

Start your dinner with 2 cups of salad greens with dressing of your choice (pages 143–144). Top with anchovies, Parmesan cheese or capers.

Here are 4 delicious entrées from which to choose:

- Mediterranean Cod (page 487)
- "Healthy Sautéed" Scallops (page 499) with ginger
- "Quick Broiled" Salmon (page 481) with rosemary
- Pinto Bean Tacos (page 607)

Entrées should be served with 2 vegetable side dishes, such as:

- 5-Minute Cauliflower with turmeric (page 201) and "Healthy Sautéed" Red Bell Peppers (page 195)
- Green Beans and almonds (page 181) and 5-Minute Mediterranean Medley (page 133)
- Mediterranean Feast (see page 276)

Dessert: 5-Minute Plums in Sweet Sauce (page 425) 5-Minute Ginger Pineapple (page 359) Raspberries or Pears with Lemon Sauce ( page 431)

## Snacks:

- Tuna Salad without Mayo (page 467) in a whole wheat tortilla spread with mustard
- Apples, pears or plums with almonds, walnuts or cashews

# week 4

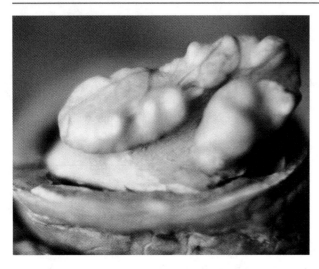

In week 4, you will be adding more heart-healthy nuts, seeds, and legumes into your "Healthiest Way of Eating." These foods are renowned as sources of fiber, healthy fats, protein, cholesterol-lowering phytosterols, and numerous minerals. I will show you how easy it is to include 1 1/2 ounces of nuts per day into your diet, as recommended by leading health organizations, by enjoying them as snacks or as toppings for many entrées. You will find it especially easy to add nuts and seeds to your "Healthiest Way of Eating" because they don't require any preparation.

This week you will also be eating more fiber-rich beans, which are low in calories and a versatile and inexpensive source of protein. So, it makes good sense to include them as part of your meals at least 4 to 5 times per week (1/2 cup is considered a serving size). I will share with you how you can enjoy beans, peas and lentils without any cooking. Healthy canned beans are readily available, easy to use, and save a lot of time.

There are 8 different nuts and seeds and 8 different legumes from which to choose on the list of the World's Healthiest Foods. Read about nuts and seeds on page 501 and legumes on page 587.

## Breakfast:

Healthier Lifestyle Tea

Great ways to add nuts and seeds to your energizing breakfast:

- 10-Minute Energizing Oatmeal (page 667) with 2 TBS sunflower seeds
- Strawberry Smoothie (page 347) made with 2 TBS almond or peanut butter
- 10-Minute Huevos Rancheros (page 612)

Serve with orange or grapefruit slices

## Lunch:

Healthier Lifestyle Tea

Here are some meal suggestions from which to choose:

- Healthy Chef's Salad (page 144) made with 4 cups of salad greens and Creamy Vinaigrette (page 143)
- Arugula Salad with Walnut Croutons (page 531) topped with 4 oz cooked chicken or canned tuna
- Spinach Salad (page 102) topped with canned salmon, goat cheese and sunflower seeds

Combine 4 cups of salad greens and Healthy Vinaigrette (page 143) with:

- Chicken Salad (page 579) and cashews
- Greek Salad (page 289) and garbanzo beans

Dessert: Papaya Fruit Cup (page 377) or 5-Minute Ginger Pineapple (page 359)

## Dinner:

Healthier Lifestyle Tea

Start your dinner with 2 cups of mixed green salad with dressing of your choice (pages 143–144). Top with cashews, pumpkin seeds or 1/2 cup garbanzo beans or black beans.

Here are 4 delicious entrées from which to choose:

- Sweet Firecracker Tofu (page 621) with shiitake mushrooms and green beans
- Sesame Chicken (page 519) with buckwheat soba noodles
- Black Bean Chili (page 613) with brown rice, dollop of plain yogurt and Quick Salsa (page 168)
- Salmon in Dill Sauce (page 481)
- Thai Shrimp with Cashews (page 549) with brown rice

Entrées should be served with 2 vegetable side dishes such as:

- Zorba the Greek Swiss Chard (page 111) with "Healthy Sautéed" Red Bell Peppers (page 195)
- Shiitake mushrooms (page 319) and Green Beans (page 181) or Mediterranean Feast (see page 276)
- Red Cabbage with Apples (page 226) and Garden Peas (page 217)

Dessert: 5-Minute Raspberry Almond Parfait (page 351) Blueberries with Cashew Almond Sauce (page 407)

## Snacks:

- Fruit such as apples, pears or plums and almonds
- Pears with Lemon Sauce (page 451)
- Egg Salmon Salad (page 481) with celery and zucchini sticks

# BENEFITS OF
# phase one

In these 4 weeks, by eating foods that support your immune system, fight free radicals, curb inflammation and promote a healthy heart, and avoiding sugar and white flour, you will not only look and feel better but have increased energy and become more mentally alert. Below, you will find how individual foods benefit you in the initial 4 weeks of the "Healthiest Way of Eating" Plan.

## Week 1 of the "Healthiest Way of Eating" Plan Provides Powerful Antioxidant Protection

Besides emphasizing fruits, Week 1 focused on vegetables. Both are especially important defenders of health since they deliver a wide array of nutrients that are essential for healthy cellular function, enhance the body's ability to detoxify potentially harmful substances, and neutralize free radicals. The spectrum of these vital nutrients in fruits and vegetables includes not only vitamins and minerals, but also many types of phytonutrients, including the plant pigments that provide their radiant hues and can provide us with radiant health.

Researchers agree that antioxidant compounds in our foods (see page 735) play an especially important role in keeping us healthy. That's because antioxidants quench free radicals, which, if left unchecked, cause damage to our blood vessels, joints, brain cells, genetic material and more. Excessive free radical activity has been linked to the development and progression of virtually all chronic health conditions.

## Week 2 of the "Healthiest Way of Eating" Plan Focuses on Supporting Your Immune System

Besides more vegetables (especially shiitake mushrooms and garlic) and salads, Week 2 continues to emphasize the fruits and omega-3-rich fish that support the immune system. Whole foods that are concentrated sources of the nutrients especially important for immune function (see page 508) help protect you from colds and flus. In addition, the "Healthiest Way of Eating" Plan boosts immunity by avoiding processed foods whose lack of necessary nutrients and inclusion of ingredients—including refined sugar, white flour and additives—actually compromise your immune system's ability to protect your health.

## Week 3 of the "Healthiest Way of Eating" Plan Features Anti-Inflammatory Benefits

In addition to more cold-water fish, Week 3 emphasized flaxseeds, dark leafy green vegetables, fruits rich in antioxidants, walnuts, flaxseeds, turmeric, ginger and rosemary, all of which also deliver nutrients effective in fighting inflammation. One important aspect of dietary strategies related to inflammation involves the omega-6 and omega-3 fatty acids (see page 456). Omega-6 fatty acids, when consumed excessively in proportion to omega-3 fats, promote inflammation. The good news is that by eating more omega-3 rich foods, such as salmon, sardines, tuna, other cold-water fish, walnuts and flaxseeds—all foods featured in the "Healthiest Way of Eating" Plan—you can easily shift the balance back to optimal health and help reduce inflammatory processes. Chronic inflammation has been linked to degenerative conditions such as heart disease, diabetes, asthma and arthritis.

## Week 4 of the "Healthiest Way of Eating" Plan Promotes Heart Health

In Week 4, you enjoy not only more nuts, seeds and beans, but other heart-healthy foods such as fish, fruits, vegetables, oats and olive oil; you also eat less foods high in saturated fats, cholesterol and trans fats. This powerful combination of delivering a lot more of what you need and a lot less of what you don't is the reason the "Healthiest Way of Eating," which reflects the principles of the Mediterranean Diet, is such a heart-healthy diet.

Black beans, garbanzo beans, split peas, lentils, and other legumes are concentrated sources of soluble fiber and phytosterols, which reduce LDL cholesterol. Legumes' contribution to heart health is amazing; in fact, one large-scale study found that those who ate the most legumes reduced their risk of heart disease by an impressive 82%!

Public health experts agree that enjoying a daily handful of nuts and seeds helps prevent heart disease. And that's not all—the numerous antioxidants found in fruits, vegetables, and olive oil all work together to prevent the oxidation of LDL cholesterol, a primary step in the development of atherosclerosis.

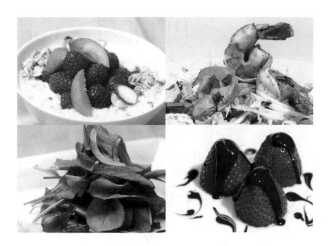

# PHASE TWO
# eating for a healthier lifestyle

Phase One helped show you how easy it is to incorporate the World's Healthiest Foods into your "Healthiest Way of Eating." Phase Two will show you how easy it is to eat healthy for a lifetime.

## How to Start Phase Two

Phase Two requires no planning as I provide you with 2 weeks' worth of different menus for breakfast, lunch, dinner and snacks. By repeating these 2 weeks, you will be all set for a month of the "Healthiest Way of Eating." After that, you can use these menu plans as a basis for building meal ideas any day of the year.

Phase Two takes all of the features of the different weeks in Phase One and combines them. Instead of just focusing on one food group, it offers you balanced menus featuring all of the food groups you began to incorporate in Phase One. These are the foods that will help you. With the "Healthiest Way of Eating" Plan, you will maximize your potential for a lifetime of vibrant health and energy.

To fulfill your nutritional needs you should include at least 5 servings of vegetables, 4 servings of fruits, 2.5–4 grams of omega-3 fatty acids (preferably from fish) and 1.5 ounces of nuts and seeds per day. You should also have a serving of legumes at least 4 to 5 times per week.

# WEEK 1 – DAY 1

## BREAKFAST:

Start your day with Healthier Lifestyle Tea
- 10-Minute Energizing Oatmeal (page 667) topped with ground flaxseeds and blueberries
- 1/2 large grapefruit

**SNACK:** Banana with cashew butter*

## LUNCH:

- 4 cups of Quick and Healthy Caesar Salad (page 144) topped with cooked chicken, cucumbers, tomatoes, avocados, and crumbled feta cheese*

**DESSERT:** 5-Minute Raspberry Almond Parfait (page 351)

**SNACK:** Apple slices spread with almond butter*

## DINNER:

Salad made with 2 cups of mixed greens. Dress with your favorite vinaigrette (page 143).
- Salmon with Dill Sauce (page 481)
- Serve with "Healthy Sautéed" Asparagus (page 125) and "Heathy Steamed" Winter Squash (page 243) topped with grated Parmesan*

**DESSERT:** 5-Minute Grapes in Honey Lemon Sauce (page 399)

* Optional (only the one food with an asterick)

# WEEK 1 – DAY 2

## BREAKFAST:

Start your day with Healthier Lifestyle Tea
- Salmon Frittata (page 482)
- 1/2 cantaloupe

**SNACK:** Hummus (page 617) with red bell pepper and carrot sticks

## LUNCH:

- Mixed green salad (4 cups) topped with avocado chunks, tomatoes, chicken or turkey slices, and Blue Cheese Dressing (page 144)

**DESSERT:** kiwifruit with Lemon Sauce (page 365)

**SNACK:** Pear or apple

## DINNER:

Salad made with 2 cups of arugula. Top with feta cheese and red bell pepper slices. Dress with your favorite vinaigrette (page 143)
- Mediterranean Cod (page 487)
- Serve with Creamy Curry Spinach (page 103) and Crimini Mushrooms (page 119)

**DESSERT:** Blueberries with Cashew-Almond Sauce (page 407)

# WEEK 1 - DAY 3

## BREAKFAST:

Start your day with Healthier Lifestyle Tea

- Whole grain bagel or whole wheat bread, low-fat cheese, tomato and avocado slices
- 1/2 large grapefruit or 1/2 papaya with lime

**SNACK:** Raisins and walnuts*

## LUNCH:

- Spinach (4 cups) with "Quick Broiled" Tuna Salad (page 469) and crumbled feta cheese and olives served with your favorite vinaigrette (page 143)

**DESSERT:** 5-Minute Apple Treats (page 437)

**SNACK:** Navy Bean Pesto (page 627) with whole wheat crackers or carrots and celery

## DINNER:

Salad made with 2 cups of mixed greens. Top with 1/4 cup garbanzo beans and 2 TBS goat cheese.* Dress with Red Pepper Vinaigrette (page 143)

- Spicy Shrimp Asian (page 475) with "Healthy Sautéed" Asparagus (page 125) and "Healthy Sautéed" Red Bell Peppers (page 195) or Mediterranean Feast (see page 276)

**DESSERT:** 10-Minute Strawberries with Chocolate Crème (page 347)

# WEEK 1 - DAY 4

## BREAKFAST:

Start your day with Healthier Lifestyle Tea

- Fruit bowl with bananas, berries, walnuts, ground flaxseeds and vanilla yogurt

**SNACK:** Orange wedges

## LUNCH:

- Mixed green salad (4 cups) with Healthy Vinaigrette Dressing (page 143) topped with 2 cups Waldorf Salad (page 143)

**DESSERT:** Sliced pear

**SNACK:** Fig and Almond Treat (page 445)

## DINNER:

Salad made with 2 cups of spinach topped with sliced fennel, walnuts, and orange sections, and served with French Healthy Vinaigrette (page 143).

- 3-Minute "Healthy Sautéed" Scallops (page 499)
- Serve with 2 servings of 5-Minute Mediterranean Medley (page 137) or Mediterranean Feast (see page 276)

**DESSERT:** 5-Minute Plums in Sweet Sauce (page 425)

# WEEK 1 - DAY 5

## BREAKFAST:

Start your day with Healthier Lifestyle Tea

- High Energy Breakfast Shake (page 347) with 2 TBS ground flaxseeds
- 1/2 large grapefruit

**SNACK:** Tropical Banana Treat (page 419)

## LUNCH:

- Healthy Chef's Salad made with 4 cups of salad greens served with walnuts* and French Dressing (page 144)

**DESSERT:** Raspberries with Yogurt and Chocolate (page 351)

**SNACK:** Fresh fruit such as grapes, pears or tangerines

## DINNER:

Salad made with 2 cups of mixed greens. Top with pumpkin seeds* and black beans or garbanzo beans. Dress with your favorite vinaigrette (page 143)

- 7-Minute "Quick Broiled" Miso Salmon (page 481)
- Serve with Nutty Brussels Sprouts (page 177) and Garden Peas (page 217) or Mediterranean Feast (see page 276)

**DESSERT:** 5-Minute Grapes in Honey Lemon Sauce (page 399) with chopped walnuts*

# WEEK 1 - DAY 6

## BREAKFAST:

Start your day with Healthier Lifestyle Tea

- Classic Tofu Scramble (page 621) topped with premade salsa, sesame seeds and avocado slices
- Orange slices

**SNACK:** Dried cranberries and almonds*

## LUNCH:

- Mixed green salad (4 cups) topped with "Quick Broiled" Salmon (page 481) with grated ginger, sesame seeds* and green onion. Dress with Asian Vinaigrette (page 143)

**DESSERT:** Kiwi with Lemon (page 365)

**SNACK:** 10-Minute Apricot Bars (page 387)

## DINNER:

Salad made with 2 cups of arugula. Top with feta cheese* and red bell pepper. Dress with Healthy Vinaigrette (page 143)

- 7-Minute "Healthy Sautéed" Chicken with Asparagus (page 578) served with "Healthy Steamed" Broccoli (page 133), pumpkin seeds* and brown rice

**DESSERT:** Blueberries with Cashew-Almond Sauce (page 407)

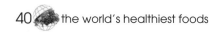

# WEEK 1 – DAY 7

## BREAKFAST:
Start your day with Healthier Lifestyle Tea
- 10-Minute Huevos Rancheros (page 612)
- Orange slices

**SNACK:** 5-Minute Apple Treat (page 437)

## LUNCH:
- Salad of mixed greens (4 cups) and sunflower seeds* topped with Shrimp Salad (page 475). Dress with Ginger Healthy Vinaigrette (page 143)

**DESSERT:** Sliced plums or apricots

**SNACK:** Cantaloupe with Lime and Mint (page 355)

## DINNER:
Cold Asparagus Salad (page 125)
- "Quick Broiled" Salmon with Ginger Mint Salsa (page 481)
- Serve with Onions, Potatoes and Olives (page 273) and "Healthy Steamed" Green Beans (page 181) with almonds* or Mediterranean Feast (see page 276)

**DESSERT:** Raspberries with Balsamic Vinegar or Raspberries with Lemon Sauce (page 351)

# WEEK 2 – DAY 1

## BREAKFAST:
Start your day with Healthier Lifestyle Tea
- High Energy Breakfast Shake (page 347) with 2 TBS ground flaxseeds
- Melon slices

**SNACK:** Hummus (page 617) with crisp vegetables such as celery or bell pepper

## LUNCH:
- Salad of 4 cups mixed greens with Healthy Vinaigrette (page 143). Topped with Curry Chicken Salad (page 578) or Pineapple Chicken Salad (page 359) with cashews*

**DESSERT:** kiwifruit slices

**SNACK:** Cranberry Trail Mix (page 413)

## DINNER:
Salad made with 2 cups of mixed greens. Top with orange sections and slivered almonds*. Dress with your favorite vinaigrette (page 143)
- Rosemary Lamb Chops (page 573) or Miso Salmon (page 481)
- Serve with "Healthy Steamed" Broccoli and Red Onions (page 133) topped with tamari (soy sauce) and sesame seeds* or Mediterranean Feast (see page 276)

**DESSERT:** 10-Minute Apple Sundae (page 437)

# WEEK 2 – DAY 2

## BREAKFAST:
Start your day with Healthier Lifestyle Tea
- Poached Eggs (page 637) with shiitake mushrooms, spinach and whole wheat toast
- 1/2 large grapefruit

**SNACK:** Carrot Cashew Paté (page 548) with red bell pepper and cauliflower florets

## LUNCH:
Mixed green salad (4 cups) with tomatoes, cucumbers and goat cheese* topped with:
- "Quick Broiled" Salmon (page 481) and French Healthy Vinaigrette (page 143)

**DESSERT:** Papaya with Lime (page 377)

**SNACK:** Pears with Lemon Sauce (page 451)

## DINNER:
Salad made with 2 cups of mixed greens. Top with garbanzo beans or Parmesan cheese*. Dress with your favorite vinaigrette (page 143)
- Turkey with Ravigote Sauce (page 585) or Black Bean Chili (page 613) and brown rice
- Serve with "Healthy Steamed" Green Beans (page 181) and "Healthy Sautéed" Bell Peppers with feta cheese (page 195) or almonds*

**DESSERT:** 10-Minute Strawberries and Chocolate Crème (page 347)

# WEEK 2 – DAY 3

## BREAKFAST:
Start your day with Healthier Lifestyle Tea
- Orange French Toast (page 371) spread with almond butter and sprinkled with strawberries
- Cantaloupe Fruit Salad (page 355)

**SNACK:** 5-Minute Banana Treat (page 419)

## LUNCH:
- Citrus Spinach Salad (page 102) topped with Quick Boiled Shrimp (page 473)

**DESSERT:** Kiwi with Lemon Sauce (page 365)

**SNACK:** Cranberry Trail Mix (page 413)

## DINNER:
Salad made with 2 cups of mixed greens. Top with tomato, sunflower seeds or Parmesan cheese*. Dress with your favorite vinaigrette (page 143)
- 7-Minute Poached Salmon (page 482) with tamari (soy sauce) and fresh grated ginger and brown rice
- Serve with "Healthy Sautéed" Shiitake Mushrooms, (page 319) and Red Bell Peppers (page 319)

**DESSERT:** 5-Minute Plums in Sweet Sauce (page 425)

# WEEK 2 – DAY 4

## BREAKFAST:
Start your day with Healthier Lifestyle Tea
- High fiber cereal with bananas, nuts and soymilk
- 10-Minute Grapefruit Sunrise (page 393)

**SNACK:** Tahini served with vegetable crudités (cucumber, red bell pepper)

## LUNCH:
- Egg-Salmon Salad (page 481) on 4 cups mixed greens with your favorite Healthy Vinaigrette Dressing (page 143)

**DESSERT:** Grapes

**SNACK:** 5-Minute Rye Raisin Snack (page 403)

## DINNER:
Salad made with 2 cups of mixed greens. Top with shredded carrots and pumpkin seeds*. Dress with your favorite vinaigrette (page 143)
- Thai Shrimp with Cashews (page 549) on brown rice
- Serve with 5-Minute "Healthy Sautéed" Red Cabbage (page 225) and "Healthy Sautéed" Shiitake Mushrooms (page 319) or Mediterranean Feast (page 276)

**DESSERT:** Strawberries and Mint (page 347) or Raspberries with Balsamic Vinegar (page 351)

# WEEK 2 – DAY 5

## BREAKFAST:
Start your day with Healthier Lifestyle Tea
- 10-Minute Energizing Oatmeal, topped with yogurt and ground flaxseeds
- Sliced pears and walnuts*

**SNACK:** Bananas with cashew butter*

## LUNCH:
- Healthy Chef's Salad (page 144) made with 4 cups of salad greens and Blue Cheese Dressing (page 144)

**DESSERT:** Plums or grapes

**SNACK:** Apple slices topped with almond butter*

## DINNER:
Salad made with 2 cups of mixed greens. Top with cucumber and red bell pepper. Dress with French Dressing (page 144)
- Salmon with Dill Sauce (page 481) or Quick Eggplant Parmesan (page 257)
- Serve with "Healthy Sautéed" Asparagus (page 125) and "Heathy Steamed" Winter Squash (page 243) topped with pumpkin seeds or grated Parmesan cheese* or Mediterranean Feast (see page 276)

**DESSERT:** 5-Minute Grapes in Honey Lemon Sauce (page 399)

# WEEK 2 – DAY 6

## BREAKFAST:
Start your day with Healthier Lifestyle Tea
- Poached Eggs on Steamed kale or collards (page 635) with whole grain bagel
- 1/2 large grapefruit

**SNACK:** 5-Minute Energy Bars (page 445)

## LUNCH:
- Mexican Cheese Salad (page 651) made with 4 cups salad greens, 1 cup cooked chicken breast and Healthy Vinaigrette (page 143)

**DESSERT:** Grapes or apricots

**SNACK:** Yogurt with honey and walnuts*

## DINNER:
Salad made with 2 cups of mixed greens. Top with pear slices and Parmesan cheese or walnuts*. Serve with your favorite vinaigrette (page 143)
- 2-Minute "Quick Broiled" Tuna (page 469) with tamari (soy sauce) and quinoa (page 675)
- Serve with Creamy Curry Spinach (page 103) and crimini mushrooms (page 119) or Mediterranean Feast (see page 276)

**DESSERT:** 10-Minute Orange Treat (page 371)

# WEEK 2 – DAY 7

## BREAKFAST:
Start your day with Healthier Lifestyle Tea
- Breakfast Power Smoothie (page 419)
- Orange and kiwi slices

**SNACK:** Tuna Salad without Mayonnaise (page 467) wrapped in a tortilla with mustard

## LUNCH:
- 4 cups lettuce or spinach mixed with Niçoise Salad (page 144) and French Healthy Vinaigrette (page 143)

**DESSERT:** Sliced apple

**SNACK:** English muffin with almond butter and banana slices

## DINNER:
Salad made with 2 cups of mixed greens. Top with feta cheese or kalamata olives*, tomatoes and cucumbers. Dress with your favorite vinaigrette (page 143)
- 7-Minute "Quick Broiled" Salmon with Ginger Mint Salsa (page 481)
- Serve with "Healthy Sautéed" Bok Choy (page 226) and "Healthy Sautéed" Snap Peas (page 216) tossed with sesame seeds, rice vinegar and tamari (soy sauce) or Mediterranean Feast (see page 276)

**DESSERT:** 5-Minute Blueberries with Yogurt (page 407)

*(See NOTES and BEVERAGES on Page 42)*

(Continued from Page 41)

## BEVERAGES FOR THE "HEALTHIEST WAY OF EATING" PLAN:

- Mineral water
- Green tea (hot or cold)
- Healthier Lifestyle Tea
- Herbal teas
- Spring water with or without lemon
- Red wine in moderation (with meals)

## NOTE:

It is good to sprinkle sea vegetables on your salad or vegetables everyday because they provide essential nutrients that are difficult to find elsewhere.

If you can't tolerate dairy, shrimp or any foods on this menu, substitute with comparable foods that will agree with your personal needs. For example, calcium-enriched tofu for dairy, fish rather than shrimp, etc.

## Week 1 - Day 1 Nutritional Analysis

| NUTRIENT | AMOUNT | % DAILY VALUE | NUTRIENT | AMOUNT | % DAILY VALUE |
|---|---|---|---|---|---|
| Calories | 1844 | 93% | Folate | 814.64 mcg | 204% |
| Calories from Fat | | 30% | Vitamin K | 340.87 mcg | 379% |
| Protein | 88.78 g | 195% | Pantothetic Acid | 6.21 mg | 124% |
| Carbohydrates | 255.70 g | 93% | | | |
| Dietary Fiber | 43.91 g | 158% | **Minerals** | | |
| Cholesterol | 155.14 mg | 52% | Calcium | 971.34 mg | 97% |
| Omega-3 Fatty Acids | 4.71 g | | Copper | 1.91 mg | 212% |
| | | | Iron | 17.74 mg | 99% |
| **Vitamins** | | | Magnesium | 596.76 mg | 186% |
| Vitamin A | 45,643.49 IU | 1304% | Potassium | 5160.21 | 110% |
| Beta Carotene | 21,241.88 mcg | | Selenium | 86.69 mcg | 158% |
| B1 Thiamin | 1.51 mg | 137% | Zinc | 8.00 | 100% |
| B2 Riboflavin | 1.63 mg | 148% | | | |
| B3 Niacin | 30.09 mg | 215% | | | |
| Vitamin B6 | 2.82 mg | 217% | | | |
| Vitamin B12 | 4.04 mcg | 169% | | | |
| Biotin | 26.35 mcg | 88% | | | |
| Vitamin C | 237.13 mg | 316% | | | |
| Vitamin E IU | 22.23 IU | | | | |

Each day of the Phase Two "Healthiest Way of Eating" Plan is based on 1,800 calories and approximates 100% of the daily values for most vitamins and minerals.

Calculations were based on using 1 tsp of extra virgin olive oil in the Mediterranean Dressing and various salad dressing.

## DINNER FOR TWO IN 15 MINUTES:

It may seem that the "Healthiest Way of Eating" Plan will involve a lot of time since many meals feature cooked recipes. But let me assure you that with the quick-and-easy recipes I developed and some simple steps, you can enjoy preparing dinner in no more than 15 minutes.

I do it all the time, and you can, too. You just need to follow the easy steps I use. Let me share with you what I do to make a four-course meal in just 15 minutes.

As an example, let's prepare a meal of broiled salmon, a fresh green salad, vegetables, and a dessert.

Place a stainless steel skillet under the broiler for 5 minutes. While the skillet is heating, cut a lemon in half and sprinkle your salmon with freshly squeezed juice, then season with salt and pepper.

Slice carrots and cut broccoli florets into quarters. Let them rest for 5 minutes while you bring water to boil in a steamer. Add carrots, broccoli florets, and steam just 5 minutes or use one of the Healthy Sautéed Mediterranean Feast recipes on page 277.

By the time you've put the broccoli in the steamer, the skillet under the broiler will be hot enough to cook the salmon. Place the salmon on the skillet and "Quick Broil" for 7 minutes (For more on "Quick Broil," see page 61).

While the salmon and vegetables are cooking, wash a bag of pre-packed salad greens and remove excess water by using a salad spinner or by patting dry. Toss the salad with an easy-to-prepare dressing made of salt, pepper, extra virgin olive oil and lemon right before you serve to prevent the salad from getting too soggy or serve with your favorite vinaigrette such as balsamic or raspberry vinaigrette. You will still have enough time to wash blueberries for dessert.

Remove the salmon from the broiler. Dress the broccoli and carrots with extra virgin olive oil, garlic and lemon. Season with salt and pepper. Grated fresh ginger is a great addition for extra flavor on both fish and vegetables or to use in sauces for fish such as dill sauce or Asian teriyaki sauce. For dessert, top your blueberries with a dollop of vanilla flavored yogurt. Dinner is served!

## Q What are the least expensive foods?

A Price alone may not be the best way to look for a bargain! Although fruits and vegetables may appear

*(Continued on Page 732)*

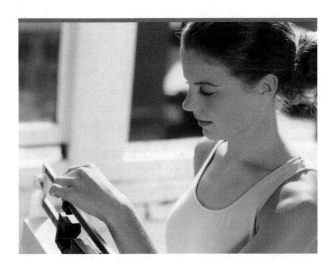

# the world's healthiest foods for healthy weight loss

Study after study shows the most effective way to be slim and healthy is to eat nutrient-rich foods—foods that will provide you with the maximum number of nutrients without empty calories. The World's Healthiest Foods meet the criteria to make them among the best foods to promote healthy weight loss. As part of the "Healthiest Way of Eating," enjoying these delicious foods will easily put you on the right track to healthy weight loss.

Regardless of how much weight you want to lose, enjoying the World's Healthiest Foods is an effective way to successfully lose weight and keep it off. You will not only be enjoying flavorful nutrient-rich foods but increasingly vibrant health and energy. You don't want just a thin body; you want a lean, energized body with glowing skin, clear eyes, strong nails and thick glossy hair. Only nutrient-rich foods, like the World's Healthiest Foods, can give you the body that expresses all you are meant to be.

By making the World's Healthiest Foods and the "Healthiest Way of Eating" the foundation of a lifestyle approach geared at healthy weight loss, you won't feel that you are dieting or that you are depriving yourself to shed extra pounds. You'll eat abundant amounts of foods that taste great and leave you satiated, not hungry.

## World's Healthiest Foods Contain Only What's Essential— Great Foods for Healthy Weight Loss

The World's Healthiest Foods are whole foods. Whole foods contain all of the nutrients that nature provides to ensure the health and life of the plant or animal. When we eat whole foods, especially when they are organically grown, we enjoy the protective qualities nature has supplied; nothing is contained in these foods that doesn't need to be there. The recipes I have created for this book and the whfoods.org website use only whole foods: no fillers, added sugars, refined flours or added saturated fats that contribute additional calories. Because the World's Healthiest Foods provide what is essential and leave out what it unnecessary, they are custom tailored for weight management.

## A Wealth of Nutrients to Support Optimal Metabolism

In order for you to lose weight, you must support for your metabolism with the nutrients that it needs. If you don't have enough nutrients to support your metabolism, you will not be able to optimize your weight loss.

Yet, you can meet your optimal nutrient needs while still staying within your caloric goals by eating nutrient-rich foods since they give you the most nutrients for your calories. These foods are your best friends when it comes to an active and healthy metabolism that can translate your food choices into successful weight loss. There are numerous examples of how getting your nutrients from nutrient-rich foods is clearly the way to go when it comes to losing weight or maintaining a healthy weight. One of my favorite examples is the difference between the energy-producing and metabolism-supporting nutrients you get from whole grain and white bread, which I discuss on page 25."

## Avoidance of Compounds that Challenge Metabolism

When you eat nutrient-rich foods, you'll find that you are so satisfied that you don't really desire other foods, namely nutrient-poor foods. Nutrient-poor foods—including those that contain refined sugar, refined grains and trans fats—can contribute to ill health and premature aging. They do not provide you with the nutrients your body needs to optimally function (and therefore optimally lose weight). At the same time, they can engender health—refined sugars can lead to reduced immune system function, refined grains can lead to blood sugar elevations and trans fats can lead to heart health problems.

The "Healthiest Way of Eating" takes into consideration each person's biochemical individuality and suggests that you examine whether you may be allergic or sensitive to different foods. I have included extensive information about this topic in the book (in the Biochemical Considerations section of each food chapter, Biochemical Individuality chapter on page 717, and Food Sensitivity Elimination Plan on page 821) so that you can see how you can structure your eating to best support your health and optimal weight loss.

### Examples of World's Healthiest Foods Support Healthy Weight

As more and more attention is given to the "Healthiest Way of Eating," scientific researchers are finding more specific examples of how nutrient-rich foods can lead to healthy weight loss.

For example, whole foods high in fiber such as beans and legumes are an important factor in weight control because not only do they provide essential nutrients, but they also keep you from feeling hungry. Beans and legumes are so slow to digest that many people find them to be natural appetite suppressants. With their low glycemic index (discussed in detail later in this article), they keep blood sugar on an even keel and stave off hunger pains.

As you'll see, throughout the book—including in the "Healthiest Way of Eating" Plan and the recipes—I emphasize "healthy fat" foods such as extra virgin olive oil, nuts and seeds. Not only are they good for promoting overall health, but they are important for healthy weight maintenance. For example, in addition to its hefty supply of polyphenol antioxidants, studies have found that extra virgin olive oil can lead to a small, but significant, loss of both body weight and fat mass. Additionally, research has shown that people who snack on nuts and seeds (in moderation) tend to be slimmer than those who don't consume these delicious foods.

And, of course, when it comes to the most nutrient-rich of all foods, vegetables take the prize. As you'll notice, vegetables comprise almost one-third of all of the World's Healthiest Foods. One look on the Nutrient-Richness Chart on page 21 will show you why: with their low calorie content and high nutrient concentration, vegetables are more nutrient-rich than any other food group. This not only bears well for optimal health but for optimal weight loss. I've dedicated a lot of time and energy to creating Healthiest Way of Cooking techniques and delicious, easy-to-make recipes for each vegetable so that you can enjoy more of these foods that will allow you to enjoy easier-to-achieve weight loss.

### Low-Glycemic Index Foods are Key to Healthy Weight Loss

Since the glycemic index (GI), the scientific ranking of foods based on how much they increase your blood sugar levels after eating, is so integral to healthy weight loss and maintenance, I have placed a lot of emphasis on it in this book. In each chapter, you'll find that food's GI in its Nutrient-Richness chart. Also, beginning on page 342, you'll find a detailed article on the subject, plus a food GI chart.

There are many reasons that GI is so integral to healthy weight. If you have balanced blood sugar, you won't experience hypoglycemic episodes that will cause you to binge on a food just to give yourself some energy and get your blood sugar level back up to normal. Plus, without fluctuating blood sugar, your release of insulin will be more steady, which will help with promoting weight loss. I recommend that you focus the majority of your food choices on foods that have a GI 60 or less.

### "Healthiest Way of Eating" Plan— A Great Tool for Healthy Weight Loss

The "Healthiest Way of Eating" Plan on page 29 is a guide that I created to help you to learn how to more easily and more enjoyably incorporate nutrient-rich foods into your lifestyle. You can use the Plan as a good foundation for a healthy eating approach to weight loss as it features the important factors inherent to healthy weight maintenance.

I'd suggest using the Plan as a map from which you can make adjustments in food choices that best support you. For example, if you know you are allergic to certain foods, substitute others. You'll notice that the Plan seems to offer you a lot of food each day. Yet, these foods are so nutrient-rich that they don't contain the level of calories that they would seem to on first glance. Also, the nutrient-richness of the Plan's meals make the menus so satiating that you can cut your portion sizes and still feel fulfilled.

An example of a great dietary component of the Plan that can help with weight loss is the recommendation to enjoy a salad (two cups of romaine lettuce contain only 16 calories) with at least one meal each day. Enjoying a low-calorie salad before

(Continued on Page 575)

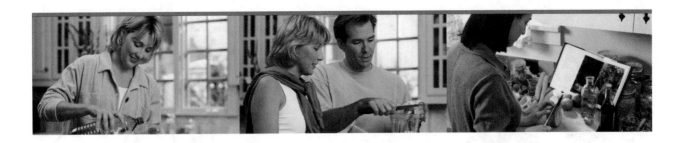

## PART 3

# healthiest
# way
# of
# cooking

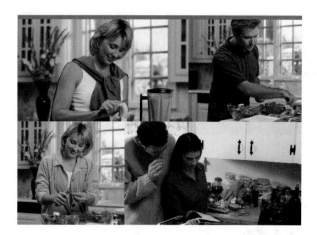

# what is the healthiest way of cooking?

**W**hile I knew that research studies had revealed that many nutrients are delicate and can be easily damaged, I was shocked when I found out exactly how many nutrients were lost due to over-cooking. Traditional ways of cooking, such as boiling certain vegetables, can deplete water-soluble vitamins, such as vitamin C and the B vitamins, as well as flavonoid phytonutrients. When I found out that up to 80% of the folic acid in carrots and 66% of the flavonoids in broccoli are destroyed through boiling for extended periods of time, I realized how important it was to develop better alternatives to traditional cooking methods that would not only enhance flavor but also preserve vitamins, minerals and antioxidants. I call these methods the "Healthiest Way of Cooking."

## The Problem with Traditional Cooking

Traditional cooking methods oftentimes involve long cooking times. This results in overcooked foods that are soft, mushy and devoid of much of their natural flavor. It was once believed that cooking for long periods of time helped to develop the flavor of food. Although this may be good practice for root vegetables used in soups and stews, it is not good for leafy greens and other vegetables. For example, many people boil broccoli until it's soft. No wonder broccoli doesn't rank high on their list of favorites—waterlogged bland food wouldn't be a favorite for anyone. The long cooking times frequently used in traditional cooking methods have another drawback. Not only does overcooking take the enjoyment out of food, it destroys vitamins, minerals, antioxidants and many other nutrients as well.

## What is the "Healthiest Way of Cooking?"

The realization that overcooking was the problem with traditional cooking methods inspired me to create the "Healthiest Way of Cooking." The "Healthiest Way of Cooking" includes a variety of methods designed to maximize retention of the beneficial vitamins, minerals, antioxidants and other nutrients found in food, which can easily be destroyed if care is not taken in preparation and cooking.

Plus, the techniques, recipes and tips that I will share with you will also help enhance the flavor of your food. No matter how nutrient-rich a food may be, if it doesn't taste delicious, you're not going to enjoy it. And what's the point of food if it doesn't bring you pleasure? I believe that eating nutrient-rich foods should be a celebration and an enjoyable experience of knowing that you are doing something wonderful for yourself.

## How Does the "Healthiest Way of Cooking" Preserve Antioxidants?

Many nutrients provide antioxidant protection against free radical activity, that can negatively affect cellular structures and DNA. These include vitamins such as A, C and E as well as phytonutrients such as the carotenoids, beta-carotene and lycopene, and flavonoids such as phenols, quercetin and rutin. Studies have found that cooking in general, the length of cooking time and the amount of water used during cooking can impact the concentration of antioxidants found in your vegetables.

You may be surprised to find that according to recent research some vegetables, such as carrots and tomatoes, actually offer greater availability of antioxidants after they have been cooked. Carotenoids are usually hooked together with proteins or locked into their own crystal-like structure when found in their natural state. Heating helps break down these structures and free carotenoids for digestion and absorption into our cells. The release of carotenoids through cooking can be measured. In carrots, for example, about 40% more carotenoids are released and made available through cooking.

Studies on the effects of cooking on the phenolic phytonutrients in zucchini, beans and carrots found that these antioxidants are best retained if cooked in small amounts of water. Dr. Anne Nugent, a nutrition scientist at the British Nutrition Foundation, has noted that it is the presence of water, rather than the cooking process itself, which makes the difference in the preservation of antioxidants. "In other words, the antioxidants would be lost upon boiling rather than steaming. . . . . it is important not to overcook . . . . as this will result in excess antioxidant loss," according to Dr. Nugent.

Since the "Healthiest Way of Cooking" methods include light steaming or "Healthy Sautéing" for a minimal amount of time, the "Healthiest Way of Cooking" methods used in the recipes are the ones I recommend to cook the different World's Healthiest Foods—not only to maximize the retention of their antioxidants, but also to enhance their flavor, texture and color.

## Testing Until I Got it Right

Finding the best way to prepare each of the World's Healthiest Foods took time. I repeatedly tested the preparation of each of the World's Healthiest Foods until I found the best cooking method to use for each food. This is how I discovered that cauliflower tastes best when "Healthy Sautéed," broccoli is best quickly steamed to retain its moisture, and "Quick Broiled" fish is the most moist and tender. I prepared some of the foods over 100 times until I got it precisely right. I tested the recipes until I was satisfied that their flavor, nutritional value or ease of preparation couldn't be improved.

I tried to make the recipes quick and easy using not only the right techniques, but a minimal number of ingredients. At first glance, the methods may seem too simple and quick to develop flavor or use too few ingredients to highlight the taste. But once you prepare them, you will see that they work really well and bring out the best flavor of your food. Believe it or not, it is actually much more difficult to create a great tasting, nutrient-rich, 5-minute recipe than to come up with a recipe that has lots of ingredients and takes many hours to prepare. I've literally put the methods and recipes in this book to the test, so I know they will work well for you.

## How the "Healthiest Way of Cooking" is Different

Most cookbooks tend to concentrate on the flavor of food and ignore the loss of nutrients that can accompany prolonged cooking times. One of the reasons this book is special is that the recipes and preparation methods focus not only on bringing out the best flavor of your food, but also on preserving the maximum number of nutrients.

You will quickly see that the way you prepare foods can not only maximize their health benefits but optimize their taste, and therefore your enjoyment. "The Healthiest Way of Cooking" is easy, and its rewards are numerous.

The Step-by-Step "Healthiest Way of Cooking" recipes in each food chapter offer maximum benefits with minimal cooking. They are easy to follow (each recipe has only a few steps), and they don't take much time to prepare. In fact, 95% of the recipes take less than 7 minutes! Since they require a minimal number of ingredients and you only need a steamer or skillet and just a few utensils, cleanup is also minimal. These recipes are great for people who don't know how to cook or don't have time to cook.

Since you won't enjoy food if it doesn't taste good, my philosophy is not just to eat nutritious foods, but to also enjoy them by preparing them properly. By following my recipes, you will not only have great tasting food but will have fun preparing it. Preparing food this way will help you build a relationship with your food. Food is essential to life; we all have to eat to live, so why not eat great tasting, nutritious food that adds to your enjoyment of life!

In the remainder of this chapter, you will find a lot of valuable information that addresses numerous aspects of cooking. I discuss the benefits of cooked and raw food, a topic on many people's minds today. Additionally, I cover how you can best preserve the nutritional value of foods with the "Healthiest Way of Cooking." Many readers of the World's Healthiest Foods' website, www.whfoods.org, have written to me asking about cooking with oils, so I have also addressed this here. Details on the cooking methods that serve as the foundation of the "Healthiest Way of Cooking" are presented, along with recommendations for the best cookware to use. Finally, you'll read about high temperature cooking and the impact it has on the nutritional value of food.

---

**HIGHLIGHTS OF THE STEP-BY-STEP "HEALTHIEST WAY COOKING" RECIPES**

- Minimal number of ingredients
- Easy directions with only a few steps to follow
- Short cooking times – 95% of the recipes take 7 minutes or less
- Flavor Tips on how to enhance the flavor of the recipe
- Minimal number of utensils required
- Only 1 pan/pot used per recipe
- Minimal cleaning

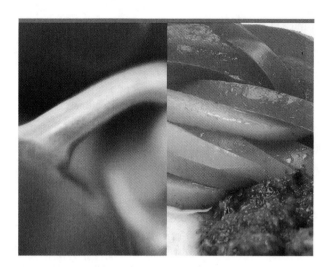

# cooked versus raw: which is better?

## Do You Have to Eat Foods Raw to Attain Their Full Nutritional Benefits?

Few human cultures have evolved or been sustained without incorporating some cooked foods, including cooked vegetables, into their eating practices. I believe that it is possible to get the full nutritional benefits from a food that has been cooked, provided that the cooking method is uniquely matched to the food and exposes the nutrients in the food to minimal damage.

### We Cook Food for Four Reasons:

- To make it easier to digest
- To increase the availability of nutrients for assimilation
- To enhance its flavor
- To preserve food safety

Here are more details on the benefits you will enjoy by cooking foods for short periods of time using the "Healthiest Way of Cooking" methods:

### "Healthiest Way of Cooking" Makes Foods Easier to Digest

Cooking vegetables quickly softens their cellulose and hemicellulose. This makes them easier to digest and allows their health-promoting nutrients to become more readily available for absorption.

### "Healthiest Way of Cooking" Helps Increase Nutrient Availability

In the case of some vegetables, cooking can actually increase the variety of nutrients that get released inside our digestive tract. Cooking onions is a good example. Onions are a member of the *Allium* family of vegetables. Most vegetables in this family have unusual amounts of sulfur-containing compounds that help protect our health. Heating onions for five minutes increases the variety of sulfur-containing substances the onions provide since it triggers chemical reactions that create variations in those sulfur compounds.

The carotenoid phytonutrient, lycopene, which is found in tomatoes, is another example of how a nutrient's bioavailability can increase when the food is heated. Heating disrupts the cellular matrix in tomatoes, which increases lycopene's availability for absorption. Heating is important in increasing the availability of lycopene because it not only disrupts the cell matrix but also converts the "trans" form of lycopene found in tomatoes into the more bioavailable "cis" form. This means that your body absorbs the lycopene in cooked tomatoes more easily than the lycopene found in raw tomatoes. (For more on *Tomatoes*, see page 164.)

### "Healthiest Way of Cooking" Enhances Flavor

I recommend cooking vegetables *al denté*. Vegetables cooked *al denté* are lightly cooked and are tender on the outside and firm on the inside. The "Healthiest Way of Cooking" vegetables is a great way to enhance their flavor as well as retain their maximum number of nutrients. By softening the texture just a bit, cooking vegetables *al denté* makes their inherent flavors come to the forefront. This is quite different than with traditional cooking methods, which usually lead to overcooking that causes flavors to dissolve or evaporate rather than come to life (for more on *Al Denté*, see page 92).

## "Healthiest Way of Cooking" Helps To Promote Food Safety

For some foods, especially animal foods, cooking temperature and duration are associated with the elimination of potentially disease-causing bacteria. Meat and poultry are cooked to avoid exposure to *E. coli* bacteria. Eggs are cooked to avoid *Salmonella*-caused food poisoning. Formerly, *Salmonella* bacteria were found only in eggs with cracked shells, but now they may be found even in clean, uncracked eggs. To destroy *Salmonella*, eggs must be cooked at high enough temperatures for a sufficient length of time.

Less known, but equally as important, is that some beans must be cooked to eliminate toxins. For example, raw kidney beans contain a naturally occurring compound called haemaglutin that causes red blood cells to clump together and inhibits their ability to take up oxygen; cooking deactivates this compound. Soybeans contain a trypsin inhibitor that prevents the assimilation of the essential amino acid, methionine, if not deactivated with heat.

Some foods should always be cooked or processed (sprouted, soaked or fermented) and never eaten raw:

**DRIED BEANS:** Potential toxins found in raw beans are decreased by cooking, soaking and sprouting.

**GRAINS:** Contain phytic acids that can partially block the availability of minerals. Grains should be cooked, soaked or sprouted to help reduce their phytic acid content.

**EGGS:** May contain *Salmonella* bacteria and therefore should always be cooked. Also, the iron and biotin found in eggs are not as well absorbed if eggs are not cooked. Raw egg whites contain a glycoprotein called avidin that binds to biotin very tightly, preventing its absorption. Cooking the egg whites changes avidin and makes it susceptible to digestion and unable to interfere with the intestinal absorption of biotin.

## Enjoy Both Raw and Cooked Foods

While I encourage you to enjoy vegetables prepared using the "Healthiest Way of Cooking" methods, I believe both raw and cooked vegetables can play important roles in your "Healthiest Way of Eating." Most animals thrive on diets consisting almost exclusively of raw, uncooked food, but raw foods require more careful and thorough chewing than cooked foods. Over 80 of the World's Healthiest Foods do not require any cooking. These include the fruits, nuts, seeds, dairy products, herbs and spices, and most of the vegetables. You can find recipes and tips for these foods in the different food chapters.

By chewing well and savoring the tastes and textures of raw food and by following the cooking suggestions for each of the World's Healthiest Foods, you will receive the unique nutritional benefits from both raw and cooked foods!

Here is a question that I received from a reader of the whfoods.org website about fresh versus frozen food:

## Q *Is fresh always better than frozen?*

A Actually, fresh is not always better than frozen. The reason is very simple: "better" depends on quality.

Suppose, for example, we chose the highest quality food source: an organically grown food, grown during its natural season and in its native habitat. In this case, would the fresh version always be better than the frozen one? Yes! Freezing would decrease the overall nutrient content of the food (although in some cases, only slightly). So fresh in this circumstance would always be better.

But imagine a second example, where the fresh food—let's say, fresh broccoli—was grown out of season, in a non-hospitable habitat, with the use of artificial fertilizers and pesticides. And to continue on in our example, let's say the frozen broccoli was grown organically in its native habitat in season. In this case, the frozen broccoli would make a better choice than the fresh broccoli because of its higher quality. Research studies have shown organically grown broccoli to have higher nutrient content than conventionally grown broccoli and to have virtually no pesticide residues.

Particularly when foods are not in season, or when organically grown products are not available, frozen organic alternatives make good sense. When fresh, organically grown foods are available, however, they always top the nourishment chart!

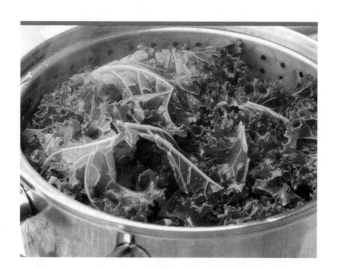

# how to preserve nutrients when cooking

## How the "Healthiest Way of Cooking" Methods Help to Preserve Nutrients

With the very precise and short cooking times used in the "Healthiest Way of Cooking" methods, you're unlikely to get a nutrient loss of more than 5–10%. This range is dramatically lower than the losses that occur in food processing or in most restaurants and cafeterias where food is routinely overcooked. Processed foods often have nutrient losses in the 50–80% range—as much as 10 times the amount that occurs with the "Healthiest Way of Cooking." While there is a 5–10% nutrient loss that occurs with careful, minimized heat and water exposure it is accompanied by other changes in the food that support our health. These other changes include improved digestibility and the conversion of nutrients into forms that are more easily absorbed.

The way that food is cooked is absolutely essential for avoiding unnecessary nutrient loss. Five minutes can make an enormous difference in the nutritional quality of a meal. (This is about the time it takes to walk away from the stove, answer the phone and say that you can't talk right now because you are in the middle of cooking.) In addition, every food is unique and should be treated that way when it comes to cooking temperatures and times. That is why I don't recommend boiling spinach for more than one minute or steaming broccoli for longer than five minutes.

The traditional rules about heat, water, time and nutrient loss are all true. The longer a food is exposed to heat, the greater the nutrient loss. Being submerged in hot water (boiling) creates more nutrient loss than steaming (surrounding with steam rather than water) if all other factors are equal. The lower nutrient loss from steaming is the main reason I recommend it so often in the recipes. I just can't think of any valid reason to expose a food to high heat and boiling water for any prolonged period of time.

Here are some questions I have received from readers of www.whfoods.org about How to Preserve Nutrients When Cooking.

**Q** *Why do overcooked vegetables lose their bright green color?*

**A** One of the primary reasons for the change in color when green vegetables are cooked is the change in chlorophyll.

Chlorophyll has a chemical structure that is quite similar to hemoglobin, which is found within our red blood cells. A basic difference is that chlorophyll contains magnesium at its center, while hemoglobin contains iron. When plants (e.g., green vegetables) are heated and/or exposed to acid, the magnesium gets removed from the center of this ring structure and replaced by an atom of hydrogen. In biochemical terms, the chlorophyll $a$ gets turned into a molecule called pheophytin $a$, and the chlorophyll $b$ gets turned into pheophytin *b*. With this one simple change, the color of the vegetable changes from bright green to olive-gray as the pheophytin *a* provides a green-gray color, and the pheophytin *b* provides an olive-green color. This color change is one of the reasons I have established the relatively short cooking times for green vegetables using the "Healthiest Way of Cooking" methods. These cooking methods are designed to preserve the unique concentrations of chlorophyll found in these vegetables.

**Q** *If many nutrients are lost in the boiling or steaming of vegetables, is pouring the remaining liquid into a glass and drinking it a good idea?*

**A** Using the water in which vegetables have been steamed or boiled is a excellent idea! Broths of this kind are a great way to salvage nutrients, especially minerals that would otherwise be lost. Covering vegetables while steaming (or a soup while cooking), instead of open-top simmering, can help retain more of the water-soluble nutrients in the cooking water.

When you boil or steam vegetables, not all of the lost nutrients end up in the water. Some evaporate into the air, and some are changed in form so that they no longer have their same health-supportive properties. But many of the lost nutrients do end up in the water, so keeping and consuming the water is definitely worthwhile.

There are exceptions, though. I would not use the cooking water from spinach, Swiss chard or beet greens, because these vegetables are high in bitter-tasting acids (including oxalic acid), that will have been extracted to the water in which they were boiled or steamed.

**Q** *Is the nutritional value of protein lost through cooking and storing of food just as vitamins are lost? For example, is the protein value still good in cooked fish that has been stored in the refrigerator for two days?*

**A** Proteins are not lost during cooking as easily as vitamins; however, overcooking and cooking at extremely high temperatures will denature proteins found in food. When cooked or agitated (as occurs when egg whites are beaten), proteins undergo physical changes called denaturation and coagulation. Denaturation changes the shape of the protein, thereby decreasing the solubility of the protein molecule. Coagulation causes protein molecules to clump together, as occurs when making scrambled eggs. Overcooking foods containing protein can destroy heat-sensitive amino acids (for example, lysine) or make the protein resistant to digestive enzymes. Refrigerating cooked foods will not further denature the proteins.

**Q** *When I pickle or marinate vegetables at home, do they lose nutrients to the pickling liquid?*

**A** Some nutrient loss occurs when you pickle or marinate vegetables. The exact nutrients that are lost and the exact percentage depends on (1) the liquids you use to pickle and marinate and (2) the length of time you keep the vegetables in the solution before consuming them. A certain percentage of some water-soluble nutrients, like vitamin C, can naturally transfer to the pickling liquid over time.

For example, 80 calories of fresh cucumber contain about 30 mg of vitamin C while 80 calories worth of pickled cucumber contains about 20 mg, for a loss of about 33%. Pickled cucumbers also lose 40–50% of their folic acid. Many of the minerals in cucumber are contained in the skins, so keeping the skins on when pickling would be important if you wanted to maintain the mineral content. (Of course, I would highly recommend organic cucumbers, especially when leaving on the skins, since it's the skin that gets the most exposure to potentially toxic sprays.)

I don't object to the pickling of vegetables and think they definitely can have a place in your "Healthiest Way of Eating." However, I do see them as significantly different (in terms of nutritional value) from both raw vegetables and minimally steamed or sautéed vegetables.

**Q** *Are vitamins like vitamin C completely destroyed when these vegetables are cooked?*

**A** In general, cooking does reduce the amount of nutrients in food, although while they may be reduced, they will not necessarily be completely destroyed. The amount of nutrient loss will be affected by a few factors including heat, time and the amount of water. For example, cooking of vegetables and fruits for longer periods of time (10–20 minutes) can result in a loss of over 50% of the total vitamin C content. The nutrient loss that can occur with cooking is the reason that I emphasize short cooking times with minimal exposure to water. These cooking methods help to create vegetables that have enhanced taste and texture and the best preserved nutrient content.

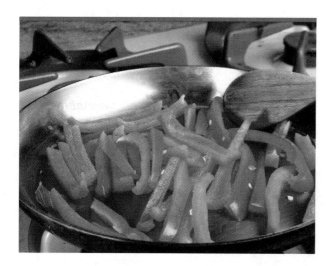

# cooking without oils

## Why it is Important to Cook Without Heated Oils

Food companies have come a long way in their ability to improve the properties of vegetable oils at the manufacturing level. There are refined and conditioned oils in the marketplace, including oils from plant hybrids that are high in certain types of fat such as monounsaturated fatty acids, which are less susceptible to damage from heating (high-oleic safflower oil is one example). If you are going to cook with oils, your best bet are these organically produced, high quality oils that have been specifically adapted for use in high heat cooking or oils that have naturally high smoke points, like avocado oil. But I believe you have an even better option—cooking without oils!

### Heating Oils

When you heat a highly unsaturated oil like safflower or sunflower oil, it will start to smoke at a fairly low heat—in the vicinity of 225°F (107°C); this is called its smoke point. When manufacturers refine these oils, they can increase the smoke point by about 100–125°F (38–52°C). In the case of refined safflower or sunflower oil, the heated oils won't smoke until about 325–350°F (163–175°C).

With a monounsaturated oil like canola oil, however, refinement can raise the smoke point to about 400°F (204°C). Manufacturers of extra virgin olive oil claim smoke points of anywhere from 200°F (93°C) to 405°F (207°C), depending on the degree of refinement and original condition of the oil. Refined avocado oil—an oil that is naturally 12% saturated and 72% monounsaturated—has one of the highest smoke points of all vegetable oils at 520°F (271°C).

When you heat an oil to its smoke point, you have definitely inflicted a good bit of damage to the oil. This damage comes in several form.

**DAMAGE TO NUTRIENTS IN THE OIL**

- Heating causes loss of available nutrients contained in oils, including fat-soluble vitamins like vitamin E and the phytonutrients that give oils their characteristic colors, smells and flavors.

- Heating oils can cause the formation of free radicals, highly reactive molecules that can damage the oil further by triggering unwanted oxidative reactions. Oil manufacturers actually assign a value (called a peroxide value, or PV) to the oils based on the amount of oxidative reactions occurring.

- Formation of unwanted aromatic substances (like polycyclic aromatic hydrocarbons, or PAHs) in the oil that can increase our risk of chronic health problems including cancer.

The smoke point is a natural property of unrefined oils, reflecting their chemical composition. When oil is refined, the process increases the oil's smoke point; in fact, raising the smoke point is one of the reasons why the refining process is used. To get a better idea of how refining increases the smoke point of oil, look at Table 1 on the next page, which shows several examples.

| TABLE 1 | |
|---|---|
| **OIL TYPE** | **SMOKE POINT** |
| Canola oil, unrefined | 225°F (107°C) |
| Canola oil, semirefined | 350°F (175°C) |
| Canola oil, refined | 400°F (204°C) |
| Safflower oil, unrefined | 225°F (107°C) |
| Safflower oil, semirefined | 320°F (160°C) |
| Safflower oil, refined | 450°F (232°C) |
| Soy oil, unrefined | 320°F (160°C) |
| Soy oil, semirefined | 350°F (175°C) |
| Soy oil, refined | 450°F (232°C) |
| Sunflower oil, unrefined | 225°F (107°C) |
| Sunflower oil, semirefined | 450°F (232°C) |
| Sunflower oil, refined high-oleic | 450°F (232°C) |

## Olive Oil and its Smoke Point

You will see various types of olive oil on the market:

- **EXTRA VIRGIN:** derived from the first pressing of the olives and has the lowest acidity level.

- **FINE VIRGIN:** also created from the first pressing of the olives, but it has an acidity level more than double that of extra virgin oil.

- **REFINED:** unlike extra-virgin and fine virgin olive oils, which only use mechanical means to press the oil, refined oil is created by using chemicals to extract the oil from the olives.

- **PURE:** a bit of a misnomer, it indicates oil that is a blend of refined and virgin olive oils.

Unlike the information presented in Table 1, the information on olive oil's smoke points is, unfortunately, not very clear or consistent since different companies list different smoke points for their olive oil products; this variability most likely reflects differences in degree of processing.

Generally, the smoke point of olive oil falls in the range of 220–437°F (104–225°C). Most commercial producers list their pure olive smoke points in the range of 425–450°F (218–232°C), while "light" olive oil products—which have undergone more processing—are listed at 468°F (242°C). Manufacturers of extra virgin oil list their smoke points in a range that starts just under 200°F (93°C) and extends all the way up to 406°F (208°C). Again, the variability here is great and most likely reflects differences in the degree of processing.

In principle, organic, unrefined, cold-pressed extra virgin olive oil should have the lowest smoke point of all forms of olive oil since it is the least refined and most nutrient-rich, containing the largest concentration of fragile nutritive components. For a natural, very high-quality extra virgin olive oil, I believe the 200–250°F (93–121°C) range reflects the most likely upper limit for heating without excessive damage. In other words, this would allow the use of extra virgin olive oil for making sauces but not for 350°F (175°C) baking or higher temperature cooking.

On my last visit to Italy, I visited many homes and restaurants to find how extra virgin olive oil was used in cooking. What I found was they don't use extra virgin olive oil for cooking; they use safflower oil or refined olive oil because of their high smoke point.

## Cooking Without Heated Oils— "Healthy Sauté"

If damage to oils only occurred at smoke point, I might be more comfortable with the idea of using oils when cooking. However, oil can be damaged from heat long before its smoke point is reached. Exactly when does damage start to occur? The research is not entirely clear about this point. Very low heating of soy oil, for example, at temperatures below 160°F (71°C), does not appear to cause many oxidative reactions even if prolonged for the course of an entire day. However, 160°F (71°C) is hardly hot enough for stovetop cooking. Water boils at 212°F (100°C). Damage seems to vary between 175°F (79°C) and the oil's smoke point—depending on the specific oil and its processing. However, even with a refined and relatively saturated oil, nutrient changes and oxidative reactions begin to occur well before the smoke point is reached.

For the reasons above, I believe it is best not to cook with heated oils. While steaming is a popular cooking method that doesn't use oils, I have created another low-heat alternative that I call "Healthy Sauté." This method was developed specifically to avoid unnecessary heating of vegetable oils by using broth instead of oil.

I have been using this technique for over 10 years with great results. Adding extra virgin olive oil to vegetables, sauces and soups after they have been cooked not only prevents the oil's exposure to high heat but allows you to enjoy more of the oil's wonderful flavor. All of the recipes in this book cook foods without the use of heated oils. I think you'll like the results in terms of flavor as well as nourishment! (For more on *"Healthy Sauté,"* see page 57.)

Here are questions that I received from the readers of the whfoods.org website about oil:

## Q *Is oil a whole food?*

A Extracting the oil from a nut or seed is a partitioning of the food. We're dividing the food up into parts and consuming only a portion. The nut or seed from which we obtain a vegetable oil is the oil's natural home. The oil is fragile and susceptible to damage from light, air and heat. The nut and seed protect it from these elements. The antioxidants that protect the oil from oxidation are contained within the nuts and seeds. When we extract the oil, we leave far too many of these antioxidants behind. That's why artificial preservatives—like BHT, for example— have to be added to some vegetable oils. These oils have lost their natural antioxidant protection. High quality manufacturers do not add BHT, of course. But they still have to add something. Vitamin E is the most common high quality ingredient added back into the oil, but some companies also use extracts from thyme, rosemary or other herbs.

There are cultures throughout the world that actually rub the nuts or the seeds directly onto their heated cooking surfaces to season and lubricate these surfaces for food preparation. Technologically, they may be a step ahead of us in understanding the natural balance found in the whole food. Yet, while I always emphasize the importance of whole foods, I still think that oil can play a part in your "Healthiest Way of Eating," as long as you use high quality, healthy oils such as organic extra virgin olive oil since it is so rich in important nutrients.

## Q *What is the difference between saturated versus unsaturated oils?*

A The susceptibility of oil to heat damage depends in part on the nature of the oil itself. There are many types of oils, but all of them can be divided into two groups: saturated and unsaturated.

The more saturated an oil, the closer the oil gets to becoming a solid instead of a liquid at room temperature. Highly saturated oils tend to be at least "semi-solid" at room temperature. Placed into the refrigerator—where oils should be stored for long-term use—highly saturated oils become difficult to pour because they take on a more solid texture. Few vegetable oils are highly saturated. This short list primarily includes coconut oil, palm oil and palm kernel oil. (Most of the highly saturated fats come from animals instead of plants. Examples would include butter, lard, chicken fat and mutton tallow.)

At the other end of the spectrum are the highly unsaturated oils. They have many ("poly") spots where they are unsaturated, so they are often referred to as the polyunsaturated oils. Most plant oils fall into this category including sunflower, safflower, soy, corn and cottonseed. These oils keep their liquid form even in the refrigerator. Today, a version of safflower oil is available called "high-oleic" safflower oil. (Oleic acid is a monounsaturated fatty acid, and it's less susceptible to heat damage than the polyunsaturated fatty acids normally found in safflower oil.) This version of safflower oil can indeed withstand higher heats and is better for use with high heats than ordinary safflower oil.

In the middle are the monounsaturated oils—oils that have a little saturated fat, a little polyunsaturated fat, and a lot of the "middle ground" fat that is only moderately unsaturated. Olive oil (about 75% monounsaturated) and canola oil (about 60% monounsaturated) are the most popular oils in this category. Olive oil is sufficiently saturated (in a healthy way) to make it semi-solid in the fridge.

## Q *While I rarely stir-fry, when I do, I use olive oil. Is this the best choice?*

A While I have included extra virgin olive oil as one of the World's Healthiest Foods owing to its wonderful nutrition and health benefits, I don't recommend cooking with it because heat can destroy the precious polyphenolic antioxidants it contains as well as cause potential oxidative damage to the oil.

Additionally, I purposely avoid cooking with oil in recipes because, unfortunately, any oil is going to undergo some damage during these cooking processes. However, if you are going to cook with oil, here is the approach I would recommend.

In general, oils become more susceptible to damage the more unsaturated they are in their chemical composition. A highly unsaturated oil (called a polyunsaturated oil) is more susceptible to damage than a minimally unsaturated oil (like a monounsaturated oil). Saturated fats are least susceptible to damage; however, they are not typically liquid at room temperature and not found in oil form. Butter, for example, is about two-thirds saturated and one-third monounsaturated and takes heat fairly well. Coconut oil is another example of a food that contains a high proportion of saturated fats.

Olive oil and canola oil are the most monounsaturated of the commonly used oils. Avocado oil is another primarily monounsaturated oil, although less commonly available.

Olive oil is about 75% monounsaturated, and canola oil is about 60% monounsaturated. Avocado oil is about 70% monounsaturated. The problem with using olive oil in high heat situations, however, is that the beneficial polyphenols in olive oil are highly susceptible to heat damage.

Corn oil, safflower oil, sunflower oil and soy oil are all more than 50% polyunsaturated. Some companies make high-oleic versions of sunflower and safflower oil. Oleic acid is the primary monounsaturated fat found in olive oil. These high-oleic versions of polyunsaturated oils make them less susceptible to heat damage and better choices for stir-frying or sautéing.

Given the above options, it makes sense to me to go with a high-oleic version of sunflower or safflower oil when frying foods. Alternatively, you could use an oil like avocado oil that is naturally monounsaturated, has a high smoke point and may not have the same kind of polyphenol composition as olive oil, which is so sensitive to high heat.

## Q Are there "good" and "bad" oils?

A While some fats are always "bad" for your health, such as those that contain trans fatty acids or high levels of saturated fats, I feel that what oftentimes makes the differentiation between "good" and "bad" is not the oil itself, but how the oil is used. Different oils have different cooking applications; an oil may be "good" if used properly but not as good if not used properly. For example, flaxseed oil is good for use in salad dressings, dips and other non-cooking applications, but it should not be heated; its fat structure is too delicate and therefore highly prone to oxidation when heated. For this reason, while flaxseed is a healthful or "good" oil when used properly, its use in a heated cooking application would be "bad."

This rationale also holds for extra virgin olive oil, which is such a "good" oil that it is included as one of the World's Healthiest Foods. It is rich in heart-healthy oleic acid, vitamin E and antioxidant polyphenolic phytonutrients. Yet, it is also very delicate and shouldn't be used in cooking. Therefore, its goodness declines if it is heated, as it can oxidize and its polyphenols can degrade.

One way to therefore consider which oil is best is to think about how you will be using it. Oils that are more delicate and have a lower smoke point are best used for dressings, non-heating cooking applications or added to foods after they are cooked; those with higher smoke points can be used at different ranges of temperature. I purposely don't cook in oil to avoid damage because, unfortunately, any oil is going to undergo some damage during these cooking processes. But if you are going to cook with oil, I would recommend high-oleic versions of sunflower and safflower oil or an oil like avocado oil. Additionally, you may want to consider a high-quality coconut oil because it is highly saturated and more stable to heat; its saturated fat is mostly medium-chain fatty acids, which do not have the health drawbacks associated with long chain saturated fats, like those found in animal fats.

## Q What do you think about coconut oil?

A Recent studies have supported the potential benefits of coconut oil. While it is true that coconuts contain saturated fats, it turns out that not all types of saturated fats are bad for you. Of the saturated fat found in coconut oil, only 9% is palmitic acid—the long-chain saturated fat most connected with increased risk of heart disease. Two-thirds of the fat in coconut oil falls into the category called "medium-chain" saturated fat; coconut oil contains caprylic and capric fatty acids, but more importantly, a very large amount of lauric acid, which has increasingly gained in its reputation as a heart-protective fatty acid.

In clinical healthcare, medium-chain fatty acids like the ones found in coconut have long-term and widespread use in the form of a product called MCT oil. ("MCT" stands for medium-chain triglyceride.) MCT oil has been widely used in clinical treatment of patients with digestion and absorption problems as well as other health conditions. The reason for use of MCT oil is its relative ease of digestion and absorption. About 30% of the MCT oil fats can be taken up from the digestive tract and into the blood without much metabolic work of any kind. This ease of absorption is very different from the absorption of long-chain fatty acids, which require much more processing. Since coconut oil, like MCT oil, contains a very high percentage of medium chain fatty acids, it can provide some of these same digestive benefits.

I have noticed that coconut oil is a very well promoted subject on the Internet, with many claims for its health benefits, notably for its antiviral activity. But from the research I have seen, many of these conclusions seem preliminary given that there has not been that much research published on this subject and that which has been conducted has often been done with individual fatty acid components of coconut oil (like monolaurin), not with coconut oil itself. Yet, at the moment it looks pretty good for coconuts and coconut oil in terms of the role that they can play in supporting health in general. But I will continue to look at the research results as they come in.

Unrefined coconut oil has a smoke point of about 350°F (170°C). Refined coconut oil has a smoke point of about 450°F (232°C).

## Q What do you think about palm oil?

A Palm oil has received a lot of media attention, and I feel that some of the information is unclear and can cause confusion. Some of the confusion has to do with the issue of the name. There are two "palm oils"—palm fruit oil and palm kernel oil—the first may be health supportive, while the second is not.

Palm fruit oil is the oil derived from the fruit of the African palm tree (*Elaeis guineensis*). Extracting the oil from the palm fruit has been practiced in Africa for thousands of years. The oil, which is a richly colored red-orange, is an integral ingredient in West African cuisine. Palm kernel oil, on the other hand, is derived from the nuts of the African palm tree.

While their names are similar, and they come from the same tree, they are actually very different. Palm kernel oil contains over 80% saturated fat, while palm fruit oil contains about 50% saturated fat (45% palmitic acid and 5% stearic acid), 40% monounsaturated fat (oleic acid) and 10% polyunsaturated fat (linolenic acid). There is also another important difference between the two—palm kernel oil requires high heat and chemical extraction in its processing, while palm fruit oil is manually expressed at low temperature (usually not exceeding 100°F/38°C).

Several studies have, in fact, shown beneficial effects on cholesterol levels by including palm fruit oil in the diet. Additionally, extracts of palm fruit have been found to exert antioxidant activity. Currently, palm fruit oil is available in some natural shortening products, which can be great baking alternatives to conventional shortenings that contain trans fatty acids. However, most of the palm oil you see on the ingredient list of processed foods is palm kernel oil. This is yet another reason why it is important to carefully read food labels.

## Q Are the fats in flaxseeds damaged when these seeds are included in baked goods such as breads, muffins or cereals?

A Fats (such as the omega-3s in flaxseed) do not get destroyed in baking because the water in the recipe, which boils at 212°F (100°C), keeps the fats cooler.

## Q What are cold pressed oils?

A The best oils are cold pressed. The oil is obtained through pressing and grinding fruit or seeds with the use of heavy granite millstones or modern stainless steel presses, which are found in large commercial operations. Although pressing and grinding produces heat through friction, the temperature must not rise above 120°F (49°C) for any oil to be considered cold pressed. Cold pressed oils are produced at even lower temperatures. Cold pressed oils retain all of their flavor, aroma, and nutritional value. Olive, peanut and sunflower are among the oils that are obtained through cold pressing.

## Q I heard that flaxseed oil taken with certain foods will enhance the value of the flaxseed oil. Is this true?

A As far as I know, the only way to naturally enhance the value of flaxseed oil would be to consume the whole flaxseed (ground) itself rather than the extracted oil. The seed contains a wider variety of nutrients than the oil, and they are uniquely combined in the seed in a natural way. I would not advise taking flaxseed oil or any oil on an empty stomach. Alongside of a balanced meal would usually be the best time to take flaxseed, although I am not aware of any special foods that could be consumed along with the oil to improve its benefits.

## Q Is it better to use olive oil or corn oil for deep frying, shallow frying and making curries?

A In general, I do not recommend frying in oil. No matter what oil you use, you are going to damage some of the fatty acids in the oil. If you are going to fry, you want to use an oil that has more monounsaturated fat than usual and less polyunsaturated fat than usual. Olive oil is about 75% monounsaturated, and that would make it the better candidate based on fat quality alone. However, frying will damage the valuable polyphenols in the olive oil. Corn oil is about 61% polyunsaturated. That would make it a worse choice based on the fat content. A third possibility would be a high-oleic oil like high-oleic sunflower or safflower oil that should be better able to withstand the higher heat and does not have the same polyphenol levels as olive oil.

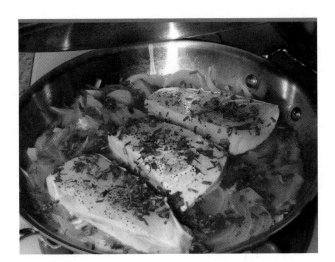

# healthiest way of cooking methods

"Healthy Sauté," "Healthy Steaming," "Quick Broil," poaching, roasting and healthiest way to grill are the healthiest methods I have found to enhance the flavor and retain the maximum number of nutrients of the World's Healthiest Foods.

## "Healthy Sauté"

"Healthy Sauté" is a very special way of preparing foods because it has the benefits of three methods in one. It is a sauté that uses vegetable or chicken broth in place of heated oils; I am particularly conscious of creating recipes that do not use heated oils because they can potentially have negative effects on your health. It is like stir-fry because it brings out the robust flavor of foods but cooks them at a lower temperature. It is like steaming because there is enough moisture to soften the cellulose and hemicellulose, which aids digestibility. "Healthy Sauté" requires just a small amount of liquid to make vegetables moist and tender. Vegetables such as cauliflower and asparagus, which only require a small amount of liquid to tenderize them, are especially good candidates for "Healthy Sauté" because steaming and boiling dilute their flavor.

---

**"Healthy Sauté," Step-by-Step**

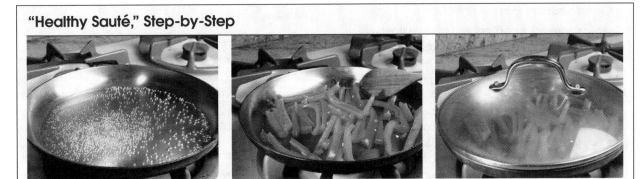

❶ Heat broth in a stainless steel skillet. ❷ When broth begins to steam add vegetables. ❸ Cover if necessary and sauté for recommended period of time.

## How to "Healthy Sauté"

Heat broth in a stainless steel skillet. When the broth begins to steam, add vegetables and cover. Sauté for the recommended amount of time. Some vegetables require cooking uncovered for several minutes before serving. "Healthy Sauté" will concentrate both the flavor and nutrition of your vegetables.

## More About Broth

Broth, a staple ingredient in "Healthy Sauté," usually contains about 1% fat, which helps bring out the flavor of the food. This small amount of fat also helps coat the food and the bottom of the pan, which helps protect the food from sticking to the pan. Yet, if some sticking occurs (let's say your "Healthy Sautéed" onions stick to the pan a little), don't worry. Just add a little more broth to your pan and stir; it will release what little is stuck, actually adding extra flavor to your dish. If your vegetables look like they are burning, simply turn the heat down and continue to sauté.

Since the broth does not require the high heat used in stir-fry and because "Healthy Sauté" does not use heated oils, this method of cooking avoids the formation of carcinogenic compounds created when oils are heated to high temperatures. Be sure to use a stainless steel skillet when "Healthy Sautéing."

If you do not have broth, a little hot water with a small amount of yeast extract would be a good substitute. Plain hot water also works although the broth adds a little extra flavor, and its minimal fat content helps to keep the vegetables from

---

### VEGETABLE AND CHICKEN BROTH

Since homemade broth takes time to prepare, for my recipes I usually use premade organic chicken or vegetable broth. If you can't find organic broth, just buy the one that contains the least amount of additional ingredients such as extra salt or MSG.

Aseptic packed cartons of chicken or vegetable broth are preferable to cans. Canned products are traditionally heated for one hour for sterilization. Aseptic packaging uses a flash heating method that preserves both flavor and nutrients. After opening, aseptic packed broth will last for up to two weeks; canned broth will last for about five days. I don't recommend bouillon cubes as they are very salty, and most contain MSG. Read labels for undesirable ingredients, especially in dried forms of broth.

Broth can be frozen and used as required. Ice cube trays are a good way to store broth; one cube contains about one to two tablespoons.

---

sticking. If you are not on an extremely salt-restrictive diet, another easy-to-make broth that I like to use and is made by adding 1 teaspoon of miso paste to 1/4 cup of warm water. Mix until it is well dissolved.

Here is a question that I received from a reader of whfoods.org about how to store broth:

**Q** *My problem with broth is that you have to open a big can of broth in order to use a tablespoon for cooking purposes. What do you do with the rest of the can? Is there a good way to keep broth fresh for an extended period of time?*

**A** You can make soup out of the remaining broth—just add chopped vegetables. You can transfer the rest of the broth from the open can into an airtight glass jar and keep it in the refrigerator for about five days after opening. Freezing the remaining broth in an ice cube tray is a very convenient way to use small amounts of broth as desired.

## "Healthy Steaming"

"Healthy Steaming" is one of the best cooking methods for retaining flavor and nutrients in foods. Foods simply steamed and flavored with fresh herbs, lemon and olive oil can be very satisfying and delicious, especially when the vegetables themselves have so much taste. It is also a way to cook that can be done in one pot on the stove, so there is very little mess and cleanup required.

A study published in the *Journal of the Science of Food and Agriculture* found that light steaming was the clear winner when comparing different types of cooking methods and their effects on the retention of phytonutrients, such as carotenoids and flavonoids that act as powerful antioxidants. Light steaming resulted in almost no loss of these health-promoting minerals nutrients.

What I have gleaned from many scientific studies is that if you cook your vegetables *al denté*, you will maximize nutrient retention, losing only around 5–10% of vitamins, while the loss of minerals and other nutrients is even less. Overcooking can destroy more than 50% of some vegetables' nutrients.

Even small variations in cooking techniques can affect how many nutrients you preserve. When you steam or boil vegetables, look at the color of the cooking water to see the difference in nutrient loss. The color of the water used to steam vegetables changes very little; this indicates very little nutrient loss.

However, if you steam for a long time, the color of the water will deepen, reflecting the loss of a large number of nutrients.

One way to preserve water-soluble nutrients like vitamin C when steaming vegetables *al denté* is to make sure the water is boiling rapidly and the steam is very hot (rolling) before you put the vegetables in the steamer. The heat of the rolling steam neutralizes enzymes that can destroy vitamin C, which otherwise doesn't stand up to heat as well as other nutrients. Up to 20% of vitamin C can be lost within the first two minutes of cooking if you're not careful!

My "Healthy Steaming" method allows you to cook your vegetables to preserve their nutrients, bring out their color and enhance their flavor. Steaming for a minimal amount of time produces vegetables cooked *al denté*, crisp inside and tender outside, and is an ideal way to maximize their nutritional value. Commonly, vegetables are steamed for much too long, causing them to lose their flavor, color and nutrients. Be sure to note the time I have recommended for steaming in the recipes. Because temperatures vary on stoves, watch to make sure your vegetables are still brightly colored and a little crisp in the center when you remove them from the heat; reduce the time they are steamed if necessary.

## How to "Healthy Steam"

Put 2 inches of water in the bottom of the pot. This will ensure that you will have enough water to avoid burning the pot. I am sharing this with you because I have burned many pots by using too little water trying to build up steam too quickly. It just takes a few seconds more with the extra amount of water.

In "Healthy Steaming," you want to make sure the water is at a rapid boil before adding your vegetables to the steamer basket. This is so the heat will be consistent throughout cooking time. Steaming cooks the vegetables with even,

moist heat. Once the water is at a rapid boil, turn the heat to a medium temperature and place the vegetables in the steamer basket. You want to make sure the steamer has a tight-fitting lid.

If you are "Healthy Steaming" more than one vegetable at a time, place the vegetables in the steamer basket in layers. There are two ways of doing this:

- Place all the vegetables in the steamer basket at once, putting the denser vegetables that need more heat on the bottom. Layer the vegetables, putting the lighter ones, such as greens, on top.

- Place the denser vegetables that take longer in the steamer basket and cook with the lid on for 2–4 minutes. Then add another layer of vegetables that take a little less time to cook and continue to steam. This can be done in several layers, ending up with all of your vegetables done to perfection at the end of cooking time. See Mediterranean Feast, page 277.

You can also "Healthy Steam" vegetables and fish together by steaming a variety of vegetables with a nice piece of salmon or other fish on top. You can make a simple Mediterranean dressing and drizzle it over everything when done. It is a perfect way to make a simple, healthy meal in one pot in a very short amount of time.

Remember that steam can be deceiving. It is still very hot and can burn you easily, so it is important to remember to open the lid on your steamer facing away from your body. This will prevent the steam from burning your face or arms as you lift the lid.

## Why I Like "Healthy Steaming"

You may think of "Healthy Steaming" as a high-heat way of cooking, but in comparison to most other ways, it isn't.

### "Healthy Steaming," Step-by-Step

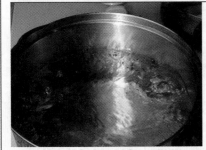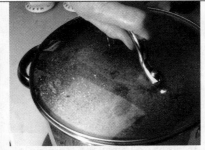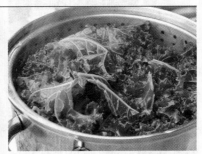

❶ Fill bottom of steamer with 2 inches of water (so you don't burn the pot) and bring to boil. Add vegetables to steamer. ❷ Cover steamer. ❸ Steam for the recommended time.

Since water boils at 212°F (100°C) and transforms into steam, steam actually cooks food at a lower temperature than most oven-based and stove-top cooking methods, which range from 350°F (175°C) to 450°F (232°C). When compared with boiling, steaming is a better way of avoiding nutrient loss since the food is surrounded by water dispersed in air, rather than being completely submerged in the water itself. The decreased contact of water with the surface of the food results in decreased nutrient loss. If a food is sliced or chopped into sufficiently small sections, steaming can get it into a tender and tasty form long before most other heating methods. Even butternut squash can be steamed in less than 10 minutes.

## Cover the Pot

It may sound silly, but covering the pot while "Healthy Steaming" can help preserve the nutritional quality of the food. When a pot is covered, the contact of the steam with the food is more consistent, allowing the steaming process to be completed in the least amount of time. In addition, light-sensitive nutrients—like vitamin B2—will not be leached out of the food so easily. As an added benefit, since many water-soluble nutrients pass out into the steam, if the pot is covered, they will drop back down into the water below the steamer basket. Save this water! It can be used as a base for soups and sauces or at the very minimum allowed to cool and used to water plants in the garden.

# "Quick Broil"

Healthy cooking methods are essential to getting all the value of the food we eat. When focusing on creating quick and easy recipes especially for the warm weather months, I have found that the "Quick Broil" method is one that I am using a lot.

---

### BENEFITS OF MARINADES

Marinades that include antioxidant-rich ingredients can help offset the formation of cancer-causing heterocyclic amines. Spices, seasonings and other marinade components with known antioxidant properties include turmeric, curry blends, rosemary, garlic and onion. The piperine in black pepper has direct antioxidant and free-radical-protective properties as does the vitamin C in lemons and oranges.

---

## How to "Quick Broil"

To "Quick Broil," you first want to preheat the broiler (on high). It heats up very quickly, so you don't have to have the broiler on for very long. I place a shallow metal pan under the heat of the broiler for 10 minutes. For fish, I usually put the rack right beneath the heat. For chicken, I put the rack closer to the middle of the oven, so it doesn't burn the top of the chicken before cooking all the way through. It is important that the pan is metal, preferably stainless steel.

Let the pan get very hot under the heat. The time of preheating the broiler and pan can be used to prepare your ingredients. Season chicken or fish with lemon juice, salt and pepper. Season red meats with salt and pepper. Once the pan is very hot, place your seasoned meat or fish on the hot pan. You do not need any oil in the pan for this cooking method. Because the pan is so hot, it immediately seals the meat on the bottom to retain the juices and keeps the meat or fish from sticking.

Return the pan with the meat or fish to under the broiler. The meat or fish is now cooking rapidly from both sides. It does not need to be turned, and it is done very quickly. For some fish fillets, the cooking time can be as quick as 1 to 2 minutes,

---

### "Quick Broil," Step-by-Step

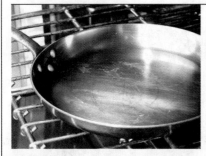 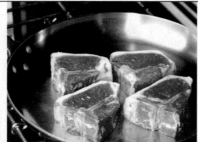 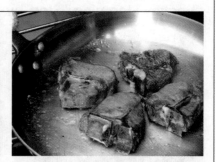

❶ Preheat broiler on high and place an empty, all stainless steel skillet under flame to get very hot, about 10 minutes. ❷ When pan is very hot, add meat or fish and place pan back under the broiler. ❸ Cook for recommended period of time.

depending on the thickness. Salmon fillets can be cooked in 5 to 7 minutes. For chicken, I have found that leaving the skin on the breast helps to keep the meat nice and juicy, and it can be cooked in as little as 15 minutes. Simply remove the skin before eating. I have found "Quick Broil" to be a very quick and healthy way of cooking meat and chicken.

## "Quick Boil"

Although very short cooking at 212°F (100°C) in boiling water produces relatively little nutrient loss, once boiling goes on for anything more than a few minutes, the nutrient loss becomes significant. Up to 80% of the folic acid in carrots, for example, can be lost from boiling. The same is true for the amount of vitamin B1 lost in boiled soybeans.

There are only three vegetables I recommend boiling: Swiss chard, spinach and beet greens. The reason I boil these vegetables is to help reduce their oxalic acid content. Spinach is "Quick Boiled" for only 1 minute, and Swiss chard and beet greens are boiled for only 3 minutes.

### How to "Quick Boil"

Use a large pot (3 quart) and fill it three-quarters full of water. Make sure the water is at a rapid boil before adding the greens. When the water is at full boil, place the greens into the pot. Do not cover. Cooking uncovered helps the acids escape into the air. Cook for the recommended time; begin timing as soon as you drop the greens into the boiling water. When vegetables are done, place a mesh strainer in the sink. Empty the contents of the pot into the strainer to drain the water from the vegetables.

## Poaching Fish

Poaching is one of the easiest and most gentle ways of cooking fish and also provides a delicious broth that can be used for soup.

### How to Poach

Chop onions and chop or press garlic and let them sit for 5 minutes. Place onion, garlic, celery, parsley, 4 cups cold water or broth and 1/2 tsp salt into a 2-quart pan. A few drops of sherry will also enhance the flavor. Cover and bring to a boil.

Cut fish fillets in half and place in the boiling liquid. Be sure that the fish is covered with the liquid. Lower heat to medium, cover and cook for 5 minutes depending on thickness. I love poached fish dressed with olive oil, lemon juice, garlic, and salt and pepper. For a Mediterranean flavor, I top the fish with a little chopped fresh basil, thyme or parsley.

## Roasting

Roasting is done with dry heat in an open pan in a hot oven, about 450°F (232°C) or higher. It crisps up the exterior of the meat or vegetables while slow cooking the inside.

### How to Roast

Roast root vegetables at 450°F (232°C) for about 30 minutes without oil; stir once in a while to distribute natural juices. The temperature for roasting nuts is much lower—use a 160–170°F (70–75°C) oven for 15–20 minutes—to preserve the heart-healthy oils in nuts. (For instructions on *Roasting Turkey*, see page 585.)

## Healthiest Way to Grill

Grilled foods have a unique flavor and texture and are synonymous with summertime and cooking outdoors.

### How to Grill

- Grill on an area without a direct flame as the temperatures directly above or below the flame can reach as high as 500°F (260°C) to 1000°F (538°C).

---

### "Quick Boiling," Step-by-Step

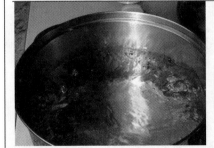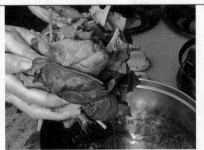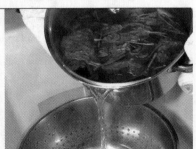

❶ Fill a 3-quart pot three-quarters full with water and bring to boil. ❷ Add vegetables, but **do not cover**. Begin cooking time as soon as you drop vegetables into the water. ❸ Strain and serve.

- Be sure not to overcook or burn your food; this helps prevent the formation of toxic compounds.

- Marinate in a mixture that includes antioxidant-rich ingredients such as lemon, onions, rosemary or black pepper.

- If you do choose to grill foods and use an oil to coat them, use an oil that has a high smoke point, such as avocado oil or high-oleic safflower oil, to lessen the amount of oxidative damage that will occur in the oil itself.

The principles of nutrient loss from charcoaled or gas-grilled foods are very similar to the principles of all cook-ing: the shorter the time of exposure to heat and the lower the heat, the less the nutrient loss.

---

# Cooking Measurement Equivalents and Conversions

## Recipe Equivalents
1 tablespoon (TBS) = 3 teaspoons (tsp)
1 cup (c)= 16 tablespoon (TBS)
1 cup (c) = 8 fluid ounces (oz)
1 pint (pt) = 2 cups (c) = 16 fluid ounces (oz)
1 quart (qt) = 2 pints (pt) = 32 fluid ounces (oz)
1 gallon (gal) = 4 quarts (qt) = 64 fluid ounces (oz)
1 pound (lb) = 16 ounces (oz-wt)

## Metric Measurements
**VOLUME**
1 teaspoon (tsp) = 5 ml
1 tablespoon (TBS) = 15 ml
1 fluid ounce (oz) = 30 ml
1 cup (c) = 240 ml
1 pint (pt) = 470 ml
1 quart (qt) = 940 ml
1 gallon (gal) = 3.8 liters

**WEIGHT**
1 ounce (oz-wt) = 28 grams
1 pound (lb) = 454 grams

**TEMPERATURE**
Throughout the book, both Fahrenheit (°F) and Celsius (°C) temperatures are provided. Should you need to convert Fahrenheit to Celsius, subtract 32 and then multiply by 5/9. Should you need to convert Celsius to Fahrenheit, multiply by 9/5 and then add 32.

---

## Poaching Fish with Vegetables, Step-by-Step

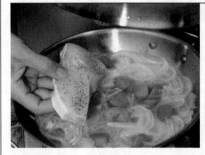 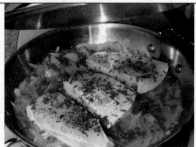 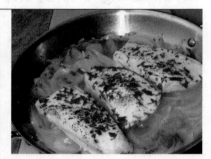

❶ Simmer vegetables, starting with cold water, for about 5 minutes. ❷ Place fish on top of vegetables and **cover**. ❸ Cook for about 5 minutes, depending on thickness of fish.

Here are some questions that I received from readers of whfoods.org about "Healthiest Way of Cooking" methods.

## Q Do you lose the nutritional value of food when using a pressure cooker?

A Pressure cooking—particularly when you keep the liquid when using the vegetables in a soup—can be a healthy approach to food preparation. But I believe it can be a little more difficult to avoid overcooking when pressure cooking than when steaming—and avoiding overcooking is one of my key concerns. You can usually tell by color and texture whether or not a food has been overcooked. Sometimes the difference between optimal heating and overheating is less than two minutes. Cooking at higher pressure can allow for shortening of cooking times with certain foods, such as beans.

Some nutrients become more available with light heating, and some become less. In general, however, it's overcooking that's the problem. Therefore, my main concern with the pressure cooker would be avoiding overcooking. If you experiment with your technique and the colors and textures of your foods are being preserved, you are probably doing a good job with your pressure cooker. If your foods are coming out discolored, limp and mushy, you are definitely losing nutrients in comparison with the light steaming technique I use for most vegetables.

## Q What type of cookware should I avoid?

A First, in spite of its convenient, lightweight and break-proof nature, plastic is not a good choice for your kitchen. Very small amounts of plastic pass from the container to the food, even at refrigerator temperatures, and even when foods are not acidic. Vinyl chloride, for example, has been shown to migrate from PVC (polyvinyl chloride) water bottles into the water itself. The worst places to use plastic are in the microwave or in a pot of boiling water (for example, in the case of "boil-in-the-bag" foods). As a general rule, you are safest microwaving in unleaded ceramic or tempered glass containers (like Pyrex®) but not in plastic, even if the plastic is a harder, polycarbonate variety (number 7 on the recycling logo). Storage of food in plastic is not as much a problem as cooking in plastic, but even in this situation, glass containers with plastic lids would be safer than containers made entirely of plastic.

On the stovetop, aluminum pots and pans are the equivalent of plastic in the microwave and should be avoided. Many anodized aluminum pans look more like stainless steel than aluminum, so check to be sure. You may need to contact the store, or the manufacturer in some cases, to determine exactly what materials your pot or pan contains.

According to a 2005 report by a scientific advisory panel at the U.S. Environmental Protection Agency (EPA), a substance derived from Teflon® (known as PFOA) was classified as a "likely carcinogen." This report set the basis for the EPA regulation of this product, most famous for its use as the original "non-stick" cookware surface. Teflon is relatively ubiquitous with pots, pans, woks, waffle makers, pancake griddles, deep fryers, slow cookers, bread makers, coffee makers, electric skillets, cooking utensils and hot air popcorn poppers, just a few of the kitchen items that may contain Teflon coatings. Although PTFE (polytetrafluoroethylene) the key susbstance found in Teflon, does not break down into PFOA (perfluorooctanoic acid) until a temperature of about 464°F (240°C) on the stovetop, this risk seems completely unnecessary to me and I recommend avoiding all PFTE non-stick cookware, including Teflon-coated cookware, for this reason.

---

*(Continued from Page 180)*
lose not only their texture and flavor, but also their nutrients. Overcooking Green Beans will significantly decrease their nutritional value: as much as 50% of some nutrients can be lost. (For more on *Al Denté*, see page 92.)

## Cooking Methods
## Not Recommended for Green Beans

### BOILING OR COOKING WITH OIL

I do not recommend boiling Green Beans because boiling increases their water absorption, causing them to become soggy and lose much of their flavor along with many of their nutrients including minerals, water-soluble vitamins (such as C and the B-complex vitamins) and health-promoting phytonutrients. I also don't recommend cooking Green Beans in oil because high temperature heat can damage delicate oils and potentially create harmful free radicals.

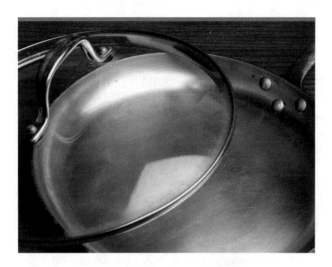

# best cookware for the healthiest way of cooking

## What is the Best Cookware?

The quality of the food you eat depends in part on the quality of your cookware, and high-quality meals require high-quality cookware.

Stainless steel, porcelain-coated, cast iron and tempered glass (if used on low heat to avoid damaging the glass) pots would be my first choices on the stovetop. Inside the oven, I would go with these same materials, although the rubber and plastic on lids and handles of cast-iron cookware can be a problem in the oven. Extra care must also be taken not to get burned by the hot iron. Glass, iron and porcelain ceramics consist of primarily natural substances, in stark contrast to a coating like Teflon®, which contains fluorocarbons not formed in the natural world. With stainless steel, I do recommend careful cleaning that avoids harsh scouring, which can release too much nickel and/or chromium from the cookware.

## Cookware to Avoid

### ALUMINUM AND PLASTIC COOKWARE

Aluminum pots and pans clearly release aluminum into foods. Even though aluminum is very lightweight and convenient on the stovetop, and plastic is very lightweight and convenient in the microwave, I suggest you steer clear of these products. Except for convenience, there is simply no reason for you to face the potential health risks associated with migration of aluminum or plastics (like polyvinyl chloride)—even in very small amounts—from the kitchenware into your food.

### TEFLON-COATED COOKWARE

In June 2005, a scientific advisory panel working at the Environmental Protection Agency (EPA) in Washington, D.C., drafted a report that described Teflon as a "likely carcinogen" and set the basis for EPA regulation of this widely used product. In the cooking world, of course, Teflon is most famous as the original "non-stick" cookware surface, introduced into the marketplace shortly after World War II. Not only pots and pans, but also woks, waffle makers, pancake griddles, deep fryers, slow cookers, bread makers, coffee makers, non-stick rolling pins, electric skillets, cooking utensils and hot air popcorn poppers may contain Teflon coatings. So can a wide variety of other consumer products. Levi Strauss & Company even came out with a Teflon-coated version of their famous Dockers line of clothing. An estimated $40 billion dollars' worth of Teflon-coated products has been sold worldwide.

In terms of chemistry, the health risks connected with Teflon involve two substances: polytetrafluoroethylene (PTFE) and perfluorooctanoic acid (PFOA). PTFE is the primary substance in Teflon and can basically be regarded as a plastic. PTFE will decompose under high heat, and one of the substances produced is PFOA. Toxic particles and fumes containing PFOA begin to be released from a Teflon-coated pan on a stovetop at about 464°F (240°C), according to research done by the Environmental Working Group (www.ewg.org) in 2003.

The EPA scientific advisory panel named PFOA as the likely carcinogen related to Teflon, not PTFE. For this reason, the manufacturer of Teflon, DuPont, has taken the position that no PFOA is contained in its non-stick cookware, only PTFE.

This position by DuPont® has come partly in response to a $5 billion dollar class-action lawsuit filed by two Florida law firms on behalf of 14 people in 8 states who purchased and used Teflon®-coated cookware. Yet, it is important to remember that PTFE can decompose into PFOA.

## Essential Cookware Necessary for the "Healthiest Way of Cooking"

There are only two essential pieces of cookware I need in my kitchen to serve one to four people using the "Healthiest Way of Cooking" methods. Large families will require larger size cookware.

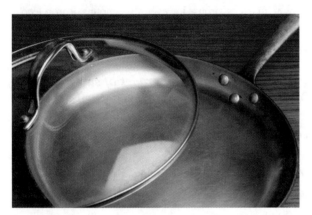

*10" Stainless Steel Skillet: For "Healthy Sauté," poaching eggs, "Quick Broil" and roasting*

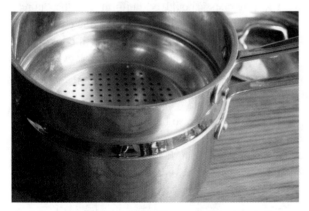

*3-Quart Steamer with a lid: For steaming and boiling vegetables and poaching fish*

I don't recomend collapsable steamers or bamboo steamers because you can easily burn your hands when using them, and they are hard to handle.

It is also important to have a battery-operated timer as well as a brush to clean the stainless steel pan. Cleaning the pan right after using it makes it much simpler to clean.

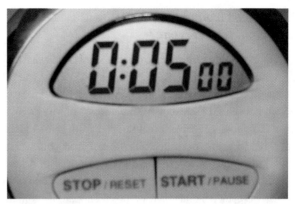

*Battery-operated timer*

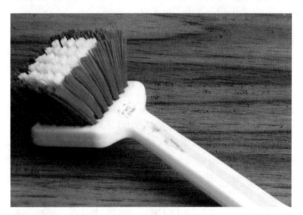

*Kitchen brush*

Here are some questions that I received from readers of whfoods.org about cookware:

**Q** *Does the small amount of aluminum released from an aluminum pot really make a difference?*

**A** It depends on a person's health status and also on a person's philosophy of health. Healthy people can ordinarily process and get rid of small amounts of toxins they encounter. This process is called detoxification. Most healthy people could detoxify the amount of aluminum released by an aluminum pot. But an unhealthy person might not be able to do so. Would that person get immediately sick? Possibly, but probably not. Would that person be using up energy and vitamins and minerals in order to get rid of the small toxic residue? Definitely. Is it reasonable for a person to keep exposing him or herself to small amounts of toxins when those toxins could be avoided? The answer to that question really depends on your philosophy of health. Since there are many inexpensive, non-toxic alternatives to aluminum pans, I always recommend those alternatives.

## Q *Is cast iron cookware good for everyone?*

A A hundred years ago, cast iron cookware was the most popular choice in U.S. households. This type of cookware is still an excellent choice, provided that no one in your household has excessive body stores of iron. While most U.S. adults receive too little iron from their meals and would benefit from cooking in cast iron cookware, some individuals have excessive body stores of iron and would be at risk of iron overload problems when cooking in cast iron. In general, men or postmenopausal women who consume beef on a daily basis are most likely to be at risk for iron overload problems.

## Q *Does seasoning my cast iron cookware with oil promote damaging free radicals to enter my body with the food?*

A Unfortunately, the answer to your question is both "yes" and "no." I'll try to provide you with the complete context. Free radicals are highly reactive molecules that can be formed under a wide variety of circumstances. They are constantly being formed in our bodies, in the bodies of most living things, and in the atmosphere itself. Free radicals aren't bad. They are neutral. Free radical reactions are necessary in order for life to continue. Excessive amounts of free radicals in the wrong place are the problem. Too many free radicals near a blood vessel wall can start to damage the blood vessel. Too many free radicals in the air can cause imbalances in the earth's atmospheric gases. But the formation of free radicals is itself a natural process.

Cast iron cookware needs to be seasoned to function properly. Not only do foods stick to cast iron when it's unseasoned, but the iron itself will leech out of the cookware more quickly. Most cast iron cookware comes with seasoning instructions. Seasoning basically involves the even application of a very light amount of oil—often less than one teaspoon—on all surfaces of the cookware, and then heating in the oven at 100–150°F (40–65°C) for 45–60 minutes. During this time, the oil seeps into the pores of the cookware and forms a protective seal. While there will be oxidation of fats during this process, the resulting coating will allow the cast iron to cook cleanly at high heats. When cast iron is properly seasoned, it needs very little oil when in use. A seasoned cast iron pot or skillet should be heated upon reuse until it begins to smoke. At that point, the surface coating of oil will have seeped back into the pores and will create an almost stick-free cooking surface.

You may have heard about the relationship between iron and free radicals. In that relationship, when too much free iron begins to accumulate in our cells, this free iron interacts with oxygen to form free radicals. Free radical formation from excess iron intake is one of the toxicity-related problems with excess iron. However, the amount of iron leeching from cast iron is not typically enough to throw a person into metabolic iron excess.

## Q *Are there different grades of cast iron? My aim is to have non-toxic cookware, and my budget is low. Do you know whether I can consider "cheap" cast iron safe?*

A As far as safety is concerned, even "cheap" cast iron should be safe. However, there are things you might want to look for when purchasing cast iron cookware:

- Although unseasoned cast iron will be rough, it shouldn't be uneven or bumpy.

- The roughness should be uniform and the "pores" small and fine. The finer the surface, the easier it will take the seasoning and the better it will cook. If it is unevenly rough, it will not heat and cook evenly.

- Check for ridges, pits, fine cracks, chips, seams and jagged edges.

- The color should also be uniformly gray with no discolored blotches or shadows; the color should be the same inside and out. If there is any variance in color, it means the metal wasn't heated evenly and may break or warp.

- The bottom of a frying pan or kettle should be smooth, without ridges, to conduct the heat evenly. This is especially important if you're going to use it on a smooth cooking surface such as an electric range.

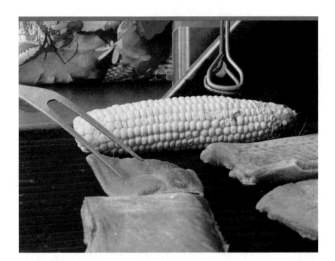

# why avoid high temperature cooking?

One of the greatest insults to nourishment in our modern, fast-paced and processed food culture is the high heat at which so much of our food is cooked. We deep fat fry at 350–450°F (177–232°C); we fry on the stovetop in shortening and vegetable oils right up to their smoke points of 375–450°F (191–232°C); and we barbecue with gas grills that can reach temperatures of over 1000°F (538°C)! This exposure of food to high heat may be convenient and quick, and it may fill the air with aromas that we savor, but it comes at a definite nutritional cost. Neither the foods nor the nutrients they contain were designed to withstand extremely high temperatures. How you prepare the foods you eat can be just as important to your health as what you eat.

## Unwanted Consequences of High-Heat Cooking

### LOSS OF NUTRIENTS

The problems with high-heat cooking are not restricted to the creation of toxic substances. High-heat cooking is also problematic when it comes to loss of nutrients. Virtually all nutrients in food are susceptible to damage from heat. Of course, whether a particular nutrient gets damaged depends on the exact nutrient in question, the degree of heat and the amount of cooking time. But in general, most of the temperatures we cook at in the oven (250–450°F/120–230°C) are temperatures at which substantial nutrient loss occurs, except for roasting turkey because it takes a long time for the heat to penetrate the meat and damage the nutrients. And although very short cooking at 212°F (100°C) in boiling water produces relatively little nutrient loss, once boiling goes on for anything more than a very short period of time (1–3 minutes), the nutrient loss becomes significant.

I've searched and searched through the nutrition research, and all of the evidence points to the same conclusion: prolonged, high-heat cooking is just not the way to go.

## Our Senses Can Tell Us a Lot

Sometimes scientific research just reminds us that we can trust our five senses and our own good judgment. This conclusion seems to apply to high-heat cooking. Almost always, there is some magical point at which our senses begin to dislike the result of the high heat. It may be a color change in the kale or collard greens, where the green ceases to become more and more vibrant and begins to take on a duller, grayer shade. It may be a change in air and aroma, as occurs when a vegetable oil starts to smoke. Vegetables oils have unique smoke points that can be more than 200 degrees apart, but the fact that they smoke is still a nice common-sense warning that high heat is doing some damage. If we expose foods to high heat for too long, our taste buds will also let us know.

## Vegetables and High-Heat Cooking

I've tried to emphasize the wonderful diversity and uniqueness of food. I've tried to pay attention to all of the little details that make each fruit, vegetable or legume nutritionally special. It should not be surprising that specific foods within any food family must be treated just as uniquely when it comes to cooking. Nevertheless, I've still found it amazing just how sensitive some foods are when it comes to high heat—especially vegetables!

When it comes to vegetables, sensitivity to high heat has to be measured in a matter of minutes! In some foods, like Swiss chard, loss of vitamin C can increase by 15% in a matter of just 4–5 minutes. Swiss chard can't be cooked as an afterthought while we are talking on the phone, setting the table or feeding the cat. Just a few minutes can change the outcome completely! Green beans will steam in about 5 minutes. During this time, their color will take on a more vibrant green hue. If you cook it longer you will notice a change in color. For example, after 7 minutes a drop in color intensity will begin to occur. By 9 or 10 minutes, the color intensity will have dropped noticeably. Just 2–3 minutes of extra steaming time can make this notable difference.

The optimal timetable for high-heat cooking will vary with a number of factors in addition to the type of vegetable. How the vegetable is sliced, for example, will change the amount of steaming it needs. Finely shredded cabbage requires less steaming (and less heat) than coarsely shredded cabbage. Because more surface of the finely shredded cabbage gets directly exposed to the steam, it takes less time for the cabbage to become tender. If you mix vegetables in the steamer basket, the topmost layers that are less directly exposed to the steam should be the vegetables needing the least steaming. The vegetables requiring longer steaming should be placed on the bottommost layer. Alternatively, vegetables that need less steaming can be added to the steamer basket later on, after the vegetables that are thicker and more dense have been added.

### HETEROCYCLIC AMINES (HCAs)

Nutritional research is just starting to catch up with the consequences of high-heat methods of cooking. We've learned, for example, that some of the most mutagenic agents formed in cooking, heterocyclic amines (HCAs), are commonly found in barbecued beef, chicken, and pork cooked at 392°F (200°C) or above. We even know what basic ingredients are required for these mutagenic agents to be produced: high temperature for more than a few minutes' duration, free amino acids (from protein), creatine (or creatinine) and sugar. Without the high temperature component, the formation of HCAs does not occur. Direct flame grilling produces another type of carcinogen called polycyclic aromatic hydrocarbons (PAHs), which might be just as harmful as the HCAs.

### ADVANCED GLYCATION END PRODUCTS (AGEs)

Researchers at Mt. Sinai Medical Hospital found that foods cooked at high temperature contain greater levels of compounds called advanced glycation end products (AGEs) that cause more tissue damage and inflammation than foods cooked at lower temperatures. AGEs irritate cells in the body, damaging tissues and increasing your risk of complications from diseases like diabetes and heart disease. These chemicals can be avoided by cooking meals at lower temperatures through "Healthy Steaming," "Healthy Sautéing" or poaching and also by cooking meats with foods containing antioxidant bioflavonoids, such as garlic, onion and pepper.

### ACRYLAMIDE

Unfortunately, we're not off the hook if we are vegetarian and don't eat beef, chicken or pork. Very recent research has discovered that a potentially toxic substance called acrylamide, which is a carcinogenic nerve-damaging compound, is also formed when certain foods are cooked at high temperature. Potato chips are a key target of research interest here, as are some other foods, including flaked breakfast cereals and roasted nuts. As is the case with HCAs, acrylamide does not appear to form when high cooking temperatures are absent.

## Food Safety

Heat is important in cooking because it can kill bacteria that can contaminate foods, especially meats and fish. The time required to kill bacteria decreases as the temperature increases. Eradication of bacteria starts at about 165°F (74°C), but as you move upward from this temperature, the time it takes to kill bacteria shortens (see table below). For some foods, like thick cuts of meat or fish, it is important to cook for however long it takes to produce a certain internal core temperature. In general, however, it takes much less than 5 minutes to kill potentially harmful bacteria on most plant foods.

## Guidelines for Final Cooking Temperatures

The table below provides the minimum recommended internal temperature needed to destroy harmful microorganisms in food that is cooked by conventional methods (i.e., heat source other than a microwave).

| FOOD PRODUCT | INTERNAL COOKING TEMPERATURE (°F OR °C) |
|---|---|
| Poultry | 165°F or 74°C |
| Stuffed Meats | 165°F or 74°C |
| Ground Beef | 165°F or 74°C |
| Ground Pork | 165°F or 74°C |
| Pork, Ham, Sausage, Bacon | 165°F or 74°C |
| Other potentially hazardous foods including eggs, fish, and seafood | 165°F or 74°C |
| Roast Beef (rare) | 165°F or 74°C |

The chart below indicates the temperatures that correspond to various cooking methods.

## METHODS OF HEATING FOOD

### WET METHODS:

| | |
|---|---|
| Low temperature sautéing | 185°F or 85°C |
| Medium temperature sautéing | 270°F to 135°C |
| High temperature sautéing | 350°–500° or 177°–260°C |
| Stewing | 185°F or 85°C |
| Simmering | 185°F or 85°C |
| Boiling, poaching and steaming | 212°F or 100°C |
| Braising | 266°–320°F or 130°–160°C |
| High temperature stir-fry | 375°–525°F or 191°–274°C |

### DRY METHODS:

| | |
|---|---|
| Stovetop | 150°–450°F or 66°–232°C |
| Baking and roasting | 350°–500°F or 177°–260°C |
| BBQ (gas powered) | 500°–1000° or 260°–538°C |
| Broiling (gas broilers) (depends on the distance of food from heat source) | 550°F or 288°C |
| Broiling (electric broilers with metal alloy coils) (depends on the distance of food from heat source) | up to 2000°F (1093°C) |
| Charcoal briquets (glowing) | up to 2000°F (1093°C) |
| Enzymes begin to denature at | 104°–122°F (40°–50°C) |

Here are questions that I received from readers of whfoods.org about high temperature cooking:

## Q What are the problems with grilling food on high heat?

A There are documented health risks associated with the char-broiling and gas grilling of foods. In general, these risks are associated with the formation of heterocyclic amines (HCAs). Most HCAs are well documented carcinogens, and keeping their levels to a minimum in your diet can decrease your cancer risk.

HCAs form most easily at high temperatures. Under 325°F, the formation of these compounds is very low. As temperatures increase above 400°F, the formation of HCAs can increase by 700%–1000%. Gas and charcoal grilling often (but not always) involve higher temperatures.

The longer a food is exposed to high heat, the greater the HCA formation. When a food like a hamburger is grilled for 10 minutes versus 6 minutes, for example, the HCA levels in the hamburger may increase by 25–30%.

Meat, fish and poultry are more likely to give rise to HCA formation because HCA formation requires the presence of amino acids (from protein) as well as the nitrogen-containing substances, creatine or creatinine. Both of these substances are plentiful in most animal foods. Since most of the research on HCAs has been done on meat, it is uncertain that the grilling of vegetables and fruits may have the same level of outcomes, notably because some of the phytonutrients found in vegetables, such as the sulforaphane in broccoli, have been found to reduce the carcinogenic effect of the HCAs in research studies.

## Q Will roasting nuts at high temperatures affect their nutritional value?

A Roasting nuts at a temperature higher than 170°F (77°C); which is usually the temperature above which they are commercially roasted, will cause a breakdown of their fats and the production of free radicals. When nuts roasted at the high temperatures used commercially are consumed, the free radicals they contain can cause lipid per-oxidation—the oxidizing of fats in your bloodstream that can trigger tiny injuries in artery walls—a first step in the buildup of plaque and cardiovascular disease.

Therefore, I don't suggest purchasing preroasted nuts. Rather if you like the taste of roasted (versus raw) nuts, I suggest that you roast them at low temperatures at home since it is safe to roast nuts *if done at a low temperature*—typically a 160–170°F (70–75°C) oven (at higher temperatures than this, research clearly shows damage to nuts' delicate fats) for 15–20 minutes will do the trick. To do so, place nuts on a cookie sheet in a single layer. To enhance the "roasted" flavor, try putting a little liquid aminos or soy sauce into a spray bottle and misting the nuts before roasting.

Because of their high content of delicate polyunsaturated fats, all nuts, whether roasted or raw, are susceptible to going rancid quickly. It is therefore important to either purchase nuts in their protective shell or, if unshelled, from a store with high turnover to ensure freshness. Store nuts in your refrigerator or freezer. Generally, if stored in the refrigerator or freezer, nuts will remain fresh for 6 to 12 months. For more detail on how long specific nuts can be stored, please check the profile for the nut of your choice that is provided on the World's Healthiest Foods website.

If nuts have been stored longer than recommended, it's a good idea to throw them out. Rancidity sets in long before they smell or taste "off" or not fresh. Like oils damaged by exposure to high cooking temperatures, rancid oils contain free radicals that can cause cell damage in your body. To protect your body, avoid damaged oils of all types.

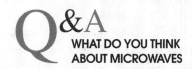

**WHAT DO YOU THINK ABOUT MICROWAVES**

### Basic Principles of Cooking and Nutrition

In a review of research, I have found that microwave heating—for the most part—impacts food nutrients in much the same way as other forms of heating. The microwaving of food creates greater nutrient loss when higher heats are created, when heating is extended over a long period of time or when food is heated while being submerged in water. Each of these principles applies to stovetop cooking as well. Surrounding a food with water and placing it in the microwave on high temperature for several minutes will result in significant nutrient loss, in a way that is parallel to boiling a food on the stovetop for several minutes.

At the other end of the heat-time-and-water spectrum, microwave heating can also be fairly protective of vitamin and mineral content if foods aren't covered with water during the microwave process and are only heated for a brief time. Heating in the microwave for a minute or less with a small amount of water (or no water) corresponds to steaming on the stovetop. It is a process that can help preserve nutrients in the same way as steaming.

Whether on the stovetop or in the microwave, soups may be one exception to the water rule that tries to keep water exposure to a minimum. Soups naturally contain large amounts of water but instead of discarding the water after heating, you consume it.

### The Case of Microwaved Broccoli

A good example of nutrient loss in the microwave can be found in the broccoli study conducted by Villejo and colleagues in 2003. They found dramatic loss of certain phytonutrients in microwaved broccoli (a loss of 97%, 74% and 87%, respectively, of its three major antioxidant compounds—flavonoids, sinapics and caffeoylquinic derivatives) and went on to recommend steaming as a preferable cooking method (since it only resulted in a loss of 11%, 0% and 8%, respectively, of the same antioxidants).

While the results may have partially been related to the amount of water used in the microwaving process, as study co-author, Dr. Cristina Garcia-Viguera explained, "Most of the bioactive compounds are water-soluble; during heating, they leach a high percentage into the cooking water. Because of this, it is recommended to cook vegetables in the minimum amount of water (as in steaming) in order to retain their nutritional benefits."

This approach matches exactly with my approach with the World's Healthiest Foods. I try to expose whole, fresh vegetables to as little heat and water as possible while still bringing out the delicious flavors and aromas of these whole, natural foods. However, I don't view the above research as "anti-microwave" so much as "anti-overcooking." Shorter microwave heating times and less water would be expected to help preserve many of the phytonutrients that were otherwise lost in the above study.

One way to avoid overcooking in a microwave oven is to treat your microwave more like a "re-heating" device than a cooking alternative to the stovetop or conventional oven. If you restrict your use of the microwave to the warming up of already-cooked foods, or the re-heating of already brewed tea or coffee, you're much more likely to end up with shorter cooking times.

### Microwave Cooking and Food Structures

There haven't been any wide-scale, peer-reviewed journal studies on the impact of micro-wave cooking on food structures. I realize that other websites have recommended avoidance of microwave cooking due to changes in food proteins. I have not seen evidence to support this recommendation.

There was one small clinical study on the effect of microwave cooking that is widely discussed on the Internet. While it was not published in a peer-reviewed journal and is not indexed on Medline, I will still report its findings. This study showed that the consumption of microwaved foods was followed by a short-term decrease in the number of white blood cells in the study participants consuming the microwaved food.

Food safety may be an issue for microwaves. One published study found the inability of microwaving to assure elimination of E. coli 0157:H7 from food. Another study found that owing to non-uniform heating of microwaves, some samples of microwaved chicken still contained the Listeria bacteria while another one found that the time needed cook mincemeat to achieve doneness, as observed by agreeable taste and texture, as insufficient to kill Salmonella and Streptococcus bacteria.

### Known Health Concerns with Microwave Cooking

I've found one basic health concern to be well documented in relationship to microwave cooking. First and foremost is the choice of food containers to be placed inside of a microwave oven. Most plastics, including film food wrap (LDPE, or low density polyethylene, displaying a Number 4 recycling symbol) and styrofoam containers (PS, or polystyrene, displaying a Number 6 recycling symbol) have been shown to migrate from plastic packaging into microwaved foods. Researchers who look at "invisible" changes occurring inside human cells (including metabolic patterns and nutrient ratios) find reason for broad-based concern about the use of plastic packaging in microwave ovens. From my perspective, there is simply no good reason to take the risk. If you do decide to use a microwave oven, I recommend using non-plastic food containers only. These containers would include glass, Pyrex and all microwave-safe ceramics.

I don't have a microwave oven in my kitchen since the "Healthiest Way of Cooking" methods are quick cooking methods that do not take much longer than cooking in a microwave. Until microwave ovens are proven safe, I am going to continue using the stovetop and oven for the "Healthiest Way of Cooking."

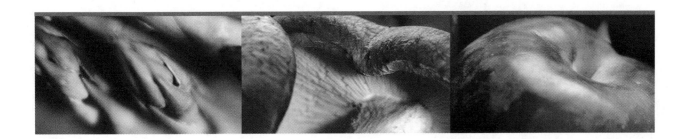

## PART 4

# the world's healthiest foods support healthy cells

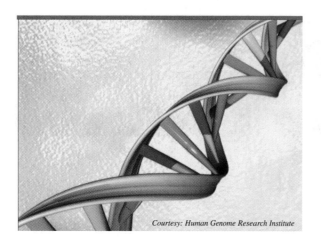

*Courtesy: Human Genome Research Institute*

# eating for healthier cells

We are in the midst of a revolution in the way we understand how the food we eat affects our health. The science of nutrition began as a study of what we need to survive in the most basic sense. Early research focused on determining the minimum amount of nutrients that we require from the food we eat in order to prevent the manifestation of obvious physical dysfunction or disease.

Today, with advanced technology and the ability to see within the body—and even within cells themselves—we are much better able to understand how these vitamins, minerals and other recently discovered nutrients nourish us. These new insights also help us understand why not having adequate intake of nutrients can lead to low energy levels, early aging and even disease. We can also see why the foods we decide to eat today affect our health not just today, but many years later in our lives.

Epidemiological studies have found that populations whose diets feature significant amounts of certain foods have a considerably lower risk of developing many chronic degenerative diseases, including cardiovascular disease, type 2 diabetes, cancer, rheumatoid arthritis, Alzheimer's disease and depression. What are these foods that are so protective of health? Insights into the answer to this question have come from studies of the Mediterranean diet, which have shown that the nutrient-rich foods people in this region enjoy—fish, olive oil, vegetables, fruits, nuts and seeds—promote health and reduce the risk of many chronic diseases. The people who live in the Mediterranean region in Europe are generally healthier and live longer lives.

Alternatively, in cultures whose diets do not focus on nutrient-rich foods, but rather on nutrient-depleted foods, the health of the population looks a lot different. Unfortunately, the United States has been a prime example. In our fast food nation, most people do not even consume five servings of fruits and vegetables per day, and highly refined foods and chemical additives comprise a common component of the average diet. Since nutrients have been shown to have a direct relationship to reducing disease risk, while chemical additives have been found to compromise physiological functioning (details on this are presented later in this chapter), it is of no surprise that the standard American diet is referred to by its well-suited acronym, S.A.D. and does not have the health-promoting reputation that others do. The clues to why the foods of the Mediterranean diet are supportive of health, while the S.A.D. is not as supportive, can be found by learning how nutrition affects our cells.

## health benefits of food have been appreciated throughout history

Although researchers' understanding about cellular nutrition is new, human beings' appreciation for the power of food to affect health is not. In fact, the belief that food plays a preeminent role in supporting health dates far back into history, with Hippocrates, the ancient Greek sage referred to as the father of modern medicine, even proclaiming, "Let food be your medicine." From treatises of ancient healing traditions to modern-day studies of cultures living throughout today's world to molecular biology investigations, all roads point to the premier role of nutrient-rich foods, such as the World's Healthiest Foods, in maintaining well-being, health and vitality.

While the understanding and appreciation of the role that food can play in attaining optimal health has ebbed and flowed throughout history, today healthcare educators and practitioners are advocating Hippocrates' perspective. They are seeing that his wise adage not only mirrors the traditional beliefs about the healing potential of food, but it also reflects the scientific evidence, which has confirmed that the power of food can provide people with the power of health.

Understanding how our cells function is at the foundation of understanding how and why the World's Healthiest Foods are so important to our health. This portion of the book is devoted to increasing both awareness and appreciation for the design and function of the human cell, and how we have the power to help maintain cellular health, prevent disease and maintain optimal health.

## The Cell—the Most Fundamental Unit of Life

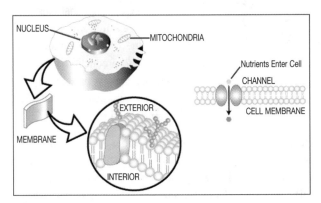

Cells are the smallest components of our bodies to be considered living organisms. They are the fundamental units of life, the building blocks from which our tissues and organs are made—heart, brain, skin, bones and muscles to name a few. In addition, they produce a host of chemical messengers, such as hormones and enzymes, which orchestrate the body's various functions. Our cells perform hundreds of thousands of activities that are responsible for keeping us functioning both physically and mentally. The functional differences between different types of cells determine their need for specific nutrients, for example:

**ALA** (alpha-linolenic acid, the omega-3 fatty acid found in many plant-based foods), which plays an important role in the structure and function of skin cells. ALA's suggested functions include controlling cells' water permeability.

**DHA** (docosahexaenoic acid, an omega-3 fatty acid found in cold-water fish) is the prominent structural fatty acid in cells in the brain and the retina.

**COENZYME Q10** is especially important for heart cells. Since the heart is essentially a large muscle that must work nonstop, heart cells have very high energy demands and a correspondingly high number of mitochondria, our cells' energy production factories. Our mitochondria are dependent upon adequate supplies of coenzyme Q10 to be able to function properly.

**GLUTAMINE** is an amino acid that is the preferred fuel for enterocytes (the cells that make up the lining of the intestines).

**VITAMIN A** (in the form of retinoic acid) is needed to maintain the normal structure and function of epithelial and mucosal tissues, which are found in the lungs, trachea, skin, oral cavity and gastrointestinal tract.

While there are about 30 trillion cells that comprise an adult body, the ones that make up our bodies today are not the ones we were born with. In fact, some of the cells that are in your body right now as you are reading this sentence weren't even there when you began reading this paragraph (1% of cells are replaced every day!). Old cells are constantly replaced with new cells. The body is in an ever-changing state of flux—it is estimated that 2.5 million red blood cells are actually created each second!

It is here, at the level of the cell, that nutrient-rich foods form the basis of good health since nutrients from the food we eat are "food" for our cells. They provide the raw materials from which new cells are created and the compounds that protect cells from the damaging effects that could endanger their ability to function properly. Therefore, you can imagine that if your diet does not provide all of the nutrients necessary for cellular health, the integrity of the cells your body can create will be compromised. For example, if the 2.5 million red blood cells produced each second don't get all the nutrients they need, they will be undernourished, unhealthy cells. This may then form the basis for reductions in physical functioning, and reduced energy and vitality can ensue, as can the onset of a host of health conditions and diseases.

On the next page is an illustration of a cell that contains the full complement of nutrients necessary to maintain health in contrast to one that is depleted of many nutrients.

While cells of different tissues or organs may vary from one another, they each contain similar components that perform specific tasks. I want to more clearly illustrate to you how food can benefit health, by first looking at how antioxidants support

## CELLULAR NUTRITION
### List of Over 50 Food Based Nutrients Needed for Cellular Health

*The numbers after each nutrient reflect the Daily Value (DV\*) for adults. DVs are based on 2000 calories.*

- Water
- Carbohydrates – *300 g*
- Fiber – *25 g*

**Water-Soluble Vitamins**
- Vitamin B1 – *1.5 mg*
- Vitamin B2 – *1.7 mg*
- Vitamin B3 – *20 mg*
- Vitamin B5 – *10 mg*
- Vitamin B6 – *2 mg*
- Vitamin B12 – *6 mcg*
- Folic Acid – *400 mcg*
- Biotin – *300 mcg*
- Vitamin C – *60 mg*

**Fat-Soluble Vitamins**
- Vitamin A – *5000 IU*
- Vitamin D – *10 mcg*
- Vitamin E – *30 IU*
- Vitamin K – *80 mcg*

**Essential Fatty Acids**
- Omega-3 Fatty Acids – *2.5 g*
- Omega-6 Fatty Acids – *12 g*
- Omega-9 Fatty Acids – *no DV*

*1mg = 1000 mcg*

**Minerals**
- Calcium – *1000 mg*
- Magnesium – *320 mg*
- Phosphorus – *1000 mg*
- Chloride – *3400 mg*
- Potassium – *3500 mg*
- Sodium – *2400 mg*

**Trace Minerals**
- Iron – *18 mg*
- Copper – *no DV*
- Iodine – *150 mcg*
- Manganese – *2 mg*
- Chromium – *120 mcg*
- Zinc – *15 mg*
- Fluorine – *no DV*
- Selenium – *70 mcg*
- Molybdenum – *75 mcg*
- Tin – *no DV*
- Silicon – *no DV*
- Vanadium – *no DV*
- Cobalt – *no DV*
- Nickel – *no DV*

**Phytonutrients**
- Carotenoids – *no DV*
- Flavonoids – *no DV*
- Other

**Essential Amino Acids**
- Arginine – *no DV*
- Histidine – *1.29 g*
- Leucine – *2.53 g*
- Isoleucine – *1.15 g*
- Lysine – *2.35 g*
- Methionine – *0.74 g*
- Phenylalanine – *1.19 g*
- Threonine – *1.24 g*
- Tryptophan – *0.32 g*
- Valine – *1.47 g*

The World's Healthiest Foods provide all nutrients the cell needs to be healthy.

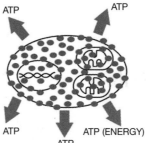

*For more details on these nutrients, including the functions and tolerable upper limits, please see page 733 and page 805.*

cellular health and then how the function of three of the cells' components—(1) the cell membrane, (2) the mitochondria and (3) DNA/genes—are affected by the foods that you consume. Once you see how food truly feeds your cells, how nutrients can positively affect cellular processes and how chemical additives can negatively impact these processes, you'll gain a deeper appreciation of the phrase "you are what you eat."

## Antioxidants Support Cellular Health

Consumption of foods rich in antioxidants is associated with reduced risk of various diseases. I will show you what antioxidants do that makes them play such a significant role in health promotion. It turns out that just how these antioxidant vitamins, minerals, phytonutrients and amino acids support health is largely due to their role in protecting the structure and function of our cells. Since each of the 30 trillion cells is barraged by 10,000 free radicals each day, we need antioxidants from food—each day—to neutralize the free radicals and guard the health of our cells.

### REACTIVE OXYGEN SPECIES (ROS)

We cannot survive without oxygen. The energy production that occurs in our cells' mitochondria requires oxygen to convert sugar, fat and protein molecules into ATP, the molecule in which energy is held for immediate use in our cells. Yet, paradoxically, oxygen is such a powerful reactant that it can disrupt cellular function and impair metabolism through the production of free radicals known as reactive oxygen species (ROS). During mitochondrial energy production, about 2% of oxygen escapes in the form of ROS, reactive molecules that bind to and break DNA chains, that directly cause mutations; ROS can also bind to and destroy proteins and fats in cell membranes.

Under normal conditions, in which you are in good health, have low toxin exposure and are eating a nutritious diet, your cells can protect themselves against these ROS free radicals. With poor nutrition or in the presence of toxins that inhibit or damage the electron transport chain (one of the stages in mitochondrial energy production), causing inadequate energy production, the amount of ROS generated in your cells exceeds the cells' ability to protect themselves against damage.

Research shows that these molecules cause cumulative oxidative damage, which is associated with many degenerative conditions, including cancer, atherosclerosis, cataracts, inflammation and autoimmune disease, lung disease, neurological disorders, aging and cell death. Proper nutrition, notably adequate intake of antioxidant nutrients, plays a critical role in neutralizing these damaging chemicals and protecting cellular health.

### ANTIOXIDANTS PROTECT AGAINST ROS DAMAGE

The protective mechanisms in your cells include antioxidant enzymes such as *superoxide dismutase* and *glutathione peroxidase*, which disable the ROS. For their production and activity, these enzymes require nutrients like the minerals manganese, selenium and copper, which are present in whole grains. Glutathione is a very important molecule that can destroy free radicals, and it can be obtained directly from

## ROS (Type of Free Radicals) Damage

CELL MEMBRANE DAMAGE

MITOCHONDRIA DAMAGE

DNA DAMAGE

ROS (Reactive Oxygen Species, type of free radicals) are toxic byproducts of energy production in the cell that can damage the cell membrane, mitochondria and DNA. This is the reason we need foods rich in antioxidants.

the diet or can be made in your body from amino acid nutrients in the diet, namely glycine, glutamic acid and the sulfur-containing amino acid cysteine, all of which are present in a variety of foods, such as broccoli, garlic and cauliflower. The enzymes involved in energy metabolism also require minerals, like iron, magnesium, copper, selenium and manganese, which can be obtained from whole foods.

Following are a few examples of the roles that individual antioxidant nutrients play in supporting cellular health and the World's Healthiest Foods that are concentrated sources of these nutrients:

### Vitamin E

The tocopherols, members of the vitamin E family, are powerful antioxidants that are able to protect both the lipid (fat) and protein components in your cell membranes from the damage caused by free radicals and other oxidative compounds. Vitamin E also protects the mitochondria from the effects of free radicals produced during ATP manufacture, while also supporting tissue retention of supplemental coenzyme Q10, a critical nutrient for energy production. Additionally, research that has shown vitamin E's ability to shield DNA from the free-radical damage caused by smoking suggests that it may play an important role in protecting our genetic material. Best sources of vitamin E include:

- Swiss chard, sunflower seeds and almonds. (For more sources of *Vitamin E*, see page 798.)

### Vitamin C

Since it plays an integral role in recycling vitamin E back to its active form, vitamin C is also critical to cellular membrane and mitochondrial health. In addition, vitamin C has been found to protect the DNA of many types of cells, including white blood cells and the eye's lens, from oxidative damage caused by free radicals and ultraviolet radiation. Best sources of vitamin C include:

- Broccoli, bell peppers, strawberries and Brussels sprouts. (For more sources of *Vitamin C*, see page 794.)

### Selenium

Selenium helps prevent oxidative stress by working together with a group of nutrients that prevent oxygen molecules from becoming overly reactive. This group of nutrients includes vitamin E, vitamin C, glutathione, selenium and vitamin B3. Best sources of selenium include:

- Crimini and shiitake mushrooms, fish, oats and barley. (For more sources of *Selenium*, see page 780.)

### Cysteine

The amino acid cysteine is a precursor for *glutathione peroxidase*, a powerful antioxidant that helps protect the mitochondria from oxidative damage. The mineral selenium serves to activate the synthesis of this important antioxidant. Best sources of cysteine include:

- Legumes, whole grains and sesame seeds. (For more sources of *Cysteine*, see page 749.)

### Carotenoids, including lycopene

Carotenoid phytonutrients can protect fat-containing portions of the cell from free-radical damage. In particular, the carotenoid lycopene, which is commonly located in cell membranes, plays an important role in preventing oxidative damage to the membrane lipids, therefore influencing the thickness, strength and fluidity of the membranes. Maintaining the integrity of cell membranes is important since they are the gatekeepers of the cell, preventing toxins from entering and facilitating the removal of cellular waste.

Best sources of carotenoids include:

- Sweet potato, spinach, kale, collard greens, carrots, Swiss chard and winter squash. (For more sources of *Carotenoids*, see page 740.)

Best sources of lycopene include:

- Tomatoes, pink watermelon, apricots and papaya. (For more sources of *Lycopene*, see page 740.)

### Flavonoids

Research supports that flavonoid phytonutrients help protect against cancer and other damage in the cell because of their powerful antioxidant activities. Vegetables and fruits contain a variety of flavonoids, which is one of the reasons why higher consumption of fruits and vegetables is associated with lower risk of a host of diseases, including cancers and many chronic degenerative diseases.

Best sources of flavonoids include:

- Apples, berries, black beans, broccoli, cabbage, green tea, onions and parsley. (For more sources of *Flavonoids*, see page 754.)

### Lipoic acid

Research on animals has suggested that lipoic acid supplementation increases the function of the mitochondrial membrane and its metabolic activity, while also reducing the potential for oxidative damage. In addition, lipoic acid functions directly as both a water- and fat-soluble antioxidant and serves as a cofactor for maintaining the active states of coenzyme Q10 and vitamin E, both of which are important to the integrity of the mitochondria. Best sources of lipoic acid include:

- Spinach, collard greens and other leafy greens. (For more sources of *Lipoic Acid*, see page 759.)

# eating for strong cell structures

## The Cell Membrane

The envelope that encapsulates the cell is referred to as the cellular membrane. The membrane fulfills many important functions. It serves as the structural boundary that encloses all of the cells' components. It acts as a semi-permeable filter through which nutrients can enter and wastes can exit. In addition, numerous molecules that allow the cell to communicate with other cells, supporting the orchestration of all of the body's physiological functions, are located in the membrane.

Following are just a few examples of the roles that individual nutrients play in supporting the health of your cells' membranes and the World's Healthiest Foods that are concentrated sources of these nutrients:

### PROTEIN

After dietary proteins are broken down into amino acids and then resynthesized into new proteins, they are used to replace the protein-containing components in the cellular membrane that have become worn out. Certain amino acids featured in protein are also used to manufacture the signaling chemicals, such as hormones, that are integral to orchestrating cell-to-cell communication. Enzymes, the compounds that catalyze important chemical reactions, which take place both on the cellular membrane surface and inside the cell itself, are made from protein. Best sources of protein include:

- Fish, lean meats, eggs, legumes, grains, nuts

and seeds. (For more sources of *Protein*, see page 778.)

### OMEGA-3 FATTY ACIDS

Omega-3 fatty acids comprise a significant percentage of the fatty acids found in phospholipids, the major form of lipid (fat) found in the cellular membrane. For example, over 35% of phospholipids in the brain and 60% in the eye's photoreceptors feature the omega-3 fatty acid, docosahexaenoic acid (DHA). Therefore, to ensure proper cellular membrane structure, it is important to provide the body with adequate levels of these important fats.

Best sources of omega-3 fatty acids include:

- Fish and seafood such as salmon, sardines and scallops; seeds and nuts such as flaxseeds and walnuts. (For more sources of *Omega-3 Fatty Acids*, see page 770.)

### CHOLINE

As a component of the cellular membrane phospholipids, choline is involved in various functions including cellular signaling. Increases in dietary choline have been found to significantly influence the concentration of membrane phospholipids and support healthy cell membranes.
Best sources of choline include:

- Egg yolks, peanuts and cauliflower. (For more sources of *Choline*, see page 744.)

# eating for vibrant energy

## Mitochondria

The mitochondria are the places where our cells produce the energy for the body from the nutrients in the food we eat. Each of our cells has several hundred to over two thousand mitochondria inside of them, depending on their need for energy. For instance,

heart cells and the cells in our skeletal muscles, which have very high energy demands to support the constant movements within our body, have up to 40% of their space taken up by mitochondria. All together, our body has over one quadrillion mitochondria, which are constantly producing energy.

Mitochondria are the body's cellular engine, converting fats, carbohydrates and some proteins into energy. Eating the World's Healthiest Foods everyday helps maintain healthy mitochondria by making them more efficient. Not only are mitochondria not as efficient when the foods you eat are less nutritious, but they also produce more damaging free radicals.

Maintaining the structural integrity of your mitochondria is essential to your overall health and well-being. If tissues and

roughly half of what you weigh in ATP, about 40 kilograms.

Approximately 90% of the oxygen you breathe will be used by your mitochondria to produce this energy. The production of energy uses a multitude of nutrients as well as many other molecules from food. Since the production of ATP requires a significant amount of oxygen, damaging ROS free radicals are also produced. Well-functioning mitochondria can control the adverse effects of the low level of free radicals normally produced by this metabolic process, but if they are not operating efficiently, damage to the mitochondria can ensue and the ATP-producing functions of the mitochondria can be compromised. The result will be a decrease in energy production affecting the whole body, particularly tissues and organs that have higher energy requirements, like the brain and the heart, that cannot function properly without adequate supplies of energy.

Following are a few examples of the roles that individual nutrients play in supporting the mitochondria and their energy production processes and the World's Healthiest Foods that are concentrated sources of these nutrients:

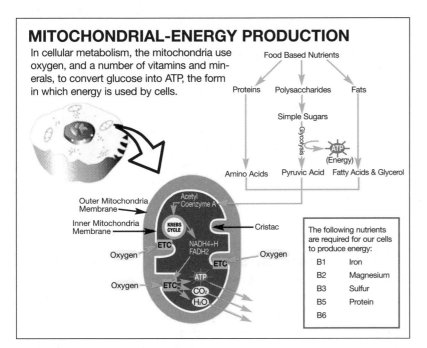

**MITOCHONDRIAL-ENERGY PRODUCTION**

In cellular metabolism, the mitochondria use oxygen, and a number of vitamins and minerals, to convert glucose into ATP, the form in which energy is used by cells.

Food Based Nutrients

Proteins    Polysaccharides    Fats

Simple Sugars

Glycolysis

ATP
(Energy)

Amino Acids    Pyruvic Acid    Fatty Acids & Glycerol

Outer Mitochondria Membrane
Inner Mitochondria Membrane
Acetyl Coenzyme A
KREBS CYCLE
NADH4+H FADH2
Cristac
ETC
Oxygen
ETC
Oxygen
Oxygen
ETC
ATP
$CO_2$
$H_2O$

The following nutrients are required for our cells to produce energy:

| | |
|---|---|
| B1 | Iron |
| B2 | Magnesium |
| B3 | Sulfur |
| B5 | Protein |
| B6 | |

organs, especially those that have higher energy requirements (like the muscle, heart and brain), do not receive adequate supplies of energy, they cannot function properly. Consequently, mitochondrial dysfunction is considered one of the major underlying factors in unhealthy aging and fatigue. Mitochondrial dysfunction is also a major factor in many chronic degenerative diseases, such as congestive heart failure, diabetes mellitus and Parkinson's disease. Along with their inability to produce energy when lacking necessary nutrients, mitochondria can become damaged with the result that they can no longer quench the free radicals that are produced as a normal byproduct of the energy production process. These damaging byproducts include reactive oxygen species (ROS), a type of free radical species that can destroy DNA, protein and fats, promoting further damage.

The mitochondria are the energy powerhouses of the cell, the place where ATP, the "fuel" that is used to drive all of the cells' (and therefore the body's) functions, is produced. On an average day in which you are not doing anything particularly strenuous, you will use the equivalent of

### VITAMIN B3 (NIACIN)

Vitamin B3 serves as a precursor to NAD+, a compound that is important in the mitochondria's production of cellular ATP. It has also been found to inhibit DNA strands from rupturing. Nicotinic acid (a form of vitamin B3) has been shown to reduce DNA damage in human white blood cells.

Best sources of vitamin B3 include:
- Crimini mushrooms, tuna, chicken and salmon. (For more sources of *Vitamin B3*, see page 768.)

### COENZYME Q10

Coenzyme Q10 serves as a component of the electron transport chain, the energy manufacturing "assembly line" of the mitochondria. It also functions as an antioxidant in the mitochondria, protecting them from free-radical damage. Coenzyme Q10 supplementation in humans and animals has been shown to beneficially affect the efficiency of mitochondrial energy production and to protect mitochondrial DNA from free-radical damage.

Best sources of coenzyme Q10 include:

- Fish, calf's liver and whole grains. (For more sources of *Coenzyme Q10*, see page 748.)

The World's Healthiest Foods are also a concentrated source of antioxidant nutrients, which help promote the integrity of the mitochondria since they protect against damage from the free radical byproducts of energy production. (For more information on *Antioxidants,* see page 735.)

# eating for healthy genes

## The DNA

Our DNA serve as the storehouse of our most personal information, the blueprint from which all of our body's proteins—those that make up our tissues, organs and chemical messengers—are designed. Our DNA resides within the cell's nucleus. Specific areas of DNA that code for individual proteins are known as genes, which are arranged in structures known as chromosomes.

Unfortunately, our DNA can easily become damaged by a host of different antagonists; therefore, it is vital to protect the integrity of our DNA since when their helix strands break and their structure becomes compromised, we are unable to make the correct types and amounts of proteins necessary for the proper functioning of our body. The effects of damage to our genetic material range from sub-optimal functioning to an array of different diseases, including cancer.

Following are a few examples of the roles that individual nutrients play in supporting healthy genes and DNA and the World's Healthiest Foods that are concentrated sources of these nutrients:

### FOLIC ACID

Folic acid is critical to our genetic integrity since a deficiency of this nutrient can cause the incorporation of an incorrect nucleotide into DNA, causing a helix strand to break. In addition, folic acid plays an important role in the process of methylation, which is necessary for proper genetic expression.

Best sources of folic acid include:
- Romaine lettuce, spinach, asparagus and mustard greens. (For more sources of *Folic Acid*, see page 756.)

### VITAMIN B6 AND VITAMIN B12

In addition to folic acid, vitamin B6 and vitamin B12 are also involved in methylation reactions that are critical for maintaining proper genetic expression. Deficiencies of these vitamins are related to increased homocysteine levels, which have been found to have a negative effect on cellular methylation and are now known to increase risk of cardiovascular and neurological disease.

Best sources of vitamin B6 include:
- Bell peppers, tuna, bananas and asparagus. (For more sources of *Vitamin B6*, see page 790.)

Best sources of vitamin B12 include:
- Calf's liver, sardines, salmon and venison. (For more sources of *Vitamin B12,* see page 792.)

### ZINC

Zinc is an integral component of many of the enzymes that are involved in DNA repair and replication.

Best sources of zinc include:
- Calf's liver, crimini mushrooms, lamb and pumpkin seeds. (For more sources of *Zinc*, see page 802.)

## Nutrition and Genes

Although we are all biochemically unique, more and more research points to the fact that our genetic tendencies are not set in stone. It's been over 50 years since Francis Watson and James Crick first proposed their model for DNA and genetics, and more than 40 years since it won them the Nobel Prize in Medicine. But it may be another 50 years before the world of food and nutrition catches up with the significance of their discovery. What we eat has a major impact on our genetics! For many of us, it's difficult to believe that genetic events can be altered by food, but the scientific evidence is plentiful and convincing.

One of the best-researched examples of this relationship between nutrition and genetics involves heart disease. Seven hundred thousand (700,000) U.S. citizens die from this condition each year, and over 23 million are diagnosed with some form of this disease. For almost 50 years, we've known about the connection between high blood cholesterol and heart disease. We've also known about several nutritional connections to high cholesterol and heart disease, including consumption of diets high in saturated fat or cholesterol and low in fiber. But only recently have we learned about an important genetic component of this story.

There's one particular spot in our genes called the apoE location (or locus). Our genetic processes can give rise to several different structures in this particular location. The most common of these structures are called E2, E3 and E4. (In science terms, all of these structures are called alleles.) When E4 structures predominate, our risk of high cholesterol goes up significantly as does our risk of heart disease. E4 alleles are genetic structures we would be much safer without in terms of heart disease risk.

What we now know is that in individuals who carry the apoE4 allele, a diet high in saturated fat virtually ensures the development of high cholesterol and cardiovascular disease. But these same individuals can avoid this outcome simply by choosing a diet low in cholesterol-rich foods and saturated fats—a diet like the Mediterranean-style diet based on the World's Healthiest Foods.

In a country like Finland, which has a very high rate of both heart disease and high cholesterol, scientists have found a definite link between the presence of the apoE4 allele, a diet high in saturated fat and cardiovascular disease. The apoE4 allele is much more frequently found in Finns, but they also have higher intake of saturated fat and, as a result, higher rates of blood cholesterol and heart disease. It is clear that our genetic susceptibilities and the unhealthy results that occur when our genes are plunged into an environment they find unhealthy contribute to the number one cause of death in the United States, and that this can be altered by how we eat.

## Nature Versus Nurture

For the past 50 years, we've been thinking about genetics as a separated part of our chemistry—a sort of secret, inner sanctum that is walled off and unaffected by everyday life. Interestingly enough, our word for describing this secret, walled-off inner sanctum is "nature"—the inner blueprint that has its own rules and regulations. We've been comparing this untouchable blueprint of nature with another world we've been calling "nurture." This word refers to everything people do day in and day out—eating, sleeping, working, playing, learning, environmental exposures—the sum total of it all. We've gotten used to thinking about things as involving either one or the other, and in the world of research, the debate continues over "nature versus nurture."

Whenever a problem comes about, whether it's a problem with a child's intelligence or a problem with some mysterious disease, we continue to ask the question, "Is it nature or is it nurture?" meaning "Is the problem something genetic that we couldn't possibly have done anything about (nature) or is it caused by the way we are doing things (nurture)?" Present-day research is fast convincing us that we've been asking the wrong question. Research has made it clear that there is no either-or, no nature versus nurture, and that virtually everything is something we can do something about, including taking steps related to our diet.

The new buzzword for this nature-nurture combination is "plastic heredity." Plastic heredity means that nothing is strictly inherited in a way that is isolated from human activity (including our diet) or from the environment. From the perspective of plastic heredity, what we inherit is only a genetic potential, tendency or propensity, but how we live and the quality of our environment determines what our genes actually express. Jeffrey Bland, a Ph.D. biochemist and author of *Genetic Nutritioneering*, likes to use the phrase "washing our genes in experience" as a way of describing how our lifestyle and environment impact genetic outcomes. The idea that we can "eat for our genes' healthiest expression" is definitely an idea whose time has come. But how do we do it? What are the steps we need to take?

## Avoiding the Food Contaminants

A first step we can take in eating for our genes is avoiding as many food contaminants as possible. By "food contaminants" I mean pesticides, heavy metals, artificial dyes and flavorings, molecules that migrate into food from plastic packaging, aluminum that leaches into food from aluminum cans, trans fats that are produced by hydrogenation of plant oils and other toxic substances that are common constituents of processed foods. When a toxic substance damages our genes that substance is referred to as "genotoxic." Genotoxic substances are substances that break apart the strands of DNA that form the structure for our genes, crosslink strands of DNA that are not meant to be linked, change the components of a DNA strand or prevent the DNA strand from being constructed in the first place.

There are literally hundreds of genotoxins in our national food supply in most every category of chemical toxin. Pesticides like pentachlorophenol (PCP) cause breaks in DNA. Benzoyl peroxide, a bleaching agent for wheat flour, can cause DNA strands to crosslink. Sodium bisulfite, the widely used preservative often added to prevent food discoloration, can cause a variety of chromosomal alterations. Heavy metals, including cadmium, lead and mercury, can cause parts of the DNA strands to become deleted.

How can we avoid these food genotoxins? We can begin by purchasing organically grown foods wherever possible. Many of the genotoxic substances found in food cannot be used in the harvesting or processing of organic crops. We can also use high quality food preparation steps in our own homes. We can cook in stainless steel, cast iron or porcelain-coated pots and pans instead of aluminum. We can also eat fresh and locally grown foods that are less likely to have been improperly processed or handled. You can find extensive information about this on whfoods.org by clicking on "All About Organic Food" in the Eating Healthy section.

## Nutritionally Supporting Our Genes

A second step we can take is to support our genetic metabolism. We need to give our bodies an optimal supply of nutrients required for genetic processing. While every year we learn more and more about the nutrients that are especially important when it comes to genetics, at this point there are three basic categories that we need to consider when eating to support our genes.

### VITAMINS

First are foods rich in the conventional vitamins, especially vitamins A and E, and perhaps to a lesser extent, vitamin C. In the past 10 years, we've learned that there are special receptors on the cell nucleus designed to link up with vitamin A and allow this vitamin to modify genetic processes. Since beta-carotene and other carotenoids can be converted into retinol, the form in which vitamin A is found in mammals, we'd be smart to include both retinol-containing foods and beta-carotene-containing foods in our "Healthiest Way of Eating." Although you're probably already aware that vegetables like carrots provide large amounts of beta-carotene, or calf's liver being rich in retinol, you may want to visit the section on Health-Promoting Nutrients for a more complete listing of vitamin A- or carotenoid-containing foods.

Vitamin E and, to a lesser extent, vitamin C, also appear to directly regulate genetic processes. Some researchers believe that the impact of E and C on gene activity involves the antioxidant function of these vitamins, but the jury is still out in this regard. It is best when vitamin E comes from food. For vitamin E, you can't do much better than green leafy vegetables like collard greens or chard, sunflower seeds and olives. For vitamin C, look for broccoli, bell peppers, strawberries and lemons as excellent sources.

### ANTIOXIDANTS

The second category of gene-supporting nutrients are the non-conventional antioxidants, including lipoic acid, flavonoids and other polyphenolic substances. You'll find a complete profile for lipoic acid in the Health-Promoting Nutrients section on page 759. This sulfur-containing nutrient is found in dark green leafy vegetables like spinach and collards and also in animal foods like beef. You'll also find a flavonoids' profile on page 754. This fascinating family of over 6,000 different pigments provides food with its diversity of color. It also provides us with much of our food-based antioxidant protection. When you eat colorfully, you are also eating for your genes because the factors that operate in gene transcription—an important early stage in genetic activity—are partly regulated by flavonoid levels.

### ESSENTIAL FATTY ACIDS

The final category of gene-supporting nutrients are the fatty acids, especially omega-3 fatty acids. Some of the recent research has looked at the unwanted genetic impact of too much linoleic acid—the omega-6 fatty acid that is found in particularly high amounts in corn oil, soy oil, peanuts, peanut oil and animal fats. You can eat for your genes by balancing your intake of linoleic acid, an omega-6 fatty acid, with intake of linolenic acid, an omega-3 alternative. A full omega-3 profile can be found on page 770 in the Health-Promoting Nutrients section.

## Eating for Healthy Genes' Expression with the World's Healthiest Foods

Considering the combined research on vitamins A, C and E, lipoic acid, flavonoids, carotenoids, omega-3 fatty acids and non-contaminated foods, what better way to eat for your genes than by enjoying the World's Healthiest Foods? Many of the specific foods I featured have been selected because they are rich in precisely these nutrients. And my emphasis on food that is organically grown, minimally processed and cooked *al denté* is a perfect blueprint for supporting your genetic processes because it minimizes your exposure to contaminants that can damage your DNA. I trust these foods will support your health, including the health of your genes!

## Latest News on How Food Affects the Health of Genes

A recent issue of Newsweek featured a fascinating cover story on the interplay between genes and diet. As research unfolds, more information about the specifics of how certain foods enhance the action of protective or harmful genes is collecting; it now appears that overwhelming evidence supports the importance of eating a healthy diet. In other words, our genetic predispositions cannot be blamed for some of our health problems. Earlier, I gave the example of heart disease as an area in which we can no longer say that a person "just got bad genes." We can no longer make that statement because we know that only when a person's genes are immersed in an unfriendly environment—for example, one in which the diet is excessively high in saturated fat—does a genetic tendency to heart disease result in actual illness. Studies have found that in most cases, a predisposition to heart disease, identified by the presence of a variety of a particular genes, can be totally neutralized by a healthy diet and lifestyle! So when all is said and done, I recommend eating more fruits and vegetables, less sugar and saturated fat, and enjoying more of the World's Healthiest Foods.

## Why Are Healthy, Whole Foods So Good for Healthy Cells?

As you can see, supporting healthy cells involves a variety of vitamins and mineral, as well as other dietary components. Providing all these nutrients to our cells means eating whole foods since they contain the fullest complement of these nutrients. As you can see from the diagram below, what you eat today impacts how you will feel tomorrow.

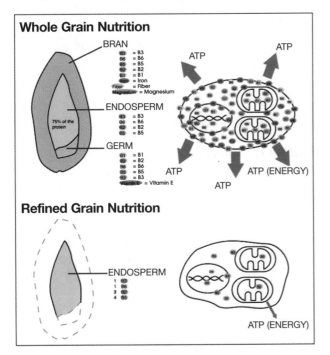

Comparing whole grains to refined grains provides a good example of why whole foods are so much better for your health. A whole grain, such as a grain of wheat, contains three main parts: the germ, or sprouting part of the grain; the endosperm, which contains the starch (calories) to support the young sprout during its early stages; and the bran, which is the protective layer encasing the sprout and its endosperm. In a whole grain food, all three parts of the grain are present; in a refined food product, like white bread and cereals made from refined grains, only the starch remains, which is why these highly processed foods cannot protect us from damage.

Each of the parts of the grain has different purposes and therefore a different complement of nutrients. The germ is rich in micronutrients to support the young sprout. It contains a high level of the vitamin E family of micronutrients, the tocopherols, and several B-vitamins.

The endosperm is the largest part of the grain. Yet, it contains the fewest micronutrients for its size because its purpose is simply to provide starch (sugar) calories for the young sprout.

The protective bran contains a host of micronutrients to protect the young sprout from damage by the sun, which can cause free radical formation, as well as other environmental damage. These same compounds protect our cells from damage, which is one reason why the bran is such a healthy food for us. The bran also contains over 60% of the minerals in grains, including their magnesium, phosphorus, potassium, iron, copper and manganese, all of which are necessary to support healthy cells.

With all of the nutrients provided by the germ and the bran, which are present in whole grains but not refined grains, it's easy to see why whole grains comprehensively protect and support healthy cells, whereas processed grain products, such as white bread and cereals made from refined grains, provide virtually no protection from damage.

## Organically Grown and Additive-Free Foods Support Cellular Health

The power of the World's Healthiest Foods to promote cellular health is related not just to what they contain—their concentration of nutrients—but to what they do not contain. The World's Healthiest Foods, by their nature, are whole foods that are free of processing chemicals. Whenever possible, the World's Healthiest Foods you choose for nourishment should be organically grown.

In addition to causing hypersensitivity (allergy) reactions in some people, certain chemical food additives that are legally allowed to be used in food processing in the United States have been identified as potentially able to damage genetic material. These include benzoyl peroxide, sodium bisulfite, butylated hydrotoluene (BHT) and butylated hydroanisole (BHA). The latter two chemicals have also been shown to cause damage to the mitochondria, reducing their ability to generate the cellular energy that runs the body's physiological processes.

Since certain agricultural chemicals may damage the structure and function of the cellular membrane, eating organically grown foods may be a vital component of a diet that protects cellular health. The insecticide endosulfan and the herbicide paraquat have been shown to oxidize lipid molecules and therefore can damage the phospholipid components of the cellular membrane. In animal studies, pesticides such as chlorpyrifos, endrin and fenthion have been shown to overstimulate enzymes involved in chemical signaling, causing an imbalance that has been linked to conditions in which inflammation is a significant contributing factor, such as atherosclerosis and psoriasis.

Eating organically grown foods also minimizes the degradation of DNA and may help to better sustain health. Recent test tube and animal research suggests that certain agricultural chemicals used in the conventional method of growing food may have the ability to cause genetic mutations that can lead to the development of cancer. An example is the chemical pentachlorophenol (PCP), which has been found to be able to cause DNA fragmentation in animals.

Several of the agricultural chemicals used in the conventional growing of foods, including paraquat, parathion, dinoseb and 2,4-D, have also been shown to have a negative effect upon mitochondrial function. They have been found to affect the mitochondria and cellular energy production in a variety of ways, including increasing membrane permeability (which exposes the mitochondria to damaging free radicals), and inhibiting *ATP synthase*, the enzyme responsible for the final step in the mitochondrial energy production process that creates ATP.

Cellular health is a complex process. It is not one nutrient but a compendium of nutrients working synergistically that determines the health of the cell and therefore the health of our bodies.

## The World's Healthiest Foods are the Foundation of Health

From ancient medical texts written thousands of years ago to scientific research presented in last week's medical journals, reports of the health-promoting effects of food are ubiquitous.

The World's Healthiest Foods provide our cells with the nutrients that serve as their building blocks and protective agents that support optimal cellular structure and function. Knowing how the nutrients in food affect the health of your cells makes it so much easier to understand not only why the World's Healthiest Foods are beneficial, but how and why a diet that features nutrient-rich, organically grown foods can best support your health. It can also show you why researchers are coming to believe that our lifestyle, including our diet, is as important, if not more important, than our genetic inheritance when it comes to living a healthy life free of chronic diseases.

Since our cells are constantly functioning and they require a concert of nutrients, it is important to consume a variety of nutrient-rich foods, like the World's Healthiest Foods, on a daily basis. These foods will nourish all of the cells of our body, providing us with health and energy.

## Further Reading

In the past few years, several books have done a great job of describing the relationship between food and genetics. Three of the books I'd like to mention are *Dependent Gene: The Fallacy of Nature vs. Nurture* by David S. Moore (WH Freeman Company, 2001); *Genetic Nutritioneering* by Jeffrey S. Bland (NTC Publishing Group, 1999); and *Genetics: The Nutrition Connection* by Ruth DeBusk (American Dietetic Association, 2003).

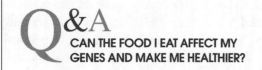

# Q&A
### CAN THE FOOD I EAT AFFECT MY GENES AND MAKE ME HEALTHIER?

The foods we eat directly affect the expression of our genes. The nutrients in the foods we consume communicate with our genes, delivering information that alters which aspects of our genes—those that promote health or those that engender dysfunction and disease—will be activated.

Research has now shown that even the genes we've inherited that render us more susceptible to various chronic diseases do not, inevitably, cause disease. Their damaging messages remain silent unless we make food, lifestyle or environmental choices that trigger them into action.

In fact, our genes are so responsive to our dietary choices that eating foods that do not provide for our genetically inherited needs is now recognized as a major factor in the development of virtually all chronic degenerative diseases, including cardiovascular disease, type 2 diabetes, arthritis, digestive disorders, loss of mental function and even many cancers.

*(Continued on Page 95)*

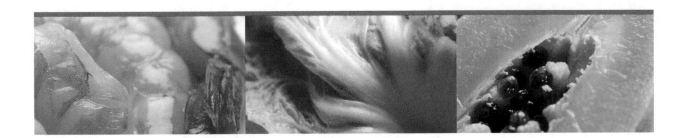

## PART 5

# 100 world's healthiest foods

*On the following pages I focus on fresh, whole, natural, nutrient-rich foods with many health-promoting benefits. Emphasis is on the value of minimally processed, non-genetically altered, and additive-free foods, which are organically grown whenever possible.*

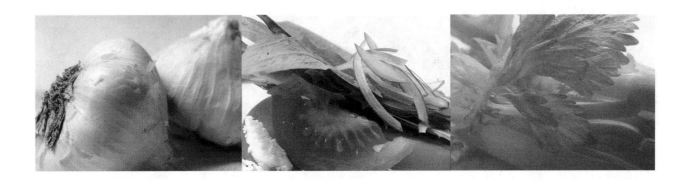

# vegetables & salads

| NUTRIENT-RICHNESS | NAME | PAGE | NUTRIENT-RICHNESS | NAME | PAGE |
|---|---|---|---|---|---|
| 65 | Spinach | 98 | 22 | Cabbage | 220 |
| 55 | Swiss Chard | 106 | 22 | Carrots | 230 |
| 47 | Crimini Mushrooms | 114 | 20 | Winter Squash | 238 |
| 43 | Asparagus | 120 | 15 | Beets / Beet Greens | 244 |
| 40 | Broccoli | 128 | 15 | Eggplant | 252 |
| 40 | Romaine Lettuce / Salads | 136 | 15 | Garlic | 258 |
| 38 | Collard Greens | 146 | 14 | Onions / Leeks | 268 |
| 34 | Kale / Mustard Greens | 154 | 13 | Sweet Potatoes | 280 |
| 34 | Tomatoes | 164 | 11 | Cucumbers | 286 |
| 33 | Brussels Sprouts | 172 | 8 | Potatoes | 292 |
| 33 | Green Beans | 178 | 7 | Avocados | 298 |
| 32 | Summer Squash | 184 | 7 | Corn | 304 |
| 29 | Bell Peppers | 190 | 7 | Sea Vegetables | 310 |
| 29 | Cauliflower | 196 | 5 | Shiitake Mushrooms | 316 |
| 25 | Celery / Fennel | 202 | 4 | Olives / Olive Oil | 322 |
| 24 | Green Peas | 212 | | | |

The numbers beside each food indicate their Total Nutrient-Richness. (For more details, see page 805.)

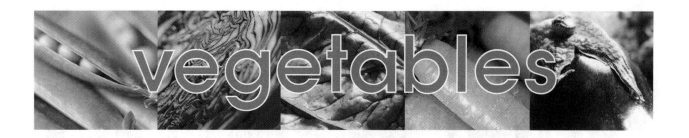

Vegetables are now taking center stage. Public health recommendations are emphasizing the importance of vegetables as the cornerstone of the "Healthiest Way of Eating." This advice is based on the wealth of scientific studies that have shown the incredible benefits of the health-promoting nutrients that vegetables contain. Including plenty of vegetables as part of your daily menu not only promotes long-term health, but provides energy and helps you look your best.

One of the primary reasons that people avoid eating vegetables is that traditional cooking methods often result in overcooked, mushy vegetables that have little flavor. Those overcooked vegetables may also have lost as much as 80% of their nutrients!

This is why I want to share with you the *al denté* "Healthiest Way of Cooking," so you will never have to eat bland-tasting, overcooked vegetables again. *Al denté* is a quick and easy way to prepare crisp, tasty, enjoyable vegetables in just minutes. In addition to improving taste, cooking vegetables *al denté* provides you with the maximum nutritional benefits.

By using the "Healthiest Way of Cooking" methods to prepare your vegetables *al denté*, you'll discover how easy it is to add vegetables to your diet. You'll experience the benefits of incorporating vegetables as a regular part of your meals, just as they have done for centuries in Asia and the Mediterranean regions of Europe where the people are renowned for their exceptional health and longevity.

All of the recipes and cooking methods for vegetables and other World's Healthiest Foods (presented in this book) have been thoroughly tested many times in my own kitchen, which is not a commercial kitchen, but one that is probably very similar to your own.

### Vegetables: Definition

Botanists describe vegetables as herbaceous (non-woody) plants that can be consumed as food. Vegetables come in many sizes and shapes and from different parts of the plant. Some are leaves (spinach, lettuce), some are roots (carrots, beets), some are stalks (celery, fennel), some are tubers (potatoes, sweet potatoes), some are inflorescents (flowering vegetables like broccoli and cauliflower) and others are bulbs (garlic, onions).

Some foods we think of as vegetables are technically fruits. It's fairly easy to tell which vegetables are actually fruits by slicing them open and seeing the seeds inside. Among these are tomatoes, peppers, squash, eggplant, avocados and cucumbers. Since they are usually considered vegetables

from a cooking perspective, however, I have included them in this section of the book.

### Why We Need to Eat Vegetables Every Day

We need to eat vegetables every day because they supply an incredible amount of health-promoting water-soluble vitamins. Our bodies require these nutrients to be supplied daily because, unlike fat-soluble vitamins (such as vitamin A, E and D) that our bodies can store for future use, the water-soluble vitamins (vitamin C and vitamins B1, B2, B3, B5, B6, B12 and folic acid) can only be stored in small amounts or not at all. Since vitamins cannot be produced by the body and can only be obtained from the food we eat, they are called "essential nutrients." Vegetables' rich concentration of water-soluble vitamins is just one reason why the U.S. government guidelines for a healthy diet recommend eating at least 2¹/₂ cups, or 5 servings, of vegetables every day.

Eating the recommended 5 servings of vegetables a day helps promote optimal health. Our bodies are very adaptive and can obviously survive on less, but not without long-term costs to our health. Negative effects may be subtle and go unnoticed for awhile as they may take a long time to fully develop. However, they can't be avoided; without adequate servings of vegetables, we deprive our bodies of excellent sources of vitamins and minerals essential to proper physiological functioning as well as dietary fiber and literally thousands of protective phytonutrients, the importance of which is just now being revealed in the scientific research. The effects of not eating enough vegetables may range from low energy levels to reduced immune function and many types of degenerative diseases. Eating vegetables every day is the way to ensure that we feel our very best.

## Why Vegetables Can Help You Stay Slim, Energized and Healthy

Vegetables are the most nutrient-rich foods. That means they are the foods that provide the most vitamins, minerals and phytonutrients (plant nutrients) for the least number of calories, so they help keep you slim and energized. The fact that vegetables are rich in nutrients and low in calories is especially significant today when obesity is the fastest growing cause of disease and death in the United States. Eating foods high in calories and low in nutrients is a leading cause of obesity and poor health. Therefore, it is especially important to include more low-calorie, nutrient-rich foods in your menu for both your long-term health and your appearance.

A recent USDA study found that people whose diets consisted of more than 55% carbohydrates from vegetables, fruits and whole grains consumed 200 to 300 fewer calories a day than those who ate the standard American diet. They also had the lowest Body Mass Index (BMI) scores. BMI is a measure of body fat based on height and weight that is used to determine whether individuals are overweight or underweight.

Eating a variety of vegetables as a regular part of your meal plan helps you to stay slim and provides the energy and vitality necessary to really enjoy daily life. All of us depend on complex carbohydrates for energy and vitality. The starchy portion of complex carbohydrates is converted into glucose, which is used to produce energy in our cells. However, the energy contained in glucose can only be released in combi-

nation with vitamins and minerals. The most important of these include all of the B vitamins, vitamin C and minerals like zinc. Vegetables are some of the best sources of these nutrients, which are essential for turning carbohydrates into energy rather than storing them as fat. So, eating plenty of vegetables rich in complex carbohydrates is a sure way to help you stay both slim and energized.

Vegetables are also one of the richest sources of calcium, a mineral that plays a host of important roles in the body, including helping to maintain bone health. (For more on *Calcium*, see page 738.)

## Vegetables, Along with Fruits, Provide More Important Phytonutrients Than Any Other Food Group

Vegetables, along with fruits, are taking the forefront in helping people to stay healthy because they are the most concentrated sources of health-promoting phytonutrients.

Phytonutrients are the compounds that not only provide vegetables with their intense colors but also help protect them as they grow and mature. Some of the more familiar phytonutrient families include flavonoids, which are found in red and purple vegetables such as beets and red cabbage, and carotenoids, which are found in yellow, orange and red vegetables such as carrots, tomatoes and winter squash. Chlorophyll phytonutrients provide plants, such as kale and Swiss chard, with their bright green color.

These phytonutrients, as well as others found in vegetables, help protect your health, just as they help protect the plants themselves. The different types of phytonutrients work together to provide powerful antioxidant protection from cellular damage in the body's cardiovascular, immune, respiratory and central nervous systems. The more vegetables you eat, the more phytonutrients you will consume, and the more you will benefit from their health-protective properties.

Lutein, beta-carotene and lycopene are just a few of the phytonutrients that researchers are now discovering have numerous health benefits. They estimate that one day up to 40,000 phytonutrients will be identified and their benefits understood. Today, the cruciferous vegetables (broccoli, cauliflower, cabbage, kale, collard greens, mustard greens and Brussels sprouts) and the *Allium* family of vegetables (onions, garlic and leeks) are among the vegetables most studied for their phytonutrient content. All of these vegetables are known for their health-promoting sulfur compounds, which have been found to reduce the risk of heart disease and cancer. (For more on *Phytonutrients*, see the

Q&A, "Are Vegetables and Fruits Equally Good for My Health?," see page 160.)

## Are Bitter Vegetables More Nutritious?

New scientific studies are now revealing fascinating findings that identify the health-promoting flavonoid phytonutrients as the compounds that give vegetables their bitter flavor. (For more, see *"Are Bitter Vegetables Better for You?"* on page 161.)

## Are Raw or Cooked Vegetables Better?

Most animals thrive on diets consisting almost exclusively of raw, uncooked foods. However, you only have to watch how grazing animals eat to realize the amount of chewing they must do to process raw foods. Few people have the time to chew their food long enough to obtain the full nutritional benefits from raw foods.

There is some concern about the destruction of enzymes when vegetables are cooked; however, enzymes aren't destroyed by cooking. Enzymes are proteins, and the proteins still remain in the food after it's cooked. Cooking deactivates enzymes so that they no longer function as enzymes, but they remain proteins that can be useful to the body. The enzymes found in vegetables may also be deactivated when they are taken out of the ground, cut off from their roots or harvested in some other way. These activities may dramatically change their metabolism.

Our primary digestive enzymes include proteases and peptidases (to digest proteins), amylases and saccharidases (to digest carbohydrates) and lipases (to digest fats). Although raw foods contain some of these enzymes to help digestion, most enzymes found in raw foods are not digestive enzymes. Our digestive tracts also have their own digestive chemistry, which also denatures enzymes. For example, our stomach is extremely acidic, and its level of acidity denatures many enzymes even more quickly than cooking.

Recent scientific research also shows that you can get more nutritional benefits from eating quickly cooked vegetables than from eating them raw. Vegetables that are cooked quickly, as in the *al denté* method of cooking (see page 92), have been found to release more nutrients inside of the digestive tract, resulting in greater assimilation of those nutrients. Other studies have shown that the amount of chlorophyll absorbed by the body is greater when the vegetables were quickly cooked. Cooking vegetables *al denté* for a short period of time can actually make food easier to digest and therefore less stressful on your digestive tract.

This does not mean that I do not support enjoying raw vegetables. Raw vegetables add color, taste and texture to our diets.

I have included many recipes showing how to enjoy vegetables raw. Raw vegetables are easy to pack in lunches, make wonderful salads and snacks and are a rich source of many nutrients. However, I feel that properly cooking vegetables can add even more flavor and nutrition to your meals.

Properly cooking vegetables (using short cooking times) plays a key role in how much you will benefit from the vegetables that you eat. Cooking aids in the digestion of vegetables by breaking down cell walls, a job your body would have to do if they were not cooked and you didn't chew thoroughly. Our digestive system has lost the ability over the last thousand years to easily digest raw vegetables. I've seen firsthand the potential benefits that can be derived from properly cooking vegetables, and I've also seen the problems that can occur from improper cooking methods. That's why I've focused much of my time and effort in coming up with methods of cooking that not only enhance the flavor and texture of vegetables but also promote good digestion and preserve as much of their original nutrient content as possible. I call this the "Healthiest Way of Cooking" (see page 45).

## What Are the Nutritional Advantages of Cooking Vegetables?

Here are some of the scientific findings that support the health benefits of eating quickly cooked foods compared to relying solely on a raw foods diet:

**MORE CAROTENOIDS:** Carotenoids are usually hooked together with proteins or locked into their own crystal-like structure when found in their natural state. Heating helps break down these structures, freeing carotenoids for digestion and absorption into our cells. Research has measured the increased availability of carotenoids after vegetables have been cooked. For example, about 40% more beta-carotene is released from carrots and made available through cooking.

**FEWER ALKALOIDS:** The alkaloid content of nightshades is problematic for some individuals. Cooking can lower the alkaloid content by as much as 40–50%. (For more on *Nightshades*, see page 723.)

**FEWER GOITROGENS:** Although research studies are limited in this area, cooking does seem to reduce goitrogens. These compounds can cause enlargement of the thyroid gland in people who are susceptible to goiters. (For more on *Goitrogens*, see page 721.)

**FEWER OXALATES:** Cooking can help reduce the oxalates found in vegetables by 5 to 15%. Although this reduction is small, it may still be beneficial for individuals needing to restrict their oxalate intake. Boiling is the best cooking method when there is concern about the oxalate content of vegetables because direct contact between the vegetable and the water helps to leach oxalates out of the vegetable and into the water. (For more on *Oxalates*, see page 725.)

**LESS *SALMONELLA* AND *E. COLI* BACTERIA:** These bacteria are sometimes found on raw sprouts because they are grown under warm and humid conditions. This is true whether they are grown commercially or in the home. The heat from cooking can help destroy the bacteria in sprouts as well as any other types of bacteria that can be found on some vegetables (see page 00).

## Overcooking Can Destroy Important Nutrients

There is a fine balance when it comes to cooking vegetables. While lightly cooking vegetables enhances their flavor and nutritional benefits, overcooking not only reduces flavor but also results in the loss of many of their health-promoting nutrients. Overcooking some vegetables can occur in as little as seven minutes.

The chart below illustrates how overcooking vegetables by boiling in water and subjecting them to very high temperatures for an extended period of time can result in substantial nutrient loss.

Overcooking can make healthy vegetables much less healthy by causing a loss of chlorophyll, magnesium and other water-soluble vitamins, minerals and phytonutrients. Overcooking vegetables by cooking for too long or at excessively high temperatures can also alter the structure of nutrients, including protein and fiber, and decrease their health benefits.

| NUTRIENT | FOOD | COOKING METHOD | % NUTRIENT LOSS |
|---|---|---|---|
| Folic acid | Carrots | Boiling | 79% |
| Folic acid | Cauliflower | Boiling | 69% |
| Folic acid | Spinach | Boiling | 51% |
| Folic acid | Broccoli | Boiling | 56% |
| Vitamin C | Mixed Vegetables | Boiling | 55% |
| Flavonoids | Broccoli | Boiling | 66% |

## What is a Serving Size of Vegetables?

The following is a list of the standard serving sizes for vegetables:

| | |
|---|---|
| Cooked or raw vegetables: | 1/2 cup |
| Leafy green raw vegetables: | 1 cup |
| Vegetable juice: | 3/4 cup |
| Fat-containing vegetables like avocado: | 1/4 cup |

## The Easy Way to Enjoy 5 Servings of Vegetables each Day

The idea of trying to eat 5 servings of vegetables a day can seem overwhelming. Yet, if you remember that one serving is only a 1/2 cup of cooked vegetables, and therefore one cup of cooked vegetables provides 2 of the recommended 5 servings, then suddenly it does not seem so difficult.

In this book, I will share with you flavorful recipes using the *al denté* method of cooking that not only make vegetables easy to prepare but so tasty that you will want to eat at least 5 servings a day because they are so enjoyable! While the U.S. Dietary Guidelines recommends including at least 5 servings of vegetables a day, there are plans to soon increase this recommendation to 13. Here are a few suggestions of how to easily include more vegetables in your diet:

### BREAKFAST
Start your day with a healthy vegetable frittata and get a serving of vegetables at breakfast or serve omega-3 rich eggs on top of a combination of spinach, mushrooms and tomatoes. (1 serving of vegetables)

### LUNCH
Start lunch with a mixed salad that contains a variety of vegetables, such as lettuce, tomatoes, avocados and cucumbers, and get 4 servings of vegetables in one dish. You can also enjoy one of the book's many salad entrées. (4 servings of vegetables)

### DINNER
Start dinner with a salad or vegetable crudités as appetizers. Have green vegetables like broccoli as a side dish and substitute vegetables such as carrots or squash for pasta or rice to accompany your fish or meat. (4 servings of vegetables)

This day's menu provides 9 servings of vegetables.

## How to Use the Individual Vegetable Chapters

Each vegetable chapter is dedicated to one of the World's Healthiest Vegetables and contains everything you need to know to enjoy and maximize its flavor and nutritional benefits. Each chapter is organized into two parts:

1. **VEGETABLE FACTS** describe each vegetable and its different varieties and peak season. It also addresses the biochemical considerations of each vegetable by describing unique compounds that may be potentially problematic for individuals with specific health problems. Detailed information of the health benefits of each vegetable can be found at the end of the chapter.

2. **THE 4 STEPS TO THE BEST TASTING AND MOST NUTRITIOUS VEGETABLES** include information on how to best select, store, prepare and cook each one of the World's Healthiest Vegetables. This section also features Step-by-Step Recipes and Flavor Tips. While specific information for individual vegetables is given in each of the specific chapters, here are the 4 Steps that can be applied to vegetables in general, including those not included in the list of the World's Healthiest Foods.

# 1. the best way to select vegetables

Adding vegetables to your "Healthiest Way of Eating" begins with selecting the best quality vegetables, which means the freshest, most nutritious vegetables—those that are organically and locally grown whenever possible. I select organically grown vegetables because they are produced without the use of pesticides and are not coated with the wax commonly found on conventionally grown varieties of vegetables such as cucumbers, tomatoes, eggplant, peppers and squash. (For more on *Organic Foods*, see page 113.)

I like to purchase locally grown vegetables whenever possible not only because they are fresher but also because they are better for the economy and the environment since they don't have to be transported over long distances, which saves fuel and contributes less to air pollution. I also recommend purchasing vegetables that are in season; studies have found that vegetables enjoyed in the height of their season contain the highest nutritional value. For example, researchers in Japan discovered that spinach contains three times more vitamin C during the peak of its season. Local, organically grown vegetables in season are the first choice of many of the most highly regarded restaurant chefs.

I also check for the maturity of my vegetables. Although vegetables do not ripen like fruits, they do reach maturity. Not only are they past their prime when they are tough, woody or show signs of decay but they have lost much of their nutritional value. In each of the vegetable chapters, I will share with you information about what features to look for to help you select the freshest, most flavorful and most nutrient-rich vegetables.

## Which Vegetables Contain the Most Pesticide Residues?

In the mid-1990s, the Environmental Working Group (EWG) developed their "Dirty Dozen" list of fruits and vegetables containing the highest levels of pesticide residue. Since then, other non-profit groups, such as Mothers and Others and the Consumer Union, have done similar analyses. In 2006, EWG updated their list. The following chart shows the World's Healthiest Vegetables that are included amongst the "Dirty Dozen" when they are conventionally grown; it also shows the World's Healthiest Vegetables that were found to have the least pesticide residues.

| HIGHEST IN PESTICIDES | LOWEST IN PESTICIDES |
|---|---|
| Bell Peppers | Onions |
| Celery | Avocados |
| Spinach | Corn |
| Lettuce | Asparagus |
| Potatoes | Cabbage |
| | Broccoli |

You can cut your pesticide intake substantially by avoiding the "Dirty Dozen."

Although I am a strong proponent of selecting organically grown vegetables and fruits whenever possible, I believe it is especially important to select the organically grown varieties of the vegetables that have been found to have the highest level of pesticide residue. If you can't find organic foods, you can cut your pesticide intake by 80% by selecting vegetables from the list of vegetables that contain the least amount of pesticides. (For more information on *Organic Foods*, see page 113.)

# 2. the best way to store vegetables

Once harvested, vegetables are much more susceptible to oxidative damage because they are no longer alive and cannot replenish their defenses. Because of this, proper storage must take the place of the ability the vegetables once had to defend themselves when they were growing. Vegetables will deteriorate much more quickly if not properly stored.

When vegetables are harvested, they have a reserve of protective nutrients. Since vegetables continue to respire after they have been picked, these nutrients are continually being used up to protect them from the oxidative effects of respiration. When these nutrients are used up, the vegetables will spoil. Thus, the key to maintaining vegetables' freshness is to minimize their respiration rate by storing them properly. Properly storing vegetables reduces their respiration rate, which helps retain their freshness, conserves their protective phytonutrient reserves and maximizes their nutrient retention.

## Respiration Rates of Vegetables

Different vegetables have different respiration rates. As noted above, this is important because the respiration rate is related to how quickly a particular vegetable will spoil. The faster a vegetable respires, the more easily it will spoil and the more important it is to store it correctly.

The following list provides the respiration rates of several different vegetables. It will help you to understand why some vegetables, such as potatoes, can be stored longer (up to one month) than others, such as green beans (two days if not refrigerated and properly stored). Rates are measured in terms of how much carbon dioxide is given off in mg (mg) per kilogram (kg) of vegetable every hour (hr) for vegetables kept at room temperature (68°F/20°C).

| VEGETABLE | MG/KG/HR |
| --- | --- |
| Onions | 8 mg/kg/hr |
| Potatoes | 17 mg/kg/hr |
| Cabbage | 42 mg/kg/hr |
| Carrots | 25 mg/kg/hr |
| Romaine Lettuce | 101 mg/kg/hr |
| Green Beans | 130 mg/kg/hr |

Refrigeration (36°–40°F/2°–4°C) is the best way to reduce the respiration rate of most vegetables and prolong their freshness. It is the most common method of storing vegetables and helps retain their vitality and nutritional value, especially their vitamin C. For example, at room temperature, cabbage can lose approximately 30% of its vitamin C in just two days.

How much the respiration rate will be reduced by refrigeration depends on the type of vegetable, the exact way it is stored in the refrigerator (in a plastic container, wrapped in plastic and/or in a storage bin are some of the best ways), and where in the refrigerator it is kept (different parts of the refrigerator differ in temperature with the back of the bottom shelf being the coolest). One study found that honeydew melons decreased in respiration rate by three times when refrigerated, while other studies have indicated that shelf life was doubled when vegetables were kept in the refrigerator.

Some plastic vegetable storage bags have tiny air holes, which reduce surface moisture while still decreasing air flow, so they minimize spoilage better than the bags provided at your local market. Tightly fitting glass or plastic storage containers are also good options as they can reduce exposure of your vegetables to air. You can also purchase specialty bags from the produce section that can keep your vegetables fresh for even longer periods of time; however, these bags can be quite expensive.

Some vegetables are best not refrigerated but are better stored in a cool dark environment at temperatures of about 50°–60°F (10°–16°C). These vegetables—including tomatoes, potatoes, avocados, onions, garlic, winter squash and eggplant—are adversely affected by refrigeration. For example, tomatoes lose their flavor, avocados will rot, the starches in potatoes will turn to sugar and garlic will get moldy and mushy. These vegetables should only be refrigerated if they have been cut.

## Vegetables Best Stored at Room Temperature

| | | |
| --- | --- | --- |
| Eggplant | Garlic | Onions |
| Potatoes | Sweet potatoes | Tomatoes |
| Winter squash | | |

## Refrigerate after Ripening

Avocados can be refrigerated after they have been ripened.

## Other Storage Tips

Do not wash vegetables before refrigeration because exposure to water will encourage them to spoil.

Vegetables should be handled with extreme care to prevent bruising. Any kind of cell damage can degrade their vitamin content, especially vitamin C.

# 3. the best way to prepare vegetables

Preparation is important. Cleaning vegetables properly is the first step in healthy preparation. Here are the best methods I have found for cleaning organic and conventionally grown vegetables:

(a) Wash organic vegetables well under cold running water.

(b) Wash conventionally grown vegetables in a solution of mild dishwashing liquid then rinse with water; this can eliminate some pesticides and fungicide residues. However, washing with soap or detergent does not remove the wax that is used to retain the moisture and increase the shelf life of conventionally grown vegetables like bell peppers, cucumbers, tomatoes, squash and eggplant. Only peeling will remove this wax.

When cleaning leafy green vegetables like spinach, I do not advise soaking them for a long period of time (more than one or two minutes) because water-soluble vitamins (such as vitamins B and C) will be lost by soaking.

(c) It is best to rinse salad greens under cold running water.

(d) It is best to cut vegetables into small pieces when using the *al denté* method of cooking because small pieces cook more quickly and therefore retain more nutrients. (For more on *Al Denté*, see below.)

For more information on washing vegetables, see page 219.

# 4. the healthiest way of cooking vegetables

When it comes to cooking vegetables, I'd like to share with you my experiences in Italy.

## Cooking *Al Denté*

When I was in Italy at the Bugialli Cooking School in Florence, I learned how to cook perfect pasta from the world's expert, Giuliano Bugialli. The term used to describe perfectly cooked pasta is *al denté*, which means tender, but not mushy, firm to the bite and retaining its shape.

Like pasta, vegetables can also easily become mushy and unappetizing. Historically, boiling vegetables until they were soft was the way they were usually cooked. They were also prepared with meats, in curries or other dishes that required a long time to cook, which also resulted in overcooked and tasteless vegetables. I became most concerned with this when I found that not only did these cooking methods cause a loss of flavor but more than half of the nutrients in the vegetables were also lost.

When I started incorporating more vegetables into my meals, I became determined to find a better way to cook them because I knew that proper cooking could make them more tasty and nutritious. So, when I learned to cook pasta *al denté*, it inspired me to also cook vegetables *al denté*. I believed that cooking vegetables *al denté* would bring out the inherently wonderful taste of vegetables and make them really enjoyable to eat. Since then, I have spent years perfecting the ways to cook vegetables *al denté* to come up with vegetables that are crisp, tender and full of flavor—appetizing vegetables that you can eat with full enjoyment. Because each vegetable is unique, and there were many variables to consider, I prepared some vegetables over 100 times until I got it right.

I always believed that if I showed people how to cook vegetables *al denté*, they would eat more vegetables because they would be more enjoyable. I avoided overcooking all of the World's Healthiest Vegetables by cooking them *al denté*. My *al denté* vegetables were my contributions to potlucks and parties where they were always one of the first dishes to disappear. My friends loved them because the vegetables tasted great, and they wanted me to teach them how to cook vegetables *al denté*. They discovered that cooking vegetables *al denté* was easy, fun and not complicated at all.

Now, with this book, you can discover this as well. You will see how *al denté* cooking brings out the best taste of vegetables yet does not require a lot of work; you just need to know your vegetables. This is the reason I have devoted a chapter to each of the World's Healthiest Vegetables and explain in detail their individual uniqueness. Not only do *al denté* vegetables taste great but this method of cooking enhances flavor, brings out color and preserves nutrients.

**ENHANCES FLAVOR:** Vegetables cooked *al denté* have the best flavor. They are crisp and flavorful with no unpleasant odors. This is because they are cooked *al denté*, just long enough to soften the cellulose and hemicellulose to make them crisp inside and tender outside, which is when their flavor is at its peak. Letting vegetables cook for as little as two minutes longer than the time required to cook them *al denté* causes them to lose their flavor and texture.

Have you ever noticed that when you cook some vegetables, they emit an unpleasant odor that negatively impacts their flavor? This is because cooking for too long results in the release and concentration of compounds that can give vegetables an unpleasant odor and taste, such as the smell of rotten eggs that comes from the hydrogen sulfide gas emitted from cruciferous vegetables when they are overcooked. When you cook vegetables *al denté*, you won't have to worry about this. The short cooking time does not allow the time for many of these compounds to form.

**BRINGS OUT COLOR:** When a green vegetable is cooked *al denté*, its color becomes a bright, vivid green. The vibrant color is a sign that its nutritional value, flavor and texture are at their peak. A fresh, uncooked vegetable has air between its cells, which masks its true bright color. Within the first minute of cooking, the air begins to disappear from the cell, causing the color of vegetables to brighten. For example, the color of broccoli continues to increase in intensity during the first 5 minutes of cooking, reflecting the peak of nutrient content. Yet, after 5 minutes, you can actually watch the loss of nutrients with your own eyes as the vegetable begins to lose its natural color. So, bringing out the color of vegetables is not only important aesthetically, it's also important nutritionally.

**PRESERVES NUTRIENTS:** It turns out that when we preserve the color of vegetables, we are preserving more than just their aesthetic value. The rainbow of colors created by phytonutrients offers a variety of health-promoting benefits as well. What I have found from scientific studies is that if you cook vegetables for a short time, as with the *al denté* method of cooking, you will bring out their color and maximize nutrient retention.

Cooking vegetables for a short period of time helps preserve and lock in nutrients, resulting in minimal loss of chlorophyll, vitamins, minerals, and health-promoting phytonutrients. There is an astonishing amount of scientific evidence supporting the relationship between how vegetables are cooked and the preservation of nutrients. For example, scientific studies have found that after 7 minutes, magnesium from the center of the chlorophyll molecule turns into a less colorful hydrogen molecule called pheophytin, and the color of vegetables turns to a drab green-gray. Just as autumn leaves change colors as they die and lose their chlorophyll, vegetables signal a significant loss of nutrients by changing color. That means you should remember to watch your cooking times to avoid losing nutrients. (For more on *Chlorophyll*, see page 183.)

## Cook Each Vegetable as an Individual Food

Vegetables are delicate foods and should be treated with care. I found that when I cook vegetables *al denté*, it is critical to treat every vegetable as a unique food with its own individual cooking requirements. Unlike meats, beans and grains, vegetables are not forgiving when you overcook them. Many foods can be cooked for 2 to 3 minutes longer than recommended without much difference in the result. But not vegetables! They are not like any other food when it comes to cooking because they are delicate, and they cook quickly. That's why in each chapter I have included the best cooking methods and optimal cooking times for each vegetable. While cooking vegetables is not complicated, it is important that you dedicate a few minutes entirely to their preparation. Don't do anything else because overcooking by 1 or 2 minutes will destroy nutrients and make an enormous difference in texture and taste.

## Timing is Essential

Since timing is essential when cooking vegetables, I started using a kitchen timer. I can't cook without it! I recommend that everyone have a timer in the kitchen because it is important to be diligent when it comes to cooking times for vegetables. You don't need any special type of timer, but I have found that battery-operated ones are best.

I use my timer to ensure that I do not cook my vegetables any longer than the recommended cooking time. And when your vegetables are finished cooking, it's not good enough to just turn off the heat. You must remove them from the pot in which they were cooking because they will continue to cook after you turn off the heat. In fact, they will continue to cook from their own heat even after you have transferred them to a bowl. So remember that although vegetables may appear to be a little more crisp than desired when you remove them from the heat, they will be just right by the time you are ready to eat.

## Vegetables Need to be Prepared Properly

I have found out that the secret to cooking *al denté* is to cut vegetables into small. equally sized pieces so that they will cook more quickly and evenly and retain the greatest amount of nutrients. Larger pieces need longer cooking time, which destroys more nutrients. For example, I cut cabbage into thin slices and broccoli florets into quarters so that they will cook more quickly. In the individual vegetable chapters,

I share with you the best ways to cut each vegetable and the benefits of using my recommended methods.

## Healthy Cooking Methods for Vegetables

Once you have selected fresh vegetables, it is important to choose the most appropriate cooking methods for the vegetables you are preparing. With each vegetable, I'll offer you the "Healthiest Way of Cooking" methods to prepare that vegetable. Because each vegetable is unique, I also recommend the method that I feel is best suited to each vegetable to help retain the greatest number of nutrients and provide you with the most flavor and enjoyment. For example, some vegetables (spinach and Swiss chard) are better boiled to reduce their acid content, some are better steamed (broccoli and kale), others are best sautéed (mustard greens and mushrooms). Using these methods will help make cooking vegetables quick and easy and ensure that you will consistently retain maximum flavor and nutritional value.

### HEALTHY SAUTÉ

An important feature of this method is that it uses no fat or oils. Heating fat or oils has been found to create free radicals and carcinogenic compounds, which are harmful to our health. "Healthy Sauté" quickly cooks vegetables in a minimal amount of time, concentrating their natural flavor and moisture. (For more on "*Healthy Sauté*," see page 57.)

### HEALTHY STEAMING

This method brings out the vibrant color of vegetables while giving them a delightful *al denté* texture. It is a gentle moist way of cooking that preserves flavor, color and nutrients. It is a quick method of cooking because, compared to boiling, you don't have to wait for as much water to come to a boil (2–3 minutes for steaming versus 10–15 minutes for boiling). It's also energy efficient. The lower nutrient loss from steaming is the main reason this method of cooking is so often recommended in the recipes in this book. (For more on "*Healthy Steaming*," see page 58.)

### QUICK BOILING

This is a commonly used cooking method but one that does dilute some of the flavor from the vegetables. Some water-soluble vitamins, such as the Bs and C, are also lost. However, it is the method I recommend using to cook spinach, beet greens and Swiss chard because some studies have shown that it helps to reduce the oxalate content of these vegetables. (For more on "*Healthy Boiling*," see page 61.)

### STOVETOP BRAISING

"Stovetop Braising" is another cooking method used for vegetables. With this method of cooking, the water-soluble nutrients that may be leached from the food can be captured in the cooking liquid and used as a broth or sauce base for the meal.

---

### DIFFERENCES IN COOKING TIMES

What I have found when cooking *al denté* is that it is important to remember that differences in temperature between different stovetops and ovens can affect the cooking time of your vegetables. The altitude where you're cooking can also have an effect on stove and oven temperatures and the time vegetables will take to cook. Individual differences in your stove or oven, the amount of water you use, how the vegetables are cut and the fact that young vegetables cook much more quickly than mature ones are just some of the reasons that vegetables may come out a little differently each time you cook them. So, use the recommended cooking time as a guideline, but be prepared to adjust for these variables. Experiment with your vegetables and have fun.

---

## The Healthiest Way of Cooking

I provide you with many recipes that cook vegetables very quickly and retain the maximum amount of nutrients. Most of them take between 3 and 7 minutes. They are featured in the "Healthiest Way of Cooking" section of each vegetable.

I found that it is very important to dress vegetables properly to enhance their flavor, increase their nutritional value and make them more enjoyable. You should dress them to your liking. I have recommended dressing all of your vegetables with extra virgin olive oil because it is a heart-healthy oil that adds antioxidants as well as flavor and also tenderizes your vegetables. It is best to dress vegetables 5 minutes before serving to make them tender. This is in sharp contrast to dressing salads. Salads are always dressed right before (or even after) serving to maintain maximum crispness.

Cutting vegetables into even smaller pieces after they are cooked and immediately after dressing them ensures that the vegetables get a good coating of dressing for a better overall flavor.

*Note:* You will find information repeated in more than one chapter when the same information applies to more than one vegetable. This is especially true in the chapters about members of the cruciferous family of vegetables including cabbage, cauliflower, kale, collard greens, mustard greens and Brussels sprouts as well as the *Allium* family, which includes garlic, onions and leeks. This repetition was intended to make it easier for you to get complete information when reading about any one vegetable.

(Continued from Page 82)

The good news is that hundreds of recent studies have provided sufficient information so that you can choose a healthy way of eating that is most likely to tell your genes to create your healthiest possible phenotype.

The research building on the results of the Human Genome Project has shown that—with the exception of a few traits like eye color and an increased potential risk for some diseases—our genetic inheritance (or genotype) holds a variety of options—not just one option as we have believed—for what will be expressed and manifest as our actual physical self (our phenotype).

### How Fruits, Vegetables, Nuts, Seeds and Whole Grains Communicate with Your Genes

Fruits, vegetables, whole grains, nuts, seeds, beans and legumes contain a lot more than carbohydrate, protein, fat, fiber, vitamins and minerals. Each and every type of plant contains thousands of protective compounds called phytonutrients (*phyto* means plant).

Phytonutrients—like flavonoids, catechins, phenols, anthocyanins, isothiocyanates, carotenoids, terpenoids and a legion of other compounds with tongue-twisting names—modify gene expression, each promoting healthy physiological function in a slightly different way.

To get the myriad benefits that occur when phytonutrients communicate with our genes, all we need to do is enjoy lots of whole, unprocessed, organically grown fruits, vegetables, nuts, seeds and whole grains:

**WHOLE:** because many phytonutrients are found in or immediately under a plant's skin (or in the grains, in the outer, fibrous layer). Processing typically removes this phytonutrient-rich outermost layer of plant foods.

**UNPROCESSED:** because some phytonutrients evaporate when exposed to heat, light and air. Others are activated when a plant's surface is cut, using up their protective energies over the next several hours or days—long before a processed food is brought home to be part of your meal.

**ORGANICALLY GROWN:** because research shows that plants produce many more phytonutrients when their needs to defend themselves are not being covered by pesticides. Also because

in conventionally grown plant foods, the pesticides and other potentially harmful agricultural chemicals used are typically concentrated in the skin. Removing the skin removes many of these toxins but also deprives us of a significant portion of the plant's phytonutrients.

For a glimpse into the abundance and complexity of nutrients whole foods deliver, let's look at oranges. When we think "oranges," we think "vitamin C," but as important as this antioxidant is to our health, it's the tip of an orange's nutrient iceberg. Oranges contain more than 170 phytonutrients, including more than 60 bioflavonoids and 20 carotenoids, all of which modify gene expression in ways that lessen inflammation, inhibit blood clot formation and activate the body's detoxification system.

And each fruit, vegetable, whole grain, nut, seed, bean and legume has developed its own unique array of phytonutrients for its personal defense and optimal growth. It's not surprising—given how evolution works—but still a most elegant serendipity that these phytonutrients in plant foods modify our gene expression in ways that help protect us against premature or unhealthy aging and chronic diseases.

Phytonutrients in whole foods interact with our genes to increase the expression of those that encode for the production of antioxidant and detoxification enzymes, while putting to sleep those that promote inflammation and the development of cancer. In doing so, phytonutrients turn up a host of protective processes in our bodies, while shutting down the damaging ones.

### What Should I Eat to Send Healthy Messages to My Genes?

While the evidence is complex, the conclusion it all points toward is simple:

A Mediterranean-style diet is the best way to send your genes the messages that will produce your optimal health. This healthy way of eating—which easily delivers between 5–10 daily servings of fruits and vegetables along with an emphasis on whole grains, nuts, cold-water fish rich in omega-3 fats and the healthy fats found in olive and flaxseed oils—will provide you with hundreds of phytonutrients, each of which will deliver its own unique health-promoting instructions to your genes.

# guide to the healthiest way of cooking vegetables

| | HEALTHY SAUTÉ | HEALTHY STEAMING | QUICK BOILING | RAW | PREPARATION | HOW TO HIGHLIGHT FLAVOR. SERVE WITH: |
|---|---|---|---|---|---|---|
| **ASPARAGUS** | 5 min | | | Ok/salads | Cut off tough stems | Toasted almonds; feta or Parmesan cheese |
| **AVOCADOS** | | | | Ok | Slice or cube | Salsa; tamari (soy sauce); lime; red onion; cilantro |
| **BEETS** | | 15 min | | Ok | Quarter | Dill; yogurt; balsamic vinegar; basil |
| **BEET GREENS** | | | 2 min | | Chop 1" thick | Tamari (soy sauce); walnuts; feta cheese |
| **BELL PEPPERS** | 7 min | | | Ok/salad (crudités) | Slice | Feta cheese; oregano; basil |
| **BOK CHOY** | 4 min | | | | Slice 1" thick ** | Tamari (soy sauce); ginger |
| **BROCCOLI** | | 5 min | | Ok | Cut florets in quarters** | Tamari (soy sauce); Parmesan or goat cheese |
| **BRUSSELS SPROUTS** | | 5 min | | | Cut in quarters** | Tamari (soy sauce); balsamic vinegar |
| **CARROTS** | | 5 min | | Ok | Slice 1/4" thick | Tarragon; cinnamon; dill; orange juice |
| **CABBAGE: RED** | 5 min | | | Ok/salad | Chop 1/4" thick ** | Ginger; tamari (soy sauce); caraway seeds; |
| **GREEN** | | 5 min | | | | cider vinegar; walnuts; red chili flakes |
| **CAULIFLOWER** | 5 min | | | Ok | Cut florets in quarters** | Turmeric; toasted almonds; nutmeg |
| **CELERY** | 5 min | | | Ok | Cut | (For raw) Hummus; almond butter |
| **COLLARD GREENS** | | 5 min | | | Chop 1/2" thick** | Tamari (soy sauce); red chili flakes; dulse flakes |
| **CORN** | | 5 min | | | Shuck and cut off ends | Chili powder; cayenne pepper; black pepper |
| **CRIMINI MUSHROOMS** | 7 min | | | | Cut into quarters | Rosemary; onions; garlic |
| **CUCUMBERS** | | | | Ok/salad | Slice | Mint; yogurt; scallion; dill; balsamic vinegar |
| **EGGPLANT** | 7 min | | | Not eaten raw | Cut into 1/2" slices | Tomatoes; Parmesan or goat cheese; oregano |
| **FENNEL** | 5 min | | | Ok /salad | Slice thin | Dill; onion; orange zest and juice |

\* *Lycopene is concentrated in the skin, so if eating tomatoes raw, choose cherry tomatoes*
\*\* *Let sit for 5–10 minutes before cooking*

- All cooking times based on a medium-size vegetable.
- All vegetables can be served with Mediterranean dressing, except olives, corn, garlic and sea vegetables.
- Mediterranean Dressing: extra virgin olive oil, lemon, garlic, and sea salt and pepper to taste.

# guide to the healthiest way of cooking vegetables

| | HEALTHY SAUTÉ | HEALTHY STEAMING | QUICK BOILING | RAW | PREPARATION | HOW TO HIGHLIGHT FLAVOR. SERVE WITH: |
|---|---|---|---|---|---|---|
| **GREEN PEAS** | 3 min | | | Ok | Shell | Carrots; mint; tamari (soy sauce) |
| **GARLIC** | 1 min | | | Ok | Chop** | |
| **GREEN BEANS** | | 5 min | | | Cut off ends | Almonds; onions; tamari (soy sauce) |
| **KALE** | | 5 min | | Ok/salad | Chop 1/2" thick** | Tamari (soy sauce); cashews; Parmesan cheese |
| **LEEKS** | 7 min | | | Ok | Slice thin ** | Dill; tarragon; mushrooms |
| **MUSTARD GREENS** | 3 min | | | Ok/Salad | Chop 1/4" thick ** | Tomatoes; onions; walnuts; tamari (soy sauce) |
| **OLIVES** | | | | Ok | Already prepared | Cucumber; tomatoes; onion; eggplant |
| **ONIONS** | 7 min | | | Ok | Chop or slice thin** | Balsamic vinegar; tamari (soy sauce) |
| **POTATOES** | | 10 min | | | Cut into 1" cubes | Parsley; chives; yogurt; red chili pepper flakes |
| **ROMAINE LETTUCE** | | | | Ok | Chop | Parmesan cheese; balsamic vinegar; anchovies |
| **SEA VEGETABLES** | | | | Ok | Already prepared*** | Miso soup; crumble over vegetables |
| **SHIITAKE MUSHROOMS** | 7 min | | | | Slice and cut stems off | Tamari (soy sauce); onions; red bell peppers |
| **SPINACH** | | | 1 min | Ok-Baby spinach | Cut off roots and cook | Tamari (soy sauce); Parmesan cheese |
| **SQUASH, SUMMER** | 3 min | | | Ok/salads | Slice 1/4" thick | Thyme; mint; tamari (soy sauce); Parmesan cheese |
| **SQUASH, WINTER** | | 7 min | | | Cut into 1" cubes | Rosemary; cinnamon; nuts or seeds; sage |
| **SWEET POTATOES** | | 10 min | | | Cut into 1" cubes | Ground pumpkin seeds; walnuts; ginger |
| **SWISS CHARD** | | | 3 min | Ok-Baby chard | Slice into 1" pieces | Tamari (soy sauce); rice vinegar |
| **TOMATOES*** | 5 min | | | Ok/salad | Chopped for sauté | Oregano; basil; feta, mozzarella or goat cheese |

\*   *Lycopene is concentrated in the skin, so if eating tomatoes raw, choose cherry tomatoes*

\*\*  *Let sit for 5–10 minutes before cooking*

\*\*\**Follow directions on package*

## NOTE: YOU CAN COOK MORE THAN ONE VEGETABLE AT A TIME.

"Healthy Sauté" for 3 minutes:     Green peas, summer squash and tomatoes

"Healthy Sauté" for 5 minutes:     Cauliflower, red cabbage, bok choy and asparagus (optional)

"Healthy Steam" for 5 minutes:     Broccoli, kale, collard greens, Brussels sprouts and carrots

"Healthy Sauté" for 7 minutes:     Bell peppers, onions, leeks and mushrooms

"Healthy Steam" for 7 minutes:     Potatoes, sweet potatoes and winter squash

For more about the information above, see Mediterranean Feast, page 277.

*HINT: To mellow the flavor of vegetables, sprinkle with a few drops of tamari (soy sauce) just before serving. Even kids will love them.*

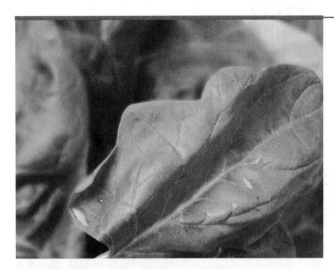

# spinach

## highlights

| | |
|---|---|
| AVAILABILITY: | Year-round |
| REFRIGERATE: | Yes |
| SHELF LIFE: | 5 days refrigerated |
| PREPARATION: | Clean well |
| BEST WAY TO COOK: | "Quick Boil" in just 1 minute |

## nutrient-richness chart

Total Nutrient-Richness: **65**  GI: **15**

One cup (180 grams) of cooked Spinach contains 41 calories

| NUTRIENT | AMOUNT | %DV | DENSITY | QUALITY |
|---|---|---|---|---|
| Vitamin K | 888.5 mcg | 1110.6 | 482.9 | excellent |
| Vitamin A | 14742.0 IU | 294.8 | 128.2 | excellent |
| Manganese | 1.7 mg | 84.0 | 36.5 | excellent |
| Folate | 262.4 mcg | 65.6 | 28.5 | excellent |
| Magnesium | 156.6 mg | 39.1 | 17.0 | excellent |
| Iron | 6.4 mg | 35.7 | 15.5 | excellent |
| Vitamin C | 17.6 mg | 29.4 | 12.8 | excellent |
| B2 Riboflavin | 0.4 mg | 24.7 | 10.7 | excellent |
| Calcium | 244.8 mg | 24.5 | 10.6 | excellent |
| Potassium | 838.8 mg | 24.0 | 10.4 | excellent |
| B6 Pyridoxine | 0.4 mg | 22.0 | 9.6 | excellent |
| Tryptophan | 0.1 g | 21.9 | 9.5 | excellent |
| Dietary Fiber | 4.3 g | 17.3 | 7.5 | very good |
| Copper | 0.3 mg | 15.5 | 6.7 | very good |
| B1 Thiamin | 0.2 mg | 11.3 | 4.9 | very good |
| Protein | 5.4 g | 10.7 | 4.7 | very good |
| Phosphorus | 100.8 mg | 10.1 | 4.4 | very good |
| Zinc | 1.4 mg | 9.1 | 4.0 | very good |
| Vitamin E | 1.7 mg | 8.6 | 3.7 | very good |
| Omega-3 Fatty Acids | 0.2 g | 6.0 | 2.6 | good |
| B3 Niacin | 0.9 mg | 4.4 | 1.9 | good |
| Selenium | 2.7 mcg | 3.9 | 1.7 | good |

**CAROTENOIDS**:

| | |
|---|---|
| Beta-Carotene | 11,318.4 mcg |
| Lutein+Zeaxanthin | 20,354.4 mcg |

Daily values for these nutrients have not yet been established.

For more on "Total Nutrient-Richness," "%DV," "Density," and The World's Healthiest Foods "Quality" Rating System, see page 805.

For more on GI, see page 342.

Spinach is a Mediterranean favorite that has been recognized as a distinctive vegetable since the Golden Age of the Renaissance back in the 16th century. When Catherine de Medici left her home in Florence, Italy, to marry the King of France, she brought cooks with her who knew how to prepare Spinach in the special way she loved best—the dish that has come to be known as Spinach *a la Florentine*. Now, you don't need special cooks from Florence to prepare your Spinach. By using the *al denté* "Healthiest Way of Cooking," you can bring out the best flavor from your Spinach while maximizing its nutritional value in just 1 minute.

It has been reported that the sale of Spinach has gone up 300% after it has become available prewashed and prepackaged.

## why spinach should be part of your healthiest way of eating

Spinach is an excellent plant-based source of iron that, in comparison to meat sources, is low in calories and virtually fat-free. It is also a rich source of phytonutrients. Carotenoid phytonutrients such as beta-carotene, lutein and zeaxanthin provide antioxidant protection against damage to cell structures. Spinach also contains at least 13 different flavonoid phytonutrients that also function as powerful antioxidants. Spinach is an ideal food to add to your "Healthiest Way of Eating" not only because it is so richly endowed with nutrients, but also because it is low in calories: one cup of cooked Spinach contains only 41 calories.

Overcooked and canned Spinach lose much of their nutrients as well as their beautiful rich green color. So, although we know Popeye made himself strong from eating Spinach, think how much stronger he would have been if he hadn't eaten it out of a can! (For more on the *Health Benefits of Spinach* and a complete analysis of its content of over 60 nutrients, see page 104.)

# varieties of spinach

Spinach *(Spinacea oleracea)* is thought to have originated in ancient Persia (Iran) and was introduced into China in the 7th century when the king of Nepal sent it as a gift to the emperor. Spinach shares a similar taste profile to Swiss chard and beet greens as they all belong to the same family of vegetables (known as "goosefoot" or *Chenopodiaceae*). Spinach can be enjoyed both cooked and raw. The varieties of Spinach are not identified at most markets; they are merely labeled as Spinach.

### CURLY OR SAVOY

This is the most popular variety of Spinach and is used for cooking. It is the variety featured in the photographs in the this chapter. Curly Spinach is usually sold in bunches and requires thorough cleaning. It has crisp, curly leaves with the root end sometimes having a reddish coloration. Because of its firm texture, this variety is usually served cooked and is not the best choice to use raw in Spinach salads.

### FLAT-LEAF SPINACH

This variety is also served cooked. Its leaves are larger, smoother, more tender and sweeter than Curly Spinach; its stems are also more tender. Flat-leaf Spinach is similar in nutritional value to Curly Spinach.

Flat-leaf Spinach is often sold in bags with stems removed. Since there is little waste when using bagged Spinach, you will generally need to purchase less bagged Spinach than Spinach sold in bunches when following recipes calling for Spinach. Although it is prewashed, it is best to rinse before using.

### BABY SPINACH

This type of Spinach is best for salads and is too tender for cooking. Baby Spinach is immature Flat-leaf Spinach that has been harvested much earlier in its lifecycle. It has a mildly sweet flavor with very tender leaves and is lower in oxalic acid (data for specific amounts is not available). Baby Spinach is usually packaged in bags or sold in bulk with the stems included, but the stems are very tender and don't need to be removed.

### NEW ZEALAND SPINACH

This native of New Zealand, Australia and Japan is not true Spinach but belongs to a different family called *Aizoaceae* and genus-species called *Tetragonia tetragoniaides*. It can be cooked in much the same way as true Spinach, is comparable in its vitamin C content and contains oxalic acid, but has slightly less beta-carotene.

### FROZEN SPINACH

Frozen Spinach is very popular. It has been well-cleaned and precooked (blanched), so all you have to do is heat it thoroughly, or just defrost it in the refrigerator if you are going to add it to a recipe. Although it is nutritionally comparable to fresh cooked Spinach, it has less flavor.

# the peak season

Spinach is available throughout the year, but its flavor is at its peak during the cold months when the frost helps to develop a sweet flavor and crisp texture. In hotter months Spinach is less tender and will require around 30 seconds additional cooking time. The flavor of Baby Spinach does not vary throughout the year as it is harvested when it is very young.

# biochemical considerations

Spinach is a highly concentrated source of oxalates, which might be of concern to certain individuals. It is one of the foods most commonly associated with allergic reactions in individuals with latex allergies. Spinach is one of the 12 foods on which pesticide residues have been most frequently found. (For more on: *Oxalates*, see page 725; *Latex Food Allergies*, see page 722; and *Pesticide Residues*, see page 726.)

# 4 steps for the best tasting and most nutritious spinach

Turning Spinach into a flavorful dish with the most nutrients is simple if you just follow my 4 easy steps:

1. The Best Way to Select
2. The Best Way to Store
3. The Best Way to Prepare
4. The Healthiest Way of Cooking

---

## new scientific findings

### HOW NUTRITIOUS ARE THE STEMS OF SPINACH?

Spinach stems are great for adding more fiber to your "Healthiest Way of Eating." They contain more fiber than the leaves while still providing the other nutrients found in the leaves but in smaller quantities. The nutrient content of the stems fluctuates dramatically and is closely related to the age and growth status of the plant since the flow of nutrients through the stems depends upon the plant's tasks at any given moment, including during its phases of growth.

# 1. the best way to select spinach

You can select the best tasting Spinach by looking for vibrant, bright green leaves with stems that look fresh and crisp. By selecting the best tasting Spinach, you will also enjoy Spinach with the highest nutritional value. As with all vegetables, I recommend selecting organically grown varieties whenever possible. (For more on *Organic Foods*, see page 113.)

Avoid Spinach that shows signs of yellowing or that has leaves that are wilted or bruised. A slimy coating on Spinach leaves is an indication of decay.

# 2. the best way to store spinach

Spinach is a delicate vegetable. Be sure to store it properly or else it can lose up to 30% of some of its vitamins as well as much of its flavor.

Spinach continues to respire even after it has been harvested; its respiration rate at room temperature (68°F /20°C) is 230 mg/kg/hr. Slowing down the respiration rate with proper storage is the key to extending its flavor and nutritional benefits. (For a *Comparison of Respiration Rates* for different vegetables, see page 91.)

### Spinach Will Remain Fresh for Up to 5 Days When Properly Stored

1. Store Spinach in the refrigerator. The colder temperature will slow the respiration rate, helping to preserve its nutrients and keep Spinach fresh for a longer period of time.

2. Place Spinach in a plastic storage bag before refrigerating. I have found that it is best to wrap the bag tightly around the Spinach, squeezing out as much of the air from the bag as possible.

3. Do not wash Spinach before refrigeration because exposure to water will encourage Spinach to spoil.

---

**COOKING INCREASES IRON ABSORPTION**

Research presented at the annual meeting of the American Chemical Society in San Francisco in 2000 by investigators at Rutgers University measured the availability of iron from several different vegetables and found an average increase of about 10–15% in the absorption of iron in cooked vegetables compared to raw vegetables.

---

# 3. the best way to prepare spinach

Properly cleaning and cutting Spinach helps ensure that the Spinach you serve will have the best flavor and retain the greatest number of nutrients.

### Cleaning Spinach
Spinach sold in bunches can often contain a large amount of soil and should be washed well. Before cleaning, reserve as much of the stem portion of the Spinach as possible by cutting only 1–2 inches off of the root end of the Spinach. You can save time by doing this in one cut before separating the bundle. Discard the outer leaves that may be tough, brown or slimy.

Place the Spinach in a large bowl of tepid water and swish the leaves around with your hands, dislodging as much of the soil as possible. To preserve nutrients, do not leave Spinach soaking or the water-soluble nutrients will leach into the water. Remove the leaves from the water, refill the bowl with fresh water and repeat this process until there is no longer any soil appearing in the water. Alternatively, once you have done this a couple of times, you can rinse it in a colander to remove any remaining soil. (For more on *Washing Vegetables*, see page 92.)

Spinach sold in bags has been pre-washed and only needs to be rinsed.

### What to Do with Stems
Spinach stems are good to eat and add extra enjoyment to your "Healthiest Way of Eating." They are usually small and tender and can be cooked along with the leaves. They give balance of flavor and texture. You may occasionally find stems that are larger and tougher than usual and require extra cooking. In this case, separate the stems from the leaves. If you would like, you can then cook them for 1–2 minutes before adding the leaves; however, I have never found it necessary to cook them separately.

# 4. the healthiest way of cooking spinach ———

Since research has shown that important nutrients can be lost or destroyed by the way a food is cooked, the "Healthiest Way of Cooking" Spinach is focused on enhancing its flavor while maximizing its vitamins, minerals and powerful antioxidants.

## The Healthiest Way of Cooking Spinach: "Quick Boiling" for just 1 Minute

In my search to find the Healthiest Way to cook Spinach, I tested every possible cooking method, and discovered that "Quick Boiling" Curly or Flat-leaf Spinach for just 1 minute produced the best result. Although 1 minute may seem like an extremely short time, I found that this is all it needs because it is a very delicate vegetable. "Quick Boiling" reduces the acids found in Spinach, brings out its mild, sweet, distinctive flavor, retains its bright green color and maximizes its nutritional profile. The Step-by-Step Recipe will show you how easy it is to "Quick Boil" Spinach.

In Mediterranean countries, where Spinach is very popular, it is usually cooked uncovered in a pot of boiling water. "Quick Boiling" is the healthiest way to cook Spinach because it frees up some of the unwanted acids and allows them to leach out into the water. While boiling is not considered the best way of cooking most vegetables, Spinach is one of only three vegetables I recommend boiling because of its acid content. The other two are Swiss chard and beet greens, which belong to the same botanical family as Spinach. After boiling any of these three vegetables, be sure to discard the cooking water. Do not drink it or use it for stock because it will contain the unwanted acids leached from the vegetables. (For more on *"Quick Boiling,"* see page 61.)

## How to Avoid Overcooking Spinach: Cook it *Al Denté*

One of the primary reasons that cooked Spinach loses its flavor and shrinks up to 80% is because it is overcooked. That is why I recommend you "Quick Boil" Spinach *al denté* for the best flavor. Spinach cooked *al denté* is tender because it is cooked just long enough to soften its cellulose and hemicellulose fibers; this makes it easier to digest and allows its health-promoting nutrients to become more readily available for absorption. Remember that testing Spinach with a fork is not an effective way to determine whether it is done.

Spinach is a delicate vegetable, so it is very important not to overcook it. Spinach cooked for as little as a minute longer than *al denté* will begin to lose its chlorophyll and its bright green color; it will take on a brownish hue, a sign that magnesium is being lost. Overcooking Spinach will cause it to become soft and mushy and significantly decrease its nutritional value: as much as 50% of some nutrients can be lost. (For more on *Al Denté*, see page 92.)

## Cooking Methods Not Recommended for Spinach

### STEAMING, SAUTÉING OR COOKING WITH OIL

I don't recommend steaming Spinach because I find steamed Spinach has a slightly bitter acid taste since it is not able to release as much of the acids as it does when it is boiled. It is best not to sauté because Spinach does not contain enough liquid to extract and reduce Spinach's acid concentration. (For more information on *Oxalates*, see page

---

### An Easy Way to Prepare Spinach, Step-by-Step

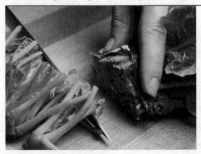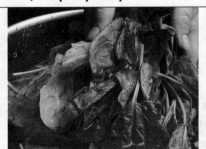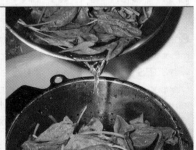

**CLEANING SPINACH**

❶ Before loosening the bundle, cut 1 to 2 inches off of the stem end. ❷ Fill bowl with tepid water and rinse Spinach. Refill the bowl with fresh water, and repeat this process until no more soil appears in water.
❸ Drain in colander.

725.) I also don't recommend cooking Spinach in oil because high-temperature heat can damage delicate oils and potentially create harmful free radicals.

### Serving Ideas From Mediterranean Countries:

Traveling through the Mediterranean region, I found that Spinach was prepared in many different ways:

In Italy, they serve Spinach with pine nuts and raisins or anchovies.

In Greece, it is cooked with rice, feta cheese and mint.

In Spain, it is cooked with garlic, onion, paprika, olive oil, vinegar and cinnamon.

In North Africa, Spinach is made spicy with the addition of chili peppers, black pepper, cumin and garlic. They also add eggs, olive oil, tomato paste and lemon juice.

In France, it is served with pine nuts, garlic and nutmeg.

In Turkey, it is made into an appetizer called *burek*, a filled pastry.

---

**Q** *I have heard that although Spinach is high in calcium, it also contains oxalates (oxalic acid) which block the calcium from being absorbed. Is there any truth to this?*

**A** Spinach does contain calcium as well as oxalates. However, in every peer-reviewed research study I've seen, the ability of oxalates to lower calcium absorption definitely exists, but is relatively small, and definitely does not outweigh the ability of oxalate-containing foods to contribute calcium to the "Healthiest Way of Eating." This relationship seems particularly true in the case of Spinach, which is incredibly calcium-rich (a cup of boiled Spinach contains over 240 mg). So while it's true that Spinach is a relatively high oxalate food, and equally true that oxalates can bind with calcium and lower its absorption, the research does not seem to support the position that Spinach is a poor choice for increasing calcium in the "Healthiest Way of Eating."

If you are still concerned about oxalates, cooking Spinach would actually be a way to reduce its oxalate content—by 5–15%—if it is cooked correctly. I recommend boiling Spinach without the top on the pot because this allows some of the oxalic acids to be liberated and therefore reduces the oxalate content of the Spinach. If you want to eat raw Spinach, use baby Spinach. Not only does baby Spinach have a sweeter flavor making it better suited for salads and other dishes where raw Spinach is called for, but it also has a lower oxalate content than mature Spinach.

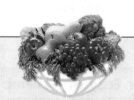

## how to enjoy fresh spinach without cooking

**Spinach Salad:** It is best to use Baby Spinach leaves rather than mature Spinach. Dress 6 cups of Baby Spinach with 3 TBS extra virgin olive oil, 1 TBS lemon juice, 1 clove chopped garlic, sea salt and pepper. The ratio of olive oil to lemon juice is 3:1. Too much dressing will wilt your Spinach. You will want the Spinach tender and not mushy.

**Wilted Mediterranean Spinach Salad:** Warm 1/4 cup of Mediterranean Dressing (page 103) and drizzle it over 6 cups of Baby Spinach. Be sure not to use too much dressing or it will cause the Spinach to become overly wilted. You can add thinly sliced black olives, boiled eggs, goat cheese, anchovies, thinly sliced red onions, cherry tomatoes and sliced mushrooms.

**Citrus Spinach Salad:** Place 6 cups of Baby Spinach in a large bowl. Add orange sections, a handful of walnuts and raisins and bits of gorgonzola or goat cheese (or pieces of chicken or turkey) for a delicious salad. To make a tasty dressing, use the juice of half an orange and half a lemon, sea salt, pepper and 3 TBS extra virgin olive oil.

STEP-BY-STEP RECIPE
## The Healthiest Way of Cooking Spinach

# 1-Minute "Quick Boiled" Spinach

*This Mediterranean way of preparing Spinach has the best flavor because it helps remove some of the acids found in Spinach and brings out its sweetness, while also enhancing its nutritional value. It tastes great served with the Mediterranean dressing.*

**1 lb fresh Spinach**

**Mediterranean Dressing:**
**3 TBS extra virgin olive oil**
**1 tsp lemon juice**
**1 medium clove garlic**
**Sea salt and pepper to taste**

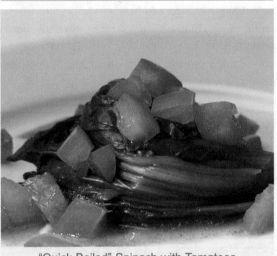
"Quick Boiled" Spinach with Tomatoes

1. Use a large pot (3 quart) with lots of water. Bring water to a rapid boil.

2. While water is coming to a boil, press or chop garlic and let it sit for at least 5 minutes. (Why?, see page 261.)

3. Wash Spinach as directed under the *The Best Way to Prepare Spinach*.

4. When water is at full boil, place Spinach into the pot. **Do not cover**. Cooking uncovered helps the acids escape into the air. Cook Spinach for 1 minute; begin timing as soon as you drop the Spinach into the boiling water. Be extremely careful to avoid burning yourself when adding Spinach to the boiling water.

5. After the Spinach has been cooking for 1 minute, (do not wait for water to return to a boil), use a mesh strainer with a handle to remove the Spinach from the pot. Press out excess liquid with fork. This will keep the Spinach from diluting the flavor of your dressing. You want the Spinach to be tender, brightly colored and not mushy when it's done. For information on *Differences in Cooking Time*, see page 94.

6. Transfer to a bowl. For more flavor, toss Spinach with the remaining ingredients while it is still hot. (Mediterranean Dressing does not need to be made separately.) Using a knife and fork, cut Spinach into small pieces. Research shows that carotenoids found in foods are best absorbed when consumed with oils.

**SERVES 2**

### COOKING TIPS:
- To prevent overcooking Spinach, I highly recommend using a timer.
- Testing Spinach with a fork is not an effective way to determine whether it is done.

## Flavor Tips: Try these 4 great serving suggestions with the recipe above. ✱

1. **Most Popular:** Add a few drops of tamari (soy sauce) to mellow the taste of Spinach and sprinkle with sesame seeds.
2. Drizzle with balsamic vinegar and crumbled goat cheese.
3. Top with kalamata olives or anchovies.

4. **Creamy Curry Spinach:** Mix 1 cup low-fat cottage cheese, 1 tsp curry powder, and sea salt and pepper to taste in a large bowl. Immediately add 1-Minute "Quick Boiled" Spinach and stir until ingredients are well combined. For a special presentation, serve in a cored tomato.

Please write (address on back cover flap) or e-mail me at info@whfoods.org with your personal ideas for preparing Spinach, and I will share them with others through our website at www.whfoods.org.

# health benefits of spinach

### Promotes Energy and Vitality

Cooked Spinach is an excellent source of iron. Boosting iron stores with Spinach is a good idea, especially because in comparison to red meat—a well-known source of iron—Spinach provides iron for a lot less calories and is virtually fat-free. Iron is an integral component of hemo-globin, which transports oxygen from the lungs to all body cells, and is also part of key enzyme systems for energy production and metabolism.

### Promotes Optimal Health

Researchers have identified at least 13 different flavonoid compounds in Spinach that function as antioxidants and as anticancer agents. (Many of these substances fall into a technical category of flavonoids known as methylene-dioxyflavonol glucuronides.) The anticancer properties of these Spinach flavonoids have been sufficiently impressive to prompt researchers to create specialized Spinach extracts that could be used in controlled studies. These Spinach extracts have been shown to slow down cell division in stomach cancer cells, and in studies with laboratory animals, to reduce skin cancers. A study on adult women also showed intake of Spinach to be inversely related to incidence of breast cancer. Spinach's chemoprotective potential may also come from its concentration of carotenoid phytonutrients; carotenoid-rich diets have been found to be associated with a reduced risk of various types of cancer. A recent study just found that a novel carotenoid, neoxanthin, found in Spinach and other leafy vegetables, not only instructs prostate cancer cells to self-destruct but is also transformed into other molecules that prevent the cancer cells' replication.

### Promotes Heart Health

For atherosclerosis and diabetic heart disease, few foods compare to Spinach in their number of helpful nutrients. Spinach is an excellent source of vitamin C and vitamin A, the latter notably through Spinach's concentration of beta-carotene. These two nutrients are important antioxidants that work to reduce the amount of free radicals in the body; vitamin C works as a water-soluble antioxidant and beta-carotene as a fat-soluble one. This water-and fat-soluble antioxidant team helps to prevent cholesterol from becoming oxidized, which can lead to the development of atherosclerosis. Spinach is also an excellent source of folic acid and vitamin B6, two B vitamins that help to keep homocysteine levels from becoming elevated. Homocysteine can directly damage artery walls and is a known risk factor for cardiovascular disease. Spinach is also an excellent source of magnesium and potassium, two minerals important for keeping blood pressure balanced.

In addition to its hefty supply of cardioprotective vitamins and minerals, a recent study revealed that an enzyme in Spinach contains protein components that inhibit *angiotensin I-converting enzyme*—the same enzyme blocked by ACE inhibitor

## Nutritional Analysis of 1 cup of cooked Spinach:

| NUTRIENT | AMOUNT | % DAILY VALUE | NUTRIENT | AMOUNT | % DAILY VALUE |
|---|---|---|---|---|---|
| Calories | 41.40 | | Pantothenic Acid | 0.26 mg | 2.60 |
| Calories from Fat | 4.21 | | | | |
| Calories from Saturated Fat | 0.68 | | **Minerals** | | |
| Protein | 5.35 g | | Boron | — mcg | |
| Carbohydrates | 6.75 g | | Calcium | 244.80 mg | 24.48 |
| Dietary Fiber | 4.32 g | 17.28 | Chloride | 0.00 mg | |
| Soluble Fiber | 0.90 g | | Chromium | 0.00 mcg | 0.00 |
| Insoluble Fiber | 3.42 g | | Copper | 0.31 mg | 15.50 |
| Sugar – Total | 0.00 g | | Fluoride | — mg | — |
| Monosaccharides | 0.00 g | | Iodine | — mcg | — |
| Disaccharides | 0.00 g | | Iron | 6.43 mg | 35.72 |
| Other Carbs | 2.43 g | | Magnesium | 156.60 mg | 39.15 |
| Fat – Total | 0.47 g | | Manganese | 1.68 mg | 84.00 |
| Saturated Fat | 0.08 g | | Molybdenum | — mcg | — |
| Mono Fat | 0.01 g | | Phosphorus | 100.80 mg | 10.08 |
| Poly Fat | 0.19 g | | Potassium | 838.80 mg | |
| Omega-3 Fatty Acids | 0.15 g | 6.00 | Selenium | 2.70 mcg | 3.86 |
| Omega-6 Fatty Acids | 0.03 g | | Sodium | 550.80 mg | |
| Trans Fatty Acids | 0.00 g | | Zinc | 1.37 mg | 9.13 |
| Cholesterol | 0.00 mg | | | | |
| Water | 164.18 g | | **Amino Acids** | | |
| Ash | 3.26 g | | Alanine | 0.26 g | |
| | | | Arginine | 0.30 g | |
| **Vitamins** | | | Aspartate | 0.45 g | |
| Vitamin A IU | 14742.00 IU | 294.84 | Cystine | 0.06 g | 14.63 |
| Vitamin A RE | 1474.20 RE | | Glutamate | 0.64 g | |
| A - Carotenoid | 1474.20 RE | 19.66 | Glycine | 0.25 g | |
| A - Retinol | 0.00 RE | | Histidine | 0.12 g | 9.30 |
| B1 Thiamin | 0.17 mg | 11.33 | Isoleucine | 0.27 g | 23.48 |
| B2 Riboflavin | 0.42 mg | 24.71 | Leucine | 0.42 g | 16.60 |
| B3 Niacin | 0.88 mg | 4.40 | Lysine | 0.33 g | 14.04 |
| Niacin Equiv | 2.08 mg | | Methionine | 0.10 g | 13.51 |
| Vitamin B6 | 0.44 mg | 22.00 | Phenylalanine | 0.24 g | 20.17 |
| Vitamin B12 | 0.00 mcg | 0.00 | Proline | 0.21 g | |
| Biotin | — mcg | — | Serine | 0.19 g | |
| Vitamin C | 17.64 mg | 29.40 | Threonine | 0.23 g | 18.55 |
| Vitamin D IU | 0.00 IU | 0.00 | Tryptophan | 0.07 g | 21.88 |
| Vitamin D mcg | 0.00 mcg | | Tyrosine | 0.20 g | 20.62 |
| Vitamin E Alpha Equiv | 1.72 mg | 8.60 | Valine | 0.30 g | 20.41 |
| Vitamin E IU | 2.56 IU | | | | |
| Vitamin E mg | 3.60 mg | | | | |
| Folate | 262.44 mcg | 65.61 | | | |
| Vitamin K | 888.50 mcg | 1110.63 | | | |

(Note: "–" indicates data is unavailable. For more information, please see page 806.)

drugs, which are used to lower blood pressure. When given to laboratory animals bred to be hypertensive, Spinach produced a blood pressure lowering effect within two to four hours.

## Promotes Brain Health

In animal studies, researchers have found that Spinach may help protect the brain from oxidative stress and may reduce the effects of age-related declines in brain function. Researchers found that feeding aging laboratory animals Spinach-rich diets significantly improved both their learning capacity and motor skills.

## Promotes Vision Health

In addition to being an excellent source of vitamin A, known as an important nutrient for eye health, Spinach is also one of the most concentrated sources of lutein and zeaxanthin, antioxidants suggested to play a very important role in promoting eye health. These carotenoid phytonutrients are thought to protect the eye from oxidative damage as well as promote the healthy distribution of epithelial tissue in the eye. Individuals who consume lutein/zeaxanthin-rich diets have been found to be at a lower risk for developing cataracts and age-related macular degeneration. Recent research has found that since these carotenoids are fat-soluble, consuming Spinach with some oil or fat-containing food like eggs or nuts may help to boost absorption of these important nutrients.

## Additional Health-Promoting Benefits of Spinach

Spinach is also a concentrated source of other nutrients providing additional health-promoting benefits. These nutrients include free-radical-scavenging manganese, copper, zinc, vitamin E and selenium; energy-producing vitamin B1, B2 and niacin; bone-building calcium and phosphorus; digestive-health-promoting dietary fiber; muscle-building protein; inflammation-reducing omega-3 fatty acids; and sleep-promoting tryptophan. Since Spinach contains only 41 calories per one cup serving, it is an ideal food for healthy weight control.

## Spinach and *E. coli*

Thorough washing of contaminated spinach cannot remove *E. coli* 0157:H7. According to the latest update statement issued by the U.S. Food and Drug Administration (FDA) on October 20, 2006, "Cooking fresh spinach at 160°F (71°C) for 15 seconds will kill any *E. coli* 0157:H7 present." The cooking method we recommend on our website for spinach — a quick boil for approximately 1 minute — greatly exceeds this safety standard.

Is certified organic spinach an option here? While we certainly cannot call it a foolproof option, there's definitely less chance of finding *E. coli* 0157:H7 bacteria in organically grown spinach than in conventionally grown spinach. The reason involves use of raw animal manure, which can be used at any time in the production of conventionally grown spinach. However, in the production of organically grown spinach, raw animal manure cannot be used less than 120 days prior to harvest if the food (like spinach) has an edible portion that comes into contact with the soil or soil surface. These restrictions on the use of raw animal manure help prevent crops like spinach from being contaminated with bacteria like *E. coli* 0157:H7.

Here is a question that I received from a reader of the whfoods.org website about Spinach:

Q *Is there a difference nutritionally between raw and cooked Spinach? How about between regular size and Baby Spinach?*

A There is little difference in the nutritional value between raw and cooked Spinach when "Quick Boiled" as I recommend since it is cooked for only a minute, and so there is little loss in vitamin content. However, Spinach is among a small number of foods that contain any measurable amount of oxalic acid, and cooking can help to reduce the oxalic acid content. This may be of importance to those who are sensitive to this compound, including those with certain kidney or gallbladder problems. If you do not have any of these health concerns, eating raw Spinach should present no problem.

When I want to enjoy Spinach raw, I usually choose Baby Spinach. From my understanding, Baby Spinach has a similar nutritional profile to regular Spinach, with one significant difference — it is lower in oxalic acid. Not only is this helpful to individuals concerned about intake of this compound, but the reduced acid content gives Baby Spinach a much sweeter taste. I also prefer the texture of raw Baby Spinach — it is more delicate and less chalky than mature Spinach. It also makes a nice presentation in salads because you can see the whole leaf compared to just a cut part of the leaf.

Baby Spinach is so convenient to use since it is widely available prewashed in bags at the grocery store. Using prewashed Spinach can really cut down the time it takes to prepare a quick and easy salad.

If you like Baby Spinach as I do, you'll be happy to know that it is becoming easier to find at restaurants. More and more restaurants are offering Baby Spinach on their menus, whether it be as part of a side or entrée salad or as an offering on their salad bars.

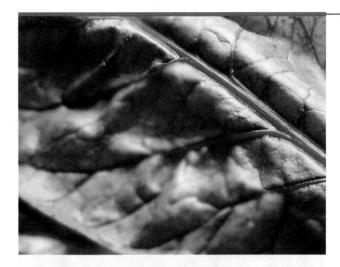

# swiss chard

## highlights

| | |
|---|---|
| AVAILABILITY: | Year-round |
| REFRIGERATE: | Yes |
| SHELF LIFE: | 5 days refrigerated |
| PREPARATION: | Minimal |
| BEST WAY TO COOK: | "Quick Boil" in just 3 minutes |

## nutrient-richness chart

Total Nutrient-Richness: **55**          GI: **15**

One cup (175 grams) of cooked Swiss Chard contains 35 calories

| NUTRIENT | AMOUNT | %DV | DENSITY | QUALITY |
|---|---|---|---|---|
| Vitamin K | 572.8 mcg | 716.0 | 368.2 | excellent |
| Vitamin A | 5493.3 IU | 109.9 | 56.5 | excellent |
| Vitamin C | 31.5 mg | 52.5 | 27.0 | excellent |
| Magnesium | 150.5 mg | 37.6 | 19.4 | excellent |
| Manganese | 0.6 mg | 29.0 | 14.9 | excellent |
| Potassium | 960.8 mg | 27.4 | 14.1 | excellent |
| Iron | 4.0 mg | 22.0 | 11.3 | excellent |
| Vitamin E | 3.3 mg | 16.6 | 8.5 | excellent |
| Dietary Fiber | 3.7 g | 14.7 | 7.6 | excellent |
| Copper | 0.3 mg | 14.5 | 7.5 | very good |
| Calcium | 101.5 mg | 10.2 | 5.2 | very good |
| Tryptophan | 0.03 g | 9.4 | 4.8 | very good |
| B2 Riboflavin | 0.2 mg | 8.8 | 4.5 | very good |
| B6 Pyridoxine | 0.2 mg | 7.5 | 3.9 | very good |
| Protein | 3.3 g | 6.6 | 3.4 | very good |
| Phosphorus | 57.8 mg | 5.8 | 3.0 | good |
| B1 Thiamin | 0.1 mg | 4.0 | 2.1 | good |
| Zinc | 0.6 mg | 3.9 | 2.0 | good |
| Folate | 15.1 mcg | 3.8 | 1.9 | good |
| Biotin | 10.5 mcg | 3.5 | 1.8 | good |
| B3 Niacin | 0.6 mg | 3.1 | 1.6 | good |
| B5 Pantothenic Acid | 0.3 mg | 2.9 | 1.5 | good |

| CAROTENOIDS: | | |
|---|---|---|
| Alpha-Carotene | 79.0 mcg | Daily values for these nutrients have not yet been established. |
| Beta-Carotene | 6,391.0 mcg | |
| Lutein+Zeaxanthin | 19,276.0 mcg | |

For more on "Total Nutrient-Richness," "%DV," "Density," and The World's Healthiest Foods "Quality" Rating System, see page 805.

For more on GI, see page 342.

S wiss Chard has been renowned for its health-promoting properties since the time of the ancient Greeks and Romans. In fact, the Greek philosopher Aristotle wrote about Chard as early as the fourth century BC Swiss Chard is not native to Switzerland as its name might imply but was named by a 19th century Swiss botanist in honor of his homeland. While Chard remains one of the most popular vegetables in the Mediterranean region, it is still coming into its own in the United States. To help increase your appreciation for Swiss Chard, I want to share with you the "Healthiest Way of Cooking" *al denté* Chard. In just 3 minutes you can bring out its best flavor while maximizing the nutritional profile of this Mediterranean favorite. Its delicious, hearty flavor and many nutritional benefits make Swiss Chard a great substitute for spinach.

## why swiss chard should be part of your healthiest way of eating

Calorie for calorie, Swiss Chard is one of the most nutritious vegetables around, featuring impressive concentrations of vitamins and minerals. Recent studies also show that Swiss Chard is a rich source of many newly discovered phytonutrients (plant nutrients). It is a concentrated source of carotenoids, such as beta-carotene, lutein and zeaxanthin. These carotenoids, along with its flavonoid phytonutrients, including anthocyanins, provide powerful antioxidant protection. Research suggests that the high concentration of chlorophyll found in Swiss Chard is also health protective. Swiss Chard is an ideal food to add to your "Healthiest Way of Eating" not only because it is high in nutrients, but also because it is low in calories: one cup of cooked Swiss Chard contains only 35 calories. (For more on the *Health Benefits of Swiss Chard* and a complete analysis of its content of over 60 nutrients, see page 110.)

# varieties of swiss chard

The term "Chard" describes a tall, leafy vegetable with a thick, crunchy stem to which wide, fan-like green leaves are attached. Swiss Chard (*Beta vulgaris*), along with kale, mustard greens and collard greens, are often referred to as "leafy greens," and are among some of the most nutritious and health-promoting vegetables. Swiss Chard belongs to the same botanical family as beets and spinach. It is characterized by a bitter flavor with acidic undertones (due to its oxalic acid content), a full-bodied texture and an abundance of nutrients. Varieties of Swiss Chard can have either smooth or curly leaves with stems that are white, red, orange, purple, pink or yellow in color.

### RAINBOW CHARD

The stems of this variety come in a rainbow of colors such as white, red, orange, purple, magenta, pink and yellow. This is the most popular variety of Swiss Chard and is the one featured in the photographs in this chapter. The mixture of colors in Rainbow Chard provides a good balance of flavors, with white-stemmed and yellow-stemmed Swiss Chard having a milder flavor than those with red stems. The leaves are tender and sweet, and I recommend enjoying the white stems along with the leaves. The colored stems are not edible; the red stems are exceptionally tough.

### FORDHOOK

This variety of Swiss Chard has crinkly leaves and is widely available. The white stems of this variety are tender, succulent and enjoyable to eat.

### BRIGHT YELLOW

This yellow-stemmed variety has a more bitter flavor than white-stemmed Chard but less than red-stemmed Swiss Chard.

### RUBY RED OR RHUBARB

Slightly stronger tasting than the Fordhook variety, this is a crinkly-leafed Swiss Chard with thin stems. The stems of this red variety are too tough to eat.

### BABY SWISS CHARD

This is immature Swiss Chard harvested early in its life cycle. Its small, mildly sweet, tender leaves are usually found in salad mixes and not sold on their own.

### SILVER BEET

Silver Beet is a British/Australian term for Swiss Chard.

# the peak season

Swiss Chard is available throughout the year, but its flavor is at its peak during the cold months when the frost helps to develop a sweet flavor and crisp texture. In hotter months, Swiss Chard is less tender and will require 1–2 minutes additional cooking time.

# biochemical considerations

Swiss Chard is a concentrated source of oxalates, which might be of concern to certain individuals. (For more on *Oxalates*, see page 725.)

# 4 steps for the best tasting and most nutritious swiss chard

Turning Swiss Chard into a flavorful dish with the most nutrients is simple if you just follow my 4 easy steps:

1. The Best Way to Select
2. The Best Way to Store
3. The Best Way to Prepare
4. The Healthiest Way of Cooking

# 1. the best way to select swiss chard ————

You can select the best tasting Swiss Chard by looking for leaves that have a vibrant, bright green color and crisp stems. I have found that Swiss Chard that has been stored in a chilled display has a crunchier texture and sweeter taste. By selecting the best tasting Swiss Chard, you will also enjoy the highest nutritional value. As with all vegetables, I recommend selecting organically grown varieties whenever possible. (For more on *Organic Foods*, see page 113.)

Avoid Swiss Chard with stems that are blemished or leaves that show signs of browning, yellowing, or wilting or that have tiny holes that may have been caused by insects.

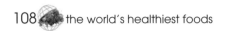

## 2. the best way to store swiss chard

Swiss Chard is not as delicate as its cousin spinach; however, it will lose its freshness if not stored properly. If you are not planning to use Swiss Chard immediately after bringing it home from the market, be sure to store it properly or else it can lose up to 30% of some of its vitamins as well as much of its flavor.

Swiss Chard continues to respire even after it has been harvested. Slowing down the respiration rate with proper storage is the key to extending its flavor and nutritional benefits. (For a *Comparison of Respiration Rates* for different vegetables, see page 91.)

### Swiss Chard Will Remain Fresh for Up to 5 Days When Properly Stored

1. Store Swiss Chard in the refrigerator. The colder temperature will slow the respiration rate, helping to preserve its nutrients and keep Swiss Chard fresh for a longer period of time.

2. Place Swiss Chard in a plastic storage bag before refrigerating. I have found that it is best to wrap the bag tightly around the Swiss Chard, squeezing out as much of the air from the bag as possible.

3. Do not wash Swiss Chard before refrigeration because exposure to water will encourage Swiss Chard to spoil.

## 3. the best way to prepare swiss chard

Properly cleaning and cutting Swiss Chard helps to ensure that the Swiss Chard you serve will have the best flavor and retain the greatest number of nutrients.

### Cleaning Swiss Chard

It is best to rinse Swiss Chard under cold running water just before cutting. To preserve nutrients, do not soak Swiss Chard or the water-soluble nutrients will leach into the water. Remove any part of leaves that may be brown, slimy or have holes. (For more on *Washing Vegetables*, see page 92.)

### What to Do with the Stems

In many parts of the world, Fordhook Swiss Chard (the type with white stems) is highly regarded with recipes created especially for its use. Unfortunately, most people in this country throw the stems away. I highly recommend enjoying the stems of Fordhook Chard together with the leaves because their flavors complement each other well. Stems from other varieties of Swiss Chard (especially those that are red) are tougher and not as succulent; I don't recommend eating them.

### Cutting Swiss Chard

Slicing Swiss Chard helps it to cook more quickly. The thinner you slice it, the more quickly it will cook. Stack the leaves and cut them into 1-inch slices until you reach the stems. If you are using Fordhook Chard, cut the stems into thinner slices (1/2-inch). Discard the bottom inch of the stems.

Depending on their width, the stems may require longer cooking time than the leaves. If the stems are not over 1-inch wide, you can cook them together with the leaves for the same length of time. However, if the stems are wider than 1 inch, you may want to cook them for 2 minutes before adding the leaves.

## 4. the healthiest way of cooking swiss chard

Since research has shown that important nutrients can be lost or destroyed by the way a food is cooked, the "Healthiest Way of Cooking" Swiss Chard is focused on enhancing its best flavor while maximizing its retention of vitamins, minerals and powerful antioxidants.

### The Healthiest Way of Cooking Swiss Chard: "Quick Boiling" for just 3 Minutes

In my search to find the healthiest way to cook Swiss Chard, I tested every possible cooking method and discovered that "Quick Boiling" all varieties of Swiss Chard (including Rainbow, Fordhook, Bright Yellow and Ruby Red) for just 3 minutes delivered the best result. "Quick Boiling" brings out the mild, sweet, distinctive flavor of Swiss Chard and retains its bright green color while maximizing its nutrient profile. The Step-by-Step Recipe will show you how easy it is to "Quick Boil" Swiss Chard.

"Quick Boiling" is the healthiest way to cook Swiss Chard because it frees up some of the unwanted acids and allows them to leach out into the water. I've observed that in Mediterranean countries, where Swiss Chard is very popular, it is cooked uncovered in a pot of boiling water. While boiling is not considered the best way of cooking most vegetables, Swiss Chard is one of only three vegetables I recommend boiling because of its acid content. The other two are spinach and beet greens. After boiling any of these three vegetables, be sure to discard the cooking water. Do not drink it or use it for stock because it will contain the unwanted acids leached from the vegetables. (For more on "*Quick Boiling,*" see page 61.)

## How to Avoid Overcooking Swiss Chard: Cook it *Al Denté*

One of the primary reasons for the loss of flavor when cooking Swiss Chard is overcooking. The traditional way of boiling Swiss Chard for 5–10 minutes, as is often recommended in cookbooks, is much too long. It not only destroys the color, flavor and texture of Swiss Chard, but most of its nutrients as well. That is why I recommend "Quick Boiling" Swiss Chard *al denté* for the best flavor. Swiss Chard cooked *al denté* is tender outside and slightly firm inside. Plus, Swiss Chard cooked *al denté* is cooked just long enough to soften its cellulose and hemicellulose fibers, which makes it easier to digest and allows its health-promoting nutrients to become more readily available for absorption. Remember that testing Swiss Chard with a fork is not an effective way to determine whether it is done.

Swiss Chard is a relatively delicate vegetable, so it is very important not to overcook it. Swiss Chard cooked for as little as a minute longer than *al denté* will begin to lose it chlorophyll and its bright green color; this is a sign that magnesium is being lost with the color of Swiss Chard slowly changing to a brownish hue. Overcooking Swiss Chard will cause it to become soft and mushy and significantly decrease its nutritional value: as much as 50% of some nutrients can be lost. (For more on *Al Denté*, see page 92.)

## Cooking Methods Not Recommended for Swiss Chard

### STEAMING OR COOKING WITH OIL

I don't recommend steaming Swiss Chard because I find steamed Swiss Chard has a slightly bitter acid taste. This is because steaming does not immerse the Swiss Chard in water, which releases the acids. I also don't recommend cooking Swiss Chard in oil because high-temperature heat can damage delicate oils and potentially create harmful free radicals.

## Serving Ideas from Mediterranean Countries:

Traveling through the Mediterranean region, I discovered that Swiss Chard is prepared in many different ways:

In Italy, both the stems and leaves of Swiss Chard are served with olive oil and tomatoes; it is also a popular addition to minestrone soup.

In Greece, Swiss Chard is prepared with leeks and dill.

In Spain, the stems and leaves of Swiss Chard are served with olive oil, garlic, pine nuts and raisins.

In Lebanon, Swiss Chard is served with hummus; the stems are used for dipping.

In France (especially in Nice, a city in the south of France, which is considered to be the Swiss Chard capital), the stems and leaves of Chard are incorporated into many dishes throughout the day. Even some French desserts contain Swiss Chard; one example is *tourte de blettes*, which is made with Swiss Chard, raisins, pine nuts, apples and eggs.

## An Easy Way to Prepare Swiss Chard, Step-by-Step

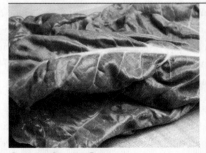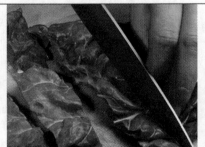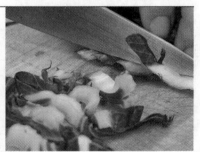

### SLICED SWISS CHARD

❶ Stack Swiss Chard leaves one on top of the other. ❷ Slice leaves into 1-inch slices. ❸ Slice white stems into 1/2-inch slices, discarding the last 1 inch of the stems.

# health benefits of swiss chard

## Promotes Digestive Health

Both the leaves and the roots of Swiss Chard have been the subject of fascinating health studies. Its combination of vitamins, minerals, phytonutrients (particularly anthocyanins), and dietary fiber may be protective in preventing digestive tract cancers. Several research studies on Swiss Chard have focused specifically on colon cancer, where the incidence of precancerous lesions in laboratory animals has been found to be significantly reduced following dietary intake of Swiss Chard extracts or fibers. Preliminary animal research also suggests that Swiss Chard may confer a protective effect on the kidneys of those with diabetes through reducing serum urea and creatinine levels.

Swiss Chard is an excellent source of vitamin C, the primary water-soluble antioxidant in the body. Vitamin C disarms free radicals and prevents oxidative damage, including damage to DNA, which can lead to cancer. Especially in areas of the body where cellular turnover is especially rapid, such as the digestive system, preventing DNA mutations translates into preventing cancer. This is why a good intake of vitamin C is associated with a reduced risk of colon cancer.

Swiss Chard is also an excellent source of dietary fiber, which can bind to cancer-causing chemicals, keeping them away from the cells lining the colon, providing yet another line of protection from colon cancer. The fiber in Swiss Chard also provides bulk that helps to keep people "regular."

## Promotes Bone Health

Swiss Chard is a very good non-dairy source of calcium, a mineral essential for optimal bone health. Swiss Chard is also an excellent source of vitamin K, which also plays an important role in maintaining bone health since it activates osteocalcin, the major non-collagen protein in bone. Magnesium, yet another nutrient of which Swiss Chard is an excellent source, is also necessary for healthy bones. About two-thirds of the magnesium in the human body is found in our bones. Some helps give bones their physical structure, while the rest is found on the surface of the bone where it is stored by the body to be drawn upon as needed.

## Promotes Vision Health

Swiss Chard is an excellent source of vitamin A because of its concentration of beta-carotene. Once inside the body, beta-carotene can be converted into vitamin A, so when you eat Swiss Chard, it's like getting both of these beneficial nutrients at once.

Both vitamin A and beta-carotene are important vision nutrients. In a study of over 50,000 women, those who consumed the highest dietary amount of vitamin A had a 39% reduced risk of developing cataracts.

Swiss Chard is also a concentrated source of the carotenoids

(Continued on Page 112)

### Nutritional Analysis of 1 cup of cooked Swiss Chard:

| NUTRIENT | AMOUNT | % DAILY VALUE |
|---|---|---|
| Calories | 35.00 | |
| Calories from Fat | 1.26 | |
| Calories from Saturated Fat | 0.19 | |
| Protein | 3.29 g | |
| Carbohydrates | 7.25 g | |
| Dietary Fiber | 3.68 g | 14.72 |
| Soluble Fiber | — g | |
| Insoluble Fiber | — g | |
| Sugar – Total | 0.70 g | |
| Monosaccharides | 0.70 g | |
| Disaccharides | 0.00 g | |
| Other Carbs | 2.87 g | |
| Fat – Total | 0.14 g | |
| Saturated Fat | 0.02 g | |
| Mono Fat | 0.03 g | |
| Poly Fat | 0.05 g | |
| Omega-3 Fatty Acids | 0.01 g | 0.40 |
| Omega-6 Fatty Acids | 0.04 g | |
| Trans Fatty Acids | 0.00 g | |
| Cholesterol | 0.00 mg | |
| Water | 162.14 g | |
| Ash | 2.21 g | |
| **Vitamins** | | |
| Vitamin A IU | 5493.25 IU | 109.86 |
| Vitamin A RE | 549.50 RE | |
| A – Carotenoid | 549.50 RE | 7.33 |
| A – Retinol | 0.00 RE | |
| B1 Thiamin | 0.06 mg | 4.00 |
| B2 Riboflavin | 0.15 mg | 8.82 |
| B3 Niacin | 0.63 mg | 3.15 |
| Niacin Equiv | 1.16 mg | |
| Vitamin B6 | 0.15 mg | 7.50 |
| Vitamin B12 | 0.00 mcg | 0.00 |
| Biotin | 10.50 mcg | 3.50 |
| Vitamin C | 31.50 mg | 52.50 |
| Vitamin D IU | 0.00 IU | 0.00 |
| Vitamin D mcg | 0.00 mcg | |
| Vitamin E Alpha Equiv | 3.31 mg | 16.55 |
| Vitamin E IU | 4.93 IU | |
| Vitamin E mg | 3.31 mg | |
| Folate | 15.05 mcg | 3.76 |
| Vitamin K | 572.80 mcg | 760.00 |

| NUTRIENT | AMOUNT | % DAILY VALUE |
|---|---|---|
| Pantothenic Acid | 0.29 mg | 2.90 |
| **Minerals** | | |
| Boron | — mcg | |
| Calcium | 101.50 mg | 10.15 |
| Chloride | — mg | |
| Chromium | — mcg | — |
| Copper | 0.29 mg | 14.50 |
| Fluoride | — mg | — |
| Iodine | — mcg | — |
| Iron | 3.96 mg | 22.00 |
| Magnesium | 150.50 mg | 37.63 |
| Manganese | 0.58 mg | 29.00 |
| Molybdenum | — mcg | — |
| Phosphorus | 57.75 mg | 5.78 |
| Potassium | 960.75 mg | |
| Selenium | 1.58 mcg | 2.26 |
| Sodium | 313.25 mg | |
| Zinc | 0.58 mg | 3.87 |
| **Amino Acids** | | |
| Alanine | 0.00 g | |
| Arginine | 0.21 g | |
| Aspartate | 0.00 g | |
| Cystine | 0.00 g | 0.00 |
| Glutamate | 0.00 g | |
| Glycine | 0.00 g | |
| Histidine | 0.07 g | 5.43 |
| Isoleucine | 0.27 g | 23.48 |
| Leucine | 0.24 g | 9.49 |
| Lysine | 0.18 g | 7.66 |
| Methionine | 0.04 g | 5.41 |
| Phenylalanine | 0.20 g | 16.81 |
| Proline | 0.00 g | |
| Serine | 0.00 g | |
| Threonine | 0.15 g | 12.10 |
| Tryptophan | 0.03 g | 9.38 |
| Tyrosine | 0.00 g | 0.00 |
| Valine | 0.20 g | 13.61 |

(Note: "—" indicates data is unavailable. For more information, please see page 806.)

STEP-BY-STEP RECIPE
# The Healthiest Way of Cooking Swiss Chard

## 3-Minute "Quick Boiled" Swiss Chard

*"Quick Boiling" Swiss Chard is tastier and more nutritious because it helps remove some of the acids found in Swiss Chard and brings out its sweet flavor. Make sure that the water is at a rapid boil before adding the Swiss Chard.*

**1 lb Swiss Chard**

**Mediterranean Dressing:**
**3 TBS extra virgin olive oil**
**1 tsp lemon juice**
**1 medium clove garlic**
**Sea salt and pepper to taste**

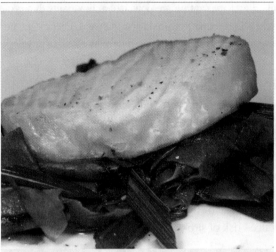

"Quick Boiled" Swiss Chard with Salmon

1. Use a large pot (3 quart) with lots of water. Make sure the water is at a rapid boil before adding Swiss Chard.

2. While water is coming to a boil, press or chop garlic, and let it sit for at least 5 minutes. (Why?, see page 261.)

3. Wash Swiss Chard as directed under *The Best Way to Prepare Swiss Chard.* Slice leaves 1-inch wide, slice white stems 1/2-inch wide. If using Swiss Chard with colored stems, discard stems.

4. When water is at full boil, place Swiss Chard and stems into the pot. **Do not cover.** Cook Swiss Chard for 3 minutes; begin timing as soon as you drop the Swiss Chard into the boiling water. Be extremely careful to avoid burning yourself when adding Swiss Chard to the boiling water. For more information on *Differences in Cooking Time,* see page 94.

5. After the Swiss Chard has been cooking for 3 minutes (do not wait for water to return to boil), use a mesh strainer with a handle to remove Swiss Chard from the pot. Press out excess liquid with fork. This will keep the Swiss Chard from diluting the flavor of your dressing. You want the Swiss Chard to be tender, brightly colored and not mushy when it's done.

6. Transfer to a bowl. For more flavor, toss Swiss Chard with the remaining ingredients while it is still hot. (Mediterranean Dressing does not need to be made separately.) Using a knife and fork, cut Swiss Chard into small pieces. Research shows that carotenoids found in foods are best absorbed when consumed with oils.

**SERVES 2**

## COOKING TIPS:
- To prevent overcooking Swiss Chard, I highly recommend using a timer.
- Testing Swiss Chard with a fork is not an effective way to determine whether it is done.

## Flavor Tips: Try these 5 great serving suggestions with the recipe above. ✳

1. **Most Popular: Zorba the Greek Swiss Chard.** Combine 1 medium chopped tomato, 6 chopped black olives (kalamata), 1/2 cup crumbled feta cheese and 1 tsp fresh or 1/2 tsp dried oregano. 3Add the hot 3-Minute "Quick Boiled" Swiss Chard recipe and gently toss together.

2. Top with grated Parmesan or Romano cheese and walnuts.

3. Add a few drops of tamari (soy sauce) to mellow the flavor of Swiss Chard.

4. Top with balsamic vinegar and crumbled goat cheese.

5. **Swiss Chard Lasagna:** For lasagna without pasta, prepare 3-Minute "Quick Boiled" Swiss Chard with Mediterranean Dressing. Place half of the Chard in a baking dish and top with plain low-fat cottage cheese mixed with dried basil, oregano, salt and pepper. Top with remaining Chard and cover with prepared tomato sauce and grated Parmesan. Place in 400°F (204°C) oven for 5 minutes to heat.

Please write (address on back cover flap) or e-mail me at info@whfoods.org with your personal ideas for preparing Swiss Chard, and I will share them with others through our website at www.whfoods.org.

*(Continued from Page 110)*

lutein and zeaxanthin, which are pivotal eye health nutrients. Lutein and zeaxanthin are powerful antioxidants that protect the lens and retina from oxidative damage. Dietary intake of these carotenoids has been found to reduce risk of developing cataracts and age-related macular degeneration.

## Promotes Heart Health

Swiss Chard is packed with nutrients that are good for your heart. Magnesium and potassium, two minerals of which Swiss Chard is an excellent source, are both important for regulating healthy blood pressure. One study found that men who ate diets higher in potassium-rich foods, as well as foods high in magnesium and fiber—also well provided by Swiss Chard—had a substantially reduced risk of stroke.

Swiss Chard is also a concentrated source of the ACE antioxidants—vitamin A, vitamin C and vitamin E. These nutrients help to protect cholesterol from being oxidized, therefore reducing its potential to form plaques that can lead to atherosclerosis and stroke.

## Promotes Energy Production

Swiss Chard is an excellent source of iron, a mineral so vital to the health of the human body that it is found in every human cell. Iron is primarily linked with protein to form the oxygen-carrying molecule hemoglobin, which is why insufficient iron can quickly translate into anemia. Iron enhances oxygen distribution throughout your body, keeps your immune system healthy and helps your body produce energy. Swiss Chard is also an excellent source of manganese, which protects the energy-producing mitochondria in your cells from being damaged by free radicals. In addition, Swiss Chard is also a very good source of vitamin B2 and a good source of vitamin B1, vitamin B6, niacin, biotin and phosphorus, nutrients that are all necessary for energy production.

## Additional Health-Promoting Benefits of Swiss Chard

Swiss Chard is also a concentrated source of other nutrients providing additional health-promoting benefits. These nutrients include free-radical-scavenging copper and zinc, heart-healthy folic acid, muscle-building protein, and sleep-promoting tryptophan. Since cooked Swiss Chard contains only 35 calories per one cup serving, it is an ideal food for healthy weight control.

---

Here are questions that I received from readers of the whfoods.org website about Swiss Chard, and weight-management, nutrient-rich foods and the immune system:

Q *Swiss Chard is often referred to as having an acid-sweet taste. What kind of acid is in Swiss Chard?*

A There are dozens of different organic acids, including carboxylic acids, which give Swiss Chard its delightful acidic bite. Additionally, Swiss Chard is a concentrated source of oxalic acid.

Q *What is the relationship between weight-management, nutrient-rich foods and the immune system?*

A Research and clinical observations suggest that obesity is associated with immune dysfunction. For example, increases in the incidence of infectious illness and infection-related mortality are found in obese people. An increase in inflammation has also been seen with an increase in weight in individuals. Some studies have shown an association between high cholesterol and susceptibility to infections as well. Therefore, maintaining a healthy weight and healthy cholesterol levels may also be beneficial to your immune system's functioning.

Eating nutrient-rich whole foods is one way to provide your body with the full spectrum of nutrients it needs while keeping calorie intake to a healthy level. The World's Healthiest Foods are analyzed for their nutrient-richness. Foods such as Swiss chard, crimini mushrooms, mustard greens, asparagus and romaine lettuce provide a broad spectrum of the key micronutrients that support healthy immune function and are therefore recommended as part of an immune-enhancing diet.

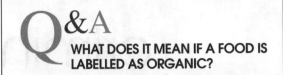

## Q&A
### WHAT DOES IT MEAN IF A FOOD IS LABELLED AS ORGANIC?

### OVERVIEW

Organic refers to an "earth-friendly" and health-supportive method of farming and processing foods. Weeds and pests are controlled using environmentally sound practices that sustain our personal health and the health of our planet. Use of renewable resources is a key principle in all organic production. The term "organic" applies to both animal and plant foods.

### WHAT ARE THE BASIC ORGANIC STANDARDS FOR PLANT CROPS?

Organically produced crops must be grown on land which has been free of prohibited substances for three years prior to harvest. The Organic Foods Production Act covers organic agricultural methods and materials in great detail, including management of soil fertility, when and how manure may be applied to crops, crop rotation and composting. Organic farmers do not use chemicals (pesticides, fungicides or fertilizers) in an environmentally harmful manner. In fact, most conventional pesticides and fertilizers are totally prohibited in the cultivation of organic food. Instead, a blend of old and new technologies and scientific research is used to avoid disrupting the earth's natural ecosystem.

Examples of organic farming methods include:

- Rotating crops. By alternating crops from year to year on any given piece of land, it is possible for one type of crop to restore nutrients to the soil that another type of crop has removed. It is also possible to interrupt the growth cycle of micro-organisms or pests like insects that might cause damage to crops.

- Planting select bushes and flowers to attract beneficial insects, which ward off unwanted pests.

Organic farming produces nutrient-rich, fertile soil, which nourishes the plant and keeps chemicals off the land to protect water quality and wildlife. Organic farming also gives us food that is safer to eat and much more likely to keep us healthy.

### WHAT ARE THE BASIC ORGANIC STANDARDS FOR LIVESTOCK (ANIMALS)?

Quite simply, organic livestock must be fed organic feed. The National Organic Standards Board recommends that conventional feed be allowed only if the organic feed supply has been compromised by a national, state or local weather emergency, or by fire or flood on an organic farm. Growth promoters and hormones, and plastic pellets for roughage in feed are prohibited. Antibiotics, wormers and other medications may not be used routinely as preventive measures.

Synthetic vitamins and minerals are allowed. Healthy living conditions and attentive care are considered first steps in the prevention of illness. Therefore, animals must not be overcrowded and must be allowed periodic access to the outdoors and direct sunlight.

### WHAT DOES THE "ORGANIC" LABEL MEAN?

The U.S. Department of Agriculture (USDA) sets, defines and regulates the use and meaning of "Organic" on food labels. It is the term used to describe raw or processed agricultural products and ingredients that have been (a) organically grown (farmed) and (b) handled in compliance with the standards of April 2001, which have been fully enforced since October 2002. These standards prohibit the use of:

- Most synthetic fertilizers and pesticides
- Sewer sludge fertilizers
- Genetic engineering
- Growth hormones
- Ionizing radiation (irradiation)
- Antibiotics
- Artificial ingredients

So, when you see foods that have the word "organic" on the packaging label, you can be assured that they meet these strict standards that were established for organic foods.

### WHAT ARE THE FEDERALLY MANDATED LABELS THAT IDENTIFY "ORGANIC" PRODUCTS?

100% organic: A raw or processed agricultural product that contains (by weight or fluid volume, excluding water and salt) 100% organically produced ingredients.

Organic: A raw or processed agricultural product that contains (by weight or fluid volume, excluding water and salt) not less than 95% organically produced or organically processed agricultural products. Any time that the word "organic" is used to describe an entire product on the front of packaging, this requirement must be met.

Made with (specified) organic ingredients: A multi-ingredient agricultural product must contain at least 70% organically produced ingredients (by weight or fluid volume, excluding water and salt) that have been handled according to USDA organic standards. An example of this labeling requirement would be "Made with organic tomatoes."

Organic ingredients listed individually: In a multi-ingredient agricultural product containing less than 70% organically produced ingredients, each organically produced ingredient can be identified as such on the side or back of the packaging; these ingredients cannot be advertised as organic on the front of the packaging.

USDA Organic Seal: The green USDA organics seal cannot be displayed on a product unless the 95% rule described above has been met.

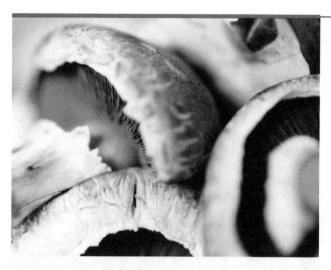

# crimini mushrooms

| | |
|---|---|
| AVAILABILITY: | Year-round |
| REFRIGERATE: | Yes |
| SHELF LIFE: | 5 days refrigerated |
| PREPARATION: | Wipe clean |
| BEST WAY TO COOK: | "Healthy Sauté" in just 7 minutes |

## nutrient-richness chart

Total Nutrient-Richness: **47**  GI: **n/a**

One cup (142 grams) of Crimini Mushrooms contains 31 calories

| NUTRIENT | AMOUNT | %DV | DENSITY | QUALITY |
|---|---|---|---|---|
| Selenium | 36.9 mcg | 52.6 | 30.4 | excellent |
| B2 Riboflavin | 0.7 mg | 40.6 | 23.4 | excellent |
| Copper | 0.7 mg | 35.5 | 20.5 | excellent |
| B3 Niacin | 5.4 mg | 26.9 | 15.6 | excellent |
| Tryptophan | 0.1 g | 25.0 | 14.4 | excellent |
| B5 Pantothenic Acid | 2.1 mg | 21.3 | 12.3 | excellent |
| Potassium | 635.0 mg | 18.1 | 10.5 | excellent |
| Phosphorus | 170.1 mg | 17.0 | 9.8 | excellent |
| Zinc | 1.6 mg | 10.4 | 6.0 | very good |
| Manganese | 0.2 mg | 10.0 | 5.8 | very good |
| B1 Thiamin | 0.1 mg | 8.7 | 5.0 | very good |
| B6 Pyridoxine | 0.2 mg | 8.0 | 4.6 | very good |
| Protein | 3.5 g | 7.1 | 4.1 | very good |
| Folate | 19.9 mcg | 5.0 | 2.9 | good |
| Dietary Fiber | 0.9 g | 3.4 | 2.0 | good |
| Magnesium | 12.8 mg | 3.2 | 1.8 | good |
| Iron | 0.6 mg | 3.2 | 1.8 | good |
| Calcium | 25.5 mg | 2.6 | 1.5 | good |

For more on "Total Nutrient-Richness," "%DV," "Density," and
The World's Healthiest Foods "Quality" Rating System, see page 805.

For more on GI, see page 342.

Ever since ancient times, people have thought of Mushrooms as being endowed with special powers. The Egyptians believed that they granted immortality, and since only the pharaohs were felt to be worthy of this gift, the common people were not even allowed to touch Mushrooms, let alone eat them. The ancient Romans described them as "foods of the Gods" and believed they were created by the lightning bolts thrown to Earth during thunderstorms by the god Jupiter. Mushrooms are delicious, and their natural *umami* flavor enhances the taste of any food with which they are cooked. Proper preparation of Crimini Mushrooms is the key to bringing out their best flavor and maximizing their nutritional benefits. That is why I want to share with you the secret of the "Healthiest Way of Cooking" Crimini Mushrooms. In just 7 minutes, you will have a dish that complements many of your favorite entrées.

## why crimini mushrooms should be part of your healthiest way of eating

Although Crimini Mushrooms are highly regarded as a side dish or salad addition, they are rarely acknowledged as a source of many health-promoting nutrients. Today, scientific research continues to discover why Mushrooms were once considered "food of the gods," and the nutritional profile of Crimini Mushrooms clearly shows why they are included among the list of the World's Healthiest Foods. Crimini Mushrooms have also been found to contain newly discovered, health-promoting polysaccharide phytonutrients, which function as powerful antioxidants, protecting against oxidative damage to cell structures and DNA. Crimini Mushrooms are an ideal food to add to your "Healthiest Way of Eating" not only because they are high in nutrients, but also because they are low in calories: one cup of Crimini Mushrooms contains only 31 calories. (For more on the *Health Benefits of Crimini Mushrooms* and a complete analysis of their content of over 60 nutrients, see page 118.)

# varieties of mushrooms

Although Mushrooms are often considered a vegetable and are prepared like one, they are actually a fungus, a special type of living organism that has no roots, leaves, flowers or seeds. Crimini Mushrooms are one variety of button Mushrooms (*Agaricus bisporus*), which generally look like small cartoon umbrellas with a dense parasol-like cap attached to a stem that can be short and thick or thin and slightly curvy. Button Mushrooms have been growing wild since prehistoric times and were consumed as food by the early hunter-gatherers. Today, hunting for wild Mushrooms is a popular recreational activity, but you must be well informed and know which ones to pick as some types are poisonous.

### CRIMINI MUSHROOMS

Crimini Mushrooms look very similar in shape and size to the white Button Mushrooms commonly found at your local market, but they have a darker coffee color and a deeper "Mushroomy" flavor. Crimini Mushrooms are especially good for making stuffed Mushrooms. These are the Mushrooms featured in the photographs in this chapter.

### PORTOBELLO MUSHROOMS

The Portobello Mushroom, whose large size and meaty flavor make it a wonderful vegetarian entrée, is an overgrown Crimini Mushroom. They are especially good for grilling and roasting.

### WHITE BUTTON MUSHROOMS

White Button Mushrooms are cousins of Crimini Mushrooms. These cream-colored Mushrooms are readily available, inexpensive and the variety most commonly found in markets. They are often served raw in salads and are especially good when combined with Crimini or Portobello Mushrooms.

### PORCINI

Known as the "king of the wild Mushrooms" because of its popularity among wild Mushroom hunters, this Mushroom has a long, fleshy stalk and round, convex fleshy cap. Their distinguishing feature is the presence of vertical tube-like pores, instead of gills, on the underside of the cap. They have a woodsy aroma with a meaty texture and delicious flavor.

### OYSTER

White, cream, yellow or reddish brown in color, they have a tender, velvety texture and mild flavor.

## the peak season available year-round.

## biochemical considerations

Crimini mushrooms are a concentrated source of purines, which might be of concern to certain individuals. (For more on *Purines*, see page 727.)

# 4 steps for the best tasting and most nutritious crimini mushrooms

Turning Crimini Mushrooms into a flavorful dish with the most nutrients is simple if you just follow my 4 easy steps:

1. The Best Way to Select
2. The Best Way to Store
3. The Best Way to Prepare
4. The Healthiest Way of Cooking

Here are questions I received from readers of the whfoods.org website about Crimini Mushrooms:

**Q** *I eat a lot of Portobello Mushrooms and was wondering whether they are considered a healthy food. I love every type of Mushroom, but I recently heard that Mushrooms aren't good for you.*

**A** Portobello Mushrooms are actually overgrown Crimini Mushrooms, the brown Mushrooms readily available in supermarkets. Many people don't realize this because they have such a unique flavor. Portobello Mushrooms' size and flavor make them so versatile in cooking—they can be used as meat substitutes for sandwiches, fajitas and more. Just like the smaller Crimini Mushroom, they are incredibly rich in vitamins and minerals. In addition, they contain powerful phytonutrients, such as lentinan, which are suggested to protect our DNA from damage. So yes, I would say that Portobello Mushrooms are a very healthy food.

While there are a variety of different edible Mushrooms, there are also some wild Mushrooms that are toxic like those that you find wild in nature, those that you may come across during a hike. Unless you are with an experienced Mushroom forager, are absolutely certain about identification of Mushrooms, and know for sure which Mushrooms are safe to eat, it is always advised not to pick wild Mushrooms.

**Q** *I currently live in the UK, and I have not been able to find Crimini Mushrooms in the stores. Is it possible that they are labeled with a different name?*

**A** Crimini Mushrooms are a variety of the common button Mushroom but instead of being white or cream in color, they have a brownish tone to them. If you identify them this way to your local grocer, he or she may be better able to locate them for you. I have noticed the term "portobellini" Mushroom used in some areas in Europe, so if you see Mushrooms by this name, they may in fact be Criminis. This name undoubtedly is in reference to a small Portobello Mushroom, since Portobello Mushrooms are none other than overgrown Criminis.

# 1. the best way to select crimini mushrooms ——

You can select the best tasting Crimini Mushrooms by looking for Mushrooms that are firm, plump and clean. If your recipe calls only for Mushroom caps, you can avoid waste by selecting Mushrooms that have short stems.

Young Crimini Mushrooms that have been harvested before maturity have a membrane that extends from the edge of the cap to the stem covering the gills that line the underside of the cap. These Crimini Mushrooms have a delicate taste. As they are stored, the membrane will open exposing the gills. The gills become increasingly dark the longer the Crimini Mushrooms are stored. Crimini Mushrooms with dark gills have a deep, rich flavor but must be used right away. Their robust flavor makes them a good choice for making soups and sauces.

By selecting the best tasting Crimini Mushrooms, you will also be getting Mushrooms with the highest nutritional value. I recommend selecting organically grown Mushrooms whenever possible; however, they are not readily available. (For more on *Organic Foods*, see page 113.)

Avoid Crimini Mushrooms that are wrinkled or have wet slimy spots.

# 2. the best way to store crimini mushrooms ——

Crimini Mushrooms do not store well and lose their freshness quickly if not stored properly, which can result in their losing their flavor and up to 30% of some of their vitamins.

Crimini Mushrooms continue to respire even after they have been harvested; their respiration rate at room temperature (68°F/20°C) is 313 mg/kg/hr. Slowing down the respiration rate with proper storage is the key to extending their flavor and nutritional benefits. (For a *Comparison of Respiration Rates* for different vegetables, see page 91.)

### Crimini Mushrooms Will Remain Fresh for Up to 5 Days When Properly Stored

1. Store Crimini Mushrooms in the refrigerator. The colder temperature will slow the respiration rate, helping to preserve their nutrients and keeping Crimini Mushrooms fresh for a longer period of time.

2. Unlike many other vegetables, Crimini Mushrooms should not be stored in a plastic storage bag since this does not allow them to respire well. Instead, place them in a paper bag, which will allow for optimal respiration.

3. Do not wash Crimini Mushrooms before refrigeration because exposure to water will encourage Crimini Mushrooms to spoil.

4. While loose Crimini Mushrooms will stay fresh for up to 5 days, those that are prepackaged will last longer, about 7–10 days before the package is opened. That is because most of these packages have been vacuum sealed.

### How to Store Dried Mushrooms

Dried Mushrooms should be stored in a tightly sealed container in either the refrigerator or freezer where they will stay fresh for six months to one year.

# 3. the best way to prepare crimini mushrooms ——

Properly cleaning and cutting Crimini Mushrooms helps to ensure that the Mushrooms you serve will have the best flavor and retain the greatest number of nutrients.

### Cleaning Mushrooms: Wipe—Do Not Wash

Mushrooms are very porous and will quickly absorb water and become soggy if washed. The best way to clean Mushrooms, without sacrificing their texture and taste, is to clean them without water. To do this, simply wipe them well with a damp paper towel. You can also use a Mushroom brush, which you can find at most stores that sell kitchenware.

### Cutting Mushrooms

Cutting Mushrooms into equal size pieces will help them to cook more evenly. Since the smaller you cut them, the more quickly they will cook, I recommend cutting Mushrooms into quarters or slicing them. The stems are also edible, so slice off the stem tip, and slice the rest of the stem along with the cap.

Dried Mushrooms must be reconstituted. Place 1 ounce of dried Mushrooms in 1 cup of hot water for 30 minutes. Most of the flavor will end up in the liquid, so be sure to save and substitute it for other liquids in the recipe. To retain more of the flavor in the Mushrooms, soak in cold water overnight.

# 4. the healthiest way of cooking crimini mushrooms

Since research has shown that important nutrients can be lost or destroyed by the way a food is cooked, the "Healthiest Way of Cooking" Crimini Mushrooms is focused on bringing out their best flavor while maximizing their vitamins, minerals and powerful antioxidants.

## The Healthiest Way of Cooking Crimini Mushrooms: "Healthy Sautéing" for just 7 Minutes

In my search to find the healthiest way to cook Crimini Mushrooms, I tested every possible cooking method looking for the ways to bring out their best flavor and maximize the amount of their nutrients and discovered that "Healthy Sautéing" them for just 7 minutes delivered the best result. "Healthy Sautéed" Crimini Mushrooms are tender, have the best flavor and are extremely rich in nutrients. The Step-by-Step Recipe will show you how easy it is to "Healthy Sauté" Crimini Mushrooms. (For more on "*Healthy Sauté*," see page 57.)

## Grilled or Broiled Mushrooms

While grilled or broiled Crimini Mushrooms taste great, make sure they do not burn. It is best to grill Mushrooms on an area without a direct flame as the temperatures directly above or below the flame can reach as high as 500°F to 1000°F (260° to 538°C). When using a broiler, keep the Mushrooms about 4–5 inches away from the flame. Coating with olive oil before cooking will also produce harmful free radicals, so brush with extra virgin olive oil immediately after they are cooked. (For more on *Grilling*, see page 61.)

## How to Avoid Overcooking Crimini Mushrooms

One of the primary reasons Crimini Mushrooms lose their flavor is because they are often overcooked. For the best flavor, I recommend "Healthy Sautéing" Crimini Mushrooms for 7 minutes. "Healthy Sautéed" Crimini Mushrooms are tender and cooked just long enough to soften their cellulose and hemicellulose fiber; this makes them easier to digest and allows their health-promoting nutrients to become more readily available for absorption.

Crimini Mushrooms cooked for as little as a couple of minutes longer than the recommended cooking time will begin to lose not only their texture and flavor, but also their nutrients. Overcooking Crimini Mushrooms will significantly decrease their nutritional value: as much as 50% of some nutrients can be lost.

## Cooking Methods Not Recommended for Crimini Mushrooms

### BOILING, STEAMING OR COOKING WITH OIL

I do not recommend boiling or steaming Crimini Mushrooms because these methods cause the Mushrooms to become watery and lose much of their flavor along with many of their nutrients; these include minerals, water-soluble vitamins (such as C and the B-complex vitamins) and powerful antioxidants unique to fruits and vegetables. I also don't recommend cooking Crimini Mushrooms in oil because high-temperature heat can damage delicate oils and potentially create harmful free radicals.

---

## An Easy Way to Prepare Crimini Mushrooms, Step-By-Step

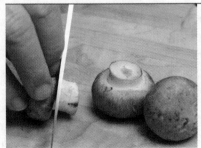 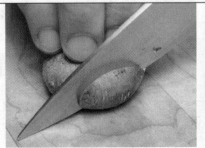 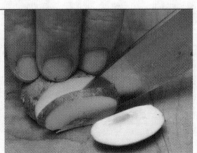

### SLICING CRIMINI MUSHROOMS

❶ Cut off the stem. The stem can be sliced either lengthwise or widthwise. ❷ Starting at an end, cut a slice in the cap. ❸ Carefully continue to slice the rest of the cap.

# health benefits of crimini mushrooms

## Promote Optimal Health

Preliminary research suggests that Crimini Mushrooms may be an important food in a diet that is geared towards protecting against cancer. Extracts of Crimini Mushrooms have been found to protect DNA from oxidative damage;

oxygen radicals attacking our genetic material is a cause of mutations that can lead to cancer development. In addition, these Mushrooms may prevent circulating levels of estrogen in the body from becoming excessive by inhibiting the *aromatase* enzyme; excessive estrogen can spark the development of breast cancer in certain women.

Crimini Mushrooms' ability to promote optimal health may come not only from their powerful lentinan phytonutrients, but also from their impressive array of antioxidant minerals, including selenium of which they are an excellent source. Selenium is a necessary cofactor of one of the body's most important internally produced antioxidants, *glutathione peroxidase* and also works with vitamin E in numerous vital antioxidant systems throughout the body. Selenium is involved in DNA repair, which is yet another way in which adequate intake of this mineral is associated with a reduced risk for cancer.

## Promote Energy Production

Crimini Mushrooms are an excellent source of riboflavin, pantothenic acid and niacin, as well as a very good source of thiamin and vitamin B6, and a good source of folic acid; all of these B vitamins are necessary for carbohydrate, protein and lipid metabolism.

Riboflavin (vitamin B2) plays at least two important roles in the body's production of energy. It is part of a molecule that allows oxygen-based energy production to occur. It is also necessary for the recycling of glutathione, an antioxidant that protects the energy-producing mitochondria from oxidative damage.

Pantothenic acid (vitamin B5) also plays an important role in the prevention of fatigue since it supports the function of the adrenal glands, particularly in times of stress. Niacin (vitamin B3) is necessary for the conversion of the body's proteins, fats and carbohydrates into usable energy.

## Additional Health-Promoting Benefits of Crimini Mushrooms

Crimini Mushrooms are also a concentrated source of other nutrients providing additional health-promoting benefits. These nutrients include free-radical-scavenging zinc, copper and manganese; heart-healthy dietary fiber, magnesium and potassium; energy-producing iron; bone-building calcium and phosphorus; muscle-building protein; and sleep-promoting tryptophan. Since 5 ounces of raw Crimini Mushrooms contain only 31 calories, they are an ideal food for healthy weight control.

### Nutritional Analysis of 5 ounces of Crimini Mushrooms:

| NUTRIENT | AMOUNT | % DAILY VALUE | NUTRIENT | AMOUNT | % DAILY VALUE |
|---|---|---|---|---|---|
| Calories | 31.19 | | Pantothenic Acid | 2.13 mg | 21.30 |
| Calories from Fat | 1.28 | | | | |
| Calories from Saturated Fat | 0.18 | | **Minerals** | | |
| Protein | 3.54 g | | Boron | — mcg | |
| Carbohydrates | 5.84 g | | Calcium | 25.52 mg | 2.55 |
| Dietary Fiber | 0.85 g | 3.40 | Chloride | — mg | |
| Soluble Fiber | — g | | Chromium | — mcg | — |
| Insoluble Fiber | — g | | Copper | 0.71 mg | 35.50 |
| Sugar – Total | 2.44 g | | Fluoride | — mg | — |
| Monosaccharides | — g | | Iodine | — mcg | — |
| Disaccharides | — g | | Iron | 0.57 mg | 3.17 |
| Other Carbs | 2.55 g | | Magnesium | 12.76 mg | 3.19 |
| Fat – Total | 0.14 g | | Manganese | 0.20 mg | 10.00 |
| Saturated Fat | 0.02 g | | Molybdenum | — mcg | — |
| Mono Fat | 0.00 g | | Phosphorus | 170.10 mg | 17.01 |
| Poly Fat | 0.06 g | | Potassium | 635.04 mg | |
| Omega-3 Fatty Acids | — g | — | Selenium | 36.85 mcg | 52.64 |
| Omega-6 Fatty Acids | — g | | Sodium | 8.51 mg | |
| Trans Fatty Acids | — g | | Zinc | 1.56 mg | 10.40 |
| Cholesterol | 0.00 mg | | | | |
| Water | 130.84 g | | **Amino Acids** | | |
| Ash | 1.39 g | | Alanine | 0.27 g | |
| | | | Arginine | 0.17 g | |
| **Vitamins** | | | Aspartate | 0.32 g | |
| Vitamin A IU | 0.00 IU | 0.00 | Cystine | 0.01 g | 2.44 |
| Vitamin A RE | 0.00 RE | | Glutamate | 0.61 g | |
| A - Carotenoid | 0.00 RE | 0.00 | Glycine | 0.16 g | |
| A - Retinol | 0.00 RE | | Histidine | 0.09 g | 6.98 |
| B1 Thiamin | 0.13 mg | 8.67 | Isoleucine | 0.14 g | 12.17 |
| B2 Riboflavin | 0.69 mg | 40.59 | Leucine | 0.22 g | 8.70 |
| B3 Niacin | 5.39 mg | 26.95 | Lysine | 0.36 g | 15.32 |
| Niacin Equiv | 6.71 mg | | Methionine | 0.07 g | 9.46 |
| Vitamin B6 | 0.16 mg | 8.00 | Phenylalanine | 0.14 g | 11.76 |
| Vitamin B12 | 0.14 mcg | 2.33 | Proline | 0.25 g | |
| Biotin | — mcg | — | Serine | 0.16 g | |
| Vitamin C | 0.00 mg | 0.00 | Threonine | 0.16 g | 12.90 |
| Vitamin D IU | — IU | — | Tryptophan | 0.08 g | 25.00 |
| Vitamin D mcg | — mcg | — | Tyrosine | 0.08 g | 8.25 |
| Vitamin E Alpha Equiv | 0.16 mg | 0.80 | Valine | 0.16 g | 10.88 |
| Vitamin E IU | 0.24 IU | | | | |
| Vitamin E mg | 0.16 mg | | | | |
| Folate | 19.85 mcg | 4.96 | | | |
| Vitamin K | — mcg | — | | | |

Note: "—" indicates data is unavailable. For more information, please see page 806.)

STEP-BY-STEP RECIPE
## The Healthiest Way of Cooking Crimini Mushrooms

# 7-Minute "Healthy Sautéed" Crimini Mushrooms

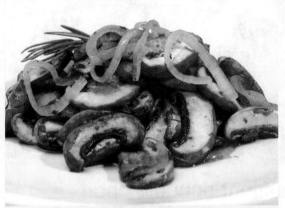

"Healthy Sautéed" Crimini Mushrooms

*If you like Crimini Mushrooms with great taste and a rich supply of nutrients, I recommend "Healthy Sautéing" them. It is fun to "Healthy Sauté," and I think you will be wonderfully surprised by the flavor.*

1 lb medium Crimini Mushrooms, sliced
3 TBS low-sodium chicken or vegetable broth

**Mediterranean Dressing:**
2 TBS extra virgin olive oil
1 tsp lemon juice
2 medium cloves garlic
Sea salt and pepper to taste

1. Chop or press garlic and let sit for at least 5 minutes. (Why?, see page 261.)

2. Heat 3 TBS broth over medium heat in a stainless steel skillet.

3. When broth begins to steam, add the sliced Mushrooms and sauté for 3 minutes. They will release liquid as they cook. Since Crimini Mushrooms are not as watery as other button Mushrooms, it is best to stir constantly for the last 4 minutes. The liquid will evaporate, and the Mushrooms will become golden brown but not burned. "Healthy Sauté" will concentrate both the flavor and nutrition of your Crimini Mushrooms. For information on *Differences in Cooking Time*, see page 94.

4. Transfer to a bowl. For more flavor, toss Crimini Mushrooms with the remaining ingredients while they are still hot. The Mediterranean Dressing does not need to be made separately.

**SERVES 2**

### COOKING TIPS:
- To prevent overcooking Crimini Mushrooms, I highly recommend using a timer.
- To mellow the flavor of garlic, add garlic to Crimini Mushrooms for the last 2 minutes of sautéing.

## Flavor Tips: Try these 8 great serving suggestions with the recipe above. ✳

1. **Most Popular:** Add 1 "Healthy Sautéed" onion (see page 273), 1/2 tsp fresh chopped rosemary and 1–2 tsp tamari (soy sauce).
2. Combine with cooked onions, fennel or peas.
3. Top with chopped pumpkin or sunflower seeds.
4. Add 7-Minute "Healthy Sautéed" Crimini Mushrooms to the beef, chicken or venison recipes of this book.
5. Add to your favorite cooked green vegetable such as broccoli or kale.
6. Add to pasta sauce.
7. **Quick Mushroom Stroganoff:** Combine the 7-Minute "Healthy Sautéed" Crimini Mushroom recipe with low-fat sour cream, dill weed, sea salt and pepper. Serve over polenta or brown rice.
8. **Crimini Mushroom Sauce:** Add onions, garlic, fresh Italian herbs and port wine to your 7-Minute "Healthy Sautéed" Crimini Mushroom recipe. It is a great sauce to serve over chicken, calf's liver or lamb.

Please write (address on back cover flap) or e-mail me at info@whfoods.org with your personal ideas for preparing Crimini Mushrooms, and I will share them with others through our website at www.whfoods.org.

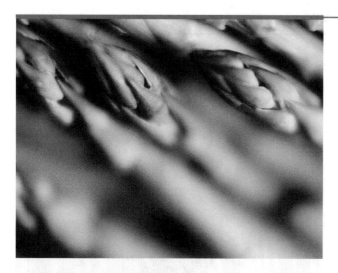

## nutrient-richness chart

Total Nutrient-Richness: **43**                    GI: **15**

One cup (180 grams) of cooked Asparagus contains 43 calories

| Nutrient | Amount | %DV | Density | Quality |
|---|---|---|---|---|
| Vitamin K | 91.8 mcg | 114.8 | 47.8 | excellent |
| Folate | 262.8 mcg | 65.7 | 27.4 | excellent |
| Vitamin C | 19.4 mg | 32.4 | 13.5 | excellent |
| Vitamin A | 970.2 IU | 19.4 | 8.1 | excellent |
| Tryptophan | 0.1 g | 15.6 | 6.5 | very good |
| B1 Thiamin | 0.2 mg | 14.7 | 6.1 | very good |
| B2 Riboflavin | 0.2 mg | 13.5 | 5.6 | very good |
| Manganese | 0.3 mg | 13.5 | 5.6 | very good |
| Dietary Fiber | 2.9 g | 11.5 | 4.8 | very good |
| B6 Pyridoxine | 0.2 mg | 11.0 | 4.6 | very good |
| Copper | 0.2 mg | 10.0 | 4.2 | very good |
| B3 Niacin | 2.0 mg | 9.8 | 4.1 | very good |
| Phosphorus | 97.2 mg | 9.7 | 4.1 | very good |
| Protein | 4.7 g | 9.3 | 3.9 | very good |
| Potassium | 288.0 mg | 8.2 | 3.4 | very good |
| Iron | 1.3 mg | 7.3 | 3.0 | good |
| Zinc | 0.8 mg | 5.1 | 2.1 | good |
| Magnesium | 18.0 mg | 4.5 | 1.9 | good |
| Selenium | 3.1 mcg | 4.4 | 1.8 | good |
| Calcium | 36.0 mg | 3.6 | 1.5 | good |

**CAROTENOIDS:**

| | |
|---|---|
| Beta-Carotene | 1,087.2 mcg |
| Lutein+Zeaxanthin | 1,387.8 mcg |
| Lycopene | 54.0 mcg |

Daily values for these nutrients have not yet been established.

**PHYTOSTEROLS:**

| | |
|---|---|
| Phytosterols–Total | 43.2 mg |

For more on "Total Nutrient-Richness," "%DV," "Density," and
The World's Healthiest Foods "Quality" Rating System, see page 805.

For more on GI, see page 342.

# asparagus

## highlights

| | |
|---|---|
| AVAILABILITY: | March through July |
| REFRIGERATE: | Yes |
| SHELF LIFE: | 7 days refrigerated |
| PREPARATION: | Cut or snap off hard bottom portion |
| BEST WAY TO COOK: | "Healthy Sauté" in just 5 minutes |

The appreciation for Asparagus's delicious flavor, as well as its medicinal properties, goes as far back as the time of ancient Rome when fleets of ships were sent to gather Asparagus for the emperors. Perhaps, this is one of the reasons it is sometimes referred to as the "aristocrat of vegetables." Today, this slender, succulent vegetable is available for you to enjoy without requiring the resources of an emperor. Because proper preparation is the key to enjoying the best flavor and the many health benefits of Asparagus, I want to share with you the secret of cooking Asparagus *al denté* using the "Healthiest Way of Cooking" method. In just 5 minutes, you will be able to enhance its flavor while maximizing its nutritional value.

## why asparagus should be part of your healthiest way of eating

Asparagus is renowned as an excellent source of folic acid, a B vitamin essential for proper cellular division and DNA synthesis as well as an essential nutrient for a healthy cardiovascular system. Asparagus also provides health-promoting carotenoid phytonutrients, such as beta-carotene, lutein and zeaxanthin, which can function as powerful antioxidants that protect cells against the oxidative damage caused by free radicals. High in nutrients and low in calories, Asparagus is an ideal food to add to your "Healthiest Way of Eating" with one cup of cooked Asparagus containing only 43 calories. (For more on the *Health Benefits of Asparagus* and a complete analysis of its content of over 60 nutrients, see page 124.)

## varieties of asparagus

Asparagus (*Asparagus officinalis*) is an almost leafless perennial belonging to the lily family. The spears are the shoots of an underground crown. It takes up to three years for the crowns to begin producing the edible shoots, after which they will continue to produce for up to 20 years.

There are over 300 varieties of Asparagus, although only 20 are edible. These fall into three categories:

### GREEN
This variety is a delicately flavored, springtime favorite that grows to be about eight inches in height and is the type of Asparagus most commonly found in local markets. It is also the one featured in the photographs in this chapter.

### WHITE
White Asparagus is much more expensive than other varieties because of the labor required to produce it. The spears are kept covered and out of the sunlight while they are growing, which prevents the formation of chlorophyll that gives Green Asparagus its color. While White Asparagus is more tender than its green or purple counterparts, it is also less flavorful; however, some chefs prefer it to make their dishes more unique and special.

### PURPLE
One to three inches in height, this variety is almost fiber-free, and some say it is best enjoyed raw. It cooks quickly, has a fruity flavor and provides additional health-promoting benefits from phytonutrients called anthocyanins that give it its purple color. The purple color will disappear with prolonged cooking.

## the peak season

The first Asparagus crops of the year are ready in California as early as February, with the peak of the season running from April through May. The growing season in the Midwest and East extends through July. These are the months when Asparagus' concentration of nutrients and flavor are highest, and its cost is at its lowest. Although you can find imported Asparagus from South America in the fall and winter, it is more expensive then, and not as fresh as, locally grown varieties.

## biochemical considerations

Asparagus is a concentrated source of purines, which might be of concern to certain individuals. (For more on *Purines,* see page 727.)

## 4 steps for the best tasting and most nutritious asparagus

Turning Asparagus into a flavorful dish with the most nutrients is simple if you just follow my 4 easy steps:

1. The Best Way to Select
2. The Best Way to Store
3. The Best Way to Prepare
4. The Healthiest Way of Cooking

---

### scientific findings

Sulfur odor: Four in ten people notice that their urine has a strong sulfur odor after eating Asparagus. A variety of chemicals—many that fall within the thiol chemical family—are responsible for the "Asparagus smell." Different people form different amounts of these compounds after eating Asparagus. These compounds have no adverse effects on the body.

---

# 1. the best way to select asparagus ————

You can select green Asparagus with the best flavor and most nutrients by looking for spears that are firm with a bright green color and tips that are closed. As with all vegetables, I recommend selecting organically grown Asparagus whenever possible. (For more on *Organic Foods*, see page 113.)

Avoid yellowish spears that appear to be on the verge of flowering and those with stems that are dried out and cracked at the base or are wrinkled and feel hollow; that is because this usually indicates they are old and have begun to lose their nutritional value. I also always check that the Asparagus smells fresh and does not have a questionable odor.

I am often asked whether Asparagus is best when the shoots are small and thin or large and thick. I actually find that medium-size Asparagus (about 1/2-inch in diameter, the thickness of your little finger) is the best. Very thin spears can be easily overcooked. Very thick spears are woody, tough and stringy and often require peeling and more time to prepare. If you are using thick-stemmed Asparagus, peel them and cut them in half lengthwise to help cook them in the recommended amount of time. Spears should be as uniform in size as possible so they will cook evenly.

# 2. the best way to store asparagus

Asparagus will become limp and decline in quality if not stored properly. Make sure to follow proper storage guidelines in order to preserve its flavor and nutrients (it can quickly lose up to 30% of some of its vitamins if not stored correctly).

Asparagus continues to respire even after it has been harvested; its respiration rate at room temperature (68°F/20°C) is 270 mg/kg/hr. Slowing down the respiration rate with proper storage is the key to extending its flavor and nutritional benefits. (For a *Comparison of Respiration Rates* for different vegetables, see page 91.)

## Asparagus Will Remain Fresh for Up to 7 Days When Properly Stored

1. Store fresh Asparagus in the refrigerator. The colder temperature will slow the respiration rate, helping to preserve its nutrients and keeping Asparagus fresh for a longer period of time.
2. Place Asparagus in a plastic storage bag before refrigerating. I have found that it is best to wrap the bag tightly around the Asparagus, squeezing out as much of the air from the bag as possible.
3. Do not wash Asparagus before refrigeration because exposure to water will encourage Asparagus to spoil.

# 3. the best way to prepare asparagus

Asparagus is very easy to prepare. Properly cleaning and cutting Asparagus will help ensure that the Asparagus you serve will have the best flavor and retain the greatest number of nutrients.

## Cleaning Asparagus
Rinse well under cold running water before cutting. (For more on *Washing Vegetables*, see page 92.)

## Peeling Asparagus
Thin Asparagus does not require peeling. Asparagus with thick stems requires extra work to prepare. Thick Asparagus requires peeling because the stems are usually tough and stringy. Remove the tough outer skin of the bottom portion of the stem (not the tips) with a vegetable peeler.

## Cutting Asparagus
You can have fun by snapping off the bottom of each individual stalk. They tend to break naturally where the woody portion of the spear ends and the tender part begins. This is usually where the color changes from white to green.

You can also remove the bottom part of all of the Asparagus stems at one time by cutting with a knife while the Asparagus is still in a bunch. You can use the tough woody ends to make broth for soup.

Thick Asparagus stems should be sliced in half lengthwise. This provides greater surface area, which will help it cook more quickly.

## Healthy Cooking Tip for Asparagus
If you want to make limp Asparagus more crisp before cooking, cut off the woody ends and place the spears in a glass of ice water for a few minutes before you cook them.

# 4. the healthiest way of cooking asparagus

Since research has shown that important nutrients can be lost or destroyed by the way a food is cooked, the "Healthiest Way of Cooking" Asparagus is focused on bringing out its best flavor while maximizing its vitamins, minerals and powerful antioxidants.

## The Healthiest Way of Cooking Asparagus: "Healthy Sautéing" for Just 5 Minutes
In my search to find the healthiest way to cook Asparagus, I tested every possible cooking method and discovered that "Healthy Sautéing" Asparagus for just 5 minutes delivered the best result. "Healthy Sautéed" Asparagus has a mild, sweet

flavor and has retained the maximum number of nutrients. I recommend using medium-size Asparagus because Asparagus with thick stems requires peeling, and very thin stems can be easily overcooked. Asparagus absorbs just enough moisture from the broth to make it tender. The Step-by-Step Recipe will show you how easy it is "Healthy Sauté" Asparagus. (For more on "*Healthy Sauté*," see page 57.)

## Grilling and Broiling Asparagus
It takes virtually no time to grill or broil Asparagus. Before grilling or broiling, sprinkle with lemon, sea salt and pepper to help protect against the formation of harmful

compounds. Grilling gives Asparagus a delicious sweet and smokey flavor. To make sure that it does not burn, be careful not to place the Asparagus too close to the flame. The temperatures directly above or below the flame can reach as high as 500°F to 1000°F (260° to 538°C). When using a broiler, keep it about 4–5 inches away from the flame. Coating with oil before cooking will produce harmful free radicals, so brush with extra virgin olive oil or your favorite vinaigrette right after it is cooked.

## How to Avoid Overcooking Asparagus: Cook it *Al Denté*

One of the primary reasons Asparagus loses its flavor is because it is often overcooked. For the best flavor, I recommend that you cook Asparagus *al denté*. Asparagus cooked *al denté* is tender outside and slightly crisp inside. Plus, Asparagus cooked *al denté* is cooked just long enough to soften its cellulose and hemicellulose, which makes it easier to digest and allows its health-promoting nutrients to become more readily available for absorption.

It is very important not to overcook Asparagus. Asparagus cooked for as little as a couple of minutes longer than *al denté* will begin to lose not only its texture and flavor, but also its nutrients. In purple varieties, you can see the purple color fade when it is overcooked, a reflection of the loss of its anthocyanin antioxidants. Overcooking Asparagus will significantly decrease its nutritional value: as much as 50% of some nutrients can be lost. (For more on *Al Denté*, see page 92.)

## Cooking Methods Not Recommended for Asparagus

**BOILING, STEAMING, BAKING OR COOKING WITH OIL**
Boiling or steaming Asparagus increases its water absorption, causing it to become soggy and lose much of its flavor along with many of its nutrients; these include minerals, water-soluble vitamins (such as C and the B-complex vitamins) and health-promoting phytonutrients. Baked Asparagus gets mushy. I don't recommend cooking Asparagus in oil because high-temperature heat can damage delicate oils and potentially create harmful free radicals.

Here is a question that I received from a reader of the whfoods.org website about Asparagus:

**Q** *I heard that you should cook Asparagus in oil in order to retain its water-soluble nutrients and flavor. Is that true?*

**A** While it is true that you will lose some water-soluble vitamins when cooking Asparagus in water, I don't recommend cooking it in oil because heating oil can create undesirable free radicals that can compromise health. For more on *Cooking with Oils*, see page 52.

I have developed alternative methods to sautéing, a method that traditionally uses oil, by replacing the oil with broth. This "Healthy Sauté" method (page 57) is an excellent way to prepare Asparagus without the use of oil. It is quick and easy, and I believe that you will really enjoy the flavor and texture of Asparagus cooked this way.

As you point out, Asparagus, like other vegetables, contains water-soluble vitamins including vitamin C and the B vitamins. By "Healthy Sautéing," for a short time you will lose no more than 5–10% of these vitamins and a minimal amount of minerals (less than 5%) while retaining the flavor and crispness of perfectly cooked Asparagus. This is because of the small amount of liquid used and the short cooking time.

---

### An Easy Way to Prepare Asparagus—Step-By-Step

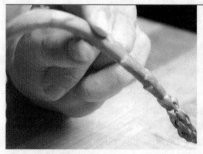 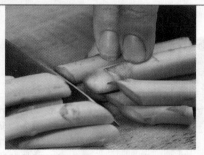 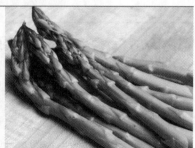

**CUTTING ASPARAGUS**

❶ Snap off the bottom of each Asparagus stalk. ❷ Or cut off the bottom fourth of Asparagus and discard as it is tough and stringy. To save time, this can be done with one cut while Asparagus is still in a bunch.
❸ Asparagus stalks are good cooked whole if you have an Asparagus steamer.

# health benefits of asparagus

## Promotes Digestive Health

Asparagus contains a special kind of carbohydrate called inulin that we don't digest, but the health-promoting friendly bacteria in our large intestine do. When our diet contains good amounts of inulin, the growth and activity of these friendly bacteria increase. And when populations of health-promoting bacteria are large, it is much more difficult for unfriendly bacteria to gain a hold in our intestinal tract. Asparagus is also a very good source of dietary fiber, which promotes intestinal regularity and may help protect against the development of colon cancer.

## Natural Diuretic Properties

Asparagus is a very good source of potassium and quite low in sodium. Its mineral profile, combined with the amino acid asparagine it contains, gives Asparagus a strong diuretic effect. Historically, Asparagus has been used to treat problems involving swelling, such as arthritis and rheumatism, and may also be useful for PMS-related water retention.

## Promotes Heart Health

Asparagus is an excellent source of folic acid and a very good source of vitamin B6, nutrients essential for a healthy
cardiovascular system through their beneficial effect on homocysteine levels. When levels of these B vitamins are low, blood levels of homocysteine rise—a situation that significantly increases the risk for heart disease. Homocysteine promotes atherosclerosis by reducing the integrity of blood vessel walls and by interfering with the formation of collagen. Elevations in homocysteine are found in approximately 20–40% of patients with heart disease. It is estimated that consumption of 400 mcg of folic acid daily would reduce the number of heart attacks suffered by Americans each year by 10%. Asparagus is also rich in other heart-health-promoting nutrients, including dietary fiber, potassium, magnesium and calcium.

## Promotes Fetal Health

Especially if you're thinking about becoming pregnant or are in the early stages of pregnancy, you may want to consider making Asparagus a frequent addition to your meals. That's because the folic acid in Asparagus is essential for proper cellular division since it is necessary in DNA synthesis. Without folic acid, the fetus' nervous system cells do not divide properly. Inadequate folic acid during pregnancy has been linked to several birth defects, including neural tube defects like spina bifida. Despite folic acid's wide availability in food (its name comes from the Latin word *folium*, meaning "foliage," because it's found in green leafy vegetables), folic acid deficiency is the most common vitamin deficiency in the world.

## Promotes Bone Health

Asparagus is also rich in bone-building nutrients. It is an excellent source of vitamin K and a good source of calcium and magnesium. In addition to its role in activating osteocalcin, which anchors calcium molecules inside of the bone, vitamin K is also important to maintaining proper blood coagulation.

## Promotes Energy Production

Asparagus is a very good source of manganese, a trace mineral that is an essential cofactor of *superoxide dismutase*, an enzyme which disarms free radicals produced within the mitochondria and keeps energy production flowing. Asparagus is also a very good source of thiamin, riboflavin and niacin, three B vitamins that are essential for the conversion of the body's proteins, fats and carbohy-

*(Continued on Page 126)*

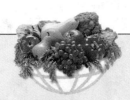

## how to enjoy fresh asparagus without cooking

Add thinly sliced pieces of Asparagus to your cold vegetable salad.

Serve raw Asparagus with extra virgin olive oil, garlic, lemon juice, sea salt and pepper, and sprinkle with Parmesan cheese or enjoy stalks of raw Asparagus with your favorite vegetable dip.

Add to vegetable sushi or your favorite wrap.

**Marinated Asparagus Salad:** Make a dressing of 1 part balsamic vinegar, 2 parts extra virgin olive oil, fresh herbs (rosemary, basil, dill, parsley) and sea salt and pepper to taste. Marinate Asparagus, red bell pepper slices, red onion slices, olives and feta cheese chunks (optional) in the dressing for 2–8 hours. Great side dish for chicken or fish!

STEP-BY-STEP RECIPE
## The Healthiest Way of Cooking Asparagus

# 5-Minute "Healthy Sautéed" Asparagus

*"Healthy Sauté" allows you to enjoy all of the great taste and health-promoting nutrients of Asparagus while the easy Mediterranean dressing enhances its delicate flavor.*

**1 lb of Asparagus**
**3 TBS low-sodium chicken or vegetable broth**

**Mediterranean Dressing:**
**3 TBS extra virgin olive oil**
**2 medium cloves garlic**
**2 tsp lemon juice**
**Sea salt and pepper to taste**

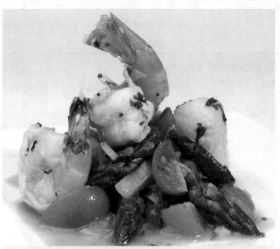
"Healthy Sautéed" Asparagus with Seafood

1. Chop or press garlic and let it sit for at least 5 minutes, (Why?, see page 261.)
2. Heat 3 TBS broth over medium heat in a stainless steel skillet.
3. While broth is heating, snap off the woody bottom of Asparagus stems, then cut the spears into 2-inch lengths. Cutting them into short pieces of equal length ensures quick, even cooking.
4. When broth begins to steam, add Asparagus. **Cover** and cook for 5 minutes. The outside will be tender, and the inside will be crisp. Thinner spears will take about 3 minutes. "Healthy Sauté" will concentrate both the flavor and nutrition of Asparagus. For information on *Differences in Cooking Time*, see page 94.
5. Transfer to a bowl. For more flavor, toss Asparagus with the remaining ingredients while it is still hot. (Mediterranean Dressing does not need to be made separately.) Research shows that carotenoids found in foods are best absorbed when consumed with oils.

OPTIONAL: To mellow the flavor of garlic, add garlic to Asparagus for the last 2 minutes of cooking.

**SERVES 2**

### COOKING TIPS:
- To prevent overcooking Asparagus, I highly recommend using a timer.
- Testing Asparagus with a fork is not an effective way to determine whether it is done.

## Flavor Tips: Try these 6 great serving suggestions with the recipe above. ✳

1. **Most Popular: Asparagus with Dijon Caper Sauce.** In a small bowl, combine the Mediterranean dressing recipe above with 1 TBS Dijon mustard, 1 tsp capers and 2 tsp minced fresh basil or parsley. Pour over hot Asparagus.
2. Top with grated sharp cheese such as Parmesan or Romano, fresh minced basil, parsley or oregano and lemon zest.
3. Add a few drops of tamari (soy sauce) to mellow the flavor of Asparagus.
4. Asparagus and omega-3 enriched eggs make a wonderful combination.
5. **"Healthy Sautéed" Asparagus with Seafood:** Combine 5-Minute "Healthly Sautéed" Asparagus recipe with "Healthy Sautéed" shrimp or fish, quartered cherry tomatoes, onions and mushrooms. Increase the Mediterranean Dressing as needed. Garnish with chopped parsley or cilantro (pictured above).
6. **Cold Asparagus Salad:** Asparagus as a cold vegetable salad is quick, easy and tastes great. Refrigerate the 5-Minute "Healthy Sautéed" Asparagus. Add other vegetables, such as roasted red peppers, and toss with your favorite vinaigrette and a small amount of pressed garlic.

Please write (address on back cover flap) or e-mail me at info@whfoods.org with your personal ideas for preparing Asparagus, and I will share them with others through our website at www.whfoods.org.

*(Continued from Page 124)*

drates into usable energy. Asparagus is a very good source of phosphorus, which is an essential component of ATP, the fuel that cells use for energy. Additionally, it is also a good source of iron, a critical component of hemoglobin, a protein in blood that helps to transport oxygen throughout the body.

## Promotes Optimal Antioxidant Status

Asparagus is an excellent source of vitamin C and vitamin A (through its concentration of carotenoids) and a good source of zinc and selenium. These nutrients help promote optimal health through their potent antioxidant activity, protects cells from free radical oxidative damage. Uncontrolled free radical activity has been linked to increased risk of chronic degenerative diseases, including cardiovascular disease, arthritis and certain forms of cancer.

## Additional Health-Promoting Benefits of Asparagus

Asparagus is also a concentrated source of other nutrients providing additional health-promoting benefits. These nutrients include muscle-building protein, free-radical-scavenging copper and sleep-promoting tryptophan. Since Asparagus contains only 43 calories per one cup serving, it is an ideal food for healthy weight control.

Here is a question that I received from a reader of the whfoods.org website about Asparagus:

## Q *Why do overcooked vegetables lose their bright green color?*

One of the primary reasons for the change in color when green vegetables are cooked is the change in chlorophyll. Chlorophyll has a chemical structure that is quite similar to hemoglobin, which is found within our red blood cells. A basic difference is that chlorophyll contains magnesium at its center, while hemoglobin contains iron. When plants (e.g., green vegetables) are heated and/or exposed to acid, the magnesium gets removed from the center of this ring structure and replaced by an atom of hydrogen. In biochemical terms, the chlorophyll *a* gets turned into a molecule called pheophytin *a*, and the chlorophyll *b* gets turned into pheophytin *b*. With this one simple change, the color of the vegetable changes from bright green to olive-gray as the pheophytin a provides a green-gray color, and the pheophytin b provides an olive-green color. This color change is one of the reasons I have established the relatively short cooking times for green vegetables in the "Healthiest Way of Cooking" methods. These cooking methods are designed to preserve the unique concentrations of chlorophyll found in these vegetables.

## Nutritional Analysis of 1 cup of cooked Asparagus:

| NUTRIENT | AMOUNT | % DAILY VALUE | NUTRIENT | AMOUNT | % DAILY VALUE |
|---|---|---|---|---|---|
| Calories | 43.20 | | Pantothenic Acid | 0.29 mg | 2.90 |
| Calories from Fat | 5.02 | | | | |
| Calories from Saturated Fat | 1.15 | | **Minerals** | | |
| Protein | 4.66 g | | Boron | — mcg | |
| Carbohydrates | 7.61 g | | Calcium | 36.00 mg | 3.60 |
| Dietary Fiber | 2.88 g | 11.52 | Chloride | 198.00 mg | |
| Soluble Fiber | 1.15 g | | Chromium | — mcg | — |
| Insoluble Fiber | 1.73 g | | Copper | 0.20 mg | 10.00 |
| Sugar – Total | 2.88 g | | Fluoride | — mg | — |
| Monosaccharides | 2.52 g | | Iodine | — mcg | — |
| Disaccharides | 0.36 g | | Iron | 1.31 mg | 7.28 |
| Other Carbs | 1.85 g | | Magnesium | 18.00 mg | 4.50 |
| Fat – Total | 0.56 g | | Manganese | 0.27 mg | 13.50 |
| Saturated Fat | 0.13 g | | Molybdenum | — mcg | — |
| Mono Fat | 0.02 g | | Phosphorus | 97.20 mg | 9.72 |
| Poly Fat | 0.24 g | | Potassium | 288.00 mg | |
| Omega-3 Fatty Acids | 0.01 g | 0.40 | Selenium | 3.06 mcg | 4.37 |
| Omega-6 Fatty Acids | 0.23 g | | Sodium | 19.80 mg | |
| Trans Fatty Acids | 0.00 g | | Zinc | 0.76 mg | 5.07 |
| Cholesterol | 0.00 mg | | | | |
| Water | 165.96 g | | **Amino Acids** | | |
| Ash | 1.19 g | | Alanine | 0.22 g | |
| | | | Arginine | 0.22 g | |
| **Vitamins** | | | Aspartate | 0.54 g | |
| Vitamin A IU | 970.20 IU | 19.40 | Cystine | 0.06 g | 14.63 |
| Vitamin A RE | 97.20 RE | | Glutamate | 0.77 g | |
| A - Carotenoid | 97.20 RE | 1.30 | Glycine | 0.15 g | |
| A - Retinol | 0.00 RE | | Histidine | 0.07 g | 5.43 |
| Thiamin B1 | 0.22 mg | 14.67 | Isoleucine | 0.17 g | 14.78 |
| Riboflavin B2 | 0.23 mg | 13.53 | Leucine | 0.20 g | 7.91 |
| Niacin B3 | 1.95 mg | 9.75 | Lysine | 0.22 g | 9.36 |
| Niacin equiv | 2.70 mg | | Methionine | 0.05 g | 6.76 |
| Vitamin B6 | 0.22 mg | 11.00 | Phenylalanine | 0.11 g | 9.24 |
| Vitamin B12 | 0.00 mcg | 0.00 | Proline | 0.25 g | |
| Biotin | 0.72 mcg | 0.24 | Serine | 0.18 g | |
| Vitamin C | 19.44 mg | 32.40 | Threonine | 0.13 g | 10.48 |
| Vitamin D IU | 0.00 IU | 0.00 | Tryptophan | 0.05 g | 15.63 |
| Vitamin D mcg | 0.00 mcg | | Tyrosine | 0.07 g | 7.22 |
| Vitamin E Alpha Equiv | 0.68 mg | 3.40 | Valine | 0.18 g | 12.24 |
| Vitamin E IU | 1.02 IU | | | | |
| Vitamin E mg | 1.80 mg | | | | |
| Folate | 262.80 mcg | 65.70 | | | |
| Vitamin K | 91.80 mcg | 114.75 | | | |

(Note: "—" indicates data is unavailable. For more information, please see page 806.)

# Q&A

## WHY ARE ORGANIC FOODS NUTRITIONALLY SUPERIOR TO CONVENTIONALLY GROWN FOODS?

Proof of their superiority has been demonstrated in numerous studies. In 1998, a review of 34 studies comparing the nutritional content of organic versus conventionally grown was published in the peer-reviewed, MEDLINE-indexed journal, *Alternative Therapies* (Vol. 4, No. 1, pgs. 58–69). In this review, organic food was found to have higher protein quality in all comparisons, higher levels of vitamin C in 58% of all studies and 5–20% higher mineral levels for all but two minerals. In some cases, the mineral levels were dramatically higher in organically grown foods—as much as three times higher in one study involving iron content.

Organic foods may also contain more flavonoids than conventionally grown foods, according to Danish research published in the August 2003 issue of the *Journal of Agricultural and Food Chemistry*. In this study, 16 healthy nonsmoking participants ranging in age from 21–35 years were given either a diet high in organically grown or conventionally grown fruits and vegetables for 22 days, after which they were switched over to the other diet for another 22 days. After both dietary trials, the researchers analyzed levels of flavonoids and other markers of antioxidant defenses in the food and in the participants' blood and urine samples. Results indicated a significantly higher content of the flavonoid quercitin in the organic produce and in the subjects' urine samples when on the organic produce diet; the subjects' urinary levels of another flavonoid, kaempferol, were also much higher when on the organically grown diet compared to the conventionally grown diet.

A review of 41 studies comparing the nutritional value of organically grown to conventionally grown fruits, vegetables and grains also indicates organic crops provide substantially more of several nutrients, including:

- 27% more vitamin C
- 21% more iron
- 29% more magnesium
- 14% more phosphorus

The review also found that while five servings of organically grown vegetables (lettuce, spinach, carrots, potatoes and cabbage) provided the daily recommended intake of vitamin C for men and women, their conventionally grown counterparts did not. Plus, organically grown foods contained 15% less nitrates than conventionally grown foods. Nitrates, a major

constituent of chemical fertilizers, bind to hemoglobin and, particularly in infants, can significantly reduce the body's ability to carry oxygen.

In another study whose findings are based on pesticide residue data collected by the U.S. Department of Agriculture, organic fruits and vegetables were shown to have only one-third as many pesticide residues as their conventionally grown counterparts. Study data, which covered more than 94,000 food samples from more than 20 crops, showed 73% of conventionally grown foods sampled had residue from at least one pesticide, while only 23% of organically grown samples had any residues. More than 90% of USDA's samples of conventionally grown apples, peaches, pears, strawberries and celery had residues.

When it comes to choosing between organic or conventionally grown foods, size is definitely not everything, suggests another study published in *Science Daily Magazine*. Chemistry professor Theo Clark and undergraduate students at Truman State University in Mississippi found organically grown oranges contained up to 30% more vitamin C than those grown conventionally. Reporting the results at the June 2, 2002, meeting of the American Chemical Society, Clark said he had expected the conventionally grown oranges, which were twice as large, to have twice the vitamin C as the organic versions. Instead, chemical isolation combined with nuclear magnetic resonance spectroscopy revealed the much higher level in organic oranges.

Why the big difference? Clark speculated that "with conventional oranges, (farmers) use nitrogen fertilizers that cause an uptake of more water, so it sort of dilutes the orange. You get a great big orange, but it is full of water and doesn't have as much nutritional value."

Eating organic may also help protect against chronic inflammation, a major factor in both cardiovascular disease and colon cancer. Another study, published in the *European Journal of Nutrition*, found that organic soups sold in the United Kingdom contain almost six times as much salicylic acid as non-organic soups. Salicylic acid, the compound responsible for the anti-inflammatory action of aspirin, has been shown to help prevent hardening of the arteries as well as bowel cancer. Researchers compared the salicylic acid content of 11 brands of organic soup to that found in non-organic varieties. The average level of salicylic acid in 11 brands of organic vegetable soup was 117 nanograms per gram, compared with 20 nanograms per gram in 24 types of non-organic soup. The highest level (1,040 nanograms per gram) was found in an organic carrot and coriander soup. Four of the conventional soups had no detectable levels of salicylic acid.

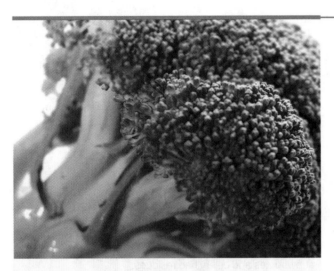

# broccoli

## highlights

| | |
|---|---|
| AVAILABILITY: | Year-round |
| REFRIGERATE: | Yes |
| SHELF LIFE: | 10 days refrigerated |
| PREPARATION: | Cut and let sit for 5 minutes |
| BEST WAY TO COOK: | "Healthy Steamed" in just 5 minutes |

## nutrient-richness chart

Total Nutrient-Richness: **40**    GI: **15**
One cup (156 grams) of cooked Broccoli contains 44 calories

| NUTRIENT | AMOUNT | %DV | DENSITY | QUALITY |
|---|---|---|---|---|
| Vitamin C | 123.4 mg | 205.7 | 84.8 | excellent |
| Vitamin K | 155.2 mcg | 194.0 | 79.9 | excellent |
| Vitamin A | 2280.7 IU | 45.6 | 18.8 | excellent |
| Folate | 93.9 mcg | 23.5 | 9.7 | excellent |
| Dietary Fiber | 4.7 g | 18.7 | 7.7 | excellent |
| Manganese | 0.3 mg | 17.0 | 7.0 | very good |
| Tryptophan | 0.05 g | 15.6 | 6.4 | very good |
| Potassium | 505.4 mg | 14.4 | 6.0 | very good |
| B6 Pyridoxine | 0.2 mg | 11.0 | 4.5 | very good |
| B2 Riboflavin | 0.2 mg | 10.6 | 4.4 | very good |
| Phosphorus | 102.8 mg | 10.3 | 4.2 | very good |
| Magnesium | 39.0 mg | 9.8 | 4.0 | very good |
| Protein | 4.7 g | 9.3 | 3.8 | very good |
| Omega-3 Fatty Acids | 0.2 g | 8.0 | 3.3 | good |
| B5 Pantothenic Acid | 0.8 mg | 7.9 | 3.3 | good |
| Iron | 1.4 mg | 7.6 | 3.1 | good |
| Calcium | 74.7 mg | 7.5 | 3.1 | good |
| B1 Thiamin | 0.1 mg | 6.0 | 2.5 | good |
| B3 Niacin | 0.9 mg | 4.7 | 1.9 | good |
| Zinc | 0.6 mg | 4.1 | 1.7 | good |
| Vitamin E | 0.8 mg | 3.8 | 1.5 | good |

**CAROTENOIDS:**

| | |
|---|---|
| Beta-Carotene | 1,840.8 mcg |
| Lutein+Zeaxanthin | 2,366.5 mcg |

**FLAVONOIDS:**

| | |
|---|---|
| Kaempferol | 2.2 mg |
| Quercetin | 1.7 mg |

Daily values for these nutrients have not yet been established.

For more on "Total Nutrient-Richness," "%DV," "Density," and The World's Healthiest Foods "Quality" Rating System, see page 805.
For more on GI, see page 342.

Broccoli originated in the Mediterranean region of Europe, and today is one of the most popular green vegetables in the United States because of its unique flavor and incredible nutritional value. It is one of those cruciferous vegetables that continues to make headlines as a superfood as more and more scientific research verifies its benefits. Proper preparation of Broccoli is the key to bringing out its best flavor and maximizing its nutritional benefits. That is why I want to share with you the secret of the "Healthiest Way of Cooking" Broccoli *al denté*. In just 5 minutes, you will be able to transform Broccoli into a flavorful vegetable while maximizing its nutritional value.

## why broccoli should be part of your healthiest way of eating

Scientific studies now show that cruciferous vegetables, like Broccoli, are included among the vegetables that contain the largest concentrations of health-promoting sulfur compounds, such as sulforaphane and isothiocyanates (see page 153), which increase the liver's ability to produce enzymes that neutralize potentially toxic substances. Broccoli is also rich in the powerful phytonutrient antioxidants lutein and zeaxanthin, carotenoids that are concentrated in the lens of the eye. Along with vitamins A and C, which provide powerful antioxidant protection, Broccoli is a rich source of folic acid, an important nutrient for a healthy heart. Broccoli is an ideal food to add to your "Healthiest Way of Eating" not only because it is high in nutrients, but also because it is low in calories: one cup of cooked Broccoli contains only 44 calories. (For more on the *Health Benefits of Broccoli* and a complete analysis of its content of over 60 nutrients, see page 134.)

## varieties of broccoli

Broccoli is a member of the cruciferous *(Brassica)* family of vegetables that also includes cauliflower, kale, collard greens, cabbage, mustard greens and Brussels sprouts. Broccoli dates back to ancient Rome, when it was developed from wild Broccoli, a plant that resembled collard greens more than the Broccoli with which we are familiar today. Its name comes from the Italian word *brachium*, which means "branch." Varieties of Broccoli include:

### GREEN BROCCOLI
#### (ALSO KNOWN AS ITALIAN GREEN OR CALABRESE)

The most popular variety of Broccoli, this is the one most commonly found in your local market. It is the variety featured in the photographs in this chapter. Named after the Italian province of Calabria where it first grew, it has light green stalks topped with clusters of dark green, purplish florets.

### BROCCOLINI

A baby Broccoli that is a cross between Broccoli and kale, this is the best type of Broccoli to serve raw.

### BROCCOFLOWER

This is a cross between Broccoli and cauliflower, but it is more like cauliflower than Broccoli.

### BROCCOLI RAAB

This variety has an intense flavor with pleasantly bitter and peppery highlights. Compared to Green Broccoli, it has more leaves and a longer stem. The stem is tender and does not need to be peeled, just cut into 1-inch thick slices and cook with the leaves and florets. Enjoy all but the bottom 2-inches of the stem, which is tough and woody and should be discarded. Broccoli Raab can be used in place of Green Broccoli in most recipes.

### BROCCOLI SPROUTS

Sprouts from Broccoli seeds that have recently become popular for their high concentration of health-promoting phytonutrients (see page 153).

## the peak season

Broccoli is available throughout the year, but its flavor is at its peak during the cold months when the frost helps to develop a sweet flavor. In hotter months, Broccoli is less tender and will require around 1 minute additional cooking time.

## biochemical considerations

Broccoli is a concentrated source of goitrogens, which might be of concern to certain individuals. (For more on *Goitrogens*, see page 721.)

## 4 steps for the best tasting and most nutritious broccoli

Turning Broccoli into a flavorful dish with the most nutrients is simple if you just follow my 4 easy steps:

1. The Best Way to Select
2. The Best Way to Store
3. The Best Way to Prepare
4. The Healthiest Way of Cooking

Here is a question that I received from a reader of the whfoods.org website about Broccoli:

Q *Which has more nutrients— the stems or florets of Broccoli?*

A The florets and stems of Broccoli are very similar in their nutrient content. The amount of most B vitamins, minerals, and fiber is very similar in the two parts of the plant (on an ounce-for-ounce basis). The largest difference we've seen documented in the research literature involves beta-carotene, which is about seven times more plentiful in the florets than in the stems. On an ounce-for-ounce basis, the darker green florets also contain more chlorophyll than the lighter green stalks. Stalks can take a little longer to steam than florets and should usually be started a little earlier in the steaming process for this reason.

Broccoli leaves are also excellent sources of nutrients. They are actually higher in beta-carotene than the florets of the Broccoli plant, and they can contain other phytonutrients that aren't found in the stems and florets.

# 1. the best way to select broccoli ——————

You can select the best tasting Broccoli by looking for tightly closed floret clusters that are dark green or purplish in color. Dark green Broccoli contains more chlorophyll, beta-carotene and vitamin C, while purple-colored heads of Broccoli contain higher concentrations of flavonoids. Stalks and stems should be firm, and the leaves should be attached, vibrant and not wilted. By selecting the best tasting Broccoli, you will also enjoy Broccoli with the highest nutritional value. As with all vegetables, I recommend selecting organically grown varieties whenever possible. (For more on *Organic Foods*, see page 113.)

Avoid Broccoli with florets that are not compact or uniformly colored. They should not be yellow, bruised or have yellow blossoms, an indication that they are overly mature.

Do not purchase Broccoli with stalks that are too wide, woody or hollow, and be sure to check for areas that may be spoiled or have a sour smell.

# 2. the best way to store broccoli

If not stored properly, Broccoli will become limp, start to turn yellow and become bitter. If you are not going to enjoy Broccoli immediately after bringing it home from the market, be sure to store it properly to maintain its optimal flavor and nutrient concentration.

Broccoli continues to respire even after it has been harvested; its respiration rate at room temperature (68°F/20°C) is 300 mg/kg/hr. Slowing down the respiration rate with proper storage is the key to extending its flavor and nutritional benefits. (For a *Comparison of Respiration Rates* for different vegetables, see page 91.)

### Broccoli Will Remain Fresh for Up to 10 Days When Properly Stored

1. Store fresh Broccoli in the refrigerator. The colder temperature will slow the respiration rate, helping to preserve its nutrients and keeping Broccoli fresh for a longer period of time.

2. Place Broccoli in a plastic storage bag before refrigerating. I have found that it is best to wrap the bag tightly around the Broccoli, squeezing out as much of the air from the bag as possible.

3. Do not wash Broccoli before refrigeration because exposure to water will encourage Broccoli to spoil.

### How to Store a Partial Head of Broccoli

If you need to store a partial head of Broccoli, place it in a container with a well-sealed lid, or a plastic bag, and refrigerate. Since the vitamin C content starts to quickly degrade once the Broccoli has been cut, it is best to use the remainder within a couple of days.

# 3. the best way to prepare broccoli

I want to share with you the best way to prepare Broccoli. Properly cleaning and cutting Broccoli helps to ensure that the Broccoli you serve will have the best flavor and retain the greatest number of nutrients.

### Cleaning Broccoli

Before cutting Broccoli, rinse well under cold running water. To preserve nutrients, do not soak Broccoli or the water-soluble nutrients will leach into the water. (For more on *Washing Vegetables*, see page 92.)

### Cutting Broccoli

Cutting Broccoli florets into equal size pieces will help them to cook more evenly. The smaller you cut the florets, the more quickly they will cook. I recommend cutting florets into quarters. Cutting florets into smaller pieces also helps maximize the formation of health-promoting compounds when you let them sit for 5 minutes before cooking.

### What to Do with Stem and Leaves

I usually include the stems and leaves when I prepare Broccoli. They are not only nutritious and taste great, but you will also get more Broccoli for your money if you enjoy them along with the florets. Stems and leaves provide a good balance of flavors.

There are several ways to peel the Broccoli stem: (1) peel the entire stalk with a knife by beginning at the top of the stalk and removing long strips of the peel, similar to removing the string from celery; (2) remove the florets, cut the stems into shorter lengths and peel with a sharp knife by standing them on end and cutting downward to remove the tough outer skin; or (3) peel the Broccoli stems with a vegetable peeler.

Slice the stems into 1/4-inch slices, and cook both the stems and leaves along with the florets.

# 4. the healthiest way of cooking broccoli ———

Since research has shown that important nutrients can be lost or destroyed by the way a food is cooked, the "Healthiest Way of Cooking" Broccoli is focused on enhancing its best flavor while maximizing its vitamins, minerals and powerful antioxidants.

## The Healthiest Way of Cooking Broccoli: "Healthy Steaming" for just 5 Minutes

In my search to find the healthiest way to cook Broccoli, I tested every possible cooking method and discovered that "Healthy Steaming" all varieties of Broccoli for just 5 minutes delivered the best results. "Healthy Steaming" provides the moisture necessary to make Broccoli tender, bring out its peak flavor, retain its bright green color and maximize its nutritional profile. The Step-by-Step Recipe will show you how easy it is to "Healthy Steam" Broccoli. (For more on "*Healthy Steaming*," see page 58.)

## How to Avoid Overcooking Broccoli: Cook it *Al Denté*

One of the primary reasons people do not enjoy Broccoli is because it is often overcooked. For the best flavor, I recommend cooking Broccoli *al denté*. Broccoli cooked *al denté* is tender outside and slightly crisp inside. Plus, Broccoli cooked *al denté* is cooked just long enough to soften its cellulose and hemicellulose fiber; this makes it easier to digest and allows its health-promoting nutrients to become more readily available for absorption.

Although Broccoli is a hearty vegetable, it is very important not to overcook it. Broccoli cooked for as little as a couple of minutes longer than *al denté* will begin to lose not only its texture and flavor but also its nutrients.

Overcooking Broccoli will significantly decrease its nutritional value: as much as 50% of some nutrients can be lost. (For more on *Al Denté*, see page 92.)

## How to Prevent Strong Smells from Forming

Cutting Broccoli florets into quarters and cooking them *al denté* for only 5 minutes is my secret for preventing the formation of smelly compounds often associated with cooking Broccoli. When I cook my Broccoli, it never develops a strong smell. After 5 minutes of cooking, the texture of Broccoli, like all other cruciferous vegetables, begins to change, becoming increasingly soft and mushy. At this point, it also starts to lose more and more of its chlorophyll, causing its bright green color to fade and a brownish hue to appear. This is a sign that magnesium has been lost. This is when it starts to release hydrogen sulfide, the cause of the "rotten egg smell," which also affects the flavor. After 7 minutes of cooking, Broccoli develops a more intense flavor, with the amount of strong smelling hydrogen sulfide doubling in quantity.

While it is important not to overcook Broccoli, cooking for less than 5 minutes is also not recommended because it takes about 5 minutes to soften its fibers and help increase its digestibility.

## Cooking Methods Not Recommended for Broccoli

### BOILING, BAKING, BROILING, GRILLING, ROASTING OR COOKING WITH OIL

Boiling Broccoli increases its water absorption, causing it to become soggy and mushy. It then loses much of its flavor along with many of its nutrients, including minerals,

---

### An Easy Way to Prepare Broccoli, Step-by-Step

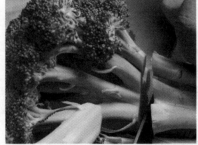 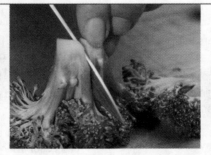 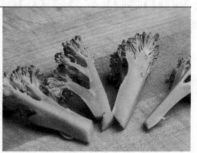

**CUTTING BROCCOLI**
❶ For larger florets, cut just above the thick stem so the smaller stems are free to separate. For smaller florets, cut closer to the head of each smaller stem. ❷ Most florets will fall away into smaller pieces. For those that don't, use knife a to separate. ❸ Cut florets into quarters.

water-soluble vitamins (such as C and the B-complex vitamins) and health-promoting phytonutrients. I don't recommend baking, broiling, grilling or roasting Broccoli as they will cause it to dry up and shrivel. I don't recommend cooking Broccoli in oil because heating oils to high temperatures can damage delicate oils and potentially create harmful free radicals.

### Serving Ideas from Mediterranean Countries:

Traveling through the Mediterranean region, I found Broccoli was prepared in many different ways:

---

### HOW TO BRING OUT THE HIDDEN HEALTH BENEFITS OF BROCCOLI

The latest scientific studies show that cutting Broccoli into small pieces breaks down cell walls and enhances the activation of an enzyme called *myrosinase* that slowly converts some of the plant nutrients into their active forms, which have been shown to contain health-promoting properties. So, to get the most health benefits from Broccoli, let it sit for a minimum of 5 minutes, optimally 10 minutes, after cutting, before eating or cooking.

Since ascorbic acid (vitamin C) increases *myrosinase* activity, you can sprinkle a little lemon juice on the Broccoli before letting it sit, in order to further enhance its beneficial phytonutrient concentration.

Heat will inactivate the effect of *myrosinase*, which is why it is important to allow the Broccoli to sit for 5–10 minutes before cooking to give the enzyme ample opportunity to enhance the concentration of active phytonutrients in your Broccoli. Cooking at low or medium heat for short periods of time (up to 15 minutes) should not destroy the active phytonutrients since once they are formed, they are fairly stable.

---

In Italy, Broccoli is served with anchovies, onions or Romano cheese.

In Greece, Broccoli is served with grated cheese.

---

Here is a question I received from a reader of the whfoods.org website about Broccoli:

**Q** *What are the special phytonutrients for which Broccoli and other cruciferous vegetables have become famous?*

**A** Broccoli, and other cruciferous vegetables, are replete with a host of different phytonutrients that contribute to their amazing health-promoting potential. Included in these are carotenoids and flavonoids as well as sulfur-containing phytonutrients that have been garnering a lot of recent attention for their cancer-prevention properties. Included among these sulfur-containing nutrients are glucosinolate, indole-3-carbinol and a group classified by their chemical family name, isothiocyanates.

While some health researchers group glucosinolate, isothiocyanates and indole-3-carbinol together and call them "indoles," only the latter actually fits that classification. (The term "indole" refers to a chemical structure that some compounds have, featuring two specifically shaped carbon rings with an attached amino group. Other well-known indoles include the amino acid tryptophan and the neurotransmitters serotonin and melatonin.) Since glucosinolate, isothiocyanates, and indole-3-carbinol are technically classified in different chemical families, I think that the best way to refer to them collectively is by calling them "sulfur-containing phytonutrients."

---

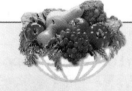

# how to enjoy fresh broccoli without cooking

Raw Broccoli florets cut into quarters are a great addition to virtually any vegetable salad.

For a quick appetizer, serve raw Broccoli florets cut into quarters as crudités. Dip into extra virgin olive oil mixed with sea salt and freshly ground pepper.

**Chopped Broccoli Salad:**
An easy way to enjoy Broccoli raw. Serves 2
INGREDIENTS:

| | |
|---|---|
| 1 cup of Broccoli florets | 1 medium carrot |
| 1/2 medium avocado, diced | 1 tomato, diced |
| 12 kalamata olives, pitted and chopped | |

DRESS WITH MEDITERRANEAN DRESSING:
2 medium cloves garlic, 2 TBS lemon juice, 3 TBS extra virgin olive oil and salt and pepper to taste

OPTIONAL: diced chicken or turkey breast

DIRECTIONS:
1. Mince Broccoli and carrots using a knife or food processor. Place in a large salad bowl.
2. Add diced tomato, avocado and olives to the bowl and toss with dressing until well mixed. For a main course, add chicken or turkey.

STEP-BY-STEP RECIPE
## The Healthiest Way of Cooking Broccoli

# 5-Minute "Healthy Steamed" Broccoli

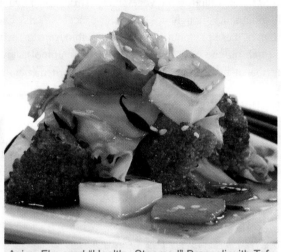

Asian-Flavored "Healthy Steamed" Broccoli with Tofu

*"Healthy Steaming" is a gentle way to prepare Broccoli that enhances it flavor, brings out its color, makes it tender and preserves most of its nutrients. It tastes best when served the Mediterranean way with this easy dressing.*

**1 lb Broccoli**

**Mediterranean Dressing:**
**3 TBS extra virgin olive oil**
**2 tsp lemon juice**
**2 medium cloves garlic**
**Sea salt and pepper to taste**

1. Fill bottom of steamer with 2 inches of water.
2. While steam is building up in steamer, cut Broccoli florets into quarters and let them sit, as described in *How to Bring out the Hidden Health Benefits of Broccoli*. Also cut stems into 1/4-inch pieces.
3. Press or chop garlic and let it sit for at least 5 minutes. (Why?, see page 261.)
4. For *al denté* Broccoli, steam florets and stems for no more than 5 minutes. If stems are cut thicker than 1/4-inch, they will require 1–2 minutes of cooking before adding the florets. For information on *Differences in Cooking Time*, see page 94.
5. Transfer to a bowl. For more flavor, toss Broccoli with the remaining ingredients while it is still hot. (Mediterranean Dressing does not need to be made separately.) Research shows that carotenoids found in foods are best absorbed when consumed with oils.

OPTIONAL: To mellow the flavor of garlic, add garlic to Broccoli for the last 2 minutes of steaming.

**SERVES 2**

**COOKING TIPS:**
- To prevent overcooking Broccoli, I highly recommend using a timer.
- Testing Broccoli with a fork is not an effective way to determine whether it is done.

## Flavor Tips: Try these 8 great serving suggestions with the recipe above. ✱

1. **Most Popular:** Add 1 TBS oil packed sundried tomatoes, 3 TBS crumbled feta cheese and 6 kalamata olives to the 5-Minute "Healthy Steamed" Broccoli recipe.
2. Sprinkle with grated Parmesan, goat or feta cheese.
3. For a different flavor replace lemon juice with 2 tsp balsamic or rice vinegar.
4. Add a few drops of tamari (soy sauce) to mellow the flavor of Broccoli.
5. Steam red onions with Broccoli and add chopped olives.
6. **Asian-Flavored Broccoli with Tofu:** Prepare 5-Minute "Healthy Steamed" Broccoli with the Mediterranean Dressing. Add cooked carrots, tofu cubes, rice vinegar, tamari (soy sauce), grated ginger and red pepper flakes to taste (pictured above).

7. **Broccoli with Mustard Tarragon Sauce**: Prepare the 5-Minute "Healthy Steamed" Broccoli recipe adding 1 TBS Dijon mustard (or your favorite mustard) and 1 TBS fresh or 1/2 tsp dried tarragon to the Mediterranean Dressing.
8. **5-Minute Mediterranean Medley:** Ingredients include: 2 cups Broccoli florets cut into quarters, 2 cups chopped curly kale, 1 medium carrot sliced into 1/2-inch rounds, 2 cloves garlic (chopped or pressed), 3 TBS extra virgin olive oil, 2 tsp fresh lemon juice, and sea salt and pepper to taste. Bring steaming water to a boil. Add Broccoli, kale and carrots, cover, and steam for 5 minutes. Add garlic to the vegetables for the last 2 minutes of steaming. Transfer to a bowl and toss with remaining ingredients while vegetables are still hot.

Please write (address on back cover flap) or e-mail me at info@whfoods.org with your personal ideas for preparing Broccoli, and I will share them with others through our website at www.whfoods.org.

# health benefits of broccoli

## Promotes Optimal Health

Like other cruciferous vegetables, Broccoli contains phytonutrients thought to have anti-cancer effects. One group of these phytonutrients are the isothiocyanates, with research on one of its members, indole-3-carbinol, showing that it helps deactivate a potent estrogen metabolite (4-hydroxyestrone) that promotes tumor growth, especially in estrogen-sensitive breast cells. Indole-3-carbinol has been shown to suppress not only breast tumor cell growth but also cancer cell metastasis (the movement of cancerous cells to other parts of the body). Broccoli also contains the phytonutrient glucoraphanin, which is converted into sulforaphane in the body. Scientists have found that sulforaphane boosts the liver's detoxification enzymes, helping to clear potentially carcinogenic substances more quickly. Animal research suggests that sulforaphane may protect against tumor development by inducing cancer cell apoptosis (programmed cell suicide).

New research has uncovered another way *Brassica* family vegetables such as Broccoli may help prevent cancer. When these vegetables are cut, chewed or digested, a sulfur-containing compound called sinigrin is brought into contact with the enzyme *myrosinase*, resulting in the release of special compounds, including isothiocyanates. Not only are these sulfur-containing phytonutrients potent inducers of liver enzymes that detoxify carcinogens, but recent research shows one of these compounds, allyl isothicyanate, also inhibits cell division and stimulates apoptosis in human tumor cells.

Broccoli sprouts definitely prove the adage, "Good things come in small packages." Broccoli sprouts concentrate phytonutrients found in mature Broccoli; researchers estimate that Broccoli sprouts contain 10–100 times the power of mature Broccoli to boost enzymes that detoxify potential carcinogens!

## Promotes Heart Health

Broccoli has been singled out as one of the small number of vegetables and fruits that contributed to the significant reduction in heart disease risk seen in a recent meta-analysis of seven prospective studies. Of the more than 100,000 individuals who participated in these studies, those whose diets most frequently included Broccoli, onions, apples and tea—the richest sources of flavonoids, such as quercetin—experienced a 20% reduction in their risk of heart disease. Animal studies suggest that eating Broccoli sprouts may also have a beneficial effect since their concentration of the phytonutrient glucoraphanin helps to quench free radicals and allay the inflammation that contributes to cardiovascular problems. In addition, Broccoli is a concentrated source of many other heart-healthy nutrients including dietary fiber, folic acid, vitamin B6, vitamin E, niacin, magnesium, potassium and omega-3 fatty acids.

## Nutritional Analysis of 1 cup of cooked Broccoli:

| NUTRIENT | AMOUNT | % DAILY VALUE | NUTRIENT | AMOUNT | % DAILY VALUE |
|---|---|---|---|---|---|
| Calories | 43.68 | | Pantothenic Acid | 0.79 mg | 7.90 |
| Calories from Fat | 4.91 | | | | |
| Calories from Saturated Fat | 0.76 | | **Minerals** | | |
| Protein | 4.66 g | | Boron | — mcg | |
| Carbohydrates | 8.19 g | | Calcium | 74.72 mg | 7.47 |
| Dietary Fiber | 4.68 g | 18.72 | Chloride | — mg | |
| Soluble Fiber | 2.03 g | | Chromium | — mcg | — |
| Insoluble Fiber | 2.65 g | | Copper | 0.07 mg | 3.50 |
| Sugar – Total | 3.12 g | | Fluoride | — mg | — |
| Monosaccharides | 2.03 g | | Iodine | — mcg | — |
| Disaccharides | 0.47 g | | Iron | 1.37 mg | 7.61 |
| Other Carbs | 0.39 g | | Magnesium | 39.00 mg | 9.75 |
| Fat – Total | 0.55 g | | Manganese | 0.34 mg | 17.00 |
| Saturated Fat | 0.08 g | | Molybdenum | — mcg | — |
| Mono Fat | 0.04 g | | Phosphorus | 102.80 mg | 10.28 |
| Poly Fat | 0.26 g | | Potassium | 505.44 mg | |
| Omega-3 Fatty Acids | 0.20 g | 8.00 | Selenium | — mcg | — |
| Omega-6 Fatty Acids | 0.06 g | | Sodium | 42.12 mg | |
| Trans Fatty Acids | 0.00 g | | Zinc | 0.62 mg | 4.13 |
| Cholesterol | 0.00 mg | | | | |
| Water | 141.49 g | | **Amino Acids** | | |
| Ash | 1.48 g | | Alanine | 0.18 g | |
| | | | Arginine | 0.23 g | |
| **Vitamins** | | | Aspartate | 0.33 g | |
| Vitamin A IU | 2280.72 IU | 45.61 | Cystine | 0.03 g | 7.32 |
| Vitamin A RE | 228.07 RE | | Glutamate | 0.58 g | |
| A - Carotenoid | 228.07 RE | 3.04 | Glycine | 0.15 g | |
| A - Retinol | 0.00 RE | | Histidine | 0.08 g | 6.20 |
| B1 Thiamin | 0.09 mg | 6.00 | Isoleucine | 0.17 g | 14.78 |
| B2 Riboflavin | 0.18 mg | 10.59 | Leucine | 0.20 g | 7.91 |
| B3 Niacin | 0.94 mg | 4.70 | Lysine | 0.22 g | 9.36 |
| Niacin Equiv | 1.70 mg | | Methionine | 0.05 g | 6.76 |
| Vitamin B6 | 0.22 mg | 11.00 | Phenylalanine | 0.13 g | 10.92 |
| Vitamin B12 | 0.00 mcg | 0.00 | Proline | 0.18 g | |
| Biotin | — mcg | — | Serine | 0.16 g | |
| Vitamin C | 123.40 mg | 205.67 | Threonine | 0.14 g | 11.29 |
| Vitamin D IU | 0.00 IU | 0.00 | Tryptophan | 0.05 g | 15.63 |
| Vitamin D mcg | 0.00 mcg | | Tyrosine | 0.10 g | 10.31 |
| Vitamin E Alpha Equiv | 0.75 mg | 3.75 | Valine | 0.20 g | 13.61 |
| Vitamin E IU | 1.11 IU | | | | |
| Vitamin E mg | 0.75 mg | | | | |
| Folate | 93.91 mcg | 23.48 | | | |
| Vitamin K | 155.20 mcg | 194.00 | | | |

(Note: "—" indicates data is unavailable. For more information, please see page 806.)

## Promotes Digestive Health

Research suggests that the phytonutrients contained in Broccoli and Broccoli sprouts may eradicate *Helicobacter pylori*, the bacterium not only responsible for most peptic ulcers but one that has also been found to increase a person's risk of getting stomach cancer three to six-fold. In a recent animal study, sulforaphane completely eliminated *H. pylori* in 8 of 11 laboratory animals infected with bacterium. A follow-up human study found that daily consumption of 100 grams (about 3 ounces) of Broccoli sprouts over a two month period greatly suppressed *H. pylori* growth and markedly decreased pepsinogen (an indicator of stomach damage).

## Promotes Vision Health

Broccoli and other leafy green vegetables contain powerful phytonutrient antioxidants in the carotenoid family called lutein and zeaxanthin, both of which are concentrated in large quantities in the lens of the eye. In a large-scale study involving over 30,000 individuals, those who ate Broccoli more than twice a week were found to have a 23% lower risk of cataracts compared to those who consumed this antioxidant-rich vegetable less than once a month. In addition to the antioxidant potential of Broccoli's carotenoids, recent research has suggested that sulforaphane may also have antioxidant potential, being able to protect human eye cells from free radical stressors.

## Promotes Bone Health

When it comes to building strong bones, Broccoli's got it all for less. One cup of steamed Broccoli contains 74 mg of calcium, plus 123 mg of vitamin C, which significantly improves calcium's absorption; all this for a total of only 44 calories with negligible amounts of fats. Dairy products, long touted as the most reliable source of calcium, contain no vitamin C, but do contain saturated fat. A glass of 2% milk contains 121 calories, and 42 of those calories come from fat.

## Promotes Healthy Pregnancy

Especially if you are pregnant, be sure to eat Broccoli, an excellent source of folic acid, a B-vitamin essential for proper cellular division and DNA synthesis. Without folic acid, the fetus' nervous system cells do not divide properly. Deficiency of folic acid during pregnancy has been linked to several birth defects, including neural tube defects like spina bifida. Despite folic acid's widespread occurrence in food (its name comes from the Latin word *folium*, meaning 'foliage' because it's found in green leafy vegetables), folic acid deficiency is the most common vitamin deficiency in the world. Folic acid has other benefits including supporting heart health through keeping homocysteine levels balanced.

## Additional Health-Promoting Benefits of Broccoli

Broccoli is also a concentrated source of many other nutrients providing additional health-promoting benefits. These nutrients include energy-producing iron, vitamin B1, vitamin B2, vitamin B5 and phosphorus; free-radical-scavenging vitamin A, manganese and zinc; muscle-building protein; and sleep-promoting tryptophan. Since Broccoli contains only 44 calories per one cooked cup serving, it is an ideal food for healthy weight control.

---

Here is a question that I received from a reader of the whfoods.org website about Broccoli.

**Q** *I've recently fallen in love with Broccoli raab. Is it as healthy as Broccoli?*

**A** Broccoli raab is definitely a great vegetable to have fallen in love with. Not only is it delicious, but it is also a highly concentrated source of nutrients.

Like its cousin Broccoli, Broccoli raab (*Brassica rapa*) is a member of the *Brassica* family of vegetables. It is sometimes spelled Broccoli rabe and is also known as rapini. Like other *Brassica* vegetables, Broccoli raab contains health-promoting sulfur-containing phytonutrients such as glucosinolates and isothiocyanates, which have been found to help the liver detoxify chemicals that can act as carcinogens.

In addition to these phytonutrients, Broccoli raab is also a concentrated source of many vitamins and minerals. For example, 100 grams (about 3.5 ounces) provides an incredible 118 mg of calcium, 1.3 grams of iron, 2.5 mg of vitamin E, and 4533 IU of vitamin A, all for only 33 calories. In fact, on an equal weight basis, Broccoli raab actually provides significantly more calcium, iron, B vitamins, vitamin A and vitamin E than does Broccoli (although it does contain less vitamin C).

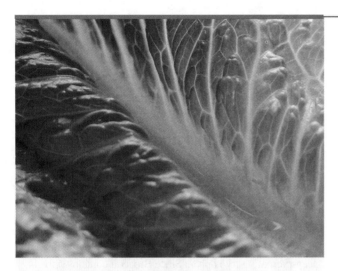

# romaine lettuce

| | |
|---|---|
| AVAILABILITY: | Year-round |
| REFRIGERATE: | Yes |
| SHELF LIFE: | 7 days refrigerated |
| PREPARATION: | Minimal, no need to cook |

## nutrient-richness chart

Total Nutrient-Richness: **40**  GI: **15**

Two cups (112 grams) of Romaine Lettuce contains 16 calories

| NUTRIENT | AMOUNT | DV(%) | DENSITY | QUALITY |
|---|---|---|---|---|
| Vitamin K | 114.8 mcg | 143.5 | 164.7 | excellent |
| Vitamin A | 2912.0 IU | 58.2 | 66.9 | excellent |
| Vitamin C | 26.9 mg | 44.8 | 51.4 | excellent |
| Folate | 152.0 mcg | 38.0 | 43.6 | excellent |
| Manganese | 0.7 mg | 35.5 | 40.8 | excellent |
| Chromium | 15.7 mcg | 13.1 | 15.0 | excellent |
| Potassium | 324.8 mg | 9.3 | 10.7 | very good |
| Molybdenum | 6.7 mcg | 9.0 | 10.3 | very good |
| Dietary Fiber | 1.9 g | 7.6 | 8.7 | very good |
| B1 Thiamin | 0.1 mg | 7.3 | 8.4 | very good |
| Iron | 1.2 mg | 6.8 | 7.8 | very good |
| B2 Riboflavin | 0.1 mg | 6.5 | 7.4 | very good |
| Phosphorus | 50.4 mg | 5.0 | 5.8 | very good |
| Calcium | 40.3 mg | 4.0 | 4.6 | good |
| Protein | 1.8 g | 3.6 | 4.2 | good |
| Omega-3 Fatty Acids | 0.1 g | 3.2 | 3.7 | good |
| Tryptophan | 0.01 g | 3.1 | 3.6 | good |
| B3 Niacin | 0.6 mg | 2.8 | 3.2 | good |
| B6 Pyridoxine | 0.1 mg | 2.5 | 2.9 | good |

| **CAROTENOIDS:** | | |
|---|---|---|
| Beta-Carotene | 3,902.1 mcg | |
| Lutein+Zeaxanthin | 2,589.4 mcg | |

Daily values for these nutrients have not yet been established.

For more on "Total Nutrient-Richness," "%DV," "Density," and The World's Healthiest Foods "Quality" Rating System, see page 805.

For more on GI, see page 342.

The cultivation of Lettuce may date as far back as 4,500 BC Depictions of Lettuce have been found on ancient Egyptian tombs, and it is believed that Lettuce was held in high esteem by the Greeks and Romans, both as a food and for its medicinal properties. The Chinese consider Lettuce a source of good luck and serve it on birthdays, New Year's Day and other special occasions. In the West, Lettuce has become an important low-calorie food that is great for weight control. Think crisp leafy Lettuce and refreshing salads come to mind. And by combining a Lettuce salad with chicken, fish, beans, nuts and seeds, you can create a great meal that is limited only by your imagination.

## why romaine lettuce should be part of your healthiest way of eating

Although Lettuce comes in many shapes, sizes and colors, Romaine Lettuce is one of the most nutritious. Highly regarded for its crunchy texture and low calorie count, its impressive nutritional profile is often overlooked. It is an excellent source of heart-healthy folic acid and chromium, a hard-to-find mineral that is important for maintaining healthy blood sugar levels. Additionally, Romaine Lettuce is a concentrated source of carotenoid phytonutrients, such as beta-carotene, lutein and zeaxanthin, which have powerful antioxidant properties. Nutrient-rich and low in calories, Romaine Lettuce is great for weight control and an ideal food to add to your "Healthiest Way of Eating"—two cups of fresh Romaine Lettuce contain only 16 calories! (For more on the *Health Benefits of Romaine Lettuce* and a complete analysis of its content of over 60 nutrients, see page 138.)

## varieties of lettuce

Most varieties of Lettuce exude small amounts of a white, milky liquid when their leaves are broken. This "milk" gives Lettuce its slightly bitter flavor and its scientific name, *Lactuca sativa*, derived from the Latin word for milk. Lettuce is described as head Lettuce or leaf Lettuce. (For more on varieties of Lettuce, see *Salads,* page 141.)

## the peak season

Most of the domestic harvest of Romaine Lettuce and other salad greens comes from California; they are available throughout the year.

## biochemical considerations

Lettuce is one of the 12 foods on which pesticide residues have been most frequently found. (For more on *Pesticide Residues*, see page 726.)

## 3 steps for the best tasting and most nutritious romaine lettuce

Turning Romaine Lettuce into a flavorful dish with the most nutrients is simple if you just follow my 3 easy steps:

1. The Best Way to Select
2. The Best Way to Store
3. The Best Way to Prepare

# 1. the best way to select romaine lettuce

You can select the best tasting Romaine Lettuce by looking for compact heads with crisp leaves. By selecting the best tasting Romaine Lettuce, you will also enjoy Romaine Lettuce with the highest nutritional value. As with all vegetables, I recommend selecting organically grown varieties whenever possible. (For more on *Organic Foods*, see page 113.)

Avoid Lettuce with wilted leaves that may have dark or slimy spots. The edge of the leaves should not have brown or yellow discoloration, and the stem ends should not be too brown.

# 2. the best way to store romaine lettuce

Romaine Lettuce is a delicate vegetable, and if not stored properly, it will become limp and lose not only its freshness, but also up to 30% of some of its vitamins.

Romaine Lettuce continues to respire even after it has been harvested; its respiration rate at room temperature (68°F/ 20°C) is 101 mg/kg/hr. Slowing down the respiration rate with proper storage is the key to extending its flavor and nutritional benefits. (For a *Comparison of Respiration Rates* for different vegetables, see page 91.)

### Romaine Lettuce Will Remain Fresh for Up to 7 Days When Properly Stored

1. Store fresh Romaine Lettuce in the refrigerator. The colder temperature will slow the respiration rate, help-

ing to preserve its nutrients and keeping Romaine Lettuce fresh for a longer period of time.

2. Place Romaine Lettuce in a plastic storage bag before refrigerating. I have found that it is best to wrap the bag tightly around the Romaine Lettuce, squeezing out as much of the air from the bag as possible.

3. Do not wash Romaine Lettuce before refrigeration because exposure to water will encourage Romaine Lettuce to spoil.

4. Romaine hearts are usually more durable and will last longer in your refrigerator than the other leaves. If you're uncertain about consuming your Romaine Lettuce within 7 days, you might want to purchase the romaine hearts.

# 3. the best way to prepare romaine lettuce

Properly cleaning and cutting Romaine Lettuce helps ensure that the Romaine Lettuce you serve will have the best flavor and retain the greatest number of nutrients.

### Cleaning Lettuce

Rinse well under cold running water to remove any soil before cutting. A salad spinner works best to remove excess water; spin the Lettuce after it has been chopped. If

you don't have a spinner, pat leaves dry to remove excess water before chopping. To preserve nutrients, do not soak Lettuce or its water-soluble nutrients will leach into the water. (For more on *Washing Vegetables*, page 92.)

I recommend washing prepackaged Lettuce even if the package label says that it has been prewashed.

# health benefits of romaine lettuce

## Promotes Healthy Weight Control

Due to its extremely low calorie content and high water volume, Romaine Lettuce is often overlooked in the nutrition world as a very nutritious food. It is delicious, versatile and very filling, making it a very nutritious addition to a "Healthiest Way of Eating" geared towards healthy weight control.

### Nutritional Analysis of 2 cups of Romaine Lettuce:

| NUTRIENT | AMOUNT | % DAILY VALUE |
|---|---|---|
| Calories | 15.68 | |
| Calories from Fat | 2.02 | |
| Calories from Saturated Fat | 0.26 | |
| Protein | 1.81 g | |
| Carbohydrates | 2.65 g | |
| Dietary Fiber | 1.90 g | 7.60 |
| Soluble Fiber | 0.89 g | |
| Insoluble Fiber | 1.01 g | |
| Sugar–Total | 0.53 g | |
| Monosaccharides | 0.00 g | |
| Disaccharides | — g | |
| Other Carbs | 0.22 g | |
| Fat–Total | 0.22 g | |
| Saturated Fat | 0.03 g | |
| Mono Fat | 0.01 g | |
| Poly Fat | 0.12 g | |
| Omega-3 Fatty Acids | 0.08 g | 3.20 |
| Omega-6 Fatty Acids | 0.03 g | |
| Trans Fatty Acids | 0.00 g | |
| Cholesterol | 0.00 mg | |
| Water | 106.30 g | |
| Ash | 1.01 g | |
| **Vitamins** | | |
| Vitamin A IU | 2912.00 IU | 58.24 |
| Vitamin A RE | 291.20 RE | |
| A - Carotenoid | 291.20 RE | 3.88 |
| A - Retinol | 0.00 RE | |
| B1 Thiamin | 0.11 mg | 7.33 |
| B2 Riboflavin | 0.11 mg | 6.47 |
| B3 Niacin | 0.56 mg | 2.80 |
| Niacin Equiv | 0.78 mg | |
| Vitamin B6 | 0.05 mg | 2.50 |
| Vitamin B12 | 0.00 mcg | 0.00 |
| Biotin | 2.13 mcg | 0.71 |
| Vitamin C | 26.88 mg | 44.80 |
| Vitamin D IU | 0.00 IU | 0.00 |
| Vitamin D mcg | 0.00 mcg | |
| Vitamin E Alpha Equiv | 0.49 mg | 2.45 |
| Vitamin E IU | 0.73 IU | |
| Vitamin E mg | 0.84 mg | |
| Folate | 151.98 mcg | 37.99 |
| Vitamin K | 114.80 mcg | 143.50 |

| NUTRIENT | AMOUNT | % DAILY VALUE |
|---|---|---|
| Pantothenic Acid | 0.19 mg | 1.90 |
| **Minerals** | | |
| Boron | 0.09 mcg | |
| Calcium | 40.32 mg | 4.03 |
| Chloride | 63.84 mg | |
| Chromium | 15.68 mcg | 13.07 |
| Copper | 0.04 mg | 2.00 |
| Fluoride | 0.00 mg | 0.00 |
| Iodine | 3.70 mcg | 2.47 |
| Iron | 1.23 mg | 6.83 |
| Magnesium | 6.72 mg | 1.68 |
| Manganese | 0.71 mg | 35.50 |
| Molybdenum | 6.72 mcg | 8.96 |
| Phosphorus | 50.40 mg | 5.04 |
| Potassium | 324.80 mg | |
| Selenium | 0.22 mcg | 0.31 |
| Sodium | 8.96 mg | |
| Zinc | 0.28 mg | 1.87 |
| **Amino Acids** | | |
| Alanine | 0.08 g | |
| Arginine | 0.10 g | |
| Aspartate | 0.20 g | |
| Cystine | 0.02 g | 4.88 |
| Glutamate | 0.25 g | |
| Glycine | 0.08 g | |
| Histidine | 0.03 g | 2.33 |
| Isoleucine | 0.12 g | 10.43 |
| Leucine | 0.11 g | 4.35 |
| Lysine | 0.12 g | 5.11 |
| Methionine | 0.02 g | 2.70 |
| Phenylalanine | 0.08 g | 6.72 |
| Proline | 0.07 g | |
| Serine | 0.05 g | |
| Threonine | 0.08 g | 6.45 |
| Tryptophan | 0.01 g | 3.13 |
| Tyrosine | 0.04 g | 4.12 |
| Valine | 0.10 g | 6.80 |

(Note: "–" indicates data is unavailable. For more information, please see page 806.)

## Promotes Vision Health

Romaine Lettuce contains nutrients that are good for your eyes. It is an excellent source of vitamin A, which is necessary for the production of rhodopsin, a pigment that allows the eyes to detect small amounts of light. Additionally, Romaine Lettuce is a concentrated source of lutein and zeaxanthin, carotenoid phytonutrients that are thought to protect eyes from light-induced oxidative damage. Studies have found that higher dietary intake of lutein and zeaxanthin is related to a reduced risk of cataracts and age-related macular degeneration.

## Promotes Balanced Blood Sugar Levels

Romaine Lettuce is an excellent source of chromium, an important mineral for blood sugar regulation. Chromium is a component of glucose tolerance factor (GTF), which helps to sensitize cells to the actions of insulin, the hormone that signals cells to allow glucose to enter. Most people don't get enough chromium in their diet since food processing methods remove the naturally-occurring chromium in commonly consumed foods.

## Promotes Heart Health

A recent study found that animals fed a Lettuce-rich diet received a beneficial effect upon cholesterol metabolism and antioxidant status. This may be no surprise when we reflect upon the wealth of heart-healthy nutrients contained in Lettuce. For example, Romaine Lettuce is also an excellent source of folic acid; if folic acid is deficient, it can lead to elevated levels of homocysteine, which damages artery walls, leading to atherosclerosis. Romaine Lettuce is also a good source of vitamin B6, which is also important in maintaining proper homocysteine levels. Romaine Lettuce is a concentrated source of other heart-healthy nutrients including dietary fiber, potassium, calcium, omega-3 fatty acids and niacin.

## Additional Health-Promoting Benefits of Romaine Lettuce

Romaine Lettuce is also a concentrated source of many other nutrients providing additional health-promoting benefits. These nutrients include energy-producing iron, phosphorus, vitamin B1 and vitamin B2; muscle-building protein; free-radical-scavenging manganese; sulfite-detoxifying molybdenum; and sleep-promoting tryptophan. Since a two cup serving of Romaine Lettuce contains only 16 calories, it is an ideal food for healthy weight control.

STEP-BY-STEP RECIPE
## The Healthiest Way to Enjoy Romaine Lettuce

# 10-Minute Romaine Salad

*It just takes minutes to make this refreshing salad, which is a great accompaniment to almost any main dish. For a complete meal, you can add chicken, turkey or shrimp.*

1 head Romaine Lettuce, chopped
1/2 medium avocado, diced
1 medium tomato, diced
2 TBS goat cheese, crumbled
2 TBS toasted walnuts, chopped
1 TBS fresh lemon juice
3 TBS extra virgin olive oil
1 tsp honey
Sea salt and pepper to taste

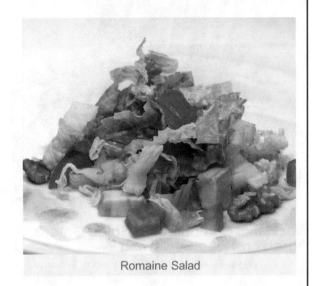
Romaine Salad

1. Combine Romaine Lettuce, avocado and tomato in a large bowl.
2. Top with crumbled goat cheese and chopped walnuts.
3. Whisk dressing ingredients in a small bowl until well combined.
4. Toss dressing and salad ingredients together right before serving.

**SERVES 2**

## Flavor Tips: Try these 4 great serving suggestions with the recipe above. ✱

1. Add chopped anchovies or garlic.
2. Top with grated Parmesan cheese.
3. **Romaine Turkey Salad:** Add to 10-Minute Romaine recipe: 1 carrot diced, 3 stalks celery diced, and 1/2 cup sliced turkey pieces. Top with grated Parmesan cheese.
4. **Spicy Caesar Dressing:** Substitute this dressing for the dressing in the recipe: In a blender, combine 4 cloves garlic, the flesh of a deseeded jalapeño pepper, 1 TBS Dijon mustard, 1 TBS vinegar, 1/2 cup extra virgin olive oil, 2 TBS lemon juice and 2 anchovies (optional). Blend at high speed for 1 minute. Add 2 TBS Parmesan cheese and capers (optional) to the salad.

**ADDITIONAL WAYS TO ENJOY ROMAINE LETTUCE:**
- Add shredded Romaine Lettuce to tacos and burritos.
- Use Romaine leaves as a wrap instead of tortillas.

## An Easy Way to Prepare Romaine Lettuce, Step-by-Step

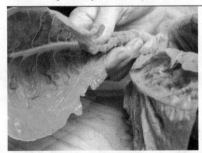 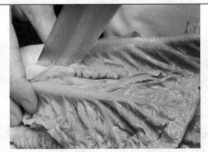 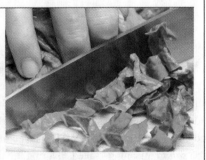

### SHREDDED LETTUCE

❶ Remove outer leaves from the head and discard as they are usually wilted and discolored. Cut tip off Romaine Lettuce head and discard as it is tough and bitter. ❷ Make a cut lengthwise through the entire head of Romaine Lettuce. Turn cut side of head to the side and cut again, so that the head has been cut into fourths leaving root end intact. ❸ Slice thinly up to the root end and discard hard end portion.

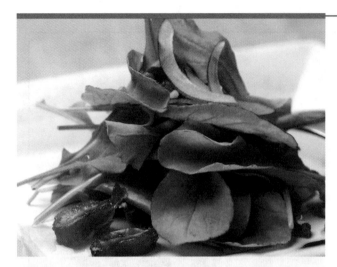

## Nutritional Comparison of Salad Greens
**Based on 1 cup = 1 serving**

| SALAD GREENS | CALORIES | VITAMIN A (IU) | VITAMIN C (MG) | CALCIUM (MG) | POTASSIUM (MG) |
|---|---|---|---|---|---|
| Romaine Lettuce | 8 | 1456 | 13 | 20 | 65 |
| Leaf Lettuce | 10 | 1064 | 10 | 38 | 148 |
| Butterhead (Bibb and Boston) | 7 | 534 | 4 | 18 | 141 |
| Arugula | 5 | 480 | 3 | 32 | 74 |
| Mixed Green Salad (prepackaged) | 9 | 1495 | 9 | 30 | 174 |
| Baby Spinach | 7 | 1200 | 8 | 20 | – |
| *Iceberg Lettuce | 7 | 182 | 2 | 10 | 87 |

*Iceberg lettuce is included for comparison only. It is not one of my favorites, and I don't recommend it. As you can see above, romaine lettuce has eight times more vitamin A and six times more vitamin C than iceberg lettuce.

– Indicates data not available.

Native to the eastern Mediterranean region and western Asia, the cultivation of lettuce is thought to date back to at least 4,500 BC In fact, depictions of lettuce appeared in ancient Egyptian tombs. Both the ancient Greeks and Romans held lettuce in high regard both as a food and for its therapeutic medicinal properties. The word "Salad" comes from the Latin word *salata*, meaning "salted." During the time of the Roman Empire, a common meal consisted of vegetables that had been seasoned with brine, olive oil and vinegar; it was called *herba salata*, or "salted vegetables." I like this original meaning of the word "Salad" because I think that vegetables are such an important part of what Salads are all about!

# salads and dressings

## why salads should be part of your healthiest way of eating

A Salad containing a wide variety of vegetables—including root vegetables, green leafy vegetables, stalks, stems and flowers—makes a great foundation upon which to build a complete meal.

The use of seeds, nuts, and beans in Salads is extremely helpful in contributing protein, fiber, minerals and omega-3 fatty acids to the meal. Small amounts of "garnish" ingredients—like a tablespoon of pumpkin seeds or a sprinkling of walnuts—are a very worthwhile addition in terms of nutrients. Trace minerals and small amounts of high-quality omega-3 fats are nutrients of which most U.S. adults don't get nearly enough, and it doesn't take many pumpkin seeds or walnuts to bring at least some of these vital nutrients into the day's meal plan.

A variety of lettuce and greens provide health-promoting phytonutrients. For example, different Salad greens offer distinct flavonoid phytonutrients. Green leaf varieties have the flavonoid quercetin, but you'll need red leaves to get any of the cyanidin flavonoids. To get good supplies of kaempferol, you may want to include some endive. The different colors in the leaves may not seem significant, but each shading represents a different combination of flavonoids and other pigments; researchers are continually learning about different ways in which these flavonoids and pigments help prevent disease.

## what makes a nutritious salad?

The best Salad includes a variety of different types of lettuce. Not only will including a variety of lettuces in your meal plan allow you to enjoy a host of different flavors and textures, but you can also enjoy the range of nutrients that each lettuce variety has to offer. And offer nutritional value they do! In fact, many lettuces really pack a punch when it comes to their vitamin and mineral content. As you see from the chart on the previous page, the different varieties are nutritionally distinct.

Fortunately, there's an amazing variety to choose from. Lettuce can usually be divided into four basic varieties:

### ROMAINE

Also known as Cos, this variety of head-forming lettuce has deep green, long leaves with a crisp texture and robust flavor. Paris Island is the most popular variety featuring a semi-dark green, stiff, upright leaf. Green Towers, with slightly larger leaves, and Cimmaron, an unusual dark red Cos type, are also available in some areas.

### BUTTERHEAD

This type of lettuce features tender large leaves, which form a loosely arranged head that is easily separated from the stem. It has a sweet flavor and a soft texture. The best known varieties of Butterhead lettuce include Boston and Bibb.

### LEAF LETTUCE

A favorite of many home gardeners. Featuring broad, curly leaves that are green and/or red, the leaf lettuces offer a delicate taste and a mildly crisp texture. This variety is much more delicate than the crisp-head variety and also much more diverse and flavorful. Best known varieties of leaf lettuce include green leaf and red leaf. Green leaf lettuces include Black-seeded Simpsons, Grand Rapids and Oak Leaf lettuce. Red leaf varieties include Red Fire, Red Sails and Ruby.

### PREPACKAGED MIXED GREENS

These prewashed and ready-to-use greens save a lot of time. Organic mixed greens come in three varieties: Salad mix, spring mix and herb mix. They have a longer shelf life because packages are sealed so that the greens have no contact with the air.

Special names for mixed greens are, in fact, part of the everyday language in France and Italy. For the French, mixed greens are often described under the heading of "mesclumo." Mesclumo is part of the Niçois dialect and means "mixture." In the United States, mesclumo is usually referred to as "mesclun mix."

The idea of a greens mix in France is not simply to get any old mixture of greens. The idea is to combine four basic flavor types through a careful mixing of greens: mild, bitter/tart, piquant and pepper/spicy. For the mild component, a leaf lettuce will typically be included. For the piquant, perhaps mustard greens. For the bitter/tart flavor, either radicchio, escarole, mizuna or curly endive. To round out the peppery/spicy component, usually included is either arugula or watercress.

## Sprouts

Sprouts can make great toppings for Salads. They are also a great addition to sandwiches.

In the life of a plant, sprouting is a moment of great vitality and energy. The seed, after having remained quiet, often for a long period of time, becomes more and more active and begins its journey up through the topsoil and into the open air. When it sprouts, a healthy seed activates many different metabolic systems. It converts some of its sugar content into vitamin C to act as an antioxidant in the new open air environment. It also begins to synthesize a variety of new enzymes, many of them necessary to handle oxygen metabolism in the world above the soil. On a gram for gram basis, sprouts are richer in vitamin C than the older, more mature plants they eventually become because this moment in their lifecyle calls for a high level of vitality. Sprouts can definitely be good for you!

For you to get the benefit of healthy sprouts, the sprouts need to be very fresh and carefully refrigerated and handled. Most any kind of seed could also be sprouted at home, using one part seed to three parts water, a wide-mouth glass jar and a screened lid. Many health food stores and natural foods groceries have sprouting starter kits that make the process easy to understand and complete. It's worth noting here that seeds are smart, and some will not do much sprouting in polluted tap water, making a cleaner water source (like bottled spring water or filtered water) a better choice when sprouting. Although mung bean sprouts and alfalfa sprouts are the most common commercially available sprouts, equally easy-to-sprout and healthy are red clover, radish, mustard, lentil, adzuki, garbanzo, pumpkin seeds and sunflower seeds. One word of caution about alfalfa: this seed has higher than usual amounts of an amino acid called canavanine, and some research studies have associated canavanine with worsening of inflammatory conditions including rheumatoid arthritis and systemic lupus erythematosus. Individuals with chronic inflammatory conditions, including autoimmune conditions, may want to avoid alfalfa sprouts for this reason.

If you decide to include raw sprouts in your "Healthiest Way of Eating" for their health benefits, here are some steps you can take to help make sure that they are safe to eat:

- Wash all sprouts thoroughly with filtered water before eating them.

- Look for the International Sprout Growers Association (ISGA) seal on the package. If you are buying bulk, ask your grocery if the sprouts are ISGA-approved.

- If the sprouts are prepackaged, only purchase if the sell-by date is current or even a few days ahead.

- If you're buying in bulk, ask your grocery about the sell-by date.

- Examine the sprouts to make sure the roots are clean. If the stem color is not white or creamy, do not purchase them. Do not purchase sprouts if the buds are no longer attached, if they are dark in color or have a musty smell.

- Keep the sprouts refrigerated.

- After 2 days, compost them rather than consuming them yourself.

- If you are sprouting seeds at home, follow the same guidelines described above. Learn about the source of your seeds, their ISGA certification, and either have your grocery confirm high-quality standards for seed production or obtain contact information for the seed source and contact that company yourself.

- Follow the above guidelines regardless of the type of seeds you are sprouting, i.e., apply the guidelines to mung, alfalfa, radish, broccoli, lentil, sunflower and all other types of sprouts.

## how to make a tasty salad

It is easy to make a tasty Salad. Salad greens are often pre-mixed and prewashed (although I always like to wash them again). Since conventionally grown lettuce has been found to have a high concentration of pesticide residues, always try to buy organically grown varieties.

To make a good tasting Salad, I always start with crisp, vibrantly colored lettuce with no signs of yellowing or wilting. Cleaning lettuce and greens is pretty simple. If you are using a head variety lettuce, first remove the outer leaves. For all lettuces, you can slice off the tips of the leaves, since they tend to be bitter, and discard the bottom root portion. Chop the remaining lettuce, rinse and pat dry or use a Salad spinner, if you have one available, to remove the excess water.

Wash loose Salad greens like you would spinach. Trim their roots and separate the leaves, placing them in a large bowl of tepid water and swishing them around with your hands. This will allow any sand to become dislodged. Remove the leaves from the water, empty the bowl, refill with clean water and repeat this process until no dirt remains in the water (usually two or three times will do the trick).

Drying Salad greens well helps to prevent diluting your dressing. Dry Salad greens require less dressing and therefore will create a Salad that contains fewer calories and more flavor. To dry Salad greens, I love to use a Salad spinner.

## Salad Spinners

One obstacle to eating fresh, raw vegetables is the time it takes to clean and chop them. Using a Salad spinner can help you throw together a fresh, nutritious Salad, even when you are in a hurry. Salad spinners are available at kitchen shops (a $25–$30 investment); make sure to get one with a tight fitting lid. All Salad spinners have the same basic design elements including an inner basket that fits into a larger bowl with gears that are connected to a mechanism on the lid. Turning or pumping a handle on the top of the lid causes the inner basket to spin rapidly; the resulting centrifugal force pulls the greens to the side of the basket and the water on the leaves into the outer bowl. The different types of spinners seem to work equally well for drying greens; using a Salad spinner definitely beats patting greens with a towel!

Chop or shred the lettuce into bite-size pieces and place the lettuce into the inner bowl of your spinner. Carefully wash the lettuce with cold water, and then return the inner bowl to fit inside the outer bowl and spin the lettuce dry in the Salad spinner. The spinning process only takes about one minute. Next, empty the liquid in the bottom of the Salad spinner—you can either keep it and use it for soup stock or just discard it into your vegetable garden. Then replace the lid on the spinner and put the whole container in the refrigerator until you are ready for Salad. When stored in your Salad spinner, this clean, chopped lettuce will keep in the refrigerator for two days.

With a bowl full of already washed and chopped lettuce, you'll enjoy eating Salad with more and more meals. (One side note: if you decide to try spinning vegetables in your Salad spinner along with the lettuce, make sure you stick with the more solid, less watery type of vegetable. For example, green pepper slices and carrot slices can spin right along with the lettuce, but cucumbers and tomatoes can't—their watery nature cannot withstand the pressure of the spinner, and they will break apart in the process.)

STEP-BY-STEP RECIPE
## The Healthiest Way to Make Salad

# 5-Minute Green Salad with Healthy Vinaigrette

My preferred Salad dressing is made of one part freshly squeezed lemon juice to three parts extra virgin olive oil. I prefer lemon to vinegar because it is less acidic. Sea salt and freshly ground black pepper are good additions.

**4 cups Salad greens (romaine, green leaf, red leaf, Boston, prepackaged mixed greens)**

**Healthy Vinaigrette Dressing:**
**3 TBS extra virgin olive oil**
**1 TBS fresh lemon juice or balsamic vinegar**
**Sea salt and pepper to taste**

1. Combine lemon juice or balsamic vinegar, extra

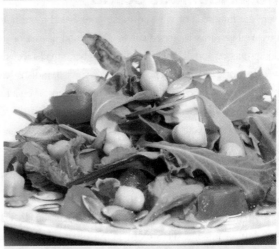

Green Salad with Healthy Vinaigrette

virgin olive oil and salt and pepper. Whisk in the olive oil a little at a time for a more well integrated dressing.

2. Toss Salad greens with dressing just before serving.

**SERVES 2**

### 10 VARIATIONS for HEALTHY VINAIGRETTE DRESSING:

1. **French:** add 1 tsp of Dijon mustard
2. **Asian:** add a few drops of tamari (soy sauce)
3. **Ginger:** add 1/2 tsp of grated ginger
4. **Parsley:** add 1 TBS parsley
5. **Chives:** add 1 tsp of chives
6. **Garlic:** add 1 clove pressed garlic
7. **Basil:** add 6 leaves of fresh chopped basil
8. **Italian Herb:** add 2 tsp chopped fresh rosemary and 1 tsp chopped fresh oregano
9. **Anchovy/Capers:** add 5 anchovy fillets and 1 tsp capers
10. **Creamy:** add 2 TBS low-fat plain yogurt

### HOW TO KEEP YOUR SALAD CRISP:

Because the ingredients in the dressing pull the moisture from your Salad greens, which causes them to wilt, I always like my dressing on the side, so I don't have to dress my entire Salad at one time. Dressing only small sections of Salad at any one time prevents the lettuce from wilting and avoids using excessive amounts of dressing, which adds extra calories to your meal. Cold plates also help keep Salads crisp. Research shows that the carotenoids found in foods are best absorbed when consumed with oils.

## Flavor Tips: Try these 11 great serving suggestions with the recipe above. ✱

1. To boost the flavor, add arugula, watercress, endive, radicchio, dandelion, fennel, chicory, sprouts and escarole to your Salad greens.
2. Add herbs such as basil, cilantro, mint, rosemary or oregano.
3. For even more flavor, add tomatoes, cucumbers, red bell peppers, summer squash, peas, radishes, scallions, carrots, fennel, celery, mushrooms, beets or avocado.
4. You can also add vegetables such as baby spinach, Swiss chard, kale, napa cabbage or mustard greens.

**For a complete meal:**
5. Add beans, such as garbanzo beans or kidney beans.
6. Add grains, such as rice, barley, couscous or bulgur.
7. Add nuts, such as walnuts, peanuts, sliced almonds or cashews.
8. Add seeds, such as sunflower, pumpkin or ground flaxseeds.
9. Add shrimp, scallops, salmon, turkey or grilled chicken.
10. Add cheese, olives or eggs.
11. Add apricots, apples, raisins, pears, oranges, grapefruit or figs.

# How to Make a Most Nutritious Salad

There are hundreds of ways to make your Salad more nutritious. You can mix in grated carrots, beets and jicama or just add sprouts on top. Thin slices of cucumber, small pieces of sweet red or green bell pepper, summer squash, radish, scallions, cherry tomatoes, a sprinkling of nuts or seeds, even a few freshly washed berries…any and all make tasty colorful additions. Make sure your Salad has a rainbow of colors to maximize not only eye appeal, but flavor and nutritional value. Here are several ideas for healthy salads and dressings.

## Quick and Healthy Caesar Salad:

In a small bowl, combine 1 clove pressed garlic, 2 TBS fresh lemon juice, 2 TBS extra virgin olive oil, 2 minced anchovies, 1 TBS Parmesan cheese, and salt and pepper to taste. Toss 4 cups of romaine lettuce with dressing. Top with 1/4 cup walnuts.

## Waldorf Salad:

Combine in a mixing bowl: 1 cup cooked diced chicken breast, 1 diced apple, 1 diced celery stalk, 1/4 cup chopped walnuts, 2 TBS chopped parsley, 3 TBS extra virgin olive oil, 2 TBS fresh lemon juice and sea salt and pepper to taste.

## Minted Greek Salad:

Combine 4 cups Salad greens, 2 TBS chopped mint, 3 TBS crumbled feta cheese, 2 TBS chopped olives, and salt and pepper to taste. Toss with 3 TBS extra virgin olive oil and 1 TBS red wine vinegar. For a variation of this salad, see page 289.

## Salad Niçoise:

This Salad is made with ingredients you have on hand. Be creative. Here are the basic ingredients: 2 cups of Salad greens, canned tuna, sliced tomatoes, chopped anchovies, chopped olives, chopped onions and capers. Top with your favorite vinaigrette. For more details, see page 181.

## Tomato-Mozzarella Salad:

Slice 2 large, ripe tomatoes and arrange on a platter. Add one slice of fresh buffalo mozzarella cheese and one basil leaf to each tomato slice. Whisk together 1/4 cup extra virgin olive oil, 2 TBS balsamic vinegar, 2 cloves pressed garlic, and sea salt and pepper to taste. Drizzle dressing over tomato, cheese and basil mixture.

## Healthy Chef's Salad:

Top 4 cups of chopped mixed greens (spinach, romaine, arugula) with 4 oz chicken or turkey slices, 4 oz grated low-fat cheese (cheddar, goat cheese or blue cheese), and 1/4 cup each of cucumbers, tomatoes, bell peppers and celery. Sprinkle with 3 TBS walnuts and your favorite Healthy Vinaigrette (see page 143).

## Blue Cheese Dressing and Dip:

| | |
|---|---|
| 8 oz blue cheese, crumbled | 1 TBS fresh lemon juice |
| 1/2 cup low-fat yogurt | 1/2 tsp fresh thyme |
| 1 cup low-fat buttermilk | Salt and pepper to taste |

Put everything, except blue cheese, in blender and blend until smooth. Add blue cheese and pulse 2–3 times.

## French Dressing:

| | |
|---|---|
| 1/2 cup extra virgin olive oil | 2 TBS honey |
| 1 TBS onion, chopped fine | 1 tsp paprika |
| 4-1/2 tsp red wine vinegar | 1/2 tsp celery seeds |
| 2 tsp tomato paste | Salt and pepper to taste |
| 1 tsp dried mustard | |

In a blender, blend all ingredients except olive oil and salt and pepper until smooth. With blender running, slowly pour in olive oil until emulsified. Season to taste with sea salt and pepper.

*(Continued from Page 145)*

The following essential nutrients are not found in spinach but are important in our diet.

| NUTRIENT | AMOUNT | % DAILY VALUE | * DAILY VALUE | WHAT WILL IT DO FOR YOU | SUGGESTS YOU NEED MORE |
|---|---|---|---|---|---|
| **Vitamin B12** | | | 6 mcg | Prevents anemia; Allows nerve cells to develop properly; Helps cells metabolize protein, carbohydrates and fats | Tingling or numbness in feet; Red or sore tongue Depression; Nervousness; Memory problems |
| **Vitamin D** | | | 400 IU | Helps keep bones and teeth strong and healthy Helps prevent excessive inflammatory immune-related activity | Thinning bones; Frequent bone fractures / soft bones Lack of exposure to sunlight; Bone deformities in children |
| **Iodine** | | | 150 mcg | Helps insure proper thyroid function | Goiter; Depression; Fatigue; Weight gain |

* DV are for 4+years.

Scientific studies show that nutrients in foods work synergistically to provide vibrant health and energy. Example: For bone health, you need more than just calcium. You also need vitamin K, magnesium, copper, phosphorus, vitamin D and other phytonutrients to absorb calcium and help promote strong bones.

# Q&A
## WHY IS IT IMPORTANT TO EAT NUTRIENT-RICH FOODS LIKE THE WORLD'S HEALTHIEST FOODS?

The World's Healthiest Foods are concentrated in important nutrients that the body needs to promote optimal health. As an example, the chart below shows the nutrient richness of spinach and describes the essential functions of each nutrient and how it contributes to energy, health and vitality.

1 cup of boiled spinach: **(180 grams): 41 calories**

| NUTRIENT | AMOUNT | % DAILY VALUE | * DAILY VALUE | WHAT WILL IT DO FOR YOU | SUGGESTS YOU NEED MORE |
|---|---|---|---|---|---|
| **Vitamin K*** | 888.5 mcg | 1110.6 | 80 mcg | Allows blood to clot normally; Helps absorption of calcium and prevents osteoporosis | Excessive bruising and bleeding Digestion, liver and gallbladder problems |
| **Vitamin A** | 14,742.0 IU | 294.8 | 5,000 IU | Preserves and improves eyesight Fights viral infections/colds and flu | Goose bumps appear on skin Frequent infections; Night blindness |
| **Manganese** | 1.7 mg | 84.0 | 2 mg | Protects from free-radical damage; Keeps bones strong and healthy; Supports thyroid gland and nerves | High blood sugar level; Excessive bone loss Loss of hair color; Skin rash; Low cholesterol levels |
| **Folic Acid** | 262.4 mcg | 65.5 | 400 mcg | Supports red blood cell production; Supports heart health; Allows nerves to function properly | Depression; Irritability; Mental fatigue Confusion; Forgetfulness; Insomnia |
| **Magnesium** | 156.6 | 39.1 | 400 mg | Relaxes nerves and muscles Builds and strengthens bones | Muscle weakness, tremors or spasms Elevated blood pressure; Headaches |
| **Iron** | 6.5 mg | 35.7 | 18 mg | Enhances oxygen distribution in body; Keeps immune system healthy; Helps energy production | Fatigue and weakness; Hair loss/brittle nails Headache/dizziness; Decrease ability to concentrate |
| **Vitamin C** | 17.6 mg | 29.4 | 60 mg | Helps protect cells from free-radical damage Improves iron absorption; Lowers cancer risk | Frequent colds and infections Lung-related problems; Poor wound healing |
| **B2 Riboflavin** | .0.4 mg | 24.7 | 1.7 mg | Helps protect cells from oxygen damage Supports cellular energy production | Sensitivity to light; Tearing, burning, itching of eyes; Soreness around lips, mouth and tongue Cracking of the skin in corners of the mouth |
| **Calcium** | 244.8 mg | 24.5 | 1,000 mg | Maintains healthy strong bones Supports proper functioning of nerves and muscles | Tingling and numbness of hands and feet Muscular pain and spasms |
| **Potassium** | 838.8 mg | 24.0 | 3,500 mg | Lowers risk of high blood pressure Helps maintain pH balance | Muscular weakness; Confusion; Irritability Fatigue; Heart problems; Chronic diarrhea |
| **B6 Pyrodoxine** | 0.4 mg | 22.0 | 2 mg | Supports nervous system health; Promotes proper breakdown of sugar and starches | Fatigue; Anemia Skin disorders including eczema and dermatitis |
| **Tryptophan** | 0.1 g | 29.9 | 3.5 mg/kg | Promotes better sleep Helps regulate appetite; Elevates mood | Overeating or carbohydrate cravings Depression; Anxiety; Inability to concentrate |
| **Dietary Fiber** | 4.3 g | 17.3 | 25 g | Supports bowel regularity; Helps maintain normal cholesterol and blood sugar levels | Constipation; Hemorrhoids; High blood sugar levels; High cholesterol levels |
| **Copper** | 0.3 mg | 15.5 | 2 mg | Maintains the health of bones and connective tissue; Keeps thyroid gland functioning normally | Blood vessels that rupture easily Frequent infections; Loss of hair or skin color |
| **B1 Thiamin** | 0.2 mg | 11.3 | 1.5 mg | Maintains your energy supplies Supports proper heart function | Pins and needles sensations; Feeling of numbness, especially in legs; Muscular tenderness |
| **Protein** | 5.4 g | 10.7 | 50 g | Maintains healthy skin, hair and nails Keeps immune system functioning properly | Weight loss; Muscle wasting Fatigue and weakness; Frequent infections |
| **Phosphorus** | 100.8 mg | 10.1 | 1,000 mg | Helps form bones and teeth Vital for energy production | Weakness; Weight loss; Irritability; Anxiety Increased incidence of hypertension |
| **Zinc** | 11.4 mg | 9.1 | 15 mg | Helps balance blood sugar; Supports optimal sense of smell and taste | Frequent colds and infections; Depression Impaired sense of taste and smell |
| **Vitamin E** | 1.7 mg | 8.6 | 30 IU | Prevents cell damage from free radicals Protects skin from ultra violet lights | Tingling or loss of sensation in arms, hands, legs and feet; Digestive system problems (malabsorption) |
| **Omega-3 Fatty Acids** | 0.2 g | 6.0 | 2.5 g | Reduces inflammation throughout body Keeps blood from clotting excessively | Dry, itchy skin; Brittle hair and nails; Fatigue Depression; Inability to concentrate; Joint pain |
| **B3 Niacin** | 0.9 mg | 4.4 | 20 mg | Stabilizes blood sugar levels; Helps lower cholesterol levels; Helps body process fat | Muscular weakness; Skin infections Lack of appetite; Digestive problems |
| **Selenium** | 2.7 mcg | 3.9 | 70 mcg | Protects cells from free-radical damage Enables thyroid hormone production | Whitening of fingernail beds; Weakness and pain in muscles; Discoloration of hair and skin |
| **Beta-carotene** | 11,318.4 mcg | | Not established | Protects cells from radicals Promotes eye and lung health Enhances functioning of immune system | Low intake of fruits and vegetables Smoking Regular alcohol consumption |
| **Lutein+ zeaxanthin** | 20,354.4 mcg | | | | |

* For more information on the individual nutrients, see page 733.

For more on *Daily Values* see page 805.

*(Chart continues on Page 144)*

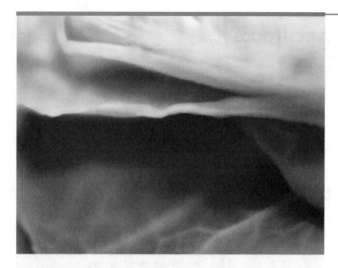

## nutrient-richness chart

Total Nutrient-Richness: **38**  GI: **15**

One cup (190 grams) of cooked Collard Greens contains 49 calories

| NUTRIENT | AMOUNT | %DV | DENSITY | QUALITY |
|---|---|---|---|---|
| Vitamin K | 704.0 mcg | 880.0 | 320.6 | excellent |
| Vitamin A | 5945.1 IU | 118.9 | 43.3 | excellent |
| Vitamin C | 34.6 mg | 57.6 | 21.0 | excellent |
| Manganese | 1.1 mg | 53.5 | 19.5 | excellent |
| Folate | 176.7 mcg | 44.2 | 16.1 | excellent |
| Calcium | 226.1 mg | 22.6 | 8.2 | excellent |
| Dietary Fiber | 5.3 g | 21.3 | 7.8 | excellent |
| Tryptophan | 0.1 g | 15.6 | 5.7 | very good |
| Potassium | 494.0 mg | 14.1 | 5.1 | very good |
| B6 Pyridoxine | 0.2 mg | 12.0 | 4.4 | very good |
| B2 Riboflavin | 0.2 mg | 11.8 | 4.3 | very good |
| Vitamin E | 1.7 mg | 8.3 | 3.0 | good |
| Magnesium | 32.3 mg | 8.1 | 2.9 | good |
| Protein | 4.0 g | 8.0 | 2.9 | good |
| Omega-3 Fatty Acids | 0.2 g | 7.2 | 2.6 | good |
| B3 Niacin | 1.1 mg | 5.5 | 2.0 | good |
| B1 Thiamin | 0.1 mg | 5.3 | 1.9 | good |
| Zinc | 0.8 mg | 5.3 | 1.9 | good |
| Phosphorus | 49.4 mg | 4.9 | 1.8 | good |
| Iron | 0.9 mg | 4.8 | 1.8 | good |
| B5 Pantothenic Acid | 0.4 mg | | | |

### CAROTENOIDS:

| | | |
|---|---|---|
| Alpha-Carotene | 171.0 mcg | |
| Beta-Carotene | 9,146.6 mcg | |
| Beta-Cryptoxanthin | 38.0 mcg | |
| Lutein+Zeaxanthin | 14,618.6 mcg | |

Daily values for these nutrients have not yet been established.

For more on "Total Nutrient-Richness," "%DV," "Density," and The World's Healthiest Foods "Quality" Rating System, see page 805.

For more on GI, see page 342.

# collard greens

## highlights

| | |
|---|---|
| AVAILABILITY: | Year-round |
| REFRIGERATE: | Yes |
| SHELF LIFE: | 5 days refrigerated |
| PREPARATION: | Cut and let sit for 5 minutes |
| BEST WAY TO COOK: | "Healthy Steamed" in just 5 minutes |

Collard Greens are native to the Mediterranean and were popular with both the ancient Greeks and Romans. Their smoky flavor and meaty texture have long made them a staple in the Southern United States, and they are now becoming increasingly popular throughout the rest of the country. If you are not familiar with Collard Greens, I highly recommend you try them. Proper preparation of Collard Greens is the key to bringing out their best flavor and maximizing their nutritional benefits. That is why I want to share with you the secret of the "Healthiest Way of Cooking" Collard Greens *al denté*. In just 5 minutes, you will be able to serve Collard Greens with the most flavor and the maximum nutritional value.

## why collard greens should be part of your healthiest way of eating

Although cultivated since ancient times, Collard Greens' many nutritional benefits have only been recently identified. Scientific studies now show that cruciferous vegetables, like Collard Greens, are included among the vegetables that contain the largest concentrations of health-promoting sulfur compounds such as glucosinolates and the methyl cysteine sulfoxides (see page 153), which increase the liver's ability to produce enzymes that neutralize potentially toxic substances. Collard Greens are also an exceptional source of the powerful phytonutrient antioxidants lutein and zeaxanthin. And if you want to increase your calcium intake, Collard Greens are one of the best plant-based sources of this important mineral. Collard

Greens are an ideal food to add to your "Healthiest Way of Eating" not only because they are high in nutrients, but also because they are low in calories: one cup of cooked Collard Greens contains only 49 calories. (For more on the *Health Benefits of Collard Greens* and a complete analysis of their content of over 60 nutrients, see page 150.)

## varieties of collard greens

Collard Greens (*Brassica Oleracea* var. *viridis*) are one of the non-head forming members of the cruciferous family of vegetables, which also includes broccoli, cauliflower, kale, cabbage, mustard greens and Brussels sprouts. While Collard Greens and kale share the same botanical name, they each have their own distinctive qualities. The most popular and widely available variety of Collard Greens features dark, relatively broad, blue-green leaves, which are smooth in texture and lack the frilled edges characteristic of their cousin, kale. This is the variety featured in the photographs in this chapter.

## the peak season

Collard Greens are available throughout the year, but their flavor is at its peak during the cold months when the frost helps to develop a sweet flavor. In hotter months, Collard Greens are less tender and will require around 1 minute additional cooking time.

## biochemical considerations

Collard Greens are a concentrated source of goitrogens and oxalates, which might be of concern to certain individuals. (For more on: *Goitrogens,* see page 721; and *Oxalates*, see page 725.)

## 4 steps for the best tasting and most nutritious collard greens

Turning Collard Greens into a flavorful dish with the most nutrients is simple if you just follow my 4 easy steps:

1. The Best Way to Select
2. The Best Way to Store
3. The Best Way to Prepare
4. The Healthiest Way of Cooking

# 1. the best way to select collard greens

You can select the best tasting Collard Greens by looking for varieties that have firm, fresh leaves with a vivid, bright, deep green color. I have found that Collard Greens with smaller leaves are usually the best because they are more tender and have a milder flavor. By selecting the best tasting Collard Greens, you will also enjoy those with the highest nutritional value. As with all vegetables, I recommend selecting organically grown varieties whenever possible. (For more on *Organic Foods*, see page 113.)

Avoid Collard Greens that show signs of yellowing or browning.

# 2. the best way to store collard greens

Collard Greens are delicate and will wilt and turn yellow if not stored properly. If care is not taken with their storage, they can also lose much of their flavor and up to 30% of some of their vitamins.

Collard Greens continue to respire even after they have been harvested. Slowing down the respiration rate with proper storage is the key to extending their flavor and nutritional benefits. (For a *Comparison of Respiration Rates* for different vegetables, see page 91.)

### Collard Greens Will Remain Fresh for Up to 5 Days When Properly Stored

1. Store Collard Greens in the refrigerator. The colder temperature will slow the respiration rate, helping to preserve their nutrients and keeping Collard Greens fresh for a longer period of time.

2. Place Collard Greens in a plastic storage bag before refrigerating. I have found that it is best to wrap the bag tightly around the Collard Greens, squeezing out as much of the air from the bag as possible.

3. Do not wash Collard Greens before refrigeration because exposure to water will encourage Collard Greens to spoil.

# 3. the best way to prepare collard greens

Whether you are going to enjoy Collard Greens raw or cooked, as a side dish or part of a main dish, I want to share with you the best way to prepare Collard Greens. Properly cleaning and cutting Collard Greens helps to ensure that the Collard Greens you serve will have the best flavor and retain the greatest number of nutrients.

### Cleaning Collard Greens

Discard damaged and discolored leaves. Rinse well under cold running water before cutting. To preserve nutrients, do not soak Collard Greens or their water-soluble nutrients will leach into the water. (For more on *Washing Vegetables*, see page 92.)

### Cutting Collard Greens

Separating the stems from leaves and throwing the stems away was the old method of preparing Collard Greens; I encourage you to eat the stems as they are juicy, succulent and enjoyable to eat. You can cut both the stems and leaves at the same time by using one of two methods. You can either stack the leaves or roll the entire bunch of Collard Greens

and then cut the leafy portion into 1/2-inch slices. Cut crosswise as well. To get the best flavor and texture, it is important to cut Collard Greens into small pieces.

When you reach the point where there is no more of the leafy portion to slice and only the stems remain, begin cutting thinner slices (1/4-inch) and continue cutting to within the bottom inch of the stem; discard the last bottom inch as it is fibrous. Let sit for at least 5 minutes after cutting.

Slicing Collard Greens thin will help them to cook more quickly. The thinner you slice them, the more quickly they will cook. Cutting the stems thinner than the leaves helps them to cook at the same rate and, unless the stems are very thick, allows you to cook them together. The stems and leaves provide a good balance of flavors.

### What To Do with Thick Stems

If the stem portions below the leaf are thick, you may want to cook them for 2–3 minutes before adding the leaf portion of the Collard Greens. Discard stems that are woody and hollow.

# 4. the healthiest way of cooking collard greens

Since research has shown that important nutrients can be lost or destroyed by the way a food is cooked, the "Healthiest Way of Cooking" Collard Greens is focused on bringing out their best flavor while maximizing retention of their vitamins, minerals and powerful antioxidants.

### The Healthiest Way of Cooking Collard Greens: "Healthy Steaming" for Just 5 Minutes

In my search to find the healthiest way to cook Collard Greens, I tested every possible cooking method and discovered that "Healthy Steaming" for just 5 minutes delivered the best result. "Healthy Steaming" provides the moisture necessary to make Collard Greens tender and brings out their peak flavor, retains their bright color and maximizes their nutritional profile. The Step-by-Step Recipe will show you how easy it is to "Healthy Steam" Collard Greens. (For more on *"Healthy Steaming,"* see page 58.)

### How to Avoid Overcooking Collard Greens: Cook Them *Al Denté*

One of the primary reasons people do not enjoy Collard Greens is because they are often overcooked. For the best flavor and texture, I recommend cooking Collard Greens *al denté*. Collard Greens cooked *al denté* are tender outside and slightly firm inside. Plus, Collard Greens cooked *al denté* are cooked just long enough to soften their cellulose and hemicellulose; this makes them easier to digest and allows their health-promoting nutrients to become more readily available for assimilation. Remember that testing Collard Greens with a fork is not an effective way to determine whether they are done.

Although Collard Greens are a hearty vegetable, it is very important not to overcook them. Collard Greens cooked for as little as a couple of minutes longer than *al denté* will begin to lose not only their texture and flavor but also their nutrients. Overcooking Collard Greens will significantly decrease their nutritional value: as much as 50% of some nutrients can be lost. (For more on *Al Denté*, see page 92.)

## How to Prevent Strong Smells from Forming

Slicing Collard Greens thin (1/2-inch) and cooking them *al denté* for only 5 minutes is my secret for preventing the formation of smelly compounds often associated with cooking Collard Greens. When I cook my Collard Greens, they never develop a strong smell. After 5 minutes of cooking, the texture of Collard Greens, like all other cruciferous vegetables, begins to change, becoming increasingly soft and mushy. At this point, they also start to lose more and more of their chlorophyll, causing their bright green color to fade and a brownish hue to appear. This is a sign that magnesium has been lost. This is when they start to release hydrogen sulfide, the cause of the "rotten egg smell," which also affects their flavor. After 7 minutes of cooking, Collard Greens develop a more intense flavor, with the amount of strong smelling hydrogen sulfide doubling in quantity.

While it is important not to overcook Collard Greens, cooking for less than 5 minutes is also not recommended because it takes about 5 minutes to soften their fibers and help increase their digestibility.

## Cooking Methods Not Recommended for Collard Greens

### SAUTÉING", BOILING, BAKING OR COOKING WITH OIL

You will not get good results by "Healthy Sautéing" Collard Greens. They have a low moisture content, which causes them to dry out when sautéed and become scorched before they become tender. I do not recommend boiling Collard Greens because boiling increases their water absorption causing them to become soggy and lose much of their flavor along with many of their nutrients, including minerals, water-soluble vitamins (such as C and the B-complex vita-mins) and health-promoting phytonutrients. Baking Collard Greens will cause them to dry up and shrivel.

I also don't recommend cooking Collard Greens in oil because high temperature heat can damage delicate oils and potentially create harmful free radicals.

---

### HOW TO BRING OUT THE HIDDEN HEALTH BENEFITS OF COLLARD GREENS

The latest scientific studies show that cutting Collard Greens into thin slices breaks down cell walls and enhances the activation of an enzyme called *myrosinase* that slowly converts some of the plant nutrients into their active forms, which have been shown to contain health-promoting properties. So, to get the most health benefits from Collard Greens, let them sit for a minimum of 5 minutes, and optimally 10 minutes, after cutting, before eating or cooking.

Since ascorbic acid (vitamin C) increases *myrosinase* activity, you can sprinkle a little lemon juice on the Collard Greens before letting them sit in order to further enhance their beneficial phytonutrient concentration.

Heat will inactivate the effect of *myrosinase*, which is why it is important to allow the Collard Greens to sit for 5–10 minutes before cooking to give the enzyme ample opportunity to enhance the concentration of active phytonutrients in your Collard Greens. Cooking at low or medium heat for short periods of time (up to 15 minutes) should not destroy the active phytonutrients since once they are formed, they are fairly stable.

---

## An Easy Way to Prepare Collard Greens, Step-By-Step

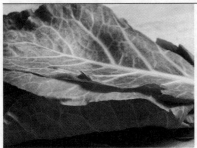 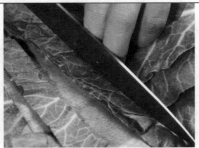 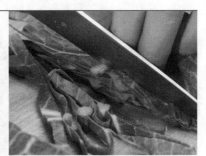

### CHOPPED COLLARD GREENS

❶ Stack Collard Greens, and either roll them or leave them stacked on top of each other. ❷ Cut into 1/2-inch slices until you reach the stem. ❸ Cut stem portion into 1/4-inch slices.

# health benefits of collard greens

## Promote Optimal Health

As a *Brassica* vegetable, Collard Greens stand out as a food that has important health-promoting qualities. The organosulfur compounds in Collard Greens that have been the main subject of phytonutrient research are the glucosinolates and the methyl cysteine sulfoxides. Although there are over 100 different glucosinolates in plants, only 10–15 are present in Collard Greens and other *Brassicas*. Yet these 10–15 glucosinolates appear able to reduce the risk of a wide variety of cancers, including breast and ovarian cancers. Exactly how Collard Greens' sulfur-containing phytonutrients prevent cancer is not clear, but several researchers point to the ability of the glucosinolates and cysteine sulfoxides to activate detoxifying enzymes in the liver that help neutralize potentially carcinogenic substances.

## Promote Bone Health

If you are concerned about building or maintaining strong bones, Collard Greens are a great food for you. They are a dairy-free alternative for those seeking foods rich in calcium (they are an excellent source of this important nutrient). In addition, Collard Greens are also an excellent source of folic acid and a very good source of vitamin B6, nutrients that reduce levels of homocysteine; while homocysteine is usually associated with heart disease risk it has also been found to be damaging to bone structure as well.

## Promote Antioxidant Protection

Collard Greens qualify as an excellent source of vitamin C and vitamin A (through their concentration of beta-carotene) and a very good source of vitamin E. While water-soluble vitamin C protects all aqueous environments both inside and outside cells, the fat-soluble antioxidants, vitamin E and beta-carotene, cover all fat-containing molecules and structures. They are also rich in manganese and zinc, two minerals that have important antioxidant properties.

## Promote Vision Health

Collard Greens contain an abundance of lutein and zeaxanthin. In fact, they are the fourth most concentrated source of these carotenoids of all of the World's Healthiest Foods. Lutein and zeaxanthin are powerful antioxidants that protect the eye from free-radical damage. Consumption of these carotenoids has been found to be associated with reduced risk of cataracts and age-related macular degeneration. Additionally, Collard Greens' vitamin A also has vision health benefits, including promoting the eye's adaptation to dark and light.

## Additional Health-Promoting Benefits of Collard Greens

Collard Greens are also a concentrated source of many other nutrients providing additional health-promoting benefits. These nutrients include heart-healthy dietary fiber,

*(Continued on Page 152)*

---

### New Scientific Finding

**HOW NUTRITIOUS ARE THE STEMS OF COLLARD GREENS?**

Collard Greens' stems are great for adding more fiber to your "Healthiest Way of Eating." They contain more fiber than the leaves, while still providing the other nutrients found in the leaves, but in smaller quantities. The nutrient content of the stems fluctuates dramatically and is closely related to the age and growth status of the plant since the flow of nutrients through the stems depends upon the plant's tasks at any given moment (including growth).

---

# how to enjoy fresh collard greens without cooking

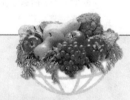

**Marinated Collard Green Salad:** Stack 3 Collard Green leaves. Tightly roll lengthwise and slice across in 1/8-inch strips. Place in a serving bowl. Toss with 1 TBS lemon juice, 3 TBS extra virgin olive oil, 1 tsp honey, and dill weed, sea salt and white pepper to taste. Let marinate 1 hour to overnight in the refrigerator. Garnish with chopped ripe olives and chopped ripe tomatoes. You will be surprised how tender Collard Greens can become.

Use fresh Collard Green leaves in place of tortillas for a low-carb wrap.

**The Healthiest Way of Cooking Collard Greens**

# 5-Minute "Healthy Steamed" Collard Greens

*Traditionally, Collard Greens are overcooked, resulting in loss of flavor and nutritional value. "Healthy Steaming" retains their bright color, crisp texture and maximum number of nutrients. Their flavor is enhanced by the easy to prepare Mediterranean Dressing.*

**1 lb Collard Greens**

**Mediterranean Dressing:**
**3 TBS extra virgin olive oil**
**1 tsp lemon juice**
**1 medium clove garlic**
**Sea salt and pepper to taste**

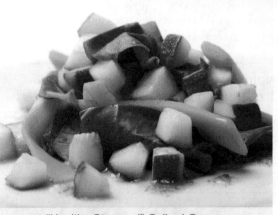

"Healthy Steamed" Collard Greens
with Carrots and Zucchini

1. Fill bottom of steamer with 2 inches of water.

2. While steam is building up, slice Collard Greens leaves into 1/2-inch slices, and cut again crosswise. Cut stems into 1/4-inch slices, and let sit as directed under the *How to Bring out the Hidden Health Benefits of Collard Greens (page 149).*

3. Chop or press garlic and let sit for at least 5 minutes. (Why?, see page 261.)

4. For *al denté* Collard Greens steam for no more than 5 minutes. (For information on *Differences in Cooking Time*, see page 91.)

5. Transfer to a bowl. For more flavor, toss Collard Greens with the remaining ingredients while they are still hot. (Mediterranean Dressing does not need to be made separately.) Research shows that carotenoids found in foods are best absorbed when consumed with oils.

OPTIONAL: To mellow the flavor of garlic, add garlic to Collard Greens for the last 2 minutes of steaming.

**SERVES 2**

**Flavor Tips:** Try these 5 great serving suggestions with the recipe above.

1. **Most Popular:** Cook Collard Greens with onions (cook onions 2 minutes before adding Collard Greens) and add some tamari (soy sauce) to mellow the flavor.

2. Add onions to the "Healthy Steamed" Collard Greens recipe (cook onions 2 minutes before adding Collard Greens). Add hot sauce to the dressing.

3. Add Cajun spices such as cayenne, chopped chili peppers or hot sauce.

4. Serve with steamed sweet potatoes, sesame seeds, and dulse (sea vegetables) flakes.

5. **Thai-Style Collard Greens:** Heat 1 small can of coconut milk, 1 tsp grated ginger, 1 clove pressed garlic, a large pinch of red pepper flakes and tamari (soy sauce) or sea salt to taste. Add hot 5-Minute "Healthy Steamed" Collard Greens (omit the dressing).

Please write (address on back cover flap) or e-mail me at info@whfoods.org with your personal ideas for preparing Collard Greens, and I will share them with others through our website at www.whfoods.org.

*Continued from Page 150)*

omega-3 fatty acids, magnesium and potassium; energy-producing vitamin B1, vitamin B2, vitamin B5, niacin, phosphorus and iron; muscle-building protein; and sleep-promoting tryptophan. Since cooked Collard Greens contain only 49 calories per one cup serving, they are an ideal food for healthy weight control.

## Nutritional Analysis of 1 cup of cooked Collard Greens:

| NUTRIENT | AMOUNT | % DAILY VALUE | NUTRIENT | AMOUNT | % DAILY VALUE |
|---|---|---|---|---|---|
| Calories | 49.40 | | Pantothenic Acid | 0.41 mg | 4.10 |
| Calories from Fat | 6.16 | | | | |
| Calories from Saturated Fat | 0.80 | | **Minerals** | | |
| Protein | 4.01 g | | Boron | — mcg | |
| Carbohydrates | 9.31 g | | Calcium | 226.10 mg | 22.61 |
| Dietary Fiber | 5.32 g | 21.28 | Chloride | — mg | |
| Soluble Fiber | 2.39 g | | Chromium | — mcg | — |
| Insoluble Fiber | 2.93 g | | Copper | 0.06 mg | 3.00 |
| Sugar - Total | 0.19 g | | Fluoride | — mg | — |
| Monosaccharides | — g | | Iodine | — mcg | — |
| Disaccharides | — g | | Iron | 0.87 mg | 4.83 |
| Other Carbs | 3.80 g | | Magnesium | 32.30 mg | 8.07 |
| Fat - Total | 0.68 g | | Manganese | 1.07 mg | 53.50 |
| Saturated Fat | 0.09 g | | Molybdenum | — mcg | — |
| Mono Fat | 0.05 g | | Phosphorus | 49.40 mg | 4.94 |
| Poly Fat | 0.33 g | | Potassium | 494.00 mg | |
| Omega-3 Fatty Acids | 0.18 g | 7.20 | Selenium | 2.09 mcg | 2.99 |
| Omega-6 Fatty Acids | 0.14 g | | Sodium | 17.10 mg | |
| Trans Fatty Acids | 0.00 g | | Zinc | 0.80 mg | 5.33 |
| Cholesterol | 0.00 mg | | | | |
| Water | 174.53 g | | **Amino Acids** | | |
| Ash | 1.44 g | | Alanine | 0.17 g | |
| | | | Arginine | 0.21 g | |
| **Vitamins** | | | Aspartate | 0.31 g | |
| Vitamin A IU | 5945.10 IU | 118.90 | Cystine | 0.04 g | 9.76 |
| Vitamin A RE | 594.70 RE | | Glutamate | 0.33 g | |
| A - Carotenoid | 594.70 RE | 7.93 | Glycine | 0.15 g | |
| A - Retinol | 0.00 RE | | Histidine | 0.08 g | 6.20 |
| Thiamin - B1 | 0.08 mg | 5.33 | Isoleucine | 0.16 g | 13.91 |
| Riboflavin - B2 | 0.20 mg | 11.76 | Leucine | 0.25 g | 9.88 |
| Niacin - B3 | 1.09 mg | 5.45 | Lysine | 0.19 g | 8.09 |
| Niacin equiv | 1.95 mg | | Methionine | 0.05 g | 6.76 |
| Vitamin B6 | 0.24 mg | 12.00 | Phenylalanine | 0.14 g | 11.76 |
| Vitamin B12 | 0.00 mcg | 0.00 | Proline | 0.17 g | |
| Biotin | — mcg | — | Serine | 0.13 g | |
| Vitamin C | 34.58 mg | 57.63 | Threonine | 0.14 g | 11.29 |
| Vitamin D IU | 0.00 IU | 0.00 | Tryptophan | 0.05 g | 15.63 |
| Vitamin D mcg | 0.00 mcg | | Trosine | 0.11 g | 11.34 |
| Vitamin E alpha equiv | 1.67 mg | 8.35 | Valine | 0.20 g | 13.61 |
| Vitamin E IU | 2.49 IU | | | | |
| Vitamin E mg | 1.67 mg | | **(Note: "—" indicates data is unavailable. For more information, please see page 806.)** | | |
| Folate | 176.70 mcg | 44.17 | | | |
| Vitamin K | 704.00 mcg | 880.00 | | | |

Here are questions I received from readers of the whfoods.org website about Collard Greens:

**Q** *Is it true that eating dark green veggies such as Collards, spinach and kale will have a negative effect if you are on blood thinning medication?*

**A** Large amounts of food high in vitamin K, such as Collards, spinach and kale, as well as other members of the *Brassica* family, may change the way blood thinning medications work. It is sometimes recommended to keep the amount of these foods in your diet about the same from week to week. Ask you physician whether you need to limit your intake of vitamin K-concentrated foods if you are on blood-thinning medications.

**Q** *Can you freeze cooked Collard Greens?*

**A** Unfortunately, unlike many other vegetables, Collard Greens do not freeze well.

**Q** *Does cooking vegetables alter their fiber amount or structure so as to impact blood sugar levels or digestibility?*

**A** Cooking does alter the structure of the fiber content in foods. For example, one research study found that raw carrots' soluble fiber has higher viscosity than blanched and microwaved carrots; this may be related to the finding that the raw carrots raised blood sugar less than their cooked counterparts. The changes in their fiber content and structure may be related to your varying response to cooked and raw vegetables.

When the cells are heated up, cellulose and other substances in the cell walls soften. The vegetable cell walls eventually collapse, opening up their structure and releasing water and other substances. That is why excessive cooking makes vegetables soft and mushy; for most vegetables, this happens within 10 minutes of heating at 98°C (about 209°F, just below boiling). That is why we recommend cooking most vegetables for about 5 minutes. Properly cooking vegetables can soften the cellulose and hemicellulose fiber just enough to make them easier to digest and allow health-promoting nutrients to become more readily available for absorption.

Plants also contain starch granules inside their cells, which they use to help store energy they capture from the sun. Starch swells when cooked in water—a process which is known as "gelatinization."

## Q&A
### WHAT ARE THE BENEFITS OF INCLUDING CRUCIFEROUS VEGETABLES IN MY "HEALTHIEST WAY OF EATING"?

Did you know that a study presented at the 4th Annual Conference on Frontiers in Cancer Prevention Research (October 30–November 2, 2005) found that Polish women emigrating to the United States increased their risk of breast cancer by 300% once they left their native country?

And did you know that one of the most important food habits they left behind was eating cabbage? Yes, cabbage, that seemingly simple and plain-looking food that's found so often in the form of slaw or kraut and gets so little nutritional fanfare.

Cabbage was eaten to the tune of almost 30 pounds per year by these women growing up in Poland, but its consumption dropped to less than one-third of that amount when the women emigrated to the U.S. Along with this huge drop in cabbage consumption came a very significant increase in their risk of breast cancer.

Cabbage turns out to be one of many lesser-heralded vegetables that are actually grand champions of our health. It belongs to a family known as the "cruciferous vegetables," and you are going to hear more and more about this family in the coming years as foods that have great potential for cancer prevention and other aspects of health promotion, including balancing hormones, protecting your skin and supporting heart health.

### A Diverse Family of Vegetables

You may have eaten crucifers and not even known it! This botanical family, the "cruciferous vegetables" (their name in Latin is *Cruciferae* or *Brassicaceae*), includes many shapes, colors and sizes of vegetable. It's only when these plants go to seed and flower that you might start to notice the family resemblance because when they flower, these plants produce a four-petal, cross-like design that gives them their name: *crucifer*, the Latin word for "cross-bearer."

You'll also hear this family of vegetables commonly referred to as "the mustards" or "mustard family" because mustards also belong to the *Cruciferae*.

The most important genus of plants belonging to the cruciferous family are the brassicas. (The Latin word "brassica" originally comes from the Celtic word for cabbage, *bresic*). Like mustard, cabbage is a very popular member of the crucifers, and you may also hear this group of foods referred to as "the cabbage family."

### Here is a More Extensive List of Vegetables That Belong to This Fascinating Family of Foods:

Cress, green cabbage, Napa cabbage, red cabbage, savoy cabbage, Chinese cabbage, bok choy, daikon (Chinese radish or Japanese radish), collard greens, mustard greens, mustard seeds, rutabaga, broccoli, Brussels sprouts, cauliflower, kohlrabi, turnip greens, turnip root, kale, rape (the source of rapeseed and canola oil), watercress, garden cress, horseradish, wasabi (Japanese horseradish), radish, collards, mizuna and arugula.

### Sulfur Compounds and Our Health

The vast majority of research studies on cruciferous vegetables have focused on the unique sulfur-containing compounds found in these foods. (Sometimes these compounds are also called "organosulfur" compounds.)

In chemical terms, the main subtypes of sulfur compounds found in cruciferous vegetables are:

- glucosinolates
- thiocyanates (including the isothiocyanates and their star molecule, sulforaphane)
- thiosulfinates and their breakdown products, including the dithiins
- sulfoxides, including the methyl cysteine sulfoxides
- a variety of other sulfur and thiol-containing compounds (the term "thiol" always means "sulfur-containing," and you will see it included in the chemical names of many sulfur-containing substances).

### Indole-3-Carbinol

There is some confusion in the popular press about one very important phytonutrient found in the cruciferous vegetables, namely, indole-3-carbinol (I3C). This substance does not contain sulfur, but it is made from the first subtype of sulfur compound mentioned above, the glucosinolates. (An enzyme called *myrosinase* splits off I3C from its parent compound, indole-3-glucosinolate.) So while closely related to the sulfur compounds, I3C is not technically one of them.

Prevention of breast cancer and prostate cancer has been repeatedly associated with I3C intake from cruciferous vegetables. One of the ways that it may help promote health is by beneficially supporting the metabolism of estrogen. The liver metabolizes estrogen into either 16-alpha-hydroxyestrone (16-OH) or 2-hydroxyestrogen (2-OH) with the former suggest to promote, and the latter suggested to oppose, cancer development; their ratio is used as a biomarker for the

*(Continued on Page 237)*

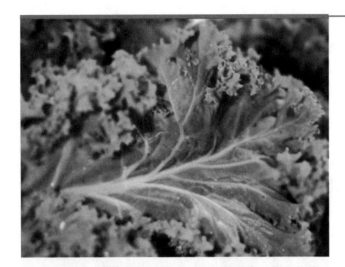

# kale

## highlights

| | |
|---|---|
| AVAILABILITY: | Year-round |
| REFRIGERATE: | Yes |
| SHELF LIFE: | 5 days refrigerated |
| PREPARATION: | Cut and let sit for 5 minutes |
| BEST WAY TO COOK: | "Healthy Steamed" in just 5 minutes |

## nutrient-richness chart

Total Nutrient-Richness: **34**  GI: **15**

One cup (130 grams) of cooked Kale contains 36 calories

| NUTRIENT | AMOUNT | %DV | DENSITY | QUALITY |
|---|---|---|---|---|
| Vitamin K | 1062.1 mcg | 1327.6 | 656.5 | excellent |
| Vitamin A | 9620.0 IU | 192.4 | 95.1 | excellent |
| Vitamin C | 53.3 mg | 88.8 | 43.9 | excellent |
| Manganese | 0.5 mg | 27.0 | 13.4 | excellent |
| Dietary Fiber | 2.6 g | 10.4 | 5.1 | very good |
| Copper | 0.2 mg | 10.0 | 4.9 | very good |
| Tryptophan | 0.03 g | 9.4 | 4.6 | very good |
| Calcium | 93.6 mg | 9.4 | 4.6 | very good |
| B6 Pyridoxine | 0.9 mg | 9.0 | 4.5 | very good |
| Potassium | 296.4 mg | 8.5 | 4.2 | very good |
| Iron | 1.2 mg | 6.5 | 3.2 | good |
| Magnesium | 23.4 mg | 5.8 | 2.9 | good |
| Vitamin E | 1.1 mg | 5.6 | 2.7 | good |
| B2 Riboflavin | 0.1 mg | 5.3 | 2.6 | good |
| Omega-3 Fatty Acids | 0.1 g | 5.2 | 2.6 | good |
| Protein | 2.5 g | 4.9 | 2.4 | good |
| B1 Thiamin | 0.1 mg | 4.7 | 2.3 | good |
| Folate | 17.3 mcg | 4.3 | 2.1 | good |
| Phosphorus | 36.4 mg | 3.6 | 1.8 | good |
| B3 Niacin | 0.7 mg | 3.3 | 1.6 | good |

| CAROTENOIDS: | | |
|---|---|---|
| Beta-Carotene | 10,624.9 mcg | Daily values for these nutrients have not yet been established. |
| Lutein+Zeaxanthin | 23,719.8 mcg | |

For more on "Total Nutrient-Richness," "%DV," "Density," and The World's Healthiest Foods "Quality" Rating System, see page 805.

For more on GI, see page 342.

Like other cruciferous vegetables, Kale is a descendent of the wild cabbage, a plant thought to have originated in Asia Minor and to have been brought to Europe around 600 BC by groups of Celtic wanderers. Both the ancient Greeks and Romans are known to have grown Kale. Although most varieties of Kale have been grown for thousands of years, there are now new varieties, such as "Lacinato" Kale, with even more robust flavor. Proper preparation is the key to enjoying the best flavor and nutritional benefits from Kale. That is why I want to share with you the secret of the "Healthiest Way of Cooking" Kale *al denté*. In just 5 minutes, you will be able to transform Kale into a flavorful vegetable while maximizing its nutritional value.

## why kale should be part of your healthiest way of eating

Scientific studies now show that cruciferous vegetables, like Kale, are included among the vegetables that contain the largest concentrations of health-promoting sulfur compounds, such as sulforaphane and isothiocyanates (see page 153), which increase the liver's ability to produce enzymes that neutralize potentially toxic substances. Kale is also rich in the powerful phytonutrient antioxidants lutein and zeaxanthin, carotenoids that protect the lens of the eye. Kale is an ideal food to add to your "Healthiest Way of Eating" not only because it is high in nutrients, but also because it is low in calories; one cup of cooked Kale contains only 36 calories, making it a great choice for weight control. (For more on the *Health Benefits of Kale* and a complete profile of its content of over 60 nutrients, see page 158.)

## varieties of kale

Kale is a member of the cruciferous family of vegetables,

which also includes broccoli, cauliflower, cabbage, collard greens, mustard greens and Brussels sprouts. Its botanical name is *Brassica oleracea*, variety *acephala*, which translates to "cabbage of the vegetable garden without a head," an appropriate description of this descendent of the wild cabbage. Kale comes in many varieties, which differ in taste, texture and appearance:

### CURLY KALE

This is the variety most widely found in your local market. The frilly edged leaves and long stems come in a wide variety of colors (including green, deep blue Russian red and black) and are sold in bunches. It has a lively bitter flavor with delicious, peppery qualities. Curly Kale grown in the cold winter months is sweeter and more tender.

### LACINATO

Lacinato Kale is also known as Tuscan Kale, Cavalo Nero (black cabbage) or Dinosaur Kale. It was developed in Italy in the late 19th century and features dark blue-green leaves that have an embossed texture and a slightly sweeter and more delicate flavor (with a peppery undertone) than Curly Kale.

### ORNAMENTAL KALE

Originally a decorative garden plant, this variety was first cultivated commercially in the 1980s in California and is oftentimes referred to as Salad Savoy. Its leaves can be green, white or purple, and its stalks coalesce to form a loosely knit head. It has a more mellow flavor, and its texture is more tender than Curly Kale.

## the peak season

Kale is available throughout the year, but its flavor is at its peak during the cold months when the frost helps to develop a sweeter flavor and crisp texture. In hotter months, Kale is less tender and will require around 30 seconds additional cooking time.

## biochemical considerations

Kale is a concentrated source of goitrogens and oxalates, which might be of concern to certain individuals. (For more on: *Goitrogens,* see page 721; and *Oxalates,* see page 725.)

## 4 steps for the best tasting and most nutritious kale

Turning Kale into a flavorful dish with the most nutrients is simple if you just follow my 4 easy steps:

1. The Best Way to Select
2. The Best Way to Store
3. The Best Way to Prepare
4. The Healthiest Way of Cooking

# 1. the best way to select kale

You can select the best tasting Kale by looking for varieties that have firm, bright, deeply colored green leaves and moist hardy stems. I have found that smaller leaves are more tender and have a milder flavor than larger leaves. By selecting the best tasting Kale, you will also enjoy Kale with the highest nutritional value. As with all vegetables, I recommend selecting organically grown varieties whenever possible. (For more on *Organic Foods*, see page 113.)

Avoid Kale that is wilted, shows signs of browning or yellowing, or has small holes.

# 2. the best way to store kale

Kale is a delicate vegetable that will become yellow and bitter if not stored properly. If you are not planning on using it immediately after bringing it home from the market, make sure to store it properly as it can lose up to 30% of some of its vitamins as well as much of its flavor.

Kale continues to respire even after it has been harvested. Slowing down the respiration rate with proper storage is the key to extending its flavor and nutritional benefits. (For a *Comparison of Respiration Rates* for different vegetables, see page 91.)

### Kale Will Remain Fresh for Up to 5 Days When Properly Stored

1. Store Kale in the refrigerator. The colder temperature will slow the respiration rate, helping to preserve its nutrients and keeping Kale fresh for a longer period of time.

2. Place Kale in a plastic storage bag before refrigerating. I have found that it is best to wrap the bag tightly around the Kale, squeezing out as much of the air from the bag as possible.

3. Do not wash Kale before refrigeration because exposure to water will encourage Kale to spoil.

# 3. the best way to prepare kale

Properly cleaning and cutting Kale helps to ensure that the Kale you serve will have the best flavor and retain the greatest number of nutrients.

## Cleaning Kale

Discard damaged and discolored leaves. Rinse Kale under cold running water before cutting. To preserve nutrients, do not soak Kale or its water-soluble nutrients will leach into the water. (For more on *Washing Vegetables*, page 92.)

## Cutting Kale

Kale's juicy, succulent stems are rich in fiber and enjoyable to eat, which is why I offer you tips on how to prepare both the leaves and the stems. Stack the leaves, cutting the leafy portion into 1/2-inch slices. When you reach the point where the leaves end and just the stems remain, make thinner slices (1/4-inch) and continue cutting to within the bottom inch of the stem; discard the last bottom inch as it is fibrous.

Slicing Kale will help it to cook more quickly. The thinner you slice it, the more quickly it will cook. Cutting the stems thinner than the leaves will help the stems and leaves cook evenly together. The combination of stems and leaves provides a good balance of flavors. After cutting, let sit for 5 minutes before cooking.

## What to Do with Thick Stems

If the stem portions below the leaves are quite thick, you may want to cook them for 2–3 minutes before adding the rest of the Kale. Discard stems that are woody and hollow.

# 4. the healthiest way of cooking kale

Since research has shown that important nutrients can be lost or destroyed by the way a food is cooked, the "Healthiest Way of Cooking" Kale is focused on bringing out its best flavor while maximizing its vitamins, minerals and powerful antioxidants.

## The Healthiest Way of Cooking Kale: "Healthy Steaming" for just 5 Minutes

In my search to find the healthiest way to cook Kale, I tested every possible cooking method and discovered that "Healthy Steaming" Kale for just 5 minutes delivered the best result. "Healthy Steaming" provides the moisture necessary to make Kale tender, bring out its peak flavor, retain its bright green color and maximize its nutritional profile. While it is important not to overcook Kale, cooking for less than 5 minutes is also not recommended because it takes about 5 minutes to soften its fibers and help increase its digestibility. The Step-by-Step Recipe will show you how easy it is to "Healthy Steam" Kale.

## How to Avoid Overcooking Kale: Cook it *Al Denté*

One of the primary reasons people do not enjoy Kale is because it is often overcooked. For the best flavor, I recommend that you cook Kale *al denté*. Kale cooked *al denté* is tender outside and slightly firm inside. Plus, Kale cooked *al denté* is cooked just long enough to soften its cellulose and hemicellulose fiber; this makes it easier to digest and allows its health-promoting nutrients to become more readily available for absorption. Remember that testing Kale with a fork is not an effective way to determine whether it is done.

Although Kale is a hearty vegetable, it is very important not to overcook it. Kale cooked for as little as a couple of minutes longer than *al denté* will begin to lose not only its texture and flavor but also its nutrients. Overcooking Kale will significantly decrease its nutritional value: as much as 50% of some nutrients can be lost. (For more on *Al Denté*, see page 92.)

## How to Prevent Strong Smells from Forming

Slicing Kale thin (1/2-inch slices) and cooking it *al denté* is my secret for preventing the formation of smelly compounds often associated with cooking Kale. When I cook my Kale, it never develops a strong smell. After 5 minutes of cooking, the texture of Kale, like all other cruciferous vegetables, begins to change, becoming increasingly soft and mushy. At this point, it also starts to lose more and more of its chlorophyll, causing its rich green color to fade and a brownish hue to appear. This is a sign that magnesium has been lost. This is when it starts to release hydrogen sulfide, the cause of the "rotten egg smell," which also affects the flavor. After 7 minutes of cooking, Kale develops a more intense flavor, with the amount of strong smelling hydrogen sulfide doubling in quantity.

## Cooking Methods
## Not Recommended for Kale

### SAUTÉING, BOILING, BAKING
### OR COOKING WITH OIL

You will not get good results by "Healthy Sautéing" Kale. Kale has a low moisture content, which causes it to dry out when sautéed, so it will become scorched before it becomes tender. Boiling Kale increases its water absorption, causing it to become soggy and lose much of its flavor along with many of its nutrients, including minerals, water-soluble vitamins (such as C and the B-complex vitamins) and health-promoting phytonutrients. I also don't recommend cooking Kale in oil because high temperature heat can damage delicate oils and create harmful free radicals.

### New Scientific Findings

#### HOW NUTRITIOUS ARE THE STEMS OF KALE?

Kale stems are great for adding more fiber to your "Healthiest Way of Eating." They contain more fiber than the leaves, while still providing the other nutrients found in the leaves, but in smaller quantities. The nutrient content of the stems fluctuates dramatically and is closely related to the age and growth status of the plant since the flow of nutrients through the stems depends upon the plant's tasks of any given moment (including growth).

Here is a question that I received from a reader of the whfoods.org website about Kale:

## Q *Can Kale be frozen?*

A Unfortunately, unlike other vegetables, fresh Kale does not freeze well. Yet, if you have prepared a Kale recipe, you can freeze it in an airtight container. It may not taste as fresh as it was when originally prepared, but at least you will still be able to enjoy it at a later date.

### HOW TO BRING OUT THE HIDDEN HEALTH BENEFITS OF KALE

The latest scientific studies show that cutting Kale into thin slices breaks down cell walls and enhances the activation of an enzyme called *myrosinase* that slowly converts some of the plant nutrients into their active forms, which have been shown to contain health-promoting properties. So, to get the most health benefits from Kale, let it sit for a minimum of 5 minutes, optimally 10 minutes, after cutting, before eating or cooking.

Since ascorbic acid (vitamin C) increases *myrosinase* activity, you can sprinkle a little lemon juice on the Kale before letting it sit in order to further enhance its beneficial phytonutrient concentration.

Heat will inactivate the effect of *myrosinase*, which is why it is important to allow the Kale to sit for 5–10 minutes before cooking to give the enzyme ample opportunity to enhance the concentration of active phytonutrients in your Kale. Cooking at low or medium heat for short periods of time should not destroy the active phytonutrients since once they are formed, they are fairly stable.

### An Easy Way to Prepare Kale, Step-By-Step

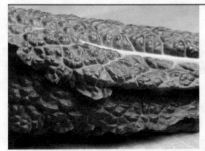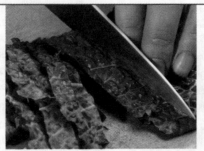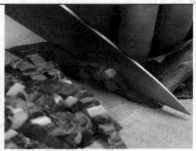

❶ Stack Kale leaves, so you can cut all the leaves at the same time. ❷ Cut widthwise into 1/2-inch slices starting from the tip until you reach the stems. ❸ Cut the stems into 1/4-inch wide slices.

# health benefits of kale

### Promotes Optimal Health

As a *Brassica* vegetable, Kale stands out as a food that may protect against cancer. Its organosulfur phytonutrient compounds, including the glucosinolates and the methyl cysteine sulfoxides, have been the main subject of *Brassica* vegetable research. Exactly how Kale's sulfur-containing phytonutrients prevent cancer is not clear, but several researchers point to the ability of these compounds to activate detoxifying enzymes in the liver that help neutralize potentially carcinogenic substances. For example, scientists have found that sulforaphane, a potent glucosinolate phytonutrient found in Kale and other *Brassica* vegetables, boosts the body's detoxification enzymes, possibly by altering gene expression, thus helping to clear potentially carcinogenic substances more quickly.

### Promotes Vision Health

Kale is the most concentrated source of the carotenoids lutein and zeaxanthin of all of the World's Healthiest Foods. These carotenoids act like sunglasses, filtering ultraviolet light and preventing damage to the eyes from excessive exposure to it. Studies have shown the protective effect of these nutrients against the risk of cataracts. In one study, people who had a diet history of eating lutein-rich foods like Kale had a 50% lower risk for new cataracts. Kale is also an excellent source of vitamin A, notably through its rich supply of beta-carotene. Vitamin A is also very important to promoting optimal vision health.

### Promotes Antioxidant Protection

In addition to being a rich source of the antioxidants lutein, zeaxanthin and beta-carotene, Kale is also an excellent source of vitamin C, the body's primary water-soluble antioxidant. Vitamin C can disarm free radicals and prevent damage in the aqueous environment both inside and outside cells. It helps protect many different bodily components from oxidative damage including our DNA as well as our cholesterol (oxidized cholesterol can lead to atherosclerosis). In addition, vitamin C helps to keep our immune system strong.

### Additional Health-Promoting Benefits of Kale

Kale is a concentrated source of many other nutrients providing additional health promoting benefits. These nutrients include free-radical-scavenging manganese and copper; heart-healthy omega-3 fatty acids, dietary fiber, folic acid, vitamin B6, vitamin E and potassium; bone-building calcium, magnesium and phosphorus; energy-producing iron, vitamin B1, vitamin B2 and niacin; muscle-building protein; and sleep-promoting tryptophan. Since Kale contains only 36 calories per one cup serving, it is an ideal food for healthy weight control.

*(See Nutritional Analysis for Kale on Page 160)*

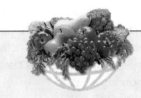

## how to enjoy fresh kale without cooking

**Kale Avocado Salad:** Combine 1 lb fresh Kale cut into 1/4-inch strips, 1 medium avocado cut into chunks, 2 tsp lemon juice, 2 TBS extra virgin olive oil and sea salt to taste. Mix thoroughly and let sit in refrigerator for 1/2 hour to tenderize. Add 2 cups chopped arugula, and mix well. Garnish with 1/2 cup chopped tomatoes.

**Kale-Apple Smoothie:** Blend 4 chopped Kale leaves, juice of 1 lemon, 2-inch piece of fresh ginger sliced thin, 2 small chopped apples or pears and 2 cups pure water for 2 minutes. Pour into a glass and enjoy. (Serves 2)

**Kale Pesto:** Ingredients: 1 bunch of Kale sliced into 1/2-inch strips, 1 clove garlic, sea salt to taste, 1/2 cup extra virgin olive oil, 2 TBS lemon juice and 1/4 cup walnuts. In a blender, drop the garlic through the feed hole while blender is running. Cover the hole with your hand while blending. Add walnuts through the feed hole one at a time. Stop blender and remove lid. Add extra virgin olive oil, lemon juice, sea salt and a small handful of Kale slices. Run blender, stopping to mix as needed. As the Kale is incorporated into the mixture, add another handful until all the Kale is incorporated and the purée is smooth. You will be surprised how tender Kale can become.

**Marinated Raw Kale:** Cut 1/2 bunch Lacinato Kale into 1/4-inch strips and cut crosswise 4–5 times. Combine with 2 TBS extra virgin olive oil, 1 TBS balsamic vinegar, 2 tsp tamari (soy sauce), 1 TBS apple juice and 1/2 tsp sea salt. Let marinate 1 hour before serving.

**STEP-BY-STEP RECIPE**
## The Healthiest Way of Cooking Kale

# 5-Minute "Healthy Steamed" Kale

*To prepare Kale with the best flavor and maximum amount of nutrients, I recommend the "Healthy Steaming" method. It is delicious with the Mediterranean Dressing.*

**1 lb Kale**

**Mediterranean Dressing:**
**3 TBS extra virgin olive oil**
**2 tsp lemon juice**
**1 medium clove garlic**
**Sea salt and pepper to taste**

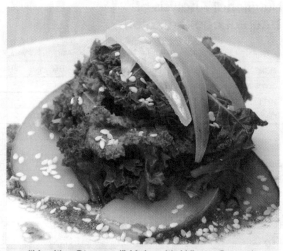

"Healthy Steamed" Kale with Winter Squash

1. Fill bottom of steamer with 2 inches of water.

2. While steam is building up, slice Kale leaves into 1/2-inch slices, and cut again crosswise. Cut stems into 1/4-inch slices, and let sit as directed under the *How to Bring out the Hidden Health Benefits of* Kale.

2. Chop or press garlic and let sit for at least 5 minutes. (Why?, see page 261.)

3. For *al denté* Kale, steam for no more than 5 minutes. (For information on *Differences in Cooking Time,* see page 94.)

4. Transfer to a bowl. For more flavor, toss Kale with the remaining ingredients while it is still hot. (Mediterranean Dressing does not need to be made separately.) Using a knife and fork, cut Kale into small pieces. Research shows that carotenoids found in foods are best absorbed when consumed with oils.

OPTIONAL: To mellow the flavor of garlic, add garlic to Kale for the last 2 minutes of steaming.

**SERVES 2**

**COOKING TIPS:**
- To prevent overcooking Kale, I highly recommend using a timer.
- Testing Kale with a fork is not an effective way to determine whether it is done.

## Flavor Tips: Try these 6 great serving suggestions with the recipe above. ✳

1. **Most Popular:** Cook with onions (cook onions 2 minutes before adding Kale) and add a few drops of tamari (soy sauce) to mellow the flavor of Kale.
2. Add 2 TBS jarred roasted red peppers and grated Parmesan cheese.
3. For a different flavor, replace lemon juice with balsamic vinegar.
4. Add soaked hijiki (sea vegetable), sesame seeds and finely chopped fresh red bell pepper.

5. Serve Kale with sweet potatoes or winter squash (like butternut squash), which provide a nice flavor complement (pictured above).
6. **Spiced Moroccan Kale:** Add 1/4 tsp allspice, 1/4 tsp ground coriander, 1/4 tsp cinnamon and a pinch of ground cloves to the 5-Minute "Healthy Steamed" Kale recipe. Top with raisins and chopped toasted almonds.

Please write (address on back cover flap) or e-mail me at info@whfoods.org with your personal ideas for preparing Kale, and I will share them with others through our website at www.whfoods.org.

*(Continued from Page 158)*

## Nutritional Analysis of 1 cup of cooked Kale:

| NUTRIENT | AMOUNT | % DAILY VALUE | NUTRIENT | AMOUNT | % DAILY VALUE |
|---|---|---|---|---|---|
| Calories | 36.40 | | Pantothenic Acid | 0.06 mg | 0.60 |
| Calories from Fat | 4.68 | | | | |
| Calories from Saturated Fat | 0.61 | | **Minerals** | | |
| Protein | 2.47 g | | Boron | — mcg | |
| Carbohydrates | 7.32 g | | Calcium | 93.60 mg | 9.36 |
| Dietary Fiber | 2.60 g | 10.40 | Chloride | — mg | |
| Soluble Fiber | 1.17 g | | Chromium | — mcg | — |
| Insoluble Fiber | 1.43 g | | Copper | 0.20 mg | 10.00 |
| Sugar – Total | 1.56 g | | Fluoride | — mg | — |
| Monosaccharides | — g | | Iodine | — mcg | — |
| Disaccharides | — g | | Iron | 1.17 mg | 6.50 |
| Other Carbs | 3.16 g | | Magnesium | 23.40 mg | 5.85 |
| Fat – Total | 0.52 g | | Manganese | 0.54 mg | 27.00 |
| Saturated Fat | 0.07 g | | Molybdenum | — mcg | — |
| Mono Fat | 0.04 g | | Phosphorus | 36.40 mg | 3.64 |
| Poly Fat | 0.25 g | | Potassium | 296.40 mg | |
| Omega-3 Fatty Acids | 0.13 g | 5.20 | Selenium | 1.17 mcg | 1.67 |
| Omega-6 Fatty Acids | 0.10 g | | Sodium | 29.90 mg | |
| Trans Fatty Acids | 0.00 g | | Zinc | 0.31 mg | 2.07 |
| Cholesterol | 0.00 mg | | | | |
| Water | 118.56 g | | **Amino Acids** | | |
| Ash | 1.13 g | | Alanine | 0.12 g | |
| | | | Arginine | 0.14 g | |
| **Vitamins** | | | Aspartate | 0.22 g | |
| Vitamin A IU | 9620.00 IU | 192.40 | Cystine | 0.03 g | 7.32 |
| Vitamin A RE | 962.00 RE | | Glutamate | 0.28 g | |
| A - Carotenoid | 962.00 RE | 12.83 | Glycine | 0.12 g | |
| A - Retinol | 0.00 RE | | Histidine | 0.05 g | 3.88 |
| B1 Thiamin | 0.07 mg | 4.67 | Isoleucine | 0.15 g | 13.04 |
| B2 Riboflavin | 0.09 mg | 5.29 | Leucine | 0.17 g | 6.72 |
| B3 Niacin | 0.65 mg | 3.25 | Lysine | 0.15 g | 6.38 |
| Niacin equiv | 1.15 mg | | Methionine | 0.02 g | 2.70 |
| Vitamin B6 | 0.18 mg | 9.00 | Phenylalanine | 0.13 g | 10.92 |
| Vitamin B12 | 0.00 mcg | 0.00 | Proline | 0.15 g | |
| Biotin | — mcg | — | Serine | 0.10 g | |
| Vitamin C | 53.30 mg | 88.83 | Threonine | 0.11 g | 8.87 |
| Vitamin D IU | 0.00 IU | 0.00 | Tryptophan | 0.03 g | 9.38 |
| Vitamin D mcg | 0.00 mcg | | Tyrosine | 0.09 g | 9.28 |
| Vitamin E alpha equiv | 1.11 mg | 5.55 | Valine | 0.14 g | 9.52 |
| Vitamin E IU | 1.65 IU | | | | |
| Vitamin E mg | 1.11 mg | | | | |
| Folate | 17.29 mcg | 4.32 | | | |
| Vitamin K | 1062.1 mcg | 1327.62 | | | |

(Note: "—" indicates data is unavailable. For more information, please see page 806.)

## Q&A
### ARE VEGETABLES AND FRUITS EQUALLY GOOD FOR MY HEALTH?

When you compare fruits and vegetables on a nutritional basis, there is no question that vegetables are more nutrient-rich and contain a much wider variety of nutrients than fruits. If you think about the lives of the plants, this difference makes sense. In the world of vegetables, we eat many parts of the plants that either grow very close to the soil (like stems and stalks) or beneath the ground itself (like roots). This closeness to the soil brings the plant into contact with the diversity of soil minerals, and almost all vegetables are richer in minerals than fruits for this reason. Fruits are also more of an end-stage occurrence: in the case of an apple tree, for example, the tree has already lived and developed for a good number of years before it produces a significant amount of edible fruit. Unlike a root, which is in charge of nutrient delivery from the soil up into the rest of the plant, the fruit—like an apple—is not nearly as active in supporting the life of the plant (although its seeds are dramatically important in allowing the tree to produce new offspring and create future generations of apple trees). Because the stems, stalks and roots are more involved in the plant's life support, they also tend to have a greater variety of vitamins, especially B-complex vitamins, than fruits.

Most fruits have a concentrated amount of sugar, and for this reason, are higher in calories and less nutrient-rich than most vegetables. Starchy root vegetables like potatoes are closer to fruits in calorie content, but green leafy vegetables are enormously lower in calories and greater in nutrient-richness.

In summary, if you had to choose between fruits and vegetables as a foundation for your health, you would do best to select vegetables because of their greater nutrient diversity and nutrient-richness. Luckily, however, it is not an either-or situation, and you can take pleasure in the delights of both fruits and vegetables while increasing your reliance on the World's Healthiest Foods!

# Q&A

### ARE BITTER VEGETABLES BETTER FOR YOU?

Bitter, a characteristic also known as pungent, is one of our four basic tastes (along with sweet, salty, and sour). We have between 20,000 and 50,000 taste buds on our tongue, and some of these taste buds—especially the ones across the back of the tongue—have receptors for bitter taste. A bitter taste can function like a warning signal and help prevent us from eating foods that would be toxic to us. But bitter foods can also be good for us.

The reason some vegetables have a bitter taste does not mean that there is anything wrong with them. Bitterness can represent something natural and healthy, and bitter vegetables can be a great addition to your "Healthiest Way of Eating"! For example, many of the health-promoting phytonutrients that act as powerful antioxidants (including glucopyranosides like salicins, some flavonoids and polyphenols) can add a bitter flavor to your vegetables. Most vegetables contain antioxidant nutrients, and most of these antioxidant nutrients are bitter.

Fresh raw vegetables are rarely bitter. Sometimes the bitter flavor of some vegetables is developed with prolonged cooking. This is the reason I recommend steaming or sautéing your vegetables, methods that cook your vegetables very quickly.

Some vegetable flavors intensify when they are overcooked. More than likely one of the reasons that the Chinese eat more vegetables than Americans is because they cook them very lightly, and doing so makes them much more enjoyable. When you overcook vegetables, they can become mushy, lose their enjoyable flavors and may become undesirably bitter. Cruciferous vegetables like broccoli, kale, Brussels sprouts and especially mustard greens are good examples how overcooking your vegetables can make them more bitter. Although mustard greens are bitter even when they are raw, overcooking will add to their bitter taste. When cruciferous vegetables are overcooked, they begin to produce sulfur compounds and emit that rotten egg smell that is closely associated with an increasingly bitter flavor.

Here are some suggestions for the 30% of the population who can't tolerate the bitter taste of vegetables:

## Young Vegetables are Less Bitter

Young vegetables are less bitter and, because they are more tender, require less cooking. Baby bok choy, baby eggplant, baby spinach, baby squash and baby carrots are examples of very young vegetables that are rarely bitter. (Most of the bagged baby carrots sold in markets are not actually baby carrots but are formed to look like baby carrots. Baby carrots can be identified since they are usually sold with their tops on.) But remember that while young vegetables are less bitter, they are also less nutritious because young vegetables are not developed fully, and they have not yet reached their peak nutritional value. Restaurants solve the bitter problem by serving baby vegetables.

## Select the Right Dressing

Selecting a dressing that satisfies your personal taste can help mellow the bitter taste of your vegetables. I have found that using dressing with extra virgin olive oil is the best way to blend the rich taste of vegetables. Olive oil makes your vegetables tasty and satisfying, especially when the olive oil binds with the flavors of lemon, garlic, salt and pepper in the favorite Mediterranean tradition. In my experience, tamari (soy sauce) also tames a bitter taste. Adding a few drops of tamari to your vegetables, especially cruciferous vegetables, gives them a mellow, sweeter flavor.

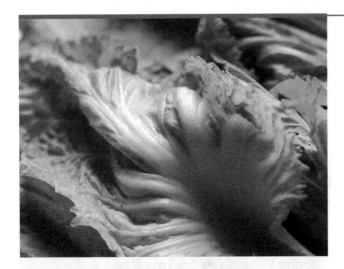

## nutrient-richness chart

Total Nutrient-Richness: **50**     GI: **15**

One cup (140 grams) of cooked Mustard Greens contains 21 calories

| NUTRIENT | AMOUNT | %DV | DENSITY | QUALITY |
|---|---|---|---|---|
| Vitamin K | 419.3 mcg | 524.1 | 449.2 | excellent |
| Vitamin A | 4243.4 IU | 84.9 | 72.7 | excellent |
| Vitamin C | 35.4 mg | 59.0 | 50.6 | excellent |
| Folate | 102.8 mcg | 25.7 | 22.0 | excellent |
| Manganese | 0.4 mg | 19.0 | 16.3 | excellent |
| Vitamin E | 2.8 mg | 14.1 | 12.0 | excellent |
| Tryptophan | 0.04 g | 12.5 | 10.7 | excellent |
| Dietary Fiber | 2.8 g | 11.2 | 9.6 | excellent |
| Calcium | 103.6 mg | 10.4 | 8.9 | excellent |
| Potassium | 282.8 mg | 8.1 | 6.9 | very good |
| B6 Pyridoxine | 0.1 mg | 7.0 | 6.0 | very good |
| Protein | 3.2 g | 6.3 | 5.4 | very good |
| Copper | 0.1 mg | 6.0 | 5.1 | very good |
| Phosphorus | 57.4 mg | 5.7 | 4.9 | very good |
| Iron | 1.0 mg | 5.4 | 4.7 | very good |
| B2 Riboflavin | 0.1 mg | 5.3 | 4.5 | very good |
| Magnesium | 21.0 mg | 5.3 | 4.5 | very good |
| B1 Thiamin | 0.1 mg | 4.0 | 3.4 | good |
| B3 Niacin | 0.6 mg | 3.0 | 2.6 | good |

| CAROTENOIDS: | | |
|---|---|---|
| Beta-Carotene | 5,311.6 mcg | Daily values for these nutrients have not yet been established. |
| Lutein+Zeaxanthin | 8,346.8 mcg | |

For more on "Total Nutrient-Richness," "%DV," "Density," and The World's Healthiest Foods "Quality" Rating System, see page 805.

For more on GI, see page 342.

S punky and soulful, Mustard Greens are native to Asia and are pungent members of the cruciferous family of vegetables with a very intense flavor. Brown seeds from this plant are used to make the condiment mustard.

# mustard greens

## highlights

| | |
|---|---|
| AVAILABILITY: | Year-round |
| REFRIGERATE: | Yes |
| SHELF LIFE: | 3 days refrigerated |
| PREPARATION: | Cut and let sit for 5 minutes |
| BEST WAY TO COOK: | "Healthy Sauté" in just 3 minutes |

## why mustard greens should be part of your healthiest way of eating

Scientific studies now show that cruciferous vegetables, like Mustard Greens, are included among the vegetables that contain the largest concentrations of health-promoting sulfur compounds, such as glucosinolates and isothiocyanates (see page 153); these phytonutrients increase the liver's ability to produce enzymes that neutralize potentially toxic substances. Mustard Greens are also rich in the powerful phytonutrient antioxidants lutein and zeaxanthin, carotenoids that are concentrated in the lens of the eye.

## varieties of mustard greens

Mustard Greens are a member of the cruciferous family of vegetables, which also includes broccoli, cauliflower, kale, collard greens, cabbage and Brussels sprouts, and are well-known for their many health-promoting properties. Mustard Greens are the leaves of the mustard plant, *Brassica juncea*. Mizuna is a Japanese Mustard Green with a jagged edge, green leaves and a mild peppery flavor. It is a popular salad green.

## the peak season available year-round.

## biochemical considerations

Mustard Greens contain goitrogens and oxalates, which might be of concern to certain individuals. (For more on *Goitrogens*, see page 721; and *Oxalates*, see page 725.)

STEP-BY-STEP RECIPE

## The Healthiest Way of Cooking Mustard Greens

# 3-Minute "Healthy Sautéed" Mustard Greens

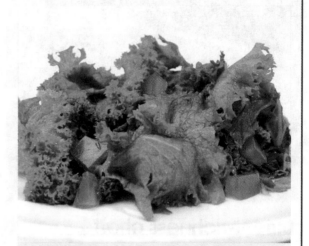

*I discovered that "Healthy Sautéing" Mustard Greens for just 5 minutes delivers the best results. "Healthy Sautéed" Mustard Greens are tender, have the best flavor and have retained the maximum number of nutrients.*

**1 lb Mustard Greens**
**1 onion (preferably yellow), sliced**
**3 TBS low-sodium chicken or vegetable broth**

**Mediterranean Dressing:**
**3 TBS extra virgin olive oil**
**2 tsp lemon juice**
**1 medium garlic clove**
**Sea salt and pepper to taste**

"Healthy Sautéed" Mustard Greens with Tomatoes

1. Chop or press garlic. Slice onion and let them sit for at least 5 minutes. (Why?, see page 261.)

2. Roll the entire bunch of Mustard Greens lengthwise, cut into 1/2-inch slices, and let sit for 10 minutes to enhance the concentration of their health-promoting phytonutrients. Stems are usually tender and do not have to separated from the leaves.

3. Heat 3 tablespoons broth over medium heat in a stainless steel skillet. (For more details on the *Differences in Cooking Time*, see page 94.)

4. When broth begins to steam, add Mustard Greens and onions and **cover**. Onions will mellow the flavor of Mustard Greens. Cook no more than 3 minutes for *al denté* Mustard Greens.

• For fuller flavor, dress Mustard Greens while they are still hot.

• To bring out the flavor and tenderize Mustard Greens, cut them into small pieces immediately after dressing.

**SERVES 2**

## Flavor Tips: Try these 5 great serving suggestions with the recipe above. ✻

1. Sprinkle with Parmesan cheese.
2. Combine with chopped olives.
3. Mustard Greens go well with tomatoes. The acid content of the tomatoes mellows the flavor of the Mustard Greens while still letting their spiciness come through (pictured above).

4. Add a few drops of tamari (soy sauce) to mellow the taste. If you add tamari, you will want to reduce the amount of sea salt.
5. Add toasted sesame seeds or sunflower seeds to cooked Mustard Greens.

Please write (address on back cover flap) or e-mail me at info@whfoods.org with your personal ideas for preparing Mustard Greens, and I will share them with others through our website at www.whfoods.org.

## An Easy Way to Prepare Mustard Greens, Step-by-Step

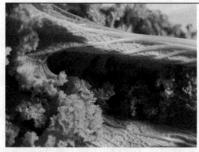 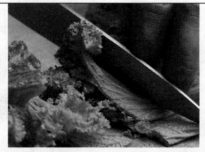 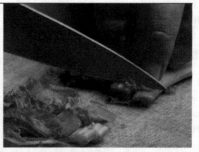

**CHOPPED MUSTARD GREENS**—You can enjoy the stems since they are succulent and tender.
❶ Roll the entire bunch of Mustard Greens. ❷ Cut into 1/2-inch slices until you reach the stem. ❸ Cut stem portion into 1/4-inch slices. To bring out the Hidden Health Benefits, see Kale (page 157).

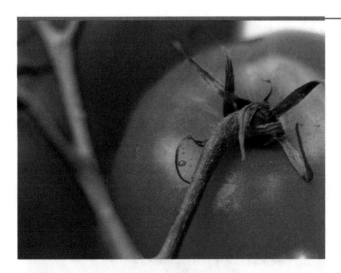

# tomatoes

| | |
|---|---|
| AVAILABILITY: | Year-round |
| REFRIGERATE: | Not recommended |
| SHELF LIFE: | 10 days |
| PREPARATION: | Minimal |
| BEST WAY TO PREPARE: | Enjoy raw or in a sauce |

## nutrient-richness chart

| Total Nutrient-Richness: | **34** | | | GI: **15** |
|---|---|---|---|---|

One cup (180 grams) of red Tomatoes contains 38 calories

| NUTRIENT | AMOUNT | %DV | DENSITY | QUALITY |
|---|---|---|---|---|
| Vitamin C | 34.4 mg | 57.3 | 27.3 | excellent |
| Vitamin A | 1121.4 IU | 22.4 | 10.7 | excellent |
| Vitamin K | 14.22 mcg | 17.8 | 8.5 | excellent |
| Molybdenum | 9.0 mcg | 12.0 | 5.7 | very good |
| Potassium | 399.6 mg | 11.4 | 5.4 | very good |
| Manganese | 0.2 mg | 9.5 | 4.5 | very good |
| Dietary Fiber | 2.0 g | 7.9 | 3.8 | very good |
| Chromium | 9.0 mcg | 7.5 | 3.6 | very good |
| B1 Thiamin | 0.1 mg | 7.3 | 3.5 | very good |
| B6 Pyridoxine | 0.1 mg | 7.0 | 3.3 | good |
| Folate | 27.0 mcg | 6.8 | 3.2 | good |
| Copper | 0.1 mg | 6.5 | 3.1 | good |
| B3 Niacin | 1.1 mg | 5.6 | 2.7 | good |
| B2 Riboflavin | 0.1 mg | 5.3 | 2.5 | good |
| Magnesium | 19.8 mg | 5.0 | 2.4 | good |
| Iron | 0.8 mg | 4.5 | 2.1 | good |
| B5 Pantothenic Acid | 0.4 mg | 4.4 | 2.1 | good |
| Phosphorus | 43.2 mg | 4.3 | 2.1 | good |
| Vitamin E | 0.7 mg | 3.4 | 1.6 | good |
| Tryptophan | 0.01 g | 3.1 | 1.5 | good |
| Protein | 1.5 g | 3.1 | 1.5 | good |

| **CAROTENOIDS:** | |
|---|---|
| Alpha-Carotene | 181.8 mcg |
| Beta-Carotene | 808.2 mcg |
| Lutein+Zeaxanthin | 221.4 mcg |
| Lycopene | 4,631.4 mcg |

| **FLAVONOIDS:** | |
|---|---|
| Kaempferol | 0.1 mg |
| Quercetin | 1.03 mg |

| **PHYTOSTEROLS:** | |
|---|---|
| Phytosterol – Total | 12.6 mg |

Daily values for these nutrients have not yet been established.

For more on "Total Nutrient-Richness," "%DV," "Density," and The World's Healthiest Foods "Quality" Rating System, see page 805.

For more on GI, see page 342.

Are Tomatoes really a vegetable or are they a fruit? The confusion arises from the fact that although Tomatoes are typically enjoyed as a vegetable, botanically they are classified as a fruit. Historically, this question caused such controversy due to a tariff dispute (different tariffs were imposed on fruits versus vegetables) that it finally took a decision by the United States Supreme Court in 1893 to declare that Tomatoes would be officially considered a vegetable! While fresh raw Tomatoes are nutritious favorites in green salads and sandwiches, scientific research is now discovering that you may derive even more health benefits from Tomatoes by enjoying them cooked. That is why I want to share with you a quick and easy way to prepare Tomatoes. By using the "Healthiest Way of Cooking" Tomatoes, you can maximize the availability of their important carotenoids and enhance their flavor in just 5 minutes!

## why tomatoes should be part of your healthiest way of eating

Tomatoes contain health-promoting carotenoid phytonutrients, including beta-carotene, lutein, zeaxanthin and lycopene, which provide antioxidant protection. In the area of food and phytonutrient research over the last five years, few nutrients have received as much attention as lycopene. While lycopene has been found to protect cells, DNA and LDL cholesterol from oxidation, as well as provide Tomatoes with their brilliant red color, it is the synergy of the entire complement of nutrients found in Tomatoes that provides them with their optimal health-promoting benefits. Additionally, they are an excellent source of both vitamins A (because of their carotenoids) and C, powerful antioxidants that provide anti-inflammatory protection and neutralize free radicals that damage cells.

Tomatoes are an ideal food to add to your "Healthiest Way of Eating" not only because they are high in nutrients, but also because they are low in calories: one cup of raw Tomatoes contains only 38 calories, so they are great for weight control. (For more on the *Health Benefits of Tomatoes* and a complete analysis of their content of over 60 nutrients, see page 168.)

## varieties of tomatoes

Although Tomatoes are closely associated with Italian cuisine, they were originally native to South America. Tomatoes are members of the *Solanaceae* (Nightshade) family of vegetables and come in shades of red, yellow, orange, green or brown. The Tomato is the fruit of the plant *Lycopersicon lycopersicum*. The leaves of the plant are inedible as they contain toxic alkaloids. There are literally thousands of different varieties of Tomatoes, but those most commonly found at local markets fall into five categories:

### CHERRY TOMATOES

Red, orange or yellow in color, these round, bite-sized Tomatoes are most often used in salads and as a garnish.

### PLUM TOMATOES OR ROMA/ITALIAN TOMATOES

These small, red, egg-shaped Tomatoes contain less juice than slicing Tomatoes, making them an ideal choice for cooking, especially if you are making Tomato sauce.

### SLICING TOMATOES

These red, round, juicy varieties are the ones most commonly found at your local market and include the flatter beefsteak Tomato. This is the variety featured in the photographs in this chapter.

### HEIRLOOM TOMATOES

Although there is no standard definition for Heirloom Tomatoes, most experts consider them to be varieties that have been passed down through several generations of a family and developed to bring out their best characteristics. Besides offering a wonderful rainbow of colors, shapes and tastes in hundreds of varieties, Heirloom Tomatoes are important because they help preserve the natural biodiversity found in nature. They are soft Tomatoes with limited shelf life, so they are not generally widely distributed, but they can be found at farmer's markets, natural food stores and supermarkets with more expansive produce sections.

### GREEN TOMATOES

Green Tomatoes are unripe Tomatoes and have less nutritional value than ripe Tomatoes because the concentrations of phytonutrients that impart the red coloration to ripe Tomatoes have not yet developed.

## the peak season

Although Tomatoes are available throughout the year, their peak season runs from July through October. These are the months when their concentration of nutrients and flavor are highest, and their cost is at its lowest.

## biochemical considerations

Tomatoes are members of the nightshade family of vegetables, which might be of concern to certain individuals. Tomatoes are also one of the foods most commonly associated with allergic reactions and are one of the foods suspected to cause a reaction in individuals with latex allergies. (For more on: *Nightshades*, see page 723; *Food Allergies*, see page 719; and *Latex Food Allergies*, see page 722.)

## 4 steps for the best tasting and most nutritious tomatoes

Turning Tomatoes into a flavorful dish with the most nutrients is simple if you just follow my 4 easy steps:

1. The Best Way to Select
2. The Best Way to Store
3. The Best Way to Prepare
4. The Healthiest Way of Cooking

# 1. the best way to select tomatoes

You can select the best tasting Tomatoes by looking for ones that are deeply and evenly colored as well as firm and heavy for their size. These are signs of a delicious tasting Tomato, and those with a rich red color have a greater supply of the health-promoting phytonutrient, lycopene. Tomatoes should be well shaped and smooth skinned. Ripe Tomatoes will yield to slight pressure and have a noticeably sweet smell.

It is impossible to ship fully ripened Tomatoes without damaging them; therefore, most Tomatoes are picked green and are exposed to ethylene gas to make them red after they have reached their destination. That is one more reason why Tomatoes from local farmers will usually have better flavor because they are not picked prematurely and are allowed to remain on the vine until ripe. By selecting the best tasting Tomatoes, you will enjoy Tomatoes with the highest nutritional value.

As with all vegetables, I recommend selecting organically grown varieties of Tomatoes whenever possible. Organically grown Tomatoes are not exposed to ethylene gas and are not covered with the wax coating used on conventionally grown Tomatoes to extend their shelf life. If you purchase conventionally grown Tomatoes, it is best to peel off the skin. (For more on *Organic Foods*, see page 113.)

Avoid pale Tomatoes with wrinkles, cracks, bruises or soft spots. I have found that ones with a puffy appearance seem to have inferior flavor and will cause excess waste during preparation.

When purchasing canned Tomatoes, it is best to purchase brands that are produced in the United States; many foreign countries do not have the same high standards for controlling the lead content of the containers. This is an especially important consideration with canned Tomatoes because their high acid content can corrode the container's metal and result in migration of lead into the food.

# 2. the best way to store tomatoes

For optimal freshness and nutrition, it is best to use Tomatoes the same day you purchase them. If you are not going to use them immediately after bringing them home from the market, be sure to store them properly as they can quickly lose their flavor as well as up to 30% of some of their vitamins.

Tomatoes continue to respire even after they have been harvested; their respiration rate at room temperature (68°F/20°C) is 35 mg/kg/hr. Slowing down the respiration rate with proper storage is the key to extending their flavor and nutritional benefits. (For a *Comparison of Respiration Rates* for different vegetables, see page 91.)

### Tomatoes Will Remain Fresh for Up to 10 Days When Properly Stored

Most Tomatoes picked in the field are green, but they will continue to ripen after they are harvested. When you bring them home, it is best to store your Tomatoes at room temperature and out of direct exposure to sunlight. They will keep for up to 10 days depending upon variety and how ripe they are when purchased.

Refrigerating unripe Tomatoes will destroy their flavor and cause them to become spongy. Tomatoes are sensitive to cold; refrigeration impedes their ripening process as well as reduces their flavor by diminishing flavor components like (2)-3-dexenal.

If Tomatoes begin to become overripe at room temperature, and you are not yet ready to eat them, you can store them in the refrigerator. If possible, place them in the butter compartment, which is the warmest part of the refrigerator, where they will keep for one or two more days. Remove them from the refrigerator about 30 minutes before using them so that they can regain their maximum flavor and juiciness.

### How to Store Tomatoes That Are Already Sliced

To store a Tomato that has been cut, place it in an airtight container or a storage bag, with all excess air removed from the bag, and refrigerate. Since the vitamin C content starts to quickly degrade once the Tomato has been cut, you should use it within one to two days.

### How to Ripen Tomatoes

To hasten the ripening process, place Tomatoes in a paper bag with a banana or apple. The ethylene gas emitted by these fruits will help speed up the ripening process. When ripening Tomatoes, it is best to place them stem side down.

# 3. the best way to prepare tomatoes

Whether you are going to enjoy your Tomatoes raw or cooked, I want to share with you the best way to prepare them. Properly cleaning and cutting your Tomatoes helps to ensure that the Tomatoes you serve will have the best flavor and retain the greatest number of nutrients.

### Cleaning Tomatoes

Rinse Tomatoes well under clear running water before cutting. (See *Washing Vegetables*, page 92.)

### Removing Pulp and Seeds

If you want to preserve the visual appeal of a broth that contains Tomatoes, remove the pulp and seeds from the Tomatoes before cooking. This will prevent the broth from turning opaque. The excess pulp can be saved to use in soup. (Details on how to remove the pulp and seeds can be found in the *Step-by-Step* on the bottom of page 169.)

## Chopping Tomatoes

Cut the Tomato into quarters or eighths and then cut across the wedges (this can be done with or without seeds and pulp removed).

## Slicing Tomatoes

With a sharp knife, cut out stem of the Tomato using a circular motion. Cut across the circumference of the Tomato into slices of desired thickness.

## Peeling Tomatoes

To peel Tomatoes, plunge them into boiling water for 20–30 seconds. The peel will come off easily after you dry them.

## Preparing Sun-Dried Tomatoes

Sun-dried Tomatoes have deep intense flavor but must be rehydrated before using. Place them in hot water for 10–15 minutes or until soft, or let them sit in extra virgin olive oil overnight.

# 4. the healthiest way of cooking tomatoes ———

For the best flavor, I recommend enjoying Tomatoes raw. They are a great addition to salads or sandwiches and can be used as a garnish or made into a salsa. However, studies are now finding that cooked Tomatoes can provide you with nutritional benefits not found in raw Tomatoes.

### The Healthiest Way of Cooking Tomatoes: "Healthy Sautéing" for just 5 Minutes

In my search to find the healthiest way to cook Tomatoes, I tested every possible cooking method and discovered that "Healthy Sautéing" Tomatoes for just 5 minutes delivered the best result. "Healthy Sautéing" retains their bright color and maximizes their nutritional profile. (For more on "*Healthy Sauté*," see page 57.)

### Cooking Methods Not Recommended for Tomatoes

#### DON'T COOK TOMATOES WITH OIL

I don't recommend cooking Tomatoes with oil because high temperature heat can damage delicate oils and potentially create harmful free radicals. My commitment to the "Healthiest Way of Cooking" includes avoiding the formation of free radicals whenever possible because they can cause inflammation. Adding extra virgin olive oil to Tomatoes immediately after they have been cooked is a wonderful way to enhance their flavor, as well as your absorption of their carotenoid phytonutrients, without increasing your exposure to free radicals. (For more on *Why It Is Important to Cook Without Heated Oils*, see page 52.)

### Serving Ideas from Mediterranean Countries:

Traveling through the Mediterranean region, I found that Tomatoes were prepared in many different ways:

In Spain, gazpacho (cold Tomato soup) is their most famous cold soup.

Italians made the Tomato sauce served on pasta famous.

In France, ratatouille (Tomato and eggplant) is a favorite dish.

In Greece, besides using them raw in salads, they like to bake Tomatoes with onions.

In Turkey, they stuff Tomatoes with rice, pine nuts and cinnamon.

### An Additional Way to Enjoy Cooked Tomatoes:

Quick Broiled Tomatoes: Cut Tomatoes in half horizontally. Sprinkle with fresh herbs, such as basil, oregano or parsley. Place them 5 inches from the broiler, with cut side up and broil for about 5 minutes. Tomatoes are done when they are tender, yet still holding their shape. Take care not to burn them. Drizzle with lemon, extra virgin olive oil, garlic, salt and pepper. Garnish with goat cheese.

---

Here is a question I received from readers of the whfoods.org website about Tomatoes:

**Q** *Aren't Tomatoes fruits and not vegetables, as you have them classified?*

**A** You are correct: from a botanical perspective, Tomatoes are considered to be fruits. Yet, like other fruits that are used in savory dishes—such as avocados and bell peppers—Tomatoes are considered vegetables from a culinary perspective. When I chose to create food categorizations for the World's Healthiest Foods, I needed to decide whether to do so based upon botanical guidelines or culinary guidelines. I chose the latter because I felt that it would be of better service to people since most people are used to thinking of food in terms of how they use it in a meal rather than in terms of scientific explanations. This is the reason that I put Tomatoes (and avocados and bell peppers) under the Vegetables category. It is also the reason that I chose to include foods such as quinoa and buckwheat, which are not botanically "grains," in the grains section as that is the way that people think of them from a culinary perspective.

# health benefits of tomatoes

### Promote Antioxidant Protection

Tomatoes are extremely rich in nutrients that have antioxidant activity. They are an excellent source of vitamin C as well as vitamin A, owing to their concentration of pro-vitamin A carotenoids such as alpha- and beta-carotene. Tomatoes also contain the carotenoids lutein, zeaxanthin and lycopene. It is because of lycopene that Tomatoes have recently been gaining center stage in the nutrition research arena as it is an important antioxidant, able to protect cells, lipoproteins and DNA from oxygen damage. Yet, while lycopene is a nutritional star on its own merits, researchers are finding out that it is not lycopene alone, but the entire array of important nutrients found in Tomatoes, which delivers the incredible health protection associated with eating Tomatoes.

### Promote Heart Health

More and more studies are finding that there is an important link between Tomatoes and heart health. Studies have found that regularly eating Tomatoes or Tomato-based products (including Tomato sauce/paste or ketchup) provides protection against LDL oxidation, one of the first steps in the progression of atherosclerosis, while also conferring a reduced risk of developing cardiovascular disease (CVD). Higher blood levels of lycopene have also been found to be protective against CVD. In addition to lycopene, Tomatoes provide numerous other heart-healthy nutrients such as beta-carotene, vitamin C, potassium, folic acid, dietary fiber and vitamin B6.

### Promote Optimal Health

Tomatoes may play an important role in cancer prevention. In a recent meta-analysis that combined the results of 21 studies, men consuming the highest amounts of raw Tomatoes were found to have an 11% reduction in their risk for prostate cancer, while those eating the most cooked Tomato products had a 19% reduction in prostate cancer risk. While lycopene seems to play a role in cancer prevention, including its suggested ability to activate cancer-preventive liver enzymes, researchers now believe that it is the whole array of health-promoting nutrients in Tomatoes, not just lycopene, which provides optimal cancer protection benefits.

*(Continued on Page 170)*

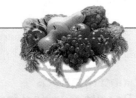

# how to enjoy fresh tomatoes without cooking

Fresh parsley, tarragon, dill and rosemary complement the flavor of Tomatoes.

**Mediterranean Tomato Salad:** This basic salad can be served as a first course. Combine 3 large ripe Tomatoes cut into chunks, 1 medium sliced red onion, 1 TBS vinegar or lemon juice, 2 minced garlic cloves, 3 TBS extra virgin olive oil, 10 fresh torn basil leaves, and sea salt and pepper to taste. You can add mozzarella cheese for extra flavor or anchovies, capers and chopped olives for more excitement.

**Seafood Tomato Salad:** For a complete meal, combine 2 medium chopped Tomatoes with 1 medium cubed avocado, 1 cup shrimp or scallops, 1 chopped medium cucumber, 1 chopped red bell pepper, 1 sliced boiled egg and 6 sliced black or Kalamata olives. Serve with your favorite vinaigrette, page 143.

**Quick Salsa:** Mix 2 diced medium Tomatoes with 1/2 medium chopped onion, 3 cloves chopped garlic, 1 medium deseeded minced jalapeño, 1 TBS fresh lime juice, 3 TBS chopped cilantro, and sea salt and pepper to taste.

**Tomato Relish:** Add a pinch of chili powder and 1 TBS vinegar to 1 large chopped Tomato and 1/2 medium chopped sweet onion. Serve with seafood or poultry.

**Fresh Tomato Dip:** Combine 2 medium Tomatoes chopped into small pieces, 3 cloves crushed garlic, 2 TBS fresh minced basil, 1 TBS sliced scallions, 3 TBS extra virgin olive oil, and sea salt and pepper to taste. Refrigerate for 1 hour. Serve with Italian bread for dipping or combine with Parmesan cheese and pour over hot pasta for a delicious fresh pasta sauce.

**No Cook Stuffed Tomato:** Cut a 1/4-inch slice off the top of 4 ripe Tomatoes and a sliver off the bottom of each. Scoop out the seeds and membrane inside. Stuff with tuna salad or low-fat cottage cheese. Top with feta cheese, chopped kalamata olives and basil leaves.

**5-Minute Tomato Salad Dressing:** Place the following ingredients in a blender and blend for 1 minute until well combined: 1 medium ripe Tomato cut into chunks, 1 tsp apple cider vinegar, 1-inch piece of ginger peeled and sliced, 1/2 medium avocado, 3 TBS extra virgin olive oil, 2 tsp fresh oregano, 2 cloves garlic, 1½ tsp tamari (soy sauce), and sea salt and pepper to taste. Serve on leafy greens or cooked grains like rice, pasta or barley.

STEP-BY-STEP RECIPE

## The Healthiest Way of Cooking Tomatoes

# Homemade Tomato Sauce

*If you know you have fully ripened Tomatoes that have not been picked green, or you have home-grown Tomatoes, you can make the best homemade Tomato sauce. It takes just minutes to prepare.*

### Ingredients:
2 TBS low-sodium chicken or vegetable broth
1/2 small onion, finely chopped
1 lb ripe Tomatoes
2 cloves garlic
1 tsp honey
1 tsp dried oregano
3 TBS extra virgin olive oil
3 TBS fresh basil leaves, minced
Sea salt and pepper to taste

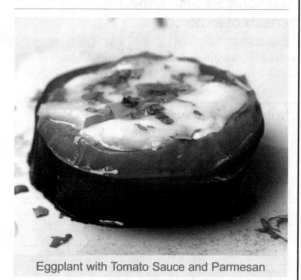

Eggplant with Tomato Sauce and Parmesan

1. Chop garlic and onions and let sit for at least 5 minutes. (Why?, see page 261.)
2. Peel, seed and dice Tomatoes as directed under *The Best Way to Prepare Tomatoes.*
3. Heat 2 TBS of broth in a stainless steel skillet over medium-low heat.
4. When broth begins to steam, add onions and sauté for 5 minutes.
5. Add Tomatoes, garlic, honey, oregano, salt and pepper.
6. Simmer **covered** until the Tomatoes are soft, about 5 minutes. (For information on *Differences in Cooking Time,* see page 94.)
7. Remove from burner. Add olive oil and fresh basil and mix well, breaking up any large pieces of Tomato. For richer flavor, you may want to add more olive oil.

**SERVES 2**

**COOKING TIP:** To prevent overcooking Tomatoes, I highly recommend using a timer.

### Flavor Tips: 5 Ways to Enjoy Homemade Tomato Sauce ✳

1. Add Parmesan cheese.
2. Add chopped olives, anchovies or capers.
3. Add "Healthy Sautéed" mushrooms and serve over pasta, chicken, fish or meat.
4. "Healthy Sauté" eggplant slices and top with Homemade Tomato Sauce and Mozzarella or Parmesan cheese (pictured above).
5. Fresh parsley, basil, dill and rosemary complement the flavor of Tomatoes.

Please write (address on back cover flap) or e-mail me at info@whfoods.org with your personal ideas for preparing Tomatoes, and I will share them with others through our website at www.whfoods.org.

## An Easy Way to Prepare Tomatoes, Step-By-Step

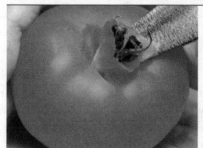
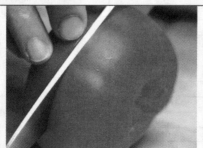
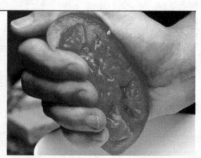

### REMOVE PULP AND SEEDS FROM TOMATOES
❶ Remove stem. ❷ Cut Tomato in half horizontally so the stem side is on one half. ❸ Gently squeeze each Tomato half to remove seeds and excess juice.

*(Continued from Page 168)*

## Additional Health-Promoting Benefits of Tomatoes

Tomatoes are also a concentrated source of other nutrients providing additional health-promoting benefits. These nutrients include bone-building vitamin K, magnesium and phosphorus; sulfite-detoxifying molybdenum; free-radical-scavenging manganese, copper and vitamin E; blood sugar-regulating chromium; energy-producing vitamin B1, vitamin B2, vitamin B5, niacin and iron; muscle-building protein; and sleep-promoting tryptophan. Since Tomatoes contain only 38 calories per one cup serving, they are an ideal food for healthy weight control.

### Nutritional Analysis of 1 cup red ripe Tomatoes:

| NUTRIENT | AMOUNT | % DAILY VALUE |
|---|---|---|
| Calories | 37.80 | |
| Calories from Fat | 5.35 | |
| Calories from Saturated Fat | 0.73 | |
| Protein | 1.53 g | |
| Carbohydrates | 8.35 g | |
| Dietary Fiber | 1.98 g | 7.92 |
| Soluble Fiber | 0.48 g | |
| Insoluble Fiber | 1.50 g | |
| Sugar – Total | 5.04 g | |
| Monosaccharides | 4.50 g | |
| Disaccharides | 0.00 g | |
| Other Carbs | 1.33 g | |
| Fat – Total | 0.59 g | |
| Saturated Fat | 0.08 g | |
| Mono Fat | 0.09 g | |
| Poly Fat | 0.24 g | |
| Omega-3 Fatty Acids | 0.01 g | 0.40 |
| Omega-6 Fatty Acids | 0.23 g | |
| Trans Fatty Acids | 0.00 g | |
| Cholesterol | 0.00 mg | |
| Water | 168.77 g | |
| Ash | 0.76 g | |
| **Vitamins** | | |
| Vitamin A IU | 1121.40 IU | 22.43 |
| Vitamin A RE | 111.60 RE | |
| A - Carotenoid | 111.60 RE | 1.49 |
| A - Retinol | 0.00 RE | |
| B1 Thiamin | 0.11 mg | 7.33 |
| B2 Riboflavin | 0.09 mg | 5.29 |
| B3 Niacin | 1.13 mg | 5.65 |
| Niacin Equiv | 1.31 mg | |
| Vitamin B6 | 0.14 mg | 7.00 |
| Vitamin B12 | 0.00 mcg | 0.00 |
| Biotin | 7.20 mcg | 2.40 |
| Vitamin C | 34.38 mg | 57.30 |
| Vitamin D IU | 0.00 IU | 0.00 |
| Vitamin D mcg | 0.00 mcg | |
| Vitamin E Alpha Equiv | 0.68 mg | 3.40 |
| Vitamin E IU | 1.02 IU | |
| Vitamin E mg | 1.67 mg | |
| Folate | 27.00 mcg | 6.75 |
| Vitamin K | 14.22 mcg | 17.77 |

| NUTRIENT | AMOUNT | % DAILY VALUE |
|---|---|---|
| Pantothenic Acid | 0.44 mg | 4.40 |
| **Minerals** | | |
| Boron | 3.06 mcg | |
| Calcium | 9.00 mg | 0.90 |
| Chloride | 108.00 mg | |
| Chromium | 9.00 mcg | 7.50 |
| Copper | 0.13 mg | 6.50 |
| Fluoride | — mg | — |
| Iodine | — mcg | — |
| Iron | 0.81 mg | 4.50 |
| Magnesium | 19.80 mg | 4.95 |
| Manganese | 0.19 mg | 9.50 |
| Molybdenum | 9.00 mcg | 12.00 |
| Phosphorus | 43.20 mg | 4.32 |
| Potassium | 399.60 mg | |
| Selenium | 0.72 mcg | 1.03 |
| Sodium | 16.20 mg | |
| Zinc | 0.16 mg | 1.07 |
| **Amino Acids** | | |
| Alanine | 0.04 g | |
| Arginine | 0.04 g | |
| Aspartate | 0.21 g | |
| Cystine | 0.02 g | 4.88 |
| Glutamate | 0.56 g | |
| Glycine | 0.04 g | |
| Histidine | 0.02 g | 1.55 |
| Isoleucine | 0.04 g | 3.48 |
| Leucine | 0.06 g | 2.37 |
| Lysine | 0.06 g | 2.55 |
| Methionine | 0.01 g | 1.35 |
| Phenylalanine | 0.04 g | 3.36 |
| Proline | 0.03 g | |
| Serine | 0.04 g | |
| Threonine | 0.04 g | 3.23 |
| Tryptophan | 0.01 g | 3.13 |
| Tyrosine | 0.03 g | 3.09 |
| Valine | 0.04 g | 2.72 |

(Note: "–" indicates data is unavailable. For more information, please see page 806.)

Here are questions I received from readers of the whfoods.org website about Tomatoes:

**Q** *Are Tomato skins good for you to eat? Do they provide any special benefits?*

**A** The skins of Tomatoes are definitely good to eat. They contain many nutrients including fiber and lycopene. Additionally, Tomato skins are a concentrated source of flavonoid phytonutrients. A recent study found that 98% of flavonols—a specific type of flavonoid—contained in Tomatoes are actually found in the skin. Extracts made from Tomato skins have also been found to have anti-allergenic properties, probably because of their concentration of another flavonoid called naringenin chalcone.

**Q** *I keep on hearing about the health benefits of lycopene. Is lycopene the reason that Tomatoes are so good for us?*

**A** Tomatoes have become well regarded for their concentration of lycopene, a carotenoid phytonutrient whose antioxidant strength is even greater than that of beta-carotene, capable of protecting cells, cholesterol and DNA from oxidative damage. Yet, recent research has suggested that the benefits of Tomatoes may be anything but lycopene-limited. Study after study shows that intake of Tomatoes or Tomato-based foods is associated with better health status, yet the results have not been as consistent for isolated lycopene, For example, in research when animals were given either lycopene or Tomatoes, those given the whole food were found to be better protected from disease.

The Tomato-lycopene link is a great example of how whole foods may be richly endowed with a particular superstar nutrient, yet it may be the food's whole matrix of nutrients, rather than just isolated ones, that provide the most benefit. So, the next time you think of taking lycopene supplements, you may want to add some sliced Tomatoes to your salad or sandwich instead.

# Q&A

## CAN ORGANIC FOODS REALLY IMPROVE MY HEALTH?

Yes. Organically grown food is your best way of reducing exposure to toxins used in conventional agricultural practices. These toxins include not only pesticides, many of which have been federally classified as potential cancer-causing agents, but also heavy metals such as lead and mercury, and solvents like benzene and toluene. Minimizing exposure to these toxins is of major benefit to your health. Heavy metals damage nerve function, contribute to diseases such as multiple sclerosis, lower IQ and also block hemoglobin production, causing anemia. Solvents damage white cells, lowering the immune system's ability to resist infections. In addition to significantly lessening your exposure to these health-robbing substances, organically grown foods have been shown to contain substantially higher levels of nutrients such as protein, vitamin C and many minerals.

## How do organic foods benefit cellular health?

**DNA:** Eating organically grown foods may help to better sustain health since recent test tube and animal research suggests that certain agricultural chemicals used in the conventional method of growing food may have the ability to cause genetic mutations that can lead to the development of cancer. One example is penta-chlorophenol (PCP) that has been found to cause DNA fragmentation in animals.

**Mitochondria:** Eating organically grown foods may help to better promote cellular health since several agricultural chemicals used in the conventional growing of foods have been shown to have a negative effect upon mitochondrial function. These chemicals include paraquat, parathion, dinoseb and 2,4-D; they have been found to affect the mitochondria and cellular energy production in a variety of ways including increasing membrane permeability, which exposes the mitochondria to damaging free radicals, and inhibiting a process known as coupling that is integral to the efficient production of ATP.

**Cell Membrane:** Since certain agricultural chemicals may damage the structure and function of the cellular membrane, eating organically grown foods can help to protect cellular health. The insecticide endosulfan and the herbicide paraquat have been shown to oxidize lipid molecules and therefore may damage the phospholipid component of the cellular membrane. In animal studies, pesticides such as chlopyrifos, endrin and fenthion have been shown to overstimulate enzymes involved in chemical signaling, causing imbalance that has been linked to conditions such as atherosclerosis, psoriasis and inflammation.

## How can organic foods contribute to children's health?

The negative health effects of conventionally grown foods, and therefore the benefits of consuming organic foods, are not just limited to adults. In fact, many experts feel that organic foods may be of paramount importance in safeguarding the health of our children.

In two separate reports, both the Natural Resources Defense Council (1989) and the Environmental Working Group (1998) found that millions of American children are exposed to levels of pesticides through their food that surpass limits considered to be safe. Some of these pesticides are known to be neurotoxic, able to cause harm to the developing brain and nervous system. Additionally, some researchers feel that children and adolescents may be especially vulnerable to the cancer-causing effects of certain pesticides since the body is more sensitive to the impact of these materials during periods of high growth rates and breast development.

The concern for the effects of agricultural chemicals on children's health seems so evident that the U.S. government has taken steps to protect our nation's young. In 1996, Congress passed the Food Quality Protection Act requiring that all pesticides applied to foods be safe for infants and children.

Organic foods that are strictly controlled for substances harmful to health can play a major role in assuring the health of our children.

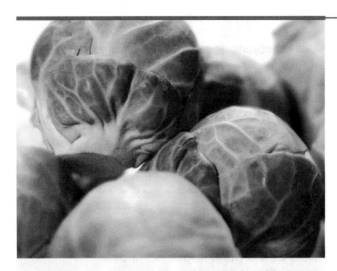

# brussels sprouts

## highlights

| | |
|---|---|
| AVAILABILITY: | Year-round |
| REFRIGERATE: | Yes |
| SHELF LIFE: | 10 days refrigerated |
| PREPARATION: | Cut and let sit for 5 minutes |
| BEST WAY TO COOK: | "Healthy Steamed" in just 5 minutes |

## nutrient-richness chart

Total Nutrient-Richness:  **33**          GI: **15**

One cup (156 grams) of cooked Brussels Sprouts contains 61 calories

| NUTRIENT | AMOUNT | %DV | DENSITY | QUALITY |
|---|---|---|---|---|
| Vitamin K | 218.8 mcg | 273.5 | 80.9 | excellent |
| Vitamin C | 96.7 mg | 161.2 | 47.7 | excellent |
| Folate | 93.6 mcg | 23.4 | 6.9 | very good |
| Vitamin A | 1121.6 IU | 22.4 | 6.6 | very good |
| Manganese | 0.4 mg | 17.5 | 5.2 | very good |
| Dietary Fiber | 4.1 g | 16.2 | 4.8 | very good |
| Potassium | 494.5 mg | 14.1 | 4.2 | very good |
| B6 Pyridoxine | 0.3 mg | 14.0 | 4.1 | very good |
| Tryptophan | 0.04 g | 12.5 | 3.7 | very good |
| B1 Thiamin | 0.2 mg | 11.3 | 3.4 | very good |
| Omega-3 Fatty Acids | 0.3 g | 10.4 | 3.1 | good |
| Iron | 1.9 mg | 10.4 | 3.1 | good |
| Phosphorus | 87.4 mg | 8.7 | 2.6 | good |
| Protein | 4.0 g | 8.0 | 2.4 | good |
| Magnesium | 31.2 mg | 7.8 | 2.3 | good |
| B2 Riboflavin | 0.1 mg | 7.1 | 2.1 | good |
| Vitamin E | 1.3 mg | 6.7 | 2.0 | good |
| Copper | 0.1 mg | 6.5 | 1.9 | good |
| Calcium | 56.2 mg | 5.6 | 1.7 | good |

**CAROTENOIDS:**

| | |
|---|---|
| Beta-Carotene | 711.4 mcg |
| Lutein+Zeaxanthin | 2,012.4 mcg |

For more on "Total Nutrient-Richness," "%DV," "Density," and
The World's Healthiest Foods "Quality" Rating System, see page 805.

For more on GI, see page 342.

Originating in northern Europe, Brussels Sprouts were named for the capital of Belgium, where they still remain an important local crop. They were introduced to England and France in the nineteenth century, and the French who settled in Louisiana brought them to the United States.

As with all vegetables, proper preparation is the key to bringing out the best flavor and nutritional benefits from Brussels Sprouts. That is why I want to share with you the secret of the "Healthiest Way of Cooking" Brussels Sprouts *al denté*. Because Brussels Sprouts are such a hearty vegetable, many people have the misconception that they take a long time to prepare, but in just 5 minutes, you can bring out their best flavor, maximize their nutritional value and transform Brussels Sprouts into a flavorful vegetable you will enjoy.

## why brussels sprouts should be part of your healthiest way of eating

Although they may look like small cabbages, Brussels Sprouts are anything but small when it comes to nutritional value. Along with vitamins C, A and E, which provide powerful antioxidant and anti-inflammatory protection, Brussels Sprouts are very rich in vitamin K and folate. Additionally, scientific studies now show that cruciferous vegetables, like Brussels Sprouts, contain large concentrations of health-promoting sulfur compounds such as glucosinolates and isothiocyanates (see page 153), which increase the liver's ability to produce enzymes that neutralize potentially toxic substances. Brussels Sprouts are also rich in the powerful phytonutrient antioxidants lutein and zeaxanthin. (For more on the *Health Benefits of Brussels Sprouts* and a complete analysis of their content of over 60 nutrients, see page 176.)

Brussels Sprouts are an ideal food to add to your "Healthiest Way of Eating" not only because they are high in nutrients, but also because they are low in calories: one cup of cooked Brussels Sprouts contains only 61 calories.

## varieties of brussels sprouts

Brussels Sprouts are a member of the cruciferous family of vegetables which also includes broccoli, cauliflower, kale, collard greens, cabbage and mustard greens. The most popular and widely available variety of Brussels Sprouts are sage green in color. This is the variety featured in the photographs in this chapter. There are also some varieties with a red hue. Although Brussels Sprouts are usually removed from the stem and sold individually, you may occasionally find them at the market still attached to the stem.

## the peak season

Brussels Sprouts are available throughout the year, but their flavor is at its peak during the cold months when the frost helps to develop a sweeter flavor. In hotter months, Brussels Sprouts are less tender and will require around 1 minute additional cooking time.

## biochemical considerations

Brussels Sprouts are a concentrated source of goitrogens, which might be of concern to certain individuals. (For more on *Goitrogens*, see page 721.)

## 4 steps for the best tasting and most nutritious brussels sprouts

Turning Brussels Sprouts into a flavorful dish with the most nutrients is simple if you just follow my 4 easy steps:

1. The Best Way to Select
2. The Best Way to Store
3. The Best Way to Prepare
4. The Healthiest Way of Cooking

# 1. the best way to select brussels sprouts ———

You can select the best tasting Brussels Sprouts by looking for ones that are firm and compact with a vibrant, bright green color. Since most Brussels Sprouts are sold off the stem, it is a good idea to select ones of comparable size so that they will cook in a similar amount of time. By selecting the best tasting Brussels Sprouts, you will also enjoy Brussels Sprouts with the highest nutritional value. As with all vegetables, I recommend selecting organically grown varieties of Brussels Sprouts whenever possible. (For more on *Organic Foods*, see page 113.)

Avoid Brussels Sprouts that are yellow or have wilted leaves. Be sure they are not puffy or soft in texture.

# 2. the best way to store brussels sprouts ———

Brussels Sprouts will turn soft, yellow and bitter if not stored properly. Make sure to store them well so that they will retain their flavor and nutrient concentrations.

Brussels Sprouts continue to respire even after they have been harvested; their respiration rate at room temperature (68°F/20°C) is 276 mg/kg/hr. Slowing down the respiration rate with proper storage is the key to extending their flavor and nutritional benefits. (For a *Comparison of Respiration Rates* for different vegetables, see page 91.)

### Brussels Sprouts Will Remain Fresh for Up to 10 Days When Properly Stored

1. Store fresh Brussels Sprouts in the refrigerator. The colder temperature will slow the respiration rate, helping to preserve their nutrients and keeping Brussels Sprouts fresh for a longer period of time.

2. Place Brussels Sprouts in a plastic storage bag before refrigerating. I have found that it is best to wrap the bag tightly around the Brussels Sprouts, squeezing out as much of the air from the bag as possible.

3. Do not wash Brussels Sprouts before refrigeration because exposure to water will encourage Brussels Sprouts to spoil.

# 3. the best way to prepare brussels sprouts

Properly cleaning and cutting Brussels Sprouts helps to ensure that the Brussels Sprouts you serve will have the best flavor and retain the greatest number of nutrients.

### Cleaning Brussels Sprouts

Before washing Brussels Sprouts, remove stems and any yellow leaves. Rinse them well under cool running water. To preserve nutrients, do not soak Brussels Sprouts or the water-soluble nutrients will leach into the water. (For more on *Washing Vegetables*, page 92.)

### Cutting Brussels Sprouts

Cutting Brussels Sprouts into equal size pieces will help them to cook more evenly. Since the smaller you cut Brussels Sprouts, the more quickly they will cook, I recommend cutting Brussels Sprouts into quarters. Cutting the Sprouts into smaller pieces helps maximize the formation of health-promoting compounds when you let them sit for at least 5 minutes before cooking.

# 4. the healthiest way of cooking brussels sprouts

Since research has shown that important nutrients can be lost or destroyed by the way a food is cooked, the "Healthiest Way of Cooking" Brussels Sprouts is focused on bringing out their best flavor while maximizing their vitamins, minerals and powerful antioxidants.

### The Healthiest Way of Cooking Brussels Sprouts: "Healthy Steaming" for Just 5 Minutes

In my search to find the healthiest way to cook Brussels Sprouts, I tested every possible cooking method and discovered that "Healthy Steaming" for just 5 minutes produced the best result. "Healthy Steaming" provides the moisture necessary to make Brussels Sprouts tender, brings out their peak flavor, retains their bright color and maximizes their nutritional profile. The Step-by-Step Recipe will show you how easy it is to "Healthy Steam" Brussels Sprouts. (For more on *"Healthy Steaming,"* see page 58.)

### How to Avoid Overcooking Brussels Sprouts: Cook Them *Al Denté*

One of the primary reasons people do not enjoy Brussels Sprouts is because they are often overcooked. For the best flavor, I recommend that you cook Brussels Sprouts *al denté*. Brussels Sprouts cooked *al denté* are tender outside and slightly firm inside. Plus, Brussels Sprouts cooked *al denté* are cooked just long enough to soften their cellulose and hemicellulose fiber; this makes them easier to digest and allows their health-promoting nutrients to become more readily available for assimilation.

Although Brussels Sprouts are a hearty vegetable, it is very important not to overcook them. Brussels Sprouts cooked for as little as a couple of minutes longer than *al denté* will begin to lose not only their texture and flavor, but also their nutrients. Overcooking Brussels Sprouts will significantly decrease their nutritional value: as much as 50% of some nutrients can be lost. (For more on *Al Denté*, see page 92.)

### An Easy Way to Prepare Brussels Sprouts, Step-By-Step

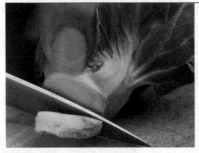 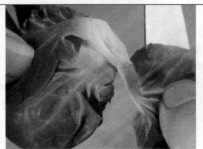 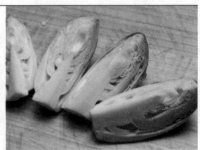

CUTTING BRUSSELS SPROUTS
❶ Remove a thin slice from bottom of Brussels Sprouts. ❷ Remove any yellow outer leaves. ❸ Cut Brussels Sprouts into quarters.

## How to Prevent Strong Smells from Forming

Cutting Brussels Sprouts into quarters and cooking them *al denté* for only 5 minutes is my secret for preventing the formation of smelly compounds often associated with cooking Brussels Sprouts. When I cook my Brussels Sprouts, they never develop a strong smell. After 5 minutes of cooking, the texture of Brussels Sprouts, like all other cruciferous vegetables, begins to change, becoming increasingly soft and mushy. At this point, they also start to lose more and more of their chlorophyll, causing their bright green color to fade and a brownish hue to appear. This is a sign that magnesium has been lost. This is when they start to release hydrogen sulfide, the cause of the "rotten egg smell," which also affects the flavor. After 7 minutes of cooking, Brussels Sprouts develop a more intense flavor, with the amount of strong smelling hydrogen sulfide doubling in quantity.

While it is important not to overcook Brussels Sprouts, cooking for less than 5 minutes is also not recommended, because it takes about 5 minutes to soften their fibers and help increase their digestibility.

## Cooking Methods
## Not Recommended for Brussels Sprouts

### BOILING, BAKING OR COOKING WITH OIL

Boiling Brussels Sprouts increases their water absorption causing them to become soggy and lose much of their flavor along with many of their nutrients, including minerals, water-soluble vitamins (such as C and the B-complex vitamins) and health-promoting phytonutrients. I don't recommend baking Brussels Sprouts as they will dry up and shrivel. I also don't recommend cooking Brussels Sprouts in oil because high temperature heat can damage delicate oils and potentially create harmful free radicals.

---

### HOW TO BRING OUT THE HIDDEN HEALTH BENEFITS OF BRUSSELS SPROUTS

The latest scientific studies show that cutting Brussels Sprouts into small pieces, such as quarters, breaks down cell walls and enhances the activation of an enzyme called *myrosinase* that slowly converts some of the plant nutrients into their active forms, which have been shown to contain health-promoting properties. So, to get the most health benefits from Brussels Sprouts, let them sit for a minimum of 5 minutes, optimally 10 minutes, after cutting, before eating or cooking.

Since ascorbic acid (vitamin C) increases *myrosinase* activity, you can sprinkle a little lemon juice on the Brussels Sprouts before letting them sit in order to further enhance their beneficial phytonutrient concentration.

Heat will inactivate the effect of *myrosinase*, which is why it is important to allow the Brussels Sprouts to sit for 5–10 minutes before cooking to give the enzyme ample opportunity to enhance the concentration of active phytonutrients in your Brussels Sprouts. Cooking at low or medium heat for short periods of time should not destroy the active phytonutrients since once they are formed, they are fairly stable.

---

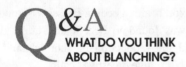

### WHAT DO YOU THINK ABOUT BLANCHING?

While blanching is often used as a preliminary step for freezing vegetables, it's important to realize that the vegetables experience nutrient loss when blanched. Commenting on her study that found that microwaving broccoli caused a great loss in flavonoids than steaming, study co-author, Dr. Cristina Garcia-Viguera, noted that "Most of the bioactive compounds in vegetables are water-soluble; during heating, they leach in a high percentage into the cooking water. Because of this, it is recommended to cook vegetables in the minimum amount of water (as in steaming) in order to retain their nutritional benefits." A second study, published in the same issue of the *Journal of the Science of Food and Agriculture*, provides similar evidence. In this study, Finnish researchers found that blanching vegetables prior to freezing caused losses of up to a third of their antioxidant content. Although slight further losses occurred during frozen storage, most bioactive compounds including antioxidants remained stable. The bottomline: how you prepare and cook your food may have a major impact on its nutrient-richness and blanching can lead to additional nutrient loss. While I would not say that you should never freeze your vegetables if you have an extra supply on hand, I think that this research further supports how fresh vegetables cooked in minimal amounts of time with the least amount of water exposure is the best way to prepare them with respect to retaining optimal nutrient concentrations.

# health benefits of brussels sprouts

## Promote Optimal Health

Plant phytonutrients found in Brussels Sprouts enhance the activity of the body's natural defense systems to protect against disease, including cancer. Scientists have found that sulforaphane, a potent compound created in the body from the glucoraphanin phytonutrient contained in

Brussels Sprouts and other *Brassica* family vegetables, boosts the body's detoxification enzymes, helping to clear potentially carcinogenic substances more quickly. Sulforaphane has been found to inhibit chemically induced breast cancers in animal studies and induce colon cancer cells to commit suicide.

In addition, men who consume Brussels Sprouts have been found to have less measured DNA damage than those who do not consume any cruciferous vegetables. Reduced DNA damage may translate to a reduced risk of cancer since mutations in DNA allow cancer cells to develop. Other beneficial sulfur-containing compounds in Brussels Sprouts include indoles and isothiocyanates.

## Promote Healthy Skin

Brussels Sprouts are an excellent source of vitamin C, the body's primary water-soluble antioxidant. Vitamin C supports immune function and the manufacture of collagen, a protein that forms the ground substance of body structures including the skin, connective tissue, cartilage, and tendons. In addition, Brussels Sprouts are a very good source of vitamin A, through their concentration of beta-carotene; both of these nutrients play important roles in defending the body against infection and promoting supple, glowing skin. Brussels Sprouts are also a good source of the omega-3 fatty acid, alpha-linolenic acid; among its many important functions, alpha-linolenic acid supports skin health.

## Promote Digestive Health

Add Brussels Sprouts to your diet, and you'll increase your intake of both soluble and insoluble fiber. Dietary fiber nourishes the cells lining the walls of your colon, which promotes colon health. Feeding Brussels Sprouts to research animals was found to beneficially affect their intestinal flora and the production of short chain fatty acids, both of which promote digestive heatlh.

## Additional Health-Promoting Benefits of Brussels Sprouts

Brussels Sprouts are also a concentrated source of many other nutrients providing additional health-promoting benefits. These nutrients include bone-building calcium, magnesium, vitamin K, copper and manganese; heart-healthy folate, vitamin B6, potassium and vitamin E; energy-producing iron, vitamin B1, vitamin B2 and phosphorus; muscle-building protein; and sleep-promoting tryptophan. Since Brussels Sprouts contain only 61 calories per serving, they are an ideal food for healthy weight control.

### Nutritional Analysis of 1 cup of cooked Brussels Sprouts:

| NUTRIENT | AMOUNT | % DAILY VALUE | NUTRIENT | AMOUNT | % DAILY VALUE |
|---|---|---|---|---|---|
| Calories | 60.84 | | Pantothenic Acid | 0.39 mg | 3.90 |
| Calories from Fat | 7.16 | | | | |
| Calories from Saturated Fat | 1.47 | | **Minerals** | | |
| Protein | 3.98 g | | Boron | — mcg | |
| Carbohydrates | 13.53 g | | Calcium | 56.16 mg | 5.62 |
| Dietary Fiber | 4.06 g | 16.24 | Chloride | — mg | |
| Soluble Fiber | 1.87 g | | Chromium | — mcg | — |
| Insoluble Fiber | 2.18 g | | Copper | 0.13 mg | 6.50 |
| Sugar – Total | 6.21 g | | Fluoride | — mg | — |
| Monosaccharides | 0.00 g | | Iodine | — mcg | — |
| Disaccharides | — g | | Iron | 1.87 mg | 10.39 |
| Other Carbs | 3.26 g | | Magnesium | 31.20 mg | 7.80 |
| Fat – Total | 0.80 g | | Manganese | 0.35 mg | 17.50 |
| Saturated Fat | 0.16 g | | Molybdenum | — mcg | — |
| Mono Fat | 0.06 g | | Phosphorus | 87.36 mg | 8.74 |
| Poly Fat | 0.41 g | | Potassium | 494.52 mg | |
| Omega-3 Fatty Acids | 0.26 g | 10.40 | Selenium | 2.34 mcg | 3.34 |
| Omega-6 Fatty Acids | 0.12 g | | Sodium | 32.76 mg | |
| Trans Fatty Acids | 0.00 g | | Zinc | 0.51 mg | 3.40 |
| Cholesterol | 0.00 mg | | | | |
| Water | 136.22 g | | **Amino Acids** | | |
| Ash | 1.48 g | | Alanine | 0.00 g | |
| | | | Arginine | 0.24 g | |
| **Vitamins** | | | Aspartate | 0.00 g | |
| Vitamin A IU | 1121.64 IU | 22.43 | Cystine | 0.02 g | 4.88 |
| Vitamin A RE | 112.32 RE | | Glutamate | 0.00 g | |
| A - Carotenoid | 112.32 RE | 1.50 | Glycine | 0.00 g | |
| A - Retinol | 0.00 RE | | Histidine | 0.09 g | 6.98 |
| Thiamin B1 | 0.17 mg | 11.33 | Isoleucine | 0.16 g | 13.91 |
| Riboflavin B2 | 0.12 mg | 7.06 | Leucine | 0.18 g | 7.11 |
| Niacin B3 | 0.95 mg | 4.75 | Lysine | 0.18 g | 7.66 |
| Niacin equiv | 1.68 mg | | Methionine | 0.04 g | 5.41 |
| Vitamin B6 | 0.28 mg | 14.00 | Phenylalanine | 0.12 g | 10.08 |
| Vitamin B12 | 0.00 mcg | 0.00 | Proline | 0.00 g | |
| Biotin | — mcg | — | Serine | 0.00 g | |
| Vitamin C | 96.72 mg | 161.20 | Threonine | 0.14 g | 11.29 |
| Vitamin D IU | 0.00 IU | 0.00 | Tryptophan | 0.04 g | 12.50 |
| Vitamin D mcg | 0.00 mcg | | Tyrosine | 0.00 g | 0.00 |
| Vitamin E Alpha Equiv | 1.33 mg | 6.65 | Valine | 0.18 g | 12.24 |
| Vitamin E IU | 1.98 IU | 12.24 | | | |
| Folate | 93.60 mcg | 23.40 | | | |
| Vitamin K | 218.80 mcg | 273.50 | | | |

(Note: "–" indicates data is unavailable. For more information, please see page 806.)

STEP-BY-STEP RECIPE
## The Healthiest Way of Cooking Brussels Sprouts

# 5-Minute "Healthy Steamed" Brussels Sprouts

*Cooking whole Brussels Sprouts takes a long time and can produce a strong smell. I discovered that cutting them in quarters and steaming them helps to make them sweeter with no odor. The easy Mediterranean Dressing enhances their flavor.*

**1 lb Brussels Sprouts**

**Mediterranean Dressing:**
**3 TBS extra virgin olive oil**
**2 tsp lemon juice**
**2 medium cloves garlic**
**Sea salt and black pepper to taste**

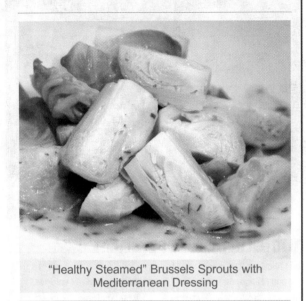

"Healthy Steamed" Brussels Sprouts with Mediterranean Dressing

1. Fill the bottom of the steamer with 2 inches of water.

2. While steam is building up in steamer, cut Brussels Sprouts into quarters and let sit as directed under *How to Bring out the Hidden Health Benefits of Brussels Sprouts.*

3. Chop or press garlic and let sit for at least 5 minutes. (Why?, see page 261.)

4. Steam Brussels Sprouts for 5 minutes. (For information on *Differences in Cooking Time,* see page 94.)

5. Transfer to a bowl. For more flavor, toss Brussels Sprouts with the remaining ingredients while they are still hot. (Mediterranean Dressing does not need to be made separately.) Research shows that carotenoids found in foods are best absorbed when consumed with oils.

OPTIONAL: To mellow the flavor of garlic, add garlic to Brussels Sprouts for the last 2 minutes of steaming.

**SERVES 2**

## COOKING TIPS:

- To prevent overcooking Brussels Sprouts, I highly recommend using a timer.
- Testing Brussels Sprouts with a fork is not an effective way to determine whether they are done.

## Flavor Tips: Try these 7 great serving suggestions with the recipe above. ✱

1. **Most Popular: Brussels Sprouts with Dijon Caper Sauce.** In a small bowl, combine the Mediterranean dressing recipe above with 1 TBS Dijon mustard, 1 tsp capers and 2 tsp minced fresh basil or parsley. Pour over hot Brussels Sprouts.
2. Sprinkle with chopped, toasted nuts or sunflower seeds.
3. Drizzle with balsamic vinegar, basil and goat cheese.
4. **Spicy Brussels Sprouts:** Cook the 5-Minute "Healthy Steamed" Brussels Sprouts with diced onions. Add raw red pepper strips and red pepper flakes. Toss with your favorite vinaigrette (see page 143 for ideas).

5. **Brussels Sprouts and Apples:** Cook the 5-Minute "Healthy Steamed" Brussels Sprouts with chopped onions and combine with finely chopped raw apples and toasted walnuts.
6. **Nutty Brussels Sprouts:** Combine the 5-Minute "Healthy Steamed" Brussels Sprouts with grated Parmesan cheese and chopped toasted almonds.
7. **Asian Sauce:** Whisk together 1 TBS tamari (soy sauce), 1 TBS honey, 1 TBS rice vinegar, 2 tsp sesame seeds and 1 tsp grated ginger. Toss with 5-Minute "Healthy Steamed" Brussels Sprouts.

Please write (address on back cover flap) or e-mail me at info@whfoods.org with your personal ideas for preparing Brussels Sprouts, and I will share them with others through our website at www.whfoods.org.

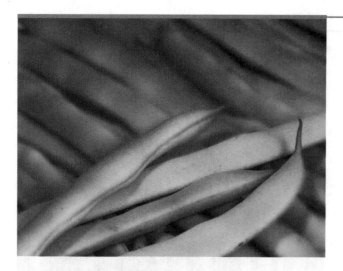

# nutrient-richness chart

| Total Nutrient-Richness: | **33** | | GI: **15** |

One cup (125 grams) of cooked Green Beans contains 44 calories

| NUTRIENT | AMOUNT | %DV | DENSITY | QUALITY |
| --- | --- | --- | --- | --- |
| Vitamin K | 20.0 mcg | 25.0 | 10.3 | excellent |
| Vitamin C | 12.1 mg | 20.2 | 8.3 | excellent |
| Manganese | 0.4 mg | 18.5 | 7.6 | excellent |
| Vitamin A | 832.5 IU | 16.6 | 6.9 | very good |
| Dietary Fiber | 4.0 g | 16.0 | 6.6 | very good |
| Potassium | 373.8 mg | 10.7 | 4.4 | very good |
| Folate | 41.6 mcg | 10.4 | 4.3 | very good |
| Tryptophan | 0.03 g | 9.4 | 3.9 | very good |
| Iron | 1.6 mg | 8.9 | 3.7 | very good |
| Magnesium | 31.3 mg | 7.8 | 3.2 | good |
| B2 Riboflavin | 0.1 mg | 7.1 | 2.9 | good |
| Copper | 0.1 mg | 6.5 | 2.7 | good |
| B1 Thiamin | 0.1 mg | 6.0 | 2.5 | good |
| Calcium | 57.5 mg | 5.8 | 2.4 | good |
| Phosphorus | 48.8 mg | 4.9 | 2.0 | good |
| Protein | 2.4 g | 4.7 | 1.9 | good |
| Omega-3 Fatty Acids | 0.1 g | 4.4 | 1.8 | good |
| B3 Niacin | 0.8 mg | 3.9 | 1.6 | good |

| **CAROTENOIDS:** | | |
| --- | --- | --- |
| Beta-Carotene | 525.0 mcg | Daily values for these nutrients have not yet been established. |
| Lutein+Zeaxanthin | 886.3 mcg | |

For more on "Total Nutrient-Richness," "%DV," "Density," and The World's Healthiest Foods "Quality" Rating System, see page 805.

For more on GI, see page 342.

G reen Beans are one of only a few varieties of beans that can be eaten fresh. They are delicious and versatile—great as a side dish, incorporated into a salad or served as crudités. Yet, while they are well known, I don't think Green

# green beans

## highlights

| AVAILABILITY: | Year-round |
| --- | --- |
| REFRIGERATE: | Yes |
| SHELF LIFE: | 7 days refrigerated |
| PREPARATION: | Minimal |
| BEST WAY TO COOK: | "Heathy Steamed" in just 5 minutes |

Beans are as well appreciated as they could be, since they are so often overcooked. Proper preparation is key to enjoying Green Beans. So, for a vibrantly colored, great tasting dish try the "Healthiest Way of Cooking" Green Beans. In just 5 minutes, you can bring out their best flavor while maximizing their nutritional value by cooking Green Beans *al denté*.

## why green beans should be part of your healthiest way of eating

Green Beans contain carotenoid phytonutrients such as beta-carotene, lutein and zeaxanthin, which provide anti-inflammatory properties. They are a concentrated source of vitamin K, which is essential for bone mineralization, and also of vitamins A and C, which provide powerful antioxidant protection and reduce the number of free radicals in the body. Green Beans are an ideal food to add to your "Healthiest Way of Eating" because they are high in nutrients and low in calories: one cup of cooked Green Beans contains only 44 calories, great for healthy weight loss. (For more on the *Health Benefits of Green Beans* and a complete analysis of their content of over 60 nutrients, see page 182.)

## varieties of green beans

Green Beans and other beans, such as kidney beans, navy beans and black beans, are all known scientifically as *Phaseolus vulgaris*. What sets Green Beans apart from their cousins is that the entire bean (pods and seeds) can be eaten. Some of the most common varieties include:

### SNAP BEANS

This is the most popular variety of Green Beans and the one featured in the photographs in this chapter. Their name was derived from the sound that occurs when the ends are snapped off to remove the tough string that runs along the seam of older varieties of Snap Beans. Most of the Snap Beans you find in the market today no longer have strings.

### CHINESE LONG BEANS

Also known as Yard-Long or Asparagus Beans, these thin Green Beans can measure up to 18 inches in length. They have a mild flavor and are a good choice for stir-fry dishes.

### HARICOT VERTS

These are a slender French version of the American Snap Bean.

### ROMANO BEANS

Also known as Italian Green Beans, they have broad, flat, bright green pods. They are most commonly found frozen.

### SCARLET RUNNER BEANS

They have broad, flat, green pods that contain scarlet seeds.

## the peak season

Although Green Beans are available throughout the year, their peak season runs from summer through early fall. These are the months when their concentration of nutrients and flavor are highest, and their cost is at its lowest.

## biochemical considerations

Green Beans are a concentrated source of oxalates, which may be of concern to some individuals. (For more on *Oxalates*, see page 725.)

## 4 steps for the best tasting and most nutritious green beans

Turning Green Beans into a flavorful dish with the most nutrients is simple if you just follow my 4 easy steps:

1. The Best Way to Select
2. The Best Way to Store
3. The Best Way to Prepare
4. The Healthiest Way of Cooking

# 1. the best way to select green beans

It is best when Green Beans are sold loose, so you can sort through them and select the best quality beans. The best tasting beans feel smooth, have a vibrant green color, are firm and "snap" when bent. I recommend selecting beans of similar size to ensure uniform cooking. By selecting the best tasting Green Beans, you will also be getting beans with the highest nutritional value. Like all vegetables, it is best to select organically grown Green Beans whenever possible. (For more on *Organic Foods*, see page 113.)

Avoid Green Beans that have brown spots or areas that are soft, bruised, wrinkled or have tough skin. Beans that are beginning to turn yellow are no longer fresh.

# 2. the best way to store green beans

Green Beans will become limp and lose their freshness if not stored properly. If you are not going to prepare them the day you bring them home from the market, store them properly so as to preserve their flavor and their nutrients.

Green Beans continue to respire even after they have been harvested; their respiration rate at room temperature (68°F/ 20°C) is 130 mg/kg/hr. Slowing down the respiration rate with proper storage is the key to extending their flavor and nutritional benefits. (For a *Comparison of Respiration Rates* for different vegetables, see page 91.)

### Green Beans Will Remain Fresh for Up to 7 Days When Properly Stored

1. Store fresh Green Beans in the refrigerator. The colder temperature will slow the respiration rate, helping to preserve their nutrients and keeping Green Beans fresh for a longer period of time.

2. Place Green Beans in a plastic storage bag before refrigerating. I have found that it is best to wrap the bag tightly around the Green Beans, squeezing out as much of the air from the bag as possible.

3. Do not wash Green Beans before refrigeration because exposure to water will encourage Green Beans to spoil.

# 3. the best way to prepare green beans

Properly cleaning and cutting Green Beans help to ensure that the Green Beans you serve will have the best flavor and retain the greatest number of nutrients.

## Cleaning Green Beans

Rinse well in a colander under running water after cutting off ends. To preserve nutrients, do not soak Green Beans or their water-soluble nutrients will leach into the water. (For more on *Washing Vegetables*, see page 92.)

## Cutting Green Beans

Most Green Beans no longer have strings; therefore, you do not have to snap off the ends of each bean individually to remove the string. To cut off the ends, take a handful of beans and align the ends by tapping them on the cutting board so that you can cut off the ends all at one time. Turn the beans around, aligning the opposite ends and cut off ends. Green Beans are best cooked whole.

# 4. the healthiest way of cooking green beans

Since research has shown that important nutrients can be lost or destroyed by the way a food is cooked, the "Healthiest Way of Cooking" Green Beans is focused on bringing out their best flavor while maximizing their vitamins, minerals and powerful antioxidants.

## The Healthiest Way of Cooking Green Beans: "Healthy Steaming" for just 5 Minutes

In my search to find the healthiest way to cook Green Beans, I tested every possible cooking method and discovered that "Healthy Steaming" Green Beans for just 5 minutes delivered the best result. "Healthy Steaming" provides the moisture necessary to make Green Beans tender, brings out their peak flavor, retains their bright color and maximizes their nutritional profile. It is best to cook Green Beans whole to ensure that they will cook evenly. The Step-by-Step Recipe will show you how easy it is to prepare "Healthy Steamed" Green Beans.

Green Beans that are cut into small pieces are more likely to become mushy because the cut ends allow more heat to penetrate the soft inner portion, which will cook more quickly than the outer skin. (For more on *"Healthy Steaming,"* see page 58.)

## How to Avoid Overcooking Green Beans: Cook Them *Al Denté*

One of the primary reasons Green Beans lose their flavor is because they are overcooked. For the best flavor, I recommend cooking Green Beans *al denté*. Green Beans cooked *al denté* are tender outside and slightly firm inside. Plus, Green Beans cooked *al denté* are cooked just long enough to soften their cellulose and hemicellulose fiber; this makes them easier to digest and allows their health-promoting nutrients to become more readily available for absorption.

Although Green Beans are a hearty vegetable, it is very important not to overcook them. Green Beans cooked for as little as a couple of minutes longer than *al denté* will begin to

*(Continued on Page 63)*

---

**An Easy Way to Prepare Green Beans, Step-by-Step**

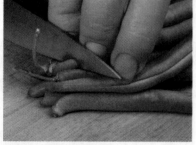 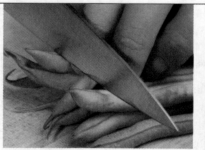 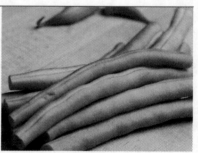

CUTTING GREEN BEANS

❶ Take a handful of Green Beans and tap the ends on cutting board to even them out. Cut ends of a handful of beans all at once. ❷ Turn beans around and tap on cutting board and cut off ends.
❸ Green Beans are best cooked whole.

**STEP-BY-STEP RECIPE**
## The Healthiest Way of Cooking Green Beans

# 5-Minute *"Healthy Steamed"* Green Beans

*The traditional method of boiling Green Beans causes a loss of many of their health-promoting nutrients, while the "Healthy Steaming" method retains the maximum number of nutrients. Combining them with the Mediterranean Dressing enhances their delicate flavor.*

**1 lb Green Beans**

**Mediterranean Dressing:**
**3 TBS extra virgin olive oil**
**2 tsp lemon juice**
**2 medium cloves garlic**
**Sea salt and ground pepper to taste**

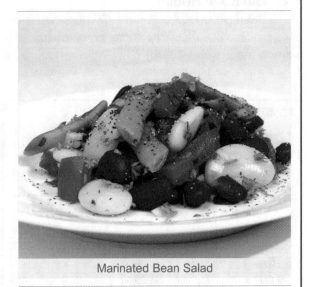
Marinated Bean Salad

1. Chop or press garlic and let sit for at least 5 minutes. (Why?, see page 261.)
2. Fill the bottom of the steamer with 2 inches of water.
3. While steam is building up in steamer, cut ends off Green Beans.
4. Steam for 5 minutes. A fork should pierce them easily when they are done. (For information on *Differences in Cooking Time*, see page 94.)

5. Transfer to a bowl. For more flavor, toss Green Beans with the remaining ingredients while they are still hot. (Mediterranean Dressing does not need to be made separately.) Research shows that carotenoids found in foods are best absorbed when consumed with oils.

OPTIONAL: To mellow the flavor of garlic, add garlic to Green Beans for the last 2 minutes of steaming.

**COOKING TIPS:**
• To prevent overcooking Green Beans, I highly recommend using a timer.

**SERVES 2**

---

## Flavor Tips:  Try these 8 great serving suggestions with the recipe above.

1. **Most Popular:** Replace the lemon juice with the juice and zest of 1 orange and top with toasted, sliced almonds.
2. Top with chopped basil, minced red bell pepper and goat cheese.
3. Add a few drops of tamari (soy sauce) to mellow the flavor of Green Beans.
4. Add "Healthy Sautéed" onions and shiitake mushrooms and tamari (soy sauce).
5. **Asian Flavored Green Beans:**  Combine 5-Minute "Healthy Steamed" Green Beans (omit dressing) with 1 TBS tamari (soy sauce), 1 TBS grated ginger, 1 TBS rice vinegar, 1 TBS honey and chopped fresh cilantro or sesame seeds.
6. **Salad Niçoise:** Combine 1 can tuna, 1/2 cup kalamata olives, 1 sliced boiled egg, 1 chopped tomato and 5-Minute "Healthy Steamed" Green Beans and dress-

ing with 1 TBS Dijon mustard and 2 TBS fresh chopped herbs, such as basil, parsley or dill.
7. **Marinated Bean Salad:** Combine 5-Minute "Healthy Steamed" Green Beans (omit dressing) with 15 oz cans of drained kidney and lima beans, 1 sliced red bell pepper and 1 cup minced red onion. Toss with 1/2 cup olive oil, 1/2 cup red wine or cider vinegar, 1 tsp sea salt, 1/2 tsp black pepper, 1/2 cup minced parsley and 3 cloves pressed garlic. Let mixture marinate overnight in refrigerator (pictured above).
8. **Indian Curry Green Beans:** In a large bowl, whisk together 2 tsp lemon juice, 1/4 cup extra virgin olive oil, 1 tsp curry powder and 2 tsp tamari (soy sauce). Toss warm 5-Minute "Healthy Steamed" Green Beans with the sauce and garnish with toasted sesame seeds and cilantro leaves.

---

Please write (address on back cover flap) or e-mail me at info@whfoods.org with your personal ideas for preparing Green Beans, and I will share them with others through our website at www.whfoods.org.

# health benefits of green beans

## Promote Bone Health

Green Beans are an excellent source of vitamin K, a nutrient important for maintaining strong bones. Vitamin K1 activates osteocalcin, the major non-collagen protein in bone, which anchors calcium molecules inside of the bone. Green Beans are also a good source of bone-building calcium, magnesium and phosphorus.

## Promote Heart Health

Green Beans provide a cornucopia of heart healthy nutrients. They are a very good source of vitamin A, notably through their concentration of beta-carotene, and an excellent source of vitamin C. These two nutrients are important antioxidants that work to reduce the amount of free radicals in the body. This water- and fat-soluble antioxidant team helps to prevent cholesterol from becoming oxidized, the first step in the process through which cholesterol becomes able to stick to and build up in blood vessels where it can cause blocked arteries, heart attack or stroke.

The magnesium and potassium found in Green Beans work together to help lower high blood pressure, while their folate is needed to convert homocysteine into other benign molecules. Since homocysteine can directly damage blood vessel walls if not promptly converted, high levels are associated with a significantly increased risk of heart attack and stroke. The fiber found in Green Beans has also been shown to help lower high cholesterol levels.

## Promote Energy Production

Green Beans are a very good source of iron, an especially important mineral for menstruating women, who are more at risk for iron deficiency. Iron is an integral component of hemoglobin, which transports oxygen from the lungs to all body cells and is also part of key enzyme systems for energy production and metabolism. Since hemoglobin synthesis also relies on copper, without this mineral, iron cannot be properly utilized in red blood cells. Fortunately, Green Beans are a good source of copper. Green beans' manganese, along with its copper, are essential cofactors of a key oxidative enzyme called *superoxide dismutase*, which disarms free radicals produced within our cells.

## Additional Health-Promoting Benefits of Green Beans

Green Beans are also a concentrated source of other nutrients providing additional health-promoting benefits. These nutrients include heart-healthy omega-3 fatty acids and potassium; energy-producing vitamin B1, vitamin B2 and niacin; muscle-building protein; and sleep-promoting tryptophan. Since Green Beans contain only 44 calories per one cup serving, they are an ideal food for healthy weight control.

### Nutritional Analysis of 1 cup of cooked Green Beans:

| NUTRIENT | AMOUNT | % DAILY VALUE | NUTRIENT | AMOUNT | % DAILY VALUE |
|---|---|---|---|---|---|
| Calories | 43.75 | | Pantothenic Acid | 0.09 mg | 0.90 |
| Calories from Fat | 3.15 | | | | |
| Calories from Saturated Fat | 0.72 | | **Minerals** | | |
| Protein | 2.36 g | | Boron | — mcg | |
| Carbohydrates | 9.86 g | | Calcium | 57.50 mg | 5.75 |
| Dietary Fiber | 4.00 g | 16.00 | Chloride | 13.75 mg | |
| Soluble Fiber | 1.63 g | | Chromium | — mcg | — |
| Insoluble Fiber | 2.38 g | | Copper | 0.13 mg | 6.50 |
| Sugar – Total | 2.38 g | | Fluoride | — mg | — |
| Monosaccharides | 1.85 g | | Iodine | — mcg | — |
| Disaccharides | 0.53 g | | Iron | 1.60 mg | 8.89 |
| Other Carbs | 3.49 g | | Magnesium | 31.25 mg | 7.81 |
| Fat – Total | 0.35 g | | Manganese | 0.37 mg | 18.50 |
| Saturated Fat | 0.08 g | | Molybdenum | — mcg | — |
| Mono Fat | 0.01 g | | Phosphorus | 48.75 mg | 4.88 |
| Poly Fat | 0.18 g | | Potassium | 373.75 mg | |
| Omega-3 Fatty Acids | 0.11 g | 4.40 | Selenium | 0.50 mcg | 0.71 |
| Omega-6 Fatty Acids | 0.07 g | | Sodium | 3.75 mg | |
| Trans Fatty Acids | 0.00 g | | Zinc | 0.45 mg | 3.00 |
| Cholesterol | 0.00 mg | | | | |
| Water | 111.53 g | | **Amino Acids** | | |
| Ash | 0.91 g | | Alanine | 0.11 g | |
| | | | Arginine | 0.10 g | |
| **Vitamins** | | | Aspartate | 0.33 g | |
| Vitamin A IU | 832.50 IU | 16.65 | Cystine | 0.02 g | 4.88 |
| Vitamin A RE | 83.75 RE | | Glutamate | 0.24 g | |
| A - Carotenoid | 83.75 RE | 1.12 | Glycine | 0.09 g | |
| A - Retinol | 0.00 RE | | Histidine | 0.04 g | 3.10 |
| Thiamin B1 | 0.09 mg | 6.00 | Isoleucine | 0.09 g | 7.83 |
| Riboflavin B2 | 0.12 mg | 7.06 | Leucine | 0.14 g | 5.53 |
| Niacin B3 | 0.77 mg | 3.85 | Lysine | 0.11 g | 4.68 |
| Niacin equiv | 1.18 mg | | Methionine | 0.03 g | 4.05 |
| Vitamin B6 | 0.07 mg | 3.50 | Phenylalanine | 0.09 g | 7.56 |
| Vitamin B12 | 0.00 mcg | 0.00 | Proline | 0.09 g | |
| Biotin | 1.00 mcg | 0.33 | Serine | 0.13 g | |
| Vitamin C | 12.13 mg | 20.22 | Threonine | 0.10 g | 8.06 |
| Vitamin D IU | 0.00 IU | 0.00 | Tryptophan | 0.03 g | 9.38 |
| Vitamin D mcg | 0.00 mcg | | Tyrosine | 0.06 g | 6.19 |
| Vitamin E Alpha Equiv | 0.18 mg | 0.90 | Valine | 0.12 g | 8.16 |
| Vitamin E IU | 0.26 IU | | | | |
| Vitamin E mg | 0.18 mg | | | | |
| Folate | 41.63 mcg | 10.41 | | | |
| Vitamin K | 20.00 mcg | 25.00 | | | |

(Note: "—" indicates data is unavailable. For more information, please see page 806.)

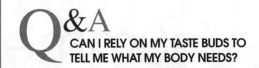

## Q&A
### CAN I RELY ON MY TASTE BUDS TO TELL ME WHAT MY BODY NEEDS?

Yes, if you work at it, you can rely on your taste buds to tell you what your body does and doesn't need. For most of us, however, trusting our taste buds is something that we will have to learn how to do, not something we can do right away. Here's why:

### Our Taste Buds Detect Four Basic Flavors

First, when it comes to our body chemistry, we don't have taste buds for avocado flavor, or olive oil flavor, or strawberry flavor. Our taste buds are designed to detect only four basic flavors: sweet, salty, sour, and bitter. (New research is suggesting that umami, the sensation of savoriness, may be the "fifth basic taste.") Because we don't have taste buds for specific food flavors, our taste buds can't tell us directly which foods we need and which ones we don't. Sometimes we might crave something sweet and find out that our bodies were telling us that our blood sugar was low, and that we needed to eat some sugar-containing food to raise our blood sugar quickly. This kind of situation, however, would be the exception and not the rule. Most of the time when we crave something sweet, our blood sugar level is normal, and we're just in the mood for a treat.

### All Our Senses Enjoy Food

Second, the taste of a food is not determined exclusively from the reaction of our taste buds. The smell of a food, the visual appearance of a food, how we expect the food to taste, and how often we've eaten it previously all affect what we actually taste. When we sit down to enjoy a meal, it's not simply a question of our taste buds detecting four basic flavors. It's all our senses that enable us to enjoy our food, not just our taste buds.

### Children Know Best

Some very interesting research studies of young, pre-school age children have tried to determine just how much our taste buds can be trusted. Children in these studies were selected because of their known, pre-existing vitamin deficiencies. For example, one study looked at children who were known to be low in vitamin D. These children were given a choice of several foods, but only one of the foods was high in vitamin D. For example, given a choice of orange juice (no vitamin D), soda pop (no vitamin D), and cod liver oil (high vitamin D), most of the kids actually chose cod liver oil! In other words, they seemed to be able to trust their taste buds. Many other studies, however, have repeatedly shown that even at a very early age, children tend to prefer the foods that their parents or brothers and sisters eat, and that the opinions of their family influence the way food tastes to them.

In addition, by the time we get to be adults, we've seen thousands of food commercials on television; we've accepted responsibilities that can make our week highly stressful; and we've had years and years of eating without trying to foster an awareness of our body's reactions to food and what it needs.

### What Adults Should Do

How can we learn, as adults, to trust our taste buds? This task requires us to get back in touch with food. We have to give our taste buds a rest from all of the artificial flavors and artificial textures that are characteristic of processed food. We can't get back in touch with food unless we know what real food actually tastes like! The recipes in this book focus exclusively on real food. They are not only free from artificial flavors of any kind, but they are also created exclusively from whole, nutrient-rich foods. These foods will get you back in touch with real food and its taste. Careful handling and preparation of all foods is also emphasized in this book. The taste of real foods can be destroyed if the foods are not handled and prepared well. Getting back in touch with food means visiting the produce section of the grocery store more often and spending more time in our own kitchens.

### Practical Tips

If you've had a hectic, stressful day where you didn't even get to sit down to lunch, and you stop at the gas station on the way home to get gas and see a bar of chocolate on the way out, you're in a very poor situation to trust your taste buds. In this kind of situation, your taste buds are going to tell you that a bar of chocolate is exactly what you need. But it isn't! What we all need is to respect ourselves and take the half hour lunch needed during our day to nourish our bodies with real food. But our taste buds can't tell us that.

At the other end of the spectrum, if we've made most of our day's food selections form the World's Healthiest Foods, and we have taken time during the day to nourish ourselves with these foods, the opinion of our taste buds becomes much more reliable.

Which sounds better? Salmon with Ginger Mint Salsa or Healthy Sautéed Cabbage? Under this different set of circumstances, if it's the salmon that tempts our taste buds, perhaps our cells are more in need of omega-3 fatty acids found in fresh salmon. If the Healthy Sautéed Cabbage sounds better, perhaps our taste buds are calling out for the sulfur compounds in the cabbage and garlic. The World's Healthiest Foods give us a starting point for trusting our taste buds. We have to do the rest by getting back in touch with these foods on a day-to-day basis.

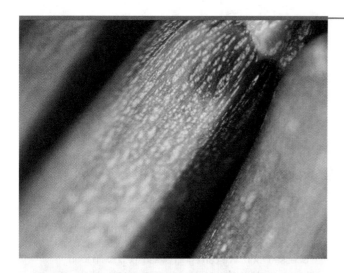

# summer squash

## nutrient-richness chart

Total Nutrient-Richness: **32**  GI: **15**

One cup (180 grams) of Summer Squash contains 36 calories

| NUTRIENT | AMOUNT | %DV | DENSITY | QUALITY |
|---|---|---|---|---|
| Manganese | 0.4 mg | 19.0 | 9.5 | excellent |
| Vitamin C | 9.9 mg | 16.5 | 8.3 | excellent |
| Magnesium | 43.2 mg | 10.8 | 5.4 | very good |
| Vitamin A | 516.6 IU | 10.3 | 5.2 | very good |
| Dietary Fiber | 2.5 g | 10.1 | 5.0 | very good |
| Potassium | 345.6 mg | 9.9 | 4.9 | very good |
| Copper | 0.2 mg | 9.5 | 4.8 | very good |
| Folate | 36.9 mcg | 9.0 | 4.5 | very good |
| Vitamin K | 6.3 mcg | 7.9 | 3.9 | very good |
| Phosphorus | 70.2 mg | 7.0 | 3.5 | very good |
| Omega-3 Fatty Acids | 0.2 g | 6.0 | 3.0 | good |
| B6 Pyridoxine | 0.1 mg | 6.0 | 3.0 | good |
| B1 Thiamin | 0.1 mg | 5.3 | 2.7 | good |
| Calcium | 48.6 mg | 4.9 | 2.4 | good |
| Zinc | 0.7 mg | 4.7 | 2.3 | good |
| B3 Niacin | 0.9 mg | 4.6 | 2.3 | good |
| B2 Riboflavin | 0.1 mg | 4.1 | 2.1 | good |
| Iron | 0.67 mg | 3.6 | 1.8 | good |
| Protein | 1.6 g | 3.3 | 1.6 | good |
| Tryptophan | 0.01 g | 3.1 | 1.6 | good |

| CAROTENOIDS: | | |
|---|---|---|
| Beta-Carotene | 228.6 mcg | |
| Lutein+Zeaxanthin | 4,048.2 mcg | |

Daily values for these nutrients have not yet been established.

For more on "Total Nutrient-Richness," "%DV," "Density," and
The World's Healthiest Foods "Quality" Rating System, see page 805.

For more on GI, see page 342.

Squash has been consumed for over 10,000 years, but it was not until it was cultivated throughout the Americas that this once bitter vegetable, with very little flesh, developed into the sweet-flavored variety we enjoy today. Summer Squash was historically distinguished from winter squash because it was available only during the summer months. While it is now available in markets throughout the year, Summer Squash remains a popular summer vegetable and an easy-to-grow favorite in summer vegetable gardens. Unlike winter squash, Summer Squash has thin edible skin, soft seeds and a high water content. Proper preparation is the key to bringing out the best flavor from Summer Squash and maximizing its nutritional benefits. That is why I want to share with you the secret of the "Healthiest Way of Cooking" Summer Squash *al denté*. By preparing Summer Squash *al denté*, you will have the best tasting, most nutritious Summer Squash in just 3 minutes!

## why summer squash should be part of your healthiest way of eating

Summer Squash is an excellent source of manganese, which helps facilitate protein and carbohydrate metabolism and activate enzymes that are responsible for the utilization of important nutrients such as biotin, thiamin and choline. Its vitamin C functions as a powerful antioxidant that has great benefits for heart health.

Summer Squash is also a notable source of the phytonutrients lutein and zeaxanthin, a pair of carotenoids that act as powerful antioxidants. It is an ideal food to add to your "Healthiest Way of Eating," especially if you are interested in losing weight or maintaining your optimal weight, because it is not only high in nutrients, but also quite low in calories: one cup of Summer Squash contains only 36 calories. (For more on the *Health Benefits of Summer Squash* and a complete analysis of its content of over 60 nutrients, see page 188.)

## varieties of summer squash

The Summer Squash (*Cucurbita pepo*) we are familiar with today developed from wild squash that grew in an area between Guatemala and Mexico. Summer Squash belongs to the *Cucurbitaceae* family and is related to both the melon and the cucumber. There are many varieties of Summer Squash that differ in shape, color, size and flavor; however, they do have one thing in common—you can enjoy the flesh, seeds and skin of all of them, so you don't have to peel them. Some even have edible flowers. The more popular varieties of Summer Squash include:

### ZUCCHINI

Probably the best-known variety of Summer Squash, it is long and narrow. It resembles a cucumber in size and shape with smooth, thin skin that is green and may be striped or speckled. Its tender flesh is creamy white in color and features numerous seeds, and its edible flowers (usually called Squash blossoms) are often used in French and Italian cooking. It is the variety featured in the photographs in this chapter.

### CROOKNECK AND STRAIGHTNECK SQUASH

Both of these varieties usually have creamy white flesh and yellow skin, although green-skinned varieties are sometimes available. Crookneck Squash is straight with a swan-like neck. It was crossbred to produce its straight neck cousin.

### PATTYPAN SQUASH

This small saucer-shaped Squash features pale green or golden yellow skin and cream-colored flesh that is denser and slightly sweeter than Zucchini. It is best to select ones that are no larger than 4 inches in diameter.

## the peak season

Although Summer Squash is now widely cultivated and available throughout the year, its peak season runs from May through July. These are the months when its concentration of nutrients and flavor are highest, and its cost is at its lowest.

## biochemical considerations

Summer Squash is a concentrated source of oxalates, which might be of concern to certain individuals. (For more on *Oxalates*, see page 725.)

## 4 steps for the best tasting and most nutritious summer squash

Turning Summer Squash into a flavorful dish with the most nutrients is simple if you just follow my 4 easy steps:
1. The Best Way to Select
2. The Best Way to Store
3. The Best Way to Prepare
4. The Healthiest Way of Cooking

# 1. the best way to select summer squash ——

You can select the best tasting Summer Squash by looking for ones that are heavy for their size, firm and have shiny, unblemished rinds. Small Zucchini that are less than 6 inches long have fewer seeds and a sweeter taste. By selecting the best tasting Summer Squash, you will also be enjoying Summer Squash with the highest nutritional value. As with all of vegetables, I recommend selecting organically grown varieties whenever possible. (For more on *Organic Foods*, see page 113.)

Avoid large, overly mature or small, immature Summer Squash. Overly mature Summer Squash has a hard outer rind with large seeds and stringy flesh. Overly small or immature Summer Squash tends to be inferior in taste.

# 2. the best way to store summer squash

Summer Squash is a delicate vegetable that stores well but will become soft, lose its flavor and up to 30% of some of its vitamins if not stored properly.

Summer Squash continues to respire even after it has been harvested; its respiration rate at room temperature (68°F/20°C) is 164 mg/kg/hr. Slowing down the respiration rate with proper storage is the key to extending its flavor and nutritional benefits. (For a *Comparison of Respiration Rates* for different vegetables, see page 91.)

### Summer Squash Will Remain Fresh for Up to 10 Days When Properly Stored

1. Store Summer Squash in the refrigerator. The colder temperature will slow the respiration rate, helping to preserve its nutrients and keeping Summer Squash fresh for a longer period of time.

2. Place Summer Squash in a plastic storage bag before refrigerating. I have found that it is best to wrap the bag tightly around the Summer Squash, squeezing out as much of the air from the bag as possible.

3. Do not wash Summer Squash before refrigeration because exposure to water will encourage Summer Squash to spoil.

# 3. the best way to prepare summer squash

Whether you are going to enjoy Summer Squash raw or cooked, I want to share with you the best way to prepare Summer Squash. Properly cleaning and cutting Summer Squash helps to ensure that it will have the best flavor and retain the greatest number of nutrients.

### Cleaning Summer Squash

Rinse Summer Squash under cold running water before cutting. It is best not to peel Summer Squash because the skin contains powerful carotenoid antioxidants, including lutein, which have many health-promoting benefits. Purchasing organically grown Summer Squash allows you to enjoy the skin without concern over pesticide residues. To preserve nutrients, do not soak Summer Squash or its water-soluble nutrients will leach into the water. (For more on *Washing Vegetables*, see page 92.)

### Cutting Summer Squash

Cutting Summer Squash into slices of equal thickness will help them to cook more evenly. Slicing them thin will help them to cook more quickly. For *al dente* Summer Squash, cut into 1/4-inch slices.

Here is a question I received from a reader of the whfoods.org website about Summer Squash:

**Q** *We have a lot of Zucchini left over from our summer garden and wondered whether we could freeze it?*

**A** Because of its high water content, raw Zucchini does not freeze well. One idea for preserving your extra Zucchini would be to prepare Zucchini-containing recipes (such as ratatouille) and freeze them.

---

### An Easy Way to Prepare Summer Squash, Step-By-Step

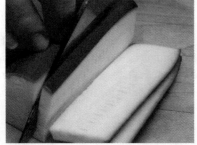 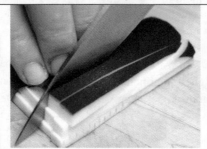 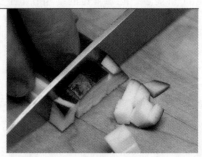

**DICED SUMMER SQUASH**
❶ Slice Summer Squash lengthwise 1/4-inch thick. ❷ Stack slices and cut lengthwise into 1/4-inch thick slices. ❸ Cut across slices at 1/4-inch intervals for 1/4-inch cubes.

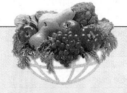

# 4. the healthiest way of cooking summer squash

Since research has shown that important nutrients can be lost or destroyed by the way a food is cooked, the "Healthiest Way of Cooking" Summer Squash is focused on bringing out its best flavor while maximizing its vitamins, minerals and powerful antioxidants.

### Healthiest Way of Cooking Summer Squash: "Healthy Sautéing" for just 3 Minutes

In my search to find the healthiest way to cook Summer Squash, I tested every possible cooking method and discovered that "Healthy Sautéing" all varieties of Summer Squash (Zucchini, Crookneck, Straightneck and Pattypan) for 3 minutes delivered the best result. "Healthy Sautéing" provides the moisture necessary to make Summer Squash tender, bring out its best flavor and brightest color and maximize its nutritional profile. The Step-by-Step Recipe will show you how easy it is to "Healthy Sauté" Summer Squash, for a vegetable with a delightful *al denté* texture. Remember that testing Summer Squash with a fork is not an effective way to determine whether it is done.

### How to Avoid Overcooking Summer Squash: Cook it *Al Denté*

One of the primary reasons that cooked Summer Squash loses its flavor is because it is overcooked. For the best flavor, I recommend cooking Summer Squash *al denté*. Summer Squash cooked *al denté* is tender and cooked just long enough to soften its cellulose and hemicellulose fiber; this makes it easier to digest and allows its health-promoting nutrients to become more readily available for absorption.

It is important not to overcook Summer Squash; if it is cooked for as little as a couple of minutes longer than *al denté*,

it will begin to lose not only its texture and flavor, but also its nutrients. Overcooking Summer Squash will significantly decrease its nutritional value: as much as 50% of some nutrients can be lost. (For more on *Al Denté*, see page 92.)

### Cooking Methods Not Recommended for Summer Squash

**BOILING, STEAMING OR COOKING WITH OIL**

Boiling and steaming Summer Squash results in excessive water absorption and the loss of much of its flavor along with many of its nutrients, including minerals, water-soluble vitamins (such as C and the B-complex vitamins) and health-promoting phytonutrients. I also don't recommend cooking Summer Squash in oil because high temperature heat can damage delicate oils and potentially create free radicals.

### Serving Ideas from Mediterranean Countries:

Traveling through the Mediterranean region, I found that Summer Squash was prepared in many different ways:

Summer Squash is very popular both raw and cooked; stuffed Summer Squash is a favorite way of serving this vegetable.

In Italy, Summer Squash is stuffed with grated cheese, tuna and tomato or with mushrooms and Parmesan cheese.

In Greece, Summer Squash is stuffed with a mixture of garlic, raisins, mint and dill.

In Turkey, Summer Squash is stuffed with a mixture of rice, raisins, mint and dill.

---

## how to enjoy fresh summer squash without cooking

Summer Squash makes great crudités served with your favorite dip. Toss grated raw Summer Squash in salads for a fresh taste and texture.

**Cool Zucchini Salad:** Grate 2 medium Zucchini and 2 medium carrots. Toss with 1 tsp each chopped fresh mint and oregano, sea salt and pepper to taste and 3 TBS extra virgin olive oil for a delicious side dish. For a creamy dressing, 1 cup low-fat plain yogurt may be added.

**Zucchini Boat:** Use Zucchini as a boat for fillings such as tuna or cottage cheese. Remove the stem, cut the

vegetable lengthwise and remove seeds with a spoon or knife. Add filling and sprinkle with your favorite herbal seasoning. Serve raw.

**Marinated Zucchini:** Slice 2 medium Zucchini in half lengthwise, then into 1/4-inch slices. In a bowl, whisk together 1/4 cup of extra virgin olive oil, 2 TBS balsamic vinegar, 1 tsp fresh chopped rosemary, 1/2 tsp crushed red pepper flakes and sea salt and pepper to taste. Let marinate for 1–3 hours.

# health benefits of summer squash

## Promotes Bone Health

When many people think of foods good for bone health, they think of dairy products and maybe nuts and seeds. Yet, vegetables, including Summer Squash, can be an important component of a diet aimed at building and maintaining healthy bones. The benefit of Summer Squash is that it supplies a wide array of many nutrients necessary to bone health, not just calcium. It is a very good source of magnesium and phosphorus, two minerals important for strengthening the bone matrix. It is also an excellent source of manganese and a very good source of copper, two trace minerals that are cofactors of enzymes necessary for bone metabolism.

## Promotes Heart Health

Summer Squash is an excellent source of vitamin C, a powerful antioxidant that has great benefits for cardiovascular health. Not only does vitamin C protect LDL cholesterol from becoming oxidized (which is the way in which it can lead to atherosclerosis), but it improves the activity of nitric oxide, a chemical important for maintaining relaxed blood vessels. Summer Squash also contains vitamin A carotenoids that help to protect LDL from oxidation. It is a very good source of magnesium and potassium, two minerals that help to keep blood pressure balanced. And there's more…while you are enjoying eating Summer Squash, your cardiovascular system will enjoy receiving its concentrations of dietary fiber, folate and vitamin B6, all necessary to keep it operating at its best.

## Promotes Healthy Weight Control

Like most vegetables, Summer Squash is a great food for people interested in losing weight or maintaining a healthy weight. One cup of this delicious vegetable contains only 36 calories, yet it is filled with nutrients, providing over 10% of the daily value for 5 nutrients—manganese, vitamin C, vitamin A, magnesium and dietary fiber.

## Additional Health-Promoting Benefits of Summer Squash

Summer Squash is also a concentrated source of other nutrients providing additional health-promoting benefits. These nutrients include anti-inflammatory omega-3 fatty acids; energy-producing vitamin B1, vitamin B2, iron and niacin; immune-supporting zinc; muscle-building protein; and sleep-promoting tryptophan. Since Summer Squash contains only 36 calories per one cup serving, it is an ideal food for healthy weight control.

### Nutritional Analysis of 1 cup of Summer Squash:

| NUTRIENT | AMOUNT | % DAILY VALUE | NUTRIENT | AMOUNT | % DAILY VALUE |
|---|---|---|---|---|---|
| Calories | 36.00 | | Pantothenic Acid | 0.25 mg | 2.50 |
| Calories from Fat | 5.02 | | | | |
| Calories from Saturated Fat | 1.04 | | **Minerals** | | |
| Protein | 1.64 g | | Boron | — mcg | |
| Carbohydrates | 7.76 g | | Calcium | 48.60 mg | 4.86 |
| Dietary Fiber | 2.52 g | 10.08 | Chloride | 46.80 mg | |
| Soluble Fiber | 0.95 g | | Chromium | — mcg | — |
| Insoluble Fiber | 1.58 g | | Copper | 0.19 mg | 9.50 |
| Sugar – Total | 3.60 g | | Fluoride | — mg | — |
| Monosaccharides | — g | | Iodine | — mcg | — |
| Disaccharides | — g | | Iron | 0.65 mg | 3.61 |
| Other Carbs | 1.64 g | | Magnesium | 43.20 mg | 10.80 |
| Fat – Total | 0.56 g | | Manganese | 0.38 mg | 19.00 |
| Saturated Fat | 0.12 g | | Molybdenum | — mcg | — |
| Mono Fat | 0.04 g | | Phosphorus | 70.20 mg | 7.02 |
| Poly Fat | 0.24 g | | Potassium | 345.60 mg | |
| Omega-3 Fatty Acids | 0.15 g | 6.00 | Selenium | 0.36 mcg | 0.51 |
| Omega-6 Fatty Acids | 0.09 g | | Sodium | 1.80 mg | |
| Trans Fatty Acids | 0.00 g | | Zinc | 0.70 mg | 4.67 |
| Cholesterol | 0.00 mg | | | | |
| Water | 168.66 g | | **Amino Acids** | | |
| Ash | 1.39 g | | Alanine | 0.09 g | |
| | | | Arginine | 0.07 g | |
| **Vitamins** | | | Aspartate | 0.20 g | |
| Vitamin A IU | 516.60 IU | 10.33 | Cystine | 0.02 g | 4.88 |
| Vitamin A RE | 52.20 RE | | Glutamate | 0.17 g | |
| A - Carotenoid | 52.20 RE | 0.70 | Glycine | 0.06 g | |
| A - Retinol | 0.00 RE | | Histidine | 0.04 g | 3.10 |
| B1 Thiamin | 0.08 mg | 5.33 | Isoleucine | 0.06 g | 5.22 |
| B2 Riboflavin | 0.07 mg | 4.12 | Leucine | 0.10 g | 3.95 |
| B3 Niacin | 0.92 mg | 4.60 | Lysine | 0.09 g | 3.83 |
| Niacin Equiv | 1.16 mg | | Methionine | 0.02 g | 2.70 |
| Vitamin B6 | 0.12 mg | 6.00 | Phenylalanine | 0.06 g | 5.04 |
| Vitamin B12 | 0.00 mcg | 0.00 | Proline | 0.05 g | |
| Biotin | — mcg | — | Serine | 0.07 g | |
| Vitamin C | 9.90 mg | 16.50 | Threonine | 0.04 g | 3.23 |
| Vitamin D IU | 0.00 IU | 0.00 | Tryptophan | 0.01 g | 3.13 |
| Vitamin D mcg | 0.00 mcg | | Tyrosine | 0.04 g | 4.12 |
| Vitamin E Alpha Equiv | 0.22 mg | 1.10 | Valine | 0.07 g | 4.76 |
| Vitamin E IU | 0.32 IU | | | | |
| Vitamin E mg | 0.25 mg | | | | |
| Folate | 36.18 mcg | 9.04 | | | |
| Vitamin K | 6.30 mcg | 7.88 | | | |

(Note: "−" indicates data is unavailable. For more information, please see page 806.)

STEP-BY-STEP RECIPE

## The Healthiest Way of Cooking Summer Squash

# 3-Minute "Healthy Sautéed" Summer Squash

*For delicately flavored Summer Squash, try "Healthy Sautéing" to retain its crisp texture and maximum amount of nutrients. The easy Mediterranean Dressing adds extra flavor.*

**1 lb of medium Summer Squash**
**3 TBS low-sodium chicken or vegetable broth**

**Mediterranean Dressing:**
**3 TBS extra virgin olive oil**
**2 tsp lemon juice**
**2 medium cloves garlic**
**Sea salt and pepper to taste**

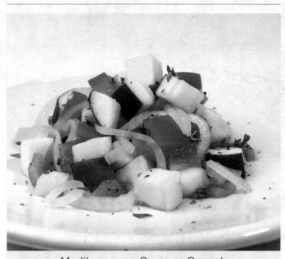

Mediterranean Summer Squash

1. Chop garlic and let it sit for at least 5 minutes. (Why?, see page 261.)

2. Heat broth over medium heat in a stainless steel skillet.

3. While broth is heating, wash and cut Summer Squash in half lengthwise, then into 1/4-inch slices.

4. When broth begins to steam, add Summer Squash and cook for 3 minutes. "Healthy Sautéed" Summer Squash will be tender. If it becomes translucent, it is overcooked. (For information on *Differences in Cooking Time*, see page 94.)

5. Transfer to a bowl. For more flavor, toss Summer Squash with the remaining ingredients while it is still hot. (Mediterranean Dressing does not need to be made separately.) Research shows that carotenoids found in foods are best absorbed when consumed with oils.

OPTIONAL: To mellow the flavor of garlic, add garlic to Summer Squash for the last 2 minutes of sautéing.

**SERVES 2**

## COOKING TIPS:

• To prevent overcooking Summer Squash, I highly recommend using a timer.

## Flavor Tips: Try these 4 great serving suggestions with the recipe above. ✳

1. **Most Popular:** Top with grated Parmesan cheese and minced fresh basil.

2. Top with a mixture of 8 kalamata olives, 1 chopped tomato, 1/2 cup red bell pepper and 1/4 cup red onion (both thinly sliced) and 1 tsp dried Italian herbs.

3. Basil, dill, oregano and rosemary complement the flavor of Summer Squash.

4. **Mediterranean Summer Squash:** Prepare the 3-Minute "Healthy Sautéed" Summer Squash recipe using yellow and green Summer Squash. Combine with "Healthy Sautéed" onions and red bell pepper. Make the Mediterranean Dressing using 4–5 TBS of olive oil, 3 cloves garlic, 4 tsp lemon juice and sea salt and pepper to taste. Toss the vegetables with dressing while they are still hot and sprinkle with chopped fresh basil or oregano (pictured above).

Please write (address on back cover flap) or e-mail me at info@whfoods.org with your personal ideas for preparing Summer Squash, and I will share them with others through our website at www.whfoods.org.

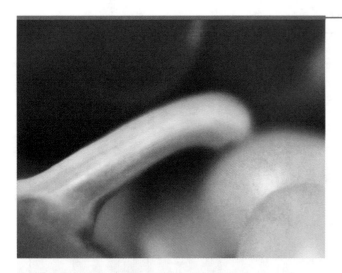

# bell peppers

| | |
|---|---|
| AVAILABILITY | Year-round |
| REFRIGERATE: | Yes |
| SHELF LIFE: | 7 days refrigerated |
| PREPARATION: | Minimal |
| BEST WAY TO COOK: | "Healthy Sauté" in just 7 minutes |

## nutrient-richness chart

Total Nutrient-Richness: **29**      GI: **40**

One cup (92 grams) of raw Bell Peppers contains 25 calories

| NUTRIENT | AMOUNT | %DV | DENSITY | QUALITY |
|---|---|---|---|---|
| Vitamin C | 174.8 mg | 291.3 | 211.1 | excellent |
| Vitamin A | 5244.0 IU | 104.9 | 76.0 | excellent |
| B6 Pyridoxine | 0.2 mg | 11.5 | 8.3 | excellent |
| Dietary Fiber | 1.8 g | 7.4 | 5.3 | very good |
| Molybdenum | 4.6 mcg | 6.1 | 4.4 | very good |
| Vitamin K | 4.51 mcg | 5.6 | 4.1 | very good |
| Manganese | 0.1 mg | 5.5 | 4.0 | very good |
| Folate | 20.2 mcg | 5.1 | 3.7 | very good |
| Potassium | 162.8 mg | 4.7 | 3.4 | good |
| B1 Thiamin | 0.1 mg | 4.0 | 2.9 | good |
| Vitamin E | 0.6 mg | 3.1 | 2.3 | good |
| Tryptophan | 0.01 g | 3.1 | 2.3 | good |
| Copper | 0.1 mg | 3.0 | 2.2 | good |

**CAROTENOIDS:**

| | |
|---|---|
| Alpha-Carotene | 29.8 mcg |
| Beta-Carotene | 2013.8 mcg |
| Beta-Cryptoxanthin | 730.1 mcg |
| Lutein+Zeaxanthin | 76.0 mcg |
| Lycopene | 458.9 mcg |

Daily values for these nutrients have not yet been established.

**FLAVONOIDS:**

| | |
|---|---|
| Luteolin | 0.9 mg |

For more on "Total Nutrient-Richness," "%DV," "Density," and The World's Healthiest Foods "Quality" Rating System, see page 805.

For more on GI, see page 342.

Like many other foods native to South America, Bell Peppers were introduced to the rest of the world by Spanish and Portuguese explorers. Bell Peppers are easy to cultivate, versatile and add a beautiful range of colors to your table. They are the essential flavoring for Louisiana Creole dishes, have become a staple in central Europe where they are dried for paprika and are a key ingredient in both Mexican and Portuguese cooking. I would to like to share with you how raw Bell Peppers make a wonderful, crunchy, colorful and healthy addition to green salads as well as how to enjoy cooked Bell Peppers. The key to enjoying the best flavor and maximizing the nutritional benefits of cooked Bell Peppers is proper preparation. That is why I want to share with you the secret of the "Healthiest Way of Cooking" Bell Peppers *al denté*. And it only takes 7 minutes!

## why bell peppers should be part of your healthiest way of eating

The splash of color that Bell Peppers add to your meals is not only a feast for your eyes, but also for your health as well. Bell Peppers are a concentrated source of carotenoid phytonutrients that are responsible for their variation in color as well as providing powerful antioxidant protection against the oxidative damage to cells caused by free radicals. The lycopene and beta-cryptoxanthin found in red Bell Peppers are associated with promoting a healthy heart and lungs, while their lutein and zeaxanthin promote vision health. Bell Peppers are also rich in numerous other nutrients, including vitamin C. Bell Peppers are an ideal food to add to your "Healthiest Way of Eating" not only because they are high in nutrients, but also because they are low in calories: one cup of raw Red Bell Peppers contains only 25 calories. (For more on the *Health Benefits of Bell Peppers* and a complete analysis of their content of over 60 nutrients, see page 194.)

## varieties of bell peppers

Bell Peppers *(Capsicum annuum)* are members of the nightshade family of vegetables along with potatoes, tomatoes and eggplants. Like chili peppers, Bell Peppers originated in South America where seeds of a wild variety are believed to date back to 5,000 BC The various colored Bell Peppers all come from the same plant, but differ in their level of maturity:

### GREEN PEPPERS

Green Bell Peppers are harvested before they are fully ripe, one reason they are less expensive than other varieties. Green Bell Peppers will continue to first turn yellow and then red if they are left on the plant to mature. They have a slightly bitter flavor and will never have the sweet taste of their red, yellow and orange counterparts.

### ORANGE AND YELLOW PEPPERS

More mature than Green Bell Peppers, Orange and Yellow Peppers have a fruity taste but are not as commonly found in local markets as Green and Red Bell Peppers. Yellow ones are rich in lutein and zeaxanthin carotenoids while orange ones are rich in alpha- and gamma-carotene

### RED PEPPERS

These are more mature than Green, Orange or Yellow Bell Peppers. They are rich in carotenoid phytonutrients and contain almost 11 times more beta-carotene than green Bell Peppers as well as one and a half times more vitamin C. Red Bell Peppers have a sweet, almost fruity taste. Pimento and paprika are both prepared from Red Bell Peppers.

## the peak season

Although Bell Peppers are available throughout the year, their peak season runs through the summer months. These are the months when their concentration of nutrients and flavor are highest, and their cost is at their lowest.

## biochemical considerations

Bell Peppers are a concentrated source of oxalates and a member of the nightshade family of vegetables, which might be of concern to certain individuals. Conventionally grown Bell Peppers often have a wax coating to help protect their surface and increase their shelf life. Bell Peppers are also among the 12 foods on which pesticide residues have been most frequently found. (For more on: *Oxalates*, see page 725; *Nightshades*, see page 723; *Wax Coatings*, see page 732; and *Pesticide Residues*, see page 726.)

## 4 steps for the best tasting and most nutritious bell peppers

Turning Bell Peppers into a flavorful dish with the most nutrients is simple if you just follow my 4 easy steps:

1. The Best Way to Select
2. The Best Way to Store
3. The Best Way to Prepare
4. The Healthiest Way of Cooking

**COMPARISON BETWEEN GREEN, YELLOW AND RED BELL PEPPERS**

|  | GREEN | YELLOW | RED |
|---|---|---|---|
| Vitamin A | 12% DV | 4% DV | 105% DV |
| Vitamin C | 137% DV | 282% DV | 291% DV |
| Beta-Carotene | 340 mcg | 110 mcg | 2014 mcg |

*Most other vitamins and minerals are comparable for the three varieties. All quantities and % Daily Values (DV) are based on 1 cup (92g) of raw Bell Peppers. No Daily Values for beta-carotene are currently available.

# 1. the best way to select bell peppers ───

You can select the best tasting Bell Peppers by looking for ones that have deep, vivid colors and taut skin. The stems should be green and fresh looking. I have found that the best Bell Peppers are heavy for their size and firm. By selecting the best tasting Bell Peppers, you will also be getting Bell Peppers with the highest nutritional value. As with all vegetables, I recommend selecting organically grown Bell Peppers whenever possible. You can enjoy the nutrient-rich skin of organically grown varieties without concern about consuming the wax coatings that are often used on conventionally grown

Bell Peppers to reduce moisture loss and increase shelf life. (For more on *Organic Foods*, see page 113.)

Avoid Bell Peppers that have signs of decay, including injuries to the skin or water-soaked areas. Be sure they are free of soft spots, wrinkles, blemishes and darkened areas.

It is good to consider the shape when you are purchasing Bell Peppers, even though it does not generally affect the quality. Oddly shaped peppers may not be suitable for certain recipe preparations or may result in excessive waste.

## 2. the best way to store bell peppers

Bell Peppers will start to become soft and bitter if not stored properly. Since they can lose their flavor and up to 30% of some of their vitamins, make sure to store them properly.

Bell Peppers continue to respire even after they have been harvested. Slowing down the respiration rate with proper storage is the key to extending their flavor and nutritional benefits. (For a *Comparison of Respiration Rates* for different vegetables, see page 91.)

### Bell Peppers Will Remain Fresh for Up to 7 Days When Properly Stored

1. Store Bell Peppers in the refrigerator. The colder temperature will slow the respiration rate, helping to preserve their nutrients and keeping Bell Peppers fresh for a longer period of time.

2. Place Bell Peppers in a plastic storage bag before refrigerating. I have found that it is best to wrap the bag tightly around the Bell Peppers, squeezing out as much of the air from the bag as possible.

3. Do not wash Bell Peppers before refrigeration because exposure to water will encourage Bell Peppers to spoil.

### How to Store Cut Bell Peppers

Store cut Bell Peppers in a container with a well-sealed lid or wrapped tightly in a plastic bag and refrigerate. Since the vitamin C content degrades quickly once the Bell Peppers have been cut, it is best to use the remainder within a day or two.

## 3. the best way to prepare bell peppers

Whether you are going to enjoy Bell Peppers raw or cooked, I want to share with you the best way to prepare them. Properly cleaning and cutting Bell Peppers helps to ensure that the Bell Peppers you serve will have the best flavor and retain the greatest number of nutrients.

### Cleaning Bell Peppers

It is best to rinse Bell Peppers under cold running water before cutting. To preserve nutrients, do not soak Bell Peppers or their water-soluble nutrients will leach into the water. (For more on *Washing Vegetables*, see page 92.)

### Cutting Bell Peppers

Cutting Bell Peppers into equal size pieces will help them to cook more evenly. Cutting them into smaller pieces will make them cook more quickly. I recommend slicing Bell Peppers into 1/4-inch strips or dicing them into 1/4-inch squares to cook them *al denté*.

You don't need to remove the stem and seeds before you cut Bell Peppers. Just stand the Bell Pepper on a cutting board, and carefully cut it on all four sides. You'll end up with four pieces that, once you cut away the rib on the inside of each, can be cut into the size and shape of your choice. The stem and seed cavity can be discarded. For more details, see the *Step-by-Step* below.

### An Easy Way to Prepare Bell Peppers, Step-by-Step

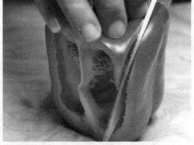 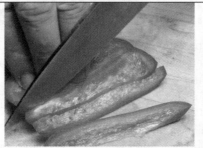 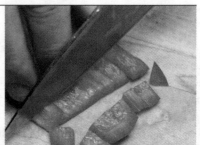

DICING BELL PEPPERS

❶ Cut pepper lengthwise on all four sides, so you end up with four pieces, then cut the rib out of the inside of each piece. ❷ Cut the pieces into thin 1/4-inch strips. ❸ Cut across the strips every 1/4-inch to end up with small 1/4-inch squares. You can use this same process for any size pieces.

# 4. the healthiest way of cooking bell peppers —

Since research has shown that important nutrients can be lost or destroyed by the way a food is cooked, the "Healthiest Way of Cooking" Bell Peppers is focused on bringing out their best flavor while maximizing their vitamins, minerals and powerful antioxidants.

## The Healthiest Way of Cooking Bell Peppers: "Healthy Sautéing" for just 7 Minutes

In my search to find the healthiest way to cook Bell Peppers, I tested every possible cooking method and discovered that "Healthy Sautéing" Bell Peppers for just 7 minutes delivered the best result. "Healthy Sautéing" concentrates their sweet flavor and retains the greatest number of nutrients. The Step-by-Step Recipe will show you how easy it is to "Healthy Sauté" Bell Peppers. (For more on *Healthy Sauté*, see page 57.)

## Easy Roasting

For rich flavor I recommend roasting Bell Peppers. It makes the flesh become very tender. The heat makes the skin darker and causes it to dry out, which enables you to easily remove it after it is finished roasting. To roast, preheat the oven to 500°F (260°C) and place whole Bell Peppers in a roasting dish and roast for 30 to 40 minutes or until they collapse. When they are finished cooking, peel away skin and remove the seeds.

## Broiling That Takes Only 15 Minutes

Quartered Red Bell Peppers can be broiled without turning or using any oil. Place Bell Peppers about 4 inches from the heat source. You want the skin to be somewhat darkened, but not burnt, and you don't want the flesh to become overcooked. Broil for about 15 minutes, but keep an eye on them to make sure they are not cooking too much. After broiling, place the Bell Peppers in a bowl covered with plastic wrap (making sure the plastic does not touch the peppers) for about 15 minutes. This allows them to steam and the skins to slip away easily. Dress with extra virgin olive oil, garlic, lemon juice, and sea salt and pepper to taste.

## How to Avoid Overcooking Bell Peppers: Cook Them *Al Denté*

One of the primary reasons people do not enjoy cooked Bell Peppers is because they are often overcooked. For the best flavor, I recommend cooking Bell Peppers until they are tender. Tender Bell Peppers have been cooked just long enough to soften their cellulose and hemicellulose fiber; this makes them easier to digest and allows their health-promoting nutrients to become more readily available for absorption.

It is important not to overcook Bell Peppers. Bell Peppers cooked for as little as a couple of minutes longer than the recommended cooking time will begin to lose not only their texture and flavor but also their nutrients. Overcooking Bell Peppers will significantly decrease their nutritional value: as much as 50% of some nutrients can be lost.

## Cooking Methods Not Recommended for Bell Peppers

### BOILING, STEAMING OR COOKING WITH OIL

I do not recommend boiling or steaming Bell Peppers because these methods increase their water absorption causing them to become soggy and lose much of their flavor along with many of their nutrients including minerals, water-soluble vitamins (such as C and the B-complex vitamins) and health-promoting phytonutrients. I also don't recommend cooking Bell Peppers in oil because high temperature heat can damage delicate oils and potentially create harmful free radicals.

# how to enjoy fresh bell peppers without cooking

Bell Peppers make a wonderful addition to salads; red, orange and yellow varieties are easier to digest than green and are therefore best to use when eating raw Bell Peppers.

Serve Red Bell Peppers as crudités. Dip into a mixture of extra virgin olive, sea salt and pepper.

**Red Pepper Vinaigrette**: In a blender, combine a seeded sweet Red Bell Pepper, 2 TBS lemon juice, 1/2 cup extra virgin olive oil, 3 cloves garlic, a pinch of cayenne, 1/2 tsp sea salt and 1/3 cup water. Blend for 1 minute. Add more water as needed to keep the blender vortex going so that the dressing becomes creamy. Serve on your favorite green salad.

# health benefits of bell peppers

### Promote Vision Health

Bell Peppers may have a protective effect against cataracts, possibly due to their vitamin C and beta-carotene content. When researchers compared the diets of those with and without cataracts, they found that eating certain vegetables, including Bell Peppers, significantly reduced the risk of needing cataract surgery. Red Bell Peppers also contain the carotenoid phytonutrients lutein and zeaxanthin, which have been found to protect against macular degeneration, the main cause of blindness in the elderly.

### Promote Heart Health

Bell Peppers are an excellent source of vitamin B6 and a very good source of folate. These two nutrients are essential for reducing high levels of homocysteine, a compound that can cause damage to blood vessels and is associated with a greatly increased risk of heart attack and stroke. Bell Peppers are also a very good source of dietary fiber, which can help lower high cholesterol levels, another risk factor for heart attack and stroke. Additionally, Red Bell Peppers are one of the few foods that are a concentrated source of lycopene. This carotenoid phytonutrient is believed to play a role in the prevention of heart disease through its ability to inhibit free-radical damage to LDL cholesterol, which, if allowed to progress, can lead to atherosclerosis. Bell Peppers are also a good source of potassium, a mineral important for maintaining normal blood pressure.

### Promote Optimal Health

Bell Peppers are rich sources of some of the best health-promoting nutrients available, including those with powerful antioxidant activity. Bell Peppers are excellent sources of vitamin C, good sources of vitamin E and the red varieties have the added benefit of supplying large quantities of carotenoids. Both vitamin C and beta-carotene are powerful antioxidants that work together to effectively neutralize free radicals, which can travel through the body causing damage to cells. Over time, this damage can manifest in a variety of diseases including cardiovascular disease, asthma, arthritis and cancer.

Two other nutrients found specifically in Red Bell Peppers—the carotenoids lycopene and beta-cryptoxanthin—may also help to promote optimal cellular health. Recent studies suggest that individuals whose diets are low in lycopene-rich foods are at greater risk for developing cancer of the prostate, cervix, bladder and pancreas. Red Bell Peppers' beta-cryptoxanthin is suggested to offer protection against the development of lung cancer.

### Additional Health-Promoting Benefits of Bell Peppers

Bell Peppers are a concentrated source of many other nutrients providing additional health benefits. These nutrients include bone-building vitamin K, energy-producing vitamin B1 and vitamin B2, free radical scavenging manganese and copper, and sulfite-detoxifying molybdenum. Since Bell Peppers contain only 25 calories per one cup serving, they are an ideal food for healthy weight control.

## Nutritional Analysis of 1 cup of raw Red Bell Peppers

| NUTRIENT | AMOUNT | % DAILY VALUE | NUTRIENT | AMOUNT | % DAILY VALUE |
|---|---|---|---|---|---|
| Calories | 24.84 | | Pantothenic Acid | 0.07 mg | 0.70 |
| Calories from Fat | 1.57 | | | | |
| Calories from Saturated Fat | 0.23 | | **Minerals** | | |
| Protein | 0.82 g | | Boron | — mcg | |
| Carbohydrates | 5.92 g | | Calcium | 8.28 mg | 0.83 |
| Dietary Fiber | 1.84 g | 7.36 | Chloride | 22.08 mg | |
| Soluble Fiber | 0.74 g | | Chromium | — mcg | — |
| Insoluble Fiber | 1.10 g | | Copper | 0.06 mg | 3.00 |
| Sugar – Total | 2.39 g | | Fluoride | — mg | — |
| Monosaccharides | — g | | Iodine | 0.92 mcg | 0.61 |
| Disaccharides | — g | | Iron | 0.42 mg | 2.33 |
| Other Carbs | 1.68 g | | Magnesium | 9.20 mg | 2.30 |
| Fat – Total | 0.17 g | | Manganese | 0.11 mg | 5.50 |
| Saturated Fat | 0.03 g | | Molybdenum | 4.60 mcg | 6.13 |
| Mono Fat | 0.01 g | | Phosphorus | 17.48 mg | 1.75 |
| Poly Fat | 0.09 g | | Potassium | 162.84 mg | |
| Omega-3-Fatty Acids | 0.01 g | 0.40 | Selenium | 0.28 mcg | 0.40 |
| Omega-6-Fatty Acids | 0.09 g | | Sodium | 1.84 mg | |
| Trans Fatty Acids | 0.00 g | | Zinc | 0.11 mg | 0.73 |
| Cholesterol | 0.00 mg | | | | |
| Water | 84.81 g | | **Amino Acids** | | |
| Ash | 0.28 g | | Alanine | 0.03 g | |
| | | | Arginine | 0.04 g | |
| **Vitamins** | | | Aspartate | 0.12 g | |
| Vitamin A IU | 5244.00 IU | 104.88 | Cystine | 0.02 g | 4.88 |
| Vitamin A RE | 524.40 RE | | Glutamate | 0.11 g | |
| A - Carotenoid | 524.40 RE | 6.99 | Glycine | 0.03 g | |
| A - Retinol | 0.00 RE | | Histidine | 0.02 g | 1.55 |
| B1 Thiamin | 0.06 mg | 4.00 | Isoleucine | 0.03 g | 2.61 |
| B2 Riboflavin | 0.03 mg | 1.76 | Leucine | 0.04 g | 1.58 |
| B3 Niacin | 0.47 mg | 2.35 | Lysine | 0.04 g | 1.70 |
| Niacin Equiv | 0.64 mg | | Methionine | 0.01 g | 1.35 |
| Vitamin B6 | 0.23 mg | 11.50 | Phenylalanine | 0.02 g | 1.68 |
| Vitamin B12 | 0.00 mcg | 0.00 | Proline | 0.04 g | |
| Biotin | — mcg | — | Serine | 0.03 g | |
| Vitamin C | 174.80 mg | 291.33 | Threonine | 0.03 g | 2.42 |
| Vitamin D IU | 0.00 IU | 0.00 | Tryptophan | 0.01 g | 3.13 |
| Vitamin D mcg | 0.00 mcg | | Tyrosine | 0.02 g | 2.06 |
| Vitamin E Alpha Equiv | 0.63 mg | 3.15 | Valine | 0.03 g | 2.04 |
| Vitamin E IU | 0.95 IU | | | | |
| Vitamin E mg | 0.68 mg | | | | |
| Folate | 20.24 mcg | 5.06 | | | |
| Vitamin K | 4.51 mcg | 5.64 | | | |

(Note: "–" indicates data is unavailable. For more information, please see page 806.)

STEP-BY-STEP RECIPE
## The Healthiest Way of Cooking Bell Peppers

# 7-Minute "Healthy Sautéed" Bell Peppers

*"Healthy Sauté" is a great way to bring out the delicate, sweet flavor of Red Bell Pepper while maximizing the number of nutrients. The easy-to-prepare Mediterranean Dressing adds even more flavor and nutrition.*

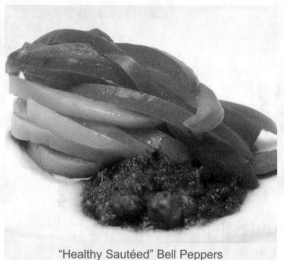
"Healthy Sautéed" Bell Peppers

**1 lb Red Bell Peppers (3–4 medium peppers)**
**3 TBS + 2 TBS low-sodium chicken or**
 **vegetable broth**

**Mediterranean Dressing:**
**3 TBS extra virgin olive oil**
**2 tsp lemon juice**
**2 medium garlic cloves**
**Sea salt and pepper to taste**

1. Chop garlic and let it sit for at least 5 minutes. (Why?, see page 261.)

2. Heat 3 TBS of broth over medium heat in a stainless steel skillet.

3. While broth is heating, slice Red Bell Peppers 1/4-inch thick. (Don't use Green Bell Peppers since they become bitter when cooked.)

4. When broth begins to steam, add Red Bell Peppers and **cover**.

5. After 3 minutes, stir and add 2 TBS broth, then cook **uncovered** on low heat for another 4 minutes. If the pan starts to scorch, add a little more liquid. (For information on *Differences in Cooking Time,* see page 94.)

6. Transfer to a bowl. For more flavor, toss Bell Peppers with the remaining ingredients while they are still hot. (Mediterranean Dressing does not need to be made separately.) Research shows that carotenoids found in foods are best absorbed when consumed with oils.

OPTIONAL: To mellow the flavor of garlic, add garlic to Bell Peppers for the last 2 minutes of sautéing. You may need to add a little more liquid to keep garlic from sticking to pan.

**SERVES 2**

**COOKING TIP:** • To prevent overcooking Bell Peppers, I highly recommend using a timer.

## Flavor Tips: Try these 5 great serving suggestions with the recipe above. ✳

1. **Most Popular:** Top 7-Minute "Healthy Sautéed" Bell Peppers with fresh basil and crumbled goat or feta cheese. Sprinkle with a few drops of balsamic vinegar.

2. Top chicken, fish or meat with "Healthy Sautéed" Bell Peppers.

3. "Healthy Sauté" Bell Peppers with onions.

4. Goat and feta cheese complement the flavor of Bell Peppers.

5. **Healthy Fajita:** Add sliced onions to your 7-Minute "Healthy Sautéed" Bell Pepper recipe. During the last minute of cooking, add strips of cooked chicken or tofu, 1 tsp chili powder, 1 tsp cumin and sea salt to taste. Heat thoroughly. Add Mediterranean Dressing, using lime juice instead of lemon juice, immediately after removing the vegetables from the heat. Wrap in a whole wheat tortilla with fresh chopped cilantro.

Please write (address on back cover flap) or e-mail me at info@whfoods.org with your personal ideas for preparing Bell Peppers, and I will share them with others through our website at www.whfoods.org.

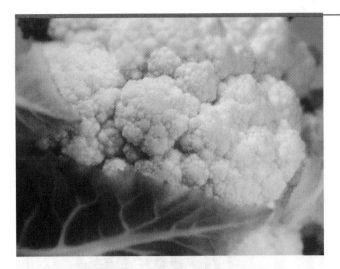

# cauliflower

## highlights

| | |
|---|---|
| AVAILABILITY: | Year-round |
| REFRIGERATE: | Yes |
| SHELF LIFE: | 7 days refrigerated |
| PREPARATION: | Cut and let sit for 5 minutes |
| BEST WAY TO COOK: | "Healthy Sauté" in just 5 minutes |

## nutrient-richness chart

Total Nutrient-Richness: **29**          GI: **30**
One cup (124 grams) of cooked Cauliflower contains 29 Calories

| NUTRIENT | AMOUNT | %DV | DENSITY | QUALITY |
|---|---|---|---|---|
| Vitamin C | 54.9 mg | 91.5 | 57.8 | excellent |
| Vitamin K | 11.2 mcg | 14.0 | 8.8 | excellent |
| Folate | 54.6 mcg | 13.6 | 8.6 | excellent |
| Dietary Fiber | 3.4 g | 13.4 | 8.5 | excellent |
| B6 Pyridoxine | 0.2 mg | 10.5 | 6.6 | very good |
| Tryptophan | 0.03 g | 9.4 | 5.9 | very good |
| Manganese | 0.2 mg | 8.5 | 5.4 | very good |
| Omega-3 Fatty Acids | 0.2 g | 8.4 | 5.3 | very good |
| B5 Pantothenic Acid | 0.6 mg | 6.3 | 4.0 | very good |
| Potassium | 176.1 mg | 5.0 | 3.2 | good |
| Protein | 2.3 g | 4.6 | 2.9 | good |
| Phosphorus | 39.7 mg | 4.0 | 2.5 | good |
| B2 Riboflavin | 0.1 mg | 3.5 | 2.2 | good |
| B1 Thiamin | 0.1 mg | 3.3 | 2.1 | good |
| Magnesium | 11.2 mg | 2.8 | 1.8 | good |
| B3 Niacin | 0.5 mg | | | |
| **CAROTENOIDS:** | | Daily values for these nutrients have not yet been established. | | |
| Beta-Carotene | 8.7 mcg | | | |
| Lutein+Zeaxanthin | 36.0 mcg | | | |

For more on "Total Nutrient-Richness," "%DV," "Density," and
The World's Healthiest Foods "Quality" Rating System, see page 805.
For more on GI, see page 342.

Originating in the Mediterranean region of Europe, Cauliflower is a versatile vegetable that can be eaten raw in a salad or as a snack, cooked as a side dish, or combined with other foods in a variety of different recipes. Ribbed, coarse green leaves protect the Cauliflower head from sunlight, preventing the production of the chlorophyll that makes vegetables green. Although Cauliflower may lack the bright green color of broccoli and its other cruciferous cousins, it is far from lacking in nutritional value or flavor. Proper preparation of Cauliflower is the key to bringing out its best flavor and maximizing its nutritional benefits. That is why I want to share with you the secret of the "Healthiest Way of Cooking" Cauliflower *al denté*. In just 5 minutes, you will be able to transform Cauliflower into a flavorful vegetable while maximizing its nutritional value.

## why cauliflower should be part of your healthiest way of eating

Scientific studies now show that cruciferous vegetables, like Cauliflower, are included among the vegetables that contain the largest concentrations of health-promoting sulfur compounds, such as sulforaphane and isothiocyanates (see page 153), which increase the liver's ability to produce enzymes that neutralize potentially toxic substances. Cauliflower is also rich in vitamin C; one cup contains almost as much as a medium orange. Cauliflower is an ideal food to add to your "Healthiest Way of Eating" not only because it is high in nutrients, but also because it is low in calories and good for weight control: one cup of cooked Cauliflower contains only 29 calories. (For more on the *Health Benefits of Cauliflower* and a complete analysis of its content of over 60 nutrients, see page 200.)

## varieties of cauliflower

Cauliflower (*Brassica oleracea* var. *botcytis*) is a member of the cruciferous family of vegetables, which also includes broccoli, kale, collard greens, cabbage, mustard greens and Brussels sprouts. Its ancestry can be traced back to the wild cabbage, which looked more like kale or collard greens than the Cauliflower we are familiar with today. Cauliflower comes in a few different varieties:

### WHITE

This is the most widely available and most commonly used variety of Cauliflower. It is the one featured in the photographs in this chapter.

### LIGHT GREEN, PURPLE OR ORANGE

These are newly developed varieties of Cauliflower that are becoming increasingly popular and easier to find in your local market.

### BROCCOFLOWER

This recently developed variety is a cross between Cauliflower and its close relative, broccoli. Its curd (compact head) is green and less dense than White Cauliflower, and it has a milder taste and cooks more quickly.

## the peak season

Cauliflower is available throughout the year, but its flavor is at its peak during the cold months when the frost helps to develop a sweeter flavor.

## biochemical considerations

Cauliflower is a concentrated source of goitrogens and purines, which might be of concern to certain individuals. (For more on: *Goitrogens*, see page 721; and *Purines,* see page 727.)

## 4 steps for the best tasting and most nutritious cauliflower

Turning Cauliflower into a flavorful dish with the most nutrients is simple if you just follow my 4 easy steps:

1. The Best Way to Select
2. The Best Way to Store
3. The Best Way to Prepare
4. The Healthiest Way of Cooking

# 1. the best way to select cauliflower

You can select the best tasting Cauliflower by looking for heads that are clean, with creamy white, compact curds, and bud clusters that are not separated. I have found that heads that are surrounded by many thick green leaves are better protected and are usually fresher. Since size is not related to the quality of Cauliflower, choose one that best suits your needs. By selecting the best tasting Cauliflower, you will also enjoy Cauliflower with the highest nutritional value. As with all vegetables, I recommend selecting organically grown varieties whenever possible. (For more on *Organic Foods*, see page 113.)

Avoid Cauliflower heads that have brown spots, dull coloration or small flowers; these are indications that the Cauliflower is old and no longer fresh.

# 2. the best way to store cauliflower

Cauliflower is a sturdy vegetable that can keep well if stored properly. If not, it will become soft, lose its freshness and flavor and up to 30% of some of its vitamins.

Cauliflower continues to respire even after it has been harvested; its respiration rate at room temperature (68°F/20°C) is 79 mg/kg/hr. Slowing down the respiration rate with proper storage is the key to extending its flavor and nutritional benefits. (For *Comparison of Respiration Rates* for different vegetables, see page 91.)

### Cauliflower Will Remain Fresh for Up to 7 Days When Properly Stored

1. Store Cauliflower in the refrigerator. The colder temperature will slow the respiration rate, helping to preserve its nutrients and keeping Cauliflower fresh for a longer period of time.

2. Place Cauliflower in a plastic storage bag before refrigerating. I have found that it is best to wrap the bag tightly around the Cauliflower, squeezing out as much of the air from the bag as possible.

3. Do not wash Cauliflower before refrigeration because exposure to water will encourage Cauliflower to spoil.

### How to Store a Partial Head of Cauliflower

If you need to store a partial head of Cauliflower, place it in a container with a well-sealed lid, or a plastic bag, and refrigerate. Since the vitamin C content starts to quickly degrade once Cauliflower has been cut, you should use it within a couple of days.

# 3. the best way to prepare cauliflower

Whether you are going to enjoy Cauliflower raw or cooked, I want to share with you the best way to prepare Cauliflower. Properly cleaning and cutting Cauliflower helps ensure that the Cauliflower you serve will have the best flavor and retain the greatest number of nutrients.

## Cleaning Cauliflower

Remove any brown discolored areas and rinse well under cold running water before cutting. To preserve nutrients, do not soak Cauliflower or its water-soluble nutrients will leach into the water. (For more on *Washing Vegetables*, see page 92.)

## Cutting Cauliflower

Discard the outer leaves. Cutting Cauliflower florets into equal size pieces will help them to cook more evenly. The smaller you cut the Cauliflower florets, the more quickly they will cook, so I recommend cutting the florets into quarters. Cutting florets into quarters will also help maximize the formation of health-promoting compounds when you let them sit for a minimum of 5 minutes before cooking.

## What to do with the Core

Discard the core of the Cauliflower because it is usually hard and inedible.

# 4. the healthiest way of cooking cauliflower

Since research has shown that important nutrients can be lost or destroyed by the way a food is cooked, the "Healthiest Way of Cooking" Cauliflower is focused on bringing out its best flavor while maximizing its vitamins, minerals and powerful antioxidants.

## The Healthiest Way of Cooking Cauliflower: "Healthy Sautéing" for just 5 Minutes

In my search to find the healthiest way to cook Cauliflower, I tested every possible cooking method looking for the ways to bring out its best flavor and preserve the maximum amount of nutrients and discovered that "Healthy Sautéing" Cauliflower for just 5 minutes delivered the best result. "Healthy Sautéing" Cauliflower brings out its mild, sweet, creamy, almost nutty flavor and maximizes its nutritional profile. Cauliflower absorbs just enough moisture from the broth to make it creamy and tender. The Step-by-Step Recipe will show you how easy it is to "Healthy Sauté" Cauliflower.

## How to Avoid Overcooking Cauliflower: Cook It *Al Denté*

One of the primary reasons people do not enjoy Cauliflower is because it is often overcooked. For the best flavor, I recommend that you cook Cauliflower *al denté*. Cauliflower cooked *al denté* is tender outside and slightly crisp inside. Plus, Cauliflower cooked *al denté* is cooked just long enough to soften its cellulose and hemicellulose fiber; this makes it easier to digest and allows its health-promoting nutrients to become more readily available for assimilation.

Although Cauliflower is a sturdy vegetable, it is very important not to overcook it. Cauliflower cooked for as little as a couple of minutes longer than *al denté* will begin to lose not only its texture and flavor but also its nutrients. Overcooking Cauliflower will significantly decrease its nutritional value: as much as 50% of some nutrients can be lost. (For more on *Al Denté*, see page 92.)

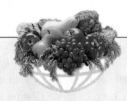

## how to enjoy fresh cauliflower without cooking

Add minced Cauliflower to tossed salads.

For an appetizer, serve raw Cauliflower as crudités. Dip into extra virgin olive oil, sea salt and pepper. Sprinkle with Parmesan cheese.

Cauliflower goes well with creamy dips.

**Marinated Cauliflower:** Mince Cauliflower finely, and mix with 2 parts extra virgin olive oil, 1 part rice vinegar and 1 part tamari (soy sauce). Marinate 4–8 hours.

## How to Prevent Strong Smells from Forming

Cutting Cauliflower florets into quarters and cooking them *al denté* is my secret for preventing the formation of smelly compounds often associated with cooking Cauliflower. When I cook my Cauliflower, it never develops a strong smell. After 5 minutes of cooking, the texture of Cauliflower, like all other cruciferous vegetables, begins to change, becoming increasingly soft and mushy. This is when it starts to release hydrogen sulfide, the cause of the "rotten egg smell," which also affects its flavor. After 7 minutes of cooking, Cauliflower develops a more intense flavor, with the amount of strong smelling hydrogen sulfide doubling in quantity.

While it is important not to overcook Cauliflower, cooking for less than 5 minutes is also not recommended because it takes about 5 minutes to soften its fibers and help increase its digestibility.

## Cooking Methods Not Recommended for Cauliflower

### BOILING, STEAMING, BAKING OR COOKING WITH OIL

Boiling and steaming Cauliflower increases its water absorption, causing it to become soggy and lose much of its flavor along with many of its nutrients, including minerals, water-soluble vitamins (such as C and the B-complex vitamins) and health-promoting phytonutrients. I don't recommend baking, broiling, grilling or roasting Cauliflower because these methods will cause it to dry up and shrivel. I also don't recommend cooking Cauliflower in oil as high temperature heat can damage delicate oils and potentially create harmful free radicals.

## Serving Ideas from Mediterranean Countries:

Traveling through the Mediterranean region, I found Cauliflower was prepared in many different ways:

In Italy, Cauliflower is served with anchovies, onions or Romano cheese.

In Greece, Cauliflower is served with grated Parmesan cheese.

---

### HOW TO BRING OUT THE HIDDEN HEALTH BENEFITS OF CAULIFLOWER

The latest scientific studies show that cutting Cauliflower florets into small pieces, such as quarters, breaks down cell walls and enhances the activation of an enzyme called *myrosinase* that slowly converts some of the plant nutrients into their active forms, which have been shown to contain health-promoting properties. So, to get the most health benefits from Cauliflower, let it sit for a minimum of 5 minutes, optimally 10 minutes, after cutting, before eating or cooking.

Since ascorbic acid (vitamin C) increases *myrosinase* activity, you can sprinkle a little lemon juice on the Cauliflower before letting it sit in order to further enhance its beneficial phytonutrient concentration.

Heat will inactivate the effect of *myrosinase*, which is why it is important to allow the Cauliflower to sit for 5–10 minutes before cooking to give the enzyme ample opportunity to enhance the concentration of active phytonutrients in your Cauliflower. Cooking at low or medium heat for short periods of time should not destroy the active phytonutrients since once they are formed, they are fairly stable.

---

## An Easy Way to Prepare Cauliflower, Step by Step

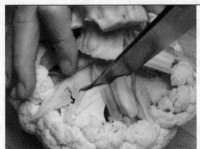 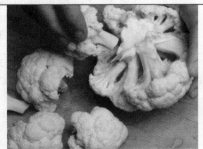 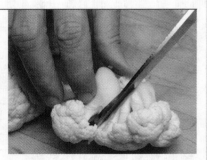

### CAULIFLOWER FLORETS

❶ Remove the leaves from the Cauliflower. Cut around the underside of the head, removing most of the core. ❷ Detach the florets where they join at the center. Separate the florets by cutting through the base to make smaller florets. ❸ Cut Cauliflower florets in quarters and let sit for 5 minutes before eating or cooking.

# health benefits of cauliflower

## Promotes Optimal Health

Epidemiological studies have long suggested a connection between *Brassica* vegetables, like Cauliflower, and resistance to cancer. However, only in the past decade have we begun to understand how the *Brassica* vegetables exert their protective effects.

### Nutritional Analysis of 1 cup of cooked Cauliflower:

| NUTRIENT | AMOUNT | % DAILY VALUE | NUTRIENT | AMOUNT | % DAILY VALUE |
|---|---|---|---|---|---|
| Calories | 28.52 | | Pantothenic Acid | 0.63 mg | 6.30 |
| Calories from Fat | 5.02 | | | | |
| Calories from Saturated Fat | 0.78 | | **Minerals** | | |
| Protein | 2.28 g | | Boron | — mcg | |
| Carbohydrates | 5.10 g | | Calcium | 19.84 mg | 1.98 |
| Dietary Fiber | 3.35 g | 13.40 | Chloride | — mg | |
| Soluble Fiber | 1.07 g | | Chromium | — mcg | — |
| Insoluble Fiber | 2.28 g | | Copper | 0.03 mg | 1.50 |
| Sugar – Total | 1.64 g | | Fluoride | — mg | — |
| Monosaccharides | — g | | Iodine | — mcg | — |
| Disaccharides | — g | | Iron | 0.41 mg | 2.28 |
| Other Carbs | 0.11 g | | Magnesium | 11.16 mg | 2.79 |
| Fat – Total | 0.56 g | | Manganese | 0.17 mg | 8.50 |
| Saturated Fat | 0.09 g | | Molybdenum | — mcg | — |
| Mono Fat | 0.04 g | | Phosphorus | 39.68 mg | 3.97 |
| Poly Fat | 0.27 g | | Potassium | 176.08 mg | |
| Omega-3 Fatty Acids | 0.21 g | 8.40 | Selenium | 0.62 mcg | 0.89 |
| Omega-6 Fatty Acids | 0.06 g | | Sodium | 18.60 mg | |
| Trans Fatty Acids | 0.00 g | | Zinc | 0.22 mg | 1.47 |
| Cholesterol | 0.00 mg | | | | |
| Water | 115.32 g | | **Amino Acids** | | |
| Ash | 0.74 g | | Alanine | 0.12 g | |
| | | | Arginine | 0.11 g | |
| **Vitamins** | | | Aspartate | 0.27 g | |
| Vitamin A IU | 21.08 IU | 0.42 | Cystine | 0.03 g | 7.32 |
| Vitamin A RE | 2.48 RE | | Glutamate | 0.30 g | |
| A - Carotenoid | 2.48 RE | 0.03 | Glycine | 0.07 g | |
| A - Retinol | 0.00 RE | | Histidine | 0.05 g | 3.88 |
| Thiamin - B1 | 0.05 mg | 3.33 | Isoleucine | 0.09 g | 7.83 |
| Riboflavin - B2 | 0.06 mg | 3.53 | Leucine | 0.13 g | 5.14 |
| Niacin - B3 | 0.51 mg | 2.55 | Lysine | 0.12 g | 5.11 |
| Niacin equiv | 1.00 mg | | Methionine | 0.03 g | 4.05 |
| Vitamin B6 | 0.21 mg | 10.50 | Phenylalanine | 0.08 g | 6.72 |
| Vitamin B12 | 0.00 mcg | 0.00 | Proline | 0.10 g | |
| Biotin | 1.61 mcg | 0.54 | Serine | 0.12 g | |
| Vitamin C | 54.93 mg | 91.55 | Threonine | 0.08 g | 6.45 |
| Vitamin D IU | 0.00 IU | 0.00 | Tryptophan | 0.03 g | 9.38 |
| Vitamin D mcg | 0.00 mcg | | Tyrosine | 0.05 g | 5.15 |
| Vitamin E Alpha Equiv | 0.05 mg | 0.25 | Valine | 0.11 g | 7.48 |
| Vitamin E IU | 0.07 IU | | | | |
| Vitamin E mg | 0.10 mg | | | | |
| Folate | 54.56 mcg | 13.64 | | | |
| Vitamin K | 11.17 mcg | 13.90 | | | |

(Note: "–" indicates data is unavailable. For more information, please see page 806.)

Cauliflower and other cruciferous vegetables, such as broccoli, cabbage and kale, contain compounds that may help prevent cancer. These compounds—including both glucosinolates and thiocyanates (such as sulforaphane)—appear to stop enzymes from activating cancer-causing agents in the body, and they increase the activity of liver enzymes that disable and eliminate carcinogens.

If potentially toxic molecules are not properly and rapidly detoxified in the liver, they can damage cell membranes and molecules, such as DNA within the cell nucleus. Such damage can start a chain reaction that may eventually lead to carcinogenesis—cell deregulation and uncontrolled growth.

Many enzymes found in Cauliflower also help with the detoxifying process. These enzymes include *glutathione transferase, glucuronosyl transferase* and *quinone reductase*. Plus, both animal and human studies show increased detoxification enzyme levels from diets providing high levels of the glucosinolates found in Cauliflower.

## Promotes Heart Health

Cauliflower is a great food to add to your "Healthiest Way of Eating" if you are looking to support your heart. It is an excellent source of folic acid and a very good source of vitamin B6, two nutrients necessary for properly metabolizing homocysteine and therefore preventing levels of this dangerous compound from rising in the bloodstream; homocysteine can damage arterial walls and high blood levels are associated with increased risk of cardiovascular disease. Cauliflower can also make a great contribution to your daily dietary fiber goals since it is an excellent source of this important nutrient. Fiber has numerous benefits, including its ability to keep cholesterol levels in check. Cauliflower is also a very good source of the omega-3 essential fatty acid, alpha-linolenic acid, a nutrient that has been found to help reduce biomarkers of cardiovascular disease. Dietary intake of alpha-linolenic acid has also been associated with reduced risk of heart disease. Cauliflower is a low-calorie source of other heart-friendly nutrients as well, including vitamin C, potassium, magnesium and niacin.

## Additional Health-Promoting Benefits of Cauliflower

Cauliflower is also a concentrated source of many other nutrients providing additional health-promoting benefits. These nutrients include energy-producing vitamin B1, vitamin B2, vitamin B5 and phosphorus; free-radical-scavenging manganese; muscle-building protein; and sleep-promoting tryptophan. Since steamed Cauliflower contains only 29 calories per one cup serving, it is an ideal food for healthy weight control.

STEP-BY-STEP RECIPE

## The Healthiest Way of Cooking Cauliflower

# 5-Minute "Healthy Sautéed" Cauliflower

*If you normally steam Cauliflower, I highly recommend trying the "Healthy Sauté" method. I think you will be wonderfully surprised by the extra flavor and nutrition you will enjoy when you "Healthy Sauté."*

**1 lb Cauliflower**
**5 TBS low-sodium chicken or vegetable broth**

**Mediterranean Dressing:**
**3 TBS extra virgin olive oil**
**2 tsp lemon juice**
**2 medium cloves garlic**
**Sea salt and pepper to taste**

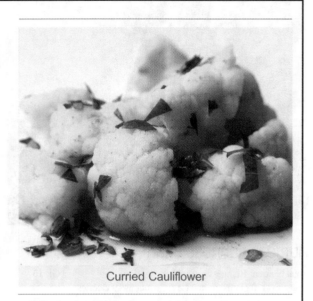

Curried Cauliflower

1. Cut Cauliflower florets into quarters and let sit as directed under *How to Bring out the Hidden Health Benefits of Cauliflower.*
2. Press or chop garlic and let sit for at least 5 minutes. (Why?, see page 261.)
3. Heat 5 TBS broth in a stainless steel skillet on medium high.
4. When broth begins to steam, add Cauliflower and **cover**. For *al denté* Cauliflower, cook for no more than 5 minutes. (For more information on *Differences in Cooking Time,* see page 94.)
5. Transfer to a bowl. For more flavor, toss Cauliflower with the remaining ingredients while it is still hot. (Mediterranean Dressing does not need to be made separately.) Research shows that carotenoids found in foods are best absorbed when consumed with oils.

OPTIONAL: To mellow the flavor of garlic, add garlic to Cauliflower for the last 2 minutes of sautéing. You may need to add a little more liquid to keep garlic from sticking to pan.

**SERVES 2**

### COOKING TIPS:
- To prevent overcooking Cauliflower, I highly recommend using a timer.
- Testing Cauliflower with a fork is not an effective way to determine whether it is done.

---

### Flavor Tips: Try these 4 great serving suggestions with the recipe above. ✳

1. **Most Popular: Curried (Turmeric) Cauliflower.** Nothing enhances the flavor of Cauliflower better than curry or turmeric. They give it a creamy, rich flavor. Sprinkle curry or turmeric (curry is usually spicier) over Cauliflower after it is added to the steaming broth. Top with cilantro (pictured above).
2. **Savory Cauliflower:** In a small bowl, whisk 1 TBS Dijon mustard and 2 TBS olive oil until well combined. Pour over cooked 5-Minute "Healthy Sautéed" Cauliflower, and garnish with 1 TBS capers or minced anchovies. Reduce the amount of olive oil if desired.
3. **Mashed Cauliflower:** Mash 5-Minute "Healthy Sautéed" Cauliflower with a potato masher or blend in a food processor until it attains the consistency of mashed potatoes. Sprinkle with finely sliced scallions or minced parsley and Parmesan cheese.
4. **Creamy Cauliflower Soup:** Combine 1 cup of the 5-Minute "Healthy Sautéed" Cauliflower recipe with 1 cup warm low-fat milk (or coconut milk) and 2 TBS grated Parmesan cheese in a blender until smooth. Place in a serving bowl and garnish with grated Parmesan cheese and minced parsley for a filling soup.

---

Please write (address on back cover flap) or e-mail me at info@whfoods.org with your personal ideas for preparing Cauliflower, and I will share them with others through our website at www.whfoods.org.

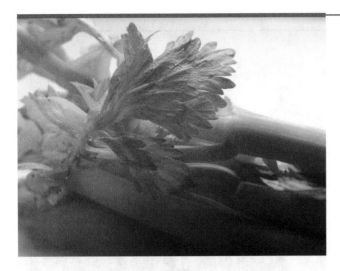

# celery

| | |
|---|---|
| AVAILABILITY: | Year-round |
| REFRIGERATE: | Yes |
| SHELF LIFE: | 2 weeks refrigerated |
| PREPARATION: | Minimum |
| BEST WAY TO COOK: | "Healthy Sauté" in just 5 minutes |

## nutrient-richness chart

Total Nutrient-Richness: **25**  GI: **15**

One cup (120 grams) of raw Celery contains 19 calories

| NUTRIENT | AMOUNT | %DV | DENSITY | QUALITY |
|---|---|---|---|---|
| Vitamin K | 35.3 mcg | 44.1 | 41.3 | excellent |
| Vitamin C | 8.4 mg | 14.0 | 13.1 | excellent |
| Potassium | 344.4 mg | 9.8 | 9.2 | very good |
| Folate | 33.6 mcg | 8.4 | 7.9 | very good |
| Dietary Fiber | 2.0 g | 8.2 | 7.7 | very good |
| Molybdenum | 6.0 mcg | 8.0 | 7.5 | very good |
| Manganese | 0.1 mg | 6.0 | 5.6 | very good |
| B6 Pyridoxine | 0.1 mg | 5.0 | 4.7 | very good |
| Calcium | 48.0 mg | 4.8 | 4.5 | good |
| B1 Thiamin | 0.01 mg | 4.0 | 3.8 | good |
| Magnesium | 13.2 mg | 3.3 | 3.1 | good |
| Vitamin A | 160.8 IU | 3.2 | 3.0 | good |
| Tryptophan | 0.01 g | 3.1 | 2.9 | good |
| Phosphorus | 30.0 mg | 3.0 | 2.8 | good |
| B2 Riboflavin | 0.1 mg | 2.9 | 2.8 | good |
| Iron | 0.5 mg | 2.7 | 2.5 | good |

| CAROTENOIDS: | |
|---|---|
| Beta-Carotene | 334.8 mcg |
| Lutein+Zeaxanthin | 350.9 mcg |

| FLAVONOIDS: | |
|---|---|
| Apigenin | 5.7 mg |
| Luteolin | 1.6 mg |
| Quercetin | 4.3 mg |

Daily values for these nutrients have not yet been established.

| PHYTOSTEROLS: | |
|---|---|
| Phytosterols – Total | 7.4 mg |

For more on "Total Nutrient-Richness," "%DV," "Density," and The World's Healthiest Foods "Quality" Rating System, see page 805.

For more on GI, see page 342.

Celery has a long and prestigious history of use, first as a medicine and later as a food. The initial mention of the medicinal properties of Celery leaves appeared in *The Odyssey*, the famous epic by the Greek poet, Homer, which dates back to the 9th century BC Celery's use as a food began with the ancient Romans, who used it as a seasoning because of its distinct aromatic flavor. This tradition has been carried on to this day as we continue to enjoy Celery as a flavor enhancer in soups and stews. Today, raw Celery is also very popular. It adds crunch to a favorite salad and is great served as crudités with a favorite dip or as a convenient low-calorie snack for those watching their weight. When cooking Celery, it is important to prepare it properly to obtain the best flavor and maximize its nutritional value; that is why I want to share with you the "Healthiest Way of Cooking" Celery for a tasty 5-minute dish that will complement almost any meal.

## why celery should be part of your healthiest way of eating

Today, science is discovering why Celery has long been considered such a health-promoting vegetable. Calorie for calorie, Celery provides a surprising number of nutrients. Its low-calorie count (19 calories per cup) combined with its high-fiber content, which helps provide a feeling of satiation, make Celery an excellent food for promoting weight control. Celery also contains antioxidant compounds known as coumarins, which support the immune system's ability to eliminate potentially harmful cells, and pthalides, which may help reduce blood pressure. It also contains flavonoids, such as apigenin, luteolin and quercetin, which promote optimal health. (For more on the *Health Benefits of Celery* and a complete analysis of its content of over 60 nutrients, see page 206.)

## varieties of celery

Celery (*Apium graveolens*) is thought to have its origins in the Mediterranean regions of northern Africa and southern Europe. It is also native to areas extending east to the Himalayas. Unlike the Celery we are familiar with today, the original wild Celery had fewer stalks and more leaves.

Celery is a biennial vegetable that belongs to the *Umbelliferae* family, which also includes fennel, parsley and dill. Celery grows to a height of 12 to 16 inches and is composed of leaf-topped stalks that are arranged in a conical shape and joined at a common base. The stalks have a crunchy texture and a delicate, but mildly salty, taste. The stalks in the center are called the heart and are the most tender portion of the Celery. Varieties of Celery include:

### PASCAL CELERY

This is the well-known green variety found in most supermarkets and the one featured in the photographs in this chapter.

### WHITE CELERY

In addition to green Celery, Europeans enjoy a variety that is white in color. Similar to white asparagus, white Celery is grown in an environment shaded from direct sunlight. This inhibits the production of the chlorophyll that would otherwise make it green.

### CHINESE CELERY

Typically found in Asian markets, this variety looks like a cross between parsley and Celery and is very flavorful.

### CELERIAC

This variety, also known as Celery root, is eaten raw or cooked and puréed.

## the peak season

Although Celery from California and Florida is available year-round, locally grown Celery is harvested during the summer months. The months when Celery is in season are the months when its concentration of nutrients and flavor are highest, and its cost is at its lowest.

## biochemical considerations

Celery is a concentrated source of oxalates, which might be of concern to certain individuals. It is one of the 12 foods on which pesticide residues have been most frequently found and is one of the foods most commonly associated with allergic reactions in individuals with latex allergies. (For more on *Oxalates,* see page 725; *Pesticide Residues,* see page 726; and *Latex Food Allergies,* see page 722.)

## 4 steps for the best tasting and most nutritious celery

Turning Celery into a flavorful dish with the most nutrients is simple if you just follow my 4 easy steps:

1. The Best Way to Select
2. The Best Way to Store
3. The Best Way to Prepare
4. The Healthiest Way of Cooking

# 1. the best way to select celery

You can select the best tasting Celery by looking for ones with stalks that are relatively tight, compact and do not splay out. The stalks should be crisp and look like they would snap easily when pulled apart; the leaves should be green in color. By selecting the best tasting Celery, you will also enjoy Celery with the highest nutritional value. As with all vegetables, I recommend selecting organically grown varieties whenever possible. (For more on *Organic Foods,* see page 113.)

Avoid Celery with stalks that have yellow or brown patches. Dry stalks become stringy. I have found Celery with seedstems are often more bitter in flavor (seedstems are a round stem in the place of the smaller tender stalks usually found in the center of the Celery). It is also good to separate the stalks and check for brown or black discoloration, which may indicate a condition caused by insects called "blackheart." Avoid bruised or damaged Celery or Celery that has any evidence of rot.

Q *Celery has a reputation among some persons as being a high-sodium vegetable, vegetable, so how much impact does it have on sodium intake and raising blood pressure?*

A There are approximately 100 mg of sodium in a full cup of chopped celery—that's about 2 stalk's worth.

The U.S. Food and Drug Administration's Daily Value for sodium intake is 2,400 mg—the equivalent of about 24 cups, or 48 stalks of celery. Since two stalks of celery only provide about 4% of the sodium DV, most individuals would be able to include two or even more (Continued on Page 208)

# 2. the best way to store celery

Celery is a sturdy vegetable, but it will become yellow and lose its crispness if not stored properly. Be sure to store Celery properly as it can quickly lose up to 30% of some of its vitamins as well as much of its flavor.

Celery continues to respire even after it has been harvested; its respiration rate at room temperature (68°F/20°C) is 71 mg/kg/hr. Slowing down the respiration rate with proper storage is the key to extending its flavor and nutritional benefits. (For a *Comparison of Respiration Rates* for different vegetables, see page 91.)

## Celery Will Remain Fresh for Up to 2 Weeks When Properly Stored

1. Store Celery in the refrigerator. The colder temperature will slow the respiration rate, helping to preserve vitamins and keeping Celery fresh for a longer period of time.

2. Place Celery in a plastic storage bag before refrigerating. I have found that it is best to wrap the bag tightly around the Celery, squeezing out as much of the air from the bag as possible.

3. Do not wash Celery before refrigeration because exposure to water will encourage Celery to spoil.

# 3. the best way to prepare celery

Whether you are going to enjoy Celery raw or cooked, I want to share with you the best way to prepare Celery. Properly cleaning and cutting Celery helps to ensure that the Celery you serve will have the best flavor and retain the greatest number of nutrients.

## Cleaning Celery

To clean Celery, cut off the base and leaves, and wash the stalks under cold running water. To preserve nutrients, do not soak Celery or the water-soluble nutrients will leach into the water. (For more on *Washing Vegetables*, see page 92.)

## How to Remove Celery's Strings

Remove any strings in Celery before eating. Pull the strings down along the length of the stalk. You can use a knife or vegetable peeler to peel and remove strings from the outer surface of Celery. Young Celery is not as stringy as old Celery.

## Cutting Celery

Cut off bottom 1-inch portion of the Celery stalks and discard. Cut off tips and leaves; tips are bitter and usually dry. Diagonally cut Celery into 1-inch pieces.

# 4. the healthiest way of cooking celery

Since research has shown that important nutrients can be lost or destroyed by the way a food is cooked, the "Healthiest Way of Cooking" Celery is focused on bringing out its best flavor while maximizing its vitamins, minerals and powerful antioxidants.

## The Healthiest Way of Cooking Celery: "Healthy Sautéing" for just 5 Minutes

In my search to find the healthiest way to cook Celery, I tested every possible cooking method looking for the ways to bring out its best flavor and preserve the maximum amount of nutrients and discovered that "Healthy Sautéeing" Celery for just 5 minutes delivered the best results. "Healthy Sautéed" Celery has a mild flavor and retains the maximum number of nutrients. The Step-by-Step Recipe will show you how easy it is to "Healthy Sauté" Celery.

## How to Avoid Overcooking Celery: Cook it *Al Denté*

One of the primary reasons people do not enjoy cooked Celery is because it is often overcooked. For the best flavor, I recommend that you cook Celery *al denté*. Celery cooked *al denté* is tender and is cooked just long enough to soften its cellulose and hemicellulose fiber; this makes it easier to digest and allows its health-promoting nutrients to become more readily available for absorption.

Although Celery is a hearty vegetable, it is very important not to overcook it. Celery cooked for as little as a couple of minutes longer than *al denté* will begin to lose not only its texture and flavor but also its nutrients. Overcooking Celery will significantly decrease its nutritional value: as much as 50% of some nutrients can be lost. (For more on *Al Denté*, see page 92.)

## Celery in Soups and Stews

Celery is also a popular flavor enhancer in soups and stews. When making soups and stews, you want to transfer the flavors into the liquid, and the way to do this is to start cooking your Celery in cold water. Cold water that is heated up gradually allows the pores of Celery to remain open and most of its nutrients and flavor to leach into the water. That is why Celery cooked this way has little flavor and is usually discarded once the flavor has been extracted.

## Cooking Methods
## Not Recommended for Celery

### BOILING, STEAMING, BROILING, GRILLING OR COOKING WITH OIL

I do not recommend boiling or steaming Celery because these methods increase its water absorption, causing the Celery to become soggy and mushy. Celery then loses much of its flavor along with many of its nutrients including minerals, water-soluble vitamins (such as C and the B-complex vitamins) and health-promoting phytonutrients. Broiling or grilling Celery also results in a loss of much of Celery's flavor. I don't recommend cooking Celery in oil because high temperature heat can damage delicate oils and potentially create harmful free radicals.

Here are questions I received from readers of the whfoods.org website about Celery:

### Q *What are Celery seeds?*

A Celery seeds are the dried fruit of a plant known as *Apium graviolens*. While the Celery that we eat is also known botanically by the same name, they are not the same plant, but rather relatives. Celery seeds are small in size and green-brown in color and, not surprisingly, have a Celery-like flavor. Celery seeds are often used in tomato dishes, curries, breads and pickling blends. Preliminary research suggest that they may have health-promoting properties, including antioxidant and anti-inflammatory activity.

### Q *Is juicing Celery as healthy as eating it raw?*

A In general, juicing Celery (or other vegetables) is not nearly as healthy as eating it raw. That's because juicers usually separate the juice from the solids in the leaves or stems or stalks (which some people call the pulp), all of which are then discarded. Unfortunately, these portions of the vegetable often contain a majority—and even a large majority—of the total nutrients, including fiber, and many phytonutrients including certain carotenoids and flavonoids.

# how to enjoy fresh celery without cooking

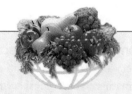

Add diced Celery whenever you want your tuna, shrimp or chicken salad to have an extra crunch.

Raw Celery is great in salads and as crudités for a healthy appetizer or a between-meal snack.

Serve as crudités dressed with extra virgin olive oil, sea salt and pepper.

Fill Celery stalks with your favorite soft cheese or low-fat cottage cheese and sprinkle with Celery sea salt .

Serve Celery sticks with 3-Minute Avocado Dip (see page 301) or Garlic Dip (see page 263).

**Most Popular: Nut Butter Celery Snacks:** Fill the Celery stalk with nut butter and then cut into 2-inch pieces. Dot with raisins and enjoy!

**Celery Salad:** Combine 3 stalks of sliced Celery, 1 medium cubed pear or apple, 2 TBS chopped walnuts, 1 tsp lemon juice, 1 TBS Parmesan cheese, 1 TBS extra virgin olive oil, and sea salt and pepper to taste.

**Refreshing Celery Salad with Yogurt:** Combine 1 cup low-fat yogurt, 1 cup chopped Celery, 1/2 cup chopped cucumber, 1 medium chopped tomato and 1 tsp each minced mint and basil.

**Celery Relish:** Combine 2 cups diced Celery, 1/2 cup diced red bell peppers, 1/4 cup chopped scallions and 1 TBS capers. Mix with 3 TBS extra virgin olive oil, 1 TBS cider vinegar, and sea salt and pepper to taste.

# health benefits of celery

## Promotes Heart Health

Celery's ability to reduce blood pressure has long been recognized by Chinese medicine practitioners. Celery contains compounds called phthalides, which relax the muscles of the arteries that regulate blood pressure and allow the vessels to dilate. When researchers injected phthalides into test animals, they found that the animals' blood pressure dropped 12 to 14 percent. In addition, Celery is a very good source of potassium, a mineral that is necessary for maintaining healthy blood pressure. Celery is also a very good source of folate and vitamin B6, which can reduce cardiovascular disease risk through their role in guarding against elevated levels of homocysteine. Diets high in fiber-rich foods, like Celery, have been associated with reduced levels of heart disease.

Celery's suggested ability to lower cholesterol has been demonstrated in animals bred to have high cholesterol levels. Water-based solutions of Celery (such as Celery juice) fed to these animals for eight weeks significantly lowered their total cholesterol by increasing the secretion of bile acid, which helps to remove cholesterol from the body.

Celery is an excellent source of vitamin C, a nutrient that may help to protect against chronic disease. In one large-scale study, researchers found that men with the highest vitamin C levels in their blood (a reflection of dietary intake) had a 71% reduced risk of dying from heart disease, while women with the highest levels had a 59% reduced risk.

## Promotes Optimal Health

Celery also contains antioxidant compounds called coumarins, which enhance the activity of certain white blood cells, immune defenders that target and eliminate potentially harmful cells, including cancer cells. In addition, compounds in Celery called acetylenics have been shown to stop the growth of tumor cells.

## Diuretic Activity

Traditionally, the seeds of wild Celery, which first grew around the Mediterranean, were widely used as a diuretic. Today, we understand how the potassium and sodium found in Celery help regulate fluid balance, stimulate urine production and rid the body of excess fluid.

## Additional Health-Promoting Benefits of Celery

Celery is also a concentrated source of many other nutrients providing additional health-promoting benefits. These nutrients include bone-building calcium and magnesium; sulfite-detoxifying molybdenum; free-radical-scavenging vitamin A and manganese; energy-producing vitamin B1, vitamin B2, phosphorus and iron; and sleep-promoting tryptophan. Since Celery contains only 19 calories per one cup serving, it is an ideal food for healthy weight control.

*(See Page 208 for Nutritional Analysis Chart)*

---

Here is a question I received from a reader of the whfoods.org website about Celery:

**Q** *Does Chinese Celery also contain phthalides?*

**A** Your question is a very good one—and one for which, unfortunately, I do not have a full answer. I tried to find measurements of the phthalides in the Celery

*(Continued on Page 208)*

---

### An Easy Way to Prepare Celery, Step-by-Step

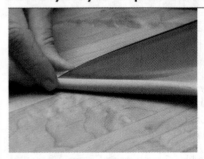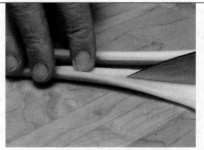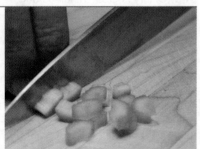

**DICED CELERY**

❶ Cut each stalk in half lengthwise. ❷ Cut each half and make thin strips about 1/4-inch wide. ❸ Turn and cut slices crosswise about 1/4-inch apart, ending up with small 1/4-inch square pieces.

STEP-BY-STEP RECIPE
## the Healthiest Way of Cooking Celery

# 5-Minute "Healthy Sautéed" Celery

*"Healthy Sauté" tenderizes Celery, brings out its mellow taste and produces a richly flavored broth. It is a great side dish for your favorite entrée.*

**4 large stalks Celery**
**1/4 cup low-sodium vegetable broth**

**Mediterranean Dressing:**
**1 TBS extra virgin olive oil**
**1 clove garlic**
**1 tsp lemon juice**
**Sea salt and pepper to taste**

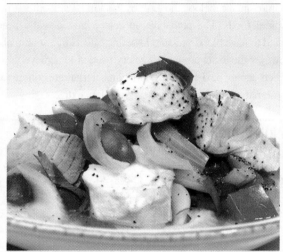

"Healthy Sautéed" Cod with Celery & Olives

1. Press or chop garlic. Let sit for at least 5 minutes. (Why?, see page 261.)

2. Heat broth in a stainless steel skillet over medium heat until it begins to steam.

3. While broth is heating, cut Celery into 1-inch slices as directed under *The Best Way to Prepare Celery.*

4. Add Celery and cook for 5 minutes over medium heat. (For information on *Differences in Cooking Time*, see page 94.)

5. Transfer to a bowl. For more flavor, toss Celery with the remaining ingredients while it is still hot. (Mediterranean Dressing does not need to be made separately.) Research shows that carotenoids found in foods are best absorbed when consumed with oils.

OPTIONAL: To mellow the flavor of garlic, add garlic to Celery for the last 2 minutes of "Healthy Sautéing."

**SERVES 2**

## COOKING TIPS:
- To prevent overcooking Celery, I highly recommend using a timer.
- Testing Celery with a fork is not an effective way to determine whether it is done.

## Flavor Tips: Try these 3 great serving suggestions with the recipe above. ✽

1. **Most Popular: "Healthy Sautéed" Cod with Celery & Olives**—(see recipe on next page).

2. **Sicilian Celery**: Toss the 5-Minute "Healthy Sautéed" Celery recipe with 6 mashed anchovies and 2 additional TBS of extra virgin olive oil.

3. **Celery with Shiitake Mushrooms**: Add 1 cup cooked and sliced shiitake mushrooms, 1 TBS tamari and 1 TBS grated ginger to the 5-Minute "Healthy Sautéed" Celery recipe.

Please write (address on back cover flap) or e-mail me at info@whfoods.org with your personal ideas for preparing Celery, and I will share them with others through our website at www.whfoods.org.

*(Continued from Page 203)*

stalks of celery in a day's diet while keeping their total sodium intake below the DV by sticking with other low-sodium foods. The phthalides in celery have actually been found to have blood pressure lowering effects in test animals, however the exact amount of celery needed to achieve these effects cannot be determined until clinical trials are conducted on humans using the food instead of celery extracts.

*(Continued from Page 206)*

that we are familiar with in the West as well as Chinese Celery and could not find any resources that had this information. Yet, that being said, I am pretty confident that Chinese Celery would have these phytonutrients since Celery for hypertension has a long and revered place in traditional Chinese medicine, and I assume they were using the Chinese version.

## Nutritional Analysis of 1 cup of raw Celery:

| NUTRIENT | AMOUNT | % DAILY VALUE | NUTRIENT | AMOUNT | % DAILY VALUE |
|---|---|---|---|---|---|
| Calories | 19.20 | | Pantothenic Acid | 0.22 mg | 2.20 |
| Calories from Fat | 1.51 | | | | |
| Calories from Saturated Fat | 0.40 | | **Minerals** | | |
| Protein | 0.90 g | | Boron | — mcg | |
| Carbohydrates | 4.38 g | | Calcium | 48.00 mg | 4.80 |
| Dietary Fiber | 2.04 g | 8.16 | Chloride | — mg | |
| Soluble Fiber | 0.55 g | | Chromium | — mcg | — |
| Insoluble Fiber | 1.49 g | | Copper | 0.04 mg | 2.00 |
| Sugar – Total | 1.20 g | | Fluoride | — mg | — |
| Monosaccharides | 1.08 g | | Iodine | — mcg | — |
| Disaccharides | 0.24 g | | Iron | 0.48 mg | 2.67 |
| Other Carbs | 1.14 g | | Magnesium | 13.20 mg | 3.30 |
| Fat – Total | 0.17 g | | Manganese | 0.12 mg | 6.00 |
| Saturated Fat | 0.04 g | | Molybdenum | 6.00 mcg | 8.00 |
| Mono Fat | 0.03 g | | Phosphorus | 30.00 mg | 3.00 |
| Poly Fat | 0.08 g | | Potassium | 344.40 mg | |
| Omega-3 Fatty Acids | 0.00 g | 0.00 | Selenium | 1.08 mcg | 1.54 |
| Omega-6 Fatty Acids | 0.08 g | | Sodium | 104.40 mg | |
| Trans Fatty Acids | 0.00 g | | Zinc | 0.16 mg | 1.07 |
| Cholesterol | 0.00 mg | | | | |
| Water | 113.57 g | | **Amino Acids** | | |
| Ash | 0.98 g | | Alanine | 0.03 g | |
| | | | Arginine | 0.03 g | |
| **Vitamins** | | | Aspartate | 0.15 g | |
| Vitamin A IU | 160.80 IU | 3.22 | Cystine | 0.00 g | 0.00 |
| Vitamin A RE | 15.60 RE | | Glutamate | 0.12 g | |
| A - Carotenoid | 15.60 RE | 0.21 | Glycine | 0.03 g | |
| A - Retinol | 0.00 RE | | Histidine | 0.02 g | 1.55 |
| B1 Thiamin | 0.06 mg | 4.00 | Isoleucine | 0.03 g | 2.61 |
| B2 Riboflavin | 0.05 mg | 2.94 | Leucine | 0.04 g | 1.58 |
| B3 Niacin | 0.39 mg | 1.95 | Lysine | 0.03 g | 1.28 |
| Niacin Equiv | 0.59 mg | | Methionine | 0.01 g | 1.35 |
| Vitamin B6 | 0.10 mg | 5.00 | Phenylalanine | 0.03 g | 2.52 |
| Vitamin B12 | 0.00 mcg | 0.00 | Proline | 0.02 g | |
| Biotin | 0.12 mcg | 0.04 | Serine | 0.03 g | |
| Vitamin C | 8.40 mg | 14.00 | Threonine | 0.03 g | 2.42 |
| Vitamin D IU | 0.00 IU | 0.00 | Tryptophan | 0.01 g | 3.13 |
| Vitamin D mcg | 0.00 mcg | | Tyrosine | 0.01 g | 1.03 |
| Vitamin E Alpha Equiv | 0.43 mg | 2.15 | Valine | 0.04 g | 2.72 |
| Vitamin E IU | 0.64 IU | | | | |
| Vitamin E mg | 0.88 mg | | | | |
| Folate | 33.60 mcg | 8.40 | | | |
| Vitamin K | 35.26 mcg | 44.1 | | | |

(Note: "–" indicates data is unavailable. For more information, please see page 806.)

## "Healthy Sautéed Cod with Celery & Olives

(Pictured on page 207.)

*Recipe takes about 25 minutes to prepare.*

**2 TBS + 1/2 cup low-sodium chicken or vegetable broth**
**1 medium onion**
**6 cloves garlic**
**2 cups celery, cut into 1-inch pieces on the diagonal**
**1 15-oz can diced tomatoes, drained**
**3/4 cup green olives, sliced**
**1 lb cod, cut into 2-inch pieces**
**1 TBS lemon juice**
**Pinch red chili flakes**
**Sea salt and pepper to taste**
**Extra virgin olive oil**
**Chopped cilantro**

1. Slice onion into thin strips and slice garlic. Let sit for 5 minutes. (Why? See page 276.)

2. Heat 2 TBS broth in a stainless steel sauté pan. Add onion and sauté, **covered**, over medium heat for 5 minutes.

3. Add sliced garlic and celery and sauté **covered** for 1 minute.

4. Add tomatoes, olives and remaining broth. Simmer **covered** on medium-low for 15 minutes.

5. Add cod, lemon juice, chili flakes and salt and pepper to top of celery mixture. **Cover** and continue cooking on medium for 5 minutes or until fish is cooked.

6. Transfer to a serving dish and drizzle with olive oil and cilantro.

SERVES **2**

# Homemade
# VEGETABLE BROTH

*Many recipes in this book call for vegetable broth. It's easy to make your own broth that is full of flavor and nutrients. Make a double batch and freeze it for later use. It's best to use organic vegetables for this recipe.*

- **1 LARGE CARROT, scrubbed and cut into** 1/2-inch slices
- **3 LARGE CELERY STALKS, cut into 1/2-inch slices**
- **1 MEDIUM YELLOW ONION, cut into large pieces**
- **2 LARGE BAY LEAVES**
- **10 FRESH PARSLEY SPRIGS (1 small bunch),** left whole
- **8 CUPS FILTERED WATER**

**OPTIONAL: 4–5 whole cloves garlic, smashed**
1/2 tsp sea salt
1/2 cup tomato sauce (for tangy broth)

1. Place vegetables, herbs and any optional ingredients desired in a large stock pot with water.

2. Cover pot and bring to a boil. It's important to cover the vegetables with water before heating it, so that the nutrients from the vegetables go into the water.

3. When broth boils, reduce heat to low and continue cooking, covered, for 45 minutes to 1 hour. It's important to keep the pot covered during this time so the broth won't evaporate.

4. Strain out vegetables and herbs and discard. The broth is now ready to use or store. Broth will store in the refrigerator for a week to 10 days. If longer than 10 days, you can store broth in the freezer in ice cube trays; this makes it very convenient to use.

Many recipes in this book call for vegetable broth. Cans and aseptic packages of broth are widely available in food markets; if possible look for ones that are organic and/or don't include additives.

---

**Q** *Can you please tell me about broth? What can I use as a substitute? Can I use hot water with a small amount of yeast extract added?*

**A** "Healthy Sauté" is a cooking method that does not use heated fats or oils. I have discovered that you can have the wonderful flavor of sautéed foods by cooking with chicken or vegetable broth.

By testing recipes many times using many different cooking methods I have found that chicken broth is an excellent substitute for fats and oils. Good chicken broth has a nice flavor and aroma and enhances the flavor of your food. Here are some tips to help select the best chicken broth:

- Look for low-sodium versions without MSG.

- Aseptically packaged cartons of chicken broth are preferable to cans of broth. Canned products are traditionally heated for 1 hour for sterilization. Aseptic packaging uses a flash heating method that better preserves both flavor and nutrients. After opening, aseptic packages of broth will last for up to 2 weeks; canned broth will last for 5–6 days.

- Chicken flavored bouillon cubes are very salty and most contain MSG.

- Read labels for undesirable ingredients especially in dried forms of broth.

- Homemade chicken broth is the best. You can freeze it and use it as required. Ice cube trays are a good way to store broth; one cube contains about 1–2 tablespoon.

Vegetable broth is good if you want to make a vegetarian dish. You can find vegetable broth in cartons, cans and in the form of bouillon cubes; once again, I prefer the aseptically packaged cartons. Vegetable broth is sweet, cloudy and thin and has a tendency to be very salty so I prefer to buy the low- or no-sodium variety. For selecting vegetable broth, use the same tips listed above for chicken broth.

If you do not have either of these on hand, a little hot water with a small amount of yeast extract or 1 teaspoon of miso paste would be a great substitute. Plain hot water also works but, of course, the broth adds a little extra flavor.

# fennel

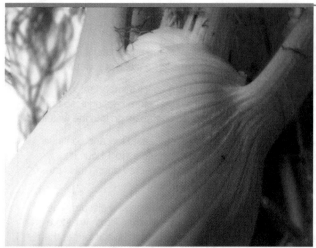

| | |
|---|---|
| AVAILABILITY: | Year-round |
| REFRIGERATE: | Yes |
| SHELF LIFE: | 7 days refrigerated |
| PREPARATION: | Minimal |
| BEST WAY TO COOK: | "Healthy Sautéed" in just 7 minutes |

## nutrient-richness chart

Total Nutrient-Richness: **20**    GI: **n/a**

One cup (87 grams) of raw sliced Fennel contains 27 calories

| NUTRIENT | AMOUNT | %DV | DENSITY | QUALITY |
|---|---|---|---|---|
| Vitamin C | 10.4 mg | 17.4 | 11.6 | excellent |
| Dietary Fiber | 2.7 g | 10.8 | 7.2 | very good |
| Potassium | 360.2 mg | 10.3 | 6.9 | very good |
| Manganese | 0.2 mg | 8.0 | 5.3 | very good |
| Folate | 23.5 mcg | 5.9 | 3.9 | very good |
| Molybdenum | 4.3 mcg | 5.8 | 3.9 | very good |
| Phosphorus | 43.5 mg | 4.3 | 2.9 | good |
| Calcium | 42.6 mg | 4.3 | 2.8 | good |
| Magnesium | 14.8 mg | 3.7 | 2.5 | good |
| Iron | 0.6 mg | 3.6 | 2.4 | good |
| Copper | 0.1 mg | 3.0 | 2.0 | good |
| B3 Niacin | 0.6 mg | 2.8 | 1.9 | good |
| **CAROTENOIDS:** | | | Daily values for this nutrient have not yet been established. | |
| Beta-Carotene | 67.9 mcg | | | |

For more on "Total Nutrient-Richness," "%DV," "Density," and
The World's Healthiest Foods "Quality" Rating System, see page 805.
For more on GI, see page 342.

D uring medieval times, Fennel meant "flattery." Some believe it earned that name because monks in the Middle Ages cooked with Fennel, and it won their dishes great praise. Fennel seeds are actually the fruits of the Fennel plant. They are available year-round and can be stored the same way as celery seeds.

Fennel is a member of the *Umbellifereae* family of plants, which also includes celery, parsley, dill and coriander. Fennel is also a relative of anise (licorice), with which it is often confused because of its similarity in appearance and aroma.

## why fennel should be part of your healthiest way of eating

Science has discovered that Fennel contains many health-promoting antioxidant phytonutrients, such as quercetin, kaempferol and rutin, which protect cells from oxidative damage. One of Fennel's unique phytonutrients, anethole, is the primary component of its volatile oil and functions not only as an antioxidant, but also as an anti-inflammatory compound. The vitamin C found in Fennel bulb has antimicrobial properties and is also needed for the proper function of the immune system.

## how to enjoy fresh fennel without cooking

- Sliced raw Fennel is a great addition to green salads.

- Cut Fennel bulb into thin strips and add to citrus salads.

- Thinly sliced Fennel bulb is a wonderful addition to sandwiches, such as tuna, or avocado, lettuce and tomato.

- In the Mediterranean region, Fennel is served in salads with anchovy fillets and olives.

- **BEET FENNEL SALAD:** Combine Fennel with steamed beets. Toss with dressing made with equal parts fresh lemon juice and extra virgin olive oil, complemented with sea salt and black pepper to taste.

- **APPLE FENNEL SALAD:** Combine 1 tsp fresh lemon juice, 1 TBS of honey, 1 TBS Dijon mustard, 1 tsp Fennel seeds, 3 TBS extra virgin olive oil and sea salt and pepper to taste in a large mixing bowl. Add 1 very thinly sliced medium-size apple and thinly sliced Fennel bulb, including the fine leaves. Toss until well coated.

STEP-BY-STEP RECIPE
## The Healthiest Way of Cooking Fennel

# 7-Minute "Healthy Sautéed" Fennel

*In my search to find the healthiest way to cook Fennel, I discovered that "Healthy Sautéing" Fennel for just 7 minutes delivered the best results.*

**1 Fennel bulb, sliced thin (1/4-inch)**
**2 + 2 TBS low-sodium chicken or vegetable broth**

**Mediterranean Dressing:**
**3 TBS extra virgin olive oil**
**2 tsp lemon juice**
**2 medium cloves garlic**
**Sea salt and black pepper to taste**

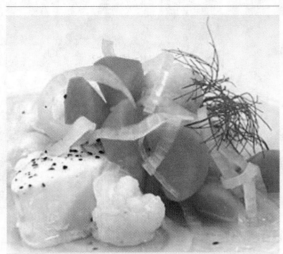
Fish with "Healthy Sautéed" Fennel and Carrots

1. Chop garlic and let it sit for at least 5 minutes. (Why?, see page 261.)
2. Heat 2 TBS broth over medium heat in a stainless steel skillet.
3. Slice Fennel bulb thin (1/4-inch) to cook *al denté*.
4. When broth begins to steam, add Fennel, **cover** and sauté for 4 minutes. Remove cover, stir and add 2 TBS of broth, and cook **uncovered** for 3 more minutes over medium heat. (For information on *Differences in Cooking Time,* see page 94.)
5. Transfer to a bowl. For more flavor, toss Fennel with the remaining ingredients while it is still hot. (Mediterranean Dressing does not need to be made separately.) Research shows that carotenoids found in foods are best absorbed when consumed with oils.

**SERVES 2**

---

## Flavor Tips: Try these 3 great serving suggestions with the recipe above. ✳

1. **Most Popular:** "Healthy Sautéed" Fennel with sliced red bell peppers and top with feta or grated parmesan cheese.
2. **Fennel Mashed Potatoes:** Combine 7-Minute "Healthy Sautéed" Fennel with 2 steamed potatoes, 2 TBS extra virgin olive oil and 2 TBS fresh dill in the food processor. Add salt and pepper to taste.
3. **Fish with Sautéed Fennel and Carrots:** Combine 7-Minute "Healthy Sautéed" Fennel recipe with cooked fish pieces (cod, tuna or salmon) and cooked carrots and cauliflower (pictured above).

---

Please write (address on back cover flap) or e-mail me at info@whfoods.org with your personal ideas for preparing Fennel, and I will share them with others through our website at www.whfoods.org.

## An Easy Way to Prepare Fennel, Step-By-Step

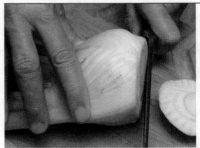 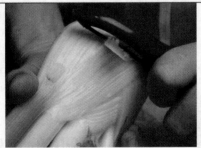 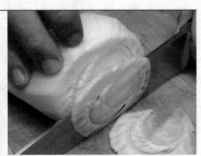

**SLICED FENNEL BULB**—Rinse Fennel under cold running water before cutting.
❶ Take a thin slice off of the bottom end of the Fennel bulb. ❷ Peel the outer part of the bulb with a potato peeler if it is tough. ❸ For *al denté* be sure to slice thin (about 1/4-inch), starting at the root end and cutting up to the stalks. Save stalks for use in vegetable broth. Use leaves as garnish.

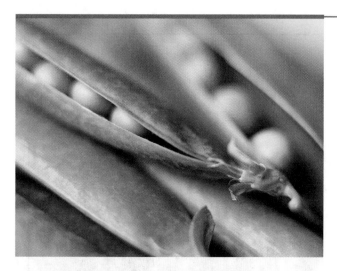

# green peas

## garden, snow and sugar snap peas

### highlights

| | |
|---|---|
| AVAILABILITY: | Year-round |
| REFRIGERATE: | Yes |
| SHELF LIFE: | 10 days refrigerated |
| PREPARATION: | Minimal |
| BEST WAY TO COOK: | "Healthy Sauté" in just 3 minutes |

## nutrient-richness chart

Total Nutrient-Richness: **24**          GI: **40**

One cup (160 grams) of cooked Garden Peas contains 134 calories

| NUTRIENT | AMOUNT | %DV | DENSITY | QUALITY |
|---|---|---|---|---|
| Vitamin K | 41.4 mcg | 51.8 | 6.9 | very good |
| Manganese | 0.8 mg | 42.0 | 5.6 | very good |
| Vitamin C | 22.7 mg | 37.9 | 5.1 | very good |
| Dietary Fiber | 8.8 g | 35.2 | 4.7 | very good |
| B1 Thiamin | 0.4 mg | 27.3 | 3.7 | very good |
| Folate | 101.3 mcg | 25.3 | 3.4 | very good |
| Vitamin A | 955.2 IU | 19.1 | 2.6 | good |
| Tryptophan | 0.1 g | 18.8 | 2.5 | good |
| Phosphorus | 187.2 mg | 18.7 | 2.5 | good |
| B6 Pyridoxine | 0.4 mg | 17.5 | 2.3 | good |
| Protein | 8.6 g | 17.2 | 2.3 | good |
| B3 Niacin | 3.2 mg | 16.1 | 2.2 | good |
| Magnesium | 62.4 mg | 15.6 | 2.1 | good |
| B2 Riboflavin | 0.2 mg | 14.1 | 1.9 | good |
| Copper | 0.3 mg | 14.0 | 1.9 | good |
| Iron | 2.5 mg | 13.7 | 1.8 | good |
| Zinc | 1.90 mg | 12.7 | 1.7 | good |
| Potassium | 433.6 mg | 12.4 | 1.7 | good |

**CAROTENOIDS:**

| | | |
|---|---|---|
| Alpha-Carotene | 35.2 mcg | Daily values for these nutrients have not yet been established. |
| Beta-Carotene | 752 mcg | |
| Lutein+Zeaxanthin | 4,148.8 mcg | |

For more on "Total Nutrient-Richness," "%DV," "Density," and The World's Healthiest Foods "Quality" Rating System, see page 805.

For more on GI, see page 342.

Peas date as far back as Biblical times. Archeologists have found them in Egyptian tombs, and they are known to have been prized by the ancient Greeks and Romans. But it was not until tender varieties were developed in the 16th century that Green Peas were popularized by the French King Louis XIV. Today, you too can enjoy Green Peas fit for a king by using the "Healthiest Way of Cooking" Green Peas *al denté*. Cooking Green Peas *al denté* will not only help maximize their nutritional value but will bring out their best flavor and vibrant green color for a great tasting dish that only takes 3 minutes to prepare!

## why green peas should be part of your healthiest way of eating

Green Peas are an especially rich source of B vitamins, including B1, B2, B3, B6 and folate, which are essential for the proper metabolism of fats, proteins and carbohydrates. They are also rich in health-protective carotenoid phytonutrients, including lutein and zeaxanthin, which provide antioxidant protection against the oxidative damage to cellular structures that can be caused by free radicals. (For more on the *Health Benefits of Green Peas* and a complete profile of their content of over 60 nutrients, see page 216.)

## varieties of green peas

Peas (*Pisum Sativum*) are a member of the legume family of plants. Legumes bear fruit in the form of pods enclosing the fleshy seeds we know as beans. Peas are one of the few legumes that are sold and cooked as fresh vegetables. All varieties of Green Peas are available as fresh or frozen. Frozen Peas are often sweeter than fresh Peas because they are frozen at the peak of their freshness.

There are two types of Green Peas: fresh shelled Garden Peas and Peas with edible pods such as Snow Peas and Snap Peas.

### GARDEN PEAS

Garden Peas need to be shelled before eating. Fresh Garden Peas have rounded pods that are usually slightly curved in shape with a smooth texture and vibrant green color. This is the variety of Green Peas featured in the photographs in this chapter. Inside Garden Peas are green rounded Pea seeds that are sweet and starchy in taste and can be eaten raw or cooked. Garden Peas have more nutrients and more calories than Snow Peas or Sugar Snap Peas. However, they require more work to prepare because they must be shelled before eating. As most people do not want to spend the extra time to shell their Peas, the demand for fresh Garden Peas is very low, and they can be more difficult to find than other varieties of Peas. Garden Peas are sweet and succulent for three to four days after they are picked but tend to become mealy and starchy very quickly if they are not cooked soon after harvesting.

Ninety-five percent of Garden Peas are sold either frozen or canned. Frozen Garden Peas are a good substitute for fresh Garden Peas. They are already shelled, and because they are blanched before freezing, they take no time to prepare—just heat and serve. They also retain their flavor and nutritional value because they are frozen soon after they are picked. Frozen Peas are more flavorful, contain less sodium and have more nutritional value than canned Peas.

### SNOW PEAS OR CHINESE PEA PODS

Sometimes called Chinese Pea Pods, this variety is usually used in stir-fries. Snow Peas are flat with edible pods through which you can usually see the shadows of the flat Pea seeds inside; they are never shelled. Overall, they are not as nutritious as Garden Peas, but they do have a higher concentration of vitamin C and fewer calories. Fresh and frozen Snow Peas are available.

### SUGAR SNAP PEAS

A cross between the Garden and Snow Pea, they have plump edible pods with a crisp, snappy texture; they are not shelled. Both Snow Peas and Snap Peas feature a slightly sweeter and cooler taste than the Garden Pea. Like Snow Peas, Snap Peas have fewer nutrients and calories than Garden Peas. Fresh and frozen Sugar Snap Peas are available.

## the peak season

Fresh Garden Peas are generally available from spring through the beginning of winter. Fresh Snow Peas can usually be found throughout the year in Asian markets and from spring through the beginning of winter in supermarkets. Fresh Sugar Snap Peas are generally only available from late spring through early summer. The times when they are in season are when their concentration of nutrients and flavor are highest, and their cost is at its lowest.

## biochemical considerations

Green peas are a concentrated source of purines, which might be of concern to certain individuals. (For more on *Purines,* see page 727.)

## 4 steps for the best tasting and most nutritious green peas

Turning Green Peas into a flavorful dish with the most nutrients is simple if you just follow my 4 easy steps:

1. The Best Way to Select
2. The Best Way to Store
3. The Best Way to Prepare
4. The Healthiest Way of Cooking

# 1. the best way to select green peas ⸻

### Garden Peas

You can select the best tasting fresh Garden Peas in the shell by looking for ones that are firm, velvety and smooth with a lively medium-green color. It is best if they have been stored in the refrigerated section of your market because warm temperatures hasten the conversion of their sugars to starch, which reduces their flavor.

Avoid Garden Peas that have shells that are exceptionally light or dark green in color or that are yellow, whitish or speckled with gray. They should not be puffy, water-soaked or have mildew residue. I have also found that pods that make a slight rattling sound when shaken are more likely to contain fewer Pea seeds inside.

### Snow Peas

Unlike the rounded pods of Garden Peas, the pods of Snow Peas are flat. If you can see the shape of the Peas through the non-opaque shiny pod and the pods snap when you bend them in half, you will be selecting the freshest Snow

Peas with the best flavor. I also find that smaller Snow Peas tend to be sweeter.

### Sugar Snap Peas

The best tasting Sugar Snap Peas are fresh, bright green, firm and plump. To test for freshness of Snap Peas, snap one open to see whether it is crisp.

By selecting the best tasting, sweetest, fresh Green Peas you will also be enjoying Peas with the highest nutritional value. Like all vegetables, I recommend selecting organically grown varieties whenever possible. (For more on *Organic Foods*, see page 113.)

# 2. the best way to store green peas

Green Peas lose their freshness quickly if not stored properly, which can result in their losing their flavor and up to 30% of some of their vitamins.

Green Peas continue to respire even after they have been harvested; their respiration rate at room temperature (68°F/20°C) is 313 mg/kg/hr. Slowing down the respiration rate with proper storage is the key to extending their flavor and nutritional benefits. (For a *Comparison of Respiration Rates* for different vegetables, see page 91.)

Frozen Peas can be kept in the freezer for about 1 year.

### Green Peas Will Remain Fresh for Up to 10 Days When Properly Stored

1. Store fresh Green Peas in the refrigerator. The colder temperature will slow the respiration rate, helping to preserve vitamins and keeping Green Peas fresh for a longer period of time.

2. Place Green Peas in a plastic storage bag before refrigerating. I have found that it is best to wrap the bag tightly around the Green Peas, squeezing out as much of the air from the bag as possible.

3. Do not wash Green Peas before refrigeration because exposure to water will encourage your Green Peas to spoil.

# 3. the best way to prepare green peas

Whether you are going to enjoy Green Peas raw or cooked, in a salad, as a side dish or part of a main dish, I want to share with you the best way to prepare Green Peas. Properly preparing Green Peas helps ensure that they will have the best flavor and retain the greatest number of nutrients.

### Cleaning and Shelling Green Peas

It is best to rinse Garden Peas, Snow Peas and Sugar Snap Peas under cold running water before cooking. To preserve nutrients, do not soak Green Peas or their water-soluble nutrients will leach into the water. (See *Washing Vegetables*, page 92.)

#### GARDEN PEAS

Rinse Garden Peas briefly under running water before

removing them from their pods. To shell them easily, snap off the top and bottom of the pod, and then gently pull off the "thread" that lines the seam of most pods. For those that do not have "threads," carefully cut through the seam, making sure not to cut into the Pea seeds. Gently open the pods to remove the seeds; the seeds do not need to be washed since they have been encased in the pod.

The Pea pods are edible. They can be steamed and enjoyed as part of the vegetable, or you can save them to make soup stock.

#### SNOW PEAS AND SUGAR SNAP PEAS

Most Snow Peas do not have strings, but if you find yours do, it is best to remove them before cooking. Sugar Snap Peas do not have strings.

# 4. the healthiest way of cooking green peas

Since research has shown that important nutrients can be lost or destroyed by the way a food is cooked, the "Healthiest Way of Cooking" Green Peas is focused on bringing out their best flavor while maximizing their vitamins, minerals and powerful antioxidants.

### The Healthiest Way of Cooking Green Peas: "Healthy Sauté" for just 3 Minutes

In my search to find the healthiest way to cook Green Peas, I tested every possible cooking method and discovered that "Healthy Sautéing" all varieties of Green Peas (Garden

Peas, Snow Peas and Sugar Snap Peas) for just 3 minutes delivered the best result. "Healthy Sautéed" Green Peas are tender, have sweet flavor and have retained the maximum number of nutrients. The Step-by-Step Recipe will show you how easy it is to "Healthy Sauté" Green Peas. (For more on *"Healthy Sauté,"* see page 57.)

## How to Avoid Overcooking Green Peas: Cook Them *Al Denté*

One of the primary reasons Green Peas lose their flavor is because they are overcooked. For the best flavor, I recommend that you cook Green Peas *al denté*. Green Peas cooked *al denté* are tender and cooked just long enough to soften their cellulose and hemicellulose fiber; this makes them easier to digest and allows their health-promoting nutrients to become more readily available for absorption. Remember that testing Green Peas with a fork is not an effective way to determine whether they are done.

Green Peas are a delicate vegetable, so it is very important not to overcook them. Green Peas cooked for as little as a couple of minutes longer than *al denté* will begin to lose not only their texture and flavor, but also their nutrients. Overcooking Green Peas will significantly decrease their nutritional value: as much as 50% of some nutrients can be lost. (For more on *Al Denté*, see page 92.)

## Cooking Methods Not Recommended for Green Peas

### BOILING, STEAMING OR COOKING WITH OIL

I don't recommend boiling or steaming Green Peas because these methods increase water absorption, causing them to become soggy and mushy. They then lose much of their flavor along with many of their nutrients including minerals, water-soluble vitamins (such as C and the B-complex vitamins) and health-promoting phytonutrients. I don't recommend cooking Green Peas in oil because high temperature heat can damage delicate oils and potentially create harmful free radicals.

## Healthy Cooking Tips for Green Peas

• If you are using frozen Peas for your recipe, a 10 ounce package of Peas will equal $1^1/2$ pounds of fresh shelling Peas in the pod.

• Pea pods are edible and can be steamed for 2–5 minutes or used for soup stock.

Here is a question I received from a reader of the whfoods.org website about Green Peas:

Q *I prepare Peas by microwaving frozen ones with a little water. Is this an OK way to prepare them from a nutritional perspective?*

A Cooking, no matter what the method, can alter the nutrient profile of vegetables including Green Peas. The actual change depends upon the nutrient itself, how long the food is cooked, and how much water is used. The fact that microwaving takes less time than boiling, for example, doesn't necessarily mean that microwaved Peas would contain an enhanced nutrient content. Research seems to indicate that microwaving decreases the phytonutrient content of vegetables, and using excessive amounts of water when microwaving results in a large loss of vitamins and minerals. At this point, I have not seen adequate comparative information to tell you for certain the quantitative differences by nutrient for microwaving compared to boiling or steaming Peas. A good clue to nutrient retention is to enjoy Peas that maintain a vibrant green color and *al denté* texture; In other words, be sure they are not overcooked.

## An Easy Way to Prepare Green Peas, Step-By-Step

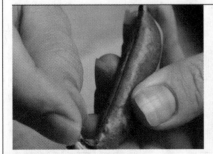 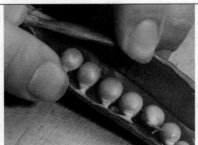 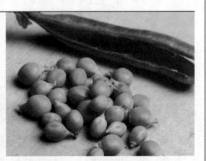

### SHELLING GREEN PEAS
❶ Snap off top and bottom ends of pod, and gently pull off the string (if they have a string). ❷ Open pods.
❸ Remove Peas.

# health benefits of green peas

## Promote Bone Health

Green Peas provide nutrients that are important for maintaining bone health. They are a very good source of vitamin K1, which activates osteocalcin, the major non-collagen protein in bone. When osteocalcin levels are inadequate, bone mineralization is impaired. Green Peas also serve as a very good source of folate and a good source of

vitamin B6. These two nutrients help to reduce the buildup of a metabolic by-product called homocysteine, a dangerous molecule that can obstruct collagen cross-linking, resulting in poor bone matrix and osteoporosis.

## Promote Heart Health

In addition to affecting bone health, homocysteine contributes to atherosclerosis through its ability to damage the blood vessels, keeping them in a constant state of injury. Therefore, the folic acid and vitamin B6 in Green Peas are supportive of cardiovascular health as well as helpful in maintaining bone health. Yet, the contributions of Green Peas to heart health do not stop there; the vitamin K featured in Green Peas is instrumental to the body's healthy blood clotting ability, while their potassium and magnesium help regulate blood pressure, and their dietary fiber helps to keep cholesterol levels in check.

## Promote Vision Health

Green Peas can be an important part of a diet aimed at promoting eye health. They are a good source of vitamin A through their concentration of beta-carotene. Additionally, they are rich in the carotenoids lutein and zeaxanthin, antioxidant phytonutrients that promote eye cell health by protecting against oxidative damage. Studies have found that those who consume lutein- and zeaxanthin-rich diets have less risk of developing cataracts and age-related macular degeneration.

## Promote Energy Production

Green Peas provide nutrients that help support the energy-producing cells and systems of the body. Green Peas are a very good source of vitamin B1, and a good source of vitamin B2, vitamin B6 and niacin, nutrients that are necessary for carbohydrate, protein and lipid metabolism. They are also a good source of iron, a mineral necessary for normal blood cell formation and function, whose deficiency results in anemia, fatigue, decreased immune function and learning problems.

*(Continued on Page 218)*

---

### 3-Minute "Healthy Sautéed" Snow Peas or Sugar Snap Peas

*For the best flavor and maximum amount of nutrients, "Healthy Sauté" your Snow Peas and Sugar Snap Peas.*

**1 lb Snow Peas or Sugar Snap Peas, unshelled**
**1 TBS low-sodium chicken or vegetable broth**

**Mediterranean Dressing:**
**2–3 TBS extra virgin olive oil**
**1–2 medium cloves garlic**
**1 tsp lemon juice**
**Sea salt and pepper to taste**

1. Chop or press garlic and let sit for at least 5 minutes. (Why?, see page 261.)
2. Prepare Snow Peas or Sugar Snap Peas as directed under *The Best Ways to Prepare*.
3. Heat 1 TBS broth over medium high heat until steam begins to rise.
4. Add Snow Peas or Sugar Snap Peas and stir frequently for 3 minutes. Peas will remain fresh and crisp. "Healthy Sauté" will concentrate both the flavor and nutrition of Peas.
5. Transfer to a bowl and toss with the Mediterranean Dressing while Peas are still hot.

OPTIONAL: To mellow the flavor of garlic, add garlic to Peas for the last 2 minutes of sautéing.

**SERVES 2**

---

# how to enjoy fresh green peas without cooking

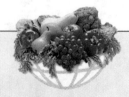

All varieties of Peas can be eaten raw. Just rinse under cool water and enjoy.

Fresh Garden Peas are a great addition to green salads.
Snap Peas are a delicious addition to a crudités platter.

STEP-BY-STEP RECIPE
## The Healthiest Way of Cooking Garden Peas

# 3-Minute "Healthy Sautéed" Garden Peas

*Garden Peas have to be shelled and come both fresh or frozen. If you like Garden Peas with a mildly sweet flavor and the maximum amount of nutrients, I recommend "Healthy Sautéing" your Peas.*

**1 lb fresh or frozen Garden Peas**
**3 TBS low-sodium chicken or vegetable broth**

**Mediterranean Dressing:**
**3 TBS extra virgin olive oil**
**2 tsp lemon juice**
**2 medium cloves garlic**
**Sea salt and pepper to taste**

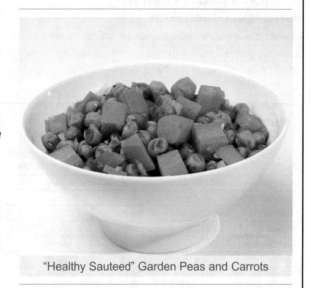

"Healthy Sauteed" Garden Peas and Carrots

1. Chop or press garlic and let sit for at least 5 minutes. (Why?, see page 261)

2. If using fresh Garden Peas, prepare as directed under *The Best Way to Prepare Green Peas*.

3. Heat 3 TBS broth in a stainless steel skillet over medium heat until steam begins to rise.

4. Add fresh or frozen Garden Peas. Cook fresh Peas for only 3 minutes so that they will remain bright green and crisp. Frozen Peas just take 1–2 minutes as they have already been blanched. (For information on *Differences in Cooking Time*, see page 94.)

5. Transfer to a bowl. For more flavor, toss Garden Peas with the remaining ingredients while they are still hot. (Mediterranean Dressing does not need to be made separately.) Research shows that carotenoids found in foods are best absorbed when consumed with oils.

OPTIONAL: To mellow the flavor of garlic, add garlic to Garden Peas for the last 2 minutes of sautéing. You may need to add a little more liquid to keep the garlic from sticking to the pan.

**SERVES 2**

**COOKING TIP:**
• To prevent overcooking Garden Peas, I highly recommend using a timer.

## Flavor Tips: Try these 9 great serving suggestions with the recipe above. ✱

1. **Most Popular: Asian Peas and Shiitakes.** "Healthy Sauté" Garden Peas with onion, garlic, ginger and shiitake mushrooms. Sprinkle with rice vinegar and tamari (soy sauce) to serve.

2. Thyme and mint are perfect matches for Peas.

3. Add rice vinegar, grated ginger and sesame seeds.

4. Add a few drops of tamari (soy sauce).

5. Garden Peas combine well with mushrooms, lamb, chicken, fish or rice.

6. **"Healthy Sautéed" Garden Peas and Carrots:** "Healthy Sauté" diced carrots and onions for 5 minutes. Add "Healthy Sautéed" Garden Peas and sauté 1 minute (pictured above).

7. **Peas and Chicken Salad:** Add shredded carrots to the 3-Minute "Healthy Sautéed" Garden Peas recipe. Add to Chicken Salad (page 579) and season with chopped fresh tarragon.

8. **3-Minute Garden Pea Soup:** Heat 1 cup low-fat milk with 2 cups "Healthy Sautéed" Garden Peas. Blend until creamy. Garnish with minced fresh mint. Serve immediately.

9. **Honey-Mustard Sauce:** Whisk together 1 TBS honey, 1 TBS Dijon mustard, 1 tsp grated ginger, 1 tsp lemon juice, 3 TBS extra virgin olive oil, 1 TBS water, and sea salt and white pepper to taste in a small bowl. Serve over 3-Minute "Healthy Sautéed" Garden Peas. Omit Mediterranean Dressing.

Please write (address on back cover flap) or e-mail me at info@whfoods.org with your personal ideas for preparing Green Peas, and I will share them with others through our website at www.whfoods.org.

*(Continued from Page 216)*

## Additional Health-Promoting Benefits of Green Peas

Green Peas are also a concentrated source of many other nutrients providing additional health-promoting benefits. These nutrients include free-radical-scavenging vitamin C, manganese and copper, energy-promoting phosphorus, muscle-building protein, immune-supportive zinc, and sleep-promoting tryptophan.

Here are questions I received from readers of the whfoods.org website about Green Peas:

**Q** *Are Green Peas considered a starch, vegetable or protein?*

**A** Green Peas are considered a vegetable, although one with a good amount of protein. One cup of boiled Green Peas supplies 17% of the daily value (DV) for protein. It also provides 9% of the DV for carbohydrates.

**Q** *I usually see dried Peas listed as a purine-containing food. What about fresh Peas?*

**A** From my understanding, both fresh garden Peas and dried Peas contain purines. Many individuals with gout are counseled to limit their intake of purines.

**Q** *How does freezing affect the nutritional quality of foods, such as Green Peas?*

**A** While you do lose some flavor when food is frozen, freezing can be a very good way to preserve the nutritional value, texture and flavor of many foods. The initial quality of the food and the length of time between harvest and freezing are important factors. As long as the food was grown in a high-quality way (for example, organically grown) and was fairly fresh at the time of freezing, the overall nutrient retention in a frozen food can be quite high. In other words, many of the vitamins and minerals will keep fairly well in frozen foods.

While some of the phytonutrients found in food may also keep fairly well, one of the main concerns for nutrient loss associated with freezing seems to be related to the blanching process that oftentimes occurs prior to freezing. About 25% of the vitamin C and a greater percentage of folate are lost during the blanching process that occurs before foods are frozen. About 10% of thiamin (vitamin B1) is also lost during blanching. It's important to remember that these percentages of nutrient loss are very general and can be different with different foods.

Since we have seen some research that suggests that thawing degrades part of the vitamin C content, you may want to avoid this step when cooking frozen vegetables. Storing frozen foods properly for no more than 6 months will also help maintain the nutritional value of frozen foods.

### Nutritional Analysis of 1 cup of cooked Green Peas:

| NUTRIENT | AMOUNT | % DAILY VALUE |
|---|---|---|
| Calories | 134.40 | |
| Calories from Fat | 3.17 | |
| Calories from Saturated Fat | 0.56 | |
| Protein | 8.58 g | |
| Carbohydrates | 25.02 g | |
| Dietary Fiber | 8.80 g | 35.20 |
| Soluble Fiber | 2.40 g | |
| Insoluble Fiber | 6.40 g | |
| Sugar - Total | 9.28 g | |
| Monosaccharides | 0.48 g | |
| Disaccharides | 8.00 g | |
| Other Carbs | 6.94 g | |
| Fat - Total | 0.35 g | |
| Saturated Fat | 0.06 g | |
| Mono Fat | 0.03 g | |
| Poly Fat | 0.16 g | |
| Omega-3 Fatty Acids | 0.03 g | 1.20 |
| Omega-6 Fatty Acids | 0.13 g | |
| Trans Fatty Acids | 0.00 g | |
| Cholesterol | 0.00 mg | |
| Water | 124.59 g | |
| Ash | 1.47 g | |

| **Vitamins** | | |
|---|---|---|
| Vitamin A IU | 955.20 IU | 19.10 |
| Vitamin A RE | 96.00 RE | |
| A - Carotenoid | 96.00 RE | 1.28 |
| A - Retinol | 0.00 RE | |
| B1 Thiamin | 0.41 mg | 27.33 |
| B2 Riboflavin | 0.24 mg | 14.12 |
| B3 Niacin | 3.23 mg | 16.15 |
| Niacin Equiv | 4.22 mg | |
| Vitamin B6 | 0.35 mg | 17.50 |
| Vitamin B12 | 0.00 mcg | 0.00 |
| Biotin | 0.64 mcg | 0.21 |
| Vitamin C | 22.72 mg | 37.87 |
| Vitamin D IU | 0.00 IU | 0.00 |
| Vitamin D mcg | 0.00 mcg | |
| Vitamin E Alpha Equiv | 0.62 mg | 3.10 |
| Vitamin E IU | 0.93 IU | |
| Vitamin E mg | 0.80 mg | |
| Folate | 101.28 mcg | 25.32 |
| Vitamin K | 41.40 mcg | 51.8 |

| NUTRIENT | AMOUNT | % DAILY VALUE |
|---|---|---|
| Pantothenic Acid | 0.24 mg | 2.40 |

| **Minerals** | | |
|---|---|---|
| Nutrient | amount | %DV |
| Boron | — mcg | |
| Calcium | 43.20 mg | 4.32 |
| Chloride | 12.80 mg | |
| Chromium | — mcg | — |
| Copper | 0.28 mg | 14.00 |
| Fluoride | — mg | — |
| Iodine | 3.20 mcg | 2.13 |
| Iron | 2.46 mg | 13.67 |
| Magnesium | 62.40 mg | 15.60 |
| Manganese | 0.84 mg | 42.00 |
| Molybdenum | 8.00 mcg | 10.67 |
| Phosphorus | 187.20 mg | 18.72 |
| Potassium | 433.60 mg | |
| Selenium | 3.04 mcg | 4.34 |
| Sodium | 4.80 mg | |
| Zinc | 1.90 mg | 12.67 |

| **Amino Acids** | | |
|---|---|---|
| Alanine | 0.38 g | |
| Arginine | 0.68 g | |
| Aspartate | 0.78 g | |
| Cystine | 0.05 g | 12.20 |
| Glutamate | 1.17 g | |
| Glycine | 0.29 g | |
| Histidine | 0.17 g | 13.18 |
| Isoleucine | 0.31 g | 26.96 |
| Leucine | 0.51 g | 20.16 |
| Lycine | 0.50 g | 21.28 |
| Methionine | 0.13 g | 17.57 |
| Phenylalanine | 0.32 g | 26.89 |
| Proline | 0.27 g | |
| Serine | 0.29 g | |
| Threonine | 0.32 g | 25.81 |
| Tryptophan | 0.06 g | 18.75 |
| Tyrosine | 0.18 g | 18.56 |
| Valine | 0.37 g | 25.17 |

(Note: "—" indicates data is unavailable. For more information, please see page 806.)

## Q&A

**DO ALL VEGETABLES AND SALAD GREENS NEED WASHING— EVEN ORGANIC?**

To keep your family's food safe to eat, you need to wash all fruits and vegetables thoroughly. Even if there is no visible soil clinging to your produce, bacteria can be present. Once ingested, that bacteria could cause illness. It's a good idea to always wash your hands and produce before preparing any meal or snack.

### Washing Technique

The good news is, you do not need to spend money on a special rinse to make your produce safe to eat— but you do need to use proper techniques. The goal of washing is to remove any potentially harmful organisms such as bacteria, soil and spray residue. Washing does not remove toxins that may have been absorbed by the plant while growing.

There are several options for washing lettuce and leafy green vegetables:

1. You can gently rub each leaf while holding it under a strong stream of water, washing both sides.

2. You can put the separated leaves in a sink full of water (make sure the sink has been cleaned and rinsed thoroughly first). Swish the greens around, lift out of the sink and rinse. Do not let the water drain out of the sink with the greens still in the water, as they will fall to the bottom and pick up sand and dirt that may be left as the water drains away.

3. Using a salad spinner is a great way to clean greens. Remove the inner basket from the spinner. Tear or cut greens into pieces, placing them in the inner basket and rinse them with water for a minute or so, then replace the inner basket and spin dry.

You can get rid of bacteria on fruits and vegetables other than leafy greens by holding them under a strong stream of water and using the appropriate scrub brush. Don't skimp here, trickling water does not have enough force to help dislodge and wash away offending bacteria. Scrub produce while holding it under the water and then give it a final rinse. Use a soft brush for tender items, such as summer squash, so you don't damage the skin. Use a firm brush for tougher items, such as apples and melons.

It is also very important to wash produce with thick skins, such as citrus fruit, melons and winter squashes, with their skin or rind still intact. Bacteria from the soil, fieldworkers' hands and other shopper's hands can accumulate on the skin.

If you peel an orange and eat it without washing it or your hands after peeling, you run the risk of ingesting bacteria. If you slice into a melon, the knife blade can carry potentially harmful bacteria into the center of the melon, which makes a perfect growing medium for bacteria, especially if left at room temperature. So always wash produce, even the fruits and vegetables you plan to peel.

Very fragile items, such as berries, should be washed in a colander or strainer, using a moderate flow of water while gently tossing the fruits. To avoid rapid spoilage, wait to rinse berries until right before using and do not rinse beforehand.

If you use a mild detergent to wash conventionally grown produce, don't use too much. Detergent residue, consumed in large enough quantities, can cause gastrointestinal upset or diarrhea.

Many conventionally grown produce items have a thin layer of wax applied to prevent them from drying out— check out the list of waxed produce at your grocery store; it is often posted near the door to the back room of the produce department. Although washing will not remove wax or any bacteria trapped beneath it, waxed produce is washed before the wax is applied. The most effective way to remove the wax is to peel the produce. If you choose to do this, use a peeler that takes only a thin layer of skin, as many healthy vitamins and minerals lie right below the skin.

### EVEN ORGANIC?

Even organic fruits and vegetables need a good washing, as described above, so it is a good idea to get in the habit of washing your fruits and vegetables under a strong stream of running water. All soil contains bacteria. In addition, the natural fertilizers used in organic agricultural may also contain bacteria. Properly aged manure no longer harbors harmful bacteria, but why take the chance that some of the natural fertilizers coming into contact with your produce may not have been aged long enough?

Although organically grown salad mixes in bags often are prewashed, they still need to be rinsed. It's always a good idea to rinse all produce, even "prewashed" greens, under a strong stream of running water, then toss or spin dry. The process only takes a minute, and you'll be certain your greens have been properly cleaned. To ensure the produce you eat delivers only the building blocks of good health into your body even your organic fruits and vegetables should be washed thoroughly.

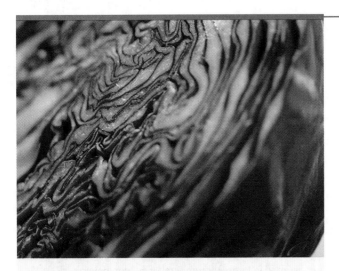

# cabbage

## highlights

| | |
|---|---|
| AVAILABILITY: | Year-round |
| REFRIGERATE: | Yes |
| SHELF LIFE: | 7 to 10 days refrigerated |
| PREPARATION: | Cut and let sit for 5 minutes |
| BEST WAY TO COOK: | "Healthy Sauté" in just 5 minutes |

## nutrient-richness chart

Total Nutrient-Richness: **22**       GI: **15**
One cup (150 grams) of shredded cooked Green Cabbage contains 33 calories

| NUTRIENT | AMOUNT | %DV | DENSITY | QUALITY |
|---|---|---|---|---|
| Vitamin K | 73.4 mcg | 91.7 | 50.0 | excellent |
| Vitamin C | 30.2 mg | 50.3 | 27.4 | excellent |
| Dietary Fiber | 3.5 g | 13.8 | 7.5 | very good |
| Manganese | 0.2 mg | 9.0 | 4.9 | very good |
| B6 Pyridoxine | 0.2 mg | 8.5 | 4.6 | very good |
| Folate | 30.0 mcg | 7.5 | 4.1 | very good |
| Omega-3 Fatty Acids | 0.2 g | 6.8 | 3.7 | very good |
| B1 Thiamin | 0.1 mg | 6.0 | 3.3 | good |
| B2 Riboflavin | 0.1 mg | 4.7 | 2.6 | good |
| Calcium | 46.5 mg | 4.7 | 2.5 | good |
| Potassium | 145.5 mg | 4.2 | 2.3 | good |
| Vitamin A | 198.0 IU | 4.0 | 2.2 | good |
| Tryptophan | 0.01 g | 3.1 | 1.7 | good |
| Protein | 1.5 g | 3.1 | 1.7 | good |
| Magnesium | 12.0 mg | 3.0 | 1.6 | good |

| Carotenoids: | | |
|---|---|---|
| Alpha-Carotene | 30.0 mcg | Daily values for these nutrients have not yet been established. |
| Beta-Carotene | 111.0 mcg | |
| Lutein+Zeaxanthin | 379.5 mcg | |

For more on "Total Nutrient-Richness," "%DV," "Density," and The World's Healthiest Foods "Quality" Rating System, see page 805.

For more on GI, see page 342.

Native to the Mediterranean region of Europe, Cabbage has been cultivated for more than 4,000 years. Chinese scrolls dating as far back as 1,000 BC mentioned the health benefits of Cabbage. Today, one of the most popular vegetables in the world, Cabbage is considered the national food of Russia where they eat seven times more Cabbage than the average North American. Many Chinese could not imagine a stir-fry without Cabbage, and in Germany, people eat so much sauerkraut that they have often been referred to as "Krauts." If Green Cabbage is not your favorite, try Red Cabbage, which you will find to have more flavor. Proper preparation of Cabbage is the key to bringing out its best flavor and maximizing its nutritional benefits. That is why I want to share with you the secret of the "Healthiest Way of Cooking" Cabbage *al denté*. In just 5 minutes, you will be able to transform Cabbage into a flavorful vegetable while maximizing its nutritional value.

## why cabbage should be a part of your healthiest way of eating

Long before scientists discovered vitamin C, sauerkraut (a dish made from fermented Cabbage) was prized by Dutch sailors, who consumed it during extended exploration voyages as they knew it would prevent scurvy and save many lives. Scientific studies now show that cruciferous vegetables, like Cabbage, are included among the vegetables that contain the largest concentrations of health-promoting sulfur compounds, such as sulforaphane and isothiocyanates (see page 153), which increase the liver's ability to produce enzymes that neutralize potentially toxic substances. (For more on the *Health Benefits of Cabbage* and a complete analysis of its content of over 60 nutrients, see page 228.)

Cabbage is an ideal food to add to your "Healthiest Way of Eating" not only because it is high in nutrients, but also because it is low in calories making it great for weight control: one cup of cooked Cabbage contains only 33 calories.

## varieties of cabbage

The cruciferous (*Brassica*) family of vegetables, which includes Cabbage, broccoli, cauliflower, kale, collard greens and Brussels sprouts, originated from the wild cabbage and is well-known for its many health-promoting properties. Unlike the varieties we are familiar with today, wild Cabbage looked more like collard greens or kale having leaves that did not form a head. The name Cabbage comes from *caboche*, the French word for head.

Although there are hundreds of varieties of Cabbage, the five most popular are listed below:

### RED CABBAGE

Red Cabbage contains almost twice the vitamin C as Green Cabbage and is rich in anthocyanins, powerful antioxidants that are responsible for its vibrant reddish-purple color. It has 23 mg of anthocyanins per 100 grams while Green Cabbage has virtually none. One hundred grams also contains 190 mg polyphenous versus the 45 mg found in Green Cabbage. Red Cabbage has a deep hearty flavor that I highly recommend.

### GREEN CABBAGE

This is the most popular cruciferous vegetable and ranges in color from pale to dark green. It has smooth textured leaves. Since the inner leaves are protected from sunlight, they are often lighter in color. Green Cabbage is an excellent source of powerful antioxidants that help protect against harmful free radicals.

### SAVOY CABBAGE

Distinguished by its frilly ruffled leaves that are yellow-green in color, Savoy Cabbage contains more beta-carotene than either Red or Green Cabbage and has a more delicate texture and superior flavor. Unfortunately, Savoy Cabbage is not as readily available as Red or Green Cabbage.

### CHINESE (OR NAPA) CABBAGE

Napa Cabbage is my favorite choice for salads. Oblong in shape with pale green ruffled leaves, Napa Cabbage stalks join in a milky white base. Not only is it slightly softer in texture than other varieties, but it has a really wonderful, delicate flavor. It is a great choice for those who prefer a milder tasting variety of Cabbage. Napa also boasts the highest concentration of the B vitamin, folate, and incredible amounts of zinc; one cup of cooked Napa cabbage contains over 4 grams (27% DV) for this important mineral.

### BOK CHOY/BABY BOK CHOY

This variety is characterized by a loose, bulbous cluster of dark green leaves with firm stems. Bok Choy has a very mild flavor and a higher concentration of beta-carotene and vitamin A than any other variety of Cabbage. Baby Bok Choy has a lower concentration of nutrients because it is harvested when it is still immature.

## the peak season

Red, Green and Napa Cabbage, as well as Bok Choy, are available throughout the year. Savoy Cabbage is less common and is most widely available from September through December. The flavor of Cabbage is at its peak during the cold months when the frost helps to develop a sweet flavor and crisp texture. In hotter months, Cabbage is less tender and will require an additional minute of cooking time.

## biochemical considerations

Cabbage is a concentrated source of goitrogens, which might be of concern to certain individuals. (For more on *Goitrogens*, see page 721.)

## 4 steps for the best tasting and most nutritious cabbage

Turning Cabbage into a flavorful dish with the most nutrients is simple if you just follow my 4 easy steps:

1. The Best Way to Select
2. The Best Way to Store
3. The Best Way to Prepare
4. The Healthiest Way of Cooking

# 1. the best way to select cabbage

You can select the best tasting Cabbage by choosing heads that have a vibrant, bright color and are firm, heavy and dense. Only a few of the outer leaves should be loose, and they should still be attached to the stem; leaves that are detached from the stem usually have undesirable texture and taste. By selecting the best tasting Cabbage, you will also enjoy the highest nutritional value. As with all vegetables, I recommend selecting organically grown Cabbage whenever possible. (For more on *Organic Foods*, see page 113.)

Avoid purchasing Cabbage that is cracked, bruised or blemished. Severe damage to the outer leaves often indicates damage from worms or decay that may also infest the inner core. I don't recommend purchasing precut halves or shredded Cabbage because Cabbage begins to lose its valuable vitamin content as soon as it is cut.

# 2. the best way to store cabbage

Although Cabbage is a hearty vegetable, it will become limp and begin to lose its freshness if not stored properly. If you are not planning to use Cabbage the day you purchase it, make sure to store it properly as it can lose up to 30% of some of its vitamins as well as much of its flavor.

Cabbage continues to respire even after it has been harvested; its respiration rate at room temperature (68°F/ 20°C) is 42 mg/kg/hr. Slowing down the respiration rate with proper storage is the key to extending its flavor and nutritional benefits.

While whole-head Cabbage can be stored for 7 to 10 days, a partly cut head of Cabbage should be tightly covered and kept for no more than 3–5 days

### Cabbage Will Remain Fresh for Up to 7 to 10 Days When Properly Stored

1.  Store Cabbage in the refrigerator. The colder temperature will slow the respiration rate, helping to preserve its nutrients and keeping Cabbage fresh for a longer period of time.

2.  Place Cabbage in a plastic storage bag before refrigerating. I have found that it is best to wrap the bag tightly around the Cabbage, squeezing out as much of the air from the bag as possible.

3.  Do not wash Cabbage before refrigeration because exposure to water will encourage Cabbage to spoil.

# 3. the best way to prepare cabbage

Whether you are going to enjoy your Cabbage raw or cooked, I want to share with you the best way to prepare Cabbage. Properly cleaning and cutting your Cabbage helps to ensure that the Cabbage you serve will have the best flavor and retain the greatest number of nutrients.

### Cleaning Cabbage
Although you don't need to wash head Cabbage because it has never been exposed to the outside environment and is clean inside, it is a good idea to remove the outer leaves. However, if you prefer to wash all your vegetables, rinse head Cabbage under running water after cutting. (For more on *Washing Vegetables,* see page 92.)

### Cutting Cabbage
Cutting your Cabbage into slices of equal thickness will help it to cook more evenly. Because thinly sliced Cabbage cooks more quickly, I recommend cutting Cabbage into 1/4-inch slices to cook it *al denté*. Let sit for 5–10 minutes before cooking. (See bottom of next page for details.)

### Preparing Bok Choy
Bok Choy should be rinsed well under cold running water before cutting. To preserve nutrients, do not soak Bok Choy or its water-soluble nutrients will leach into the water.

Cut off and discard the tough bottom inch of the bunch of Bok Choy. Wash the individual leaves, which will now be separated. Stack the leaves and cut into 1/4-inch slices; cut stems into 3/4-inch pieces. Put the leaves in one bowl and the stems in another; they require different cooking times. Let the cut Bok Choy sit for 5 minutes to increase its health-promoting benefits before cooking. Bok Choy doesn't shrink down as much as some other green leafy vegetables. You can enjoy both the stalks and leafy green portions of Bok Choy.

### How to Store a Partial Head of Cabbage
If you need to store a partial head of Cabbage, place it in a container with a well-sealed lid or a plastic bag and refrigerate. Since the vitamin C content starts to quickly degrade once the Cabbage has been cut, you should use the remainder within a couple of days.

---

### HOW TO BRING OUT THE HIDDEN HEALTH BENEFITS OF CABBAGE

The latest scientific studies show that cutting Cabbage into thin slices breaks down cell walls and enhances the activation of an enzyme called *myrosinase* that slowly converts some of the plant nutrients into their active forms, which have been shown to contain health-promoting properties. So, to get the most health benefits from Cabbage, let it sit for a minimum of 5 minutes, optimally 10 minutes, after cutting, before eating or cooking.

Since ascorbic acid (vitamin C) increases *myrosinase* activity, you can sprinkle a little lemon juice on the Cabbage before letting it sit in order to further enhance its beneficial phytonutrient concentration.

Heat will inactivate the effect of *myrosinase*, which is why it is important to allow the Cabbage to sit for 5–10 minutes before cooking to give the enzyme ample opportunity to enhance the concentration of active phytonutrients. Cooking at low or medium heat for short periods of time should not destroy the active phytonutrients since once they are formed, they are fairly stable.

# 4. the healthiest way of cooking cabbage

Since research has shown that important nutrients can be lost or destroyed by the way a food is cooked, the "Healthiest Way of Cooking" Cabbage is focused on bringing out its best flavor while maximizing its vitamins, minerals and powerful antioxidants.

### The Healthiest Way of Cooking Cabbage: "Healthy Sautéing" for just 5 Minutes

In my search to find the healthiest way to cook Cabbage, I tested every possible cooking method, and I discovered that "Healthy Sautéing" Red Cabbage and Bok Choy concentrated their flavor and "Healthy Steaming" Green Cabbage and Savoy Cabbage made them the most tender. Both methods will give you delicious *al denté* Cabbage in just 5 minutes. Cabbage cooked *al denté* is succulent with a mild sweet flavor and bright color. The Step-by-Step Recipe will show you how easy it is to "Healthy Sauté" Cabbage. (For more on *"Healthy Sautéing,"* see page 57 and for *"Healthy Steaming,"* see page 58.)

### How to Avoid Overcooking Cabbage: Cook It *Al Denté*

One of the primary reasons people do not enjoy cooked Cabbage is because it is often overcooked. For the best flavor and texture, I recommend that you cook your Cabbage *al denté*. Cabbage cooked *al denté* is tender outside and slightly crisp inside. Plus, Cabbage cooked *al denté* is cooked just long enough to soften its cellulose and hemicellulose; this makes it easier to digest and allows its health-promoting nutrients to become more readily available for assimilation.

Although Cabbage is a hearty vegetable, it is very important not to overcook it. Cabbage cooked for as little as a couple of minutes longer than *al denté* will begin to lose not only its texture and flavor but also its nutrients. Overcooking Cabbage will significantly decrease its nutritional value: as much as 50% of some nutrients can be lost. (For more on *Al Denté*, see page 92.)

### Cooking Methods Not Recommended for Cabbage

**BOILING, BAKING, BROILING, GRILLING, ROASTING OR COOKING WITH OIL**

Boiling Cabbage increases its water absorption, causing it to become soggy and lose much of its flavor along with many of its nutrients, including minerals, water-soluble vitamins (such as C and the B-complex vitamins) and health-promoting phytonutrients. I don't recommend baking, broiling, grilling or roasting Cabbage because

---

**CABBAGE TASTES SWEET WHEN COOKED *AL DENTÉ***

Raw Cabbage is a naturally sweet-tasting vegetable, which can be enjoyed as coleslaw or in Chinese chicken salad. Cooking your Cabbage *al denté* will help you retain the sweetness of raw Cabbage and increase its digestibility. The strong smell and unpleasant taste often associated with cooked Cabbage (the reasons I believe to be responsible for its decline in popularity in the U.S.) can also be avoided by cooking it *al denté*. Cabbage is a great tasting, inexpensive and nutritious vegetable. I highly recommend enjoying Cabbage as part of your "Healthiest Way of Eating" at least once a week.

---

### An Easy Way to Prepare Cabbage, Step-By-Step

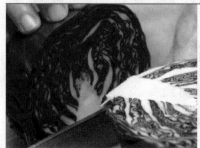 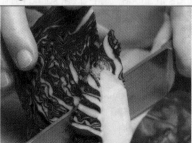 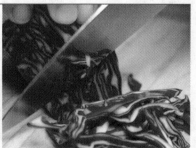

❶ Remove outer leaves of Cabbage head as they are usually bitter and discolored. Cut in half.
❷ Cut head into quarters and cut out core. ❸ Slice into 1/4-inch slices and let sit for 5 minutes.

these methods will cause it to dry up and shrivel. I also don't recommend cooking Cabbage in oil because high temperature heat can damage delicate oils and create harmful free radicals.

## How to Prevent Strong Smells from Forming

Cutting Cabbage thin (1/4-inch) slices and cooking it *al denté* for only 5 minutes is my secret for preventing the formation of smelly compounds often associated with cooking Cabbage. When I cook my Cabbage, it never develops a strong smell. After 5 minutes of cooking, the texture of Cabbage, like all other cruciferous vegetables, begins to change, becoming increasingly soft and mushy. At this point, it also starts to lose more and more of its chlorophyll, causing its bright green or purple color to fade and a brownish hue to appear. This is a sign that

magnesium has been lost. This is when it starts to release hydrogen sulfide, the cause of the "rotten egg smell," which also affects the flavor. After 7 minutes of cooking, Cabbage develops a more intense flavor, with the amount of strong smelling hydrogen sulfide doubling in quantity.

While it is important not to overcook Cabbage, cooking for less than 5 minutes is also not recommended because it takes about 5 minutes to soften its fibers and help increase its digestibility.

## Healthy Cooking Tips

Pots containing iron, tin and non-anodized aluminum turn the chlorophyll in Cabbage from green to brown. Pots containing copper preserve the vivid green, but copper can leach into food, and too much copper in the diet is not advisable. I recommend cookware lined with stainless steel.

Use only stainless steel knives when cutting Cabbage; a knife made from carbon steel will discolor your Cabbage.

## Baby Bok Choy

You do not need to separate leaves and stems. Slice 1/2-inch thick. "Healthy Sauté" for 3 minutes.

## Chinese (or Napa) Cabbage

Chinese (Napa) Cabbage has a crisp, crunchy texture with a slightly sweet flavor and is best used in salads.

*(Continued on Page 227)*

### COMPARING THE NUTRITIONAL VALUE OF CABBAGE VARIETIES

|  | GREEN | RED | SAVOY | NAPA | BOK CHOY |
|---|---|---|---|---|---|
| Vitamin C | 38% DV | 66% DV | 36% DV | 43% DV | 53% DV |
| Folate | 8% DV | 4% DV | 14% DV | 15% DV | 11% DV |
| Fiber | 6% DV | 6% DV | 9% DV | 9% DV | 3% DV |
| Vitamin A | 2% DV | 1% DV | 14% DV | 18% DV | 42% DV |
| Calcium | 33 mg | 3 mg | 25 mg | 59 mg | 74 mg |
| Beta-Carotene | 55 mcg | 16 mcg | 420 mcg | 547 mcg | 1250 mcg |

*All quantities and % daily values (DV) are based on 1 cup of raw shredded Cabbage.

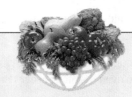

# how to enjoy fresh cabbage without cooking

**Mayonnaise-Free Coleslaw:** Shred half of a medium head of Red or Green Cabbage and 2 carrots in a food processor. In a large bowl, mix together with 2 TBS vinegar, 4 TBS extra virgin olive oil, sea salt to taste and 1 TBS chopped fresh dill. Sprinkle with diced scallions and caraway seeds to make a great alternative to the usual coleslaw made with mayonnaise.

**Marinated Cabbage Salad:** Green Cabbage makes a delicious salad. Shred 1/2 of a medium head of Cabbage and 1 medium carrot. Dress with 3 TBS extra virgin olive oil, 2 TBS rice vinegar, 1/2 cup chopped cilantro, 1 TBS sesame seeds, sea salt and a touch of honey. Let marinate for 1/2 hour in refrigerator.

**Cabbage Spring Roll:** Napa Cabbage leaves make a great spring roll wrapper! First make a sauce by combining 1 TBS peanut or almond butter, 1 tsp honey or maple syrup, 1 tsp tamari (soy sauce), 1 tsp lemon juice and a dash of cayenne in a small bowl. Spread on 2 large Napa Cabbage leaves. Add shredded carrots, thinly sliced cucumbers, cubed avocados and sprouts. Roll as a wrap.

**Chinese Cabbage Salad:** Dress 4 cups thinly sliced Napa Cabbage with 3 TBS extra virgin olive oil, 2 TBS rice vinegar, 1 tsp tamari, 1 TBS minced fresh ginger, 1 medium clove garlic (pressed) and 2 TBS chopped cilantro. For Chinese Chicken Salad, add cooked chicken pieces.

Use finely grated Cabbage on tacos in place of lettuce.

STEP-BY-STEP RECIPE
## The Healthiest Way of Cooking Cabbage

# 5-Minute "Healthy Sautéed" Red Cabbage

*Even if sautéing is not the way you would usually prepare Cabbage, I suggest you try it. It is fun to "Healthy Sauté" Cabbage, and I think you will be wonderfully surprised by the extra flavor. The easy to prepare Mediterranean Dressing will enhance its rich sweet flavor.*

**1 small head of Red Cabbage**
**5 TBS low-sodium chicken or
    vegetable broth**

**Mediterranean Dressing:**
**3 TBS extra virgin olive oil**
**1 TBS + 1 TBS lemon juice**
**1 medium clove garlic**
**Sea salt and pepper to taste**

1. Quarter Cabbage, slice into 1/4-inch strips and let sit as directed under the *How to Bring out the Hidden Health Benefits of Cabbage*. You should have approximately 4 cups of sliced Red Cabbage.

2. Chop or press garlic and let sit for at least 5 minutes. (Why?, see page 261.)

3. Sprinkle Cabbage with 1 TBS lemon juice before cooking to prevent it from turning blue.

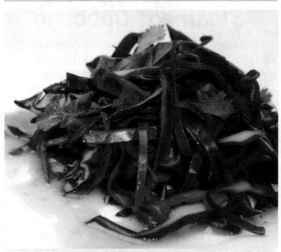
"Healthy Sautéed" Red Cabbage

4. Heat 5 TBS broth over medium heat in a stainless steel skillet. When broth begins to steam, add Cabbage and **cover**. For *al denté* Red Cabbage, cook for no more than 5 minutes. (For information on *Differences in Cooking Time*, see page 94.)

5. Transfer to a bowl. For more flavor, toss Cabbage with the remaining ingredients while it is still hot. (Mediterranean Dressing does not need to be made separately.) Research shows that carotenoids found in foods are best absorbed when consumed with oils.

OPTIONAL: To mellow the flavor of garlic, add garlic to Cabbage for the last 2 minutes of sautéing.

**SERVES 4**

---

## Flavor Tips:  Try these 3 great serving suggestions with the recipe above.

1. **Most Popular:** Prepare 5-Minute "Healthy Sautéed Red Cabbage and add grated ginger, rice or cider vinegar, tamari (soy sauce) and sesame seeds or toasted sunflower seeds.

2. Add goat cheese or feta cheese to cooked Cabbage.

3. **Caraway Cabbage:** Place 5-Minute "Healthy Sautéed" Red Cabbage recipe in a large bowl with 1 tsp caraway seeds and 1 TBS Dijon mustard. Stir until well coated.

**ADDITIONAL WAYS TO COOK CABBAGE:**

**Easy Spicy Burrito:** Lightly steam whole Cabbage leaves for 2 minutes. Stuff with black beans, rice, chopped cilantro, and salt and pepper to taste. Place on a dish and cover with spicy salsa.

**Stuffed Cabbage Leaves:**  Lightly steam whole Cabbage leaves and stuff them with your favorite rice and vegetable mixture. Top with ready-made tomato sauce and grated Parmesan cheese. Place under broiler for 5 minutes.

---

Please write (address on back cover flap) or e-mail me at info@whfoods.org with your personal ideas for preparing Cabbage, and I will share them with others through our website at www.whfoods.org.

## 5-Minute "Healthy Steamed" Cabbage

*When I was in Russia, I discovered that Cabbage was their most popular vegetable. If you are looking for the best flavor from Green or Savoy Cabbage, I recommend trying the "Healthy Steaming" method. It only takes 5 minutes and is a gentle, moist way of cooking Cabbage that enhances its flavor, brings out its color, keeps it tender and preserves most of its nutrients.*

**1 small head of Green or Savoy Cabbage**
**2-3 TBS extra virgin olive oil**
**1 TBS lemon juice**
**1 medium clove garlic**
**Sea salt and pepper, to taste**

1. Add 2 inches of water to the bottom of the steamer.

2. While steam is building up in steamer, slice Cabbage thin (1/4-inch) and let sit as directed under *How to Bring out the Hidden Health Benefits of Cabbage*. You should have about 4 cups of Cabbage.

3. Chop or press garlic and let sit for at least 5 minutes. (Why?, see page 261.)

4. When water is at a full boil, add Cabbage to steamer and **cover**.

5. Cook Green or Savoy Cabbage for no more than 5 minutes for *al denté* Cabbage.

Dress with olive oil, lemon juice, garlic, and sea salt and pepper to taste. For added flavor, you may want to add more olive oil.

For fuller flavor, dress Cabbage while it is still hot, and cut into small pieces.

**SERVES 4**

## 5-Minute "Healthy Sautéed" Red Cabbage with Apples

*"Healthy Sautéing" Red Cabbage with apples for just 5 minutes will not only preserve many nutrients but adds great flavor to your Cabbage.*

**1 small head of Red Cabbage**
**1/2 Jonathan or Granny Smith apple, cored with skin on**
**5 TBS chicken or vegetable broth**
**1 tsp lemon juice**
**1 TBS apple cider vinegar**
**2 TBS honey**
**2-3 TBS extra virgin olive oil**
**Sea salt to taste**

1. Slice Cabbage thin (1/4-inch) and let sit as directed under the *How to Bring out the Hidden Health Benefits of Cabbage*. You should have about 4 cups of Cabbage. Sprinkle Red Cabbage with lemon juice before cooking to prevent it from turning blue.

2. Slice apple into 1/2-inch slices.

3. Heat 5 TBS broth in stainless steel skillet over medium heat.

4. When broth begins to steam, add Cabbage and apples, top with vinegar and honey. Mix, **cover** and cook for 5 minutes.

5. Dress with extra virgin olive oil and sea salt and cut Cabbage into small pieces.

**SERVES 4**

## 4-Minute "Healthy Sautéed" Bok Choy

*"Healthy Sauté" will concentrate both the flavor and nutrition of your Bok Choy.*

**1 medium bunch of Bok Choy**
**3 TBS low-sodium chicken or vegetable broth**
**2-3 TBS extra virgin olive oil**
**1 tsp lemon juice**
**1 medium clove garlic**
**Sea salt and pepper to taste**

1. Cut the leafy portion into 1/4-inch slices to ensure they cook *al denté*. Cut stems into 3/4-inch slices because if they are cut too thin, they will become watery. Let stems and leaves sit as directed under *How to Bring out the Hidden Health Benefits of Cabbage*.

2. Chop or press garlic, and let sit for at least 5 minutes. (Why?, see page 261.)

3. Heat 3 TBS broth over medium heat in a stainless steel skillet.

4. When broth begins to steam, add stems and cook **uncovered** for 1 minute. Add leaves, **cover** and continue cooking for 3 more minutes.

Stems will become creamy, and the leaves will develop a robust flavor. The outside will be tender while the inside will be crisp.

If stems become translucent or watery, you know you have overcooked them. For more enjoyment, you may want to add more olive oil.

For best flavor, dress Bok Choy while it is still hot.

**SERVES 2**

*(Continued from Page 224)*

## Red Cabbage

I highly recommend incorporating Red Cabbage into your "Healthiest Way of Eating." It has a deep full flavor and a brilliant color that reflects its concentration of health-promoting anthocyanin phytonutrients. Anthocyanins are red, blue and violet pigments that have potent antioxidant properties, which have been shown to protect against free-radical damage to cell structures and DNA.

### HOW TO KEEP CABBAGE RED

If you want to keep Red Cabbage red, add one teaspoon of lemon juice or vinegar per cup of cooking liquid, or cook the Cabbage with an apple to increase its acid content. If you are steaming or sautéing Red Cabbage, sprinkle it with lemon juice or vinegar before cooking. If you forget to do this, you can add the lemon juice or vinegar after cooking, and it will return to its red color. Don't forget that Red Cabbage may take a minute longer to cook than other varieties of Cabbage because it has a sturdier structure. But what's a minute when it comes to great flavor, color and nutrition?

### WHY RED CABBAGE CHANGES ITS COLOR WHEN IT IS COOKED

The different colors of the anthocyanin pigments reflect differences in pH. The red pigments are enhanced in the more acid environment of raw Red Cabbage. As Red Cabbage is cooked, the acids begin to evaporate, the pH increases, and the Cabbage becomes more alkaline. This results in the decline of red anthocyanin pigments and an increase in the blue and violet pigments.

## Enjoy Sauerkraut

Sauerkraut is fermented and can be eaten raw or lightly warmed. But please, don't cook sauerkraut. Cooking will destroy the friendly *lactobacilli* added during the fermentation process that transformed the Cabbage into sauerkraut. Called probiotics (meaning life-supporting), these *lactobacilli* are responsible for many of the important health benefits of sauerkraut: they help aid digestion, increase the availability of vitamins, produce a variety of enzymes beneficial to the body and promote the growth of healthy flora throughout the digestive tract.

The best sauerkraut is usually found in jars rather than in cans; look for jars that do not contain preservatives and are located in the refrigerated section of your market. If possible, purchase sauerkraut that is sold in bulk because it will not contain preservatives and is fresher than packaged varieties. You can rinse sauerkraut to help reduce its salt content.

## Serving Ideas from Mediterranean Countries

Traveling through the Mediterranean region, I found that Cabbage was prepared in many different ways:

In Spain, Cabbage is served with chestnuts.

In Italy, Cabbage leaves are stuffed with mozzarella cheese and cooked in tomato sauce.

In Greece, shredded Cabbage is flavored with yogurt and dill.

In France, Cabbage leaves are stuffed with rice, peas and tomatoes.

Here is a question I received from a reader of the whfoods.org website about Cabbage:

**Q** *I recently heard that Cabbage juice is very good for me. What can you tell me about this?*

**A** Cabbage juice has a long history of use for promoting wellness, and research has supported its effectiveness in the treatment of peptic ulcers. Human clinical trials conducted by Dr. Garnett Cheney at Stanford University's School of Medicine in 1952 demonstrated that fresh Cabbage juice (1 liter daily) is highly beneficial in healing peptic ulcers with measurable effects usually seen in less than 7 days. Attempting to explain why, researchers initially dubbed what was then a mysterious anti-ulcer. I would recommend that anyone thinking of using Cabbage juice therapeutically discuss it with his or her physician. You can juice either Green or Red Cabbage. To do so, just cut it into pieces small enough to fit into the feed of your juicer. Cabbage juice has a nice, sweet taste. As with all of my vegetables, I prefer to use organically grown Cabbage.

# health benefits of cabbage

## Promotes Optimal Health

Reviewing 94 studies that evaluated the relationship between *Brassica* vegetables and cancer, researchers found that in 67% of the case control studies, eating these vegetables was associated with a reduced risk of cancer. In 70% of the studies, Cabbage consumption was associated with a lower risk of cancer, especially of the lung, stomach and colon. Cabbage is an excellent source of vitamin C, an antioxidant that helps protect cells from harmful free radicals.

## Promotes Women's Health

Much research has focused on the beneficial phytonutrients in Cabbage, particularly its indole-3-carbinole (I3C) and sulforaphane. These compounds help activate and stabilize the body's antioxidant and detoxification mechanisms that dismantle and eliminate cancer-producing substances. I3C has been shown to improve estrogen detoxification and to reduce the incidence of breast cancer. In one small human study, researchers found that after I3C was given for 7 days, the rate at which estrogen was broken down through the liver's detoxification pathway increased nearly 50%. In addition, recent research is showing that it's not only how much estrogen a woman has that puts her at risk for breast cancer, but also how her estrogen is metabolized. The route of estrogen metabolism via 2-OH (2-hydroxylation), 4-OH or 16-OH pathways determines how active, and possibly mutagenic, a woman's estrogen actually is. I3C has been shown to promote the formation of the most benign estrogen metabolite, the 2-OH form.

A recent case control study confirmed that women who eat more *Brassica* family vegetables have a much lower risk of breast cancer. In this study in China (where *Brassica* vegetables such as Chinese Cabbage are frequently consumed), the women's urinary levels of isothiocyanates (a type of beneficial compound found in *Brassica* vegetables) directly correlated with their breast cancer risk. Those women with the highest isothiocyanate levels (i.e., those women consuming the most *Brassica* vegetables) had a 45% lower risk for breast cancer compared to those with the lowest levels of isothiocyanates.

This significant protective effect is not all that surprising considering that the isothiocyanates provided by *Brassica* vegetables, such as Cabbage, are capable of numerous breast cancer-inhibiting actions. These include activating liver enzymes that remove carcinogenic compounds from the body, inducing cancer cells to self-destruct and affecting the way that steroid hormones, such as estrogen, are metabolized as well as the way that estrogen receptors on cells respond to the hormone.

Sulforaphane, potentially by altering gene expression, increases the production of antioxidants and detoxification enzymes, both of which help eliminate carcinogenic compounds, thus preventing tumors. A recent laboratory study

## Nutritional Analysis of 1 cup of cooked shredded Cabbage:

| NUTRIENT | AMOUNT | % DAILY VALUE | NUTRIENT | AMOUNT | % DAILY VALUE |
|---|---|---|---|---|---|
| Calories | 33.00 | | Pantothenic Acid | 0.21 mg | 2.10 |
| Calories from Fat | 5.80 | | | | |
| Calories from Saturated Fat | 0.72 | | **Minerals** | | |
| Protein | 1.53 g | | Boron | — mcg | |
| Carbohydrates | 6.69 g | | Calcium | 46.50 mg | 4.65 |
| Dietary Fiber | 3.45 g | 13.80 | Chloride | — mg | |
| Soluble Fiber | 1.59 g | | Chromium | — mcg | — |
| Insoluble Fiber | 1.86 g | | Copper | 0.02 mg | 1.00 |
| Sugar - Total | 2.50 g | | Fluoride | — mg | — |
| Monosaccharides | — g | | Iodine | — mcg | — |
| Disaccharides | — g | | Iron | 0.26 mg | 1.44 |
| Other Carbs | 0.73 g | | Magnesium | 12.00 mg | 3.00 |
| Fat - Total | 0.65 g | | Manganese | 0.18 mg | 9.00 |
| Saturated Fat | 0.08 g | | Molybdenum | — mcg | — |
| Mono Fat | 0.04 g | | Phosphorus | 22.50 mg | 2.25 |
| Poly Fat | 0.29 g | | Potassium | 145.50 mg | |
| Omega-3 Fatty Acids | 0.17 g | 6.80 | Selenium | 0.90 mcg | 1.29 |
| Omega-6 Fatty Acids | 0.13 g | | Sodium | 12.00 mg | |
| Trans Fatty Acids | 0.00 g | | Zinc | 0.14 mg | 0.93 |
| Cholesterol | 0.00 mg | | | | |
| Water | 140.40 g | | **Amino Acids** | | |
| Ash | 0.73 g | | Alanine | 0.05 g | |
| | | | Arginine | 0.09 g | |
| **Vitamins** | | | Aspartate | 0.15 g | |
| Vitamin A IU | 198.00 IU | 3.96 | Cystine | 0.01 g | 2.44 |
| Vitamin A RE | 19.50 RE | | Glutamate | 0.34 g | |
| A - Carotenoid | 19.50 RE | 0.26 | Glycine | 0.03 g | |
| A - Retinol | 0.00 RE | | Histidine | 0.03 g | 2.33 |
| B1 Thiamin | 0.09 mg | 6.00 | Isoleucine | 0.08 g | 6.96 |
| B2 Riboflavin | 0.08 mg | 4.71 | Leucine | 0.08 g | 3.16 |
| B3 Niacin | 0.42 mg | 2.10 | Lysine | 0.07 g | 2.98 |
| Niacin Equiv | 0.67 mg | | Methionine | 0.01 g | 1.35 |
| Vitamin B6 | 0.17 mg | 8.50 | Phenylalanine | 0.05 g | 4.20 |
| Vitamin B12 | 0.00 mcg | 0.00 | Proline | 0.30 g | |
| Biotin | — mcg | — | Serine | 0.09 g | |
| Vitamin C | 30.15 mg | 50.25 | Threonine | 0.05 g | 4.03 |
| Vitamin D IU | 0.00 IU | 0.00 | Tryptophan | 0.01 g | 3.13 |
| Vitamin D mcg | 0.00 mcg | | Tyrosine | 0.03 g | 3.09 |
| Vitamin E Alpha Equiv | 0.16 mg | 0.80 | Valine | 0.06 g | 4.08 |
| Vitamin E IU | 0.23 IU | | | | |
| Vitamin E mg | 2.55 mg | | | | |
| Folate | 30.00 mcg | 7.50 | | | |
| Vitamin K | 73.35 mcg | 50.00 | | | |

(Note: "—" indicates data is unavailable. For more information, please see page 806.)

shows sulforaphane even helps stop the proliferation of breast cancer cells in the later stages of their growth.

## Promotes Digestive Health

Raw Cabbage juice is documented as being effective in treating peptic ulcers. In one study, 1 liter of the fresh juice per day, taken in divided doses, resulted in total ulcer healing in an average of 10 days. Cabbage's high content of glutamine, an amino acid that is the preferred fuel for the cells that line the stomach and small intestine, is likely the reason for Cabbage juice's efficacy in healing ulcers.

Additionally, *Brassica* vegetables like Cabbage may also provide protection from colon cancer. This may come not only from it being a very good source of dietary fiber but also from some of its unique phytonutrients. When Cabbage is cut, chewed or digested, a sulfur-containing compound called sinigrin is brought into contact with the enzyme *myrosinase*, resulting in the release of isothiocyanates. Isothiocyanates are not only potent inducers of the liver's Phase II enzymes, which detoxify carcinogens, but recent laboratory research suggests that they may be able to inhibit cell division of colon cancer cells.

## Additional Health-Promoting Benefits of Cabbage

Cabbage is also a concentrated source of many other nutrients providing additional health-promoting benefits. These nutrients include bone-building calcium, magnesium and manganese; heart-healthy folic acid, vitamin B6, omega-3 fatty acids, potassium and vitamin A; energy-producing vitamin B1 and vitamin B2; muscle-building protein; and sleep-promoting tryptophan. Since steamed Cabbage contains only 33 calories per one cup serving, it is an ideal food for healthy weight control.

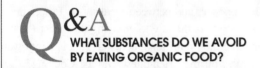

## Q&A
### WHAT SUBSTANCES DO WE AVOID BY EATING ORGANIC FOOD?

Over 3,000 high-risk toxins routinely present in the U.S. food supply are, by law, excluded from organic food, including:

**Pesticides:** By far the largest group of toxins to be largely prohibited from organically grown foods are synthetic pesticides, which are found virtually everywhere else in the food supply. Several hundred different chemicals and several thousand brand-name pesticide products are legally used in commercial food production under the U.S. Act of 1992; the Environmental Protection Agency has classified 73 pesticides authorized for agricultural use as potential carcinogens (cancer-causing agents). And pesticides don't just remain where they are applied. A 1996 study by the Environmental Working Group found 96% of all water samples taken from 748 towns across the U.S. contained the pesticide atrazine, and at least 20 different chemical pesticides are routinely present in municipal tap water across the U.S.

**Heavy metals:** The toxic metals cadmium, lead and mercury enter the food supply through industrial pollution of soil and groundwater and through machinery used in food processing and packaging. Cadmium, which can be concentrated in plant tissues at levels higher than those in soil, has been linked to lung, prostate and testicular cancers. Despite lead's long-recognized serious adverse impact on health, especially that of young children, lead solder is still used to seal tin cans, imparting the lead residues found in many canned foods. Even low levels of lead are harmful and are associated with decreased intelligence, impaired neurobehavioral development, decreased stature and growth, and impaired hearing. Mercury is toxic to brain cells and has been linked to autism and Alzheimer's disease.

**Solvents:** Used to dissolve food components and produce food additives, solvents are also virtually omnipresent in commercially processed food. Solvents, such as benzene and toluene, have been linked to numerous cancers. Benzene, specifically, has been repeatedly associated with rheumatoid arthritis—an auto-immune condition involving pain and degeneration in the joints that affects over 2 million adults in the U.S.

Not only are these toxic substances harmful singly, but when combined, as they are in commercially grown and processed food and in the human body where they accumulate, their effects have been found to be magnified as much as a 1,000-fold.

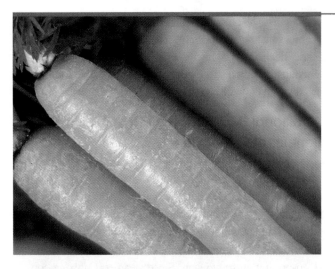

# carrots

## highlights

| | |
|---|---|
| AVAILABILITY: | Year-round |
| REFRIGERATE: | Yes |
| SHELF LIFE: | 2 weeks refrigerated |
| PREPARATION: | Minimal |
| BEST WAY TO COOK: | "Healthy Steamed" in just 5 minutes |

## nutrient-richness chart

Total Nutrient-Richness: **22**     GI: **66**

One cup (122 grams) of raw Carrots contains 52 calories

| NUTRIENT | AMOUNT | %DV | DENSITY | QUALITY |
|---|---|---|---|---|
| Vitamin A | 34317.4 IU | 686.3 | 235.5 | excellent |
| Vitamin K | 16.1 mcg | 20.1 | 6.9 | excellent |
| Vitamin C | 11.4 mg | 18.9 | 6.5 | very good |
| Dietary Fiber | 3.7 g | 14.6 | 5.0 | very good |
| Potassium | 394.1 mg | 11.3 | 3.9 | very good |
| B6 Pyridoxine | 0.2 mg | 9.0 | 3.1 | good |
| Manganese | 0.2 mg | 8.5 | 2.9 | good |
| Molybdenum | 6.1 mcg | 8.1 | 2.8 | good |
| B1 Thiamin | 0.1 mg | 8.0 | 2.7 | good |
| B3 Niacin | 1.1 mg | 5.6 | 1.9 | good |
| Phosphorus | 53.7 mg | 5.4 | 1.8 | good |
| Magnesium | 18.3 mg | 4.6 | 1.6 | good |
| Folate | 17.1 mcg | 4.3 | 1.5 | good |

| CAROTENOIDS: | |
|---|---|
| Alpha-Carotene | 3,605.8 mcg |
| Beta-Carotene | 7,390.7 mcg |
| Beta-Cryptoxanthin | 99.8 mcg |
| Lutein+Zeaxanthin | 265.0 mcg |
| Lycopene | 2.6 mcg |

Daily values for these nutrients have not yet been established.

| FLAVONOIDS: | |
|---|---|
| Quercetin | 0.1 mg |

For more on "Total Nutrient-Richness," "%DV," "Density," and The World's Healthiest Foods "Quality" Rating System, see page 805.

For more on GI, see page 342.

The earliest ancestor of our modern day Carrots can be traced back to central Asia and the Middle East and was purple in color! It was not until pre-Hellenic times that

Carrots appeared in Afghanistan where they were cultivated and developed into an early version of the orange Carrots we are familiar with today. Regardless of their color, crunchy raw Carrots have long been a convenient and healthy appetizer and between-meal snack. Proper preparation of Carrots is the key to enjoying their best flavor and maximizing their nutritional benefits. That is why I want to share with you the "Healthiest Way of Cooking" Carrots *al denté* in just 5 minutes. Lightly cooking Carrots this way not only enhances their flavor but also increases their digestibility so that we are able to more readily absorb their many health-protective nutrients.

## why carrots should be part of your healthiest way of eating

Thanks to that Carrot-eating icon, Bugs Bunny, generations of American children have grown up with the knowledge that Carrots are good for health, and one look at Carrots' nutritional profile clearly shows you why.

Carrots are one of the richest vegetable sources of the pro-vitamin A carotenoids, including alpha- and beta-carotene, which can be converted into an active form of vitamin A, a nutrient that helps support vision health and boost the immune system. The carotenoids found in Carrots not only provide this vegetable's rich orange color, but its powerful antioxidant protection as well. Easy to carry and easy to pack, nutrient-rich Carrots are an ideal food to add to your "Healthiest Way of Eating" not only because they are high in nutrients, but also because they are low in calories: one cup of raw Carrots contains only 52 calories. (For more on the *Health Benefits of Carrots* and a complete analysis of their content of over 60 nutrients, see page 236.)

## varieties of carrots

Carrots (*Daucus carota*) belong to the *Umbelliferae* family, which includes parsnips, fennel, caraway, cumin and dill. Plants in this family produce umbrella-like flower clusters from which their name is derived. Carrot roots have a crunchy texture and a sweet, minty, aromatic taste. Carrot greens are fresh-tasting and slightly bitter.

There are over 100 different varieties of Carrots varying in size and color. Carrots can be as short as 2 inches in length or as long as 3 feet, ranging in diameter from 1/2-inch to over 2 inches. While we usually think of Carrots as being bright orange in color, there are varieties that come in other colors including white, yellow, red, and purple. Varieties of Carrots include:

### COMMON ORANGE CARROTS

Long, orange and cylindrical, this is the variety of Carrots you most commonly find in your local market and is the one featured in the photographs in this chapter. They can vary greatly in length and diameter.

### BABY CARROTS

Neither the "baby Carrots" found at farmer's markets nor the bags of "baby Carrots" in the supermarkets are actually baby Carrots. The variety found at farmer's markets and specialty shops are a variety of Carrot that is fully grown but very small in size. Those found at supermarkets are pieces of regular Carrots that are sculpted into their miniature size.

### BETA III

This variety has five times more beta-carotene than regular Carrots.

### MAROON CARROTS

Sweeter than regular Carrots, this variety has a maroon exterior and a bright orange interior.

### WHITE CARROTS

This variety is mildly flavored, thin and white in color with less beta-carotene than orange Carrots.

## the peak season

Although Carrots from California are available throughout the year, locally grown Carrots are harvested in the summer and fall. These are the months when their concentration of nutrients and flavor are highest, and their cost is at its lowest.

## biochemical considerations

Carrots are one of the foods most commonly associated with allergic reactions in individuals with latex allergies. (For more on *Latex Food Allergies,* see page 722.)

### Carotenodermia

This is a condition that results from excessive consumption of carotene-rich foods. It causes the skin in parts of the body to develop a yellow or orange cast. This yellowing of the skin is presumably related to carotenemia, excessive levels of carotene in the blood. The health impact of carotenemia is not well researched. Eating or juicing large quantities of foods rich in carotene, like Carrots, may over-tax the body's ability to convert carotenes to vitamin A; as the body slowly converts carotene to vitamin A, extra carotene is stored, usually in the palms, soles of the feet or behind the ears. If the cause of the carotenodermia is a result of eating excessively large quantities of foods like Carrots, the condition will usually disappear after reducing consumption. If the condition does not improve in two to three days, a health care practitioner should be consulted.

## 4 steps for the best tasting and most nutritious carrots

Turning Carrots into a flavorful dish with the most nutrients is simple if you just follow my 4 easy steps:

1. The Best Way to Select
2. The Best Way to Store
3. The Best Way to Prepare
4. The Healthiest Way of Cooking

# 1. the best way to select carrots

You can select the best tasting Carrots by looking for ones that are firm, relatively straight and bright in color. The depth of the orange coloration reflects the amount of carotenoids present. The sugar found in Carrots is concentrated in the core, so thicker Carrots, which generally have a larger core, will also tend to be sweeter. If the greens are still attached, be sure that they are brightly colored, feathery and not wilted. By selecting the best tasting Carrots, you will also enjoy Carrots with the highest nutritional value. As with all vegetables, I recommend selecting organically grown varieties whenever possible. (For more on *Organic Foods,* see page 113.)

Avoid purchasing Carrots that are excessively cracked or forked since most of the Carrot will end up being discarded and wasted. Limp or rubbery Carrots should also be avoided as these are indications that they are past their prime. When the greens have been removed, I also check the top of the Carrots for dark coloration, an indication that they are no longer fresh.

# 2. the best way to store carrots

Carrots will begin to sprout and become bitter if not stored properly. Since they can lose their flavor and up to 30% of some of their vitamins, make sure to store them properly if you are not going to consume them right after bringing them home from the market.

Carrots continue to respire even after they have been harvested; their respiration rate at room temperature (68°F/20°C) is 25 mg/kg/hr. Slowing down the respiration rate with proper storage is the key to extending their flavor and nutritional benefits. (For a *Comparison of Respiration Rates* for different vegetables, see page 91.)

### Carrots Will Remain Fresh for Up to 2 Weeks When Properly Stored

1.  Store Carrots in the refrigerator. The colder temperature will slow the respiration rate, helping to preserve their nutrients and keeping Carrots fresh for a longer period of time.

2.  Place Carrots in a plastic storage bag before refrigerating. I have found that it is best to wrap the bag tightly around the Carrots, squeezing out as much of the air from the bag as possible.

3.  Do not wash Carrots before refrigeration because exposure to water will encourage your Carrots to spoil.

4.  Store Carrots away from apples, pears and potatoes since the ethylene gas that these foods produce will cause the Carrots to become bitter.

# 3. the best way to prepare carrots

Whether you are going to enjoy Carrots raw or cooked, I want to share with you the best way to prepare Carrots. Properly cleaning and cutting Carrots helps to ensure that the Carrots you serve will have the best flavor and retain the greatest number of nutrients.

### Cleaning Carrots

Rinse Carrots under cold running water. To preserve nutrients, do not soak Carrots or their water-soluble nutrients will leach into the water. (For more on *Washing Vegetables*, see page 92.)

### Peeling and Cutting Carrots

Most Carrots require peeling because the skin is often bitter. It is not necessary to peel them if they are young and fresh; however, they should be well scrubbed.

Make sure you have a sharp knife when cutting Carrots. Ironically, it is easier to cut yourself when cutting through a Carrot with a dull knife. Cutting your Carrots into slices of equal thickness will help them to cook more evenly. Slicing them thinly will help them to cook more quickly. For *al denté* Carrots in 5 minutes, cut into 1/4-inch slices.

If Carrots are to be eaten raw, it is best to shred them for easier digestibility.

---

### An Easy Way to Prepare Carrots, Step-by-Step

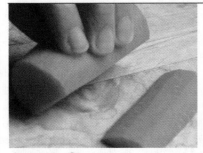 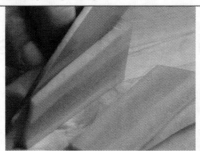 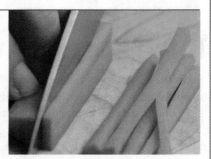

**JULIENNED CARROTS**

❶ Cut washed and peeled Carrots into 1–2 inch sections. Slice lengthwise on one side of the Carrot. Place cut side of Carrot down, so it doesn't roll when cutting. ❷ Cut Carrot into thin slices lengthwise. ❸ Stack a few slices on top of each other and slice again lengthwise. You will end up with thin matchsticks.

# 4. the healthiest way of cooking carrots

Since research has shown that important nutrients can be lost or destroyed by the way a food is cooked, the "Healthiest Way of Cooking" Carrots is focused on bringing out the their best flavor while maximizing their vitamins, minerals and powerful antioxidants.

## The Healthiest Way of Cooking Carrots: "Healthy Steaming" for just 5 Minutes

In my search to find the healthiest way to cook Carrots, I tested every possible cooking method and discovered that "Healthy Steaming" Carrots for just 5 minutes delivered the best results. "Healthy Steaming" provides the moisture necessary to make Carrots tender and bring out their peak flavor. That's when their color is at its brightest and they have retained the maximum amount of nutrients. The Step-by-Step Recipe will show you how easy it is to "Healthy Steam" Carrots. (For more on "*Healthy Steaming*," see page 58.)

## How to Avoid Overcooking Carrots: Cook them *Al Denté*

One of the primary reasons people do not enjoy cooked Carrots is because they are often overcooked. For the best flavor, I recommend that you cook Carrots *al denté*. Carrots cooked *al denté* are tender outside and slightly firm inside. Plus, Carrots cooked *al denté* are cooked just long enough to soften their cellulose and hemicellulose; this makes them easier to digest and allows their health-promoting nutrients to become more readily available for absorption. Remember that testing Carrots with a fork is an effective way to determine whether they are done.

Although Carrots are a hearty vegetable, it is very important not to overcook them. Carrots cooked for as little as a couple of minutes longer than *al denté* will begin to lose their texture and flavor. Overcooking Carrots will significantly decrease their nutritional value: as much as 50% of some nutrients can be lost. (For more on *Al Denté*, see page 92.)

## Cooking Methods Not Recommended for Carrots

### BOILING, ROASTING, GRILLING OR COOKING WITH OIL

I do not recommend boiling Carrots because boiling increases their water absorption, causing them to become soggy and lose much of their flavor along with many of their nutrients, including minerals, water-soluble vitamins (such as C and the B-complex vitamins) and health-promoting phytonutrients. Roasting Carrots makes them sweeter, but the longer cooking time also results in a greater loss of nutrients. Grilling Carrots will cause them to dry up and shrivel. I also don't recommend cooking Carrots in oil because high temperature heat can damage delicate oils and potentially create harmful free radicals.

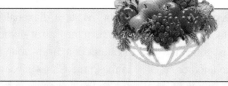

# how to enjoy fresh carrots without cooking

Raw Carrots are best to use in salads, as crudités for a healthy appetizer and as a between-meal snack.

**Mediterranean Carrot Salad:** Grate 3 medium Carrots and combine with 2 TBS minced parsley, 1 TBS extra virgin olive oil, 1 tsp lemon juice, 1 clove garlic, 1/3 cup raisins and sea salt to taste.

**Herbed Carrot Salad:** Grate 3 medium Carrots and 1 medium zucchini. Combine with 1/4 cup each sliced scallion, mint and cilantro. Toss with 2–3 TBS extra virgin olive oil and 2 tsp lemon juice. Add sea salt and pepper to taste.

**Tahini Carrot Salad:** In a small bowl, whisk 2 TBS each of tamari (soy sauce), tahini and lemon juice. Add water until the mixture is the consistency of heavy cream.

Grate 3–4 medium Carrots and place in a shallow serving dish. Pour the dressing over the Carrots and garnish with sesame seeds and minced cilantro or parsley. Serve with chicken or seafood (such as shrimp or scallops).

**Pickled Carrot Chips:** Cut 2 large Carrots into 1/8" slices cut on the diagonal. Place in bowl with 1 tsp sea salt and 1/2 cup water. Let sit for 2 hours. Drain. Add 1/2 cup vinegar, 1 tsp honey and 1 TBS fresh dill weed. Let sit for at least 2 hours. Keeps for 2 weeks in a glass jar in refrigerator. Drain to serve.

**Ginger Carrot Zinger:** Combine 1½ cups Carrot juice, 1/2 cup apple juice and 1 TBS grated ginger.

Here are questions I received from readers of the whfoods.org website about Carrots:

## Q Is it true that slightly cooked Carrots are better for you than raw Carrots?

A Cooking can make certain foods, such as Carrots, easier to digest for some people; yet, it can also reduce the amount of some of the nutrients that the food offers. Quickly cooking vegetables, such as Carrots, using the techniques that I focus on in this book, makes them more digestible but won't result in too much nutrient loss.

Yet, I would hesitate to say that cooked Carrots are better than raw since, for people who don't have any challenge digesting raw Carrots, the additional nutrients from raw Carrots would be beneficial. What I can definitely say is that lightly cooked Carrots (and all vegetables) are much better for you than Carrots (and all vegetables) cooked for a longer period of time, since cooking time is definitely related to nutrient loss.

By the way, studies have shown that carotenoids are better enhanced when carotenoid-rich foods are eaten in the presence of fat or oil. Therefore, to maximize the absorption of beta-carotene, alpha-carotene and other carotenoids in your Carrots, you may want to consider eating them with some nuts or a little flaxseed oil or olive oil dressing.

## Q How do I make "turned Carrots"? I have seen this term used in recipes and I am unsure how to prepare them.

A Here is how to cut turned Carrots: First peel and cut off ends of Carrot. Make a diagonal cut about 1/2-inch from tip of Carrot. Turn the Carrot so the diagonal cut is going the opposite direction from your knife and make another cut. Try to make the Carrot pieces a similar size. Turn the Carrot again so the diagonal cut is going the opposite way and cut again. As you approach the thicker part of the Carrot make cuts a little closer so you can still have similar size pieces.

## Q How do juice Carrots differ from regular Carrots?

A While some stores label some Carrots as "juice Carrots," in fact they are actually no different than regular Carrots, except that they are usually larger in size. Larger Carrots tend to be sweeter than smaller ones, which would be of benefit when making juice.

## Q Is there a significant difference in the nutritional value of regular Carrots vs. baby Carrots?

A Since the baby Carrots that we typically find at the market are nothing more than regular Carrots cut into small-sized pieces, ounce for ounce they should have the same nutritional profile as larger-sized Carrots. So that you can better estimate their nutrition, the weight of a cup of regular-sized Carrots is approximately the same as for 12 medium-sized baby Carrots.

## Q Can drinking Carrot juice turn the skin yellow or orange? A few months ago, I started drinking a lot of Carrot juice daily and have noticed that my skin, especially on the palms of my hands, has taken on a yellowish-orange coloration.

A You may be experiencing carotenodermia, a reversible condition that results from excessive consumption of carotene-rich foods such as Carrots and causes the skin to take on a yellow or orange hue.

It takes a good bit of carotenes (like beta-carotene) from food, however, and some time before you can see a skin change caused by diet. In studies on skin accumulation of beta-carotene, about 51 grams of beta-carotene per day are required, and up to two weeks before skin changes become visible. Since there are only 5–6 mg of beta-carotene in one carrot, we're talking about 9–10 carrots per day as the amount required, as evidenced in most studies, to see skin changes.

The impact of carotenemia, the excessive levels of carotenes in the bloodstream that causes carotenodermia, has not been well researched. Researchers suggest that the reason that the coloration occurs is that excess carotenoids may overtax the body's ability to convert it into vitamin A. The excess carotenes are stored in the body awaiting conversion and cause the Carrot-like coloration. The condition will usually disappear after a person reduces his or her intake of carotene-rich foods, so I suggest cutting back on your intake of Carrot juice and seeing if this does the trick.

STEP-BY-STEP RECIPE
## The Healthiest Way of Cooking Carrots

# 5-Minute "Healthy Steamed" Carrots

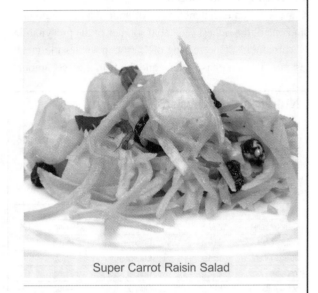
Super Carrot Raisin Salad

*Carrots don't need to take a long time to cook. By cutting them into 1/4-inch slices and "Healthy Steaming" them, they will be ready in only 5 minutes. The "Healthy Steaming" method is a gentle, moist way of preparing Carrots that enhances their flavor.*

**1 lb medium Carrots**
**3 TBS extra virgin olive oil**
**1 tsp lemon juice**
**Sea salt and pepper to taste**

1. Add 2 inches of water to the bottom of the steamer.

2. While steam is building up in steamer, cut Carrots into 1/4-inch slices. Carrots cut thicker will take longer to cook.

3. For *al denté* Carrots, steam **covered** for no more than 5 minutes. A fork will pierce them easily when they are done.

4. Transfer to a bowl. For more flavor, toss Carrots with the remaining ingredients while they are still hot. Research shows that carotenoids found in foods are best absorbed when consumed with oils.

**SERVES 2**

### COOKING TIPS:
- To prevent overcooking Carrots, I highly recommend using a timer.
- Testing Carrots with a fork is an effective way to determine whether they are done.

## Flavor Tips: Try these 4 great serving suggestions with the recipe above. ✳

1. **Most Popular: Honey Mustard Sauce**. Combine 1 TBS Dijon mustard, 2 tsp honey and 2 TBS of extra virgin olive oil. Drizzle over the 5-Minute "Healthy Steamed" Carrots recipe. Reduce amount of olive oil if desired.

2. **Orange Carrots:** Add zest and juice of 1 orange and 2 TBS fresh mint, basil or cilantro to 5-Minute "Healthy Steamed" Carrot recipe.

3. **Curried Carrot Salad**: Combine the 5-Minute "Healthy Steamed" Carrots recipe, 1 TBS capers, 1/2 minced red onion, 1 cup yogurt, 1 tsp curry, 1/2 tsp cumin, and red pepper flakes. Chill for a savory salad.

4. **Greek Carrots**: For a delicious side dish, toss the 5-Minute "Healthy Steamed" Carrots recipe with dill weed and crumbled feta cheese.

### ADDITIONAL IDEA FOR RAW CARROTS:
- **Super Carrot Raisin Salad:** Peel and shred 2–3 medium Carrots. Combine them with 1/2 cup raisins and 1/2 cup chopped fresh or canned pineapple (pictured above). Toss with "Healthy Vinaigrette" Dressing (see page 143).

Please write (address on back cover flap) or e-mail me at info@whfoods.org with your personal ideas for preparing Carrots, and I will share them with others through our website at www.whfoods.org.

# health benefits of carrots

## Promote Heart Health

Carrots are an excellent source of antioxidant compounds and one of the richest vegetable sources of the pro-vitamin A carotenoids. One serving of Carrots provides the greatest amount of alpha-carotene and the fifth greatest amount of beta-carotene compared to all of the other World's Healthiest Fruits and Vegetables. Just one cup provides a supply of carotenoids equal to roughly 680% of the DV for vitamin A.

The antioxidant compounds found in Carrots have numerous health benefits, including helping to protect against cardiovascular disease. A review of six epidemiological studies revealed that high-carotenoid diets are associated with a reduced risk of heart disease. In one study that examined the diets of more than a thousand individuals, those who had at least one serving of Carrots and/or squash each day had a 60% reduction in their risk of heart attacks compared to those who ate less than one serving of these carotenoid-rich foods per day. Carrots are also rich in other heart-healthy nutrients including vitamin C, dietary fiber, potassium, vitamin B6, niacin, magnesium and folate.

## Promote Lung Health

Vitamin A has long been known to be associated with healthy lungs. This is because it is needed to maintain the optimal structure and function of the tissues that line the lungs. Recent research has further explored the relationship between vitamin A, lung health and smoking. When experimental animals were fed a vitamin A-deficient diet, they were found to develop the lung condition emphysema. In addition, when animals were exposed to cigarette smoke, researchers found that the development of emphysema was related to a reduction in their body levels of vitamin A (it turns out that a common carcinogen in smoke, benzo(a)pyrene, causes vitamin A deficiency). In another study, smoke-exposed animals given a vitamin A-rich diet had less emphysema than those given the standard diet. This research highly suggests that vitamin A-rich foods, such as Carrots, are an important food to include in your diet if you are concerned about the health of your lungs, especially if you are a smoker or are exposed to second-hand smoke.

## Additional Health-Promoting Benefits of Carrots

Carrots are also a concentrated source of many other nutrients providing additional health-promoting benefits. These nutrients include bone-building vitamin K and phosphorus, free-radical-scavenging manganese, energy-producing vitamin B1, and sulfite-detoxifying molybdenum. Since Carrots are rich in fiber, which makes them filling, and contain only 52 calories per one cup serving, they are an ideal food for healthy weight control.

## Nutritional Analysis of 1 cup of raw Carrots:

| NUTRIENT | AMOUNT | % DAILY VALUE | NUTRIENT | AMOUNT | % DAILY VALUE |
|---|---|---|---|---|---|
| Calories | 52.46 | | Pantothenic Acid | 0.24 mg | 2.40 |
| Calories from Fat | 2.09 | | | | |
| Calories from Saturated Fat | 0.33 | | **Minerals** | | |
| Protein | 1.26 g | | Boron | 0.38 mcg | |
| Carbohydrates | 12.37 g | | Calcium | 32.94 mg | 3.29 |
| Dietary Fiber | 3.66 g | 14.64 | Chloride | — mg | |
| Soluble Fiber | 1.54 g | | Chromium | — mcg | — |
| Insoluble Fiber | 2.12 g | | Copper | 0.06 mg | 3.00 |
| Sugar – Total | 8.05 g | | Fluoride | — mg | — |
| Monosaccharides | 2.44 g | | Iodine | — mcg | — |
| Disaccharides | 4.39 g | | Iron | 0.61 mg | 3.39 |
| Other Carbs | 0.66 g | | Magnesium | 18.30 mg | 4.58 |
| Fat – Total | 0.23 g | | Manganese | 0.17 mg | 8.50 |
| Saturated Fat | 0.04 g | | Molybdenum | 6.10 mcg | 8.13 |
| Mono Fat | 0.01 g | | Phosphorus | 53.68 mg | 5.37 |
| Poly Fat | 0.09 g | | Potassium | 394.06 mg | |
| Omega-3 Fatty Acids | 0.01 g | 0.40 | Selenium | 1.34 mcg | 1.91 |
| Omega-6 Fatty Acids | 0.08 g | | Sodium | 42.70 mg | |
| Trans Fatty Acids | 0.00 g | | Zinc | 0.24 mg | 1.60 |
| Cholesterol | 0.00 mg | | | | |
| Water | 107.10 g | | **Amino Acids** | | |
| Ash | 1.06 g | | Alanine | 0.07 g | |
| | | | Arginine | 0.05 g | |
| **Vitamins** | | | Aspartate | 0.17 g | |
| Vitamin A IU | 34317.40 IU | 686.35 | Cystine | 0.01 g | 2.44 |
| Vitamin A RE | 3431.86 RE | | Glutamate | 0.25 g | |
| A - Carotenoid | 3431.86 RE | 45.76 | Glycine | 0.04 g | |
| A - Retinol | 0.00 RE | | Histidine | 0.02 g | 1.55 |
| B1 Thiamin | 0.12 mg | 8.00 | Isoleucine | 0.05 g | 4.35 |
| B2 Riboflavin | 0.07 mg | 4.12 | Leucine | 0.05 g | 1.98 |
| B3 Niacin | 1.13 mg | 5.65 | Lysine | 0.05 g | 2.13 |
| Niacin Equiv | 1.36 mg | | Methionine | 0.01 g | 1.35 |
| Vitamin B6 | 0.18 mg | 9.00 | Phenylalanine | 0.04 g | 3.36 |
| Vitamin B12 | 0.00 mcg | 0.00 | Proline | 0.04 g | |
| Biotin | 6.10 mcg | 2.03 | Serine | 0.04 g | |
| Vitamin C | 11.35 mg | 18.92 | Threonine | 0.05 g | 4.03 |
| Vitamin D IU | 0.00 IU | 0.00 | Tryptophan | 0.01 g | 3.13 |
| Vitamin D mcg | 0.00 mcg | | Tyrosine | 0.02 g | 2.06 |
| Vitamin E Alpha Equiv | 0.56 mg | 2.80 | Valine | 0.05 g | 3.40 |
| Vitamin E IU | 0.84 IU | | | | |
| Vitamin E mg | 0.73 mg | | | | |
| Folate | 17.08 mcg | 4.27 | | | |
| Vitamin K | 16.10 mcg | 20.10 | | | |

(Note: "–" indicates data is unavailable. For more information, please see page 806.)

(Continued from Page 153)
risk of developing hormone-dependent cancers such as those of the uterus and breast. I3C promotes the conversion of 2-OH and decreases the amount of 16-OH, which confers a decreased cancer risk.

There are now a few animal studies suggesting that I3C may play a role in cancer treatment as well. There is also some debate in the research as to a direct role in cancer prevention, because I3C seems to be quickly converted during the process of digestion to a doubled form of itself called diindolylmethane (DIM).

You'll see this debate in the world of dietary supplements, but not in the world of whole natural foods. Because in the food world, when we eat broccoli and cabbage and the other crucifers, we will be exposed to both sub-stances, both the I3C during digestion, and the DIM once our stomach acids create this substance from I3C.

Interestingly, the glucosinolates that provide us with both I3C and DIM were originally called "mustard oil glucosides" because of their discovery in mustard plants. Mustard seeds (which contain mustard oil) remain an excellent source of glucosinolates.

### Sulforaphane

Along with I3C, sulforaphane is one of the best-studied cancer preventive agents in the crucifers. This isothiocyanate, which seems particularly protective against stomach cancer, was first discovered in broccoli sprouts.

Sulforaphane is the compound that has recently been shown to help repair the skin damage that can be caused by excessive exposure to UV light and is likely to be protective against stomach ulcer, and perhaps stomach cancer as well.

Since sulforaphane is chemically derived from a glucosinolate (glucoraphanin), it is sometimes referred to as a glucosinolate as well as an isothiocyanate.

### Methyl Cysteine Sulfoxides

While given less attention in the popular press, these sulfur-containing compounds have been carefully studied in the cruciferous vegetables, particularly in the radishes.

These compounds appear to be created most extensively during the period of plant germination, so, like sulforaphane in broccoli sprouts, they seem to be most concentrated during the radish sprouting stage. Also like sulforaphane and I3C, their intake from food has been associated with cancer prevention and is a subject of much ongoing research interest.

### When It Comes to Cruciferous Vegetables, Where Should I Start?

One of the easiest, least expensive and most nutritious places to begin is with cabbage. This familiar crucifer is available in organic form in many supermarkets year-round, and when you purchase organic, you'll not only get all of cabbage's cancer-protective sulfur compounds, you'll get about 40% more vitamin C and increased amounts of other vitamins and minerals as well!

Whether it's Napa, Rainbow, Bozi cabbage in Asia, Galician cabbage in the Mediterranean, tender Savoy or just plain old "red" and "green" as many of us would describe what we see in the market, cabbage is universally available as a fresh cruciferous vegetable.

And recipes for this cancer-preventive food abound. In addition to dry krauts, sauerkrauts and slaws, cabbage is delicious in soups, healthy sautés and many "sweet and sour" dishes.

I also encourage you to treat cabbage as a "crucifer for all seasons." In the winter and cooler months, you can take advantage of its warmth in cabbage soups—a common practice especially in many Northern European countries. In the summer and warmer months, crisp, fresh cabbage can be used as the base for a cool, refreshing salad—such as Chinese Cabbage Salad (page 224).

From a nutritional standpoint, the beauty of taking a whole, natural food like cabbage (or any of the other cruciferous vegetables) is that it provides a full spectrum of nutrients. You don't have to worry about the difference between I3C and DIM. You can just enjoy the vibrant colors and rich flavors and be certain that your health is being optimally supported.

With the cruciferous vegetables, you also get the option of choosing from flowers and florets, leaves, stems, stalks and roots, giving you a potpourri of textures and also maximizing the dollar value of yourfood purchase.

Although research studies have confirmed the presence of sulfur-containing substances throughout these plants, you'll definitely want to follow my specific preparation instructions to get the maximum benefit from these sulfur compounds. The steps I take you through are extremely quick and simple, and don't require any unusual cookware or skills. (For details, see pages 222-227.)

You'll want to avoid overcooking any of the crucifers, but light cooking, especially my easy healthy sauté and steaming techniques, will work perfectly. As long as you remember to do a good job of chewing, these vegetables will also add excellent nutritional value to raw salads and make tasty stand-alone snacks. In every case, you'll be taking an important step toward your healthiest way of eating.

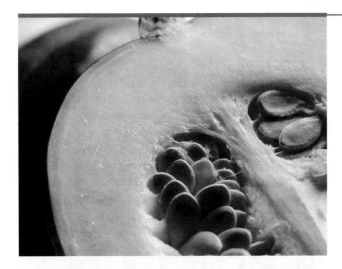

# winter squash

| | |
|---|---|
| AVAILABILITY: | Year-round |
| REFRIGERATE: | No |
| SHELF LIFE: | 3 to 4 weeks |
| PREPARATION: | Peel and cube |
| BEST WAY TO COOK: | "Healthy Steamed" in just 7 minutes |

## nutrient-richness chart

Total Nutrient-Richness: **20**  GI: **50**
One cup (205 grams) of baked Winter Squash contains 80 calories

| NUTRIENT | AMOUNT | %DV | DENSITY | QUALITY |
|---|---|---|---|---|
| Vitamin A | 7291.9 IU | 145.8 | 32.8 | excellent |
| Vitamin C | 19.7 mg | 32.8 | 7.4 | very good |
| Potassium | 895.9 mg | 25.6 | 5.8 | very good |
| Dietary Fiber | 5.7 g | 23.0 | 5.2 | very good |
| Manganese | 0.4 mg | 21.5 | 4.8 | very good |
| Folate | 57.4 mcg | 14.3 | 3.2 | good |
| Omega-3 Fatty Acids | 0.3 g | 13.6 | 3.1 | good |
| B1 Thiamin | 0.2 mg | 11.3 | 2.6 | good |
| Copper | 0.1 mg | 9.5 | 2.1 | good |
| Tryptophan | 0.03 g | 9.4 | 2.1 | good |
| Vitamin B6 | 0.2 mg | 7.5 | 1.7 | good |
| Pantothenic Acid | 0.7 mg | 7.2 | 1.6 | good |
| B3 Niacin | 1.4 mg | 7.2 | 1.6 | good |

**CAROTENOIDS:**

| | | |
|---|---|---|
| Alpha-Carotene | 2,316.0 mcg | Daily values for these nutrients have not yet been established. |
| Beta-Carotene | 9,368.0 mcg | |
| Beta-Cryptoxanthin | 6,388.0 mcg | |

For more on "Total Nutrient-Richness," "%DV," "Density," and
The World's Healthiest Foods "Quality" Rating System, see page 805.
For more on GI, see page 342.

Modern day Squash was developed from wild Squash that grew in an area between Guatemala and Mexico. The Native Americans held Winter Squash in such high regard that they buried it along with their dead to provide them nourishment on their final journey. Winter Squash was originally cultivated for its seeds because the fruit had little flesh and was very bitter, in contrast to the abundance of finely textured sweet flesh that we are familiar with today. Proper preparation of Winter Squash is the key to bringing out its best flavor and maximizing its nutritional benefits. That is why I want to share with you the secret of the "Healthiest Way of Cooking" Winter Squash, which takes only 7 minutes.

## why winter squash should be part of your healthiest way of eating

My regard for Winter Squash continues to grow as science discovers the increasing number of carotenoid phytonutrients (plant nutrients) it contains, which are not only responsible for its characteristic orange color, but many of its health-promoting benefits. These include alpha- and beta-carotene, known as "provitamin A" compounds because they can be converted into an active form of vitamin A. These carotenoid phytonutrients also function as powerful antioxidant and anti-inflammatory agents. Winter Squash is an ideal food to add to your "Healthiest Way of Eating" not only because it is high in nutrients but also because it is low in calories: one cup of cooked Winter Squash contains only 80 calories. (For more on the *Health Benefits of Winter Squash* and a complete analysis of its content of over 60 nutrients, see page 242.)

## varieties of winter squash

Winter Squash (*Cucurbita maxima*) is a member of the *Cucurbitaceae* family, a relative of both the melon and the cucumber, and comes in many different shapes and sizes. While the different varieties of Winter Squash are distinctive in both their appearance and flavor, they all share some common characteristics, including a hard protective skin that is difficult to pierce; this accounts for Winter Squash's long storage life of 3–4 weeks. They are also mildly sweet with finely textured flesh and a hollow inner cavity that contains seeds. Some of the more popular varieties include:

### BUTTERNUT SQUASH

Shaped like a large pear, this variety has cream-colored skin, deep orange-colored flesh and sweet flavor.

### ACORN SQUASH

With harvest-green skin speckled with orange patches and pale yellow-orange flesh, Acorn Squash has a unique flavor that is a combination of sweet, nutty and peppery.

### HUBBARD SQUASH

A large Squash that can be dark green, grey-blue or orange-red in color, Hubbard Squash is not as sweet as many other varieties of Winter Squash.

### TURBAN OR BUTTERCUP SQUASH

Green in color with speckles or stripes, Turban Squash has an orange-yellow flesh and a taste reminiscent of hazelnuts.

### KABOCHA

Kabocha is the generic named used for varieties of Japanese Winter Squash that are becoming increasingly available in markets throughout the United States. They have a taste similar to sweet potatoes and are richer, sweeter and creamier than other varieties of Winter Squash. Best of all, you don't have to remove the skin! It gets soft when cooked and tastes great. If you have not heard of Kabocha or have not tried this variety of Winter Squash, you are missing a special treat.

### SPAGHETTI SQUASH

Lightly sweet and yellow in color with a thin hard shell, this Winter Squash has an inside texture similar to strands of spaghetti.

### PUMPKINS

Ninety-nine percent of the Pumpkins marketed in the United States are used for Halloween jack-o-lanterns. The varieties used for this purpose are usually too stringy to eat. Sugar Pumpkins are a smaller variety that are sweeter and have close-grained flesh, which makes them a much better choice for cooking.

## the peak season

Although Winter Squash is available from August through March, its peak season is in the fall during the months of October and November. These are the months when its concentration of nutrients and flavor are highest and its cost is at its lowest.

## 4 steps to the best tasting and most nutritious winter squash

Turning Winter Squash into a flavorful dish with the most nutrients is simple if you just follow my 4 easy steps:

1. The Best Way to Select
2. The Best Way to Store
3. The Best Way to Prepare
4. The Healthiest Way of Cooking

# 1. the best way to select winter squash —

You can select the best tasting Winter Squash by looking for ones that are firm, heavy for their size and have dull (not glossy) rinds. By selecting the best tasting Winter Squash, you will also be enjoying Winter Squash with the highest nutritional value. As with all vegetables, I recommend selecting organically grown varieties whenever possible. (For more on *Organic Foods*, see page 113.)

Avoid Winter Squash with soft rinds, an indication that the Squash may be watery and lacking in flavor, and those that have water-soaked or moldy areas, which are signs of decay. Winter Squash spoils easily when damaged.

Here is a question I received from a reader of the whfoods.org website about Winter Squash:

**Q** *Do you lose a lot of nutrients when you cook Winter Squash in a microwave?*

**A** Loss of nutrients in the microwave depends on the same factors involved with loss of nutrients on the stovetop. To predict the nutrient loss, it's important to know answers to questions like: "Is the vegetable placed in water? How much water? To what temperature are the vegetable and water heated? For how long?"

I've seen studies showing minimal loss of nutrients from microwaved vegetables, and I've also seen studies showing substantial loss. In general, I much prefer stovetop steaming of Winter Squash to microwaving; it only takes 7 minutes if you cut it into cubes and therefore is a quick and easy way to prepare this great vegetable.

## 2. the best way to store winter squash

Winter Squash is a hearty vegetable and stores well. Winter Squash continues to respire even after it has been harvested. Slowing down the respiration rate with proper storage is the key to extending its flavor and nutritional benefits. (For a *Comparison of Respiration Rates* for different vegetables, see page 91.)

### Winter Squash Will Remain Fresh for Up to 3–4 Weeks When Properly Stored

The best way to store uncut Winter Squash is in a cool, dark place, away from heat and bright light. Winter Squash should not be subjected to extreme heat or extreme cold.

The ideal temperature for storing Winter Squash is between 50°F and 60°F (10°–16°C).

### How to Store Cut Winter Squash

Once it is cut, place Winter Squash in an airtight container or plastic storage bag with excess air removed, and store it in the crisper section of your refrigerator where the temperature ranges from 33°F–40°F (1°–4°C). This will limit its exposure to air flow, help reduce its respiration rate and retard spoilage; it also helps Winter Squash maintain its internal (cellular) moisture. Since the vitamin C content starts to quickly degrade once the Winter Squash has been cut, it is best to use the cut Squash within a couple of days.

## 3. the best way to prepare winter squash

Whether you are going to enjoy steaming or baking Winter Squash, I want to share with you the best ways to prepare it. Properly preparing Winter Squash helps to ensure that the Winter Squash you serve will have the best flavor and have retained the greatest number of nutrients.

### Cleaning Winter Squash

Rinse Winter Squash under cold running water before cutting. (For more on *Washing Vegetables*, see page 92.)

### Peeling Winter Squash

All varieties of Winter Squash require peeling for steaming except for Kabocha and Butternut Squash. You can peel Winter Squash with a potato peeler or a knife.

### Cubed Butternut Squash

Butternut Squash has a unique shape that requires a special approach to cutting. To cut into cubes, it is best to first cut it in half between the neck and bulb. This makes peeling it much easier. (For instructions on how to cube the neck portion of the Squash, see bottom of next page.) Cut bulb in half and scoop out seeds. Slice into 1-inch slices and make 1-inch cuts across slices for 1-inch cubes.

### Prepare Winter Squash for Baking

You don't have to peel Winter Squash when baking or slow roasting. Cut the ends off, cut the Squash in half lengthwise down the middle, scoop out the seeds and bake. Alternatively, you can leave the Squash whole, pierce a few times with a fork or tip of a paring knife, bake and scoop out the seeds after it has been cooked. You can peel cooked Squash easily with a knife and then cut into pieces of desired size.

## 4. the healthiest way of cooking winter squash

Since research has shown that important nutrients can be lost or destroyed by the way a food is cooked, the "Healthiest Way of Cooking" Winter Squash is focused on bringing out its best flavor while maximizing its vitamins, minerals and powerful antioxidants.

### The Healthiest Way of Cooking Winter Squash: "Healthy Steaming" for just 7 Minutes

In my search to find the healthiest way to cook Winter Squash, I tested every possible cooking method and discovered that "Healthy Steaming" all varieties of Winter Squash for just 7 minutes delivered the best result. "Healthy Steaming" provides the moisture necessary to make Winter Squash tender and brings out its peak flavor. While Winter Squash is a hearty vegetable, "Healthy Steaming" allows it to cook quickly, so you can enjoy it without spending too much time cooking it. "Healthy Steamed" Winter Squash is dense, firm and sweet, and has retained a maximum amount of nutrients. The Step-by-Step Recipe will show you how easy it is to "Healthy Steam" Winter Squash. (For more on "*Healthy Steaming*," see page 58.)

## How to Avoid Overcooking Winter Squash

One of the primary reasons Winter Squash loses its flavor is because it is overcooked. "Healthy Steamed" Winter Squash is tender, has the best flavor and is cooked just long enough to soften its cellulose and hemicellulose; this makes it easier to digest and allows its health-promoting nutrients to become more readily available for absorption. The shorter cooking time required for "Healthy Steamed" Winter Squash will help to keep its glycemic index low because less of the starches will have turned to sugar. Testing Winter Squash with a fork is an effective way to determine whether it is done.

## Cooking Methods Not Recommended for Winter Squash

### BOILING

I do not recommend boiling Winter Squash because boiling increases its water absorption and dilutes its flavor. It also causes the loss of many of its nutrients, including minerals, water-soluble vitamins (such as C and the B-complex vitamins) and health-promoting phytonutrients.

Here is a question I received from a reader of the whfoods.org website about Winter Squash:

## Q *Can I eat the skin of Winter Squash?*

A While from a nutritional perspective it's fine to eat the skin of Winter Squash, you may find that it is very tough and fibrous. Kabocha and Butternut Squash are the only ones I know of that have a skin enjoyable to eat. That being said, how you prepare the Squash may also have an effect on the edibility of the skin. Baking it for a long period of time may soften the outer skin enough to make it more palatable. If you are going to eat the skin, I'd strongly recommend selecting organic Squash, since the skin is the site of many potential toxic residues in the case of non-organically grown Squash. There are many nutrients in the skin of a Squash, including different types of fiber, some vitamins, some minerals and some phytonutrients.

---

### *Slow Baked Winter Squash*

*I have found that "Slow Baking" brings out the best flavor.*

1. Pierce the Squash near the stem with a knife to allow any steam to escape.

2. Place Squash in a shallow pan with a little water in the bottom to keep it from drying out and bake in a preheated 350°F (175°C) oven for about 50–60 minutes, until a knife can easily be inserted near the stem.

3. Cut Squash in half and scoop out seeds. Cut in half again (so Squash is quartered) and serve with the peel on.

- If you are short on time, you can "Slow Roast" Squash. To do so, cut squash in half, remove seeds, place the Squash (cut side down) in a baking dish and bake at 350°F (175°C) for 45 minutes.

- "Slow Roasting" Winter Squash will increase its glycemic index because starches turn into sugar.

- Seeds from all varieties of Winter Squash are edible after they have been roasted. (For more on *Roasting Seeds*, see page 508.)

---

### An Easy Way to Prepare Winter Squash, Step-by-Step

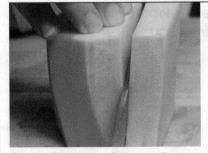 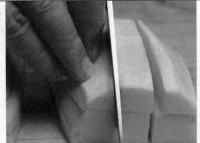 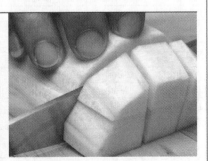

CUBED BUTTERNUT SQUASH (NECK PORTION)

❶ Follow the directions for peeling on previous page and cut neck in half. ❷ If you want 1-inch cubes, slice each half of the neck into 1-inch thick slices. Turn and make 1-inch cuts across the slices. ❸ Cut across strips for 1-inch cubes.

# health benefits of winter squash

## Promotes Heart Health

Winter Squash is one of the most concentrated vegetable sources of alpha-linolenic acid (ALA), an omega-3 essential fatty acid that is very good for heart health. Not only is it converted to EPA, the fatty acid concentrated in fish that has been found to lower triglycerides and prevent erratic heart rhythms, but recent research also suggests that dietary ALA itself reduces risk of cardiovascular disease.

Winter Squash's deep orange and yellow colors are a reflection of the carotenoid phytonutrients—alpha-carotene, beta-carotene, lutein, zeaxanthin and beta-cryptoxanthin—that it contains. In addition to being an excellent source of vitamin A through its concentration of pro-vitamin carotenoids, it is also a very good source of vitamin C. This antioxidant partnership benefits overall health, including heart health, since these nutrients can help to protect against the initiation of events that lead to atherosclerosis. Yet, its cardiovascular benefits don't stop there since Winter Squash is also a concentrated source of other nutrients that will help keep your circulatory system functioning at its best—it is a very good source of dietary fiber and potassium, and a good source of folate, vitamin B6 and niacin.

## Promotes Respiratory Health

Vitamin A is a very important nutrient for lung health since it is instrumental for the growth and development of the tissues that line this important organ. Recent research also suggests that vitamin A may play an important role in protecting the lungs from the damaging effects of smoking, as evidenced by laboratory animal studies that showed that smoking depletes vitamin A stores; animals with reduced vitamin A were more likely to develop emphysema. Additionally, certain types of Winter Squash—such as Pumpkin and Butternut—are concentrated sources of beta-cryptoxanthin, a very powerful carotenoid antioxidant found to be especially protective of lung health. A recent study just found that those who ate the most cryptoxanthin-rich foods had a significantly reduced risk of developing lung cancer.

## Additional Health-Promoting Benefits of Winter Squash

Winter Squash is also a rich source of other nutrients providing additional health-promoting benefits. These nutrients include free-radical-scavenging manganese and copper, energy-producing vitamins B1 and B5, and sleep-promoting tryptophan. Since Winter Squash contains only 80 calories per one cup serving, it is an ideal food for healthy weight control.

### Nutritional Analysis of 1 cup of Winter Squash:

| NUTRIENT | AMOUNT | % DAILY VALUE | NUTRIENT | AMOUNT | % DAILY VALUE |
|---|---|---|---|---|---|
| Calories | 79.95 | | Pantothenic Acid | 0.72 mg | 7.20 |
| Calories from Fat | 11.62 | | | | |
| Calories from Saturated Fat | 2.40 | | **Minerals** | | |
| Protein | 1.82 g | | Boron | — mcg | |
| Carbohydrates | 17.94 g | | Calcium | 28.70 mg | 2.87 |
| Dietary Fiber | 5.74 g | 22.96 | Chloride | — mg | |
| Soluble Fiber | 0.62 g | | Chromium | — mcg | — |
| Insoluble Fiber | 5.13 g | | Copper | 0.19 mg | 9.50 |
| Sugar – Total | 4.31 g | | Fluoride | — mg | — |
| Monosaccharides | — g | | Iodine | — mcg | — |
| Disaccharides | — g | | Iron | 0.68 mg | 3.78 |
| Other Carbs | 7.89 g | | Magnesium | 16.40 mg | 4.10 |
| Fat – Total | 1.29 g | | Manganese | 0.43 mg | 21.50 |
| Saturated Fat | 0.27 g | | Molybdenum | — mcg | — |
| Mono Fat | 0.10 g | | Phosphorus | 41.00 mg | 4.10 |
| Poly Fat | 0.54 g | | Potassium | 895.85 mg | |
| Omega-3 Fatty Acids | 0.34 g | 13.60 | Selenium | 0.82 mcg | 1.17 |
| Omega-6 Fatty Acids | 0.20 g | | Sodium | 2.05 mg | |
| Trans Fatty Acids | 0.00 g | | Zinc | 0.53 mg | 3.53 |
| Cholesterol | 0.00 mg | | | | |
| Water | 182.49 g | | **Amino Acids** | | |
| Ash | 1.48 g | | Alanine | 0.08 g | |
| | | | Arginine | 0.10 g | |
| **Vitamins** | | | Aspartate | 0.19 g | |
| Vitamin A IU | 7291.85 IU | 145.84 | Cystine | 0.02 g | 4.88 |
| Vitamin A RE | 729.80 RE | | Glutamate | 0.32 g | |
| A - Carotenoid | 729.80 RE | 9.73 | Glycine | 0.07 g | |
| A - Retinol | 0.00 RE | | Histidine | 0.03 g | 2.33 |
| B1 Thiamin | 0.17 mg | 11.33 | Isoleucine | 0.07 g | 6.09 |
| B2 Riboflavin | 0.05 mg | 2.94 | Leucine | 0.10 g | 3.95 |
| B3 Niacin | 1.44 mg | 7.20 | Lysine | 0.07 g | 2.98 |
| Niacin Equiv | 1.88 mg | | Methionine | 0.02 g | 2.70 |
| Vitamin B6 | 0.15 mg | 7.50 | Phenylalanine | 0.07 g | 5.88 |
| Vitamin B12 | 0.00 mcg | 0.00 | Proline | 0.07 g | |
| Biotin | — mcg | — | Serine | 0.07 g | |
| Vitamin C | 19.68 mg | 32.80 | Threonine | 0.06 g | 4.84 |
| Vitamin D IU | 0.00 IU | 0.00 | Tryptophan | 0.03 g | 9.38 |
| Vitamin D mcg | 0.00 mcg | | Tyrosine | 0.06 g | 6.19 |
| Vitamin E Alpha Equiv | 0.25 mg | 1.25 | Valine | 0.08 g | 5.44 |
| Vitamin E IU | 0.37 IU | | | | |
| Vitamin E mg | 0.25 mg | | | | |
| Folate | 57.40 mcg | 14.35 | | | |
| Vitamin K | — mcg | — | | | |

(Note: "–" indicates data is unavailable. For more information, please see page 806.)

STEP-BY-STEP RECIPE
## The Healthiest Way of Cooking Winter Squash

# 7-Minute "Healthy Steamed" Butternut Squash

*Whole Butternut Squash (or Kabocha or Hubbard) takes about one hour to cook, but I discovered that by cutting it into 1-inch cubes and using the "Healthy Steaming" method, it will cook in just 7 minutes. "Healthy Steamed" Butternut Squash also has the greatest number of nutrients.*

**2 cups Butternut Squash**
**3 TBS extra virgin olive oil**
**1 tsp lemon juice**
**Sea salt and pepper to taste**

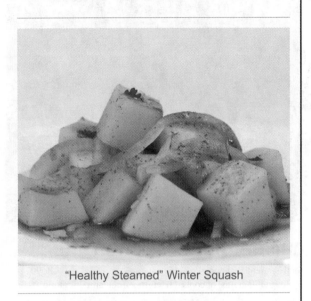
"Healthy Steamed" Winter Squash

1. Fill the bottom of the steamer with 2 inches of water.
2. While steam is building up in steamer, cut Butternut Squash into 1-inch cubes as described under *The Best to Way to Prepare Winter Squash*.
3. Steam **covered** for 7 minutes. Butternut Squash is done when it is tender, yet still firm enough to hold its shape. (For information on *Differences in Cooking Time*, see page 94.)
4. Transfer to a bowl. For more flavor, toss Butternut Squash with the oil, lemon juice, salt and pepper while it is still hot. Research shows that carotenoids found in foods are best absorbed when consumed with oils.

**SERVES 2**

**COOKING TIPS:**
• To prevent overcooking Winter Squash, I highly recommend using a timer.
• Testing Winter Squash with a fork is an effective way to determine whether it is done.

## Flavor Tips: Try these 5 great serving suggestions with the recipe above. ✳

1. **Most Popular:** Add crumbled feta and chopped fresh rosemary, sage or thyme to the 7-Minute "Healthy Steamed" Butternut Squash recipe.
2. **Pumpkin with Sea Vegetables:** Soak hijiki (sea vegetable, see page 311) for 10 minutes. Drain and combine in a large bowl with the 7-Minute "Healthy Steamed" Butternut Squash recipe (use sugar pumpkin (Kabocha) instead of butternut), 1/2 medium red onion sliced, 1 tsp tamari (soy sauce), 1 tsp ginger juice, a pinch of cayenne pepper and 1 TBS rice wine vinegar. The more ginger and cayenne, the spicier it will be. Delicious warm or cold as a salad.
3. Add 1 TBS honey and sprinkle with ground cinnamon and nutmeg.
4. **3-Minute Squash Soup:** Combine the 7-Minute Steamed Butter Squash recipe in a pan with 1 1/2 cups of chicken or vegetable broth, 3 TBS of canned premium coconut milk, 1 TBS chopped fresh ginger, 1 tsp turmeric and salt and pepper to taste. Bring it to boil. Transfer to a blender and blend for 1 minute.
5. **Mashed Butternut Squash:** Mash the 7-Minute "Healthy Steamed" Butternut Squash recipe and 2 cloves of pressed garlic with a potato masher, and serve in place of mashed potatoes. Alternatively, you can purée in a blender. Ginger or garam masala adds great flavor to mashed Butternut Squash.

Please write (address on back cover flap) or e-mail me at info@whfoods.org with your personal ideas for preparing Winter Squash, and I will share them with others through our website at www.whfoods.org

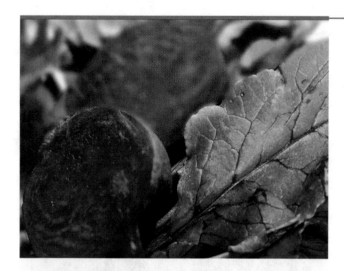

# beets and beet greens

| | |
|---|---|
| AVAILABILITY: | Year-round |
| REFRIGERATE: | Yes |
| SHELF LIFE: | 3 week refrigerated |
| PREPARATION: | Minimal |
| BEST WAY TO COOK: | "Healthy Steamed" in just 15 minutes |

## nutrient-richness chart

Total Nutrient-Richness: **15**   GI: **90**

One cup (170 grams) of cooked Beet (roots) contains 75 calories

| NUTRIENT | AMOUNT | %DV | DENSITY | QUALITY |
|---|---|---|---|---|
| Folate | 136.0 mcg | 34.0 | 8.2 | excellent |
| Manganese | 0.6 mg | 27.5 | 6.6 | very good |
| Potassium | 518.5 mg | 14.8 | 3.6 | very good |
| Dietary Fiber | 3.4 g | 13.6 | 3.3 | good |
| Vitamin C | 6.1 mg | 10.2 | 2.5 | good |
| Magnesium | 39.1 mg | 9.8 | 2.4 | good |
| Tryptophan | 0.03 g | 9.4 | 2.3 | good |
| Iron | 1.3 mg | 7.4 | 1.8 | good |
| Copper | 0.1 mg | 6.5 | 1.6 | good |
| Phosphorus | 64.6 mg | 6.5 | 1.6 | good |
| **CAROTENOIDS:** | | | Daily values for this nutrient have not yet been established. | |
| Beta-Carotene | 35.7 mcg | | | |

For more on "Total Nutrient-Richness," "%DV," "Density," and
The World's Healthiest Foods "Quality" Rating System, see page 805.

For more on GI, see page 342.

The ancient Romans were among the first to cultivate Beets for food, and the tribes that invaded Rome were responsible for introducing Beets throughout northern Europe, where they were used for animal fodder. However, it wasn't until the 16th century that Beets became popular for human consumption. Beets are a two-in-one vegetable as you can enjoy both their roots and leaves. (I will refer to Beet roots as Beets and the leaves as Beet Greens.) In fact, at one time, the Beet Greens were the preferred portion of the plant for consumption. This comes as no surprise since they are delicious, as well as nutritious, so I am always surprised when I see them discarded. Proper preparation of Beets is the key to enjoying their best flavor and maximizing their nutritional benefits. That is why I want to share with you

the secret of the "Healthiest Way of Cooking" them *al denté*. You can enjoy the creamy buttery texture of Beets by steaming or roasting.

## why beets should be part of your healthiest way of eating

Beets contain unique phytonutrient pigments. Betacyanin is the red pigment found in red Beets, and betaxanthin is the yellow pigment found in yellow Beets. Both of these pigments can provide powerful antioxidant protection. In a study comparing Beets to onions, celery, spinach, broccoli and carrots, they were found to have more polyphenolic content as well as higher antioxidant ability. Beets are also particularly rich in folate, a B vitamin important for a healthy heart and essential for normal tissue growth.

Beets are ideal to add to your "Healthiest Way of Eating" not only because they are high in nutrients, but also because they are low in calories: one cup of cooked Beets contains 75 calories. (For more on the *Health Benefits of Beets* and a complete analysis of their content of over 60 nutrients, see page 251.)

## varieties of beets

Beet consumption is thought to have originated in prehistoric times in North Africa, but wild Beets also grew along the Asian and European seashores. The sweet taste of Beets reflects their high sugar content, which makes them an important raw material in the production of refined sugar.

Beets come in a variety of colors including red, yellow and white speckled with pink. The three varieties below represent the bulk of Beets marketed today:

### TABLE BEETS

Table Beets come in red, yellow or a white/pink combination. This is the most popular variety of Beets and the ones most commonly found in local markets. Red Beets contain a health-promoting phytonutrient called betacyanin, which provides extra nutritional benefits not found in yellow or rainbow-colored Beets. This is the variety featured in the photographs in this chapter.

### SUGAR BEETS

Grown specifically for the production of refined sugar and alcohol, these large white Beets are not generally eaten as a vegetable. Their sugar content is more than twice that of red Beets (20% compared to 8% in red Beets), and they lack many of their nutritional benefits.

### MANGELWURZEL OR FODDER BEETS

A type of beet used for animal feed.

## the peak season

Although Beets are available throughout the year, their peak season runs June through October. These are the months when their concentration of nutrients and flavor are highest and their cost is at its lowest.

## biochemical considerations

Beets are a concentrated source of oxalates, which might be of concern to certain individuals. (For more on *Oxalates*, see page 725.)

### Beeturia

If you start to see red when you increase your consumption of Beets, don't be alarmed. You're just experiencing beeturia, or a red or pink color of your urine or stool. No need to panic; the condition is harmless.

## 4 steps for the best tasting and most nutritious beets

Turning Beets into a flavorful dish with the most nutrients is simple if you just follow my 4 easy steps:

1. The Best Way to Select
2. The Best Way to Store
3. The Best Way to Prepare
4. The Healthiest Way of Cooking

## 1. the best way to select beets

You can select the best tasting Beets by looking for medium-sized Beets with firm roots, smooth skin and deep color. By selecting the best tasting Beets, you will also be getting Beets with the highest nutritional value. As with all vegetables, I recommend selecting organically grown varieties of Beets whenever possible. (For more on *Organic Foods*, see page 113.)

Avoid Beets that have spots, bruises or soft, wet areas, all of which indicate spoilage. Shriveled or flabby Beets are aged, tough and fibrous.

## 2. the best way to store beets

Beets will become soft and lose their freshness if not stored properly. If you are not planning to use Beets immediately after bringing them home from the market, be sure to store them properly as they can lose up to 30% of some of their vitamins as well as much of their flavor.

Beets continue to respire even after they have been harvested; their respiration rate at room temperature (68°F/20°C) is 60 mg/kg/hr. Slowing down the respiration rate with proper storage is the key to extending their flavor and nutritional benefits. (For a *Comparison of Respiration Rates* for different vegetables, see page 91.)

### Beets Will Remain Fresh for Up to 3 Weeks When Properly Stored

1. Store fresh Beets in the refrigerator. The colder temperature will slow the respiration rate, helping to preserve their nutrients and keeping Beets fresh for a longer period of time.

2. Cut off the stems before storing Beets and then place Beets in a plastic storage bag before refrigerating. I have found that it is best to wrap the bag tightly around the Beets, squeezing out as much of the air from the bag as possible.

3. Do not wash Beets before refrigeration because exposure to water will encourage Beets to spoil.

# 3. the best way to prepare beets

Properly cleaning and cutting Beets will help to ensure that they have the best flavor and retain the greatest number of nutrients.

## Cleaning Beets

To minimize bleeding, wash Beets gently under cool running water, taking care not to tear the skin; the tough outer layer helps keep most of Beets' health-promoting pigments inside the vegetable. (See *Washing Vegetables*, page 92.)

## Peeling Beets

If you are going to roast or steam your Beets, it is best not to peel Beets until after they have been cooked. When bruised or pierced, Beets bleed, lose much of their vibrant color and turn a dull brownish-red.

Small, young Beets may be so tender after they are cooked that peeling may be unnecessary.

# 4. the healthiest way of cooking beets

Since research has shown that important nutrients can be lost or destroyed by the way a food is cooked, the "Healthiest Way of Cooking" Beets is focused on bringing out the their best flavor while maximizing their vitamins, minerals and powerful antioxidants.

## The Healthiest Way of Cooking Beets: "Healthy Steaming" for just 15 Minutes

In my search to find the healthiest way to cook Beets, I tested every possible cooking method and discovered that "Healthy Steaming" medium-size Beets (cut into pieces) for 15 minutes delivered the best result. "Healthy Steaming" makes Beets tender, brings out their rich flavor and maximizes their nutritional profile. The Step-by-Step Recipe will show you how easy it is to "Healthy Steam" Beets. (For more on "*Healthy Steaming*," see page 58.)

## How to Avoid Overcooking Beets

"Healthy Steamed" Beets are tender, have the best flavor and are cooked just long enough to soften their cellulose

and hemicellulose; this makes them easier to digest and allows their health-promoting nutrients to become more readily available for assimilation.

## Roasting Beets

Beets get sweeter and more creamy the longer they are cooked. To roast Beets, just wash and trim off the roots, cover and place in oven at 400°F (200°C) for 1 to 1 1/2 hours depending on their size. Never use aluminum foil. When cooked, rub with a paper towel to remove the skin.

## Healthy Cooking Tips for Beets

- Beet juice can stain your skin and nails. Wearing kitchen gloves is a good idea when handling Beets.

- If your hands become stained during the cleaning and cooking process, rubbing them a few times with some lemon juice will remove the stain.

- Another way to minimize your handling of the Beets is to peel cooked whole Beets while holding them with a fork.

*(Continued on Page 248)*

---

**An Easy Way to Prepare Beets, Step-By-Step**

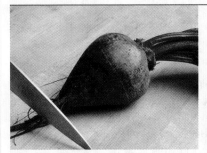 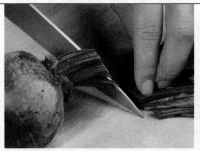 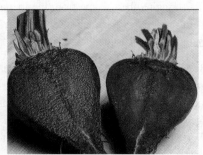

**PREPARE BEETS FOR STEAMING**
❶ Leave 1 inch of the tap root intact. ❷ Leave 1 inch of stems above the root. ❸ Cut Beets into pieces.

STEP-BY-STEP RECIPE
## The Healthiest Way of Cooking Beets

# 15-Minute "Healthy Steamed" Beets

*Boiling whole Beets takes from 1–2 hours, but I have discovered that by cutting them into quarters, they will be ready in a fraction of the time. The Mediterranean Dressing adds great flavor as well as extra nutrition.*

**1 lb medium size Beets**

**Mediterranean Dressing:**
**3 TBS extra virgin olive oil**
**2 tsp lemon juice**
**1 medium clove garlic**
**Sea salt and pepper to taste**

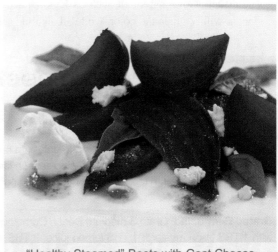

"Healthy Steamed" Beets with Goat Cheese

1. Fill the bottom of the steamer with 2 inches of water.

2. While the water is coming to a boil, chop or press garlic and let it sit for at least 5 minutes. (Why?, see page 261.)

2. Wash Beets, leaving 2 inches of tap root and 1 inch of the stem on the Beets. Cut Beets into quarters. Do not peel.

3. Steam **covered** for 15 minutes. Beets are cooked when you can easily insert a fork or the tip of a knife into the Beet. Although some of their colorful phytonutrients are lost to the steaming water, there is plenty of color and nutrients left in the Beets. (For information on *Differences in Cooking Time*, see page 94.)

4. Peel beets by setting them on a cutting board and rubbing skin off with a paper towel. Wearing kitchen gloves will help prevent staining your hands.

5. Transfer to a bowl. For more flavor, toss Beets with the remaining ingredients while they are still hot. (Mediterranean Dressing does not need to be made separately.) Research shows that carotenoids found in foods are best absorbed when consumed with oils.

OPTIONAL: To mellow the flavor of garlic, add garlic to Beets for the last 2 minutes of steaming.

**SERVES 2**

## COOKING TIPS:
- To prevent overcooking Beets, I highly recommend using a timer.
- Testing Beets with a fork is an effective way to determine whether they are done.

## Flavor Tips: Try these 7 great serving suggestions with the recipe above. ✱

1. **Most Popular:** Add 1 TBS balsamic vinegar to Mediterranean Dressing. Pour dressing over hot Beets and top with minced fresh basil and goat cheese (pictured above).

2. Top Beets with plain yogurt mixed with fresh or dried dill.

3. Serve Beets with "Healthy Sautéed" Fennel.

4. Serve Beets on a platter with cooked sliced eggs and thinly sliced red onion. Top with Mediterranean Dressing and fresh dill.

5. **Creamy Horseradish Beets:** Combine 1 tsp horseradish, 2 tsp honey, 1/2 cup plain low-fat yogurt and dill weed to taste in a mixing bowl. Add 15-Minute "Healthy Steamed" Beets recipe and toss lightly until Beets are coated with the sauce.

6. **Orange Spiced Beets:** Combine hot 15-Minute "Healthy Steamed" Beets recipe with the segments of 2 oranges, zest from 1 orange, 1 tsp fresh grated ginger, a pinch of cloves and 1 TBS honey.

7. **Mustard Beets:** Combine 1 TBS Dijon mustard, 2 tsp honey, 1/2 cup plain low-fat yogurt, 1 TBS fresh tarragon and sea salt and pepper to taste in a mixing bowl. Add 15-Minute "Healthy Steamed" Beets recipe and mix lightly until Beets are coated with sauce.

Please write (address on back cover flap) or e-mail me at info@whfoods.org with your personal ideas for preparing Beets, and I will share them with others through our website at www.whfoods.org.

*(Continued from Page 246)*

- The color of Beets can be modified during cooking. Adding an acidic ingredient such as lemon juice or vinegar will brighten the color, while an alkaline sub-stance such as baking soda will often cause them to turn a deeper purple. Salt will blunt Beets' color, so add it only at the end of cooking if desired.

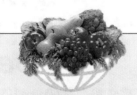

## how to enjoy fresh beets without cooking

It is best to grate Beets if you are going to eat them raw. It makes them easier to digest. For the sweetest flavor, peel before shredding. A food processor is a quick and easy way to grate Beets.

**Grated Beet Salad:** Grate 3 medium Beets. Combine with 1 TBS Dijon mustard, 1 TBS lemon juice, 3 TBS extra virgin olive oil and sea salt to taste. Place on a bed of fresh salad greens.

**Mediterranean Beets:** Grate 3 medium Beets. Place in a serving bowl and toss with 3 TBS extra virgin olive oil, 2 tsp lemon juice, 2 TBS mixed herbs (such as basil, oregano and rosemary), and sea salt and pepper to taste.

**Raw Borscht Soup:** In a blender, combine 1 peeled Beet cut into chunks, 1 cucumber cut into chunks (peel if skin is tough), 1 avocado cubed, 2 green onions sliced, juice of 1 lemon and a handful of dill. Add extra virgin olive oil, salt and pepper to taste. Blend until smooth. Add water to thin.

## *Marinated Beet Salad*

6 medium Beets, diced
1/2 medium onion, thinly sliced
1/2 cup water
1 TBS vinegar
1/4 cup walnuts, chopped
1 TBS parsley, chopped
1/2 cup extra virgin olive oil
1/4 cup cider vinegar
2 TBS Dijon mustard
2 TBS honey
1 tsp sea salt
1/2 tsp black pepper

1. "Healthy Steam" the diced Beets until tender. This will take about 15 minutes.
2. "Healthy Sauté" the thinly sliced onion in the water and vinegar for about 2 minutes.
3. Strain onion and place in a bowl with the beets. Toss with the chopped walnuts, chopped parsley, extra virgin olive oil, cider vinegar, Dijon mustard, honey, sea salt and black pepper.
4. Mix well.
5. Serve warm or chilled.

**SERVES 4–6**

Here are questions I received from readers of the whfoods.org website about Beets:

## Q Does canning affect the nutrient levels of vegetables?

A Vegetables are especially important sources of vitamins, minerals, and phytonutrients like carotenoids and flavonoids. In some cases, these particular nutrients can be very difficult to obtain from any other food group (except fruit). Vitamins and phytonutrients are especially susceptible to degradation from heat. This combination of vegetable's food group uniqueness and heat susceptibility makes the canning of vegetables a fairly high-risk process in terms of nourishment.

Because canning most often involves high heat, it can rob foods of vast amounts of nutrients. For example, in the process of canning mixed vegetables, the vitamin C loss can be as high as 67%. During the canning of tomato juice, up to 70% of the original folic acid can be lost

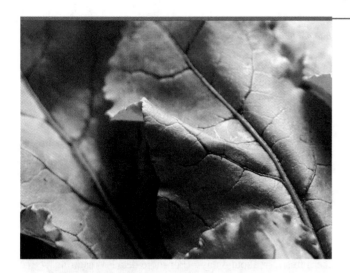

# beet greens

## highlights

| | |
|---|---|
| AVAILABILITY: | Year-round |
| REFRIGERATE: | Yes |
| SHELF LIFE: | 4 days refrigerated |
| PREPARATION: | Minimal |
| BEST WAY TO COOK: | "Quick Boil" in just 1 minute |

## nutrient-richness chart

Total Nutrient-Richness: **45**            GI: **15**

One cup (144 grams) of cooked Beet Greens contains 39 calories

| NUTRIENT | AMOUNT | %DV | DENSITY | QUALITY |
|---|---|---|---|---|
| Vitamin K | 697.0 | 871.3 | 402.1 | excellent |
| Vitamin A | 11022 | 149 | 67.7 | excellent |
| Vitamin C | 35.86 | 59.8 | 27.2 | excellent |
| Potassium | 1308.96 | 37.4 | 17 | excellent |
| Manganese | 0.74 | 37 | 16.8 | excellent |
| B2 Riboflavin | 0.42 | 24.7 | 11.2 | excellent |
| Magnesium | 97.92 | 24.5 | 11.1 | excellent |
| Copper | 0.36 | 18 | 8.2 | excellent |
| B1 Thiamin | 0.17 | 11 | 5 | excellent |
| Dietary Fiber | 4.18 | 16.7 | 8 | very good |
| Calcium | 164.2 | 16.4 | 7.4 | very good |
| Iron | 2.74 | 15.2 | 6.9 | very good |
| Pyridoxine B6 | 0.19 | 9.5 | 4.3 | very good |
| Phosphorus | 59.04 | 5.9 | 2.7 | good |
| Folate | 20.59 | 5.1 | 2.3 | good |
| Zinc | 0.72 | 4.8 | 2.2 | good |
| Pantothenic Acid | 0.47 | 4.7 | 2.1 | good |
| Niacin | 0.72 | 3.6 | 1.6 | good |

| CAROTENOIDS: | | |
|---|---|---|
| Alpha-Carotene | 5.6 mcg | Daily values for these nutrients have not yet been established. |
| Beta-Carotene | 6,609.6 mcg | |
| Lutein+Zeaxanthin | 2619.36 mcg | |

For more on "Total Nutrient-Richness," "%DV," "Density," and The World's Healthiest Foods "Quality" Rating System, see page 805.

For more on GI, see page 342.

Don't throw away the Beet Greens when preparing Beets—they are a rich source of nutrients. Beet Greens are similar in taste and texture to spinach and Swiss chard, which is not surprising since they belong to the same plant family.

## why beet greens should be part of your healthiest way of eating

Similar to spinach and Swiss chard, Beet Greens are an extremely nutritious vegetable. They are an excellent source of vitamins A and C, which provide powerful antioxidant protection from oxidative damage to cellular structures and DNA. They are also a rich source of lutein and zeaxanthin, carotenoid phytonutrients important for healthy vision. Beet Greens are an ideal food to add to your "Healthiest Way of Eating" not only because they are high in nutrients, but also because they are low in calories: one cup of cooked Beet Greens contains only 39 calories.

## varieties of beet greens

There are as many varieties of Beet Greens as there are Beets. (See "Varieties" of Beets on page 244.)

## the peak season

Beet Greens are available throughout the year; however, the peak of their season runs from June through October. These are the months when their concentration of nutrients and flavor are highest and their cost is at its lowest.

## biochemical considerations

Beet Greens are a concentrated source of oxalates, which might be of concern to certain individuals. (For more on *Oxalates*, see page 725.)

# 1. the best way to select beet greens

Beet Greens almost always come with the Beet roots; they are seldom sold separately. Although the quality of the greens does not reflect that of the roots, you can select the best tasting Beet Greens by looking for those that appear fresh, have a lively green color and are not limp. Be sure to enjoy this very nutritious part of the plant. As with all veg-etables, I recommend selecting organically grown varieties of Beet Greens whenever possible. (For more on *Organic Foods*, see page 113.)

Avoid Beet Greens that have turned yellow and are wilted as this is an indication that they have lost some nutritional value.

# 2. the best way to store beet greens

It is important to refrigerate Beet Greens. I have found that it is best to place Beet Greens in a plastic storage bag like those you get free in the vegetable section of your local market. (Beet Greens may be cut away from the roots or left attached.) Squeeze out as much of the air from the bag as possible by wrapping the bag tightly around the greens. This will help to extend the storage life of Beet Greens and keep them fresh for about 4 days. (For more details on storing, see *Spinach*, page 100.)

# 3. the best way to prepare beet greens

Rinse under cool running water. Prepare Beet Greens as you would Swiss chard by stacking the leaves and cutting them into 1-inch slices. Thin stems are sweet and tender and can be prepared with the leaves.

# 4. the healthiest way of cooking beet greens

### The Healthiest Way of Cooking Beet Greens: "Quick Boiling" for Just 1 Minute

"Quick Boiling" is the healthiest way to cook Beet Greens because it frees up some of the unwanted acids and allows them to leach out into the water. It takes only 1 minute to "Quick Boil" Beet Greens. While boiling is not considered the best way of cooking most vegetables, Beet Greens are one of only three vegetables I recommend boiling because of their acid content. The other two are Swiss chard and spinach. After boiling any of these three vegetables, be sure to discard the cooking water. Do not drink it or use it for stock because it will contain the unwanted acids leached from the vegetables. (For more on *"Quick Boiling,"* see page 61.)

Since Beet Greens can be prepared in the same way as spinach, refer to the Spinach chapter (page 98) for instructions and recipe.

Here are questions I received from readers of the whfoods.org website about Beets:

Q *Can you eat Beets raw?*

A You absolutely can eat Beets raw. Some ideas include adding julienned red Beets to a salad, adding shaved yellow Beets to coleslaw or making a "napoleon" of layered thinly sliced Beets goat cheese, chopped walnuts and chopped mint.

Q *Do "pickled" Beets still contain nutrients in them?*

A Pickled Beets provide some of the same nutritional benefits of raw Beets, including being a rich source of dietary fiber, folate, selenium and antioxidant phytonutrients such as betacyanins. For some people, the concern with pickled Beets would be that they oftentimes have a high sodium content.

# health benefits of beets and beet greens

## Promote Optimal Health

Beet roots contain a unique class of phytonutrients called betalains. Currently, betalains have only been identified in a few plant foods, and Beets are those that are the most commonly consumed. Betacyanin, a red pigment that is concentrated in red Beets, and betaxanthin, the yellow-orange pigment found in yellow Beets, are two examples of betalain phytonutrients that have been found to offer potent antioxidant protection.

These health-promoting phytonutrient pigments may be partially responsible for Beets' suggested role as a chemo-protective food. In one study, liver antioxidant enzymes increased in laboratory animals that were fed Beet fiber. Since these enzymes protect the liver from free radicals, they are thought to prevent the beginnings of cancerous activity. In another study, scientists noted that animals fed Beet fiber had an increase in their number of large intestine CD8 cells, special immune cells that detect and eliminate abnormal cells and protect animals against precancerous cellular abnormalities. In a human clinical trial, Beet juice was found to be a potent inhibitor of cell mutations that are normally caused by nitrosamines, metabolic byproducts of nitrates, which are chemical preservatives commonly used in processed meats.

It turns out that Beet Roots are not the only part of the plant offering protection against free-radical damage—Beet Greens also have amazing antioxidant potential. In one study that compared them to spinach, broccoli, carrots, onions and celery, Beet Greens were found to have the highest phenolic phytonutrient content as well as the greatest ability to absorb oxygen radicals (a marker of their antioxidant capacity).

## Promote Heart Health

Beets may be a great food when it comes to promoting heart health. Animals consuming diets high in Beet fiber were found to have 30% lower total cholesterol levels, 40% lower triglyceride levels and significantly increased HDL (beneficial cholesterol) levels. In addition to fiber, other heart-healthy nutrients concentrated in Beets include folate, potassium, magnesium and vitamin C. And owing to their antioxidant abilities, Beet phytonutrient pigments have been found to prevent the oxidation of LDL, which is one of the initiating steps in the development of atherosclerosis.

## Additional Health-Promoting Benefits of Beets

Beets are also a concentrated source of many other nutrients providing additional health-promoting benefits. These nutrients include free-radical-scavenging manganese and copper, energy-producing iron, bone-building phosphorus, and sleep-promoting tryptophan. Since Beets contain only 74 calories per one cup serving, and cooked Beet Greens contain only 39 calories per one cup serving, they are an ideal food for healthy weight control.

## Nutritional Analysis of 1 cup of cooked Beets:

| NUTRIENT | AMOUNT | % DAILY VALUE |
|---|---|---|
| Calories | 74.80 | |
| Calories from Fat | 2.75 | |
| Calories from Saturated Fat | 0.43 | |
| Protein | 2.86 g | |
| Carbohydrates | 16.93 g | |
| Dietary Fiber | 3.40 g | 13.60 |
| Soluble Fiber | 0.99 g | |
| Insoluble Fiber | 2.41 g | |
| Sugar – Total | 8.16 g | |
| Monosaccharides | — g | |
| Disaccharides | — g | |
| Other Carbs | 5.37 g | |
| Fat – Total | 0.31 g | |
| Saturated Fat | 0.05 g | |
| Mono Fat | 0.06 g | |
| Poly Fat | 0.11 g | |
| Omega-3 Fatty Acids | 0.01 g | 0.40 |
| Omega-6 Fatty Acids | 0.10 g | |
| Trans Fatty Acids | 0.00 g | |
| Cholesterol | 0.00 mg | |
| Water | 148.00 g | |
| Ash | 1.90 g | |
| **Vitamins** | | |
| Vitamin A IU | 59.50 IU | 1.19 |
| Vitamin A RE | 6.80 RE | |
| A - Carotenoid | 6.80 RE | 0.09 |
| A - Retinol | 0.00 RE | |
| B1 Thiamin | 0.05 mg | 3.33 |
| B2 Riboflavin | 0.07 mg | 4.12 |
| B3 Niacin | 0.56 mg | 2.80 |
| Niacin Equiv | 1.13 mg | |
| Vitamin B6 | 0.11 mg | 5.50 |
| Vitamin B12 | 0.00 mcg | 0.00 |
| Biotin | — mcg | — |
| Vitamin C | 6.12 mg | 10.20 |
| Vitamin D IU | 0.00 IU | 0.00 |
| Vitamin D mcg | 0.00 mcg | |
| Vitamin E Alpha Equiv | 0.51 mg | 2.55 |
| Vitamin E IU | 0.76 IU | |
| Vitamin E mg | 0.51 mg | |
| Folate | 136.00 mcg | 34.00 |
| Vitamin K | 0.34 mcg | 0.43 |

| NUTRIENT | AMOUNT | % DAILY VALUE |
|---|---|---|
| Pantothenic Acid | 0.25 mg | 2.50 |
| **Minerals** | | |
| Boron | — mcg | |
| Calcium | 27.20 mg | 2.72 |
| Chloride | — mg | |
| Chromium | — mcg | — |
| Copper | 0.13 mg | 6.50 |
| Fluoride | — mg | — |
| Iodine | — mcg | — |
| Iron | 1.34 mg | 7.44 |
| Magnesium | 39.10 mg | 9.78 |
| Manganese | 0.55 mg | 27.50 |
| Molybdenum | — mcg | — |
| Phosphorus | 64.60 mg | 6.46 |
| Potassium | 518.50 mg | |
| Selenium | 1.19 mcg | 1.70 |
| Sodium | 484.50 mg | |
| Zinc | 0.60 mg | 4.00 |
| **Amino Acids** | | |
| Alanine | 0.11 g | |
| Arginine | 0.07 g | |
| Aspartate | 0.21 g | |
| Cystine | 0.03 g | 7.32 |
| Glutamate | 0.76 g | |
| Glycine | 0.06 g | |
| Histidine | 0.04 g | 3.10 |
| Isoleucine | 0.09 g | 7.83 |
| Leucine | 0.12 g | 4.74 |
| Lysine | 0.10 g | 4.26 |
| Methionine | 0.03 g | 4.05 |
| Phenylalanine | 0.08 g | 6.72 |
| Proline | 0.07 g | |
| Serine | 0.11 g | |
| Threonine | 0.08 g | 6.45 |
| Tryptophan | 0.03 g | 9.38 |
| Tyrosine | 0.07 g | 7.22 |
| Valine | 0.10 g | 6.80 |

(Note: "—" indicates data is unavailable. For more information, please see page 806.)

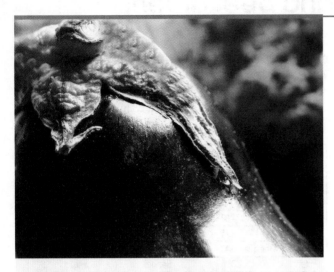

# eggplant

## highlights

| | |
|---|---|
| AVAILABILITY: | Year-round |
| REFRIGERATE: | Yes |
| SHELF LIFE: | 7 days refrigerated |
| PREPARATION: | Slice or cube |
| BEST WAY TO COOK: | "Healthy Sauté" in just 7 minutes |

## nutrient-richness chart

Total Nutrient-Richness: **15**  GI: **15**
One cup (99 grams) of cooked Eggplant contains 28 calories

| NUTRIENT | AMOUNT | %DV | DENSITY | QUALITY |
|---|---|---|---|---|
| Dietary Fiber | 2.5 g | 9.9 | 6.4 | very good |
| Potassium | 245.5 mg | 7.0 | 4.6 | very good |
| Manganese | 0.1 mg | 6.5 | 4.2 | very good |
| Copper | 0.1 mg | 5.5 | 3.6 | very good |
| B1 Thiamin | 0.1 mg | 5.3 | 3.5 | very good |
| B6 Pyridoxine | 0.1 mg | 4.5 | 2.9 | good |
| Folate | 14.3 mcg | 3.6 | 2.3 | good |
| Magnesium | 12.9 mg | 3.2 | 2.1 | good |
| Tryptophan | 0.01 g | 3.1 | 2.0 | good |
| B3 Niacin | 0.6 mg | 3.0 | 1.9 | good |

| CAROTENOIDS: | | Daily values for this nutrient have not yet been established. |
|---|---|---|
| Beta-Carotene | 21.8 mcg | |

For more on "Total Nutrient-Richness," "%DV," "Density," and
The World's Healthiest Foods "Quality" Rating System, see page 805.

For more on GI, see page 342.

E ggplant originally grew wild in India and was first culti-vated in China in the 5th century BC Although it has become an esteemed vegetable, especially in Mediterranean countries, Eggplant did not gain popularity until many centuries after its introduction to Europe because of its overly bitter taste. It was only after the development of new varieties in the 18th century that Eggplant lost both its bitter taste and bitter reputation. As with all vegetables, proper preparation of Eggplant is the key to bringing out its best flavor and maximizing its nutritional benefits. That is why I want to share with you the secret of the "Healthiest Way of Cooking"

Eggplant. In just 7 minutes, you will be able to enhance its flavor and enjoy its soft, creamy texture while maximizing its nutritional value.

## why eggplant should be part of your healthiest way of eating

In addition to the vitamins and minerals that it contains, Eggplant's health-promoting properties are also provided by an anthocyanin called nasunin; this phytonutrient provides protection from oxidative damage to cellular structures and also provides Eggplant with its deep rich color and distinctive flavor. Eggplant is an ideal food to add to your "Healthiest Way of Eating" because it is not only high in nutrients but is low in calories: one cup of cooked Eggplant contains only 28 calories. (For more on the *Health Benefits of Eggplant* and a complete analysis of its content of over 60 nutrients, see page 256.)

## varieties of eggplant

Eggplant (*Solanum melongena*) belongs to the nightshade family of vegetables, which also includes tomatoes, peppers and potatoes. While different varieties of Eggplant vary slightly in taste and texture, they can generally be described as having a pleasantly bitter taste and spongy texture. Its unique texture makes Eggplant a versatile vegetable that can be used in many different types of recipes. Eggplant is also available in a cornucopia of colors—ranging from lavender to jade green, orange, and yellow-white—and in a variety of shapes and sizes.

### AMERICAN EGGPLANT

This is the most popular variety of Eggplant in the United States, and the one featured in the photographs in this chapter. It is shaped like a cross between a pear and an egg, the characteristic form from which its name is derived. Its skin is glossy and deep purple in color, while its flesh is cream colored and spongy in consistency. Contained within the flesh are seeds arranged in a conical pattern.

### ITALIAN OR BABY EGGPLANT

A miniature variety of Eggplant that is deep purple and round or oval in shape.

### CHINESE EGGPLANT

A miniature variety of Eggplant that is slim and pale violet in color.

### ITALIAN ROSA BIANCOS

A miniature variety of Eggplant that ranges from violet to white in color.

### JAPANESE EGGPLANT

Longer and more slender than American Eggplant, it has a thinner skin and sweeter, more delicate flavor. It is most commonly purple but can range in color from lavender to pink, green and white.

## the peak season

Although Eggplant is available throughout the year, its peak season runs from August through October. These are the months when its concentration of nutrients and flavor are highest, and its cost is at its lowest.

## biochemical considerations

Eggplant is a concentrated source of oxalates and is also a member of the nightshade family of vegetables, which might be of concern to certain individuals. Conventionally grown Eggplants often have a wax coating to help protect their surface and increase their shelf life. (For more on: *Oxalates*, see page 725; *Nightshades*, see page 723; and *Wax Coatings*, see page 732.)

## 4 steps for the best tasting and most nutritious eggplant

Turning Eggplant into a flavorful dish with the most nutrients is simple if you just follow my 4 easy steps:

1. The Best Way to Select
2. The Best Way to Store
3. The Best Way to Prepare
4. The Healthiest Way of Cooking

# 1. the best way to select eggplant

You can select the best tasting Eggplant by looking for ones that are firm, feel heavy for their size and have smooth, shiny skin. There is usually a bright green stem and cap on one end of the Eggplant. Ripe Eggplants have the best flavor. I test Eggplants for ripeness by gently pressing the skin with the pad of my thumb. If it springs back, the Eggplant is ripe; if an indentation remains, it is not ripe. By selecting the best tasting Eggplant, you will also enjoy Eggplant with the highest nutritional value. As with all vegetables, I recommend selecting organically

grown varieties whenever possible. (For more on *Organic Foods*, see page 113.)

Conventionally grown Eggplants are often waxed to prevent moisture loss and increase their shelf life. Organically grown varieties allow you to enjoy the benefits found in the skin without concern about ingesting wax or any contaminants that might be trapped in the wax.

Avoid Eggplant that is shriveled, wrinkled, discolored, scarred or bruised. These are indications that the flesh beneath has become damaged or decayed.

# 2. the best way to store eggplant

Eggplant is a delicate vegetable and will become bitter and lose its freshness quickly if not stored properly and it can lose up to 30% of some of its vitamins.

Eggplant continues to respire even after it has been harvested. Slowing down the respiration rate with proper storage is the key to extending its flavor and nutritional

benefits. (For a *Comparison of Respiration Rates* for different vegetables, see page 91.)

### Eggplant Will Remain Fresh for Up to 7 Days When Properly Stored

1. Store Eggplant in the refrigerator. The colder temperature will slow the respiration rate, helping to preserve

vitamins and keeping Eggplant fresh for a longer period of time.

2. Place Eggplant in a plastic storage bag before refrigerating. I have found that it is best to wrap the bag tightly around the Eggplant, squeezing out as much of the air from the bag as possible.

3. Do not wash Eggplant before refrigeration because exposure to water will encourage Eggplant to spoil.

## How to Store Cut Eggplant

If you need to store Eggplant that has been cut, place it in a plastic bag or a container with a well-sealed lid and refrigerate. Eggplants start to quickly degrade once they have been cut, so it is best to use the remainder within a couple of days.

# 3. the best way to prepare eggplant

Properly cleaning and cutting Eggplant will help to ensure that it has the best flavor and retains the greatest number of nutrients.

## Cleaning Eggplant

Rinse under cold running water before cutting. (For more on *Washing Vegetables*, see page 92.)

## Peeling Eggplant

You do not need to peel Eggplant unless it is coated with wax. Organically grown varieties do not have a wax coating. If you want to peel Eggplant, use a vegetable peeler after cutting off the ends. Avoid peeling if possible since Eggplant's nasunin phytonutrient is found in its skin.

## Cutting Eggplant

Cut off ends and slice the remainder of the Eggplant into 1/2-inch slices. Cutting Eggplant into slices of equal thickness will help it to cook more evenly. Slicing it thin will help it to cook more quickly. It is good to brush the slices with a little lemon juice to keep them from turning brown when they are exposed to the air.

## How to Reduce Bitterness from Eggplant

After slicing the Eggplant and tossing with lemon juice, sprinkle with coarse salt (fine salt will make Eggplant too salty), and allow it to sit for about an hour to draw out excess moisture. This will also reduce bitterness. Rinse the slices to remove the excess salt. If you need to restrict sodium intake, alternative methods would be to soak the Eggplant in cool water for 10–15 minutes.

# 4. the healthiest way of cooking eggplant

Since research has shown that important nutrients can be lost or destroyed by the way a food is cooked, the "Healthiest Way of Cooking" Eggplant is focused on bringing out its best flavor while maximizing its vitamins, minerals and powerful antioxidants.

## The Healthiest Way of Cooking Eggplant: "Healthy Sauté" for just 7 Minutes

In my search to find the healthiest way to cook Eggplant, I tested every possible cooking method and discovered that "Healthy Sautéing" Eggplant for just 7 minutes retained

## An Easy Way to Prepare Eggplant, Step-By-Step

**SLICED EGGPLANT**
❶ Cut off top end of Eggplant. ❷ Turn Eggplant and cut off bottom end. ❸ Cut into 1/2-inch slices.

the best flavor and maximized its nutritional profile. The Step-by-Step Recipe will show you how easy it is to "Healthy Sauté" Eggplant. (For more on *"Healthy Sauté,"* see page 57.)

## How to Avoid Overcooking Eggplant

7-Minute "Healthy Sautéed" Eggplant is tender, has the best flavor and is cooked just long enough to soften its cellulose and hemicellulose; this makes it easier to digest and allows its health-promoting nutrients to become more readily available for absorption. It is important not to overcook Eggplant; overcooking Eggplant will significantly decrease its nutritional value (as much as 50% of some nutrients can be lost). Remember that testing Eggplant with a fork is not an effective way to determine whether it is done.

## Cooking Methods
## Not Recommended for Eggplant

STEAMING, BOILING, BROILING,
GRILLING OR COOKING WITH OIL

I do not recommend steaming or boiling Eggplant because these methods result in the Eggplant becoming soggy and losing much of its flavor along with many of its nutrients including minerals, water-soluble vitamins (such as C and the B-complex vitamins) and health-promoting phytonutrients. Broiling or grilling Eggplant will cause it to become dry and shriveled. I don't recommend cooking Eggplant in oil because high temperature heat can damage delicate oils and potentially create harmful free radicals.

According to an Australian study, Eggplant absorbs more fat in cooking than any other vegetable. When researchers deep-fried a serving of Eggplant, they found that it absorbed 83 grams of fat in just 70 seconds, four times as much as an equal portion of potatoes. That is yet another reason why the "Healthy Sauté" method of cooking is a great way to prepare Eggplant. You can enjoy the taste and health benefits of Eggplant without the use of oil.

Here are questions that I received from readers of the whfoods.org website about Eggplant:

## Q *Can you eat Eggplant raw?*

## A I have not seen any research showing that cooking is required to denature or remove any potential toxic substances in Eggplant. Like other nightshade vegetables, Eggplant contains alkaloid substances that are problematic for some individuals in terms of allergic-type reactions and

increased inflammatory response. Yet, I haven't seen any research showing differences in allergic response to cooked versus raw Eggplant. If you do consume raw Eggplant with the skin, I would highly recommend organically-grown Eggplant so that you will not be exposed to the pesticide residues found in conventionally grown Eggplant. If you want to eat raw eggplant, I would cut it into small pieces since it has a spongy texture.

## Q *What is nasunin and is Eggplant the only vegetable that contains it?*

## A Nasunin is a colorful pigment that is found in the skin of Eggplants. While I have yet to see a study positively identifying it in other foods, I would not be surprised if researchers find other foods that contain it. That's because nasunin is technically classified as an anthocyanin, a type of flavonoid pigment found in a variety of foods; this is why I would expect that there is nasunin in other fruits and vegetables. Yet, until that time, if you are looking to benefit from this powerful antioxidant, Eggplant would be your food of choice.

## Q *I eat more vegetables, and less fruit, than recommended. Should I eat fewer vegetables?*

## A No, you should not decrease your consumption of vegetables in order to eat more fruit! In fact, if I were absolutely forced to pick only one category of food, I would pick vegetables over fruit every time. Although both of these food groups contain some fantastic antioxidant nutrients, fibers, vitamin C and unique phytonutrients, you're not going to find significant protein, diverse mineral sources, diverse B vitamin sources, or many fat-soluble vitamin sources among the fruit. Alternatively, vegetables (as a group) can provide all of these nutrients in significant amounts. That being said, I would never want to choose only one of these food categories, because both can make such fantastic contributions to an optimal diet.

While fruits and vegetables contain some similar nutrients, there are ones found in each food group that are unique. Therefore, it would be optimal if you can find some fruits that you can enjoy. If you are generally healthy and are meeting your nutrient needs by your present day diet, then concerning yourself over a few daily servings of fruit while you are enjoying an abundance of vegetables may not be necessary; should you have more specific concerns about the details of your diet, we would suggest you consult with a licensed healthcare practitioner skilled in nutrition who can provide you with insights on how to best meet your individual dietary and health goals.

# health benefits of eggplant

## Promotes Heart Health

When rabbits with high cholesterol were given Eggplant juice, their blood cholesterol, the cholesterol in their artery walls and the cholesterol in their aortas (the aorta is the main artery that carries blood to the body) were significantly reduced; the walls of their blood vessels also relaxed, improving blood flow. These positive effects are supported by the many heart-healthy nutrients contained in Eggplant including dietary fiber, folate, vitamin B3, vitamin B6, magnesium and potassium. In addition, Eggplant contains many phytonutrients including nasunin, an anthocyanin phytonutrient found in its skin. Nasunin is a powerful free radical scavenger that has been shown to protect cells from oxidative damage.

## Promotes Central Nervous System Health

In animal studies, nasunin has been found to protect the lipids (fats) in brain cell membranes from oxidative damage. Cell membranes are almost entirely composed of lipids and are responsible for protecting the cell from free radicals, letting nutrients in and wastes out, and receiving instructions from messenger molecules that tell the cell which activities it should perform. If nasunin can protect brain cell membrane lipids, it may greatly help to preserve the structure and function of the brain. Eggplant may also benefit central nervous system health since it is a very good source of vitamin B1, which is an integral cofactor in the synthesis of acetylcholine, a neurotransmitter that is used by the nervous system to relay messages between the nerves and the muscles.

## Promotes Optimal Antioxidant Status

Part of nasunin's antioxidant activity may come from its being an iron chelator. Although iron is an essential nutrient and is necessary for oxygen transport, normal immune function and collagen synthesis, too much iron is not a good thing as it can increase the production of free radicals. By chelating iron, nasunin reduces free radical formation with numerous beneficial results, including protecting blood cholesterol from peroxidation, preventing cellular damage that can promote cancer and decreasing free-radical damage in joints, a primary factor in causing rheumatoid arthritis. In addition to its nasunin, Eggplant also contains other nutrients that help scavenge free radicals. It is a very good source of both manganese and copper, two minerals necessary for the function of the antioxidant enzyme *superoxide dismutase* (SOD).

## Additional Health-Promoting Benefits of Eggplant

Eggplant is also a concentrated source of other nutrients providing additional health-promoting benefits, including sleep-promoting tryptophan. Since Eggplant contains only 28 calories per one cup serving, it is an ideal food for healthy weight control.

### Nutritional Analysis of 1 cup of cooked Eggplant:

| NUTRIENT | AMOUNT | % DAILY VALUE | NUTRIENT | AMOUNT | % DAILY VALUE |
|---|---|---|---|---|---|
| Calories | 27.72 | | Pantothenic Acid | 0.07 mg | 0.70 |
| Calories from Fat | 2.05 | | | | |
| Calories from Saturated Fat | 0.39 | | **Minerals** | | |
| Protein | 0.82 g | | Boron | 0.19 mcg | |
| Carbohydrates | 6.57 g | | Calcium | 5.94 mg | 0.59 |
| Dietary Fiber | 2.48 g | 9.92 | Chloride | — mg | |
| Soluble Fiber | 0.40 g | | Chromium | — mcg | — |
| Insoluble Fiber | 2.08 g | | Copper | 0.11 mg | 5.50 |
| Sugar – Total | 4.10 g | | Fluoride | — mg | — |
| Monosaccharides | — g | | Iodine | — mcg | — |
| Disaccharides | — g | | Iron | 0.35 mg | 1.94 |
| Other Carbs | 0.00 g | | Magnesium | 12.87 mg | 3.22 |
| Fat – Total | 0.23 g | | Manganese | 0.13 mg | 6.50 |
| Saturated Fat | 0.04 g | | Molybdenum | — mcg | — |
| Mono Fat | 0.02 g | | Phosphorus | 21.78 mg | 2.18 |
| Poly Fat | 0.09 g | | Potassium | 245.52 mg | |
| Omega-3 Fatty Acids | 0.01 g | 0.40 | Selenium | 0.40 mcg | 0.57 |
| Omega-6 Fatty Acids | 0.08 g | | Sodium | 2.97 mg | |
| Trans Fatty Acids | 0.00 g | | Zinc | 0.15 mg | 1.00 |
| Cholesterol | 0.00 mg | | | | |
| Water | 90.85 g | | **Amino Acids** | | |
| Ash | 0.53 g | | Alanine | 0.04 g | |
| | | | Arginine | 0.05 g | |
| **Vitamins** | | | Aspartate | 0.13 g | |
| Vitamin A IU | 63.36 IU | 1.27 | Cystine | 0.00 g | 0.00 |
| Vitamin A RE | 5.94 RE | | Glutamate | 0.15 g | |
| A - Carotenoid | 5.94 RE | 0.08 | Glycine | 0.03 g | |
| A - Retinol | 0.00 RE | | Histidine | 0.02 g | 1.55 |
| B1 Thiamin | 0.08 mg | 5.33 | Isoleucine | 0.04 g | 3.48 |
| B2 Riboflavin | 0.02 mg | 1.18 | Leucine | 0.05 g | 1.98 |
| B3 Niacin | 0.59 mg | 2.95 | Lysine | 0.04 g | 1.70 |
| Niacin Equiv | 0.73 mg | | Methionine | 0.01 g | 1.35 |
| Vitamin B6 | 0.09 mg | 4.50 | Phenylalanine | 0.03 g | 2.52 |
| Vitamin B12 | 0.00 mcg | 0.00 | Proline | 0.03 g | |
| Biotin | — mcg | — | Serine | 0.03 g | |
| Vitamin C | 1.29 mg | 2.15 | Threonine | 0.03 g | 2.42 |
| Vitamin D IU | 0.00 IU | 0.00 | Tryptophan | 0.01 g | 3.13 |
| Vitamin D mcg | 0.00 mcg | | Tyrosine | 0.02 g | 2.06 |
| Vitamin E Alpha Equiv | 0.03 mg | 0.15 | Valine | 0.04 g | 2.72 |
| Vitamin E IU | 0.04 IU | | | | |
| Vitamin E mg | 0.03 mg | | | | |
| Folate | 14.26 mcg | 3.56 | | | |
| Vitamin K | — mcg | — | | | |

(Note: "—" indicates data is unavailable. For more information, please see page 806.)

## The Healthiest Way of Cooking Eggplant

# 7-Minute "Healthy Sautéed" Eggplant

*Eggplant can take a long time to cook, but I have found that it only takes minutes using the "Healthy Sauté" method. The Mediterranean Dressing will add even more flavor and extra nutrition to this dish.*

**1 medium Eggplant**
**3 TBS + 3 TBS low-sodium chicken or vegetable broth**

**Mediterranean Dressing:**
**3 TBS extra virgin olive oil**
**2 medium cloves garlic**
**2 tsp lemon juice**
**Sea salt and pepper to taste**

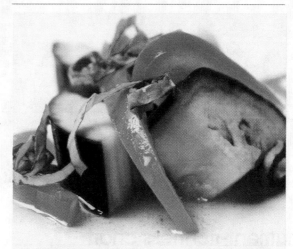

"Healthy Sautéed" Eggplant with Bell Peppers

1. Chop or press garlic and let it sit for at least 5 minutes. (Why?, see page 261.)
2. Heat 3 tablespoons broth over medium heat in a stainless steel skillet.
3. While broth is heating, cut whole Eggplant into 1/2-inch slices.
4. When broth begins to steam, add Eggplant slices, **cover** and sauté for 4 minutes. Turn Eggplant, add 3 TBS broth, reduce heat to low and sauté **uncovered** for 3 more minutes. This will result in tender, creamy, flavorful Eggplant slices. Eggplant has a texture that can substitute for meat if you want to make a recipe vegetarian. (For information on *Differences in Cooking Time*, see page 94.)
5. Transfer to a bowl. For more flavor, toss Eggplant with the remaining ingredients while it is still hot. (Mediterranean Dressing does not need to be made separately.) Research shows that carotenoids found in foods are best absorbed when consumed with oils.
OPTIONAL: To mellow the flavor of garlic, add garlic to Eggplant for the last 2 minutes of sautéing. You may need to add a little more liquid to prevent the garlic from sticking to the pan.

**SERVES 2**

## COOKING TIP:
- To prevent overcooking Eggplant, I highly recommend using a timer.

## Flavor Tips: Try these 7 great serving suggestions with the recipe above. ✳

1. **Most Popular:** After Eggplant is "Healthy Sautéed" for 4 minutes and turned, top with mozzarella cheese, a tomato slice and Parmesan and/or goat cheese. Continue cooking as directed.
2. Add a few drops of tamari (soy sauce) to mellow the taste of Eggplant. If you add tamari, you will want to reduce the amount of sea salt you use.
3. Add raisins and sliced onions while you are sautéing Eggplant. Garnish with chopped fresh parsley.
4. Add chopped fresh tomatoes, chopped black olives, minced basil and crumbled goat cheese to cooked Eggplant.
5. "Healthy Sauté" red bell peppers with your Eggplant (pictured above)—they cook in the same amount of time.
6. **Quick Eggplant Parmesan:** Combine 3–5 TBS extra virgin olive oil, 2 cloves minced garlic, 1/4 cup minced fresh basil and sea salt to taste in a small mixing bowl for a tasty basil sauce. "Healthy Sauté" Eggplant for 5 minutes. Top each slice of Eggplant with a thin slice of tomato and 1½ TBS low-fat ricotta cheese. Continue to sauté covered for 2 more minutes. Remove Eggplant from pan and arrange on a serving plate. Top each slice with 1 tsp basil sauce. Grate Parmesan cheese over it and serve.
7. **Eggplant Dip:** "Healthy Sauté" Eggplant and let cool. Purée in food processor or blender with 1–2 cloves garlic, 1 TBS tahini, 2 tsp lemon juice, sea salt to taste and 3 TBS extra virgin olive oil. Makes a great dip for vegetables or a spread for sandwiches.

Please write (address on back cover flap) or e-mail me at info@whfoods.org with your personal ideas for preparing Eggplant, and I will share them with others through our website at www.whfoods.org.

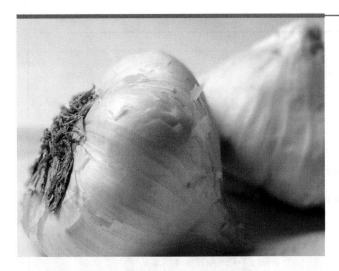

# garlic

highlights

| | |
|---|---|
| AVAILABILITY: | Year-round |
| REFRIGERATE: | Not recommended |
| SHELF LIFE: | Up to 1 month |
| PREPARATION: | Chop and let sit for 5 minutes |
| BEST WAY TO COOK: | Best as a seasoning |

## nutrient-richness chart

Total Nutrient-Richness: **15**          GI: **15**

One ounce (28 grams) of fresh Garlic (3 medium cloves) contains 42 calories

| NUTRIENT | AMOUNT | %DV | DENSITY | QUALITY |
|---|---|---|---|---|
| Manganese | 0.5 mg | 23.5 | 10.0 | excellent |
| B6 Pyridoxine | 0.4 mg | 17.5 | 7.5 | very good |
| Vitamin C | 8.9 mg | 14.8 | 6.3 | very good |
| Tryptophan | 0.02 g | 6.3 | 2.7 | good |
| Selenium | 4.0 mcg | 5.8 | 2.5 | good |
| Calcium | 51.3 mg | 5.1 | 2.2 | good |
| Phosphorus | 43.4 mg | 4.3 | 1.8 | good |
| Copper | 0.1 mg | 4.0 | 1.7 | good |
| B1 Thiamin | 0.1 mg | 4.0 | 1.7 | good |
| Protein | 1.8 g | 3.6 | 1.5 | good |

| CAROTENOIDS: | | Daily values for this nutrient have not yet been established. |
|---|---|---|
| Lutein+Zeaxanthin | 7.4 mcg | |

For more on "Total Nutrient-Richness," "%DV," "Density," and The World's Healthiest Foods "Quality" Rating System, see page 805.

For more on GI, see page 342.

The ancient Egyptians believed Garlic was not only bestowed with sacred qualities but enhanced the endurance and strength of the slaves that built the Pyramids. Throughout the millennia, Garlic has been used for both culinary and medicinal purposes. Its unique taste is like no other. It hits the palate with a hot pungency that is shadowed by a subtle background sweetness. Garlic is indispensable to almost all of the cuisines throughout the world and adds great flavor to your favorite savory dish. Its aroma fills the kitchen and adds both extra flavor and nutrition to your "Healthiest Way of Cooking."

## why garlic should be part of your healthiest way of eating

In addition to it being a rich source of many vitamins and minerals, garlic also contains unique sulfur compounds that contribute to its healthy benefits. One of its sulfur compounds is allicin, which promotes antioxidant activity and functions as a powerful antibacterial and antiviral agent that joins forces with vitamin C to help kill harmful microbes. And since it is also responsible for the strong smell of Garlic, you'll now appreciate its pungent smell as a reflection of its health-promoting properties! (For more on the *Health Benefits of Garlic* and a complete analysis of its content of over 60 nutrients, see page 265.)

## varieties of garlic

Garlic (*Allium sativum*) is native to central Asia and is one of the oldest cultivated plants in the world, dating back over 5,000 years. Although over 300 varieties of Garlic are grown worldwide, most Garlic consumed in the United States is either "early" or "late" Garlic and is grown in California, Mexico and Chile. A typical Garlic bulb is made up of 8–20 cloves. Garlic is classified under the following categories:

### SOFT NECK GARLIC

Sometimes called artichoke Garlic, this is the type most commonly found in your market. It stores well and does not have the strong pungent taste of Hard Neck Garlic. The variety of Soft Neck Garlic most commonly used in Garlic braids is called Silverskin.

### HARD NECK GARLIC

This type of Garlic has a thick, unbendable stem emerging from the center of the Garlic bulb and has a more complex and intense flavor than Soft Neck Garlic. There are several varieties of Hard Neck Garlic. The rich well-balanced flavor of Rocambole makes it one of the most popular with chefs. Garlic imported from Mexico has a reddish skin and sharp taste, while Purple-Stripe Garlic is a hard neck variety with rosy purple and white stripes on the skin. It is easy to confuse the large size and smaller number of cloves of Porcelain Garlic with Elephant Garlic; however, unlike Elephant Garlic, Porcelain Garlic has a very pungent taste.

### GREEN GARLIC

This is baby Garlic that is harvested before the cloves have formed. It does not have the same health-promoting properties as fully matured Garlic.

### ELEPHANT GARLIC

Elephant Garlic is actually not a true Garlic. It is more closely related to leeks and does not offer the full flavor or health benefits of regular Garlic.

## the peak season

Although Garlic is available throughout the year, the peak season for California Garlic begins in June and runs through December, while Garlic from Mexico becomes available shortly afterwards. These are the months when its concentration of nutrients and flavor are highest, and its cost is at its lowest.

## 4 steps for the best tasting and most nutritious garlic

To enhance the flavor and nutrients of Garlic just follow my 4 easy steps:
1. The Best Way to Select
2. The Best Way to Store
3. The Best Way to Prepare
4. The Healthiest Way of Cooking

---

### SENSITIVITY TO THE SMELL OF GARLIC

The Garlic bulb itself has little smell to most people. It is not until the cloves have been crushed, sliced or chopped that the enzymes in Garlic are activated and transform the sulfur compounds into the form assumed to be responsible for the characteristically strong odor of Garlic.

In most people, the adverse reaction to the smell of Garlic is probably related to overstimulation of the nerves involved in smell since the sulfur-containing compounds are extremely pungent. In rare cases, individuals who are overly sensitive to the smell of Garlic, as well as the smell of other compounds, may have allergies, asthma, chemical sensitivities or seasonal affective disorders.

Cooking Garlic for 30 to 50 minutes will help to eliminate most of the smell, although this will also reduce its nutritional benefits. Chewing on parsley, fennel seed and mint helps to eliminate the smell of Garlic breath after eating as does chlorophyll tablets or enjoying a scoop of lemon-lime sorbet.

---

# 1. the best way to select garlic

You can select the most flavorful and nutritionally rich Garlic by looking for bulbs that are plump. Gently squeeze the bulb between your fingers; fresh Garlic will feel firm with no trace of dampness. Select large cloves whenever possible to make peeling easier. As with all vegetables, I recommend selecting organically grown varieties whenever possible. (For more on *Organic Foods*, see page 113.)

Avoid Garlic that is soft, shriveled and moldy or has begun to sprout. These may be indications of decay that will cause excess waste and inferior flavor and texture.

Although Garlic in flake, powder or paste form may be more convenient, you will find that it has less flavor.

# 2. the best way to store garlic

Although Garlic is a sturdy vegetable, it will become soft and start to mold if not stored properly. Proper storage will help to preserve its nutrients and flavor.

Garlic continues to respire even after it has been harvested; its respiration rate at room temperature (68°F/20°C) is 20 mg/kg/hr. Slowing down the respiration rate with proper storage is the key to extending its flavor and nutritional benefits. (For a *Comparison of Respiration Rates* for different vegetables, see page 91.)

### Garlic Will Remain Fresh for Up to 1 Month When Properly Stored

1. The best way to store Garlic is in an uncovered or loosely covered container in a cool dark place away

from heat and bright light. This will minimize its respiration rate.

2. Do not refrigerate Garlic since moisture in the refrigerator will cause Garlic to spoil. Refrigerating Garlic causes it to soften and sprout, producing a bitter taste.

3. Be sure to inspect the bulb frequently and remove any cloves that appear to be dried out or moldy. Once you break the head of Garlic and use some of the cloves, its shelf life becomes greatly reduced, and it will last only up to two weeks.

# 3. the best way to prepare garlic

### Peeling Garlic

The first step to using Garlic is to separate the individual cloves. An easy way to do this is to place the bulb on a cutting board and gently, but firmly, apply pressure with the palm of your hand at an angle. This will cause the layers of skin that hold the bulb together to separate. If you prefer, you can insert a knife between the individual cloves, and they will separate from the rest of the bulb.

Place the side of a chef's knife on the Garlic clove and give it a quick whack with the palm of your hand. This loosens the skin, making it easier to remove. Or if you prefer, you can peel it with a paring knife. It is best to peel and prep Garlic as needed because stored chopped Garlic loses its volatile oils with time.

### Removing Garlic Odor

To remove the odor from your fingers, rub them on a stainless steel spoon under cold running water.

### What to Do With Sprouted Garlic?

Don't throw it away. Warm, unventilated conditions can cause Garlic to sprout. Sometimes you may not see the sprouts until you break open the bulb. The sprouts actually contain flavonoids (health-promoting phytonutrients) that also give them their bitter, and sometimes metallic, taste. But if you don't mind a little bitterness, you can use the sprouts to gain extra nutrition. If you don't want to use the sprouts, you can cut them off and just use the clove. The flavor of the cloves will mellow as the sprouts become increasingly bitter. Cooked sprouts are more bitter than raw sprouts.

If you see green spots on the surface of the cloves, it is best to cut them off as they will have a bitter flavor. If you don't mind the bitterness, go ahead and use these cloves, but I have found that it is best when you cut these areas off.

# 4. the healthiest way of cooking garlic

You will find Garlic used in many of the recipes in this book. It is an important seasoning that adds aroma to your food and extra flavor and nutrition to your meal.

Throughout the book, I suggest adding chopped or pressed fresh raw garlic to most vegetables because cooking definitely has an effect on the health benefits you derive from Garlic. Garlic is most pungent when eaten raw and milder when quickly cooked. For those individuals who cannot tolerate raw garlic, I suggest you add chopped garlic to your vegetables while they are cooking. To retain the maximum flavor and nutrition, add Garlic towards the end of the cooking process.

### An Easy Way to Prepare Garlic, Step-by-Step

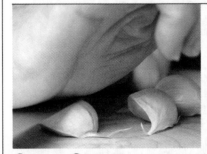 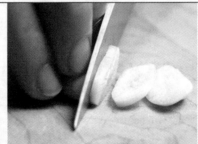 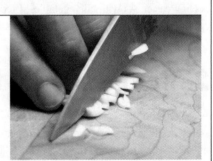

CHOPPED GARLIC
❶ Loosen the skin of garlic by whacking the side of a knife (placed on garlic clove) w/the palm of your hand.
❷ Slice Garlic. ❸ To chop, cut across the slices of Garlic using a rocking motion with your knife, chopping into the desired size. For minced Garlic, chop fine. Let sit for 5–10 minutes before cooking.

Both flavor and nutrition diminish as Garlic cooks. Too much heat for too long will reduce the activity of the health-promoting sulfur compounds that have formed when you let the Garlic sit for 5–10 minutes before cooking. It will also make the Garlic bitter. Therefore, exposing the Garlic to heat for as little time as possible (5–15 minutes) is critical to preserving the maximum amount of sulfur-containing molecules. (See *How to Bring out the Hidden Health Benefits of Garlic* below.)

## Cooking Methods
## Not Recommended for Garlic

### DON'T COOK GARLIC WITH OIL

I don't recommend cooking Garlic in oil because high-temperature heat can damage delicate oils and potentially create harmful free radicals.

### WHAT HAPPENS WHEN YOU ROAST GARLIC?

Roasting Garlic brings out its mild, sweet flavor. It is no wonder hundreds of recipes have been written describing the best ways to roast Garlic. While Garlic roasted in a 350°F oven for 45 minutes will lose its pungency and become sweeter as its starches turn to sugar, it will also lose most of its health-promoting sulfur compounds. The longer it is cooked, the more sulfur compounds it will lose.

Here are questions I received from readers of the whfoods.org website about Garlic:

### Q *How do I maximize Garlic's health benefits?*

A Garlic contains numerous nutrients that have health-promoting properties. One well-known phytonutrient in Garlic is the sulfur-containing compound alliin, which upon its conversion to the active phytonutrient allicin, has been shown to have cancer-protective properties. This conversion occurs when Garlic is chopped or pressed since this allows for the release of the enzyme *alliinase*, which serves as the catalyst for the synthesis of allicin. Therefore, to enhance the health benefits that you receive from Garlic it is

*(Continued on Page 262)*

---

## HOW TO BRING OUT THE HIDDEN HEALTH BENEFITS OF GARLIC

### Why chopping Garlic is important

The latest scientific research tells us that slicing, chopping, mincing or pressing Garlic before cooking will enhance its health-promoting properties. A sulfur-based compound called alliin and an enzyme called *alliinase* are separated in the Garlic's cell structure when it is whole. Cutting Garlic ruptures the cells and releases these elements, allowing them to come in contact and form a powerful new compound called allicin; this phytonutrient not only adds to Garlic's health-promoting benefits but is also the culprit behind its pungent aroma and gives Garlic its "bite."

By chopping Garlic more finely, more allicin may be produced. Pressing Garlic or mincing it into a smooth paste will give you the strongest flavor and may also result in an increased amount of allicin. So, the next time you chop, mince or press your Garlic, you will know that the more pungent the smell, the better it probably is for your health.

### Why you should let Garlic sit for 5–10 minutes

To get the most health benefits from Garlic, let it sit for a minimum of 5 minutes, optimally 10 minutes, after cutting and before eating or cooking. Waiting 5–10 minutes allows the health-promoting allicin to form. If you do not let it sit, allicin is never formed, so it is worth the wait.

### How cooking affects the nutrients in Garlic

Heating Garlic without letting it sit has been found to deactivate the enzyme that is responsible for the formation of allicin. However, if you have allowed your Garlic to sit for 5–10 minutes, you can cook it on low or medium heat for a short period of time (up to 15 minutes) without destroying the allicin. This is because letting it sit not only ensures the maximum synthesis of the allicin, but also makes it more stable and resistant to the heat of cooking.

Research on Garlic reinforces the validity of this practice. When crushed Garlic was heated, its ability to inhibit cancer development in animals was blocked; yet, when the researchers allowed the crushed Garlic to sit for 10 minutes before heating, its anticancer activity was preserved.

### Cooking for:

5–15 minutes: minimal loss of nutrients
15–30 minutes: moderate loss of nutrients
45+ minutes: substantial loss of nutrients

*(Continued from Page 261)*

important to chop or press the Garlic before eating it so that the maximum amount of allicin can be formed. (Chewing will also release the *alliinase* enzyme, but since most people don't chew thoroughly, I think it is better to chop it first.)

### WHY CHOPPING IS SO IMPORTANT
### WHEN YOU ARE COOKING GARLIC

While it is important to cut or press Garlic before consuming it raw, it is of even more importance to do so before cooking it. That's because heating Garlic has been found to deactivate the *alliinase* enzyme, thwarting allicin's ability to prevent against genetic damage that can lead to cancer. Yet, exciting new research has found that letting Garlic sit for 10 minutes (after chopping it and before heating it) helps to preserve much of the Garlic's cancer-protective properties. Why? Because it takes time for *alliinase* to catalyze the conversion of alliin, and allowing the Garlic to sit before heating allows for the optimal transformation to occur.

As you will notice, throughout the book I recommend letting Garlic sit for between 5–10 minutes before eating or cooking it. While 10 minutes may be ideal, 5 minutes will still allow for a substantial amount of allicin to be formed and may work better for people who have less time to cook. I also recommend this process for Garlic that is going to be used raw in a recipe so as to maximize its potential.

### THE EFFECT OF COOKING TIME
### ON SULFUR-CONTAINING PHYTONUTRIENTS

Once Garlic's active sulfur-containing phytonutrients are formed they seem to be somewhat resistant to moderate heat for a short period of time. Low-heat cooking for shorter periods of time (15–30 minutes) seems to preserve more of their activity than longer term cooking (for example, 45 minutes cooking time) where substantial loss of activity has been found to occur.

It is important to remember that when we think about the effect of heat and cooking time on Garlic, we need not limit ourselves to only considering allicin and Garlic's other sulfur-containing nutrients. Overcooking has a general effect on Garlic's nutrient content, and therefore careful preparation is the key to maintaining its overall nutritional integrity.

## Q *Do Garlic supplements provide the same benefits as eating fresh Garlic?*

A Garlic has been attributed with numerous health benefits—promoting cardiovascular health, lowering blood pressure and reducing total cholesterol, to name a few. With the wide supply of Garlic supplements on the market, many people ask me why they should eat fresh Garlic and not just take a Garlic pill. Here are my thoughts on this subject:

While Garlic supplements are promoted as containing allicin, the compound to which many of Garlic's health-promoting properties are attributed, supplements rarely contain the complement of nutrients provided in the whole food that work synergistically to promote good health. Additionally, the active compounds in Garlic are so delicate that most techniques used to create Garlic supplements don't preserve the full vitality of Garlic's compounds. This is the reason why my recommendation is to enjoy one clove of fresh Garlic per day (which usually contains from 4–12 mg of allicin) as opposed to taking Garlic supplements.

## Q *What is responsible for the pungent smell and taste of Garlic and why does it change throughout the cooking process?*

A If you notice, before you cut Garlic, its smell is pretty tempered. It is not until you start chopping it that its

*(Continued on bottom of next Page)*

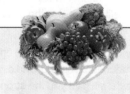

# how to enjoy fresh garlic
# without cooking

**Spicy Guacamole:** Mix together 2 cloves pressed garlic, 2 medium mashed avocados, 1 small diced tomato, 1/4 minced red onion, juice of 1/2 lime, 1/2 tsp cumin, pinch of cayenne and sea salt to taste. Serve with tortilla chips or vegetables.

**Eggplant Garlic Dip:** Remove skin from medium cooked eggplant and place flesh in a mixing bowl. Mash with a fork. For more nutrition you can leave skin on. Add 4 cloves finely minced Garlic, 2 TBS minced cured olives, salt to taste. Mash with the eggplant. Spread on a deep plate. Sprinkle generously with minced parsley and drizzle with olive oil. Serve with crudités.

STEP-BY-STEP RECIPE
## The Healthiest Ways of Using Garlic

# Garlic Dip

*This is a quick and easy dip that goes great with crudités.*

2 cups cooked or canned garbanzo beans
1 TBS fresh lemon juice
3 cloves Garlic, chopped
1/4 cup chicken or vegetable broth
3 TBS extra virgin olive oil
Sea salt and pepper to taste

1. Combine all ingredients in a blender and blend until smooth.

   Serve with carrot sticks, celery sticks or any raw vegetable of your choice.

**SERVES 8**

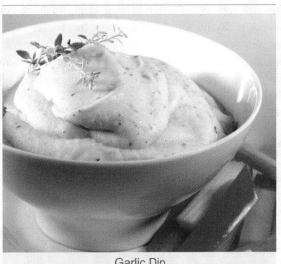
Garlic Dip

---

## Flavor Tips: 6 Ways to add Flavor and Nutrition with Garlic.

1. **Most Popular: Bruschetta.** Toast slices of whole wheat baguette or foccacia. In a bowl, combine 3–4 cloves pressed Garlic, 1 TBS chopped basil, 1 tsp oregano, 1 tsp rosemary, 1/2 cup of extra virgin olive oil and sea salt and pepper to taste. Brush tops of bread with this mixture and then top each piece with finely chopped tomatoes and feta cheese. Also try topping bruschetta with Garlic mixture and different cheeses such as Asiago or Parmesan, finely minced vegetables, or roasted red bell peppers or eggplant. Many delicious bruschetta combinations are possible using Garlic.

2. Use Garlic as a seasoning for chicken, meat, fish, pasta or your favorite vegetables because it adds great flavor to many foods.

3. To mellow the flavor of Garlic, add Garlic to whatever you are cooking for the last 2 minutes of the cooking time. To prevent overcooking Garlic, I highly recommend using a timer.

4. **Garlic Rice:** Add 1 TBS chopped Garlic and 1 TBS fresh minced ginger at the end of cooking rice.

5. **Baked Garlic Chicken:** Rub chicken with lemon juice and place sliced Garlic pieces and fresh rosemary under the skin of the chicken. Season the top of the skin with sea salt and black pepper to taste. Cover and marinate in the refrigerator for 1–12 hours. Bake or use "Quick Broil" method to cook (see page 60).

6. **Garlic Mashed Potatoes**: Press 3 medium cloves Garlic and add to 4 cups mashed potatoes, along with extra virgin olive oil, and sea salt and pepper to taste.

---

Please write (address on back cover flap) or e-mail me at info@whfoods.org with your personal ideas for preparing Garlic, and I will share them with others through our website at www.whfoods.org

---

famously penetrating odor begins to waft through the air. Here's why:

While both the sulfur-containing compound alliin and the enzyme *alliinase* are naturally found in Garlic, they reside in different cells. Therefore, they cannot interact to form the powerful phytonutrient allicin unless the cells are broken, which is accomplished through chopping, pressing or even chewing. Yet, not only is allicin responsible for many of

Garlic's health-promoting benefits, but through its conversion to other compounds, notably diallyl disulfide, it is also responsible for much of the famous smell and flavor of the "stinking rose."

### THE EFFECT OF TIME AND TEMPERATURE
Allicin, diallyl disulfide and their metabolites are fairly unstable and are affected by both time and heat. Eventually, when enough time passes, the smell of Garlic

begins to soften, reflecting that these sulfur-compounds have transformed themselves into other ones, which have different sensory properties. The volatility of these compounds is also one of the main reasons that cooking Garlic tempers its flavor since many sulfur-containing compounds, including allicin, will begin to deactivate during prolonged exposure to heat. As they deactivate and the sugars in Garlic begin to caramelize, Garlic takes on a sweeter, mellower flavor.

### THE EFFECT ON HEALTH BENEFITS

Yet, what you lose in pungent flavor, you may also lose in health benefits. That is why I suggest you only cook Garlic for short periods of time (at the very most 15 minutes). This way you will temper Garlic's bite but you will still preserve more of the benefits of these powerful sulfur-containing phytonutrients.

## Q Sometimes when I pickle Garlic, I notice that some of the pieces turn bluish-green. Can you tell me why this happens?

A I have also had this experience while pickling Garlic. I did some research, and what I found was that one of the main reasons for the appearance of this blue-green color is that it reflects the formation of a compound called copper-sulfate. The copper-sulfate is naturally formed from the copper and sulfur that are contained in the Garlic itself, with enzymes in the Garlic triggering a reaction between these two. The concentration of copper-sulfate would match the intensity of the color; therefore, a very bright-blue green color would correspond to a much higher copper-sulfate concentration than a dull blue-green. I am not aware of any health risks related to the formation of copper-sulfate during the pickling of food. The amount of copper involved would be very small and not enough to pose a risk of copper toxicity. While copper-sulfate formation may be the most likely reason for the blue-green coloration, there could be other reasons. For example, sunlight can cause Garlic to develop some green shades of color and can sometimes trigger a bitter taste in the Garlic.

## Q What can I do to preserve Garlic? Would these preservation methods affect the nutritional quality of the Garlic?

A When carefully done, freezing, drying or freeze-drying of Garlic has minimal impact on its nutritional value. The age of the Garlic that was frozen or dried would be important to consider, as food undergoes a reduction in its nutritional value over time. For example, Garlic that was frozen soon after it was purchased would feature a superior nutritional profile to Garlic that has been first stored for months at room temperature before being frozen.

### FREEZING GARLIC

There are two easy ways I know to freeze Garlic. You can chop the Garlic, wrap it tightly in a plastic freezer bag or in plastic wrap and then freeze. Or just freeze the Garlic unpeeled and remove the cloves as needed. To use, grate or break off the amount needed.

### DRYING GARLIC

Dry only fresh, firm Garlic cloves that have no bruises. To prepare, separate and peel the cloves. Cut in half lengthwise and let sit for 5 minutes (optimally 10 minutes) before drying. No additional pre-drying treatment is necessary. Dry at 140°F (60°C) for 2 hours, then reduce heat to 130°F (55°C) until completely dry or crisp. Please note that dried Garlic may have less sulfur compounds, such as allicin, than fresh Garlic.

If desired, Garlic salt may be made from dried Garlic. Powder dried Garlic by processing in a blender or food processor until fine. Add 4 parts sea salt to 1 part Garlic powder and blend 1 to 2 seconds. If blended longer, the salt will become too fine and cake together in clumps.

### STORING GARLIC IN OIL

Extreme care must be taken when preparing flavored oils with Garlic or when storing Garlic in oil. Peeled Garlic cloves may be submerged in oil and stored in the freezer for several months but definitely do not store Garlic in oil at room temperature. Garlic-in-oil mixtures stored at room temperature provide perfect conditions for producing botulism toxin. The same hazard exists for roasted Garlic stored in oil. At least three outbreaks of botulism associated with Garlic-in-oil mixtures have been reported in North America.

By law, commercially prepared Garlic in oil has been prepared using strict guidelines and must contain citric or phosphoric acid to increase the acidity. Unfortunately, there is no easy or reliable method to acidify Garlic at home. Acidifying Garlic in vinegar is a lengthy and highly variable process; a whole clove of Garlic covered with vinegar can take from 3 days to more than 1 week to sufficiently acidify. As an alternative, properly dried Garlic cloves may be safely added to flavor oils.

Here is an easy way to make a Garlic-in-oil mixture that you can store in the freezer:

Peel Garlic cloves and purée them with oil in a blender or food processor using 2 parts oil to 1 part Garlic. Place in an airtight container and place immediately in the freezer. The purée will stay soft enough in the freezer to scrape out parts to use in your recipes.

# health benefits of garlic

## Promotes Heart Health

Numerous studies have demonstrated that regular consumption of Garlic lowers blood pressure and decreases platelet aggregation, serum triglycerides and LDL-cholesterol, while increasing serum HDL-cholesterol and fibrinolysis (the process through which the body breaks up blood clots). As a result of these beneficial actions, Garlic may help prevent atherosclerosis and diabetic heart disease and reduce the risk of heart attack or stroke. Garlic's positive cardiovascular effects are probably due not only to its sulfur compounds, but its vitamin C, vitamin B6, selenium and manganese as well.

## Promotes Optimal Inflammatory Status

Garlic, like onions, contains sulfur containing phyto-nutrient compounds that inhibit *lipoxygenase* and *cyclooxygenase* (the enzymes that generate inflammatory prostaglandins and thromboxanes), thus markedly reducing inflammation. These anti-inflammatory compounds, along with Garlic's vitamin C, make it useful for helping to protect against attacks in some cases of asthma and may also help contribute to its usefulness in reducing the pain and inflammation of osteoarthritis and rheumatoid arthritis.

## Promotes Optimal Health

Allicin, one of the sulfur compounds responsible for Garlic's characteristic odor, is a powerful antibacterial and antiviral agent that joins forces with vitamin C to help kill harmful microbes. In laboratory research, allicin has been shown to be effective against common infections like colds, flu, stomach viruses and Candida yeast.

Researchers suggest that one reason Garlic may be a potent remedy against the common cold is its ability to reduce the activity of a chemical mediator of inflammation called NF-Kappa B. Recent research also supports Garlic's antibiotic potential, even among bacterial strains that have become resistant to many drugs. In one of these studies, Garlic extract was found to protect laboratory animals from infection from *methicillin-resistant Staphylococcus aureus* (*MSRA*).

Other studies have shown that as few as two or more servings of Garlic a week may help protect against colon cancer. Substances found in Garlic, such as allicin, have been shown to not only protect colon cells from the toxic effects of cancer-causing chemicals, but also to stop the growth of cancer cells once they develop. While more research is needed to confirm these effects, recent animal research also

suggests that Garlic may confer protection against the development of stomach cancer through its potential ability to decrease *H. pylori*-induced gastritis.

## Promotes Healthy Weight Control

The most potent active constituent in Garlic, allicin, has been shown to not only lower blood pressure, insulin and triglycerides in laboratory animals fed a fructose-rich diet, but also to prevent weight gain, according to a recent study.

### Nutritional Analysis of 1 ounce (about 3 medium cloves) raw Garlic:

| NUTRIENT | AMOUNT | % DAILY VALUE | NUTRIENT | AMOUNT | % DAILY VALUE |
|---|---|---|---|---|---|
| Calories | 42.24 | | Vitamin E Alpha Equiv | 0.00 mg | 0.00 |
| Calories from Fat | 1.28 | | Vitamin E IU | 0.00 IU | |
| Calories from Saturated Fat | 0.23 | | Vitamin E mg | 0.00 mg | |
| Protein | 1.80 g | | Folate | 0.88 mcg | 0.22 |
| Carbohydrates | 9.38 g | | Vitamin K | — mcg | — |
| Dietary Fiber | 0.60 g | 2.40 | Pantothenic Acid | 0.17 mg | 1.70 |
| Soluble Fiber | — g | | | | |
| Insoluble Fiber | — g | | **Minerals** | | |
| Sugar – Total | 0.45 g | | Boron | — mcg | |
| Monosaccharides | 0.00 g | | Calcium | 51.31 mg | 5.13 |
| Disaccharides | — g | | Chloride | — mg | |
| Other Carbs | 8.33 g | | Chromium | — mcg | — |
| Fat – Total | 0.14 g | | Copper | 0.08 mg | 4.00 |
| Saturated Fat | 0.03 g | | Fluoride | — mg | — |
| Mono Fat | 0.00 g | | Iodine | — mcg | — |
| Poly Fat | 0.07 g | | Iron | 0.48 mg | 2.67 |
| Omega-3 Fatty Acids | 0.01 g | 0.40 | Magnesium | 7.09 mg | 1.77 |
| Omega-6 Fatty Acids | 0.06 g | | Manganese | 0.47 mg | 23.50 |
| Trans Fatty Acids | 0.00 g | | Molybdenum | — mcg | — |
| Cholesterol | 0.00 mg | | Phosphorus | 43.38 mg | 4.34 |
| Water | 16.61 g | | Potassium | 113.68 mg | |
| Ash | 0.43 g | | Selenium | 4.03 mcg | 5.76 |
| | | | Sodium | 4.82 mg | |
| **Vitamins** | | | Zinc | 0.33 mg | 2.20 |
| Vitamin A IU | 0.00 IU | 0.00 | | | |
| Vitamin A RE | 0.00 RE | | **Amino Acids** | | |
| A - Carotenoid | 0.00 RE | 0.00 | Alanine | 0.04 g | |
| A - Retinol | 0.00 RE | | Arginine | 0.18 g | |
| B1 Thiamin | 0.06 mg | 4.00 | Aspartate | 0.14 g | |
| B2 Riboflavin | 0.03 mg | 1.76 | Cystine | 0.02 g | 4.88 |
| B3 Niacin | 0.20 mg | 1.00 | Glutamate | 0.23 g | |
| Niacin Equiv | 0.51 mg | | Glycine | 0.06 g | |
| Vitamin B6 | 0.35 mg | 17.50 | Histidine | 0.03 g | 2.33 |
| Vitamin B12 | 0.00 mcg | 0.00 | Isoleucine | 0.06 g | 5.22 |
| Biotin | — mcg | — | Leucine | 0.09 g | 3.56 |
| Vitamin C | 8.85 mg | 14.75 | | | |
| Vitamin D IU | 0.00 IU | 0.00 | (Note: "—" indicates data is unavailable. For more information, please see page 806.) | | |
| Vitamin D mcg | 0.00 mcg | | | | |

In this study, three groups of animals were fed the same diet, except that two groups were also given allicin. While those in the control group gained weight, those that received the Garlic phytonutrient were found to have either stable or slightly reduced weight levels. In addition to its unique phytonutrients, which may contribute to its healthy weight control benefits, Garlic is naturally low in calories—one ounce contains only 42 calories (one ounce equals approximately 3 medium cloves).

### Promotes Optimal Antioxidant Status

Garlic is naturally replete with vitamins and minerals that act as powerful antioxidants; these include vitamin C, selenium, manganese and copper. Additionally, its sulfur-containing phytonutrients also promote antioxidant activity. For example, animal research has shown that feeding animals the Garlic phytonutrients allicin and diallyl disulfide causes a substantial elevation in the stomach and small intestines of the critically important antioxidant *glutathione-S-transferase*.

### Additional Health-Promoting Benefits of Garlic

Garlic is also a concentrated source of other nutrients providing additional health-promoting benefits. These nutrients include bone-building calcium, energy-producing vitamin B1 and phosphorus, muscle-building protein, and sleep-promoting tryptophan.

---

## *Aglio E Olio*

*This is traditional Italian comfort food. Use whole wheat pasta and the very best olive oil for nutrition and great flavor. The optional ingredients can be used in combination and create a satisfying meal.*

**5 oz (about 1/3 lb) whole wheat spaghetti or spaghettini**
**4 TBS low-sodium vegetable broth**
**4 cloves garlic**
**Red pepper flakes to taste**
**3 TBS extra virgin olive oil or to taste**
**Sea salt and pepper to taste**

1. Cook spaghetti *al denté* according to package directions.
2. Chop or press garlic and let sit 5 minutes. (Why? see page 261.)
3. Heat broth in a stainless steel skillet over medium heat. When broth begins to steam, add garlic and red pepper flakes, **cover**, and sauté 2–3 minutes. This will mellow the garlic flavor and infuse the broth.
4. Turn off heat and add hot pasta, extra virgin olive oil, and salt and pepper to taste. Toss well and serve.

**SERVES 2**

### Flavor Tips:

**Add any combination of these ingredients to increase the flavor and nutrition of Aglio E Olio:**

1. Freshly grated Parmesan or Romano cheese.
2. Fresh baby spinach or arugula leaves (add to hot broth and garlic mixture just before adding pasta).
3. Fresh chopped tomato.
4. Chopped fresh basil and oregano leaves.
5. High quality black olives.
6. Cooked chicken or shrimp.

---

Here are questions I received from readers of the whfoods.org website about Garlic:

**Q** *Are vitamins like vitamin C completely destroyed when vegetables are cooked?*

**A** In general, cooking does reduce the amount of nutrients in food, although while they may be reduced, they will not necessarily be completely destroyed. The amount of nutrient loss will be affected by a few factors including heat, time and the amount of water. For example, cooking of vegetables and fruits for longer periods of time (10–20 minutes) can result in a loss of over one half the total vitamin C content. The nutrient loss that can occur with cooking is the reason that I emphasize short cooking times with minimal exposure to water. These cooking methods help to create vegetables that have enhanced taste and texture and the best-preserved nutrient content.

# Q&A

**CAN YOU TELL ME MORE ABOUT THE DIETARY FIBER AND RESISTANT STARCHES FOUND IN WHOLE GRAINS AND OTHER WHOLE FOODS?**

Dietary fiber and resistant starches are included among the macronutrient family called carbohydrates. Yet, unlike other types of carbohydrates, they are not used in the body for energy. Rather, they play important health-promoting roles in your gastrointestinal tract, supporting digestion and absorption and helping you eliminate toxins and waste products.

## Dietary Fiber

Since dietary fibers are classified as polysaccharides they are considered complex carbohydrates; however, the sugar units in fiber are linked (bonded) together in such a way that your body can't break the bonds and digest them. Instead, fibers transit through your small intestine and make it all the way to your large intestine intact. This ability to move through your system to your large intestine helps speed the transit time of wastes excreted from your body; for this reason, fiber helps support your health by reducing constipation and promoting the excretion of toxins and wastes.

Fibers that promote overall healthy digestion and waste excretion are found in vegetables, whole grains, and legumes and are well represented in whole foods. Often, when processed, foods have these fibers removed. For example, bran contains high levels of fibers but it is removed when grains are processed. Fruit skins are also high in fiber but are often removed when the fruit is processed for a fruit-containing product.

Much has been written about the health-promoting benefits of fiber, and ample numbers of studies support an association between high-fiber diets and a decrease in risk of many types of cancers, including colon cancer and breast cancer. Some of this benefit comes from the ability of fiber to bind and remove toxins and to promote healthy digestion. Recent research suggests, however, that fiber provides its health-protecting benefits in other ways as well, and one of the most important appears to be its ability to promote healthy intestinal-tract bacteria.

Your large intestine contains a multitude of beneficial bacteria that are required for your body's health. They are called the "friendly flora" and they support the health of your whole body by promoting healthy immune function and providing important molecules to your intestinal tract cells to promote their growth, thus sustaining overall intestinal tract integrity. These bacteria use some of the fibers you eat as fuel for their own growth and through their own metabolism produce molecules called short-chain fatty acids (SCFA). SCFA production by these "friendly flora" has been associated with a decrease in cancerous colonic cells, reduction of serum cholesterol and maintenance of healthy blood sugar levels and healthy intestinal tract cell walls.

Yet, not all fiber is fermented by the "friendly flora" in your intestinal tract. Some, as discussed above, goes through your entire system unchanged, binding toxins and waste products as it goes and promoting healthy elimination. Some fibers can be fermented by bacteria of all types while other fibers are preferentially fermented by the "friendly flora," the bacteria that are most beneficial to your body, including *Bifidobacteria* and *Lactobacillus*. When these friendly bacteria are given their favorite types of fibers, called "prebiotic fibers," they will flourish, significantly improving the health of your digestive tract. Excellent sources of these prebiotic fibers include foods such as Jerusalem artichoke, chicory, rice fiber and soy fiber.

The classical way of talking about fiber is to divide it into two types, soluble or insoluble fiber, a classification determined by how much water a type of fiber holds. New research, however, suggests that fiber has a multitude of activities besides holding water and that this classical distinction is not adequate. Providing a full range of all types of fibers, including prebiotic fibers, will support your immune system and enhance healthy digestion, absorption and the removal of wastes and toxins. In fact, the health of your gastrointestinal tract is dependent upon your consumption of the variety of fibers well represented in the World's Healthiest Foods.

## Resistant Starch

Resistant starch is another type of polysaccharide, or complex carbohydrate. It gets its name because, although it is starch, it is resistant to digestion in the small intestine. The result of this resistance is that this type of starch acts more like fiber than starch and travels through the intestinal tract until it reaches the large intestine where, like fiber, it may be fermented by the bacteria in the colon. Research has shown that resistant starch promotes the generation of SCFAs by the bacteria in the large intestine and, therefore, has many of the same health-promoting abilities as fiber. Resistant starch is found in whole grains such as brown rice, barley, whole wheat and buckwheat.

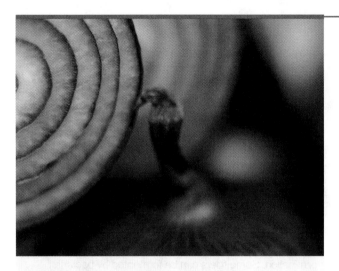

# onions

## highlights

| | |
|---|---|
| AVAILABILITY: | Year-round |
| REFRIGERATE: | Not recommended |
| SHELF LIFE: | Up to 1 month |
| PREPARATION: | Chop or slice, and let sit for 5 minutes |
| BEST WAY TO COOK: | "Healthy Sauté" in just 7 minutes |

## nutrient-richness chart

Total Nutrient-Richness: **14**   GI: **15**

One cup (160 grams) of raw Onions contains 61 calories

| NUTRIENT | AMOUNT | %DV | DENSITY | QUALITY |
|---|---|---|---|---|
| Chromium | 24.8 mcg | 20.7 | 6.1 | very good |
| Vitamin C | 10.2 mg | 17.1 | 5.1 | very good |
| Dietary Fiber | 2.9 g | 11.5 | 3.4 | very good |
| Manganese | 0.2 mg | 11.0 | 3.3 | good |
| Molybdenum | 8.0 mcg | 10.7 | 3.2 | good |
| B6 Pyridoxine | 0.2 mg | 9.5 | 2.8 | good |
| Tryptophan | 0.03 g | 9.4 | 2.8 | good |
| Folate | 30.4 mcg | 7.6 | 2.3 | good |
| Potassium | 251.2 mg | 7.2 | 2.1 | good |
| Phosphorus | 52.8 mg | 5.3 | 1.6 | good |
| Copper | 0.1 mg | 5.0 | 1.5 | good |

| **CAROTENOIDS:** | |
|---|---|
| Beta-Carotene | 1.6 mcg |
| Lutein+Zeaxanthin | 8.0 mcg |

| **FLAVONOIDS:** | |
|---|---|
| Isorhamnetin | 3.1 mg |
| Kaempferol | 0.3 mg |
| Quercetin | 21.2 mg |

Daily values for these nutrients have not yet been established.

| **PHYTOSTEROLS:** | |
|---|---|
| Phytosterols – Total | 24.0 mg |

For more on "Total Nutrient-Richness," "%DV," "Density," and The World's Healthiest Foods "Quality" Rating System, see page 805.

For more on GI, see page 342.

The ancient Egyptians had such a high regard for Onions that they were used as currency to pay the workers who built the pyramids. They were also deemed to have such great spiritual significance that they were placed in the tombs of the Pharaohs to accompany them to the afterlife. Today, these humble white, red and yellow bulbs, with their paper-thin skins, play a unique role in the cuisine of almost every region of the world. Although cutting Onions may bring a tear to your eye, they will also bring delight to your taste buds by adding their aromatic flavor to your "Healthiest Way of Eating." Proper preparation of Onions is the key to enjoying their best flavor and maximizing their nutritional benefits. That is why I want to share with you my easy and convenient "Healthiest Way of Cooking" Onions. In just 7 minutes, you can enjoy great tasting Onions with the maximum nutritional value.

## why onions should be part of your healthiest way of eating

Regular consumption of Onions has been associated with a number of health benefits including reducing risk of heart disease, lowering cholesterol levels and reducing blood pressure. Many of these benefits have been attributed to the health-promoting phytonutrients found in Onions. Sulfur-containing phytonutrients, such as allyl propyl sulfoxides, help maintain healthy blood sugar levels and are also responsible for the smell of Onions and their irritating effect on your eyes. In fact, it has been found that the stronger the smell and the more they affect your eyes, the more health-promoting nutrients they contain! Onions are also a concentrated source of flavonoid phytonutrients, such as quercetin, which have anti-inflammatory benefits and have been suggested to promote heart health. Additionally, they are a very good source of chromium, a hard-to-find mineral that is important for balancing blood sugar levels. Onions are an ideal food to add to your "Healthiest Way of Eating" not only because they are rich in nutrients, but also because they are low in calories: one cup of raw Onions contains only 61 calories. (For more on the *Health Benefits of Onions* and a complete analysis of their content of over 60 nutrients, see page 275.)

# varieties of onions

Onions *(Allium cepa)* are native to Asia and the Middle East and have been cultivated for over 5,000 years. The word Onion comes from the Latin word *unio,* meaning "single" or "one." The name helps distinguish the Onion, which produces a single bulb, from its cousin, garlic, which produces many small bulbs. The name also describes the union (also from *unio*) of the many separate, concentrically arranged layers of the Onion.

Onions range in size, color and taste depending upon their variety. There are generally two types of large, globe-shaped Onions:

### STORAGE ONIONS

These Onions are known as Storage Onions because they store for a long period of time. They are grown in colder climates; because they are dried for a period of several months after harvesting, their skin is dry and crisp. They generally have a more pungent flavor than Spring/Summer Onions and are usually named by their color: yellow, red or white. Spanish Onions also fall into this classification.

> YELLOW Storage Onions are very flavorful and the most commonly used variety of Onions. They also contain the highest concentration of the powerful antioxidant called quercetin, which gives them their yellow color.

> SPANISH Onions are large yellow Onions with a very mild taste.

> RED OR BERMUDA Onions are the hottest and sweetest of the Storage Onions. They are high in quercetin and also contain health-promoting anthocyanins, which give them their red color.

> WHITE Onions are not too sweet and have a mild taste.

> PEAR OR BOILING Onions are a smaller version of Storage Onions. Prepare pearl Onions by dropping them in boiling water for 1 minute. After they are cooked, pinch the root and the Onion will slip from the peel.

### SPRING/SUMMER ONIONS

These juicy Onions are grown in warm climates. Since they remain in the soil longer than Storage Onions, much of their carbohydrates turn to sugar, giving them their characteristically mild, sweet taste. The extended time in the soil also results in the reduction of their nutritional value due to the loss of many of their health-promoting compounds, including sulfur-containing phytonutrients. This is the reason Spring/Summer Onions do will not bring tears to your eyes like Storage Onions.

Varieties of Spring/Summer Onions include: Walla Walla, Vidalia and Maui Sweet Onions. They are generally not used in cooking but are enjoyed raw in salads and sandwiches. Unlike Storage Onions, Spring/Summer Onions do not store well, so it is best not to keep them longer than one week.

## Other Varieties of Onions:

### SCALLIONS OR GREEN ONIONS

They are bright green in color with long, narrow hollow leaves and a small, pear-shaped white bulb. Both leaves and bulb are enjoyed in cooking.

# the peak season

Although Storage Onions are available throughout the year, Spring/Summer Onions have a more limited growing season and are available only a few months out of the year:

> Maui Onions – April through June
> Vidalia Onions – May and June
> Walla Walla – July and August

# 4 steps for the best tasting and most nutritious onions

Turning Onions into a flavorful dish with the most nutrients is simple if you just follow my 4 easy steps:

1. The Best Way to Select
2. The Best Way to Store
3. The Best Way to Prepare
4. The Healthiest Way of Cooking

---

## New Scientific Findings

### WHICH ONIONS ARE THE MOST NUTRITIOUS?

Of the Storage Onions, white Onions have the least number of nutrients. Yellow and red Storage Onions are a concentrated source of quercetin, a powerful antioxidant, and have the greatest amount of health-promoting sulfur compounds. Red Onions also contain anthocyanin phytonutrients that function as powerful antioxidants. Spring/Summer Onions contain fewer nutrients than Storage Onions.

# 1. the best way to select onions

You can select the best tasting Onions by looking for ones that are clean and well shaped, have no opening at the neck and feature crisp, dry outer skins. By selecting the best tasting Onions, you will also enjoy Onions with the highest nutritional value. As with all vegetables, I recommend selecting organically grown varieties whenever possible because conventionally grown Onions are often irradiated to prevent them from sprouting. (For more on *Organic Foods*, see page 113.)

Avoid selecting Onions that are sprouting or have signs of mold. Soft spots, moisture at their neck and dark patches may be indications of decay and reflect inferior quality.

When purchasing scallions or green Onions, I look for ones that have fresh-looking green tops that appear crisp and tender. The base should have two to three inches of whitish color. Avoid green Onions and scallions that have wilted or yellowed tops.

# 2. the best way to store onions

Onions are a hearty vegetable and store well. If you are not planning to cook Onions immediately after bringing them home from the market, be sure to store them properly to preserve their vitamins and flavor.

Onions continue to respire even after they have been harvested; their respiration rate at room temperature (68°F/20°C) is 8 mg/kg/hr. Slowing down the respiration rate with proper storage is the key to extending their flavor and nutritional benefits. (For a *Comparison of Respiration Rates* for different vegetables, see page 91.)

### Onions Will Remain Fresh for Up to 1 Month When Properly Stored, Depending on Variety

The length of time you can store Onions will depend on the variety. Varieties that are more pungent in flavor, such as yellow Onions, can be stored longer than those with a sweeter taste, such as white Onions. The compounds that give yellow Onions their sharp taste also help to preserve them.

1. The best way to store Storage and Spring/Summer Onions is in a cool, dark place, away from heat and bright light. Be sure that they are well ventilated and do not put them in plastic bags. You can put them in a wire hanging basket or a perforated bowl with a raised base so that air can circulate underneath. This will minimize their respiration rate.

2. Do not refrigerate uncut Storage and Spring/Summer Onions since moisture in the refrigerator will cause Onions to spoil.

3. Be sure that all Storage and Spring/Summer Onions are stored away from potatoes, as they will absorb their moisture, and the potatoes' ethylene gas will cause the Onions to spoil more quickly.

4. Store Scallions in the refrigerator in a plastic storage bag that is wrapped tightly around them. The colder temperature will slow the respiration rate, helping to preserve their nutrients and keeping Scallions fresh for a longer period of time. Do not wash Scallions before refrigeration because exposure to water will encourage Scallions to spoil.

### How to Store Onions That Have Been Cut

The unused portion of a cut Onion should be placed in a sealed container to limit its exposure to airflow and stored in the crisper section of your refrigerator. A cut Onion should be used within a day or two since it tends to oxidize and lose its nutrient content very quickly.

# 3. the best way to prepare onions

While most people love to eat Onions, most dread cutting them since this process usually brings tears to their eyes. The compound that causes eyes to burn is a phytonutrient known as allyl sulfate, which is produced when sulfur compounds are released when the Onion is cut and the Onion's cells are ruptured.

### Cutting Onions

Cutting Onions into slices of equal thickness will help them to cook more evenly. The thinner they are sliced, the more quickly they will cook. I recommend cutting Onions into 1/4-inch slices to cook them *al denté*. Let them sit for 5 minutes before cooking.

## Preventing Onions from Irritating Your Eyes

There are a few methods you can use if cutting Onions irritates your eyes. Chilling the Onions for an hour or so before cutting will slow the activity of the enzyme that produces the allyl sulfate responsible for eye irritation. While this compound may be irritating to the eyes, it is also one of the phytonutrients most responsible for Onion's significant health benefits. Chilling is a better alternative to the more traditional method of cutting Onion under running water, which may dilute the amount of allyl sulfate.

Some people also put a slice of bread or metal spoon in their mouth while cutting Onions as they find this helps neutralize the irritating compounds.

The method I use to avoid eye irritation is to make sure my kitchen windows are open. I cut the Onion while standing, pulling my head back and keeping my eyes as far away from the Onions as possible.

If cutting Onions really makes you cry, consider wearing swimming goggles.

## To Remove Odor of Onions from Your Hands

Rubbing your fingertips on a stainless steel spoon under warm running water will help to reduce the odor that the Onions may have imparted.

# 4. the healthiest way of cooking onions

Onions are a kitchen staple and are used in more recipes than any other ingredient. They are one of the most important seasonings, adding both aroma to your meal and extra sweetness and nutrition to your dishes. Although Onions are usually used as a flavoring agent, I want to share with you ways to also enjoy them as a vegetable side dish.

Since research has shown that important nutrients can be lost or destroyed by the way a food is cooked, the "Healthiest Way of Cooking" Onions is focused on bringing out the their best flavor while maximizing their vitamins, minerals and powerful antioxidants.

## The Healthiest Way of Cooking Onions: "Healthy Sautéing" for just 5 Minutes

In my search to find the healthiest way to cook Onions, I tested every possible cooking method and discovered that "Healthy Sautéing" Onions for just 7 minutes delivered the best result. "Healthy Sautéing" Onions brings out their sweet flavor and retains the greatest amount of nutrients. The Step-by-Step Recipe will show you how easy it is to "Healthy Sauté" Onions. (For more on "Healthy Sauté," see page 57.)

### GRILLING AND BROILING ONIONS

Before grilling or broiling, sprinkle Onions with lemon juice, sea salt and pepper to help protect against the formation of harmful compounds. While grilled or broiled Onions have a nice smoky flavor, take care that they do not burn. It is best to grill Onions on an area without a direct flame as the temperatures directly above or below the flame can reach as high as 500°F to 1000°F (260° to 538°C). When using a broiler, keep the Onions about 4–5 inches away from the flame. Coating with oil before cooking will also

## An Easy Way to Prepare Onions, Step-by-Step

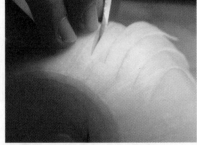 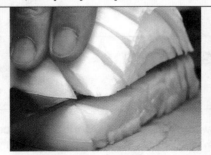 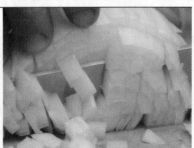

### CHOPPED ONION

❶ Place a peeled Onion half in front of you with the root end away from you, and slice the Onion from side to side just short of the root end, leaving it intact. The slices can be made large or small depending on the size cut you want to end up with. ❷ Slice horizontally through the slices, 2-3 times, again leaving the root intact. ❸ Slice the Onion crosswise down through the other cuts. The Onion will fall into pieces. Let sit for at least 5 minutes.

produce harmful free radicals, so brush with extra virgin olive oil immediately after it is cooked. (For more on *Grilling*, see page 61.)

## Avoid Overcooking Onions

Although Onions are a hearty vegetable, it is very important not to overcook them. Onions cooked for as little as a couple of minutes longer than recommended will begin to lose their nutrients. Overcooking Onions will significantly decrease their nutritional value: as much as 50% of some nutrients can be lost.

## Cooking Methods
## Not Recommended for Onions

**ROASTING, COOKING WITH OIL OR CARAMELIZING**
While Onions roasted at 350°F (175°C) for 1 to 1$^1$/2 hours will lose their pungency and become sweeter as their starches turn to sugar, they will also lose most of their health-promoting sulfur compounds. The longer they are cooked, the more sulfur compounds they will lose. I also don't recommend cooking Onions in oil because high temperature heat can damage delicate oils and potentially create harmful free radicals.

Hundreds of recipes have been written on caramelizing Onions because it tames their flavor and make them sweeter. Caramelized Onions have a beautiful brown tone and become sweet as their starch turns to sugar. While the brown coloration indicates they have lost their pungency, it also is a sign that they have become oxidized, lost many beneficial nutrients and formed free radicals that have been found to be harmful to your health. The healthiest alternative to caramelizing your Onions is using the "Healthy Sauté" method of cooking (see page 273).

---

Here are questions I received from readers of the whfoods.org website about Onions:

### Q *What gets released when Onions are sautéed—is it oil or water?*

A When Onions are sautéed, they primarily release water. Onions are virtually fat-free but are significantly endowed with water; in fact, they are about 90% water by weight. When Onions are exposed to heat during the sauté process, their cell walls break down, and the water they contain is released.

### Q *Is there anything special I need to know when preparing Onions?*

A Like their cousin garlic, Onions contain beneficial sulfur-containing compounds, although in lesser amounts. As in garlic, upon cutting and exposure to oxygen, these phytonutrients are converted into compounds that have health-promoting properties. Therefore, it would be beneficial to allow Onions to sit for about 10 minutes after you have chopped them before cooking them. This procedure will allow you to enjoy the most health benefits from one of the World's Healthiest Foods.

### Q *Do the nutritional benefits of Onions vary depending upon their color?*

A Since the groundbreaking research that found the intake of flavonoid-rich Onions to be related to reduced risk of certain chronic diseases, researchers have been testing different types of Onions to determine whether any are more richly endowed with these potent antioxidant phytonutrients. Research studies so far have found that red Onions and yellow Onions seem to contain more

*(Continued on Page 274)*

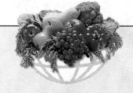

# how to enjoy fresh onions without cooking

**Onion Spinach Salad:** In a large bowl, slice half of a sweet (Spring/Summer) yellow Onion into very thin slices. Combine with the segments of 2 oranges, 2 TBS red wine vinegar, 4 TBS extra virgin olive oil, 1/2 tsp finely minced fresh rosemary, 1/4 tsp sea salt and black pepper to taste. Let sit for 1 hour and toss with 10 oz of baby spinach.

**Marinated Onions:** Cover thinly sliced onions with balsamic vinegar and 1 TBS honey and marinate 1–12 hours refrigerated. Drain and add to a green salad, to sliced cucumbers for a delicious cucumber salad or use as an accompaniment to cooked fish.

STEP-BY-STEP RECIPE
## The Healthiest Way of Cooking Onions

# 7-Minute "Healthy Sautéed" Onions

*The traditional way of sautéing Onions until brown (caramelized) destroys many of their health benefits. I discovered that "Healthy Sautéing" brings out their sweet flavor and preserves the maximum number of nutrients.*

**1 medium Onion, thinly sliced**
**2 TBS + 2 TBS low-sodium chicken or**
   **vegetable broth**
**3 TBS extra virgin olive oil**
**Sea salt and pepper to taste**

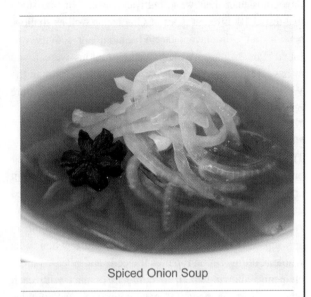
Spiced Onion Soup

1. Slice onions and let them sit for at least 5 minutes as described under *How to Bring out the Hidden Health Benefits of Onions* (page 276).

2. Heat 2 TBS broth over medium heat in a stainless steel skillet.

3. When broth begins to steam, add Onions and **cover** for 3 minutes. The Onions wil release a small amount of liquid. **Uncover**, add another 2 TBS broth and continue to stir for 4 minutes, leaving the lid off.

4. Remove from heat when Onions become translucent, about 7 minutes, depending on the thickness of the slices. If you would like your Onions more tender, cook for 2 to 3 more minutes **uncovered,** and stir frequently. (For *Differences in Cooking Time,* see page 94.)

5. Transfer to a bowl. For more flavor, toss Onions with the remaining ingredients while they are still hot.

**SERVES 2**

### COOKING TIPS:
- To prevent overcooking Onions, I highly recommend using a timer.

## Flavor Tips: Try these 6 great serving suggestions with the recipe above.

1. **Most Popular:** Add a few drops of tamari (soy sauce) to mellow the taste of the Onions. If you add tamari, you will want to reduce the amount of sea salt.

2. Sprinkle with balsamic vinegar, chopped walnuts and dill.

3. For an Asian flavor, add rice vinegar and tamari to the 7-Minute "Healthy Sautéed" Onions recipe. Serve over chicken, liver or fish.

4. Onions share the same cooking time and method as bell peppers, eggplant and shiitake mushrooms.

5. **Onions, Potatoes and Olives:** Combine the 7-Minute "Healthy Sautéed" Onions recipe with steamed cubed potatoes and cured olives.

6. **Spiced Onion Soup:** Bring the following to a boil: 3 cups chicken or vegetable broth, 1/2 inch sliced ginger, 1 star anise, 1 bay leaf and a cinnamon stick. **Cover**, reduce heat and simmer 10 minutes. "Healthy Sauté" one large thinly sliced Onion on medium heat for 15 minutes, adding broth as needed to prevent it from sticking. Keep sauté pan **covered**. Add 2 cloves sliced garlic for last 3 minutes. Strain spices out of broth and add Onions and garlic, 1 tsp tamari (soy sauce) and 1 tsp maple syrup and continue to cook 5 minutes on low (pictured above).

Please write (address on back cover flap) or e-mail me at info@whfoods.org with your personal ideas for preparing Onions, and I will share them with others through our website at www.whfoods.org.

*(Continued from Page 272)*

flavonoids than their white cultivar cousins. In one study that tested 10 different types of Onions, as well as shallots, a wide range in flavonoids and antioxidant activity was found. For example, Western Yellow Onions were found to have 11 times greater flavonoid concentrations than the Western White variety, while shallots had 6 times more phenolic content than Vidalias.

### PREPARATION FOR COOKING

The latest scientific research tells us that slicing, chopping or mincing Onions and letting them sit before cooking will enhance their health-promoting properties. A sulfur-based compound called S-alk(en)yl-L-cysteine sulfoxide and an enzyme called *sulfoxide lyase* (also known as *alliinase*) are separated in the Onion's cell structure when it is whole. Cutting Onion ruptures the cells and releases these elements, allowing them to come in contact with each other to form a powerful new compound called thiopropanal sulfoxide. This new compound not only increases Onions' health-promoting properties, but is also the culprit behind their pungent aroma and the cause of the eye irritation that results from cutting Onions.

The finer the Onion is cut, the more extensive is the transformation of the sulfur compounds. The stronger the smell and the more they affect your eyes, the more health-promoting nutrients they provide. So the next time you cut your Onions, you will have a greater appreciation of their "irritating" effects, knowing that the pungent smell that makes you cry will also make you healthy!

To get the most health benefits from Onions, let them sit for a minimum of 5 minutes, and optimally for 10 minutes, after cutting, before eating or cooking. This is to ensure the maximum synthesis of the sulfur compounds.

Heat will inactivate the effect of *alliinase*, which is why it is important to allow the Onions to sit for 5–10 minutes before cooking to give the enzyme ample opportunity to enhance the concentration of active phytonutrients in your Onions. Cooking at low or medium heat for short periods of time (up to 15 minutes), such as with methods like "Healthy Sauté," should not destroy the active phytonutrients since once they are formed, they are fairly stable.

Research on garlic, a close relative of Onion, reinforces the validity of this practice. When crushed garlic was heated, its ability to inhibit cancer development in animals was blocked; yet, when the researchers allowed the chopped garlic to 'stand' for 10 minutes before heating, its anti-cancer activity was preserved.

Here are questions I received from readers of the whfoods.org website about Onions:

**Q** *How can you guarantee that the mineral values that you report for Onions (as well as other foods) if the soil has been depleted of those minerals, as most farm soils are?*

**A** With respect to nutrient data—including mineral data—for any food (not just Onions), our website used the "gold standard" software in clinical nutrition, an application called "Food Processor" with a database published by ESHA Research, Inc. in Salem, Oregon. We are also familiar with many nutrient databases, including the USDA's SR19 foods database.

The nutrient data in any nutritional database uses statistical averages. Sometimes the averages involve testing of a very small number of food samples. Sometimes hundreds of samples are tested. These samples may take into account a variety of different growing conditions, or they may not take into account any differences in growing conditions. The only responsible way to view these database estimates is with a "ballpark" approach. At best, the data in a nutrient database give you a ballpark estimate of the nutrient contents of a particular food. Differences in soil quality definitely affect mineral content of foods.

The bottom line here is that you cannot guarantee that every serving of a food that you enjoy contains exactly the amount of nutrients that we report on our website or is reported in any nutrition database. However, you can guarantee that Onions and other of the World's Healthiest Foods are a good place to look if you are trying to increase your mineral intake.

We don't know a better place to start to up the chances of healthy soil than buying organic. The Organic Foods Production Act contains extensive soil requirements, and most of the requirements promote not only immediate soil health but soil sustainability. Soil quality is one of the reasons we support organically grown foods so strongly. There are quality requirements for fertilization and use of compost in organic farming that would give these Onions (and other foods) their best chance to provide the minerals they are naturally capable of providing.

# health benefits of onions

## Promote Blood Sugar Balance

The higher the intake of Onions, the lower the level of glucose found during glucose tolerance tests. Experimental and clinical evidence suggests that allyl propyl disulfide, one of the important sulfur-containing phytonutrients contained in Onions, is responsible for this effect and lowers blood sugar levels by increasing the amount of free insulin available. Allyl propyl disulfide does this by competing with insulin, which is also a disulphide, to occupy the sites in the liver where insulin is inactivated. This results in an increase in the amount of insulin available to usher glucose into cells, causing a lowering of blood sugar.

In addition, Onions are a very good source of chromium, the mineral component in glucose tolerance factor, a molecule that helps cells respond appropriately to insulin. Clinical studies of diabetics have shown that chromium can decrease fasting blood glucose levels, improve glucose tolerance, lower insulin levels and decrease total cholesterol and triglyceride levels while increasing good HDL-cholesterol levels.

## Promote Heart Health

The regular consumption of Onions has been shown to lower high cholesterol levels and high blood pressure, both actions that can help prevent atherosclerosis and diabetic heart disease, and reduce the risk of heart attack or stroke. These beneficial effects are likely due to Onions' sulfur compounds, chromium, folate and vitamin B6; the latter two help prevent heart disease by lowering high homocysteine levels, another significant risk factor for heart attack and stroke.

Onions are also very rich in the flavonoid phytonutrient, quercetin. In a meta-analysis of seven prospective studies, Onions were singled out as one of the small number of vegetables and fruits that contributed to a significant reduction in heart disease. Of the more than 100,000 individuals who participated in these studies, those whose diets most frequently included Onions, tea, apples and broccoli—the richest sources of flavonoids—enjoyed a 20% reduction in their risk of heart disease.

## Promote Digestive Health

The regular consumption of Onions, as little as two or more times per week, is associated with a significantly reduced risk of developing colon cancer. Onions contain a number of flavonoids, the most studied of which is quercetin, which have been shown to halt the growth of tumors in animals and protect colon cells from the damaging effects of certain cancer-causing substances. Cooking meats with Onions may help reduce the amount of carcinogens produced when meat is cooked with high-heat methods. Onions are also a very good source of dietary fiber, which is important for colonic health.

## Nutritional Analysis of 1 cup of raw Onions:

| NUTRIENT | AMOUNT | % DAILY VALUE | NUTRIENT | AMOUNT | % DAILY VALUE |
|---|---|---|---|---|---|
| Calories | 60.80 | | Pantothenic Acid | 0.17 mg | 1.70 |
| Calories from Fat | 2.30 | | | | |
| Calories from Saturated Fat | 0.37 | | **Minerals** | | |
| Protein | 1.86 g | | Boron | 0.27 mcg | |
| Carbohydrates | 13.81 g | | Calcium | 32.00 mg | 3.20 |
| Dietary Fiber | 2.88 g | 11.52 | Chloride | 40.00 mg | |
| Soluble Fiber | 1.15 g | | Chromium | 24.80 mcg | 20.67 |
| Insoluble Fiber | 1.73 g | | Copper | 0.10 mg | 5.00 |
| Sugar – Total | 9.92 g | | Fluoride | — mg | — |
| Monosaccharides | 5.92 g | | Iodine | 3.20 mcg | 2.13 |
| Disaccharides | 2.34 g | | Iron | 0.35 mg | 1.94 |
| Other Carbs | 1.01 g | | Magnesium | 16.00 mg | 4.00 |
| Fat – Total | 0.26 g | | Manganese | 0.22 mg | 11.00 |
| Saturated Fat | 0.04 g | | Molybdenum | 8.00 mcg | 10.67 |
| Mono Fat | 0.04 g | | Phosphorus | 52.80 mg | 5.28 |
| Poly Fat | 0.10 g | | Potassium | 251.20 mg | |
| Omega-3 Fatty Acids | 0.00 g | 0.00 | Selenium | 0.96 mcg | 1.37 |
| Omega-6 Fatty Acids | 0.09 g | | Sodium | 4.80 mg | |
| Trans Fatty Acids | 0.00 g | | Zinc | 0.30 mg | 2.00 |
| Cholesterol | 0.00 mg | | | | |
| Water | 143.49 g | | **Amino Acids** | | |
| Ash | 0.59 g | | Alanine | 0.05 g | |
| | | | Arginine | 0.25 g | |
| **Vitamins** | | | Aspartate | 0.10 g | |
| Vitamin A IU | 0.00 IU | 0.00 | Cystine | 0.03 g | 7.32 |
| Vitamin A RE | 0.00 RE | | Glutamate | 0.30 g | |
| A - Carotenoid | 0.00 RE | 0.00 | Glycine | 0.08 g | |
| A - Retinol | 0.00 RE | | Histidine | 0.03 g | 2.33 |
| B1 Thiamin | 0.07 mg | 4.67 | Isoleucine | 0.07 g | 6.09 |
| B2 Riboflavin | 0.03 mg | 1.76 | Leucine | 0.07 g | 2.77 |
| B3 Niacin | 0.24 mg | 1.20 | Lysine | 0.09 g | 3.83 |
| Niacin Equiv | 0.69 mg | | Methionine | 0.02 g | 2.70 |
| Vitamin B6 | 0.19 mg | 9.50 | Phenylalanine | 0.05 g | 4.20 |
| Vitamin B12 | 0.00 mcg | 0.00 | Proline | 0.06 g | |
| Biotin | 5.60 mcg | 1.87 | Serine | 0.05 g | |
| Vitamin C | 10.24 mg | 17.07 | Threonine | 0.04 g | 3.23 |
| Vitamin D IU | 0.00 IU | 0.00 | Tryptophan | 0.03 g | 9.38 |
| Vitamin D mcg | 0.00 mcg | | Tyrosine | 0.05 g | 5.15 |
| Vitamin E Alpha Equiv | 0.21 mg | 1.05 | Valine | 0.04 g | 2.72 |
| Vitamin E IU | 0.31 IU | | | | |
| Vitamin E mg | 0.50 mg | | | | |
| Folate | 30.40 mcg | 7.60 | | | |
| Vitamin K | 3.20 mcg | 4.00 | | | |

(Note: "—" indicates data is unavailable. For more information, please see page 806.)

## Promote Inflammatory Balance and Immune Health

Several anti-inflammatory agents in Onions render them helpful in reducing the severity of symptoms associated with inflammatory conditions, such as the pain and swelling of osteoarthritis and rheumatoid arthritis, the allergic inflammatory response of asthma and the respiratory congestion associated with the common cold. Onions contain compounds that inhibit *lipoxygenase* and *cyclooxygenase* (the enzymes that generate inflammatory prostaglandins and thromboxanes), thus markedly reducing inflammation. Onions' anti-inflammatory effects are due not only to their vitamin C and quercetin, but also to other active components called isothiocyanates. These compounds work synergistically to spell relief from inflammation. In addition, quercetin and other flavonoids found in Onions work with vitamin C to help kill harmful bacteria, making Onions an especially good addition to soups and stews during cold and flu season.

## Additional Health-Promoting Benefits of Onions

Onions are also a concentrated source of other nutrients providing additional health-promoting benefits. These nutrients include free-radical-scavenging manganese and copper, sulfite-detoxifying molybdenum, heart-healthy potassium, energy-promoting phosphorus and sleep-promoting tryptophan. Since Onions contain only 61 calories per one cup serving, they are an ideal food for healthy weight control.

### HOW TO BRING OUT THE HIDDEN HEALTH BENEFITS OF ONIONS

Onions are a wonderful reservoir of many important nutrients. Not only are they a concentrated source of vitamin C, vitamin B6, chromium and the flavonoid quercetin, but they also contain important phytonutrients known as allyl sulfides. These sulfur-containing phytonutrients are the compounds that give the Onions so many of their health-promoting qualities. Among these phytonutrients are those known as alliin and ajeone as well as the allyl propyl disulfides including allicin, diallyl disulfide and diallyl trisulfide.

The striking difference in flavor and aroma that exists between cooked and raw Onions is largely due to the effect of cooking on the allyl sulfide phytonutrients; not only do they contribute to the Onion's nutritional qualities, but they also give them their pungent flavor and aroma. Thanks to scientific research, we have learned tips on how we can best cook Onions so as to maximize their sulfur-containing phytonutrient profile.

The latest scientific research tells us that slicing, chopping or mincing Onions before cooking will enhance their health-promoting properties. A sulfur-based compound called alliin and an enzyme called *alliinase* are separated in the Onion's cell structure when it is whole. Cutting Onion ruptures the cells and releases these elements, allowing them to come in contact with each other to form a powerful new compound called thiopropanal sulfoxide. This new compound not only increases Onions' health-promoting properties but is also the culprit behind their pungent aroma and the cause of the eye irritation that results from cutting Onions.

The finer the Onion is cut, the more extensive is the transformation of the sulfur compounds. The stronger the smell and the more they affect your eyes, the more health-promoting nutrients they contain. So, the next time you cut your Onions, you will have a greater appreciation of their "irritating" effects, knowing that the pungent smell that makes you cry will also make you healthy!

To get the most health benefits from Onions, let them sit for a minimum of 5 minutes, optimally 10 minutes, after cutting, before eating or cooking. This will ensure the maximum synthesis of the sulfur compounds.

Heat will inactivate the effect of *alliinase*, which is why it is important to allow the Onions to sit for 5–10 minutes before cooking to give the enzyme ample opportunity to enhance the concentration of active phytonutrients in your Onions. Cooking at low or medium heat for short periods of time (up to 15 minutes) should not destroy the active phytonutrients since, once they are formed, they are fairly stable.

Heat can actually increase the breadth of sulfur-containing phytonutrients in Onions since it catalyzes some chemical reactions responsible for their creation. Yet, too much heat for too much time can also reduce the activity of the enzymes responsible for converting the sulfoxides into active sulfur-containing molecules. This is because some of these enzymes can become denatured at 158°F (70°C), which is likely to be lower than the temperatures used in most every method of cooking Onions. Therefore, exposing the Onions to the heat for as little time as possible during cooking, such as with methods like "Healthy Sauté," is critical as it will help to retain as much enzyme activity as possible while preserving the maximum amount of sulfur-containing molecules.

Research on garlic, a close relative of Onion, reinforces the validity of this practice. When crushed garlic was heated, its ability to inhibit cancer development in animals was blocked; yet, when the researchers allowed the chopped garlic to sit for 10 minutes before heating, anticancer activity was preserved.

# Mediterranean Feast in Minutes

*In Mediterranean Countries they know how to prepare tasty vegetables.
This is the reason why they enjoy them daily.*

## "Healthy Sautéed" Mediterranean Feast

*Try these great combinations of "Healthy Sautéed" vegetables that will make your meals quicker and easier to prepare because they share the same cooking time. Place the following combinations in the pan together. Toss with Mediterranean dressing, page 331 after cooking.*

- **3-MINUTE "HEALTHY SAUTÉED"**

  1 cup garden peas, 1 medium sliced summer squash (zucchini), 1 medium chopped tomato.

- **5-MINUTE "HEALTHY SAUTÉED"**

  1 medium head sliced red cabbage, 1 medium cauliflower (florets cut into quarters), 10 whole medium asparagus spears.

- **7-MINUTE "HEALTHY SAUTÉED"**

  1 medium sliced onion, 10 sliced crimini mushrooms, 1 medium sliced bell pepper. **Or** another good combination is 3 1/2-inch slices eggplant, 2 sliced leeks, 8 sliced shiitake mushrooms.

## "Healthy Steamed" Mediterranean Feast

*"Healthy Steaming" preserves the nutrients and enhances the flavor of vegetables. "Healthy Steam" these vegetables together and toss with Mediterranean dressing, page 331 after cooking.*

- **5-MINUTE "HEALTHY STEAMED"**

  1 lb broccoli, 2 medium sliced carrots, 2 cups of sliced collard greens or kale. **Or** corn on the cob, 1 medium head sliced green cabbage, 6 Brussels sprouts (cut into quarters).

  Another good combination is cooking 5-Minute "Healthy Steamed" onions, broccoli, collard greens and green beans together. If you like your onions and green beans soft, cook them 2 minutes before adding the other vegetables.

- **7-MINUTE "HEALTHY STEAMED"**

  2 cups cubed sweet potatoes or winter squash. Add 2 cups of sliced kale or collard greens for the last 5 minutes of cooking time. **SERVES 2**

## Mediterranean Feast with Seafood

*Fish and shellfish cook quickly and take only minutes to prepare depending on size and thickness. For a complete meal that takes only 3, 5 or 7 minutes, include "Healthy Sautéed" or "Healthy Steamed" seafood with your favorite Mediterranean Feast combination.*

**For 3-MINUTE** "Healthy Sautéed" or "Healthy Steamed" combinations: Use small shrimp, cod, salmon, flounder or thin sole fillets (less than 1/2-inch thick) and cook on top of 3-Minute vegetables.

**For 5-MINUTE** "Healthy Sautéed" or "Healthy Steamed" combinations: Use medium shrimp, cod, or salmon fillets (3/4-inch thick) and cook on top of 5-Minute vegetables.

**For 7-MINUTE** "Healthy Sautéed" or "Healthy Steamed" combinations: Use large Shrimp, salmon, or cod fillets (1-inch thick) and place on top of 7-Minute vegetables.

 * Make sure you **cover** the pan for the entire cooking time.

** For more details on the preparation of vegetables, see individual food chapters, page 85 or the Guide to the Healthiest Way of Cooking Vegetables, page 96.

Use any combination of vegetables that are prepared with the same cooking method to create a Feast that will suit your personal taste. If a vegetable you like requires a longer cooking time than the others, just begin by cooking it first and add the other vegetables when the appropriate number of minutes have elapsed. This is a great method to not only save time and energy but you will have all of your vegetables hot and ready to serve at the same time.

*NOTE: I recommend cutting your vegetables into equal size pieces to ensure even cooking. Also, when steaming carrots and Brussels sprouts, it is best to place them in the bottom of the steamer to help them cook evenly.*

# leeks

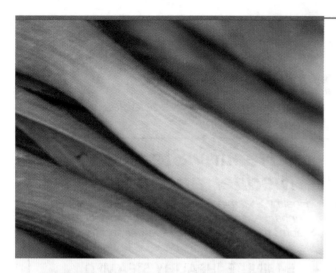

| | |
|---|---|
| AVAILABILITY: | Year-round |
| REFRIGERATE: | Yes |
| SHELF LIFE: | 7 days refrigerated |
| PREPARATION: | Cut and let sit for 5 minutes |
| BEST WAY TO COOK: | "Healthy Sautéed" in just 7 minutes |

## nutrient-richness chart

Total Nutrient-Richness: **6** GI: **15**
One-half cup (52 grams) of cooked Leeks contains 16 calories

| NUTRIENT | AMOUNT | %DV | DENSITY | QUALITY |
|---|---|---|---|---|
| Manganese | 0.1 mg | 6.5 | 7.3 | very good |
| Vitamin C | 2.2 mg | 3.6 | 4.1 | good |
| Iron | 0.6 mg | 3.2 | 3.5 | good |
| Folate | 12.6 mcg | 3.2 | 3.5 | good |
| B6 Pyridoxine | 0.1 mg | 3.0 | 3.3 | good |

For more on "Total Nutrient-Richness," "%DV," "Density," and
The World's Healthiest Foods "Quality" Rating System, see page 805.

For more on GI, see page 342.

Leeks have been cultivated in the Mediterranean region and Central Asia for thousands of years. The Greek philosopher Aristotle credited the clear voice of the partridge to a diet of Leeks, while the Roman emperor Nero supposedly ate Leeks every day to make his voice stronger.

## why leeks should be part of your healthiest way of eating

While Leeks are more delicate and milder in flavor than their cousins, onions and garlic, they are similiar to them in that they also contain health-protective, sulfur-containing phytonutrients, such as thiopropanal sulfoxides.

Although most of the research on *Allium* vegetables and their role in reducing the risk of atherosclerosis and heart disease has been conducted on onions and garlic, Leeks also appear to contain many of the same protective qualities.

## varieties of leeks

Leeks are in the same family as garlic, onions, shallots and scallions. Cultivated Leeks are the variety most commonly found in markets and the one featured in the photographs in this chapter. Ramps are wild Leeks that are a great delicacy, but they are very seasonal, only available in the spring.

## the peak season available year-round.

## biochemical considerations

Leeks are considered to have a small amount of oxalates, which might be of concern to certain individuals. (For more on *Oxalates*, see page 725.)

## the best way to select leeks

You can select the best tasting Leeks by looking for ones that are firm and straight with dark green leaves and long white necks. They should be between 1/2 and 1 inch in diameter.

Avoid Leeks that are yellow, wilted or have bulbs that are cracked or bruised. Also avoid overly large Leeks since they are generally more fibrous.

## the best way to store leeks

**LEEKS WILL REMAIN FRESH FOR UP TO 7 DAYS WHEN PROPERLY STORED**

Place Leeks in a plastic storage bag before refrigerating. I have found that it is best to wrap the bag tightly around the Leeks, squeezing out as much of the air from the bag as possible.

### Cleaning Leeks

After they are cut in half lengthwise, fan out the Leeks and rinse again. Do not wash Leeks before refrigeration because exposure to water will encourage your Leeks to spoil.

STEP-BY-STEP RECIPE

## The Healthiest Way of Cooking Leeks

# 7-Minute "Healthy Sautéed" Leeks

*In my search to find the healthiest way to cook Leeks, I tested every possible cooking method. I discovered that "Healthy Sautéing" Leeks for just 7 minutes delivered the best results.*

1 lb medium size Leeks
    (approximately 1/2 to 1 inch in diameter)
3 TBS + 2 TBS low-sodium chicken or
    vegetable broth
2 TBS extra virgin olive oil
1 tsp lemon juice
Sea salt and pepper to taste

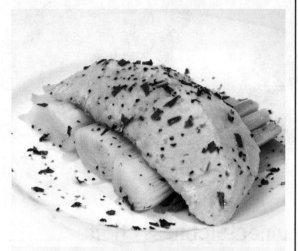

"Healthy Sautéed" Leeks with Salmon

1. Clean and slice Leeks very thin (1/8-inch), and let sit for at least 5 minutes. Do not use the green portion of the Leeks.
2. Heat 3 TBS broth over medium heat in a stainless steel skillet until it begins to steam.
3. Add Leeks, **cover**, and sauté for 4 minutes. Add 2 TBS broth, reduce heat to medium low and sauté for 3 minutes, **uncovered**, while stirring frequently. They are done when tender. "Healthy Sauté" will concentrate both the flavor and nutrition of Leeks.
4. Transfer to a bowl. For more flavor, toss Leeks with the remaining ingredients while they are still hot. Research shows that carotenoids found in foods are best absorbed when consumed with oils.

SERVES 2

**COOKING TIP:** To prevent overcooking Leeks, I highly recommend using a timer.

**Flavor Tips:** Try these 5 great serving suggestions with the recipe above. ✳

1. Top with grated Parmesan cheese.
2. Top with balsamic vinegar or your favorite vinaigrette.
3. Sprinkle with fresh grated ginger.
4. Dill and chives complement the flavor of Leeks.

5. **Quick Creamy Leek and Potato Soup:** In a blender, combine the 7-Minute "Healthy Sautéed" Leeks recipe and 1 cup steamed potatoes with 1 cup warm low-fat milk, 2 TBS Parmesan cheese and 1/2 tsp dill weed. Blend for 1 minute.

Please write (address on back cover flap) or e-mail me at info@whfoods.org with your personal ideas for preparing Leeks, and I will share them with others through our website at www.whfoods.org.

## An Easy Way to Prepare Leeks, Step-by-Step

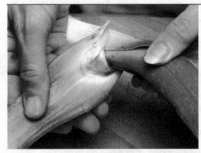
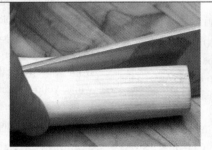
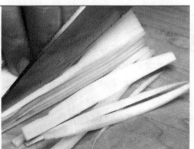

LEEKS, CUT LENGTHWISE

❶ Cut off green tops and roots of Leeks and remove outer tough leaves. ❷ Cut white, tender part of Leeks in half lengthwise. ❸ Cut the Leeks into about 2-inch lengths. Cut each 2-inch section lengthwise into very thin strips. Let them sit for 5–10 minutes to bring out *Hidden Health Benefits* (see pg 276).

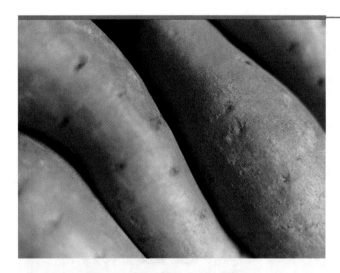

# sweet potatoes
## including yams

| | |
|---|---|
| AVAILABILITY: | Year-round |
| REFRIGERATE: | Not recommended |
| SHELF LIFE: | 1 month |
| PREPARATION: | Minimal |
| BEST WAY TO COOK: | "Healthy Steamed" in just 7 minutes |

## nutrient-richness chart

Total Nutrient-Richness: **13**          GI: **85**

One small (77 grams) baked Sweet Potato with skin contains 95 calories

| Nutrient | Amount | %DV | Density | Quality |
|---|---|---|---|---|
| Vitamin A | 13107.7 IU | 262.2 | 49.5 | excellent |
| Vitamin C | 17.1 mg | 28.4 | 5.4 | very good |
| Manganese | 0.5 mg | 26.0 | 4.9 | very good |
| Copper | 0.3 mg | 13.0 | 2.5 | good |
| Dietary Fiber | 3.1 g | 12.6 | 2.4 | good |
| B6 Pyridoxine | 0.3 mg | 12.5 | 2.4 | good |
| Potassium | 306.1 mg | 8.7 | 1.7 | good |
| Iron | 1.5 mg | 8.1 | 1.5 | good |

| CAROTENOIDS: | | |
|---|---|---|
| Alpha-Carotene | 86.0 mcg | Daily values for these nutrients have not yet been established. |
| Beta-Carotene | 23,018.0 mcg | |

For more on "Total Nutrient-Richness," "%DV," "Density," and The World's Healthiest Foods "Quality" Rating System, see page 805.

For more on GI, see page 342.

A lthough researchers have found Sweet Potato relics deep in Peruvian caves dating back 10,000 years, this delicious vegetable was not introduced to Europe until 1492 when Christopher Columbus brought it back from his voyage to the New World. Today, Sweet Potatoes are considered one of the most nutritious vegetables around. While they have become synonymous with the traditional Thanksgiving feast, I want to share with you the "Healthiest Way of Cooking" Sweet Potatoes that will not only maximize their nutritional value but also bring out the best of their unique sweet flavor, so that you will want to enjoy these great vegetables throughout the year.

## why sweet potatoes should be part of your healthiest way of eating

Sweet Potatoes are not just a sweet version of regular potatoes; they have a very different nutritional profile. Sweet Potatoes are exceptionally rich in beta-carotene, the carotenoid phytonutrient that not only provides their characteristic yellow/orange color, but also many of their health-promoting benefits. They also have unique root storage proteins that provide powerful antioxidant protection. Additionally, unlike potatoes, sweet potatoes do not belong to the nightshade family of vegetables. (For more on the *Health Benefits of Sweet Potatoes* and a complete analysis of their content of over 60 nutrients, see page 285.)

## varieties of sweet potatoes

Sweet Potatoes are native to Central America and are one of the oldest vegetables known to man. They have a characteristically starchy, sweet taste with the different varieties exhibiting unique flavor profiles. The flesh may range in color from white to yellow to orange; their skin colors may be white, yellow, orange, red or purple. Sweet Potatoes belong to the *Convolvulaceae* family of vegetables and are known by the scientific name *Ipomoea batatas*.

### BROWNISH-PURPLE-SKINNED SWEET POTATOES (OFTEN CALLED YAMS)

These Sweet Potatoes have a plump shape with soft, moist, orange-colored flesh when cooked. While they are typically called yams, they are not related to the "true yam" (members of the *Dioscoreae* family), a starchy root vegetable that plays an important role in the cuisines of South America, Africa, the Pacific Islands and the West Indies. Yams are typically the Sweet Potato varieties most commonly enjoyed at Thanksgiving. Distinct varieties include: CHRISTMAS BEAUREGARD—smooth skin and deep orange flesh; GARNETS—garnet-colored skin with orange-yellow flesh; and JEWELS—orange skin and deep orange flesh. The latter is the type of Sweet Potato featured in the photographs in this chapter.

### BEIGE-SKINNED SWEET POTATOES

These Sweet Potatoes are characterized by their yellow flesh. Varieties include NANCY HALL and JUICY YELLOW.

### PURPLE-SKINNED SWEET POTATOES

Known as Okinawan Sweet Potatoes, they are not as moist as other varieties. Their purple pigment provides extra health-promoting anthocyanin antioxidants.

## the peak season

Although Sweet Potatoes are available throughout the year, their peak season is November and December. These are the months when their concentration of nutrients and flavor are highest and their cost is at their lowest.

## biochemical considerations

Sweet Potatoes are a concentrated source of oxalates, which might be of concern to certain individuals. (For more on *Oxalates*, see page 725.)

## 4 steps for the best tasting and most nutritious sweet potatoes

Turning Sweet Potatoes into a flavorful dish with the most nutrients is simple if you just follow my 4 easy steps:

1. The Best Way to Select
2. The Best Way to Store
3. The Best Way to Prepare
4. The Healthiest Way of Cooking

# 1. the best way to select sweet potatoes ───

The best tasting Sweet Potatoes are ones that are firm and free of any cracks, bruises or soft spots. By selecting the best tasting Sweet Potatoes, you will also enjoy Sweet Potatoes with the highest nutritional value. As with all vegetables, I recommend selecting organically grown varieties whenever possible. (For more on *Organic Foods*, see page 113.)

Avoid Sweet Potatoes that are displayed in the refrigerated section of the produce department because the cold temperature negatively alters their taste. Be sure they have not sprouted and are not wrinkled.

# 2. the best way to store sweet potatoes ───

Sweet Potatoes are a sturdy vegetable that stores well. Yet, it is still important to store them properly to preserve their nutrients and flavor.

Sweet Potatoes continue to respire even after they have been harvested. Slowing down the respiration rate with proper storage is the key to extending their flavor and nutritional benefits. (For a *Comparison of Respiration Rates* for different vegetables, see page 91.)

### Sweet Potatoes Will Remain Fresh for Up to 1 Month When Properly Stored

Sweet Potatoes should not be stored in the refrigerator as they will develop an undesirable taste. The refrigerator's temperature (about 40°F, or 4°C) isn't the problem since Sweet Potatoes like temperatures ranging from 40°–45°F (4°–7,C); that's why they

are so happy in root cellars. It is the moisture of the refrigerator that can be a problem for Sweet Potatoes since it increases the conversion of some of their starches into sugars. Moisture, as well as light, will also encourage Sweet Potatoes to sprout, which is another reason why a very cool, dark, dry place like a root cellar is the perfect place for storing these root vegetables.

If you don't have a root cellar, it is best to store loose Sweet Potatoes in a cool, dark and well-ventilated cupboard where they will keep fresh for one month. Do not store in plastic bags. Exposure to sunlight or temperatures above 60°F (15°C) will cause them to sprout and ferment.

### How to Store Cooked Sweet Potatoes

Place cooked Sweet Potatoes in an airtight container in the refrigerator; they will keep for several days.

# 3. the best way to prepare sweet potatoes

Properly cleaning and cutting Sweet Potatoes will help to ensure that they have the best flavor and retain the greatest number of nutrients.

### Cleaning and Peeling Sweet Potatoes

Rinse them thoroughly under cold running water. (See *Washing Vegetables*, page 92.)

If you purchase organically grown Sweet Potatoes, you can enjoy both the flesh and skin. If you buy conventionally grown Sweet Potatoes, it is best to peel them before eating to avoid pesticide residues and the dye or wax with which they are sometimes treated.

### Prevent Sweet Potatoes From Turning Brown

To prevent Sweet Potatoes from turning brown after cutting, place them in two cups of water combined with one tablespoon of lemon juice.

### Cutting Sweet Potatoes

Cutting Sweet Potatoes into small pieces will help them to cook more quickly, while cutting them into equal size pieces will help them to cook more evenly. I recommend cutting them into 1/2-inch cubes.

# 4. the healthiest way of cooking sweet potatoes

Since research has shown that important nutrients can be lost or destroyed by the way a food is cooked, the "Healthiest Way of Cooking" Sweet Potatoes is focused on bringing out the best flavor while maximizing their vitamins, minerals and powerful antioxidants.

### The Healthiest Way of Cooking Sweet Potatoes: "Healthy Steaming" for just 7 Minutes

In my search to find the healthiest way to cook Sweet Potatoes, I tested every possible cooking method and discovered that "Healthy Steaming" 1/2-inch cubes of Sweet Potatoes for just 7 minutes delivered the best results. "Healthy Steaming" Sweet Potatoes makes them tender, brings out their best flavor and maximizes their nutritional profile. The Step-by-Step Recipe will show you how

easy it is to "Healthy Steam" Sweet Potatoes. (For more on *"Healthy Steaming,"* see page 58.)

### How to Avoid Overcooking Sweet Potatoes

Overcooked Sweet Potatoes will lose their flavor. "Healthy Steamed" Sweet Potatoes are tender, have the best flavor and are cooked just long enough to soften their cellulose and hemicellulose. This makes them easier to digest and allows their health-promoting nutrients to become more readily available for assimilation.

### Cooking Methods Not Recommended for Sweet Potatoes
**BOILING OR COOKING WITH OIL**

Boiling Sweet Potatoes increases their water absorption, (Continued on Page 284)

(Continued on Page 284)

---

**An Easy Way to Prepare Sweet Potatoes, Step-by-Step**

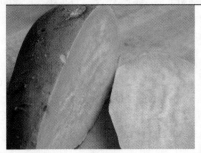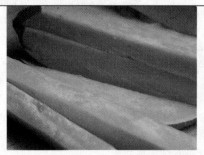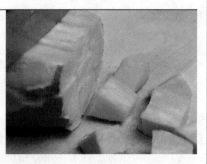

CUBED SWEET POTATOES
❶ Cut a slice lengthwise off one side of the Sweet Potato and turn it so that it lies flat. Cut it lengthwise into 1/2-inch slices.
❷ Stack a few slices on top of each other and cut the width of the Sweet Potato lengthwise again into 1/2-inch strips.
❸ Turn Sweet Potato so you can now make 1/2-inch wide cuts across the lengthwise strips to create 1/2-inch cubes.

STEP-BY-STEP RECIPE
## The Healthiest Way of Cooking Sweet Potatoes

# 7-Minute "Healthy Steamed" Sweet Potatoes

*Boiled Sweet Potatoes get watery and lose their flavor. I discovered that "Healthy Steaming" Sweet Potatoes not only takes just 7 minutes but also enhances their flavor and preserves their nutrients.*

**2 medium Sweet Potatoes**
**3 TBS extra virgin olive oil**
**2 medium cloves garlic**
**Sea salt and pepper to taste**

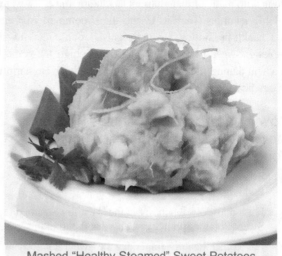
Mashed "Healthy Steamed" Sweet Potatoes

1. Fill the bottom of the steamer with 2 inches of water.
2. While steam is building up, chop or press garlic and let sit for at least 5 minutes. (Why?, see page 261.)
3. Cut Sweet Potatoes into 1/2-inch cubes.
4. Steam for 7 minutes. Sweet Potatoes are done when you can easily penetrate them with a fork. (For information on *Differences in Cooking Time,* see page 94.)

5. Transfer to a bowl. For more flavor, toss Sweet Potatoes with the remaining ingredients while they are still hot. Research shows that carotenoids found in foods are best absorbed when consumed with oils.

**OPTIONAL:** To mellow the flavor of garlic, add garlic to Sweet Potatoes for the last 2 minutes of steaming.

**SERVES 2**

**COOKING TIPS:**
• To prevent overcooking Sweet Potatoes, I highly recommend using a timer.
• Testing Sweet Potatoes with a fork is an effective way to determine whether they are done.

## Flavor Tips: Try these 6 great serving suggestions with the recipe above. ✳

1. **Most Popular:** Top with chopped fresh rosemary and ground pumpkin seeds. (Grind pumpkin seeds in coffee grinder or blender.)
2. Cinnamon, cloves and nutmeg all complement the flavor of Sweet Potatoes.
3. For spicy Sweet Potatoes, combine with 1–2 tsp mashed canned chipotle peppers.
4. **Mashed "Healthy Steamed" Sweet Potatoes:** For mashed sweet potatoes, peel potatoes before steaming. Mash cooked potatoes with potato masher, and stir in remaining ingredients (pictured above).
5. **Sweet Potatoes and Black Beans:** Combine the 7-Minute "Healthy Steamed" Sweet Potatoes recipe with one 15-oz can black beans and 1 tsp cumin powder. Top with 2 TBS goat cheese.
6. **Sweet Potato Pudding:** Make the 7-Minute "Healthy Steamed" Sweet Potatoes using two Sweet Potatoes. Omit olive oil, garlic and salt. Combine

1/4 cup honey or maple syrup, 1 tsp pumpkin pie spice, 1/2 tsp nutmeg, 3 TBS extra virgin olive oil and cooked Sweet Potatoes. Whip until creamy with a hand mixer. Put in individual dessert dishes and garnish with chopped toasted pecans.

**RICH, FLAVORFUL RECIPE FOR SWEET POTATOES**

• **"Slow Baked" Sweet Potatoes:** Wash 2 Sweet Potatoes and pierce with a fork or knife before baking to allow steam to escape and prevent the Sweet Potatoes from bursting. Place in a 400°F (200°C) degree oven for 45–60 minutes. Check for doneness by squeezing. There will be a slight give to the Sweet Potato when it is done. Dress with 3 TBS extra virgin olive oil, 1 tsp rosemary, and salt and pepper to taste. Recipe serves 2. (If you cut the Sweet Potatoes in half, the receipe will take half the time.)

Please write (address on back cover flap) or e-mail me at info@whfoods.org with your personal ideas for preparing Sweet Potatoes, and I will share them with others through our website at www.whfoods.org.

*(Continued from Page 282)*

causing them to become soggy and lose much of their flavor along with many of their nutrients including minerals, water-soluble vitamins (such as C and the B-complex vitamins) and health-promoting phytonutrients. I don't recommend cooking Sweet Potatoes in oil because high temperature heat can damage delicate oils and potentially create harmful free radicals.

### How to Include the 7-Minute "Healthy Steamed" Sweet Potatoes as Part of Your Lunch or Dinner, or Even Breakfast

- Like dessert for breakfast? Try the Sweet Potato Pudding.

- For a nutritious lunch, serve the "Healthy Steamed" Sweet Potatoes with Swiss chard and pumpkin seeds.

- For a quick healthy dinner, try the Sweet Potatoes and' Black Beans with brown rice.

Here are questions I received from readers of the whfoods.org website about Sweet Potatoes:

### Q *Are Sweet Potatoes just orange-colored regular potatoes?*

A Sweet Potatoes and regular potatoes are completely different foods. In fact, they are not even in the same botanical family; Sweet Potatoes belong to the *Convolvulaceae* plant family, while the potato belongs to the *Solanaceae* family. While each is an important vegetable, deserving of a place in a healthy diet, these two foods feature different tastes and unique nutritional benefits. Sweet potatoes are considered an "anti-diabetic food," offering a host of nutrients and an impressive array of antioxidants. They taste delicious, are easy to prepare and can be used in a variety of dishes, even in some that call for white potatoes. And, unlike regular potatoes, Sweet Potatoes are not considered a nightshade vegetable and therefore are not of the same concern for those who need to limit their consumption of these types of foods.

### Q *Is the sweetness of Sweet Potatoes a concern for those who worry about their blood sugar?*

A Actually, Sweet Potatoes may be more supportive of blood sugar regulation than regular white potatoes, even though they are sweeter. The "sweet" part of the Sweet Potato is fascinating from a health perspective. Without a doubt, cooked Sweet Potatoes taste sweeter than cooked "white" potatoes. Usually when one food tastes sweeter than another, it's because it contains more sugar, which also gives it the potential to make our blood sugar

less stable. With sweet versus regular potatoes, it's exactly the opposite. Sweet Potatoes, despite their sweetness, appear to act almost like an "anti-diabetic" food in some respects and do not appear to place our blood sugar at risk as much as their more common counterpart.

This "blood-sugar-friendly" character of Sweet Potato seems related to two aspects of its composition. First, Sweet Potatoes are about twice as high in dietary fiber as ordinary Russet Burbank white baking potatoes, and this doubled fiber slows down digestion and the release of sugar. Second, Sweet Potatoes have actually been examined in the lab for their specific "anti-diabetic" effects. In a laboratory animal study, Sweet Potatoes were shown to be comparable to a prescription drug in enhancing the effectiveness of insulin under certain circumstances.

### Q *I am trying to eat foods rich in antioxidants. Should I include Sweet Potatoes in my diet?*

A Sweet Potatoes actually feature many antioxidant nutrients. They are a concentrated source of vitamin C, as well as an excellent source of vitamin A, in the form of beta-carotene. The vitamin C and beta-carotene in the Sweet Potatoes work as powerful antioxidants to help eliminate free radicals, molecules that damage cells and cell membranes, and that are associated with the development of conditions such as colon cancer, atherosclerosis and diabetic heart disease.

Yet, the antioxidant profile of Sweet Potatoes extends even further. Some of the proteins found in Sweet Potatoes, usually referred to as root storage proteins, have been found to have antioxidant activity. In fact, one of the compounds studied has been shown to be about one-third as active as glutathione, one of the most active antioxidant compounds in the body. So yes, if you're looking to boost the antioxidant potential of your body, Sweet Potatoes would be a sweet addition.

---

### SWEET POTATOES ARE NOT A SWEET VERSION OF REGULAR POTATOES

Sweet Potatoes are an entirely different vegetable than regular potatoes. Sweet Potatoes do not contain nightshade alkaloids and belong to the *Convolvulaceae* family unlike regular potatoes, which are members of the *Solanaceae* family. Regular potatoes and their cousins, including tomatoes, eggplants and peppers, are referred to as nightshade vegetables. Individuals sensitive to the alkaloid compounds found in nightshade vegetables may find that Sweet Potatoes are a good substitute in recipes calling for regular potatoes.

# health benefits of sweet potatoes

## Promote Blood Sugar Balance

Sweet Potatoes have been recently classified as an "anti-diabetic" food. They have been given this label because of recent animal studies in which Sweet Potatoes helped stabilize blood sugar levels and lowered insulin resistance. Some of Sweet Potatoes' blood sugar regulatory properties may come from their concentration of carotenoids, such as beta-carotene. Research has suggested that physiological levels, as well as dietary intake, of carotenoids may be inversely associated with insulin resistance and high blood sugar levels. More research is needed in this area, but the stage is set for Sweet Potatoes to show unique healing properties in the area of blood sugar control.

## Promote Antioxidant Protection

Sweet Potatoes are rich in many nutrients that have antioxidant activity. They are an excellent source of vitamin A (through their concentration of beta-carotene) and a very good source of vitamin C. They are also a good source of both copper and manganese, minerals that are cofactors of *superoxide dismutase*, one of the body's most powerful antioxidant enzymes. Recent research has also found that Sweet Potatoes have unique root storage proteins that may offer protection against oxidative damage. In one study, these proteins had about one-third the antioxidant activity of glutathione—one of the body's most impressive internally produced antioxidants.

## Promote Lung Health

Vitamin A has long been known to be associated with healthy lungs. That is because it is needed to maintain the optimal structure and function of the tissues that line the lungs.

Recent research further supports this, finding a relationship between vitamin A, smoking and lung health. Experimental animals fed a vitamin A-deficient diet have been found to develop the lung condition, emphysema. When animals were exposed to cigarette smoke, not only did they develop emphysema, but their vitamin A levels decreased (it turns out that a common carcinogen in smoke, benzo(a)pyrene, causes vitamin A deficiency). In another study, smoke-exposed laboratory animals given a vitamin A-rich diet had less emphysema than those given the standard diet. From this research, all results point to the importance of vitamin A-rich foods, like Sweet Potatoes, in the diets of everyone concerned about protecting their lung health, especially smokers.

## Additional Health-Promoting Benefits of Sweet Potatoes

Sweet Potatoes are also a concentrated source of many other nutrients providing additional health-promoting benefits. These nutrients include energy-producing iron, heart-healthy vitamin B6 and potassium, and digestive-health-promoting dietary fiber.

### Nutritional Analysis of 1 small baked Sweet Potato with skin:

| NUTRIENT | AMOUNT | % DAILY VALUE | NUTRIENT | AMOUNT | % DAILY VALUE |
|---|---|---|---|---|---|
| Calories | 95.39 | | Pantothenic Acid | 0.54 mg | 5.4 |
| Calories from Fat | 0.75 | | | | |
| Calories from Saturated Fat | 0.17 | | **Minerals** | | |
| Protein | 1.76 g | | Boron | — mcg | |
| Carbohydrates | 22.38 g | | Calcium | 22.58 mg | 2.26 |
| Dietary Fiber | 3.14 g | 12.56 | Chloride | — mg | |
| Soluble Fiber | 1.01 g | | Chromium | — mcg | — |
| Insoluble Fiber | 1.46 g | | Copper | 0.26 mg | 13.00 |
| Sugar - Total | 16.34 g | | Fluoride | — mg | — |
| Monosaccharides | — g | | Iodine | — mcg | — |
| Disaccharides | — g | | Iron | 1.46 mg | 8.11 |
| Other Carbs | 2.90 g | | Magnesium | 19.29 mg | 4.82 |
| Fat - Total | 0.08 g | | Manganese | 0.52 mg | 26.00 |
| Saturated Fat | 0.02 g | | Molybdenum | — mcg | — |
| Mono Fat | 0.00 g | | Phosphorus | 50.14 mg | 5.01 |
| Poly Fat | 0.04 g | | Potassium | 306.05 mg | |
| Omega-3 Fatty Acids | 0.01 g | 0.40 | Selenium | 0.54 mcg | 0.77 |
| Omega-6 Fatty Acids | 0.03 g | | Sodium | 9.56 mg | |
| Trans Fatty Acids | 0.00 g | | Zinc | 0.26 mg | 1.73 |
| Cholesterol | 0.00 mg | | | | |
| Water | 51.77 g | | **Amino Acids** | | |
| Ash | 1.46 g | | Alanine | 0.10 g | |
| | | | Arginine | 0.08 g | |
| **Vitamins** | | | Aspartate | 0.30 g | |
| Vitamin A IU | 13107.70 IU | 262.15 | Cystine | 0.01 g | 2.44 |
| Vitamin A RE | 1310.69 RE | | Glutamate | 0.17 g | |
| A – Carotenoid | 1310.70 RE | 17.48 | Glycine | 0.08 g | |
| A – Retinol | 0.00 RE | | Histidine | 0.03 g | 2.33 |
| B1 Thiamin | 0.06 mg | 4.00 | Isoleucine | 0.09 g | 7.83 |
| B2 Riboflavin | 0.09 mg | 5.29 | Leucine | 0.13 g | 5.14 |
| B3 Niacin | 0.88 mg | 4.40 | Lysine | 0.09 g | 3.83 |
| Niacin Equiv | 1.24 mg | | Methionine | 0.04 g | 5.41 |
| Vitamin B6 | 0.25 mg | 12.50 | Phenylalanine | 0.11 g | 9.24 |
| Vitamin B12 | 0.00 mcg | 0.00 | Proline | 0.08 g | |
| Biotin | — mcg | — | Serine | 0.09 g | |
| Vitamin C | 17.06 mg | 28.43 | Threonine | 0.09 g | 7.26 |
| Vitamin D IU | 0.00 IU | 0.00 | Tryptophan | 0.02 g | 6.25 |
| Vitamin D mcg | 0.00 mcg | | Tyrosine | 0.07 g | 7.22 |
| Vitamin E Alpha Equiv | 0.17 mg | 0.85 | Valine | 0.11 g | 7.48 |
| Vitamin E IU | 0.26 IU | | | | |
| Vitamin E mg | 0.17 mg | | (Note: "–" indicates data is | | |
| Folate | 17.23 mcg | 4.31 | unavailable. For more information, | | |
| Vitamin K | — mcg | — | please see page 806.) | | |

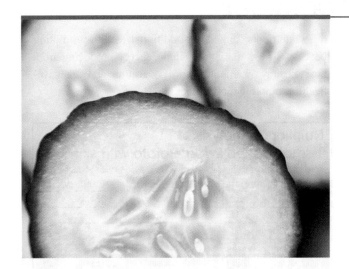

# cucumbers

## highlights

| | |
|---|---|
| AVAILABILITY: | Year-round |
| REFRIGERATE: | Yes |
| SHELF LIFE: | 10 days refrigerated |
| PREPARATION: | Minimal and needs no cooking |

## nutrient-richness chart

Total Nutrient-Richness: **11**   GI: **15**

One cup (104 grams) of raw Cucumber contains 14 calories

| NUTRIENT | AMOUNT | %DV | DENSITY | QUALITY |
|---|---|---|---|---|
| Vitamin C | 5.5 mg | 9.2 | 12.2 | very good |
| Molybdenum | 5.2 mcg | 6.9 | 9.2 | very good |
| Vitamin A | 223.6 IU | 4.5 | 6.0 | good |
| Potassium | 149.8 mg | 4.3 | 5.7 | good |
| Manganese | 0.1 mg | 4.0 | 5.3 | good |
| Folate | 13.5 mcg | 3.4 | 4.5 | good |
| Dietary Fiber | 0.8 g | 3.3 | 4.4 | good |
| Tryptophan | 0.01 g | 3.1 | 4.2 | good |
| Magnesium | 11.4 mg | 2.9 | 3.8 | good |
| **CAROTENOIDS:** | | | Daily values for this nutrient have not yet been established. | |
| Beta-Carotene | 131.0 mcg | | | |

For more on "Total Nutrient-Richness," "%DV," "Density," and
The World's Healthiest Foods "Quality" Rating System, see page 805.

For more on GI, see page 342.

Cucumbers were thought to have originated over 10,000 years ago in southern Asia and were introduced to India and other parts of Asia by early explorers and travelers. The popularity of Cucumbers dates back to the ancient civilizations of Egypt, Greece and Rome, where they were used not only as a food, but were also held in high esteem for their skin healing properties. Although it is unlikely that "cool as a Cucumber" was a popular phrase in ancient times, it is highly likely that their unique moisture levels and cooling properties were very much appreciated. Crunchy, refreshing and nutritious, Cucumbers are easy to prepare. Serve as an appetizer with your favorite dip or as an addition to almost any salad.

## why cucumbers should be part of your healthiest way of eating

High in nutrients, low in calories and very filling, Cucumbers are an ideal food to add to your "Healthiest Way of Eating," and with one cup of Cucumbers containing only 14 calories, they are also an excellent choice for healthy weight control. Scientific research has also identified phytonutrient compounds in Cucumbers, such as caffeic acid, which help soothe irritated skin and reduce swelling, confirming the ancient wisdom that Cucumbers are truly good for the skin. (For more on the *Health Benefits of Cucumbers* and a complete analysis of their content of over 60 nutrients, see page 290.)

## varieties of cucumbers

Scientifically known as *Cucumis sativus*, Cucumbers are grown to be enjoyed fresh or used for pickling. Louis XIV was very fond of Cucumbers, and it was during his reign that the greenhouse cultivation of Cucumbers originated. While it is unknown when the pickling process was developed, researchers speculate that the gherkin variety of Cucumber used for pickling was developed from a plant native to Africa.

### COMMON CUCUMBERS
### (ALSO KNOWN AS SLICING CUCUMBERS)

This variety is cultivated to be eaten fresh. They are cylindrical in shape and can vary greatly in size, although they most commonly range from six to nine inches in length and are larger in diameter than English Cucumbers. They have thick, dark green skin that may be either smooth or ridged. The flesh of the Cucumber is very pale green and has a dense, aqueous and crunchy texture. The center is comprised of numerous fleshy edible seeds. This is the variety most commonly found in markets and the one featured in the photographs in this chapter. Conventionally grown varieties are commonly waxed to extend their shelf life; organically grown Cucumbers are not waxed.

### ENGLISH CUCUMBERS
#### (ALSO KNOWN AS EUROPEAN CUCUMBERS)
Sometimes called Hothouse Cucumbers, this variety is grown in greenhouses. They are almost always seedless, have thinner skins and are longer in length (usually between 12 and 20 inches) than most other varieties. They are often referred to as "burpless" Cucumbers since people find them easier to digest than other varieties.

### PICKLING CUCUMBERS
These are commonly called gherkins. They are a smaller, squatter variety developed for pickling that have bumpy light green skins. Pickled Cucumbers have a high sodium content with 4 ounces of pickled Cucumbers containing over 1,500 mg of sodium.

### JAPANESE CUCUMBERS
They are long and slender with wart-like bumps and few seeds.

### ARMENIAN CUCUMBERS
This variety is very crisp and has pale green skin, soft seeds and curled ends.

### SFRAN CUCUMBERS
These are extra crisp, compact Cucumbers from the Persian Gulf.

## the peak season
Although Cucumbers are available throughout the year, their peak season is from May through July. These are the months when their concentration of nutrients and flavor are highest and their cost is at its lowest.

## biochemical considerations
Conventionally grown Cucumbers often have a wax coating to help protect their surface and increase their shelf life. (For more on *Wax Coatings*, see page 732.)

## 3 steps to the best tasting and most nutritious cucumbers
Turning Cucumbers into a flavorful dish with the most nutrients is simple if you just follow my 3 easy steps:

1. The Best Way to Select
2. The Best Way to Store
3. The Best Way to Prepare

# 1. the best way to select cucumbers

As Cucumbers are very sensitive to heat, it is best to select Cucumbers displayed in the refrigerated section of your local market. The best tasting Cucumbers are firm, with rounded ends (except for the Armenian variety which should have curled ends) and a bright color that ranges from medium to dark green. I have found that thinner Cucumbers generally have fewer seeds than ones that are thick. By selecting the best tasting Cucumbers, you will also enjoy Cucumbers with the highest nutritional value.

As with all vegetables, I recommend selecting organically grown varieties whenever possible. The skin is the source of many nutrients and organically grown varieties can be enjoyed without concern about ingesting wax or any chemicals that may be trapped in the skin. (For more on *Organic Foods*, see page 113.)

Avoid Cucumbers that are yellow, puffy or those that have sunken water-soaked areas or are wrinkled at their tips. These may be indications that they are old or spoiled.

# 2. the best way to store cucumbers

Cucumbers will become soft and lose their freshness if not stored properly. If you are not planning to use Cucumbers immediately after you bring them home from the market, be sure to store them properly as they can lose up to 30% of some of their vitamins as well as much of their flavor.

Cucumbers continue to respire even after they have been harvested; their respiration rate at room temperature (68°F/20°C) is 31 mg/kg/hr. Slowing down the respiration rate with proper

storage is the key to extending their flavor and nutritional benefits. (For a *Comparison of Respiration Rates* for different vegetables, see page 91.)

### Cucumbers Will Remain Fresh for Up to 10 Days When Properly Stored

1. Store Cucumbers in the refrigerator. The colder temperature will slow the respiration rate, helping to pre-

serve their nutrients and keeping Cucumbers fresh for a longer period of time.

2. Place Cucumbers in a plastic storage bag before refrigerating. I have found that it is best to wrap the bag tightly around the Cucumbers, squeezing out as much of the air from the bag as possible.

3. Do not wash Cucumbers before refrigeration because exposure to water will encourage Cucumbers to spoil.

## How to Store Cut Cucumbers

If you need to store a Cucumber that has been cut, place it in a container with a well-sealed lid, or a plastic bag, and refrigerate. Since the vitamin C content starts to quickly degrade after it has been cut, you should use the remainder within a couple of days.

# 3. the best way to prepare cucumbers

Whether you are going to enjoy Cucumbers in a salad, as an appetizer or with a dip, I want to share with you the best way to prepare Cucumbers. Properly cleaning and cutting Cucumbers help to ensure that the Cucumbers you serve will have the best flavor and retain the greatest number of nutrients.

## Cleaning Cucumbers

Rinse Cucumbers under cold running water before slicing. (For more on *Washing Vegetables*, see page 92.)

## Cutting Cucumbers

There are many different ways to cut Cucumbers, depending on how you will be serving them:

**SLICED CUCUMBERS:** Cut off and discard ends and peel Cucumbers if they are not organically grown. Cut the Cucumber widthwise to achieve the desired thickness. For some salads, you will want thicker slices than others. If your salad will be sitting in dressing for awhile, it is best to slice the Cucumbers a little thicker, so that they don't get soggy.

**DICED CUCUMBERS:** To dice Cucumbers, first cut off ends and discard, then peel if they are not organically grown. Cut in half lengthwise, and using a small spoon, carefully scoop out the seeds. Take the hollowed Cucumber and cut strips lengthwise. Depending on the size you want, you can cut these strips either 1/4-inch or 1/2-inch wide. Turn Cucumber so that you can cut across strips again either 1/4-inch or 1/2-inch wide for cubes of the same size.

**SEEDS SCOOPED OUT AND SLICED:** Cut off and discard ends, then peel Cucumber if not organically grown. Cut in half lengthwise. Scoop out seeds with a small spoon, turn over and slice.

## Salting Cucumbers

Cucumbers are sometimes salted to draw out excess liquid. I don't recommend salting Cucumbers because they become limp and overly salty.

Here is a question I received from a reader of the whfoods.org website about Cucumbers:

**Q** *Does soaking Cucumbers in vinegar take away from the quality of the vegetable?*

**A** Soaking Cucumbers in vinegar will give them nice flavor, but if soaked for more than three to four minutes, the nutrients will begin to leach out into the vinegar, and they will also lose their nice, crisp texture.

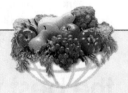

# how to enjoy fresh cucumbers in quick refreshing drinks

**Refreshing Pick-Me-Up Drink:** Combine peeled Cucumber and the flesh of your favorite melon in a blender. Blend for 1 minute. Serve in a chilled glass for a light start to the day or a mid-afternoon pick-me-up.

**Easy Summer Cooler:** In a large pitcher of water, place one whole organic lemon sliced very thin, a whole organic Cucumber sliced very thin, and a handful of mint leaves. Place in the refrigerator for 1 hour or more. You will be amazed how refreshing this is!

**Tangy Gazpacho:** Blend together until chunky: 1 Cucumber cut into large chunks, 3–4 tomatoes, 1 green bell pepper cut into chunks, 1/2 sliced red onion, 1 TBS red wine vinegar, 1/2 tsp red pepper flakes and sea salt to taste. For gazpacho that delivers extra vitamin C, add some orange or tangerine sections.

**STEP-BY-STEP RECIPE**

## The Healthiest Way of Preparing Cucumbers

# 5-Minute Cold Cucumber Salad

*Cucumbers are most often enjoyed in warm weather when they are served fresh and cold, providing refreshing enjoyment during the summer months. Cucumbers are best eaten raw in salads or served with dips.*

1 Cucumber
1 medium tomato or red bell pepper
1 small red onion

**Mediterranean Dressing:**
2 TBS extra virgin olive oil
2 tsp lemon juice or wine vinegar
1 medium clove garlic
Sea salt and pepper to taste
Optional: 2 TBS fresh or 1 tsp dried dill

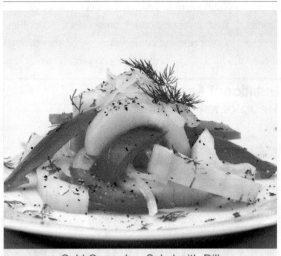

Cold Cucumber Salad with Dill

1. Slice onion, press garlic, and let sit for at least 5 minutes. (Why?, see page 276.)
2. Slice Cucumbers as described under *The Best Way to Prepare Cucumbers.*
3. Dice tomatoes, or slice bell pepper.
4. Combine onions, garlic, Cucumbers, and tomatoes or bell pepper in a bowl and dress with lemon juice or vinegar, garlic, olive oil, and salt and pepper to taste.

**SERVES 2**

---

**Flavor Tips:** Try these 6 great serving suggestions with the recipe above. ✱

1. **Most Popular: Greek Salad.** Add goat cheese or feta cheese, kalamata olives, green bell peppers and oregano to the 5-Minute Cold Cucumber Salad recipe. Increase lemon juice or vinegar and olive oil as needed. For a nutritious lunch or a quick, low-calorie dinner, serve the Greek Salad with your favorite entrée.

2. For a sweet and sour flavor replace lemon juice with 2 tsp balsamic vinegar.

3. Add 1 diced avocado to the recipe.

4. Add capers or chopped anchovies to the recipe.

5. **Asian Salad:** Replace lemon juice with rice vinegar, add 2 tsp tamari (soy sauce), 1/2 cup soaked hijiki (see page 311) and 2 TBS chopped fresh cilantro.

6. **Yogurt Cucumber Salad:** Combine the 5-Minute Cold Cucumber Salad recipe with non-fat plain yogurt, minced fresh mint, minced fennel rib, and red pepper flakes. Refrigerate for 1/2 hour. Stir and serve immediately.

---

Please write (address on back cover flap) or e-mail me at info@whfoods.org with your personal ideas for preparing Cucumbers, and I will share them with others through our website at www.whfoods.org.

---

## An Easy Way to Prepare Cucumbers, Step-by-Step

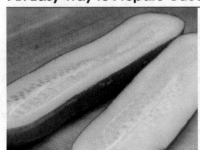 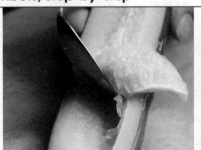 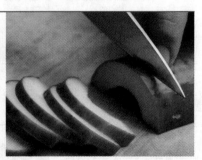

**DICED CUCUMBERS**
❶ Cut in half lengthwise. ❷ Cut off ends. Scoop out seeds using a small spoon ❸ Cut into 1/4-inch slices.

# health benefits of cucumbers

## Promote Healthy Skin

Cucumbers are known for their concentration of silica, a mineral that is an essential component of collagen. Therefore, Cucumber juice is often recommended as a source of silica to improve the complexion and health of the skin. Additionally, Cucumber's high water content makes it naturally hydrating—a must for glowing skin. Cucumbers are also used topically for various types of skin problems, including swelling under the eyes and sunburn. Two compounds in Cucumbers, vitamin C (of which they are a very good source) and the phytonutrient caffeic acid, prevent water retention; this may explain why Cucumbers applied topically are often helpful for swollen eyes, burns and dermatitis. Muscles, tendons, ligaments, cartilage and bone also have silica-containing connective tissue.

## Promote Healthy Weight Control

Like most vegetables, Cucumbers are a great food for people interested in losing weight or maintaining a healthy weight. This is because they are very nutrient rich. They contain many different nutrients but do not contain many calories—only 14 calories per cup! Since Cucumbers have such a high water content, they are satiating and refreshing.

## Promote Heart Health

Cucumbers are a good source of potassium, magnesium and fiber. When individuals following the DASH diet (low-fat dairy foods, seafood, lean meat and poultry) added more foods rich in these nutrients, their blood pressure dropped to healthier levels: they lowered their systolic blood pressure (the top number) by 5.5 points and their diastolic blood pressure (the bottom number) by 3.0 points. In addition, Cucumbers are also a good source of folate, a B vitamin critical to heart health because it helps to keep homocysteine levels in check.

## Promote Healthy Digestion

Trying to get adequate dietary fiber on a daily basis is a challenge for many Americans. Adding a crunchy, cool Cucumber to salads is an especially good way to increase fiber intake because Cucumbers come naturally prepackaged with the extra fluid needed when consuming more fiber. Fiber has many benefits including promoting healthy digestion.

## Additional Health-Promoting Benefits of Cucumbers

Cucumbers are also a concentrated source of many other nutrients providing additional health-promoting benefits. These nutrients include free-radical-scavenging vitamin A and manganese, sulfite-detoxifying molybdenum, and sleep-promoting tryptophan.

### Nutritional Analysis of 1 cup of raw Cucumbers:

| NUTRIENT | AMOUNT | % DAILY VALUE |
|---|---|---|
| Calories | 13.52 | |
| Calories from Fat | 1.22 | |
| Calories from Saturated Fat | 0.32 | |
| Protein | 0.72 g | |
| Carbohydrates | 2.87 g | |
| Dietary Fiber | 0.83 g | 3.32 |
| Soluble Fiber | 0.21 g | |
| Insoluble Fiber | 0.62 g | |
| Sugar – Total | 2.04 g | |
| Monosaccharides | 2.04 g | |
| Disaccharides | 0.00 g | |
| Other Carbs | 0.00 g | |
| Fat – Total | 0.14 g | |
| Saturated Fat | 0.04 g | |
| Mono Fat | 0.00 g | |
| Poly Fat | 0.06 g | |
| Omega-3 Fatty Acids | 0.03 g | 1.20 |
| Omega-6 Fatty Acids | 0.02 g | |
| Trans Fatty Acids | 0.00 g | |
| Cholesterol | 0.00 mg | |
| Water | 99.85 g | |
| Ash | 0.43 g | |

**Vitamins**

| NUTRIENT | AMOUNT | % DAILY VALUE |
|---|---|---|
| Vitamin A IU | 223.60 IU | 4.47 |
| Vitamin A RE | 21.84 RE | |
| A - Carotenoid | 21.84 RE | 0.29 |
| A - Retinol | 0.00 RE | |
| B1 Thiamin | 0.02 mg | 1.33 |
| B2 Riboflavin | 0.02 mg | 1.18 |
| B3 Niacin | 0.23 mg | 1.15 |
| Niacin Equiv | 0.32 mg | |
| Vitamin B6 | 0.04 mg | 2.00 |
| Vitamin B12 | 0.00 mcg | 0.00 |
| Biotin | 0.94 mcg | 0.31 |
| Vitamin C | 5.51 mg | 9.18 |
| Vitamin D IU | 0.00 IU | 0.00 |
| Vitamin D mcg | 0.00 mcg | |
| Vitamin E Alpha Equiv | 0.08 mg | 0.40 |
| Vitamin E IU | 0.12 IU | |
| Vitamin E mg | 0.26 mg | |
| Folate | 13.52 mcg | 3.38 |
| Vitamin K | — mcg | — |

| NUTRIENT | AMOUNT | % DAILY VALUE |
|---|---|---|
| Pantothenic Acid | 0.19 mg | 1.90 |

**Minerals**

| NUTRIENT | AMOUNT | % DAILY VALUE |
|---|---|---|
| Boron | — mcg | |
| Calcium | 14.56 mg | 1.46 |
| Chloride | — mg | |
| Chromium | — mcg | — |
| Copper | 0.03 mg | 1.50 |
| Fluoride | — mg | — |
| Iodine | — mcg | — |
| Iron | 0.27 mg | 1.50 |
| Magnesium | 11.44 mg | 2.86 |
| Manganese | 0.08 mg | 4.00 |
| Molybdenum | 5.20 mcg | 6.93 |
| Phosphorus | 20.80 mg | 2.08 |
| Potassium | 149.76 mg | |
| Selenium | 0.00 mcg | 0.00 |
| Sodium | 2.08 mg | |
| Zinc | 0.21 mg | 1.40 |

**Amino Acids**

| NUTRIENT | AMOUNT | % DAILY VALUE |
|---|---|---|
| Alanine | 0.02 g | |
| Arginine | 0.05 g | |
| Aspartate | 0.04 g | |
| Cystine | 0.00 g | 0.00 |
| Glutamate | 0.20 g | |
| Glycine | 0.02 g | |
| Histidine | 0.01 g | 0.78 |
| Isoleucine | 0.02 g | 1.74 |
| Leucine | 0.03 g | 1.19 |
| Lysine | 0.03 g | 1.28 |
| Methionine | 0.01 g | 1.35 |
| Phenylalanine | 0.02 g | 1.68 |
| Proline | 0.02 g | |
| Serine | 0.02 g | |
| Threonine | 0.02 g | 1.61 |
| Tryptophan | 0.01 g | 3.13 |
| Tyrosine | 0.01 g | 1.03 |
| Valine | 0.02 g | 1.36 |

(Note: "–" indicates data is unavailable. For more information, please see page 806.)

**Q** *If I use a veggie wash to clean my conventionally grown Cucumbers, will it remove the wax coating?*

**A** From my experience and understanding, the only real way to get the wax off of the the skin of Cucumbers, as well as other vegetables and fruits, is to remove the skin by peeling. While there are many produce washes and sprays available in the marketplace that make claims about removing waxes (as well as pesticides), I have yet to see any published research in the scientific literature supporting these claims. By the way, organically grown Cucumbers should not have a wax coating, so you may want to see if your market sells them.

---

## Q&A

### WHAT DO YOU DO WHEN YOU CAN'T BUY ORGANIC FOODS?

As you know, I am a strong supporter of organic farming, and I encourage you to purchase organically grown foods whenever possible. But what should you do when it's not possible to buy organic? Here are some recommendations:

1. Make sure you've exhausted all of your local options. Check farmer's markets, community-supported farms, even roadside food stands. Locally grown foods may or may not be lower in pesticides and other contaminants, but it's easy enough to ask, and you may be surprised how many local growers you'll find within driving distance and how close to organic some of their foods may turn out to be. Sometimes local growers simply don't have the money to fund an organic certification process, even though they practice organic techniques in the way they grow their crops.

2. Talk to your local grocers. You may be surprised at their willingness to experiment with new foods, particularly if you are a patron of the store. In addition, ask questions about their conventionally grown produce and conventionally raised meats. These foods may turn out to be very different in terms of their quality. What information does the buyer have from the supplier? Can the buyer get more information? Could you contact the supplier yourself?

3. Shop online. There are many websites that offer a good selection of organic foods.

4. Read the ingredient lists on all non-organic food packaging. Although you cannot trust the terms "natural" or "all natural" on the front of the package, you can trust the ingredient lists to include most of the substances added to the food. Look for the terms "artificial flavor" and "artificial color." Also look for the FD&C colorings (for example, Yellow 5). Of course, you won't find pesticides, heavy metals or other potentially toxic residues listed on ingredient lists. But watching out for other potential toxins is still very worthwhile.

5. Rinse your produce thoroughly and use a vegetable brush to help remove potential toxins found on the surface of the food. If you don't have a water filter installed on your kitchen sink, consider installing one so that you can rinse your vegetables with high quality water.

6. Peel all waxed fruits. Also peel any fruits you know or suspect to be heavily sprayed.

7. Continue to use all of the other World's Healthiest Foods' principles in your food selection. For example, continue to choose 100% whole grain products, even when they are not organic. Similarly, continue to choose cold pressed olive oil, lean meats, cold-water fish and a wide variety of natural spices and seasonings.

8. Enjoy the delicious flavors and textures of your food. Even when you aren't able to buy organic, take satisfaction in the selections you've made and recognize the benefits of nutrient-rich, minimally processed foods—one-of-a-kind foods!

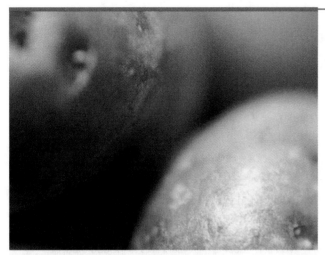

# potatoes

## highlights

| | |
|---|---|
| AVAILABILITY: | Year-round |
| REFRIGERATE: | Not recommended |
| SHELF LIFE: | 1 month for most varieties |
| PREPARATION: | Minimal |
| BEST WAY TO COOK: | "Healthy Steamed" in just 10 minutes |

## nutrient-richness chart

Total Nutrient-Richness: **8**     GI: **119**

One cup (122 grams) of baked Potato with skin contains 133 calories

| NUTRIENT | AMOUNT | %DV | DENSITY | QUALITY |
|---|---|---|---|---|
| Vitamin C | 15.7 mg | 26.2 | 3.6 | very good |
| B6 Pyridoxine | 0.4 mg | 21.0 | 2.8 | good |
| Copper | 0.4 mg | 18.5 | 2.5 | good |
| Potassium | 510.0 mg | 14.6 | 2.0 | good |
| Manganese | 0.3 mg | 14.0 | 1.9 | good |
| Tryptophan | 0.04 g | 12.5 | 1.7 | good |
| Dietary Fiber | 2.9 g | 11.7 | 1.6 | good |

| CAROTENOIDS: | | |
|---|---|---|
| Beta-Carotene | 7.3 mcg | Daily values for these nutrients have not yet been established. |
| Lutein+Zeaxanthin | 36.6 mcg | |

For more on "Total Nutrient Richness," "%DV," "Density," and The World's Healthiest Foods "Quality" Rating System, see page 805. For more on GI, see page 342.

Potatoes have been cultivated by South American Indians for over 4,000 years and have played an important role as a food source throughout history. Today, Potatoes remain relatively inexpensive and are the number one vegetable crop, not only in the United States, but throughout the world! When cooked properly, Potatoes can be surprisingly healthy, with a neutral starchy flavor that can complement many different types of food. That is why I would like to share with you the "Healthiest Way of Cooking" Potatoes. In just 10 minutes, you will have a healthy version of this popular vegetable that not only preserves its nutritional value but that features its best flavor.

## why potatoes should be part of your healthiest way of eating

Spanish explorers "discovered" that Potatoes helped prevent scurvy on their long oversea voyages, but what they did not know was that it was Potatoes' high concentration of vitamin C that prevented the disease. Today we know that vitamin C is the primary water-soluble antioxidant in the body, protecting against damage to cellular structures, including DNA. Potatoes' nutritional value, combined with their ready availability in almost any market, are among the reasons that they have been included as one of the World's Healthiest Foods. And remember that many of the health-promoting properties of Potatoes are found in the skin, so be sure to include the skin as a part of your "Healthiest Way of Eating." (For more on the *Health Benefits of Potatoes* and a complete analysis of their content of over 60 nutrients, see page 296.)

## varieties of potatoes

Potatoes (*Solanum tuberosum*) originated in the Andean mountain region of South America. The Potato belongs to the *Solanaceae* or nightshade family, which also includes tomatoes, eggplants, peppers and tomatillos. They are the swollen portion of an underground stem (called a tuber) and provide food for the green leafy portion of the plant. If allowed to flower and fruit, the Potato plant will bear an inedible fruit resembling a tomato.

There are approximately a hundred different varieties of edible Potatoes that feature a wide range of sizes, shapes, colors, starch contents and flavors. Most of those that we are familiar with belong to one of the following classifications:

### LONG RUSSETS

These are the favorite Potatoes for baking. They weigh up to 18 ounces and have a hard brown skin and starchy flesh. The RUSSET BURBANK is the most commonly grown variety of Long Russets.

### LONG WHITES

The WHITE ROSE is the most well-known of the Long Whites. They weigh up to one-half pound and have a thin waxy skin when mature.

### NEW POTATOES (OR ROUND REDS)

RED LESODA and RED PONTIAC are two varieties of New Potatoes. They are harvested before maturity and are small in size. They have smooth red skin and are good for boiling. This is the type of Potatoes featured in the photographs in this chapter.

### ROUND WHITES

These are multi-purpose Potatoes that are smaller than the Long Whites, weighing about one-third of a pound each. KATAHDIN is a popular Round White variety.

### OTHER VARIETIES

FINNISH YELLOW WAX Potatoes have a deep yellow flesh with a rich buttery flavor. The BLUE CARIB and ALL BLUE have grey-blue skin and dark blue flesh with a delicate flavor. Yellow Potatoes possess greater quantities of carotenoids, including beta-carotene, while the blue varieties contain more flavonoid anthocyanin phytonutrients.

## the peak season

Potatoes are available year-round as they are harvested somewhere in the United States every month of the year.

## biochemical considerations

Potatoes are considered to be a member of the nightshade family of vegetables, which might be of concern to certain individuals. Potatoes are also one of the 12 foods on which pesticide residues have been most frequently found and are also one of the foods most commonly associated with allergic reactions in individuals with latex allergies. Processed dehydrated and peeled raw Potatoes may contain sulfite preservatives. (For more on *Nightshades*, see page 723; *Pesticide Residues*, see page 726; *Latex Food Allergies*, see page 722; and *Sulfites*, see page 729.)

Care should be taken not to eat Potatoes that have sprouted or have a green coloration because they contain a compound known as solanine, a toxic alkaloid compound that not only imparts an undesirable taste, but may cause a host of different health conditions such as circulatory and respiratory depression, headaches and diarrhea. Cut away the affected area before preparing the Potatoes; if there is a large amount of greening and/or sprouting, discard the whole Potato.

## 4 steps for the best tasting and most nutritious potatoes

Turning Potatoes into a flavorful dish with the most nutrients is simple if you just follow my 4 easy steps:

1. The Best Way to Select
2. The Best Way to Store
3. The Best Way to Prepare
4. The Healthiest Way of Cooking

# 1. the best way to select potatoes

You can select the best tasting Potatoes by looking for ones that are firm, well-shaped and relatively smooth. I prefer to buy individually Potatoes from a bulk display rather than those that are prepackaged in plastic bags. Not only does this allow you to inspect the Potatoes for signs of decay or damage, but many times the plastic bags are not perforated, which causes a build up of moisture that can negatively affect the Potatoes. By selecting the best tasting Potatoes, you will also enjoy Potatoes with the highest nutritional value. As with all vegetables, I recommend selecting organically grown varieties whenever possible. This is especially important with Potatoes since their skin contains many nutrients. You can enjoy the skin without concern about pesticide residues and other contaminants that may remain on the skin if you select organically grown Potatoes. (For more on *Organic Foods*, see page 113.)

Avoid Potatoes that look decayed with wet or dry rot. In addition, they should not be sprouting or have green coloration since this indicates that they may contain the toxic alkaloid solanine.

New Potatoes are harvested before they are fully mature, making them much more susceptible to damage. Be especially careful when purchasing them, and look for ones that are free from discoloration and injury.

# 2. the best way to store potatoes

Although Potatoes are a hearty vegetable that store well, it is still important to use proper storage techniques in order to best preserve their flavor and nutrients.

Potatoes continue to respire even after they have been harvested. Slowing down the respiration rate with proper storage is the key to extending their flavor and nutritional benefits. (For a *Comparison of Respiration Rates* for different vegetables, see page 91.)

## Potatoes Will Remain Fresh for Up to 1 Month When Properly Stored

Potatoes should not be stored in the refrigerator as they will develop an undesirable taste. It isn't the temperature of the refrigerator (about 40°F/4°C) that's the problem since Potatoes like temperatures ranging from 40°–45°F (4°–7°C), which is why they are so happy in root cellars. The problem is the moisture in the refrigerator, which increases conversion of some of the Potatoes' starches to sugars and adversely affects their flavor. Both light and moisture will also encourage the Potatoes to sprout; once again, is why a very cool, dry, dark spot like a root cellar is the perfect place for storing Potatoes.

Place Potatoes in a burlap or paper bag, and store them in a cool, dark place. Keep them out of the light, as light will cause them to turn green. If you store them in a plastic bag, be sure that it is perforated to allow moisture to escape. It is also important not to store Potatoes near onions as the gases that they each emit will cause the degradation of both vegetables.

Check Potatoes frequently and remove any that have sprouted or shriveled since they can quickly affect the quality of the others. New Potatoes are much more perishable and will only keep for 1 week.

## How to Store Cooked Potatoes

Place cooked Potatoes in a tightly sealed container and store in the refrigerator where they will keep for several days.

# 3. the best way to prepare potatoes

Properly cleaning and cutting Potatoes will help to ensure that they have the best flavor and retain the greatest number of nutrients.

## Cleaning Potatoes

The Potato skin is a concentrated source of dietary fiber and many nutrients. If you purchase organically grown Potatoes, you can enjoy both the flesh and skin. Just scrub Potatoes under cold running water right before cooking and then remove any deep eyes or bruises with a paring knife. (For more on *Washing Vegetables*, see page 92.)

## Peeling Potatoes

If you buy conventionally grown Potatoes, it is best to not eat the peel in order to avoid pesticide residues and the dye or wax with which they are sometimes treated. If you peel them, do so carefully with a vegetable peeler, removing only a thin layer of the skin and therefore retaining the nutrients that lie just below the skin. Be sure to cut off any green portion of the Potato. But remember that even mashed Potatoes taste good with the peels, so if you use organically grown Potatoes, consider using the whole vegetable.

## Cutting Potatoes

Potatoes should be cleaned and cut right before cooking in order to avoid the discoloration that occurs with exposure to air. Be sure to remove any sprouted areas of the Potato before cutting. If you cannot cook them immediately after cutting, place them in a bowl of cold water with a little lemon juice (2 cups of water to 1 TBS of lemon juice) as this will prevent their flesh from darkening and will also help to maintain their shape during cooking.

Cutting Potatoes into small pieces will help them to cook more quickly, while cutting them into equal size pieces will help them to cook more evenly. I recommend cutting them into 1/2-inch cubes.

Here is a question I have received from a reader of the whfoods.org website about Potatoes:

**Q** *What should I do if my Potatoes start to sprout?*

**A** If Potatoes are stored for too long or not stored in ideal conditions, they can develop a green coloration or can begin to sprout. These changes reflect the accumulation of solanine, a toxic alkaloid compound that not only imparts an undesirable taste but can also cause a host of different health conditions such as circulatory and respiratory depression, headaches and diarrhea. Cut away the affected area before preparing the Potatoes; if there is a large amount of greening and/or sprouting, discard the whole Potato.

# 4. the healthiest way of cooking potatoes

Since research has shown that important nutrients can be lost or destroyed by the way a food is cooked, the "Healthiest Way of Cooking" Potatoes is focused on bringing out their best flavor while maximizing their vitamins, minerals and powerful antioxidants.

## The Healthiest Way of Cooking Potatoes: "Healthy Steaming" for Just 10 Minutes

In my search to find the healthiest way to cook Potatoes, I tested every possible cooking method and discovered that "Healthy Steaming" Potatoes (cut into 1/2-inch cubes) for just 10 minutes delivered the best result. "Healthy Steaming" makes Potatoes tender, brings out their best flavor and maximizes their nutritional profile. The Step-by-Step Recipe will show you how easy it is to "Healthy Steam" Potatoes. (For more on "*Healthy Steaming*," see page 58.)

## Slow Baked Potatoes

If you are looking for richer flavor from your Potatoes, I recommend baking. Pierce the Potato with a fork or knife before baking to allow steam to escape and prevent the Potato from bursting. Place in a 400°F (200°C) oven for 45–60 minutes. Check for doneness by squeezing. There will be a slight give to the Potato if it is done.

## How to Avoid Overcooking Potatoes

Overcooked Potatoes will lose their flavor, so for the best flavor, I recommend "Healthy Steaming" Potatoes (cut into 1/2-cubes) for just 10 minutes. "Healthy Steamed" Potatoes are tender and cooked just long enough to soften their cellulose and hemicellulose, which makes them easier to digest and allows their health-promoting nutrients to become more readily available for absorption.

## Cooking Methods Not Recommended for Potatoes

### BOILING OR COOKING WITH OIL

Boiling Potatoes increases their water absorption causing them to become soggy and lose much of their flavor along with many of their nutrients, including minerals, water-soluble vitamins (such as C and the B-complex vitamins) and health-promoting phytonutrients. I don't recommend cooking Potatoes in oil because high temperature heat can damage delicate oils and potentially create harmful free radicals.

---

### *Add Extra Flavor to Baked Potatoes*

- Liberally cover a baked Potato with spicy chili.

- Top baked Potatoes with "Healthy Sautéed" crimini mushrooms and extra virgin olive oil, instead of the usual butter and sour cream, and season with salt and pepper to taste.

- **Stuffed Potato:** Cut a cooked Potato in half and remove the flesh from each side saving the skin. In a bowl, mix the Potato flesh together with goat cheese, low-fat milk, dill weed, and sea salt and pepper to taste. Spoon back into the Potato skin and serve.

---

Here are questions I have received from readers of the whfoods.org website about Potatoes:

### Q *Are Potatoes a good food to eat for someone with blood sugar concerns?*

A Potatoes—whether they be baked, boiled or steamed—are considered to be moderately high glycemic index foods. Therefore, individuals concerned about maintaining balanced blood sugar levels should probably be careful about eating Potatoes. Potatoes should not be eaten alone or in a meal that has other high-carbohydrate foods or those that are not nutrient rich. Yet, if Potatoes are included as part of a meal that also features high-fiber, low-glycemic load foods (such as green vegetables) as well as protein foods, the impact on blood sugar of the overall meal will be less; therefore, this may be a way for people to still enjoy including some Potatoes in their Healthiest Way of Eating. For more on *Glycemic Index*, see page 342.

### Q *Can I store Potatoes in the refrigerator?*

A Potatoes are among the few vegetables that don't like to be stored in the refrigerator. It's not that the temperature of the refrigerator is the problem; in fact, Potatoes thrive in 40–45°F (4°–7°C) temperature, within the range which most refrigerators are set and the reason potatoes are so happy in a root cellar. The incompatibility between Potatoes and refrigerators has to do with the fact that refrigerators are moist environments, and the moisture increases the conversion of some of the Potato starches into sugar, giving them an undesirable taste and reducing their storage time. In addition, both moisture and light will encourage Potatoes to sprout, which is why a very cool, dark, dry place like a root cellar is the perfect place for storing Potatoes.

# health benefits of potatoes

## Ways to Promote Potatoes' Health-Promoting Benefits

Potatoes are a very popular food source. Unfortunately, most people eat Potatoes in the form of greasy French fries or Potato chips; even baked Potatoes are often loaded with fat-filled fixings. Such treatment can make even the healthy Potato—a concentrated source of vitamin B6, vitamin C, dietary fiber, potassium and many minerals—into a nemesis of good health. That's why it's important to serve Potatoes with healthy toppings.

## Promote Cellular Health

If only for its high concentration of vitamin B6—a cup of baked Potato contains about one-fifth of the daily value for this important nutrient—the Potato earns high marks as a health-promoting food. Since vitamin B6 is involved in more than 100 enzymatic reactions, it is active virtually everywhere in the body. Vitamin B6 is necessary for the synthesis of amino acids and nucleic acids (and therefore our DNA), so it is essential for the formation of new cells in the body.

## Promote Nervous System Health

Vitamin B6 is necessary for the creation of many neurotransmitters including serotonin, a lack of which is linked to depression; melatonin, the hormone needed for a good night's sleep; epinephrine and norepinephrine, hormones that help us respond to stress; and GABA, which is needed for normal brain function.

## Promote Heart Health

Vitamin B6 plays a critically important role in keeping homocysteine levels in check. Since homocysteine can directly damage blood vessel walls, greatly increasing the progression of atherosclerosis, high homocysteine levels are associated with a significantly increased risk for heart attack and stroke. Potatoes are also a good source of potassium, a mineral that is important for regulating blood pressure. In addition, they contain concentrated amounts of dietary fiber, which mostly resides in the skin. So, if you want the cholesterol-lowering (and digestive-health-promoting) effects of fiber, be sure to eat the Potato's flavorful skin as well as its creamy center.

## Promote Antioxidant Protection

If you're looking for a food with a good supply of antioxidants, don't forget about Potatoes. They are a very good source of vitamin C, providing over one-quarter of the daily value for this important nutrient. In addition, Potatoes are a good source of copper and manganese, trace minerals that are necessary for the functioning of the *superoxide dismutase* antioxidant enzyme.

## Additional Health-Promoting Benefits of Potatoes

Since a large Potato is rich in fiber, it is very filling, yet a one cup serving contains only 133 calories. Enjoyed without lots of added fat, satisfying Potatoes can play a role in a diet geared towards healthy weight control.

### Nutritional Analysis of 1 cup of baked Potato with skin:

| NUTRIENT | AMOUNT | % DAILY VALUE | NUTRIENT | AMOUNT | % DAILY VALUE |
|---|---|---|---|---|---|
| Calories | 132.98 | | Pantothenic Acid | 0.68 mg | 6.80 |
| Calories from Fat | 1.10 | | | | |
| Calories from Saturated Fat | 0.29 | | **Minerals** | | |
| Protein | 2.81 g | | Boron | — mcg | |
| Carbohydrates | 30.78 g | | Calcium | 12.20 mg | 1.22 |
| Dietary Fiber | 2.93 g | 11.72 | Chloride | — mg | |
| Soluble Fiber | 0.73 g | | Chromium | — mcg | — |
| Insoluble Fiber | 2.20 g | | Copper | 0.37 mg | 18.50 |
| Sugar – Total | 1.95 g | | Fluoride | — mg | — |
| Monosaccharides | 0.98 g | | Iodine | — mcg | — |
| Disaccharides | 0.37 g | | Iron | 1.66 mg | 9.22 |
| Other Carbs | 25.90 g | | Magnesium | 32.94 mg | 8.23 |
| Fat – Total | 0.12 g | | Manganese | 0.28 mg | 14.00 |
| Saturated Fat | 0.03 g | | Molybdenum | — mcg | — |
| Mono Fat | 0.00 g | | Phosphorus | 69.54 mg | 6.95 |
| Poly Fat | 0.05 g | | Potassium | 509.96 mg | |
| Omega-3 Fatty Acids | 0.01 g | 0.40 | Selenium | 0.98 mcg | 1.40 |
| Omega-6 Fatty Acids | 0.04 g | | Sodium | 9.76 mg | |
| Trans Fatty Acids | 0.00 g | | Zinc | 0.39 mg | 2.60 |
| Cholesterol | 0.00 mg | | | | |
| Water | 86.86 g | | **Amino Acids** | | |
| Ash | 1.42 g | | Alanine | 0.09 g | |
| | | | Arginine | 0.13 g | |
| **Vitamins** | | | Aspartate | 0.69 g | |
| Vitamin A IU | 0.00 IU | 0.00 | Cystine | 0.04 g | 9.76 |
| Vitamin A RE | 0.00 RE | | Glutamate | 0.47 g | |
| A - Carotenoid | 0.00 RE | 0.00 | Glycine | 0.08 g | |
| A - Retinol | 0.00 RE | | Histidine | 0.06 g | 4.65 |
| B1 Thiamin | 0.13 mg | 8.67 | Isoleucine | 0.11 g | 9.57 |
| B2 Riboflavin | 0.04 mg | 2.35 | Leucine | 0.17 g | 6.72 |
| B3 Niacin | 2.01 mg | 10.05 | Lysine | 0.17 g | 7.23 |
| Niacin Equiv | 2.74 mg | | Methionine | 0.04 g | 5.41 |
| Vitamin B6 | 0.42 mg | 21.00 | Phenylalanine | 0.12 g | 10.08 |
| Vitamin B12 | 0.00 mcg | 0.00 | Proline | 0.10 g | |
| Biotin | — mcg | — | Serine | 0.12 g | |
| Vitamin C | 15.74 mg | 26.23 | Threonine | 0.10 g | 8.06 |
| Vitamin D IU | 0.00 IU | 0.00 | Tryptophan | 0.04 g | 12.50 |
| Vitamin D mcg | 0.00 mcg | | Tyrosine | 0.10 g | 10.31 |
| Vitamin E Alpha Equiv | 0.06 mg | 0.30 | Valine | 0.16 g | 10.88 |
| Vitamin E IU | 0.09 IU | | | | |
| Vitamin E mg | 0.06 mg | | | | |
| Folate | 13.42 mcg | 3.35 | | | |
| Vitamin K | 4.88 mcg | 6.10 | | | |

(Note: "–" indicates data is unavailable. For more information, please see page 806.)

STEP-BY-STEP RECIPE

# The Healthiest Way of Cooking Potatoes

## 10-Minute "Healthy Steamed" Potatoes

*While boiled Potatoes become watery and lose some of their flavor, I have found that "Healthy Steaming" Potatoes enhances their flavor and preserves most of their nutrients. But hold the butter and sour cream!*

**2 medium-sized Potatoes**
**3 TBS extra virgin olive oil**
**1 medium clove garlic**
**Sea salt and pepper to taste**

1. Fill the bottom of the steamer with 2 inches of water.
2. While steam is building up in steamer, press or chop garlic and let it sit at least 5 minutes. (Why?, see page 261.)
3. Cut Potatoes into 1/2-inch cubes with skin on as described under *The Best Way to Prepare Potatoes*.
4. Steam for 10 minutes. Potatoes are done when you can easily penetrate them with a fork. (For

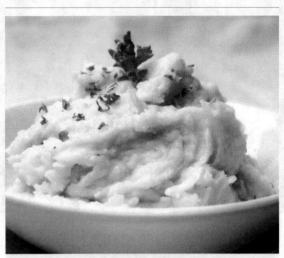

Smashed Potatoes with Garlic

information on *Differences in Cooking Time*, see page 94.)

5. Transfer to a bowl. For more flavor, toss the Potatoes with the remaining ingredients while they are still hot.

**SERVES 2**

### COOKING TIPS:
• To prevent overcooking Potatoes, I highly recommend using a timer.

### Flavor Tips: Try these 5 great serving suggestions with the recipe above. ✳

1. **Most Popular: Smashed Potatoes with Garlic.** Prepare 10-Minute "Healthy Steamed" Potatoes using peeled potatoes. Mash with 3 TBS extra virgin olive oil, 3 cloves pressed garlic, 3 TBS soy or low-fat milk, and sea salt and pepper to taste (pictured above).

2. Chopped fresh rosemary, parsley, dill and chives are wonderful additions to Potatoes.

3. Mix steamed Potatoes with the Swiss chard, spinach, broccoli or green beans recipes.

4. **Warm Potato Salad #1:** Mix 10-Minute "Healthy Steamed" Potatoes with 1 chopped boiled egg, 8–10 slices kalamata olives, 1 TBS capers, 2 TBS flat-leaf parsley, 1 TBS red wine vinegar, 2 TBS extra virgin olive oil, and salt and pepper to taste.

5. **Warm Potato Salad #2:** Mix 10-Minute "Healthy Steamed" Potatoes with 1 cup chopped celery, 1/2 cup diced green apple, 1 small shredded carrot, 1/2–1 TBS lemon juice, 1 TBS extra virgin olive oil, 1 TBS fresh dill, and salt and pepper to taste.

Please write (address on back cover flap) or e-mail me at info@whfoods.org with your personal ideas for preparing Potatoes, and I will share them with others through our website at www.whfoods.org.

## An Easy Way to Prepare Potatoes, Step-By-Step

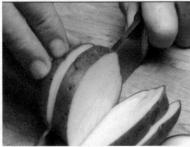
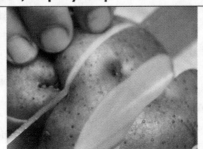
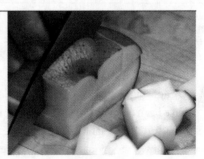

### DICED POTATOES

❶ Cut a slice lengthwise off the Potato and lay it flat on the cut side so that it doesn't roll. Cut lengthwise into 1/2-inch slices. ❷ Stack a few slices on top of each other and cut lengthwise into 1/2-inch wide pieces.
❸ Turn Potato. Cut across lengthwise every 1/2 inch. You will end up with 1/2-inch cubes.

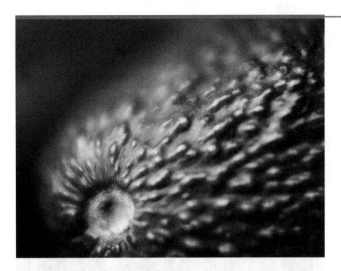

# avocados

## highlights

| | |
|---|---|
| AVAILABILITY: | Year-round |
| REFRIGERATE: | Yes, after ripening |
| SHELF LIFE: | 2 days when ripe |
| PREPARATION: | Sliced or cubed; needs no cooking |

## nutrient-richness chart

Total Nutrient-Richness: **7**      GI: **n/a**

One cup (146 grams) of Avocado slices contains 235 calories

| NUTRIENT | AMOUNT | %DV | DENSITY | QUALITY |
|---|---|---|---|---|
| Vitamin K | 29.2 mcg | 36.5 | 2.8 | good |
| Dietary Fiber | 7.3 g | 29.2 | 2.2 | good |
| Potassium | 874.5 mg | 25.0 | 1.9 | good |
| Folate | 90.4 mcg | 22.6 | 1.7 | good |
| B6 Pyridoxine | 0.4 mg | 20.5 | 1.6 | good |
| Vitamin C | 11.5 mg | 19.2 | 1.5 | good |
| Copper | 0.4 mg | 19.0 | 1.5 | good |
| **CAROTENOIDS:** | | | | |
| Alpha-Carotene | 36.0 mcg | | | |
| Beta-Carotene | 93.0 mcg | | | |
| Beta-Cryptoxanthin | 42.0 mcg | | | |
| Lutein+Zeaxanthin | 406.5 mcg | | | |
| **FLAVONOIDS:** | | | | |
| (-)-Epicatechin | 0.8 mg | | | |
| **PHYTOSTEROLS:** | | | | |
| Beta-Sitosterol | 1.1 mg | | | |
| Camposterol | 1.1 mg | | | |
| Sigmasterol | 3.0 mg | | | |

Daily values for these nutrients have not yet been established.

For more on "Total Nutrient-Richness," "%DV," "Density," and The World's Healthiest Foods "Quality" Rating System, see page 805.

For more on GI, see page 342.

Avocados are native to Central and South America and have been cultivated since 8,000 BC. Although they are usually served as vegetables, Avocados are actually a type of tropical fruit with a smooth, buttery texture and rich, distinctive flavor. Best eaten raw, Avocados can be enjoyed in a number of ways. Add them to a salad, use them as a creamy replacement for mayonnaise or prepare them as a dip that will be sure to delight both you and your friends. Proper storage and preparation are keys to enjoying the best flavor and nutritional benefits from Avocados. That is why I want to share with you the secrets to enhancing the flavor and preserving the nutrients of Avocados.

## why avocados should be part of your healthiest way of eating

While the majority of Avocados' calories do come from fat, almost two-thirds of the fats they contain are the heart-healthy monounsaturated fats, like those found in olive oil. Monounsaturated fats have been noted as one of the reasons for the healthfulness of the Mediterranean diet, which features monounsaturated-fat-rich foods such as olive oil, olives and nuts. Avocados are a great tasting and nutritious food and, when eaten in moderation, can be an important part of your "Healthiest Way of Eating." (For more on *Health Benefits of Avocados* and a complete analysis of their content of over 60 nutrients, see page 302.)

## varieties of avocados

Botanically classified as a fruit, Avocados are usually served as vegetables. Some of the most common varieties include:

### HASS

Grown in California, this variety makes up over 75% of the U.S. Avocado crop. About the size of a pear, they have pebbly, brown-black skin when ripe. Their edible, yellow-green flesh has the consistency of butter and a subtle, nutty flavor. This is the variety featured in the photographs in this chapter.

### FUERTE

These Florida-grown Avocados are larger than the Hass

variety with a more defined pear-like shape and smooth, bright green skin. Because their flesh is more watery, fibrous and contains half the fat of Hass Avocados, they are also lower in calories.

### ZUTANO AND BACON

These varieties have similar characteristics to the Fuerte, but they are less commonly available.

### COCKTAIL AVOCADO

Weighing a modest one to two ounces, these small Avocados have no pit. They are difficult to find but well worth the search.

## the peak season

The peak season for Avocados varies with the different varieties. Hass Avocados are generally available throughout the year, although the peak of their season runs from spring through summer. The season for most Fuerte Avocados extends from June to March and peaks in October. Bacon

and Zutano are available during the fall and winter months. The months they are in season are the months when their concentration of nutrients and flavor is highest, and their cost is at its lowest.

## biochemical considerations

Avocados are one of the foods most commonly associated with allergic reactions in individuals with latex allergies. (For more on *Latex Allergies*, see page 722.)

## 3 steps for the best tasting and most nutritious avocados

Turning Avocados into a flavorful dish with the most nutrients is simple if you just follow my 3 easy steps:

1. The Best Way to Select
2. The Best Way to Store
3. The Best Way to Prepare

## 1. the best way to select avocados

A friend of mine once planted an Avocado tree, and as the Avocados would grow to full size, she would let them sit on the tree, waiting and waiting for them to get soft before harvesting them; but they never got soft. The lesson: Avocados do not ripen on the tree, but only after they have been harvested. This is the reason that Avocados found at the market are often still hard and will need to be ripened after you take them home. Hard Avocados are not a sign of inferior fruit. In fact, unless you are going to be serving the Avocado immediately after purchasing, it is better to buy one that is still hard, so you can control the ripening process and have one ready when you want to consume it.

Avoid overripe Avocados and ones that have dark sunken spots or cracks. Be sure not to purchase Avocados that rattle when you shake themsaute since this is a sign that the pit has

pulled away from the flesh and it is overripe. You should not eat overripe Avocados because the brown coloration of the overripe fruit indicates the formation of free radicals.

### How Do You Know Which Avocados are Ready to Eat?

Although most of the Avocados that you find at the store are hard, some stores do carry ripe, ready-to-eat Avocados. Whether you are selecting ripe Avocados at the store or ripening them at home, you can tell that an Avocado is ripe and ready to eat when its skin has turned from green to a dark brown-green or almost black color and "gives" slightly under gentle pressure. The best tasting, ripe and ready-to-eat Avocados are slightly soft and should be eaten within a day or two.

## 2. the best way to store avocados

If you have more ripe Avocados than you can consume, it is best to refrigerate them as this will halt the ripening process. They can be kept in the refrigerator for up to 2 days. If left for longer than 2 days, they will begin to lose their flavor and they will begin to turn dark in color. Avoid slicing Avocados before refrigerating since they will turn brown after they are cut.

Avocados continue to respire even after they have been harvested; their respiration rate at room temperature (68°F/

20°C) is 190 mg/kg/hr. Slowing down the respiration rate with proper storage is the key to extending their flavor and nutritional benefits. (For a *Comparison of Respiration Rates* for different vegetables, see page 91.)

### Avocados Will Remain Fresh for Up to 7 Days When Properly Stored

If you purchase unripe (hard) Avocados, you should store

them at room temperature where they will last for up to 7 days. As they ripen, their skin color will darken. Do not refrigerate unripe Avocados as they will never ripen but merely rot in the cold environment of the refrigerator.

## How to Ripen Avocados

If you want to hasten the ripening process of Avocados, you can place them in a paper bag for several days (check on them frequently to ensure that they do not get overripe). The paper bag traps the ethylene gas produced by the Avocados; ethylene gas helps the Avocados to ripen more quickly, while the paper bag allows for healthy oxygen exchange with the environment (as opposed to plastic bags, which limit oxygen exchange and will lead to premature rotting). Keep the paper bag in a dark, cool place as excessive heat will also cause the Avocados to rot rather than ripen. If you want to speed up the ripening even more, you can add a banana or apple to the bag since it will increase the amount of ethylene produced.

# 3. the best way to prepare avocados

Avocados are easy to prepare: just slice and eat. Once they are cut, Avocados are very susceptible to oxidation, which turns them brown as they come in contact with oxygen in the air.

## How to Prevent Avocados From Turning Brown

One way to prevent cut Avocados from turning brown is to sprinkle them with lime or lemon juice. The antioxidants found in citrus fruits help prevent the oxidation responsible for the change in color. It is best to cut away and discard any areas that have turned brown before eating, as they are an indication of the formation of free radicals.

When Avocados are sprinkled with lime or lemon juice, the surface sometimes does not remain well coated with the juice, causing it to still turn brown. If you have half an Avocado to store, you can avoid this problem by gently removing the pit, placing the Avocado cut side down in a bowl that contains 1 TBS lemon juice and 1 cup of water, covering with plastic wrap and refrigerating it. The skin will protect the outer surface from browning. This technique should help reduce most, if not all, of the browning. Remove any brown areas gently with a knife before eating.

Kitchen folklore purports that leaving the pit in halved Avocados or adding the pit to mashed Avocados will prevent them from browning. Unfortunately, this only holds true for the small area surrounding the pit—the rest of the Avocado will still turn brown.

Here are questions that I received from readers of the whfoods.org website about Avocados:

**Q** *I make a dish with dark greens, broccoli, lemon juice and Avocado. I then refrigerate any leftovers I have. Is this OK even though you say on your website that refrigerated Avocado slices will turn brown?*

**A** The reason I don't recommend refrigerating sliced Avocados is because once they are cut, they become easily oxidized (causing brown coloration), which reflects the formation of free radicals in the Avocados. The lemon in your mixture should prevent the Avocados from oxidizing, and it should be fine in your refrigerator if you do not keep it for too long.

*(Questions continued on next page and page 303)*

---

### An Easy Way to Prepare Avocados, Step-By-Step

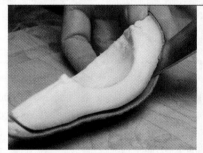 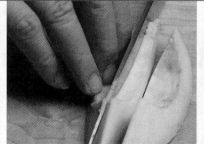 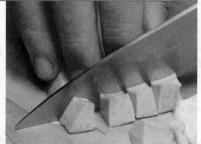

CUBED AVOCADO

❶ Cut Avocado in half and then into quarters. Remove pit and cut away peel. ❷ Cut Avocado sections lengthwise into slices about 1/4-inch or 1/2-inch wide, depending on size of desired cubes. ❸ Cut across slices to make cubes. Toss with lemon or lime juice to keep from browning.

STEP-BY-STEP RECIPE
## The Healthiest Way to Enjoy Avocados

# *3-Minute Avocado Dip*

*Avocados are best eaten raw in salads and dips as they turn bitter if they are cooked. The only place I have seen Avocados as part of a cooked dish was in Mexico where they are sliced and added to chicken soup before serving; but even then, the Avocados themselves were not cooked. Guacamole is very popular in Mexican and Southwestern cuisines. This tasty version takes only 3 minutes to make!*

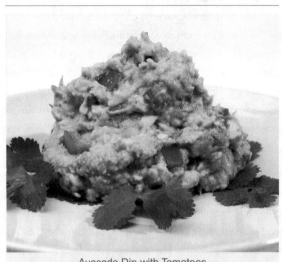

**1 medium ripe Avocado**
**1 TBS lemon or lime juice**
**1/2 cup cilantro, chopped**
**Sea salt and pepper to taste**

Avocado Dip with Tomatoes

Combine all ingredients in a blender and blend for 1 minute. Alternatively, you can mash the Avocado with a potato masher or fork and then add rest of ingredients.

**SERVES 2**

## Flavor Tips: 9 Ways to Enjoy the Avocado Dip and Avocados.

1. **Most Popular:** Add 1 small diced tomato, 2 thinly sliced scallions (green onions) and 1 tsp chopped canned chipotle peppers to Avocado Dip. Serve with baked tortilla chips or crudités (raw vegetables).

2. The creamy texture of Avocados makes them an excellent substitute for mayonnaise. Add pressed garlic to the Avocado Dip for a great spread.

3. Fill half an Avocado with tuna salad and serve with green salad for lunch.

4. Add chunks of Avocado to chicken salad.

5. Sprinkle Avocado slices with tamari (soy sauce) and lemon juice for a simple treat.

6. **Avocado Tomato Salad:** Alternate slices of tomatoes and Avocado, and drizzle with your favorite salad dressing.

7. **Quick Avocado Salad Dressing:** Mash one-quarter of a large Avocado with your favorite vinaigrette. Stir until creamy.

8. **Mexican Avocado Dressing or Dip:** In a blender, combine 3/4 cup water, juice of 1/2 lemon, 1 small diced tomato, 1 medium Avocado, 1/2 cup cilantro leaves, 1 tsp maple syrup, 1 tsp chili powder, cayenne pepper and sea salt to taste. Blend for 1 minute on high speed until creamy. Use as a salad dressing or as a dip with crudités.

9. **Papaya Avocado Salsa:** Combine 1 diced medium Avocado, 1 diced medium papaya, 1 diced small sweet onion, 1 TBS minced cilantro, 2 tsp minced fresh ginger, 1 TBS lime juice and sea salt to taste. Serve with chicken or fish.

Please write (address on the back cover flap) or e-mail me at info@whfoods.org with your favorite ideas for preparing Avocados, and I will share them with others through our website at www.whfoods.org.

**Q** *I would like to know the sugar content of Avocados. Does it vary based upon where it is grown?*

**A** According to the nutritional analysis program that we use on the website, one cup of Avocados contains 1.31 grams of sugar. While this amount may vary a little with variety and where it is grown, I feel that this is a pretty good gauge for the sugar content of Avocados. While I have not come across a glycemic index value for Avocados, it is a food that is high in fats (good fats, actually) and high in fiber; in general, these factors would suggest it should not cause a rapid rise in blood sugar levels.

# health benefits of avocados

## Promote Heart Health

Avocados are a rich source of oleic acid, with 59% of their total fat content represented by this heart-healthy monounsaturated fat. In one study of people with moderately high cholesterol levels, individuals who ate a diet rich in Avocados showed clear health improvements. After seven days on the Avocado-rich diet, they had significant decreases in total cholesterol and LDL cholesterol, along with an 11% increase in health-promoting HDL cholesterol.

Avocados are also a good source of potassium, a mineral that helps regulate blood pressure. Adequate intake of potassium can help to guard against circulatory diseases, like high blood pressure, heart disease or stroke. In fact, the U.S. Food and Drug Association has authorized a health claim that states: "Diets containing foods that are good sources of potassium and low in sodium may reduce the risk of high blood pressure and stroke."

Avocados are also good sources of two heart-healthy B-vitamins, folic acid and vitamin B6. Inadequate levels of these nutrients are related to elevated homocysteine levels. Since homocysteine can damage artery walls, promoting atherosclerosis, and is an independent risk factor for cardiovascular disease, these two B vitamins are of great importance to heart health.

Further cardiovascular protection is provided by the dietary fiber contained in Avocados. In addition to its well-known benefit to digestive health, fiber has been found to lower blood cholesterol levels.

## Promote Optimal Antioxidant Status

Avocados are a good source of copper and vitamin C. These nutrients help to promote optimal health since they provide potent antioxidant activity and therefore protect cells from free radical oxidative damage. Copper is an essential cofactor of the *superoxide dismutase* enzyme, which disarms free radicals produced in the lungs and red blood cells. Vitamin C is a powerful antioxidant that works its magic in the water-soluble components of the body. Uncontrolled free radical activity has been linked to increased risk of diseases including cardiovascular disease, arthritis and certain forms of cancer.

## Promote Blood and Bone Health

Avocados are a good source of vitamin K, which plays a role in proper blood and bone function. Vitamin K is needed to activate a variety of clotting factors in the blood; without adequate supplies, the blood may become too thin, leading to excess bleeding. Since certain bone proteins have also been found to be vitamin K-dependent, this nutrient is important in the process of bone mineralization, which creates and maintains structural integrity.

## Nutritional Analysis of 1 cup of Avocado:

| NUTRIENT | AMOUNT | % DAILY VALUE | NUTRIENT | AMOUNT | % DAILY VALUE |
|---|---|---|---|---|---|
| Calories | 235.06 | | Pantothenic Acid | 1.42 mg | 14.20 |
| Calories from Fat | 201.31 | | | | |
| Calories from Saturated Fat | 32.02 | | **Minerals** | | |
| Protein | 2.89 g | | Boron | — mcg | |
| Carbohydrates | 10.79 g | | Calcium | 16.06 mg | 1.61 |
| Dietary Fiber | 7.30 g | 29.20 | Chloride | 8.76 mg | |
| Soluble Fiber | 2.99 g | | Chromium | — mcg | — |
| Insoluble Fiber | 4.31 g | | Copper | 0.38 mg | 19.00 |
| Sugar – Total | 1.31 g | | Fluoride | — mg | — |
| Monosaccharides | 1.02 g | | Iodine | 2.92 mcg | 1.95 |
| Disaccharides | 0.15 g | | Iron | 1.49 mg | 8.28 |
| Other Carbs | 2.18 g | | Magnesium | 56.94 mg | 14.23 |
| Fat – Total | 22.37 g | | Manganese | 0.33 mg | 16.50 |
| Saturated Fat | 3.56 g | | Molybdenum | — mcg | — |
| Mono Fat | 14.03 g | | Phosphorus | 59.86 mg | 5.99 |
| Poly Fat | 2.85 g | | Potassium | 874.54 mg | |
| Omega-3 Fatty Acids | 0.16 g | 6.40 | Selenium | 0.58 mcg | 0.83 |
| Omega-6 Fatty Acids | 2.69 g | | Sodium | 14.60 mg | |
| Trans Fatty Acids | 0.00 g | | Zinc | 0.61 mg | 4.07 |
| Cholesterol | 0.00 mg | | | | |
| Water | 108.43 g | | **Amino Acids** | | |
| Ash | 1.52 g | | Alanine | 0.17 g | |
| | | | Arginine | 0.09 g | |
| **Vitamins** | | | Aspartate | 0.41 g | |
| Vitamin A IU | 893.52 IU | 17.87 | Cystine | 0.03 g | 7.32 |
| Vitamin A RE | 89.06 RE | | Glutamate | 0.30 g | |
| A - Carotenoid | 89.06 RE | 1.19 | Glycine | 0.12 g | |
| A - Retinol | 0.00 RE | | Histidine | 0.04 g | 3.10 |
| B1 Thiamin | 0.16 mg | 10.67 | Isoleucine | 0.10 g | 8.70 |
| B2 Riboflavin | 0.18 mg | 10.59 | Leucine | 0.18 g | 7.11 |
| B3 Niacin | 2.80 mg | 14.00 | Lysine | 0.14 g | 5.96 |
| Niacin Equiv | 3.32 mg | | Methionine | 0.05 g | 6.76 |
| Vitamin B6 | 0.41 mg | 20.50 | Phenylalanine | 0.10 g | 8.40 |
| Vitamin B12 | 0.00 mcg | 0.00 | Proline | 0.11 g | |
| Biotin | 5.26 mcg | 1.75 | Serine | 0.12 g | |
| Vitamin C | 11.53 mg | 19.22 | Threonine | 0.10 g | 8.06 |
| Vitamin D IU | 0.00 IU | 0.00 | Tryptophan | 0.03 g | 9.38 |
| Vitamin D mcg | 0.00 mcg | | Tyrosine | 0.07 g | 7.22 |
| Vitamin E Alpha Equiv | 1.96 mg | 9.80 | Valine | 0.14 g | 9.52 |
| Vitamin E IU | 2.92 IU | | | | |
| Vitamin E mg | 3.31 mg | | | | |
| Folate | 90.37 mcg | 22.59 | | | |
| Vitamin K | 29.20 mcg | 36.50 | | | |

(Note: "—" indicates data is unavailable. For more information, please see page 806.)

## Q If Avocados are full of fat, why are they still so good for us?

A While the majority of Avocados' calories do come from fat, almost two-thirds of the fat that they contain are the heart-healthy monounsaturated fats, like those found in olive oil. Monounsaturated fats are associated with reduced risk of heart disease and have been noted as one of the reasons for the healthfulness of the Mediterranean diet, which features foods rich in mono-unsaturated fat such as olive oil, olives and nuts. A recent study even showed that adding Avocados or Avocado oil to a salad enhanced the absorption of carotenoid phytonutri-ents from the vegetables, supporting another health benefit of this delicious food. In addition to being a storehouse of healthy fatty acids, Avocados are also a concentrated source of fiber, folic acid, vitamin B6, potassium and copper. Their wonderful nutrient profile may be the reason that researchers found that after just seven days on an Avocado-rich diet, individuals with moderately high cho-lesterol were found to have reduced levels of total and LDL cholesterol and increased levels of HDL cholesterol. Avocados are a great tasting and nutritious food and, if eaten in moderation, can be an important part of your "Healthiest Way of Eating."

## Q Why can't you grate and eat an avocado pit?

A Avocado pits are inedible. They contain tannins, which are released when the pit is grated or bitten into. These tannins interact with substances in the mouth and alter them in a way similar to the process that occurs when leather is tanned.

## Q A friend just told me that adding Avocados to salad is healthy as it has been found to enhance absorption of the nutrients from the salad greens. Is this true?

A Your friend must have heard about the study reported in the March 2005 edition of the *Journal of Nutrition*. This study found that adding Avocados to salad increased the absorption of carotenoids in the bloodstream of the lucky individuals eating the delicious salad. Compared to when they ate the Avocado-free salad, the study participants experienced a greater absorption of alpha-carotene (7.2 times), beta-carotene (15.3 times) and lutein (5.1 times) when they ate salad containing Avocado. The amount of Avocado used was 150 grams, which is about 1 cup. While

that seems like a lot of Avocado to add to your salad on a regular basis (it would contain over 230 calories), adding even some of that should have a great effect on carotenoid absorption as well.

Researchers also tested the effect of adding Avocado to tomato-containing salsa (since tomatoes are a concentrated source of the lycopene carotenoid) and found that once again the Avocado enhanced carotenoid absorption—4.4 times greater absorption of lycopene and 2.6 times greater absorption of beta-carotene was found in those eating the Avocado-enriched salsa than the Avocado-free salsa.

The reason for the Avocado's benefit on carotenoids is probably due to its fat content, since carotenoids are fat-soluble. So, the next time you make a salad, salsa or any carotenoid-containing dish, consider adding some Avocado. Not only is it filled with many important nutrients itself, but the enhancement of carotenoid absorption means more antioxidant activity hap-pening in your body, which is a great thing for health promo-tion. Not only that, but Avocados taste great too.

## Q Is is OK to eat Avocado each day?

A Whether eating avocado each day will be supportive of your health from an overall fat and caloric intake perspective really depends upon your individual fat and caloric intake goals as well as the rest of your diet. Since it is difficult to know how large your avocados are and since you are probably mashing your avocados for your sandwich I have based this answer on 1/2 cup of mashed avocado. One-half cup of mashed avocado contains 184 calories and 16.86 grams of total fat with 11.27 of these being monoun-saturated fats. So the question is whether this amount of calories fits into your overall nutritional goals and whether your diet has room for this amount of fat. Given a 2,000 calorie diet with 30% fat intake would mean that 600 of the day's calories could come from fat, which is about 67 grams. So, if these were your individual goals and the rest of your day's diet didn't exceed about 49 grams of fat then you would be in target. The other thing that would further support that eating avocado every day is health supportive would be to ensure that the rest of your diet provides you with the other nutrients in which avocadoes are not concen-trated. For example, while they are concentrated in nutrients such as folate, vitamin E, vitamin B3 and vitamin B5, there are other nutrients (for example, calcium) of which they do not necessarily contain a great concentration.

# corn

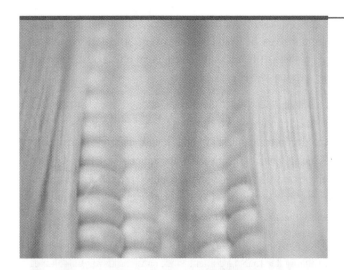

| | |
|---|---|
| AVAILABILITY: | Year-round |
| REFRIGERATE: | Yes |
| SHELF LIFE: | 2–3 days refrigerated |
| PREPARATION: | Remove husk and wipe clean |
| BEST WAY TO COOK: | "Healthy Steamed" in just 5 minutes |

## nutrient-richness chart

Total Nutrient-Richness: **7**          GI: **78**

One cup (164 grams) of cooked Corn contains 177 calories

| NUTRIENT | AMOUNT | %DV | DENSITY | QUALITY |
|---|---|---|---|---|
| B1 Thiamin | 0.4 mg | 24.0 | 2.4 | good |
| Folate | 76.1 mcg | 19.0 | 1.9 | good |
| Dietary Fiber | 4.6 g | 18.4 | 1.9 | good |
| Vitamin C | 10.2 mg | 16.9 | 1.7 | good |
| Phosphorus | 169.0 mg | 16.9 | 1.7 | good |
| Manganese | 0.3 mg | 16.0 | 1.6 | good |
| B5 Pantothenic Acid | 1.4 mg | 14.4 | 1.5 | good |

**CAROTENOIDS:**

| | | |
|---|---|---|
| Alpha-Carotene | 37.7 mcg | Daily values for these nutrients have not yet been established. |
| Beta-Carotene | 108.2 mcg | |
| Beta-Cryptoxanthin | 264.0 mcg | |
| Lutein+Zeaxanthin | 1,585.9 mcg | |

For more on "Total Nutrient-Richness," "%DV," "Density," and
The World's Healthiest Foods "Quality" Rating System, see page 805.

For more on GI, see page 342.

Corn has been a time-honored food staple for 7,000 years! It provided food, shelter, fuel and decoration for the ancient Mayan, Aztec and Incan civilizations. Today, Corn continues to play a vital role in Native American cultures and is one of the most popular summer vegetables. Any local farmer or gardener will tell you that one moment's delay from the Corn stalk to the pot results in the loss of flavor in fresh Corn. But since most of us are not able to grow our own Corn, I want to share with you the "Healthiest Way of Cooking" Corn that will help bring out its best flavor while maximizing its nutritional value.

## why corn should be part of your healthiest way of eating

Early varieties of Corn featured red, yellow, white and even black kernels, but our choices today are usually limited to white and yellow Corn. Although I enjoy the extra sweetness of white Corn, I prefer to get the extra health benefits derived from the carotenoids found in the yellow variety. Corn also provides other phytonutrients, such as phenolics, which function as powerful antioxidants and work in many different ways to promote health. In addition, Corn is a concentrated source of many other nutrients, including vitamins B1, B5 and folate. (For more on the *Health Benefits of Corn* and a complete analysis of its content of over 60 nutrients, see page 308.)

## varieties of corn

An important food plant native to the Americas, Corn is thought to have originated in either Mexico or Central America. Corn is known scientifically as *Zea mays*, a moniker that reflects its traditional name, *maize*, by which it is known throughout many areas of the world. Varieties of Corn fall under two main categories:

**SWEET CORN**

Produced for human consumption, it is tender, juicy and sweet. It comes in a variety of colors including yellow, blue, black and white.

**DENT CORN**

Mainly used to feed livestock, this variety is low in sugar and high in starch.

## the peak season

Although Corn is available throughout the year, its peak season runs from late summer to early fall when Corn is produced throughout the United States. Winter Corn from Florida is available from fall to spring. The months that it is in season are the months when its concentration of nutrients and flavor are highest, and its cost is at its lowest.

| COMPARISON OF VITAMIN A AND BETA-CAROTENE IN YELLOW AND WHITE CORN | | |
|---|---|---|
| | YELLOW CORN | WHITE CORN |
| Vitamin A | 356 IU (7% Daily Value) | 0 |
| Beta-Carotene | 108 mcg | 0 |

*All quantities and % Daily Values are based on 1 cup of cooked Corn.

## biochemical considerations

Corn is a concentrated source of oxalates and one of the foods most commonly associated with allergic reactions.

(For more on *Oxalates*, see page 725; and *Food Allergies*, see page 719.)

## 4 steps for the best tasting and most nutritious corn

Turning Corn into a flavorful dish with the most nutrients is simple if you just follow my 4 easy steps:

1. The Best Way to Select
2. The Best Way to Store
3. The Best Way to Prepare
4. The Healthiest Way of Cooking

# 1. the best way to select corn

You can select the best tasting Corn by looking for ears of Corn that are displayed in the refrigerated section of your local market since warm temperatures will change the sugars in Corn to starch and reduce their level of sweetness. If you are purchasing Corn at a farmer's market or a roadside stand, and the Corn has not been refrigerated, make sure it has at least been kept in the shade and out of direct sunlight. The husks should be fresh, bright green and envelop the ear, and the silk should be moist and flowing. You can examine the kernels by pulling back part of the husk and checking to see if they are plump and arranged tightly in rows. Corn will squirt a white milky substance if you take your fingernail and press on a kernel. This means the Corn is just right for eating. By selecting the best tasting sweet Corn, you will also enjoy Corn with the highest nutritional value.

As with all vegetables, I recommend selecting organically grown varieties of Corn whenever possible. Because most of us cannot pick our Corn straight from the stalk, the next best alternative is to purchase organically grown Corn on the same day you are planning to cook it. (For more on *Organic Foods*, see page 113.)

Avoid Corn that looks dried out, has husks that fit too loosely around the ear or silk that is dry and turning brown.

# 2. the best way to store corn

For optimal flavor and nutrition, it is best to cook Corn the same day you purchase it. If you are not planning on cooking it the same day that you bring it home from the market, make sure to store it properly so that it will retain its optimal flavor and nutrient concentration.

Fresh Corn continues to respire even after it has been harvested. Slowing down the respiration rate with proper storage is the key to extending its flavor and nutritional benefits. (For a *Comparison of Respiration Rates* for different vegetables, see page 91.)

### Corn Will Remain Fresh for Up to 2-3 Days When Properly Stored

1. Store fresh Corn in the refrigerator. The colder temperature will slow the respiration rate, helping to preserve nutrients and keeping Corn fresh for a longer period of time.

2. Place Corn in a plastic storage bag before refrigerating. I have found that it is best to wrap the bag tightly around the Corn, squeezing out as much of the air from the bag as possible.

3. Do not wash fresh Corn before refrigeration because exposure to water will encourage Corn to spoil.

# 3. the best way to prepare corn

When you are ready to cook Corn, remove the husks, then rub the ears with a damp paper towel. The silk will stick to the towel and come right off. You can leave the Corn whole and just cut off the tips or cut the ears into lengths you desire.

# 4. the healthiest way of cooking corn

Since research has shown that important nutrients can be lost or destroyed by the way a food is cooked, the "Healthiest Way of Cooking" Corn is focused on bringing out its best flavor while maximizing its vitamins, minerals and powerful antioxidants.

## The Healthiest Way of Cooking Corn: "Healthy Steaming" for just 5 Minutes

In my search for the healthiest way to cook Corn, I tested every possible cooking method and discovered that "Healthy Steaming" Corn for just 5 minutes delivered the best result. "Healthy Steaming" Corn not only brings out its sweet flavor, but it also maximizes its nutritional profile. The Step-by-Step Recipe will show you how easy it is to "Healthy Steam" Corn. (For more on "*Healthy Steaming*," see page 58.)

## Grilling or Broiling Fresh Sweet Corn

Before grilling or broiling, sprinkle Corn with lemon juice, sea salt and pepper to help protect against the formation of harmful compounds. While grilled or broiled Corn tastes great, make sure it does not burn. It is best to grill ears of Corn on an area without a direct flame as the temperatures directly above or below the flame can reach as high as 500°F to 1000°F (260°–538°C). When using a broiler, keep the Corn about 4–5 inches away from the flame. Coating with oil before cooking will produce harmful free radicals, so brush with extra virgin olive oil immediately after it is cooked. (For more on *Grilling*, see page 61.)

## How to Avoid Overcooking Corn

One of the primary reasons that Corn loses its flavor is because it is overcooked. To prevent overcooking Corn, I highly recommend using a timer. Since Corn takes only 5 minutes to cook, it is important to begin timing as soon as you place it into the steamer.

## Cooking Methods Not Recommended for Corn

### BOILING

Boiling Corn results in a loss of its flavor along with many of its nutrients, including minerals, water-soluble vitamins (such as C and the B-complex vitamins) and health-promoting phytonutrients.

## how to enjoy fresh corn without cooking

Cut kernels off the cob and add to your favorite salad or salsa.

**Seaweed Corn Salad:** Toss together kernels of 1 ear of Corn, 1 grated carrot, 3/4 cup soaked arame or hijiki sea vegetable (measure after soaking), 1 diced red bell pepper, 2 thinly sliced green onions, 1 tsp sesame seeds, 1/2 tsp toasted sesame oil, 1/2 tsp sea salt and 2 tsp rice vinegar. Serve immediately.

**Corn Salsa:** In a medium mixing bowl, combine kernels from 2 ears of Corn, 1 small diced red pepper, 1/2 diced sweet onion, 1 diced jalapeño with seeds and pith removed, 2 tsp lime juice, 1 tsp chili powder, 2 tsp extra virgin olive oil, 1 TBS chopped cilantro and sea salt to taste.

## An Easy Way to Prepare Fresh Corn, Step-By-Step

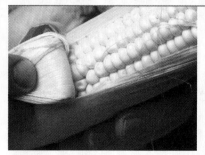 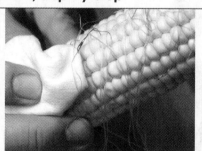 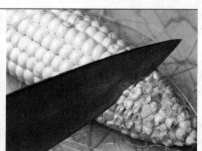

❶ Remove the husk and Corn silk. ❷ Rub the ears with a damp paper towel. ❸ Cut off the tips.

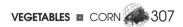

STEP-BY-STEP RECIPE
## The Healthiest Way of Cooking Corn

# 5-Minute "Healthy Steamed" Corn

*I discovered that you get the sweetest tasting Corn by "Healthy Steaming" for 5 minutes. It is a gentle, moist way of preparing Corn that enhances its flavor and retains its nutritional value. Serve with olive oil and hold the butter!*

**2 ears fresh Corn on the cob**
**1 TBS extra virgin olive oil**
**Sea salt and black pepper to taste**

1. Fill the bottom of the steamer with 2 inches of water.
2. While steam is building up, remove husk from Corn.
3. Steam Corn for 5 minutes. (For information on *Differences in Cooking Time*, see page 94.)
4. To enhance the flavor of Corn, dress with extra virgin

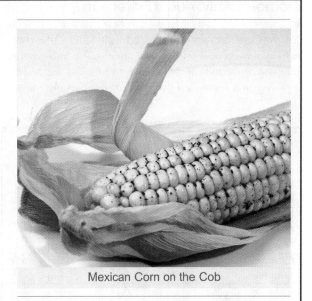

Mexican Corn on the Cob

olive oil, and sea salt and extra pepper to taste. For added flavor you may want to use more olive oil!.

**SERVES 2**

## COOKING TIPS:
• To prevent overcooking Corn, I highly recommend using a timer.

## Flavor Tips: Try these 8 great serving suggestions with the recipe above.

1. **Most Popular:** Add extra black pepper to taste and a squeeze of fresh lemon or lime juice.
2. Sprinkle with grated Parmesan cheese.
3. Brush with your favorite vinaigrette and sprinkle with 1 TBS of fresh chopped herbs such as cilantro, parsley or oregano.
4. **Mexican Corn on the Cob:** Add chili powder, cumin and a squeeze of lime.
5. **Corn, Avocado and Tomato Salad:** Combine 2 cups of cooked Corn, 1 diced avocado and 1 medium chopped tomato in a bowl. Whisk together 2 TBS extra virgin olive oil, 1 TBS lemon or lime juice, 1/2 cup chopped cilantro and sea salt and black pepper to taste. Add to Corn mixture.
6. **Corn Frittata:** Blend 1/2 cup fresh cooked Corn

kernels, 1 TBS chopped cilantro and 1 medium chopped tomato into a frittata (see page 635).

7. **Cheesy Corn Soup:** In a blender, combine cooked Corn kernels, warm low-fat milk (enough to cover the corn), low-fat Parmesan cheese and ground pepper and salt to taste. Blend on medium speed for 2 minutes.

8. **Spicy Corn Chowder:** In a blender, combine 2 cups warm low-fat milk, 1 cup of warm cooked Corn kernels, 1 TBS diced onion, 1 tsp chili powder, 1/2 jalapeño pepper (with or with out the seeds depending upon how hot you want it; seeds increase hotness) and sea salt to taste. Blend for 2 minutes on medium speed. Pour into serving bowls and garnish with finely sliced green onions, Corn kernels and a sprinkle of chili powder.

Please write (address on back cover flap) or e-mail me at info@whfoods.org with your personal ideas for preparing Corn, and I will share them with others through our website at www.whfoods.org.

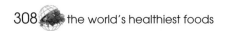

# health benefits of corn

### Promotes Antioxidant Protection

Recent research has found that whole grains, such as Yellow Corn, contain many powerful phytonutrients whose activity has gone unrecognized until this point because traditional research methods have overlooked them. This new research has found that most of the phenolic phyto-nutrients found in Corn and other whole grains are in their "bound" form versus the "free" form in which they are typically found in fruits and vegetables; most studies have only measured the "free" form of phenolics. Yet, in this new research where total antioxidant activity was measured, Corn scored on par with other fruits and vegetables. These findings may help explain why studies have shown that populations eating diets high in fiber-rich whole grains consistently have lower risk for colon cancer, yet short-term clinical trials that have focused on fiber alone in lowering colon cancer risk, often to the point of giving subjects isolated fiber supplements, yield inconsistent results. The explanation is most likely that these studies have not taken into account the interactive effects of all the nutrients in whole grains—not just their fiber, but also their many phytonutrients.

### Promotes Lung Health

Consuming foods rich in beta-cryptoxanthin, an orange-red carotenoid found in yellow Corn, may benefit lung health. An analysis that combined the results of seven different studies found that intake of beta-cryptoxanthin was inversely related to risk of developing lung cancer—the higher the beta-cryptoxanthin in the diet, the less risk for developing the disease.

### Promotes Heart Health

Corn contains significant amounts of folate, a B vitamin that helps to promote heart health through lowering levels of homocysteine, an amino acid that can directly damage blood vessels. Elevated levels of homocysteine have been found to be an independent risk factor for heart attack, stroke or peripheral vascular disease, and are found in 20–40% of patients with heart disease. Corn's ability to promote heart health also comes from its concentration of dietary fiber, which helps to reduce cholesterol levels.

### Promotes Energy Production

Corn is a good source of two B vitamins—thiamin and pantothenic acid—which are important for energy production. Its thiamin is integral to the process of converting sugar into usable energy. Its pantothenic acid is necessary for carbohydrate, protein and lipid metabolism; it is an especially valuable B-vitamin when you're under stress since it supports the function of the adrenal glands.

### Additional Health-Promoting Benefits of Corn

Corn is also a concentrated source of other nutrients providing additional health-promoting benefits. These nutrients include free-radical-scavenging vitamin C and bone-building phosphorus and manganese.

## Nutritional Analysis of 1 cup of cooked Corn:

| NUTRIENT | AMOUNT | % DAILY VALUE | NUTRIENT | AMOUNT | % DAILY VALUE |
|---|---|---|---|---|---|
| Calories | 177.12 | | Pantothenic Acid | 1.44 mg | 14.40 |
| Calories from Fat | 18.90 | | | | |
| Calories from Saturated Fat | 2.90 | | **Minerals** | | |
| Protein | 5.44 g | | Boron | — mcg | |
| Carbohydrates | 41.18 g | | Calcium | 3.28 mg | 0.33 |
| Dietary Fiber | 4.60 g | 18.40 | Chloride | — mg | |
| Soluble Fiber | 0.18 g | | Chromium | — mcg | — |
| Insoluble Fiber | 4.42 g | | Copper | 0.08 mg | 4.00 |
| Sugar – Total | 4.26 g | | Fluoride | — mg | — |
| Monosaccharides | 1.32 g | | Iodine | — mcg | — |
| Disaccharides | 2.78 g | | Iron | 1.00 mg | 5.56 |
| Other Carbs | 32.32 g | | Magnesium | 52.48 mg | 13.12 |
| Fat – Total | 2.10 g | | Manganese | 0.32 mg | 16.00 |
| Saturated Fat | 0.32 g | | Molybdenum | — mcg | — |
| Mono Fat | 0.62 g | | Phosphorus | 168.92 mg | 16.89 |
| Poly Fat | 0.98 g | | Potassium | 408.36 mg | |
| Omega-3 Fatty Acids | 0.02 g | 0.80 | Selenium | 1.32 mcg | 1.89 |
| Omega-6 Fatty Acids | 0.96 g | | Sodium | 27.88 mg | |
| Trans Fatty Acids | 0.00 g | | Zinc | 0.78 mg | 5.20 |
| Cholesterol | 0.00 mg | | | | |
| Water | 114.10 g | | **Amino Acids** | | |
| Ash | 1.18 g | | Alanine | 0.48 g | |
| | | | Arginine | 0.22 g | |
| **Vitamins** | | | Aspartate | 0.40 g | |
| Vitamin A IU | 355.88 IU | 7.12 | Cystine | 0.04 g | 9.76 |
| Vitamin A RE | 36.08 RE | | Glutamate | 1.06 g | |
| A - Carotenoid | 36.08 RE | 0.48 | Glycine | 0.22 g | |
| A - Retinol | 0.00 RE | | Histidine | 0.14 g | 10.85 |
| Thiamin B1 | 0.36 mg | 24.00 | Isoleucine | 0.22 g | 19.13 |
| Riboflavin B2 | 0.12 mg | 7.06 | Leucine | 0.58 g | 22.92 |
| Niacin B3 | 2.64 mg | 13.20 | Lysine | 0.22 g | 9.36 |
| Niacin equiv | 3.26 mg | | Methionine | 0.12 g | 16.22 |
| Vitamin B6 | 0.10 mg | 5.00 | Phenylalanine | 0.24 g | 20.17 |
| Vitamin B12 | 0.00 mcg | 0.00 | Proline | 0.48 g | |
| Biotin | — mcg | — | Serine | 0.26 g | |
| Vitamin C | 10.16 mg | 16.93 | Threonine | 0.22 g | 17.74 |
| Vitamin D IU | 0.00 IU | 0.00 | Tryptophan | 0.04 g | 12.50 |
| Vitamin D mcg | 0.00 mcg | | Tyrosine | 0.20 g | 20.62 |
| Vitamin E alpha equiv | 0.14 mg | 0.70 | Valine | 0.30 g | 20.41 |
| Vitamin E IU | 0.22 IU | | | | |
| Vitamin E mg | 0.80 mg | | (Note: "–" indicates data is unavailable. For more information, please see page 806.) | | |
| Folate | 76.10 mcg | 19.02 | | | |
| Vitamin K | 0.66 mcg | 0.83 | | | |

Here are questions I received from readers of the whfoods.org website about Corn:

## Q What do you think of Corn oil?

A While Corn oil is a concentrated source of polyunsaturated fats, almost all of them are an omega-6 fat called linoleic acid. Linoleic acid is an essential fatty acid (meaning our bodies cannot make it and we need to get it from our diets), but it is already very commonplace in our diet. Many medical researchers and healthcare practitioners advise the public that instead of increasing their intake of linoleic acid, they should limit it and increase their intake of omega-3 fatty acids, such as alpha-linolenic acid, which serves to thwart linoleic acid's potential inflammatory nature. Oils that would be good sources of alpha-linolenic acid include flax oil, walnut oil and canola oil. Thus, while I consider Corn to be one of the World's Healthiest Foods, I would not consider Corn oil to be one. Extra virgin olive oil is the only oil that I include in the World's Healthiest Foods.

## Q I am confused about high fructose Corn syrup? Do you think it is a good sweetener?

A Unfortunately, names can be deceiving. While Corn syrup may originate as Corn, its nutrient profile does not resemble Corn at all. Unfortunately, Corn syrup is basically a storehouse of calories and sugar—and not much else. It is found in so many processed foods, and some researchers feel that its commonplace role in the diets of many people may be anything but beneficial. While it is from a whole, natural food, I don't consider Corn syrup to be a whole, natural food and avoid it when I can. The body supposedly does not process high fructose Corn syrup in the same way it does cane or beet sugar. This not only affects the way that metabolic hormones function, but also causes the liver to send more fat into the bloodstream.

## Q Do the anthocyanins in blue tortilla chips survive the baking process?

A We are confident that there would be benefits in eating blue tortilla chips in relationship to their anthocyanin content, and some form of the anthocyanins clearly remain in the baked chips. The color of the chips, all by itself, indicates the presence of anthocyanins in some form. We assume that there may be some loss of anthocyanins compared to the fresh Corn, yet we are uncertain as to what that may be. Stability of anthocyanins has to do with factors such as pH and heat; according to research in other anthocyanin-containing foods, these flavonoids are very stable at temperatures between 80°–150°F (27°–66°C) while at temperatures between 150°–212°F (66°–100°C), the stability of anthocyanins in the foods studied decreases in a gradual and steady way.

## Q How is puffed Corn cereal made?

A Puffed Corn cereal is usually made from Corn starch or Corn flour and not from the whole Corn grain. Additionally, it may have other ingredients added to it as well. As such, puffed Corn would not be a whole food like whole Corn grain, which would have a superior nutrient content.

## Q Does stone ground cornmeal, like that found in some Corn tortilla chips, have the nutrients that are present in Corn?

A You will definitely get some of the benefits from consuming cornmeal that you would get from whole Corn, yet it is important to remember that a processed form of a food will never have quite the same level of nutrients as the original form. The answer to how much nutritional benefit you will get depends upon the specifics of the cornmeal used since there are various types. Some cornmeals are degermed, with some of them being enriched while others are non-enriched; the enriched one would obviously offer more nutrients. The best type of cornmeal from a nutritional perspective would be whole grain cornmeal, which hasn't been degermed.

## Q Can you tell me more about the beta-cryptoxanthin phytonutrient found in Corn and other foods?

A Beta-cryptoxanthin is one of the most abundant carotenoids in the North American diet. It is a "provitamin A" compound, one of approximately 50 carotenoids able to be converted in the body into retinol, an active form of vitamin A. Beta-cryptoxanthin has approximately one-half of the vitamin A activity of beta-carotene. It provides plants with yellow-orange coloring and, in addition to Corn, is found in foods such as oranges, carrots, papaya and apricots.

In addition to being a source of vitamin A, beta-cryptoxanthin is also a powerful antioxidant, protecting cells from free-radical damage. Researchers believe that there may be a link between beta-cryptoxanthin intake and lung health. Since carotenoids, like beta-cryptoxanthin, are fat-soluble, a very low-fat diet may lead to a deficiency. You can enhance your absorption of this and other carotenoids by consuming a little oil or fat-containing food when you eat carotenoid-rich foods; for example, research has shown that carotenoids from salad are better absorbed when the salad is accompanied by a regular salad dressing made with oil rather than with a fat-free version.

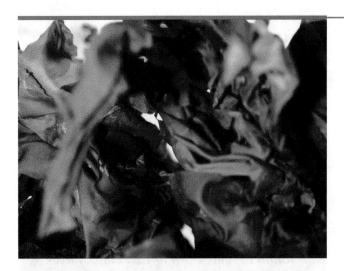

# sea vegetables

| | |
|---|---|
| AVAILABILITY: | Year-round |
| REFRIGERATE: | Not recommended |
| SHELF LIFE: | Several months |
| PREPARATION: | Minimal and no need to cook |

## nutrient-richness chart

Total Nutrient-Richness: **7**          GI: **n/a**
1/4 cup (20 grams) Kelp contains 9 calories

| NUTRIENT | AMOUNT | %DV | DENSITY | QUALITY |
|---|---|---|---|---|
| Iodine | 415.00 mcg | 276.7 | 579.1 | excellent |
| Vitamin K | 13.2 mcg | 16.5 | 34.5 | excellent |
| Folate | 36.0 mcg | 9.0 | 18.8 | very good |
| Magnesium | 24.2 mg | 6.0 | 12.7 | very good |
| Calcium | 33.6 mg | 3.4 | 7.0 | good |
| Iron | 0.6 mg | 3.2 | 6.6 | good |
| Tryptophan | 0.01 g | 3.1 | 6.5 | good |
| **CAROTENOIDS:** | | | | Daily values for this nutrient have not yet been established. |
| Beta-Carotene | 756.0 mcg | | | |

For more on "Total Nutrient-Richness," "%DV," "Density," and
The World's Healthiest Foods "Quality" Rating System, see page 805.
For more on GI, see page 342.

The consumption of Sea Vegetables (also called seaweed) enjoys a long history throughout the world. Archaeological evidence suggests that Japanese cultures have been consuming Sea Vegetables for more than 10,000 years. In ancient China, Sea Vegetables were a delicacy served to honored guests and royalty. Since Sea Vegetables are becoming increasingly popular in the West, I would like to share with you quick and easy ideas of how to add the best flavor and nutritional benefits from Sea Vegetables to your "Healthiest Way of Eating."

## why sea vegetables should be part of your healthiest way of eating

One of Nature's best sources of iodine, a mineral essential for proper thyroid function, Sea Vegetables also contain health-promoting lignans and carbohydrate-related nutri-ents called fucans, which have been studied for their anti-inflammatory and phytoestrogenic properties. Sea Vegetables are an ideal food to add to your "Healthiest Way of Eating" not only because of their unique nutritional profile, but also because 1/4 cup of Sea Vegetables, such as Kelp, contains only 9 calories and therefore can be important for healthy weight control. (For more on the *Health Benefits of Sea Vegetables* and a complete analysis of their content of over 60 nutrients, see page 312.)

## varieties of sea vegetables

Sea Vegetables grow both in saltwater oceans and freshwater lakes. They commonly grow on coral reefs or in rocky landscapes and can be found at great depths as long as the sunlight can penetrate deep enough for them to survive. They are not classified as either a plant or animal but belong to a group or organisms known as algae.

The thousands of varieties of Sea Vegetables are categorized as either red-brown or green. Not all Sea Vegetables are edible; however, there are a wide variety of edible Sea Vegetables, each having a uniquely different shape, taste and texture. The following are some of the most popular:

**DULSE**

Dulse is soft, chewy and reddish-brown in color. I find Dulse to be the easiest Sea Vegetable to incorporate into the "Healthiest Way of Eating." Just chop it and sprinkle it on your food.

**KELP**

Light brown to dark green in color, Kelp is commonly found in powder form.

**HIKIJI**

Hijiki looks like small strands of black wiry pasta and has a strong flavor.

**NORI**

Nori has a dark purple-black color that turns phosphorescent green when toasted and is famous for its role as the wrapper used in making sushi rolls.

**KOMBU**

Very dark in color and generally sold in strips or sheets that are very thick in comparison to nori, it is often used as a flavoring for soups and beans.

**WAKAME**

Very dark in color, it is commonly used in Japanese miso soup.

**ARAME**

This lacy, wiry sea vegetable is sweeter and milder in taste than many of the other varieties.

## the peak season

Sea Vegetables are available throughout the year.

## 3 steps for the best tasting and most nutritious sea vegetables

Turning Sea Vegetables into a flavorful dish with the most nutrients is simple if you just follow my 3 easy steps:

1. The Best Way to Select
2. The Best Way to Store
3. The Best Way to Prepare

# 1. the best way to select sea vegetables

Most Sea Vegetables are dried. Some are ready to eat, while others just need to be reconstituted. The best way to select them is to be sure that they come in a tightly sealed package. Sea Vegetables come in sheets, flakes or powders. Choose the form of Sea Vegetables that will best suit your taste and recipe needs. Natural foods stores and Asian markets oftentimes have the best selection of Sea Vegetables.

Avoid packages of Sea Vegetables that have evidence of excessive moisture.

# 2. the best way to store sea vegetables

Store Sea Vegetables in a tightly sealed container at room temperature where they will stay fresh for at least several months.

# 3. the best way to prepare sea vegetables

Although Sea Vegetables can be a delicious addition to cooked dishes, none of them require cooking. Sprinkling vegetables, grains or legumes with Sea Vegetables is an excellent way to increase the nutritional value of virtually any dish. Soaking Sea Vegetables (except Nori) will help reduce its sodium content.

**DULSE:** It is very simple to use dulse as it does not require any preparation. Just chop and sprinkle on vegetables, grains or legumes for extra flavor. Dulse is sold as flakes, which do not even require chopping, but I have found that their flavor is inferior.

**KELP:** Kelp is available as flakes and powder and requires no preparation. Just add to vegetables, grains or legumes.

**HIJIKI:** Soak for 10 minutes, rinse and then chop to desired size and serve on salads or vegetables. If adding to a cooked dish, be sure to add at the end of the cooking time.

**NORI:** Nori can be purchased toasted or untoasted. If it is not toasted, you can either toast it in a 350°F (175°C) oven for about 1–2 minutes or hold a sheet about 1 inch above the flame of your stove with a pair of tongs for about 2 minutes (or until it changes color). It is not necessary to toast nori to make sushi.

**KOMBU:** It makes a great soup base (it is one of the ingredients used to make the Japanese soup base known as *dashi*). Just follow the package directions for instructions on how to prepare it.

**WAKAME:** Wakame softens quickly. Soak in fresh water for 5–15 minutes and add to salads or use in vegetable dishes. It requires only 5–10 minutes of cooking when added to soups.

**ARAME:** Soak in cold water for 15 minutes. Chop and add to rice and vegetable dishes. It can also be added to soups.

### Healthy Preparation Tip for Sea Vegetables

The water in which you soak Sea Vegetables is very nutritious and can be used in the recipe you are making. Use as much soaking water as can be used in the recipe to maximize its flavor and nutritional value.

# health benefits of sea vegetables

## Promote Healthy Thyroid Function

Sea Vegetables, especially kelp, are some of nature's richest sources of iodine. Since it is a component of the thyroid hormones triiodothyronine (T3) and thyroxine (T4), iodine is essential to human life. Without sufficient iodine, your body cannot synthesize these hormones. Because these thyroid hormones regulate metabolism in every cell of the body and play a role in virtually all physiological functions, an iodine deficiency can have a devastating impact on your health and well-being. A common sign of thyroid deficiency is an enlarged thyroid gland, commonly called a goiter.

## Promote Women's Health

Sea Vegetables contain lignan phytonutrients that have phytoestrogenic activity. In fact, dried Sea Vegetables were rated second behind flaxseeds as the food that contains the highest amounts of these substances, ahead of legumes and whole grains. These lignans are converted in the body to compounds such as enterolactone and enterodiol, which have weak estrogenic activity. They can act like estrogen when the body stores of this hormone are low, like in menopause, potentially relieving associated symptoms. Additionally, they also provide benefits when estrogen levels are too high since they can weakly bind to estrogen receptors, crowding out the endogenous hormone and therefore minimizing its effects. This may have benefit in the treatment of PMS and in the prevention of breast cancer since some forms of both conditions are sparked by excess estrogen.

## Promote Optimal Health

Some Sea Vegetables have been shown to be unique sources of carbohydrate-like substances called fucans, which have numerous beneficial properties including reducing the body's inflammatory response. They are also suggested to have antithrombotic activity, the ability to inhibit blood clots. These important phytonutrients have also been found to have antiviral activity in laboratory studies. Additionally, other studies have suggested that fucans from Sea Vegetables may have the ability to inhibit the development of tumors; this may also help explain why the Sea Vegetable wakame has been found to inhibit the growth of breast cancer in experimental animals.

## Additional Health-Promoting Benefits of Sea Vegetables

Sea Vegetables are also a concentrated source of other nutrients providing additional health-promoting benefits. These nutrients include energy-producing iron, bone-building calcium and magnesium, heart-healthy folate, and sleep-promoting tryptophan. Since Sea Vegetables contain only 9 calories per 1/4 cup serving, they are an ideal food for healthy weight control.

### Nutritional Analysis of 1/4 cup Kelp Sea Vegetable:

| NUTRIENT | AMOUNT | % DAILY VALUE | NUTRIENT | AMOUNT | % DAILY VALUE |
|---|---|---|---|---|---|
| Calories | 8.60 | | Pantothenic Acid | 0.13 mg | 1.30 |
| Calories from Fat | 1.01 | | | | |
| Calories from Saturated Fat | 0.44 | | **Minerals** | | |
| Protein | 0.34 g | | Boron | 0.00 mcg | |
| Carbohydrates | 1.91 g | | Calcium | 33.60 mg | 3.36 |
| Dietary Fiber | 0.26 g | 1.04 | Chloride | 0.00 mg | |
| Soluble Fiber | 0.00 g | | Chromium | 0.00 mcg | 0.00 |
| Insoluble Fiber | 0.00 g | | Copper | 0.03 mg | 1.50 |
| Sugar – Total | 0.00 g | | Fluoride | 0.00 mg | 0.00 |
| Monosaccharides | 0.00 g | | Iodine | 415.00 mcg | 276.67 |
| Disaccharides | 0.00 g | | Iron | 0.57 mg | 3.17 |
| Other Carbs | 0.00 g | | Magnesium | 24.20 mg | 6.05 |
| Fat – Total | 0.11 g | | Manganese | 0.04 mg | 2.00 |
| Saturated Fat | 0.05 g | | Molybdenum | 1.00 mcg | 1.33 |
| Mono Fat | 0.02 g | | Phosphorus | 8.40 mg | 0.84 |
| Poly Fat | 0.01 g | | Potassium | 17.80 mg | |
| Omega-3 Fatty Acids | 0.00 g | 0.00 | Selenium | 0.14 mcg | 0.20 |
| Omega-6 Fatty Acids | 0.01 g | | Sodium | 46.60 mg | |
| Trans Fatty Acids | 0.00 g | | Zinc | 0.25 mg | 1.67 |
| Cholesterol | 0.00 mg | | | | |
| Water | 16.32 g | | **Amino Acids** | | |
| Ash | 1.32 g | | Alanine | 0.02 g | |
| | | | Arginine | 0.01 g | |
| **Vitamins** | | | Aspartate | 0.03 g | |
| Vitamin A IU | 23.20 IU | 0.46 | Cystine | 0.02 g | 4.88 |
| Vitamin A RE | 2.40 RE | | Glutamate | 0.05 g | |
| A - Carotenoid | 2.40 RE | 0.03 | Glycine | 0.02 g | |
| A - Retinol | 0.00 RE | | Histidine | 0.00 g | 0.00 |
| B1 Thiamin | 0.01 mg | 0.67 | Isoleucine | 0.02 g | 1.74 |
| B2 Riboflavin | 0.03 mg | 1.76 | Leucine | 0.02 g | 0.79 |
| B3 Niacin | 0.09 mg | 0.45 | Lysine | 0.02 g | 0.85 |
| Niacin Equiv | 0.25 mg | | Methionine | 0.01 g | 1.35 |
| Vitamin B6 | 0.00 mg | 0.00 | Phenylalanine | 0.01 g | 0.84 |
| Vitamin B12 | 0.00 mcg | 0.00 | Proline | 0.01 g | |
| Biotin | 0.00 mcg | 0.00 | Serine | 0.02 g | |
| Vitamin C | 0.60 mg | 1.00 | Threonine | 0.01 g | 0.81 |
| Vitamin D IU | 0.00 IU | 0.00 | Tryptophan | 0.01 g | 3.13 |
| Vitamin D mcg | 0.00 mcg | | Tyrosine | 0.01 g | 1.03 |
| Vitamin E Alpha Equiv | 0.17 mg | 0.85 | Valine | 0.01 g | 0.68 |
| Vitamin E IU | 0.26 IU | | | | |
| Vitamin E mg | 0.17 mg | | | | |
| Folate | 36.00 mcg | 9.00 | | | |
| Vitamin K | 13.20 mcg | 16.50 | | | |

(Note: "–" indicates data is unavailable. For more information, please see page 806.)

**STEP-BY-STEP RECIPE**
## The Healthiest Ways to Enjoy Sea Vegetables

# Hijiki Cucumber Salad

*This is a quick and easy way to add Sea Vegetables to your "Healthiest Way of Eating."*

1 TBS dried organic Hijiki
2 medium cucumbers
1/2 small red onion
1 TBS rice vinegar
2 TBS extra virgin olive oil
Sea salt and pepper to taste

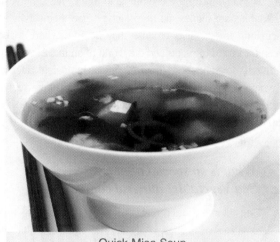

Quick Miso Soup

1. Soak Hijiki in warm water for 10 minutes while preparing rest of ingredients.
2. Slice onions thin and let sit for at least 5 minutes. (Why? See page 276.)
3. Slice cucumbers and cut in half lengthwise. Scoop out seeds with a small spoon and then cut cucumber into thin slices.
4. Whisk rest of ingredients together. Squeeze out excess water from seaweed. Chop if necessary: you don't want Hijiki pieces to be too large. Combine cucumbers with Hijiki and onions, toss with dressing and serve immediately.

## Flavor Tips: 6 Ways to Enjoy Hijiki.

1. Add tamari (soy sauce) to the salad recipe. If you add tamari, you will want to reduce the amount of sea salt you use.
2. Add ginger or cilantro to the Hijiki Cucumber Salad for a nice kick.
3. Any of the Sea Vegetables can be used as a topping on salads, mixed in rice dishes or added to soups, legumes or and vegetable dishes.
4. **Hijiki Sweet Potatoes:** Soak 2 TBS Hijiki in water for 10 minutes. In a small mixing bowl, whisk 1 tsp tamari, 3 TBS extra virgin olive oil, 2 tsp minced ginger, 2 TBS lemon juice, 2 tsp white miso, 1 TBS brown rice vinegar and sea salt to taste. Combine 2 cooked medium sweet potatoes with Hijiki and the dressing, and serve with chicken or fish.
5. **Nori Wrap:** Wrap nut spread or hummus, sprouts, grated carrot and marinated onion (page 272) in a Nori sheet. Serve with Hijiki Cucumber Salad.
6. **Quick Miso Soup:** Bring 10 oz. water to a boil and then take off heat. Add 1 TBS light-colored miso, stirring to dissolve. Add 1/4 cup soaked Arame or Hijiki and 2 TBS sliced scallions to serving bowl and then pour hot broth over. Optional: add cubed tofu and cooked soba noodles (pictured above).

\* Dulse can also be used in any of these suggestions.

Please write (address on back cover flap) or e-mail me at info@whfoods.org with your personal ideas for preparing Sea Vegetables, and I will share them with others through our website at www.whfoods.org.

## An Easy Way to Prepare Hijiki, Step-By-Step

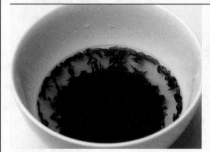 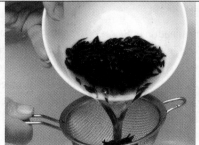 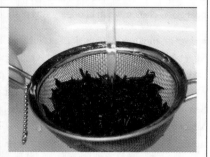

**SOAKING HIJIKI**
❶ Soak Hijiki in warm water for about 10–15 minutes. ❷ Pour off the water. ❸ Rinse under cold running water.

## Q Are Sea Vegetables plants?

A Scientists are now beginning to agree that Sea Vegetables are algae, and not plants. Algae themselves are fascinating to scientists because they lie somewhere in between the world of plants and the world of animals. As scientists learn more and more about the unique biological category in which Sea Vegetables belong, I am certain that we will learn more about their amazing nutritional qualities and that Sea Vegetables will become more popular, which will definitely be a boon for everyone's "Healthiest Way of Eating."

## Q What is so special about Sea Vegetables mineral content?

A Consider the fact that our earth, containing vast expanses of oceans, is about 60% water and that our bodies are also about 60% water (from the fluids in and around our cells and our blood). Then examine the mineral profile of the oceans, the Sea Vegetables that grow in these oceans, and our blood. It turns out that it is difficult to find any category of food that has as diverse a mineral composition as Sea Vegetables. It's also difficult to find any category of food whose overall mineral composition better matches that of human blood. It is a wonderful mineral match.

## Q Do you have to worry about contamination with Sea Vegetables like you do with fish?

A You do have to worry about contamination of Sea Vegetables just like with other food you consume. For example, during the period 2000–2005, the governments of England, New Zealand and Canada issued public health recommendations advising against consumption of hijiki sea vegetable unless verified as containing low levels of arsenic. These recommendations came after determination of high arsenic levels in hijiki harvested off the coasts of Korea and Japan. There are organic hijiki products in the marketplace with verified low levels of arsenic, and these products would be a good choice when choosing this particular sea vegetable.

However, in general, the risk of pollutant contamination of Sea Vegetables is usually less than the risks posed by fish since toxins can accumulate in fish (through a process called biomagnification) in a way that does not occur with algae, such as Sea Vegetables. If you are concerned about this, organic Sea Vegetables may be the best way to go. If you are having trouble finding these products in your area, there are resources on the Internet through which you can purchase them.

## Q Are Sea Vegetables a good source of iodine?

A No food group serves as a better iodine source than Sea Vegetables. According to the Institute of Medicine at the National Academy of Sciences, adults need 150 mcg (micrograms) of iodine each day to meet their health needs. Depending upon the specific type of Sea Vegetable, this guideline can be met by a 1–2 gram serving—the amount contained in about to 2/3–1 teaspoon.

Compared to ordinary table salt, Sea Vegetables have a higher iodine content. A gram of iodized table salt typically contains about 65 mcg of iodine. For Sea Vegetables, the range is 79–300 mcg.

| SEA VEGETABLE | AMOUNT | IODINE CONTENT |
|---|---|---|
| Kelp | 1 gram | 100–200 mcg |
| Wakame | 1 gram | 79 mcg |
| Dulse | 1 gram | 150–300 mcg |
| Iodized Salt | 1 gram | 65 mcg |

It is important to note that Sea Vegetables vary greatly in their iodine content, depending on the circumstances in which they grow. Even state-of-the-art databases, like the Food Processor Software that I used for this book and the World's Healthiest Foods website, do not provide iodine values for Sea Vegetables. The reason is simple: the iodine content of most Sea Vegetables is just too variable.

Variations in Sea Vegetables' iodine content are due to two factors. First, the iodine content of marine water undergoes much greater natural change than the iodine content of soil. And secondly, unlike other minerals, which usually get hooked onto other substances in Sea Vegetables, iodine does not hook onto other substances very readily but tends to stay in its free, water-soluble form. In studies of Pacific Sea Vegetables, for example, about 10% of the total iodine content is hooked onto other substances (usually parts of protein, called amino acids) while the other 90% remains in its free, water-soluble form. Since most of the iodine remains water-soluble, even when it's inside the Sea Vegetable, it can easily move back and forth between the ocean and the "plant." This constant movement of iodine in its water-soluble form means that some Sea Vegetables can increase or decrease their iodine content by as much as 10-fold depending on ocean conditions. For this reason, it's best to think of Sea Vegetables as providing a high amount of iodine that falls within a general range, rather than a specific, pinpoint amount.

Q *How can I incorporate more Sea Vegetables into my diet?*

A It's great that you are thinking about how to enjoy more Sea Vegetables since they are rich in many nutrients, including iodine, a mineral that is hard to find in most other foods. Here are some of my favorite ideas for enjoying more Sea Vegetables:

- Keep a shaker of granulated/ground dulse, kelp or nori (available at many natural food stores) on the table and use it instead of salt.

- Flavor soups with Sea Vegetables such as arame, kombu and wakame.

- Add strips of nori to rice or cooked vegetable dishes.

---

## Q&A
### WHAT ARE SOME ALTERNATIVES TO SALT?

Most Americans, especially those eating the Standard American Diet, love salt! We consume significant amounts of salt-laden packaged and processed foods and have grown so accustomed to the salty flavor of foods that we add it to most of our foods—even fruits and vegetables! For some people, excessive consumption of salt has very few health consequences. For others, however, excessive consumption of dietary sodium (from table salt and packaged foods), coupled with a low dietary intake of potassium, is a common cause of high blood pressure (known as the "silent killer"), especially in "salt-sensitive" individuals.

Of course, sodium is an essential mineral, necessary for maintaining proper water and electrolyte balance in the body. Therefore we do need to consume some sodium every day. Since there is enough naturally occurring sodium in vegetables, most people can get a sufficient amount of sodium without adding any extra salt to their food. But, unfortunately, only 5% of the sodium intake consumed by people living in the United States comes from the natural ingredients in food. Prepared foods contribute 45 percent of our sodium intake, 45 percent is added in cooking and another 5 percent is obtained through condiments (e.g., ketchup, mustard, relish, salad dressings).

As you begin (or continue!) your journey to discovering the wonders of the World's Healthiest Foods, you will naturally decrease the amount of salt you consume. This is because in place of table salt and other seasonings that contain sodium or monosodium glutamate you may begin to use a variety of herbs that will add tremendous flavor, freshness and zest to your food that allow you to experience the full flavor of the food itself. Increasing the amount of herbs you use in cooking provides a double benefit. Not only will you decrease your sodium intake, but the scientific community continues to uncover the powerful health benefits of herbs. Recent studies by researchers at the U.S. Department of Agriculture reveal that common herbs are loaded with antioxidants, critical for good health. They include a wide variety of plant-derived compounds that prevent cellular damage caused by an excess of free radicals, corrosive molecules produced during normal metabolic processes and which are also generated by many external sources including pesticides, smoking and exhaust fumes. Free radicals have been implicated as major contributing factors in the development of virtually all chronic and age-related diseases. Not only is the antioxidant activity of some herbs studied higher than that reported for vitamin E, these herbs even surpass foods well-known for their antioxidant content such as vegetables, berries and other fruits. In one particular study, oregano emerged the clear winner. In addition to oregano, a number of other herbs also pack a significant antioxidant punch. Among the more familiar—ranked in order—are dill, garden thyme, rosemary and peppermint. Less familiar herbs with comparable antioxidant power include rose geranium, sweet bay, purple amaranth, winter savory and Vietnamese coriander.

Sea vegetables, also among the World's Healthiest Foods, can provide a salty flavor to recipes. Sea vegetables are rich sources of a vast array of minerals and also contain lignans, plant compounds with cancer-protective properties. Kelp is commonly used as an alternative to salt as it is available in flakes that can be added easily to most foods during cooking or at the table.

So, take a step toward better health by cutting back on your salt intake, and take advantage of the flavor and health benefits of herbs and sea vegetables.

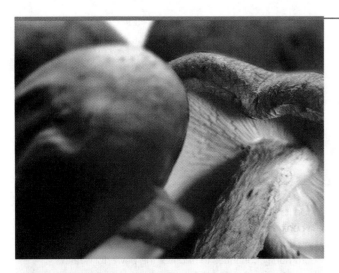

# shiitake mushrooms

## highlights

| | |
|---|---|
| AVAILABILITY: | Year-round |
| REFRIGERATE: | Yes |
| SHELF LIFE: | 5 days refrigerated |
| PREPARATION: | Wipe clean |
| BEST WAY TO COOK: | "Healthy Sauté" in just 7 minutes |

## nutrient-richness chart

Total Nutrient-Richness: **5**    GI: **n/a**
8 oz-wt (227 grams) of raw Shiitake Mushrooms contains 87 calories

| NUTRIENT | AMOUNT | %DV | DENSITY | QUALITY |
|---|---|---|---|---|
| Iron | 3.6 mg | 19.9 | 4.1 | very good |
| Vitamin C | 6.0 mg | 10.0 | 2.1 | good |
| Protein | 5.0 g | 10.0 | 2.1 | good |
| Dietary Fiber | 2.5 g | 10.0 | 2.1 | good |

For more on "Total Nutrient-Richness," "%DV," "Density," and
The World's Healthiest Foods "Quality" Rating System, see page 805.
For more on GI, see page 342.

For almost 3,000 years, people in Asia have known about the medicinal properties of Shiitake Mushrooms and have regarded them as a symbol of longevity. Ancient traditions prescribed Shiitakes to improve the life energy they called *chi*, and Chinese herbalists used them for a wide variety of health problems ranging from colds and flu to headaches, measles and liver problems. They also prescribed them for improving circulation and increasing vitality. Their name is derived from the Japanese word *shii*, the hardwood host tree under which they grow, and *take*, which means Mushroom. As Shiitake Mushrooms, with their wonderfully hearty, smoky flavor and meaty texture, are now becoming increasingly popular in the West, I want to share with you the "Healthiest Way of Cooking" them. In just 7 minutes, you will not only bring out their best flavor but maximize their nutritional value.

## why shiitake mushrooms should be part of your healthiest way of eating

While Shiitake Mushrooms are a very good source of iron and a good source of protein, extensive research has found them to have other unique health-promoting compounds that may be responsible for many of their legendary health benefits. These include eritadenine, a cholesterol-lowering compound, and lentinan, an immune-stimulating phytonutrient. Shiitake Mushrooms are an ideal food to add to your "Healthiest Way of Eating" not only because they are high in nutrients, but also because they are low in calories and can promote healthy weight control: 8 ounces (net weight) of raw Shiitake Mushrooms contains only 87 calories. (For more on the *Health Benefits of Shiitake Mushrooms* and a complete analysis of their content of over 60 nutrients, see page 320.)

## varieties of shiitake mushrooms

Shiitake Mushrooms (*Lentinus edodes*) and other Japanese mushrooms have grown wild since prehistoric times. Shiitake Mushrooms are the most popular of the Japanese specialty Mushrooms and the variety that is most easily found in local markets. Flavorful and meaty with a smoky aroma, they have slightly convex caps that range in diameter from about two to four inches.

### Other Varieties of Japanese Mushrooms

**MAITAKE**

Like Shiitakes, this variety has a delicious flavor. They grow as a cluster of brownish-colored, overlapping, fan-shaped caps and are commonly known as "Hen of the Woods."

**REISHI**

They are woody and bitter and not as enjoyable to eat; however, they are highly revered for their medicinal properties. They are usually shaped like an antler or rounded fan. They come in six different colors with the red variety being the most popular.

All varieties of Japanese specialty Mushrooms are available dried and are easily reconstituted.

## the peak season

Once grown only in Japan, Shiitake Mushrooms are now grown in the U.S. in many states and are available year-round.

## 4 steps for the best tasting and most nutritious shiitake mushrooms

Turning Shiitake Mushrooms into a flavorful dish with the most nutrients is simple if you just follow my 4 easy steps:

1. The Best Way to Select
2. The Best Way to Store
3. The Best Way to Prepare
4. The Healthiest Way of Cooking

# 1. the best way to select shiitake mushrooms

You can select the best tasting Shiitake Mushrooms by looking for ones that are firm, plump and dry. As Shiitake Mushrooms are stored, the center portion of the cap will turn darker in color, and the Mushroom will develop a richer flavor. This is also an indication that they should be used as soon as possible. By selecting the best tasting Shiitake Mushrooms, you will also enjoy Mushrooms with the highest nutritional value.

Avoid Shiitake Mushrooms that are wrinkled or have wet slimy spots.

As the popularity of Shiitake Mushrooms grows, they are becoming more common in many grocery stores. If your grocery store does not carry them, you can usually find them at natural foods stores or Asian markets.

# 2. the best way to store shiitake mushrooms

Shiitake Mushrooms are very perishable and do not store well. For optimal freshness and nutrition, it is best to cook them the same day you purchase them; but if you cannot, you should ensure that you store them properly so that they will best retain their nutrients and flavor.

Shiitake Mushrooms continue to respire even after they have been harvested. Slowing down the respiration rate with proper storage is the key to extending their flavor and nutritional benefits. (For a *Comparison of Respiration Rates* for different vegetables, see page 91.)

### Shiitake Mushrooms Will Remain Fresh for Up to 5 Days When Properly Stored

1. Store fresh Shiitake Mushrooms in the refrigerator. The colder temperature will slow the respiration rate, helping to preserve vitamins and keeping Shiitake Mushrooms fresh for a longer period of time.

2. I have found it is best to either wrap Shiitake Mushrooms in a damp cloth and place them in a loosely closed paper bag or lay them out on a glass dish and cover with a moist cloth.

3. Do not wash Shiitake Mushrooms before refrigeration because exposure to water will encourage Shiitake Mushrooms to spoil.

### How to Store Dried Shiitake Mushrooms

Dried Shiitake Mushrooms should be stored in a tightly sealed container in either the refrigerator or freezer where they will stay fresh for six months to one year.

# 3. the best way to prepare shiitake mushrooms

I want to share with you the best way to prepare Shiitake Mushrooms. Properly cleaning and cutting Mushrooms helps ensure that they will have the best flavor and retain the greatest number of nutrients.

### Cleaning Shiitake Mushrooms: Wipe but Do Not Wash

Mushrooms are very porous, so if they are exposed to too much water, they will quickly absorb the water and become soggy. Therefore, the best way to clean Mushrooms without sacrificing their texture and taste, is to clean them without water. To do this, simply wipe them well with a damp paper towel. You can also use a Mushroom brush, which you can purchase at most kitchenware stores.

## Cutting Shiitake Mushrooms

### FRESH SHIITAKE MUSHROOMS

To cut fresh Shiitake Mushrooms, lay mushrooms upside down and cut off stem, and then slice the cap. Discard stems or save for soup stock. See the Step-by-Step below for more details.

### DRIED SHIITAKE MUSHROOMS

Rinse dried Shiitakes with water. Place in a bowl with just enough hot water to cover; this water can be incorporated into the recipe you are making and will add a lot of flavor to it.

Let Mushrooms sit in the hot water for about 10 minutes or until they are soft.

Squeeze out excess water, slice Mushrooms up to the stem on all sides and discard the stem since it is usually too tough to eat (or use them to make a stock).

# 4. the healthiest way of cooking shiitake mushrooms

Since research has shown that important nutrients can be lost or destroyed by the way a food is cooked, the "Healthiest Way of Cooking" Shiitake Mushrooms is focused on bringing out their best flavor while maximizing their vitamins, minerals and powerful antioxidants.

## The Healthiest Way of Cooking Shiitake Mushrooms: "Healthy Sautéing" for just 7 minutes

In my search to find the healthiest way to cook Shiitake Mushrooms, I tested every possible cooking method and discovered that "Healthy Sautéing" Shiitake Mushrooms for 7 minutes delivered the best result. "Healthy Sautéing" provides the moisture necessary to make Shiitake Mushrooms tender, bring out their best flavor and maximize their nutritional profile. The Step-by-Step Recipe will show you how easy it is to "Healthy Sauté" Shiitake Mushrooms. (For more on "Healthy Sautéing," see page 57.)

## How to Avoid Overcooking Shiitake Mushrooms

For the best flavor, I recommend "Healthy Sautéing" Shiitake Mushrooms for 7 minutes. This method allows them to become tender and cook just long enough to soften their cellulose and hemicellulose fibers; this makes them easier to digest and allows their health-promoting nutrients to become more readily available for absorption.

## Cooking Methods Not Recommended for Shiitake Mushrooms

### BOILING, STEAMING OR COOKING WITH OIL

Boiling and steaming Shiitake Mushrooms results in excessive water absorption, which causes them to lose much of their flavor. Additionally, it leads to a reduction of many of their nutrients, including minerals, water-soluble vitamins (such as C and the B-complex vitamins) and health-promoting phytonutrients. I also don't recommend cooking Shiitake Mushrooms in oil because high temperature heat can damage delicate oils and potentially create free radicals.

---

### An Easy Way to Prepare Shiitake Mushrooms, Step-by-Step

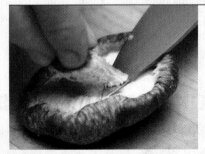 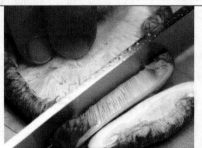 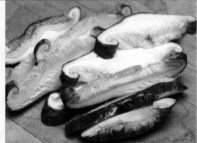

### SLICING SHIITAKE MUSHROOMS

❶ Wipe Shiitake Mushrooms and cut off stem. ❷ Lay Mushrooms upside down and slice into desired thickness. ❸ Slice entire cap but discard stem as it is too tough to eat.

**STEP-BY-STEP RECIPE**
## The Healthiest Way of Cooking Shiitake Mushrooms

# 7-Minute "Healthy Sautéed" Shiitake Mushrooms

*If you like Shiitake Mushrooms with a rich flavor, a tender and meaty texture and the maximum amount of nutrients, I recommend "Healthy Sautéing." It is fun to "Healthy Sauté," and I think you will be wonderfully surprised by the extra flavor.*

**1 lb of Shiitake Mushrooms, tough stems removed**
**3 TBS low-sodium chicken or vegetable broth**
**2 TBS extra virgin olive oil**
**2 medium cloves garlic**
**Sea salt and pepper to taste**

1. Chop garlic and let it sit for at least 5 minutes. (Why?, see page 261.)

2. Clean Mushrooms and slice as directed under *The Best Way to Prepare Shiitake Mushrooms.*

3. Heat 3 TBS broth in a stainless steel skillet over medium heat until it begins to steam.

4. Add Shiitake Mushrooms and sauté **covered** for 4 minutes. They will begin to release liquid after

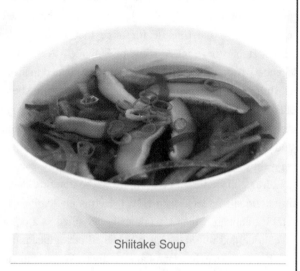
Shiitake Soup

2 minutes. After 4 minutes, reduce the heat to low, and continue to cook **uncovered** for 3 more minutes stirring constantly. (For information on *Differences in Cooking Time*, see page 94.)

5. Transfer to a bowl. For more flavor, toss Shiitake Mushrooms with the remaining ingredients while they are still hot.

OPTIONAL: To mellow the flavor of garlic, add garlic to Shiitake Mushroom for the last 2 minutes of sautéing. You may need to add a little more liquid to prevent garlic from sticking to pan.

### COOKING TIPS:

• To prevent overcooking Shiitake Mushrooms, I highly recommend using a timer.

## Flavor Tips: Try these 7 great serving suggestions with the recipe above. ✳

1. **Most Popular: Shiitakes with Onions.** "Healthy Sauté" 1 small sliced onion with Shiitake Mushrooms (these two share the same cooking time) and omit dressing. Sprinkle with tamari, rice vinegar and 3 TBS extra virgin olive oil. Add grated ginger and red pepper flakes for a spicy kick.

2. Add a few drops of tamari (soy sauce). If you add tamari, you will want to reduce the amount of sea salt.

3. Top with anchovy fillets.

4. Top with rosemary for great flavor.

5. Top with balsamic vinegar or your favorite vinaigrette.

6. For a Greek flavor, add oregano and feta cheese.

7. **Shiitake Soup:** Make Miso soup by combining 4 cups boiling water with 4 TBS miso paste. Add 7-Minute "Healthy Sautéed" Shiitake Mushrooms, (omit dressing) sautéed onion, thin strips of nori (sea vegetable) and thinly sliced green onions. Add tamari to taste (pictured above).

Please write (address on back cover flap) or e-mail me at info@whfoods.org with your personal ideas for preparing Shiitake Mushrooms, and I will share them with others through our website at www.whfoods.org.

# health benefits of shiitake mushrooms

## Promote Optimal Health

A symbol of longevity in Asia because of their health-promoting properties, Shiitake Mushrooms have been used medicinally by the Chinese for more than 6,000 years. Recent studies have traced some of Shiitake Mushrooms' legendary benefits to an active compound contained in these Mushrooms called lentinan. Among lentinan's healing benefits is the ability to power up the immune system, strengthening its ability to fight infection and disease. In test tube studies against influenza and other viruses, lentinan has been shown to be even more effective than some prescription drugs; in studies, it even improved the immune status of individuals infected with HIV, the virus that can cause AIDS. Lentinan, which is technically classified as a polysaccharide and referred to as a branched beta-glucan, has also been shown to have anti-cancer activity. When lentinan was given for human gastric cancer, special cells called reticular fibers developed in tumor sites; reticular cells are immune cells that have the ability to ingest bacteria, particulate matter and worn out or cancerous cells. When lentinan was administered, not only was there a proliferation of reticular cells in gastric tumor sites, but many T-lymphocytes (another type of immune defender) were drawn to these cancer sites with the result that the cancer cell nests were fragmented and destroyed.

## Promote Heart Health

Numerous animal studies conducted over the last ten years have shown that eritadenine, another active component in Shiitake Mushrooms, lowers cholesterol levels, regardless of the type of fat in the diet. Eritadenine has been found to lower plasma cholesterol levels in a dose-dependent manner; in other words, the more eritadenine, the more the cholesterol levels drop. Preliminary animal research also suggests that in addition to its hypocholesterolemic properties, the eritadenine in Shiitake Mushrooms may be anti-atherogenic; when animals were fed Shiitake Mushrooms, they were found to have less development of atherosclerosis on their artery walls. Shiitake Mushrooms' vitamin C and dietary fiber also offer additional heart-health benefits.

## Additional Health-Promoting Benefits of Shiitake Mushrooms

Shiitake Mushrooms are also a concentrated source of other nutrients providing additional health-promoting benefits.

These nutrients include energy-producing iron and muscle-building protein. Since an 8 ounce (net weight) serving of raw Shiitake Mushrooms contains only 87 calories, they are an ideal food for healthy weight control.

### Nutritional Analysis of 8 ounces of raw Shiitake Mushrooms:

| NUTRIENT | AMOUNT | % DAILY VALUE | NUTRIENT | AMOUNT | % DAILY VALUE |
|---|---|---|---|---|---|
| Calories | 87.23 | | Pantothenic Acid | — mg | — |
| Calories from Fat | 0.00 | | | | |
| Calories from Saturated Fat | 0.00 | | **Minerals** | | |
| Protein | 4.98 g | | Boron | — mcg | |
| Carbohydrates | 12.46 g | | Calcium | 0.00 mg | 0.00 |
| Dietary Fiber | 2.49 g | 9.96 | Chloride | — mg | |
| Soluble Fiber | — g | | Chromium | — mcg | |
| Insoluble Fiber | — g | | Copper | — mg | — |
| Sugar – Total | 2.49 g | | Fluoride | — mg | — |
| Monosaccharides | — g | | Iodine | — mcg | — |
| Disaccharides | — g | | Iron | 3.59 mg | 19.94 |
| Other Carbs | 7.48 g | | Magnesium | — mg | — |
| Fat – Total | 0.00 g | | Manganese | — mg | — |
| Saturated Fat | 0.00 g | | Molybdenum | — mcg | — |
| Mono Fat | 0.00 g | | Phosphorus | — mg | — |
| Poly Fat | 0.00 g | | Potassium | — mg | |
| Omega-3 Fatty Acids | 0.00 g | 0.00 | Selenium | — mcg | — |
| Omega-6 Fatty Acids | 0.00 g | | Sodium | 49.85 mg | |
| Trans Fatty Acids | 0.00 g | | Zinc | — mg | — |
| Cholesterol | 0.00 mg | | | | |
| Water | 207.41 g | | **Amino Acids** | | |
| Ash | 1.94 g | | Alanine | — g | |
| | | | Arginine | — g | |
| **Vitamins** | | | Aspartate | — g | |
| Vitamin A IU | 0.00 IU | 0.00 | Cystine | — g | — |
| Vitamin A RE | 0.00 RE | | Glutamate | — g | |
| A - Carotenoid | 0.00 RE | 0.00 | Glycine | — g | |
| A - Retinol | 0.00 RE | | Histidine | — g | — |
| B1 Thiamin | — mg | — | Isoleucine | — g | — |
| B2 Riboflavin | — mg | — | Leucine | — g | — |
| B3 Niacin | — mg | — | Lysine | — g | — |
| Niacin Equiv | — mg | | Methionine | — g | — |
| Vitamin B6 | — mg | — | Phenylalanine | — g | — |
| Vitamin B12 | 0.00 mcg | 0.00 | Proline | — g | |
| Biotin | — mcg | — | Serine | — g | |
| Vitamin C | 5.98 mg | 9.97 | Threonine | — g | — |
| Vitamin D IU | — IU | — | Tryptophan | — g | — |
| Vitamin D mcg | — mcg | | Tyrosine | — g | |
| Vitamin E Alpha Equiv | — mg | — | Valine | — g | — |
| Vitamin E IU | — IU | | | | |
| Vitamin E mg | — mg | | | | |
| Folate | — mcg | — | | | |
| Vitamin K | — mcg | | | | |

(Note: "—" indicates data is unavailable. For more information, please see page 806.)

Here are some questions I received from readers of the whfoods.org website about Shiitake Mushrooms:

## Q Would it make any difference if I seek out organic Shiitake Mushrooms or is it OK to buy the regular ones available at my local supermarket?

A Organically grown Shiitake Mushrooms would be superior because the strict standards employed with organic farming help to enhance soil quality. Yet, organically grown Shiitake Mushrooms are oftentimes difficult to find. While I prefer to purchase them whenever possible, I oftentimes buy conventionally grown Shiitake Mushrooms since that is what is usually available.

## Q Are dehydrated Shiitake Mushrooms as healthy as fresh ones? It is much more convenient for me to buy the dehydrated ones.

A In general, I prefer fresh foods to non-fresh foods (such as canned or dehydrated foods). Yet, that being said, dehydrated Shiitake Mushrooms are a wonderful way to enjoy this very healthy food as they still retain great nutritional value. I like to think about nutrition not just from an ideal perspective but from a realistic perspective as well. Even if the dehydrated Shiitake Mushrooms have a bit less nutritional value, if buying them in this form will enable and inspire you to use them more than if relying upon the fresh ones, than I am all for buying/using dehydrated Shiitake Mushrooms.

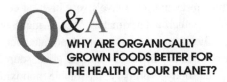

## Q&A
### WHY ARE ORGANICALLY GROWN FOODS BETTER FOR THE HEALTH OF OUR PLANET?

Organically grown foods are cultivated using farming practices that work to preserve and protect the environment.

Most conventional farming methods used today adhere to a chemical-dependent model of agribusiness. Residues from conventional farming methods use toxic chemicals that remain in the soil, leach into groundwater, and frequently end up either on the skin or become internal constituents of commercially grown foods. The predominant use of this model has resulted in adversely affecting the earth's environment and the health of its inhabitants. These methods have adversely affected soil quality, water purity, biodiversity, safety and health of farm workers, survival of small and family farms, connection to the land, and taste and quality of foods.

Organic farming is seen as the alternative to chemical farming. It is often inaccurately and simplistically described as farming without the use of pesticides. More accurately, it is a method of farming that partners with nature rather than altering or controlling natural processes that includes:

- Not applying dangerous synthetic pesticides, herbicides and chemical fertilizers
- Improving soil quality
- Conserving and keeping up water quality
- Encouraging biodiversity
- Minimalizing the health and occupational hazards to farm workers
- Maintaining a restorative and sustainable biosystem

### WHAT IS SUSTAINABLE AGRICULTURE?

Sustainable agriculture is farming practices that preserve and protect the future productivity and health of the environment. In 1992, during the UN Conference on Environment and Development, a number of non-governmental organizations (NGO) drafted their own Sustainable Agriculture Treaty that states:

"Sustainable Agriculture is a model of social and economic organization based on equitable and participatory vision of development which recognizes the environment and natural resources as the foundation of economic activity. Agriculture is sustainable when it is ecologically sound, economically viable, socially just, culturally appropriate and based on a holistic scientific approach.

Sustainable Agriculture preserves biodiversity, maintains soil, fertility and water purity, conserves and improves the chemical, physical and biological qualities of the soil, recycles natural resources and conserves energy.

Sustainable Agriculture uses locally available renewable resources, appropriate and affordable technologies, and minimizes the use of external and purchased inputs, thereby increasing local independence and self sufficiency and insuring a source of stable income for peasants, family small farmers and rural communities, and integrates humans with their environment. Sustainable Agriculture respects the ecological principles of diversity and interdependence and uses the insights of modern science to improve rather than displace the traditional wisdom accumulated over centuries by innumerable farmers around the world.

Organic farmers use sustainable agricultural practices in the production of organically grown foods."

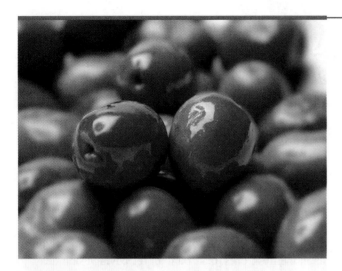

# olives

## highlights

| | |
|---|---|
| AVAILABILITY: | Year-round |
| REFRIGERATE: | Yes |
| SHELF LIFE: | 1 year refrigerated |
| PREPARATION: | Minimal |
| BEST WAY TO COOK: | No need to cook |

## nutrient-richness chart

Total Nutrient-Richness: **4**     GI: **n/a**

One cup (134 grams) of sliced Olives contains 155 calories

| NUTRIENT | AMOUNT | %DV | DENSITY | QUALITY |
|---|---|---|---|---|
| Iron | 4.4 mg | 24.7 | 2.9 | good |
| Vitamin E | 4.0 mg | 20.1 | 2.3 | good |
| Dietary Fiber | 4.3 g | 17.2 | 2.0 | good |
| Copper | 0.3 mg | 17.0 | 2.0 | good |
| **CAROTENOIDS:** | | | | |
| Beta-Carotene | 318.5 mcg | | | Daily values for these nutrients have not yet been established. |
| Beta-Cryptoxanthin | 12.1 mcg | | | |
| Lutein+Zeaxanthin | 685.4 mcg | | | |

For more on "Total Nutrient-Richness," "%DV," "Density," and The World's Healthiest Foods "Quality" Rating System, see page 805.

For more on GI, see page 342.

O lives are one of the oldest foods and are believed to have originated in Crete between 5,000 and 7,000 years ago. Since ancient times, the Olive tree has been a source of food, fuel, timber and medicine; it has been regarded as a symbol of both peace and wisdom. Olives cannot be eaten right off of the tree. Only after they have gone through special processing methods that reduce the intrinsic bitterness concentrated in their skin do they acquire their delicious taste. The length of time the Olives remain on the tree combined with the processing method used to cure them are some of the factors that determine their variety. Sour to bitter, piquant to sweet, the tangy taste of Olives is an easy and enjoyable addition to your "Healthiest Way of Eating."

## why olives should be part of your healthiest way of eating

Olives are fruits of the *Olea europaea* tree. *Olea* is the Latin word for "oil," reflecting the Olive's very high fat content (over 80%), of which approximately 75% is made up of oleic acid, a health-promoting monounsaturated fat that supports heart health. Olives are also a good source of vitamin E, the body's primary fat-soluble antioxidant, which protects cells from the oxidative damage that can be caused by free radicals. Olives contain phenolic phytonutrients (plant nutrients) including oleuropein and hydroxytyrosol, which have strong antioxidant potential, and are one of the foods that researchers feel gives the Mediterranean diet its impressive health-promoting properties. (For more on the *Health Benefits of Olives* and a complete analysis of their content of over 60 nutrients, see page 326.)

## varieties of olives

Olives can be produced from both ripe and unripe Olives. Olives are not edible before they are cured because of their high levels of oleuropein, which gives uncured Olives a very bitter flavor. Curing Olives reduces enough of the oleuropein to eliminate most of their bitterness while retaining much of oleuropein's protective antioxidant qualities. The color and taste of Olives are determined by their ripeness when picked and how they are processed, which involves fermentation and/or curing in oil, brine or salt. These methods not only cause the Olives to turn black, purple, brown, red or yellow, but they also affect their skin texture and determine whether they will be smooth or shiny. While fully ripened Olives are black in color, green unripe Olives can also turn black due to processing.

In addition to varying in size and appearance, the flavor of Olives spans a range from sour to smoky to bitter to acidic. Olives are often very salty because they are cured in salt brine. You can wash them before eating to reduce the salt content. Olives come whole with seeds, pitted or stuffed with ingredients such as almonds, garlic or pimentos. Additionally, specialty stores offer Olives that are marinated with ingredients such as lemon peel, herbs and hot peppers.

## Curing Methods Using Ripe Olives

### GREEK METHOD

Fully ripened, dark purple or black Olives are gradually fermented in brine (saltwater) to leach out their bitter taste. They are sweeter and richer with a more complex taste than other varieties. Because caustic soda solutions, which speed up the curing time, are not permitted in Greece, fermentation takes eight to ten months. KALAMATA OLIVES are cured using red wine vinegar or red wine to give them their distinctive flavor.

### DRY CURED

Fully ripened black Olives that are rubbed with coarse salt and left to cure for months, resulting in their characteristically wrinkled appearance. The salt is removed before the Olives are sold.

### SUN CURED

Fully ripe black Olives that are left on the tree to dry.

### OIL CURED

Fully ripe black Olives that are soaked in oil for a few months.

## Curing Methods Using Unripe Olives

### SPANISH METHOD

Unripe, light green Olives are soaked in a fast-acting lye solution (caustic soda) for six to sixteen hours to leach out the oleuropein, the phytonutrient that gives them their bitter taste. This method of using a lye solution to cure Olives was invented in Spain. Olives cured this way have a crisp texture and nutty flavor.

---

### WHAT ARE THE BEST OLIVES?

I believe the best Olives are those that are tree ripened because they are nutritionally mature, and their black color reflects their rich content of phytonutrients. Green Olives are less nutritious because they are not allowed to fully ripen. I believe that the best varieties are Kalamata from Greece, Liguria from Italy and Niçoise from France. All of these are carefully harvested and hand-picked, so they do not have bruises, soft spots or bitter taste, and they are never cured in lye. Be sure to read the ingredients on the label.

---

### AMERICAN METHOD

Half-ripe, yellow-red-colored Olives are soaked in an alkaline lye solution without fermentation. A flow of air bubbled through the olive-lye solution is used to oxidize the Olives and give them their characteristic black color. Cold water rinses are used after curing to remove as much of the curing solution as possible. Iron is also added (in the form of ferrous gluconate) to preserve the dark color. Some varieties of American Olives, which are produced in California, include SEVILLANO and QUEENS. MISSION Olives are dry-cured.

## Canned Olives

Canned black Olives are made from unripe Olives, which are picked green, cured in lye and pumped with oxygen to make them black. Canned Green Olives are cured in lye. Canned Olives are soft in texture and flat in flavor.

# the peak season

Olives are available throughout the year.

# 3 steps for the best tasting and most nutritious olives

Adding Olives to your favorite meal is simple if you just follow my 3 easy steps:

1. The Best Way to Select
2. The Best Way to Store
3. The Best Way to Prepare

---

Here is a question I received from a reader of the whfoods.org website about Olives:

**Q** *I was told that the peppery taste and deep color of Olives was good for my health. Is this true?*

**A** The peppery taste and rich color of olives are part of what makes Olives so good for your health. For example, the color in Green Olives comes primarily from chlorophyll in combination with various carotenoids, phytonutrients that have been shown to have health-supportive properties. The taste of Olives reflects some fairly complicated chemistry involving phytonutrients such as polyphenols, tannins and secoiridoid derivatives. Particularly in the polyphenol category, there is fairly extensive research on their health benefits. In general, the phytonutrient components of a food often provide it with its color and taste. These components also frequently function as antioxidant and anti-inflammatory compounds in our bodies after we've enjoyed the great taste of the Olives or their oil.

# 1. the best way to select olives

Olives have been traditionally sold in jars and cans, but you can now find Olives in bulk in many local markets. I find that buying Olives in bulk allows you to try many different types of Olives without having to purchase large quantities of any one kind. You can choose from whole Olives with seeds, pitted Olives or those that are stuffed with peppers, garlic or almonds. If you purchase Olives in bulk, make sure that the store has a good turnover and keeps its Olives immersed in brine or oil for freshness and moisture.

# 2. the best way to store olives

### Refrigerate

Olives remain the freshest if stored in an airtight container in the refrigerator. Make sure the Olives are stored in a liquid, such as the brine or oil in which they were preserved, so they do not dry out. If there is not enough liquid in the container in which you are storing the Olives, you can add Olive oil to increase the amount of liquid.

# 3. the best way to prepare olives

If you find Olives a bit too salty, you can rinse them under cold water them before using them.

If you want to remove the pits, use the flat side of a large heavy knife and press the Olives to crush them. This will make it easier to remove pits.

Here is a question that I received from a reader of the whfoods.org website about Olives:

**Q** *Can Olives be eaten right off the tree? And do they look the same on the tree as they do when I purchase them in a store?*

**A** Olives actually cannot be eaten right off of the tree. They require special processing to reduce their intrinsic bitterness, caused by the glycoside phytonutrient oleuropein, which is concentrated in their skin. These processing methods vary with the olive variety, cultivation region and the desired taste, texture and color to be created.

Some olives are picked green and unripe, while others are allowed to fully ripen on the tree to a black color. Yet, not all of the black olives that you may purchase actually began with a black color. Some processing methods expose unripe greens olives to the air, and the subsequent oxidation turns them a dark color. Wrinkled Olives, such as those that have been dry cured, do not start out with that raisin-like appearance; these ripened black Olives have been rubbed with coarse salt, which draws out their moisture, leaving them with their signature appearance.

---

### An Easy Way to Prepare Olives, Step-By-Step

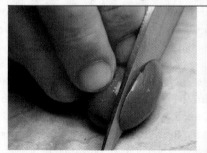 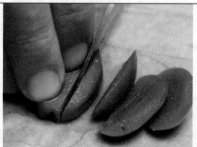 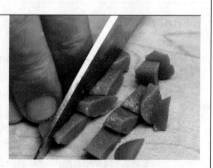

**CHOPPED OLIVES**

❶ To remove pit, cut one side of the Olive alongside the pit. ❷ Turn and do this on all four sides, removing as much meat as possible. ❸ Discard the pit. Using a rocking motion with your knife, chop meat into the desired size.

**The Healthiest Ways to Enjoy Olives**

# Olive Tapenade

*Olive Tapenade is delicious, easy to make and can be used as a dip, sandwich spread or topping for fish and poultry. Make a batch to keep in the refrigerator for enhancing your meals throughout the week.*

**8 oz Kalamata Olives,
    pitted and minced
3 garlic cloves, minced
2 TBS capers, rinsed and drained
2 TBS minced fresh Italian parsley
1 minced anchovy fillet (optional)
2 tsp minced lemon peel
Freshly ground black pepper to taste
3 TBS extra virgin Olive oil**

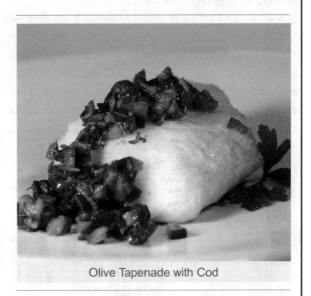

Olive Tapenade with Cod

1. In a small bowl, combine Olives, garlic, capers, parsley, anchovy, lemon peel and black pepper.

2. Add extra virgin Olive oil and mix thoroughly. Research shows that carotenoids found in foods are best absorbed when consumed with oils.

**Kitchen Hint:**

The Olives, capers, garlic and parsley may be minced at the same time in a food processor.

**Additional Ways to use Olive Tapenade:**
- Stir into vinaigrette dressing.
- Use as topping on sliced tomatoes.
- Combine with "Healthy Steamed" Broccoli or "Healthy Sautéed" Eggplant.
- Add to a wrap.
- Use as a topping on "Quick Broiled" chicken or fish.

**MAKES 1/2 CUP**

---

**Flavor Tips:** Try these 5 great serving suggestions with the recipe above. ✳

1. Blend minced Kalamata Olives into your favorite vinaigrette.

2. Add chopped Olives to your favorite tuna or chicken salad recipe.

3. **Italian Tuna Salad:** Combine 1 can of tuna, 1 diced celery stalk, 1/2 minced medium onion, 1 tsp rinsed capers, 8 chopped cured Olives, 1 clove of crushed garlic and 3 TBS extra virgin Olive oil to make a robust tuna salad.

4. **Marinated Olives:** Marinate Olives in a cup of extra virgin Olive oil, 1 tsp lemon zest, 1 tsp coriander seeds and 1 tsp cumin seeds.

5. **Appetizer:** Set out a small plate of Olives on the dinner table along with some vegetable crudités for your family to enjoy with the meal.

**ADDITIONAL RECIPES**

- **Spicy Putenesca Sauce:** In a sauce pan, combine: 1 small can of mashed anchovies, 2 large diced tomatoes, 3 cloves pressed garlic, 3 TBS capers, 3 TBS chopped cured Olives and plenty of freshly ground black pepper. Sauté for 5 minutes, stirring frequently. Mix with "Healthy Steamed" Broccoli or use on your favorite pasta or polenta.

- **Olive Crostini:** Slice Italian bread into 1/4-inch diagonal slices. Bake in a 400°F (200°C) degree oven for 3 minutes on each side. As soon as they come out of the oven, rub with a crushed garlic clove. Top with chopped Kalamata Olives, minced fresh rosemary, and crumbled feta cheese. Place back in the oven for 1 minute. Drizzle with extra virgin Olive oil and serve.

---

Please write (address on back cover flap) or e-mail me at info@whfoods.org with your personal ideas for preparing Olives, and I will share them with others through our website at www.whfoods.org.

# health benefits of olives

## Promote Cellular Health

Olives, a staple of the disease-preventive Mediterranean diet, are a concentrated source of monounsaturated fats, notably oleic acid. Monounsaturated fats are an important component of the cell membrane, and since they are less easily damaged than polyunsaturated fats, they have a protective effect on the cell and can lower the risk of cellular damage and inflammation. Olives are also a good source of vitamin E, the body's primary fat-soluble antioxidant. Vitamin E protects the cells from the damage that can be caused by free radicals in the fat-rich components of the body, which include the brain and cell membranes.

In addition to monounsaturated fats and vitamin E, Olives contain a variety of phytonutrients that have potent antioxidant activity and can therefore protect cellular health. These include the polyphenolic compounds, oleuropein and hydroxytyrosol. Research has suggested that the antioxidant potential of these phenolic phytonutrients is at least equal to that of vitamin E and vitamin C.

## Promote Heart Health

Individuals who follow the Mediterranean diet have been found to have lower risk of heart disease. While the Mediterranean Diet contains many healthful foods (including fruits, vegetables, nuts, seeds, whole grains and fish), Olives and Olive oil have been shown to play a very important role. Some of the benefit may come from the ability of antioxidant compounds in Olives to protect LDL molecules from oxidation (this is one of the first steps in the development of atherosclerosis). While vitamin E's ability to protect fat-containing molecules such as LDL cholesterol has been long known, recent research has shown that the polyphenolics, hydroxytyrosol and oleuropein, also have the same benefit.

## Promote Optimal Inflammatory Balance

Vitamin E, oleic acid, and the polyphenolic compounds, hydroxytyrosol and oleuropein, have all been found to inhibit markers of inflammation. Since health conditions such as asthma, osteoarthritis and rheumatoid arthritis have been associated with high levels of free radicals, the anti-inflammatory actions of these compounds found in Olives may help reduce the severity of these health conditions. This benefit is further supported by research showing that populations who consumed oil made from Olives had a reduced risk of rheumatoid arthritis compared to those not consuming this oil.

## Additional Health-Promoting Benefits of Olives

Olives are also a concentrated source of many other nutrients providing additional health-promoting benefits. These nutrients include energy-producing iron, free-radical-scavenging copper, and digestive-health-promoting fiber.

### Nutritional Analysis of 1 cup of Olives:

| NUTRIENT | AMOUNT | % DAILY VALUE | NUTRIENT | AMOUNT | % DAILY VALUE |
|---|---|---|---|---|---|
| Calories | 154.56 | | Pantothenic Acid | 0.02 mg | 0.20 |
| Calories from Fat | 129.19 | | | | |
| Calories from Saturated Fat | 17.12 | | **Minerals** | | |
| Protein | 1.13 g | | Boron | — mcg | |
| Carbohydrates | 8.41 g | | Calcium | 118.27 mg | 11.83 |
| Dietary Fiber | 4.30 g | 17.20 | Chloride | — mg | |
| Soluble Fiber | 0.22 g | | Chromium | — mcg | — |
| Insoluble Fiber | 4.09 g | | Copper | 0.34 mg | 17.00 |
| Sugar – Total | 4.11 g | | Fluoride | — mg | — |
| Monosaccharides | — g | | Iodine | — mcg | — |
| Disaccharides | — g | | Iron | 4.44 mg | 24.67 |
| Other Carbs | 0.00 g | | Magnesium | 5.38 mg | 1.34 |
| Fat — Total | 14.35 g | | Manganese | 0.03 mg | 1.50 |
| Saturated Fat | 1.90 g | | Molybdenum | — mcg | — |
| Mono Fat | 10.60 g | | Phosphorus | 4.03 mg | 0.40 |
| Poly Fat | 1.22 g | | Potassium | 10.75 mg | |
| Omega-3 Fatty Acids | 0.09 g | 3.60 | Selenium | 1.21 mcg | 1.73 |
| Omega-6 Fatty Acids | 1.14 g | | Sodium | 1171.97 mg | |
| Trans Fatty Acids | 0.00 g | | Zinc | 0.30 mg | 2.00 |
| Cholesterol | 0.00 mg | | | | |
| Water | 107.51 g | | **Amino Acids** | | |
| Ash | 3.00 g | | Alanine | 0.06 g | |
| | | | Arginine | 0.09 g | |
| **Vitamins** | | | Aspartate | 0.12 g | |
| Vitamin A IU | 541.63 IU | 10.83 | Cystine | 0.00 g | 0.00 |
| Vitamin A RE | 53.76 RE | | Glutamate | 0.12 g | |
| A - Carotenoid | 53.76 RE | 0.72 | Glycine | 0.07 g | |
| A - Retinol | 0.00 RE | | Histidine | 0.03 g | 2.33 |
| B1 Thiamin | 0.00 mg | 0.00 | Isoleucine | 0.04 g | 3.48 |
| B2 Riboflavin | 0.00 mg | 0.00 | Leucine | 0.07 g | 2.77 |
| B3 Niacin | 0.05 mg | 0.25 | Lysine | 0.04 g | 1.70 |
| Niacin Equiv | 0.05 mg | | Methionine | 0.02 g | 2.70 |
| Vitamin B6 | 0.01 mg | 0.50 | Phenylalanine | 0.04 g | 3.36 |
| Vitamin B12 | 0.00 mcg | 0.00 | Proline | 0.05 g | |
| Biotin | — mcg | — | Serine | 0.04 g | |
| Vitamin C | 1.21 mg | 2.02 | Threonine | 0.03 g | 2.42 |
| Vitamin D IU | 0.00 IU | 0.00 | Tryptophan | 0.00 g | 0.00 |
| Vitamin D mcg | 0.00 mcg | | Tyrosine | 0.03 g | 3.09 |
| Vitamin E Alpha Equiv | 4.03 mg | 20.15 | Valine | 0.05 g | 3.40 |
| Vitamin E IU | 6.01 IU | | | | |
| Vitamin E mg | 4.03 mg | | | | |
| Folate | 0.00 mcg | 0.00 | | | |
| Vitamin K | 1.88 mcg | 2.35 | | | |

(Note: "–" indicates data is unavailable. For more information, please see page 805.)

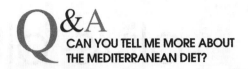

## Q&A
### CAN YOU TELL ME MORE ABOUT THE MEDITERRANEAN DIET?

## What Are the Mediterranean Food Traditions?

Many countries border along the Mediterranean Sea, and many different food traditions are represented in these countries. While several Middle Eastern and North African countries border the Mediterranean, it is usually the foods from the countries of Italy, Greece, Spain, Portugal and (southern) France that are referred to as "Mediterranean" cuisines.

## Olive Oil

If you've purchased olive oil in the grocery store, you may have noticed that virtually all of it comes from one of three countries: Italy, Spain or Greece. In fact, over 75% of all olive oil worldwide comes from the three Mediterranean countries. Olive trees are native to this area of the world, and it would be impossible to follow a Mediterranean diet tradition without including olives and their oil.

Mediterranean diets have been especially interesting to researchers in relationship to heart disease. Given the total amount of fat in many Mediterranean foods (including olives and nuts), it might seem logical to expect a higher incidence of heart disease in Mediterranean countries than actually occurs. One reason for the lower-than-expected rates of heart disease is olive oil (and olives). Olives are very high in monounsaturated fat, a type of fat that often escapes damage by free radicals and is therefore more heart healthy. Oleic acid accounts for most of the monounsaturated fat in olives, and diets containing significant amounts of this fatty acid have also been shown to help lower LDL cholesterol and homocysteine levels in the body. Both of these changes are considered protective of the heart and circulation.

Olives also contain some unique phytonutrients called polyphenols. Oleuropein is the best studied of these polyphenols. This phenolic substance in olives has been found to help lower blood fats, prevent interruption of blood flow and function as an antioxidant that helps protect the blood vessels.

## Mediterranean Climate, Vegetables and Fruits

The climate around the Mediterranean Sea is often referred to as "dry summer subtropical." This climate is ideal for a wide variety of fresh, locally grown vegetables including an abundance of tomatoes and peppers. Figs and pomegranates are also unique fruits widely available in this region. The Mediterranean climate leaves populations in this part of the world with an especially rich vegetable-and-fruit platform for building a delicious and optimally nourishing food plan.

## Fish

All of the Mediterranean countries share an active stretch of coastline along the Mediterranean Sea. For this reason, fish are a staple part of the Mediterranean diet. Bass, blue whiting, striped mullet, skate, shark, shad, sturgeon and tuna are all common to this region. Many of the fish contribute to the much better-than-average intake of omega-3 fatty acids in the Mediterranean diet. The omega-3 fatty acids are not only helpful in prevention of heart disease, but also in support of most organ systems in the body.

## Red Wine

Italy, Spain, and France are countries famous world wide for their production of red wine. Regular consumption of red wine would be considered part of most Mediterranean diets, and like olive oil, red wine supplies civilizations along the Mediterranean with ample supplies of several unique phytonutrients. Resveratrol is one of the best-studied polyphenols in red wine. This substance has been shown to improve blood flow to the brain and to help keep heart muscle flexible. Tannin and saponin glycosides are other substances in red wine that are clearly heart-protective due to their total cholesterol-lowering and HDL-cholesterol-increasing effects. The saponins in red wine also help prevent unwanted clumping together of red blood cells.

## The Rich and Authentic Taste of Real Food

Devotion to taste is one final topic that's impossible to avoid when describing the Mediterranean diet. Culture traditions in this region of the world prize the deliciousness of food in a way that is almost legendary. One of the reasons that fast food, processed food and hydrogenated oils play a smaller role in this region than in the United States is because of these cultures' reverence of the taste of fresh food. To inhabitants of the Mediterranean, there is just nothing like the spectacular taste of fresh, regionally grown foods seasoned and prepared with the utmost of care. Everything else falls short. The simplicity of good taste is a key factor in the healthiness of the Mediterranean diet. It's also one reason why there is so much overlap between this way of eating and the "Healthiest Way of Eating" I recommend based on the World's Healthiest Foods.

Fresh vegetables, fruits, extra virgin olive oil, nuts, seeds, fish...all staples of the Mediterranean diet and the World's Healthiest Foods. So enjoy the "Healthiest Way of Eating" with the World's Healthiest Foods and you'll gain benefits like those who enjoy the Mediterranean diet.

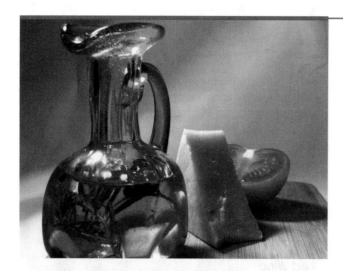

# olive oil, extra virgin

## highlights

| | |
|---|---|
| AVAILABILITY: | Year-round |
| REFRIGERATE: | No |
| SHELF LIFE: | 1 year |
| PREPARATION: | None |

## nutrient-richness chart

One TBS (14 grams) of Extra Virgin Olive Oil contains 126 calories

| NUTRIENT | AMOUNT | %DV |
|---|---|---|
| Total Fat | 14.00 g | |
| Monounsaturated Fat | 10.78 g | |
| Polyunsaturated Fat | 1.26 g | |
| Saturated Fat | 1.26 g | |
| Vitamin E | 1.96 mg | 8.7 |
| **PHYTOSTEROLS:** | | Daily values for these nutrients have not yet been established. |
| Phytosterols–Total: | 30 mcg | |

Olive trees are well suited to the region along the Mediterranean Sea where they have been cultivated since the time this area of the world was settled. Some of the olive groves in Spain are older than 1,000 years as olive trees have a very long life. So, it is no surprise that Olive Oil has long been associated with the cooking and flavors of Mediterranean food. Olive Oil comes in a wide range of colors from yellow to smoky green, each having its own unique taste. Along with its wonderful flavor, Olive Oil has been found to have many nutritional benefits and is a great addition to both cold salads and hot entrées. There are hundreds of delicious ways to include it in your "Healthiest Way of Eating."

## why olive oil should be part of your healthiest way of eating

A high-fat diet and a low rate of heart disease (in fact, the lowest of all countries studied) was the fascinating anomaly that researchers found in Crete, an island in Greece. It turns out that the major contributor of fat to the Cretan diet is Olive Oil. Research is finding that Olive Oil, with its concentration of monounsaturated fats (such as oleic acid), vitamin E and powerful antioxidant phenolic phytonutrients, can play a major role in a heart-healthy diet. The vitamin E contained in Olive Oil serves as a natural preservative, preventing the Olive Oil from going rancid. Of the different varieties of Olive Oil, Extra Virgin Olive Oil is the least refined and retains the most nutrients, including antioxidants such as oleuropein and hydroxytyrosol, from the olives from which it is pressed. (For more on the *Health Benefits of Olive Oil* and a complete analysis of its content of over 60 nutrients, see page 332.)

## varieties of olive oil

Olives were brought to America by the Spanish and Portuguese explorers during the 15th and 16th centuries and were introduced into California by the Franciscan missionaries in the late 18th century. Olive Oil is made from the crushing and then subsequent pressing of olives. The fact that olives are rich in oil is reflected in the botanical name of the olive tree — *Olea europaea* — as *oleas* means "oil" in Latin.

### EXTRA VIRGIN OLIVE OIL

"Extra virgin" is the most superior and pure form of Olive Oil and the only type that I recommend. It has the most delicate, yet complex, flavor. It also has the most abundant nutrient profile, featuring concentrated levels of polyphenolic antioxidant compounds. Extra Virgin Olive Oil is made using only mechanical or physical pressing methods. Only 1% of the oil extracted from olives can be called Extra Virgin Olive Oil. The olives are not exposed to heat, solvents or other treatments that may alter their oil's composition. Among virgin Olive Oils, extra virgin is the one that is closest to the natural state of the olive since it is made from the first pressing of the olives. It is the finest type of Olive Oil, featuring premiere quality and having the lowest level of acidity (under 1%) of all Olive Oils. As the most unrefined of all Olive Oils, it also has the lowest smoke point. (See page 52 for more on the smoke point of Extra Virgin Olive Oil.) I prefer to purchase Extra Virgin Olive Oil that is made from organically grown olives, whenever possible.

### OTHER VARIETIES OF OLIVE OIL

Many varieties of Olive Oil can be found at the market. I have included this information to provide you a comparison between the different types of Olive Oil, so you can better understand why Extra Virgin Olive Oil is the best choice and the one I recommend:

- **Virgin Olive Oil:** Virgin Olive Oil is also derived from the first pressing of the olives but contains an acidity level that can be more than double that of Extra Virgin Olive Oil. Therefore, it has a much less delicate and complex flavor. Additionally, Virgin Olive Oil has been found to have less antioxidant phytonutrients than Extra Virgin Olive Oil.

- **Pure Olive Oil:** Pure Olive oil is a refined oil. Unlike Extra Virgin and Virgin Olive Oils, which are only pressed by mechanical means, refined oil is created by using charcoal and/or chemicals to filter the oil. Refined oils are usually produced from poorer quality olives. Refined oils have a higher smoke point, approximately 438°F (225°C).

- **Light Olive Oil:** When it comes to Olive Oil, don't be fooled by the term "light." Its caloric and fat content is the same as other oils. "Light" refers to its light taste and light color; it is devoid of the peppery flavor and green color of the best Extra Virgin Olive Oils and of far inferior quality. The term is one that manufacturers have developed for marketing appeal and not one that is officially used to define Olive Oil.

**the peak season** available year-round.

## 3 steps for the best tasting and most nutritious extra virgin olive oil

Enjoying the best tasting Extra Virgin Olive Oil with the most nutrients is simple if you just follow my 3 easy steps:

1. The Best Way to Select
2. The Best Way to Store
3. The Best Way to Prepare

> **THE MORE FLAVOR IN OLIVE OIL, THE GREATER ITS HEALTH BENEFITS**
>
> The flavor of Olive Oil does more than just enhance the taste of your food. Extra Virgin Olive Oils differ in both color and flavor. Yellow-colored oils are rich in beta-carotene and have a fruity flavor. Green-colored oils are rich in health-promoting cholorophyll and polyphenolic compounds that provide antioxidant protection as well as a peppery bite to the oil. The more intense the flavor, the more health benefits they contain. I recommend selecting Extra Virgin Olive Oil because not only does additional refining of Olive Oil reduce its flavor, but it also reduces the amount of its health-promoting compounds. People of the Mediterranean region love the peppery taste and the green color of Extra Virgin Olive Oil.

## 1. the best way to select extra virgin olive oil ——

Since Extra Virgin Olive Oil is very delicate and can become rancid from exposure to light and heat, there are some important purchasing criteria to ensure buying a better quality product. I look for Extra Virgin Olive Oils that are sold in darkly tinted bottles since the packaging will help protect the oil from oxidation caused by exposure to light. I never buy Extra Virgin Olive Oil in clear or lightly tinted bottles because the oil will become rancid so much more quickly. In addition, I make sure the oil is displayed in a cool area, away from any direct or indirect contact with heat. Additionally, I never buy more than I am going to use within a 90 day period once the bottle is opened because I want to enjoy the freshest oil possible.

### What you should know about the labeling of Extra Virgin Olive Oil

Unfortunately, the United States Department of Agriculture (USDA) does not have labeling laws for Olive Oil that define what "extra virgin" means; rather, they make a differentiation for Olive Oil manufacturers using terms like "fancy" or "choice." Since there is not full agreement and worldwide adoption of Olive Oil definitions, this means that you may buy two bottles of Extra Virgin Olive Oil, and they could have been processed differently.

In order to feel confident that you are getting the highest quality product, I recommend purchasing organic Extra Virgin Olive Oil from companies that subscribe to the International Olive Oil Council's definition of "extra virgin," which will be indicated on the label. These are standards that have been adopted by most other countries for Extra Virgin Olive Oil. According to this definition, an Extra Virgin Olive Oil only undergoes cold, mechanical processing ("cold pressing") and is not made using methods that involve the use of solvents or re-esterification. Extra Virgin Olive Oil can only contain up to 0.8% free oleic acid, while Virgin Olive Oil can contain up to 2.0%. (The difference in free oleic acid relates to its overall acidity—Extra Virgin having less—rather than its mono-unsaturated fat content.) It is important to find companies that follow these standards since U.S. importers of European oils not subscribing to these definitions can label hexane-extracted oil as Extra Virgin (and hexane is certainly not a compound to which I would want the Olive Oil I consume to be exposed).

# 2. the best way to store extra virgin olive oil ——

Proper storage techniques for Extra Virgin Olive Oil are very important not only to preserve the delicate taste of the oil but also to ensure that it does not spoil and become rancid, which will have a negative effect on its nutritional profile. While it may be convenient to keep Extra Virgin Olive Oil in a container near the stove, the exposure to extra heat will increase its rate of spoilage. It is best to store Olive Oil in a darkly tinted glass container in a dark cool cupboard until opening. After that, it can be stored in the refrigerator to further preserve its freshness. It will typically remain fresh for 1 year from the time it is bottled, so it is best to follow the expiration date on the bottle.

# 3. the best way to prepare extra virgin olive oil —

Olive Oil needs little, if anything, in the way of preparation. It can be used straight from the bottle. Some people refrigerate their Olive Oil, which is a personal preference. If Olive Oil is refrigerated, it should be allowed to come to room temperature before being used as the cold temperatures of the refrigerator causes it to become thick and cloudy.

---

Here are questions that I received from readers of the whfoods.org website about Olive Oil:

**Q** *Can Olive Oil lower high cholesterol? If so, why?*

**A** Olive oil is suggested to not only reduce cholesterol levels but to protect LDL cholesterol from oxidizing; LDL oxidation is one of the first steps in the development of atherosclerosis. While many studies have found the cholesterol-lowering benefit to occur when Olive Oil replaced saturated fats in the diet, more recent studies suggest that its benefits may not be limited to this and that just adding Olive Oil to the diet may instill a benefit. Researchers believe that the benefits of Olive Oil on cholesterol and heart health come from an interplay of many of its nutrients including oleic acid (its monounsaturated fat), vitamin E and polyphenolic antioxidant phytonutrients such as hydroxytyrosol and oleuropein. For example, all help to reduce the potential of LDL cholesterol from becoming oxidized.

**Q** *I use a great deal of Extra Virgin Olive Oil. I know it is good for me but is there such a thing as too much?*

**A** Yes, there is such a thing as too much, even of something as healthy as Extra Virgin Olive Oil. Extra Virgin Olive Oil, like virtually all plant oils, contains about 250 calories per ounce and 28 grams of fat. If a person wanted his or her diet to contain about 20% fat and that person ate about 1,800 calories per day, he or she would need to consume no more than 40 grams of fat for the entire day. That level would allow for about 1.5 ounces of Olive Oil (three tablespoons) but no more fat in the entire day. In addition, those three tablespoons of Olive Oil would be providing about 375 out of 1,800 calories, or about 21% of all calories. So, think about that amount as the upper limit for a diet of that caloric and percentage fat pattern.

STEP-BY-STEP RECIPES
## The Healthiest Ways of Using Extra Virgin Olive Oil

# Mediterranean Dressing

*Time Saver: This dressing can be made ahead and used on many of the vegetable recipes in this book.*

**1 cup Extra Virgin Olive Oil**
**1/3 cup fresh lemon juice**
**4–5 cloves garlic**
**Sea salt and pepper to taste**

1. Press garlic and let sit for 5 minutes (Why?, see page 261.)

2. Whisk together the lemon juice, garlic, sea salt and pepper.

3. Slowly pour the Extra Virgin Olive Oil into the mixture while whisking constantly. The more slowly you pour and the faster you whisk, the thicker and creamier the dressing will be.

This dressing will store in the refrigerator for up to 10 days. It will solidify, so you will need to bring it back to room temperature before using.

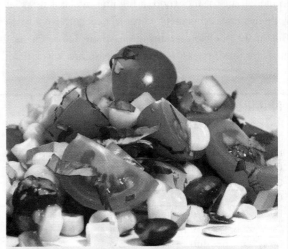

Kidney Bean Salad with Mediterranean Dressing

To add additional flavor and nutrition to the dressing, you can add any of the following: minced basil or cilantro, minced onion, curry powder, honey, finely diced avocado or red bell pepper (if using avocado or bell pepper, use dressing immediately).

**Alternative:** Dressing ingredients can be added directly to vegetables or salads without whisking.

### YIELDS ABOUT 1 1/3 CUPS

Please write (address on back cover flap) or e-mail me at info@whfoods.org with your personal ideas for preparing Extra Virgin Olive Oil, and I will share them with others through our website at www.whfoods.org.

## 10 QUICK SERVING IDEAS for EXTRA VIRGIN OLIVE OIL and MEDITERRANEAN DRESSING:

1. **Most Popular: Better than Butter Olive Oil Dip.** Instead of putting the butter dish out on the table, place Extra Virgin Olive Oil on a butter dish to use on your bread or rolls. For extra flavor, try adding a little balsamic vinegar, salt and pepper, or any of your favorite fresh herbs and spices, such as rosemary, oregano or basil.
2. Drizzle Extra Virgin Olive Oil over healthy sautéed vegetables before serving.
3. Drizzle Olive Oil on your favorite egg dish after cooking.
4. Top salmon with Extra Virgin Olive Oil, minced garlic and minced fresh ginger.
5. **Garlic Bean Dip:** Purée 5 TBS Extra Virgin Olive Oil, 3 medium cloves garlic and 2 cups of navy beans together in a food processor. Add sea salt and pepper to taste and serve as a dip or sandwich spread.
6. **Kidney Bean Salad with Mediterranean Dressing:** Combine 1 ear of raw corn kernels, 1/4 cup minced red onion, one 14 oz can kidney beans, rinsed and drained, 1 chopped medium tomato and 2 TBS minced fresh parsley or cilantro. Dress salad with 1/2 cup Mediterranean Dressing (pictured above).
7. **Healthy Tuna Salad:** Combine 1/4 cup Mediterranean Dressing recipe (above) with rinsed capers and minced parsley. Add cooked tuna chunks and coat with dressing. Serve on a bed of fresh greens.
8. **Italian Tomato Salad:** Combine 2 sliced ripe tomatoes, 2 sliced scallions, 1/4 cup chopped basil, 1 clove pressed garlic, 3 TBS Extra Virgin Olive Oil, and sea salt and pepper to taste. Best when refrigerated 1/2 hour before eating.
9. **Bruschetta:** See page 263.
10. **Herbed Potatoes with Olive Oil:** Toss "Healthy Steamed" Potatoes (page 297) with fresh parsley, basil and oregano. Mix with 5 TBS Extra Virgin Olive Oil, 1 tsp lemon juice, 1/2 tsp sea salt and 1/4 tsp pepper.

# health benefits of extra virgin olive oil

## Promotes Optimal Health

In many parts of the world, a high fat intake is associated with the development of chronic degenerative diseases. But in the Mediterranean region where Olive Oil is the main fat used, rates of chronic disease are lower than in cultures where the main fat sources are animal fats, hydrogenated fats, soy oil and corn oil. In the Mediterranean region, people who use Olive Oil regularly, especially in place of other fats, have been found to have much lower rates of heart disease, atherosclerosis, diabetes, colon cancer and asthma.

## Promotes Heart Health

Studies on Olive Oil and atherosclerosis reveal that particles of LDL cholesterol that contain the monounsaturated fats found in Olive Oil are less likely to become oxidized. Additionally, Extra Virgin Olive Oil contains polyphenolic phytonutrients—such as oleuropein and hydroxytyrosol—that further protect LDL from becoming oxidized. Since only oxidized cholesterol sticks to artery walls, preventing the oxidation of cholesterol is a good way to help prevent atherosclerosis.

## Promotes Balanced Blood Sugar

Studies in diabetic patients have shown that healthy meals that contained some Olive Oil had better effects on blood sugar than even healthy meals that were low in fat. When Olive Oil is used to enhance a low-saturated fat, high-carbohydrate diabetic diet, the diet still has beneficial effects on blood sugar control. In addition to this, a good diabetic diet with some Olive Oil added helps to keep triglyceride levels low. Triglyceride levels tend to be high in diabetic patients, which is a problem since high levels of these fat-carrying molecules also contribute to the development of heart disease.

## Anti-Inflammatory Benefits

Regular use of Olive Oil has been associated with lower rates of asthma and rheumatoid arthritis. Researchers have proposed several mechanisms for Olive Oil's anti-inflammatory benefits, including that oleic acid may inhibit the production of inflammatory compounds and that oleuropein's and hydroxytyrosol's antioxidant activity may reduce the expression of inflammation.

## Promotes Healthy Weight Control

A preliminary study focused on overweight men suggests that substituting Olive Oil, a monounsaturated fat, for saturated fat in your diet, without changing anything else about your diet or increasing your physical activity, can translate into a small but significant loss of both body weight and fat mass. Additional support for Olive Oil's fat-burning effects comes from a recent animal study that suggests that the monounsaturated fats found in Olive Oil cause an increase in the breakdown of fats in fat cells.

### Nutritional Analysis of 1 TBS of Extra Virgin Olive Oil:

| NUTRIENT | AMOUNT | % DAILY VALUE | NUTRIENT | AMOUNT | % DAILY VALUE |
|---|---|---|---|---|---|
| Calories | 126.00 | | Pantothenic Acid | — mg | — |
| Calories from Fat | 126.00 | | | | |
| Calories from Saturated Fat | 17.64 | | **Minerals** | | |
| Protein | 0.00 g | | Boron | — mcg | |
| Carbohydrates | 0.00 g | | Calcium | — mg | — |
| Dietary Fiber | 0.00 g | 0.00 | Chloride | — mg | |
| Soluble Fiber | 0.00 g | | Chromium | — mcg | — |
| Insoluble Fiber | 0.00 g | | Copper | — mg | — |
| Sugar - Total | 0.00 g | | Fluoride | — mg | — |
| Monosaccharides | 0.00 g | | Iodine | — mcg | — |
| Disaccharides | 0.00 g | | Iron | — mg | — |
| Other Carbs | 0.00 g | | Magnesium | — mg | — |
| Fat - Total | 14.00 g | | Manganese | — mg | — |
| Saturated Fat | 1.96 g | | Molybdenum | — mcg | — |
| Mono Fat | 10.78 g | | Phosphorus | — mg | — |
| Poly Fat | 1.26 g | | Potassium | — mg | |
| Omega-3 Fatty Acids | 0.10 g | 4.00 | Selenium | — mcg | — |
| Omega-6 Fatty Acids | 1.12 g | | Sodium | — mg | |
| Trans Fatty Acids | — g | | Zinc | — mg | — |
| Cholesterol | — mg | | | | |
| Water | 0.03 g | | **Amino Acids** | | |
| Ash | 0.00 g | | Alanine | 0.00 g | |
| | | | Arginine | 0.00 g | |
| **Vitamins** | | | Aspartate | 0.00 g | |
| Vitamin A IU | — IU | — | Cystine | 0.00 g | 0.00 |
| Vitamin A RE | — RE | | Glutamate | 0.00 g | |
| A - Carotenoid | — RE | — | Glycine | 0.00 g | |
| A - Retinol | — RE | | Histidine | 0.00 g | 0.00 |
| B1 Thiamin | — mg | — | Isoleucine | 0.00 g | 0.00 |
| B2 Riboflavin | — mg | — | Leucine | 0.00 g | 0.00 |
| B3 Niacin | — mg | — | Lysine | 0.00 g | 0.00 |
| Niacin Equiv | — mg | | Methionine | 0.00 g | 0.00 |
| Vitamin B6 | — mg | — | Phenylalanine | 0.00 g | 0.00 |
| Vitamin B12 | — mcg | — | Proline | 0.00 g | |
| Biotin | — mcg | — | Serine | 0.00 g | |
| Vitamin C | — mg | — | Threonine | 0.00 g | 0.00 |
| Vitamin D IU | — IU | — | Tryptophan | 0.00 g | 0.00 |
| Vitamin D mcg | — mcg | | Tyrosine | 0.00 g | 0.00 |
| Vitamin E Alpha Equiv | 1.74 mg | 8.70 | Valine | 0.00 g | 0.00 |
| Vitamin E IU | 2.59 IU | | | | |
| Vitamin E mg | 1.74 mg | | | | |
| Folate | — mcg | — | | | |
| Vitamin K | — mcg | — | | | |

(Note: "—" indicates data is unavailable. For more information, please see page 806.)

## Q&A

### CAN YOU HELP ME DIFFERENTIATE BETWEEN DIFFERENT TYPES OF FATS?

Fats are probably the most complex of the macromolecules in foods because there are so many different types. Unfortunately, fats have been given a bad reputation, in part because fat is the way we store excess calories, and in part because saturated fats, trans-fatty acids and cholesterol have been associated with health conditions like cardiovascular disease and obesity. The facts are, however, that not only are all fats not bad, some fats have been shown to be health promoting, and some fats are absolutely essential for your health. So, when you think about fats, the quality of the fat, and therefore the quality of the food from which you are getting the fat, really matters.

One extremely important role that fats play is their inclusion in all the membranes in your cells. Your cell membranes contain all different kinds of fats; however, they are needed in different amounts. Your cells primarily need polyunsaturated fats along with some monounsaturated fat to keep your membranes, and therefore your cells, flexible and moveable. When levels of saturated fat are too high, cell membranes become inflexible and don't function well, so they can't protect the internal parts of the cell, such as its DNA, as well.

### Saturated Fats and the Controversy of the "Bad" Fats

Excessive consumption of saturated fats can negatively affect your health since the fat you eat gets directly into your cell membranes. Minimizing the consumption of saturated fats is a good idea, but minimizing the consumption of all fats is not. Consider that your brain is approximately 70% fat. In addition, diets low in all types of fats have been associated with increased risk of hormone abnormalities, cardiovascular disease and decreased brain and immune function. So, the real question is not how to indiscriminately avoid all fats, but which fats, in which amounts, are good for you?

### Monounsaturated Fats

Monounsaturated fats caught the attention of research scientists after they first noticed that people who eat a traditional Mediterranean diet have a lower risk of developing cardiovascular disease, certain types of cancer and rheumatoid arthritis. Traditional Mediterranean diets contain high amounts of olive oil, which is high in oleic acid, a monounsaturated fatty acid.

Other monounsaturated fats include myristoleic and palmitoleic acids. In addition to olive oil, other food sources for monounsaturated fatty acids include avocados, almonds, cashews and canola oil. Research continues to support the theory that diets high in monounsaturated fats are health promoting.

### Polyunsaturated Fats

The polyunsaturated fats (PUFAs) are molecules that contain many unsaturated bonds, a characteristic that distinguishes them chemically from the other fats. In practical terms, this chemical structure is the reason these fats are liquid even when cold. Many different polyunsaturated fats exist, but the ones getting the most attention from research scientists are the essential fats, linoleic acid (LA) and alpha-linolenic acid (ALA), as well as the long-chain omega-3 fatty acids.

Your body can make all the different fats it needs from two starting molecules, the two essential fats: LA (an omega-6 fatty acid) and ALA (an omega-3 fatty acid). Because these are essential fats, meaning your body can't make them, you must get them from your diet. All other PUFAs can be made from these fats.

LA is plentiful in the diet of most Americans. This fat is found at high levels in oils from grains, nuts and legumes; it is often provided in your diet by sunflower, safflower, sesame, corn, soy and peanut oils. Few people are deficient in omega-6 fatty acids not only because of the high intake of vegetable oils but also because the Western diet contains a lot of meat, which is a concentrated source of the omega-6 arachidonic acid.

Long-chain omega-3 fats such as eicosapentaenoic acid (EPA) and docosahexaenoic acid (DHA) are produced in your body from the essential omega-3 fat, ALA; they have generated much interest since studies continue to show that diets low in omega-3 fats are associated with many health conditions. ALA is found in high quantities in walnuts, flaxseeds and their oil, and some leafy vegetables. EPA and DHA can be obtained directly from the diet as well. Excellent sources for EPA and DHA are fish and algae.

For good health, it is vital to consider the ratio of omega-6 to omega-3 fats in your diet. The proper balance of omega-3 to omega-6 is extremely important not only for healthy cell membranes, but also because omega-6 fats are the precursors for pro-inflammatory molecules—the molecules that promote and maintain inflammatory reactions. In order to achieve a more beneficial ratio, it is important to decrease the amount of omega-6 fatty acids in your diet, while increasing the amount of omega-3 fatty acids like EPA, DHA, and ALA.

# Q&A
### WHAT IS CHLOROPHYLL AND IN WHAT FOODS IS IT FOUND?

Although it's not very well-known in the world of nutrition, chlorophyll couldn't be more important in the world of biology and plants. All green plants contain at least one type of chlorophyll (chlorophyll *a*). Plants that evolved at a later point in history ("higher plants") also contain a second type of chlorophyll (chlorophyll *b*). There are also forms of chlorophyll called chlorophyll *c1, c2* and *c3*, as well as a chlorophyll d, but these forms are much less widely distributed in the plant world. Chlorophyll is the single most critical substance in plants that allows them to absorb light from the sun and convert that light into usable energy. (In biochemistry, it's called the primary photo-receptor pigment.)

In many vegetables, there is slightly more chlorophyll *a* than chlorophyll *b*, and this slight edge in favor of chlorophyll a tends to decrease as the plant ages. However, research studies have yet to clarify what the exact health significance is of this ratio of chlorophyll *a* to chlorophyll *b*.

## The Color of Chlorophyll

It's usually easy to tell when a food has significant amounts of chlorophyll because chlorophyll provides the green color that is found in grasses, leaves and many of the vegetables that we eat. These plants and foods would not be green without their chlorophyll, since chlorophyll pigments reflect sunlight at the exact appropriate wavelengths for our eyes to detect them as green. The chlorophyll a molecule actually reflects light in a blue-green range (about 685 nanometer wavelengths), while chlorophyll *b* reflects light in a more yellow-green color (about 735 nanometer wavelengths). The overall effect, however, is for us to see varying shades of a color we would simply call "green."

## Foods That Contain Chlorophyll

While all green plants contain chlorophyll a, and most vegetables that we eat contain both chlorophyll *a* and chlorophyll *b*, some vegetables contain particularly high amounts of total chlorophyll. Best studied of all the vegetables is spinach which contains about 300–600 mcg per ounce.

To understand how high in chlorophyll this amount turns out to be, compare the chlorophyll content of spinach to another of the World's Healthiest Foods—olives. Chlorophyll is one of the primary pigments in olives, but olives contain only 30–300 micrograms per ounce (about 1/1000th as much as spinach). Some olive oil producers deliberately allow olive tree leaves to be placed in the olive presses to increase the chlorophyll and "grassiness" of the olive oil.

All of the green vegetables in the World's Healthiest Foods—asparagus, bell peppers, broccoli, Brussels sprouts, green cabbage, celery, collard greens, green beans, green peas, kale, green olives, parsley, romaine lettuce, sea vegetables, spinach and Swiss chard among others—are concentrated sources of chlorophyll.

## Chlorophyll and Health

Research on the health benefits of chlorophyll has focused on the area of cancer (including treatment and prevention). This research got underway when damage to genes (or more precisely, to the genes' DNA) by carcinogenic substances called aflatoxins (or more precisely aflatoxin B1, or AFB1), was found to be prevented by chlorophyllin, a derivative of chlorophyll in which the magnesium in its center is removed—usually by placing it in an acid bath in a science lab—and replaced with copper. Research on the prevention and treatment of various types of cancer in relationship to chlorophyll is still in the early stages and is being investigated.

## Effect of Cooking on Chlorophyll

The jury is definitely still out on the impact of cooking on chlorophyll. On one end of the spectrum, it's totally clear that dramatic loss of chlorophyll occurs after prolonged cooking. In studies on broccoli, for example, about two-thirds of the chlorophyll was removed after 20 minutes of boiling. Researchers have also determined that there are steadily increasing losses of both chlorophyll *a* and chlorophyll *b* when the boiling time for broccoli is increased from 5 to 20 minutes. However, at cooking times less than 5 minutes, the research is not as clear, and some studies suggest that brief steaming of vegetables like spinach actually increases the amount of chlorophyll that can be absorbed into our body.

Whenever a vegetable is cooked long enough to cause a change in color from bright green to olive-gray, we know that some of the chlorophyll *a* and chlorophyll *b* has changed to pheophytins *a* and *b*. This color change is one of the reasons I have established the relatively short cooking times for green vegetables in the "Healthiest Way of Cooking" techniques! These cooking methods are designed to preserve the unique concentrations of chlorophyll found in these vegetables.

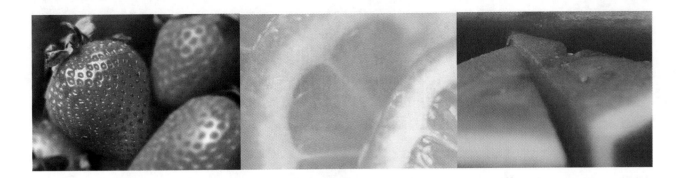

# fruits

The numbers beside each food indicate their Total Nutrient-Richness. (For more details, see page 805.)

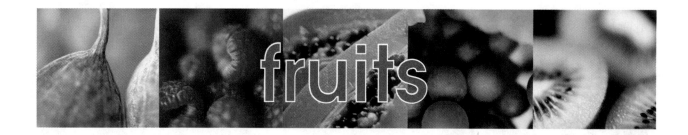

# fruits

The assortment of different types of fruit available in the marketplace has exploded in recent years. Tropical fruits like papayas, pineapple and kiwifruit, once only available at specialty stores, are now commonly found in the produce sections of many markets throughout the country. Additionally, because of improved means of transportation and global trade, fruits that have been traditionally offered only seasonally (during their local growing seasons) are now available year-round. Organically grown fruits look better, taste better and are more readily available than ever before.

Fruits are flavorful, refreshing and full of health-promoting nutrients. And most fruits are also easy to eat, requiring no preparation or utensils. Fruits are so versatile that they are no longer reserved for snacks, desserts or breakfast—they can add a sweet zest to many types of dishes including salads, sandwiches and numerous entrées.

In the vegetable chapters, I emphasized how proper cooking can improve the nutritional value of vegetables. Here in the fruits section, I will share with you the reasons why fruits are best eaten raw.

## Fruits: Definition

Fruits are distinguished from vegetables in that they contain the seeds that will produce the next generation of plants, which will flower and fruit again.

### Why You Need to Eat Fruits Everyday

We need to eat fruits everyday because we need to provide our body with water-soluble vitamins everyday, and fruits (along with vegetables) provide more of these critical nutrients than any other type of food. Unlike fat-soluble vitamins (such as vitamin A, D and E), which our bodies can store for future use, the water-soluble vitamins (vitamin C and the B vitamins—B1, B2, B3, B5, B6, B12 and folic acid), are needed every single day for our bodies to function optimally since they either can't be stored or can only be stored in very small amounts. Vitamins are called essential nutrients because our bodies cannot produce them, and the best way to obtain them is through the foods that we eat. Fruits are one of the richest sources of water-soluble vitamins, which is one reason why guidelines for a healthy diet recommend eating 3–4 servings (around 2 cups) of fruits everyday.

Fruits are rich in newly discovered health-promoting phytonutrients (plant nutrients), such as carotenoids, flavo-noids and organic acids (such as ellagic acid), which act as powerful antioxidants. For example, fruits provide us with a cornucopia of health-promoting flavonoids called anthocyanins, which give them (as well as vegetables), their red and purple coloration. Blueberries, plums, strawberries, apples, oranges, pears all have lustrous shades of red and purple signifying their high anthocyanin content. Not only do these phytonutrients give fruits their wide variety of wonderfully vibrant colors, but they also act as powerful antioxidants that help reduce the effects of harmful free-radical activity and the risk of disease. In fact, on a serving-for-serving basis, blueberries contain more anthocyanins than red wine, which has received much publicity as a rich source of these heart-healthy compounds. Fruits also contain special enzymes that can help with digestion that are not found in any other type of food. Papaya, for example, provides the enzyme *papain*, while *bromelain* is the well-known enzyme we get from pineapple.

To maintain optimal health, enjoy the recommended 3–4 servings of fruit each day. Although our bodies can obviously survive on less, and effects of deficiencies can be subtle or take a long time to fully develop, they cannot be avoided. They may range from low energy levels to reduced immune function. Without adequate servings of fruits, we are depriving our bodies of great sources of important nutrients essential to proper physiological functioning. When all is said and done, you will be taking an important step toward better health if you enjoy fresh fruits seven days a week and make them a regular part of your "Healthiest Way of Eating."

## How Fruits Help You Stay Slim, Energized and Healthy

Fruits not only look and taste good, but they provide us with energy! Enjoying a piece of fruit when we are craving a bit of sweetness is one way to stay slim and healthy.

The natural sugars and other carbohydrates in fruit provide us with a much healthier form of fuel for many of our metabolic processes than the snack bars and cookies we often grab between meals. Fruits not only satisfy our sweet tooth, but, like vegetables, they are rich in nutrients including vitamin A, vitamin C, manganese and potassium. They are also a rich source of dietary fiber, which is essential for good digestion and maintaining healthy blood cholesterol levels as well as other health benefits. (For more on *What are the Keys to Supporting Healthy Energy Production?*, see page 379.)

### FRUITS CAN BE LOW IN CALORIES

Fruits like strawberries, raspberries and cantaloupe contain only 70–100 calories per one cup serving and are very nutrient-rich. This means they provide you with the most vitamins, minerals and newly discovered phytonutrients for the least number of calories. This is very important today when we are looking for foods that will help control our weight and also provide us with maximum nutritional value. A recent USDA study has shown that people who eat more fruit and vegetables have the lowest Body Mass Index (BMI) and they consume fewer calories than people on the standard American diet.

When it comes to deciding what form of fruits to eat, I believe fresh raw fruit is the best choice since any type of processing—juicing, drying, freezing and canning—can decrease the nutritional value found in whole fresh fruit.

## Not All Fruits are Created Equal— Fruits and Blood Sugar Levels

One of the things to consider when selecting foods that are a concentrated source of carbohydrates and/or sugars is how these foods affect blood sugar levels since blood sugar regulation plays a key role in maintaining good health. While all fruits are sweet (some more than others), all fruits do not affect your blood sugar in the same way. A food's glycemic index (GI) is a value that ranks foods based on their immediate effect on blood sugar levels. It is a measure of how much your blood sugar increases over a period of two or three hours after a meal.

Sweet fruits that break down quickly during digestion have the highest glycemic index. Tropical fruits, such as pineapples, papayas and mangoes, are considered high GI foods (see chart, page 409); if consumed alone without the accompaniment of another low glycemic food, they may cause a spike in blood sugar. Other fruits, such as apples, grapefruit, pears, blueberries and plums actually have low to medium GI values. The skin of fruits not only provides extra antioxidants but is also a concentrated source of fiber, which helps slow digestion and thereby slows the release of sugar into the bloodstream. The GI for fruit juice and dried fruit is higher than for whole fresh fruit because the juice contains less pulp and skin than the whole fruit, and drying fruit concentrates its sugar content. (For more on the *Glycemic Index*, see page 342.)

## Ripe Fruit is the Best

It is best to eat fresh, ripe fruit. A ripe fruit is vibrant in color, is at its peak of flavor, has the highest nutritional value and is ready to eat!

What happens when fruits ripen? Health-promoting nutrients (vitamins and phytonutrients), which act as powerful antioxidants, are predominantly produced during the ripening process when fruits are still on the tree or vine. When fruits have been picked green, they have not had time to fully develop the power of their vitamins and phytonutrients. As fruits ripen, they turn from hard, sour and inedible to soft, sweet and juicy. Their acidic content decreases, their color becomes more brilliant and vibrant, their vitamin content increases and most of the starches change to sugars, giving them a sweet aroma and taste. So how do you know when fruits are ripe? Smell them. Ripe strawberries smell like strawberries; ripe apricots smell like apricots; ripe cantaloupe smells like cantaloupe. It's as simple as that.

When you purchase fruit that is already ripe, it is best to eat it right away as it will turn from ripe to rotten very quickly. Once fruit is ripe, it starts to decay:

- First the color turns brown
- Next the flavor deteriorates
- Then the texture softens
- And the vitamin content declines

Remember that overly "green" fruits may never ripen, and some fruits will not ripen at all after they have been picked.

## Why Fruits at the Market May Not Be Ripe

It is very difficult to find ripe fruit at the market because most fruits are picked before they are totally ripe. Fruits that are not ripe can better withstand the duress of being transported and distributed; however, because they are picked green, many of them will never develop their full flavor. That is why it is best to purchase locally grown, preferably organic, fruit in season, which is more likely to be picked closer to when it is ripe. Locally grown fruit is therefore not only tastier but also more affordable.

## The Best Way to Ripen Fruit

Bananas will fully ripen after they have been picked green. Other fruits such as apricots, apples, pears, blueberries and figs will not fully ripen but will improve in flavor after they have been picked. They will become softer, juicier and more colorful if you leave them at room temperature or place them in a paper bag kept in a dark, cool and well ventilated place. The bag traps ethylene gas produced by the fruit and helps it to soften, which I refer to as "ripening" for lack of a better word. (The quotation marks differentiate it from true ripening.) Adding an apple or banana to the bag will help speed up the "ripening" process.

Some fruits will not "ripen" at all after being picked. These include strawberries, raspberries, cherries, grapes, citrus fruits, pineapples, and melons. They are not worth buying unless they are already ripe.

More complete information on how to complete the "ripening" process is included in each of the individual fruit chapters.

## Is Fruit Juice as Good as Whole Fruit?

You'll notice that all of the fruits included among the World's Healthiest Foods are listed in their whole food form (this includes lemons and limes even thought their nutritional profile is for the juice). Fruit juice, although tasty and refreshing, is not as healthy as whole fruit. When a whole fruit is pressed or squeezed to make juice, some of the nutrients, most notably fiber and the water-soluble vitamins, are lost in the process; its GI value also increases. So, I highly recommend you enjoy the most diverse and intact collection of nutrients by consuming the whole fruit.

Orange juice provides a good example of how the nutritional value of the juice compares to that of the whole fruit. The white pulpy part of the orange is the primary source of its flavonoids, plant nutrients that support numerous metabolic processes in the body. The juicy orange-colored sections of the orange contain most of its vitamin C. In the body, flavonoids and vitamin C often work together and support health through their interaction. Since the pulpy white portion of the oranges is removed when they are juiced, the flavonoids are lost in the juicing process. This loss of flavonoids is one of the many reasons I recommend eating oranges in their whole food form (even if you only end up eating a little bit of the white pulpy part).

Additionally, many fruit juices that are sold in supermarkets contain added sweeteners (sucrose or high fructose corn syrup) and only a small percentage of real fruit juice. As a result, it is easy to consume a large amount of calories without getting any actual nutrition when you consume these beverages. Make sure you read fruit juice labels carefully! Turn the jar or bottle around and look at the ingredient list on the back. You may be surprised to see exactly how much juice is actually in the product (the order in which the foods appear in the ingredient list is the order in which they are concentrated)!

Whether fruit juice can actually be considered healthy depends upon how often it is consumed and what food it replaces. If it is the only "convenience" choice for replacing a canned soda pop, I'm all in favor of fruit juice. I would also support drinking juices that are made using a home juicer or blender that allow for close to 100% retention of the pulp and skin, which supplies the fiber and many of the nutrients found in fruit. If using a regular juicer, I suggest adding back the pulp to the juice so that you can enjoy more of the fruit's nutritional benefits. It is even better if the juice is a combination of both fruits and vegetables to help increase its nutritional value. However, for the most part, I would still consider the substitution of fruit juice for whole fruit to be at the expense of the full nutritional value and health benefits found in whole fruit.

## Is Dried Fruit as Good as Fresh Fruit?

The commercial process of drying fruit in large quantities is very hard on nutrients. Desirable components like beta-carotene, vitamin C and many other nutrients are largely lost in the drying process (although flavonoids are often conserved, and some are even enhanced). Fiber always remains, but on a cup-per-cup basis, calories and sugar go way up. A cup of cranberries has about 47 calories; a cup of dried cranberries has about 370. We're making a mistake when we routinely replace fresh fruit with its commercially dried equivalent.

With home dehydrating, however, it's a different story. A home dehydrator does nothing more than blow warm air up through the fresh fruit, so it's not nearly as harsh on

| NUTRIENT | FRESH CRANBERRIES | DRIED CRANBERRIES |
|---|---|---|
| Calories | 47 | 370 |
| Fiber | 4g | 7 g |
| Vitamin A | 44 IU | 0 |
| Beta-Carotene | 28 mcg | 0 |
| Vitamin C | 13 mg | 0.2 mg |
| Magnesium | 5 g | 6 g |
| Potassium | 67 mg | 48 mg |
| Phosphorus | 9 mg | 10 mg |

Cranberries also contain trace amounts of other vitamins and minerals. Amounts based on 1 cup.

the nutrients. The fruit is still "dried" and lasts much longer than fresh fruit, but it isn't dried in the same way as if it were commercially processed. Even though home dehydration is not a bad way to go from an overall nutrient standpoint, we all still need to be careful from the sugar and calories standpoint. Sometimes we might end up eating a lot more dehydrated apple slices than the amount of apple we would have eaten if we had a fresh, organic, whole apple. The chewing and whole experience of eating can be quite different.

## Raw Fruit versus Cooked Fruit

The healthiest way to eat fruit is the traditional way: raw. By eating fruit raw, you can enjoy its fullest flavor and gain the greatest benefits from its vast array of nutrients and digestion-aiding enzymes. When you think about the natural enzymes in fruit, it is no surprise that for millennia in Asia and those living along the Mediterranean have been eating fruit for dessert, not only as a delicious ending to a meal but as a great digestive aid as well.

One of the problems with cooking fruit is that exposing it to the high temperatures (baking at 350°F/175°C) used in cooking can destroy its naturally occurring, health-promoting enzymes; these enzymes are destroyed at 118–180°F/48°–82°C. Vitamins are also lost at temperatures above 200°F/93°C. For example, fresh apples are a good source of vitamin C, but when they are cooked, most of their vitamin C is lost, and their GI increases. The chapters on individual fruits will provide you with simple tips and recipes suggesting many ways you can incorporate more fresh raw fruits into your "Healthiest Way of Eating." The recipes are quick and easy to prepare and require no baking. If you have extra fruit on hand, freezing is a good way to store it for future use.

## The Easy Way to Eat 3 to 4 Servings (2 Cups) of Fruit Each Day

I recommend following the guidelines set by various health-promoting associations, which advise eating 3 to 4 servings of fruit each day. By enjoying different colored fruits, you will be certain to reap the nutritional benefits of their varied phytonutrient pigments as well as their rich concentration of vitamins and minerals.

Breakfast is an easy time to eat fruit: whole fruit, fruit cups, fruit smoothies and adding fruit to whole grain cereals are some quick and easy ideas.

Fruit is great as a morning and afternoon snack. Not only are they delicious, refreshing and filling, but many fruits are easy to carry with you.

Fruits eaten after lunch and dinner help aid digestion. Their concentration of digestive enzymes makes them a good choice, not only for dessert but as an evening snack.

## What is a Serving Size of Fruit?

| | |
|---|---|
| 1 medium apple, pear or orange | 1/2 cup grapes or berries |
| | 1 cup diced melon |
| 1/2 grapefruit | 1/4 cup dried fruit |
| 1 small banana | 3/4 cup juice |

## How to Use the Individual Fruit Chapters

Each fruit chapter is dedicated to one of the World's Healthiest Fruits and contains everything you need to know to enjoy and maximize its flavor and nutritional benefits. Each chapter is organized into two parts:

1. **FRUIT FACTS** describes each fruit, its different varieties and its peak season. It also addresses the biochemical considerations of each fruit by considering any of its unique compounds that may be potentially problematic to individuals with specific health problems. Detailed information of the health benefits of each fruit can be found at the end of the chapter, as can a complete nutritional profile.

2. **THE 3 STEPS TO THE BEST TASTING AND MOST NUTRITIOUS WORLD'S HEALTHIEST FRUITS** includes information about how to best select, store and prepare each of the World's Healthiest Fruits. This section also features recipes and quick serving ideas. While specific information for individual fruits is given in each of the specific chapters, here are the 3 steps that can be applied to fruits in general, including those not on the list of the World's Healthiest Foods.

# 1. the best way to select fruit

Adding fruits to your "Healthiest Way of Eating" begins with selecting ones that are vibrantly colored, fresh and ripe. Whenever possible they should also be organic, locally grown and in season. The reason I emphasize buying fruit that is ripe is because not only does it taste better, but it is at the peak of its nutritional value, offering you a wealth of vitamins, antioxidants and enzymes. In this section, I want to share with you how to select the World's Healthiest Fruits, so you can be sure to enjoy the ones that are most delicious and nutritious.

## Which Fruits Contain the Most Pesticide Residues?

In 2006, the Environmental Working Group updated their "Dirty Dozen" list of fruits and vegetables containing the highest levels of pesticide residues; other non-profit groups such as Mothers and Others and the Consumer Union have done similar analysis. (For more information on the "*Dirty Dozen,*" see page 726.)

Below are two lists of fruits: one consists of fruits that contain the most pesticide residue and are included among the "Dirty Dozen," while the other list notes those fruits that have been found to have the least pesticide residues. Although I always try to select organically grown whenever possible, I believe it is especially important to choose only organically grown varieties of those on the list of fruits with the "most" pesticide residues.

| Most Pesticides | Least Pesticides |
| --- | --- |
| Peaches | Pineapples |
| Strawberries | Mangoes |
| Apples | Bananas |
| Nectarines | Kiwifruit |
| Pears | Papayas |
| Cherries | |
| Grapes (imported) | |

## Organically Grown

I find it is best to eat fruit that is organically grown. One of the many benefits of eating organically grown fruits is that you can enjoy the peel and the many nutrients it contains. The peel of conventionally grown fruits can contain many pesticides. Conventionally grown fruits are also often coated with wax. Citrus fruits, apples and pears are fruits that are commonly waxed to keep in moisture, extend their shelf life and make them shiny and more appealing. Fruits such as bananas and oranges may also be sprayed with ethylene gas to force the ripening process. (For more on *Organic Foods,* see page 113.)

## Seasonal and Locally Grown Fruits

It is best to buy fruits in season and locally grown whenever possible, even though it is becoming increasingly easy to find fruits in local markets that are out of season. Fruits that are in season and locally grown require less processing and handling, resulting in fruit with a much more robust flavor and better texture. Fruits that have not been locally grown may need to be picked while they are still "green" and immature and before they have developed their full sweetness and flavor profile; this allows them to withstand the conditions to which they are exposed while traveling so that they can arrive at your market looking fresh and ready to eat. Add this to the fact that locally grown, seasonally available fruits are usually less expensive, and you have another reason why seasonal, locally grown fruits are your best bet.

## Heirloom Fruits

There are a number of heirloom fruit varieties from which to choose. Heirloom fruits are, generally speaking, old-time varieties that were developed decades ago as opposed to the newer varieties that have been more recently bred. In addition to the wonderful rainbow of colors, shapes and tastes they offer, heirloom fruits, with their hundreds of varieties, are also important because they help preserve the biodiversity found in nature. Although not generally available at most supermarkets, heirloom fruits can be found at farmer's markets, natural food stores and supermarkets with more expansive produce sections.

# 2. the best way to store fruit

Since every fruit is unique, each one has different storage needs. Fruits last for different time periods and require different storage approaches because of various factors including their nutrient composition, their texture and shape, and how they were handled before and after harvesting.

Properly storing your fruits will help them retain their flavor and nutritional value and enable you to keep them fresh for a longer period of time. Fruits are still respiring when you bring them home from the market. Different fruits have different respiration rates. This is important because the respiration rate is related to how quickly a particular fruit will spoil. Since the faster the fruit respires, the more easily it will spoil, it is important to store fruits correctly since this will slow down their respiration rate.

The chart below shows the respiration rate of six different fruits at room temperature of 68°F (20°C). Notice the range in respiration rates, which is a reflection of the difference in storage times for different fruit:

| FRUIT | MG/KG/HR 68°F (20°C) |
|---|---|
| APPLES | 20 |
| GRAPES | 27 |
| ORANGES | 28 |
| PAPAYAS | 80 |
| RASPBERRIES | 125 |
| BANANAS (RIPE) | 280 |

Fruit respire at different rates at different temperatures. Lower temperatures help slow down the respiration rate, which is why refrigeration helps to extend shelf life. The chart in the next column shows the respiration rate of raspberries at five different temperatures, ranging from 32°F (0°C) to 68°F (20°C).

While refrigeration may help slow down the respiration rate, there are other factors to consider. For example, while tropical fruits, such as pineapple, may have a slower respiration rate when refrigerated, they will experience chill

| RESPIRATION RATES OF RASPBERRIES | | |
|---|---|---|
| 32°F | (0°C) | 17 |
| 41°F | (5°C) | 23 |
| 48°F | (10°C) | 35 |
| 59°F | (15°C) | 42 |
| 68°F | (20°C) | 125 |

injury and lose their flavor when exposed to the refrigerator's cold temperature. For these types of fruit, I always recommend purchasing them close to the time you are going to consume them, since they are really best when eaten within a day or two of purchase. Unlike other foods, most fruits cannot really be stored for very long. That is because they are very perishable and lose their flavor, texture and optimal nutrition relatively quickly. Yet, there are several fruits—including citrus fruits, apples, pears and bananas—that can actually be stored for a longer period of time (about a week or so).

Some fruits thrive when stored in the refrigerator, while others are better when left at room temperature. Still others like to be at room temperature but can be put in the refrigerator a few hours before being eaten to make them crisper and more fresh-tasting; watermelon is a good example as it is better to keep watermelon at room temperature, but you'll want to refrigerate it before eating so that its refreshing and cooling flavor can be enhanced.

# 3. the best way to prepare fruit

Preparing your fruit properly will help enhance its flavor, texture and enjoyment.

## How to Wash Your Fruit

Rinse all of your fruit under cold running water. For all conventionally grown fruit, I recommend washing in a solution of water and a mild dishwashing liquid since this usually can eliminate at least 30% of pesticide and fungicide residues. However, washing with soap or detergent does not remove the wax that is used to retain the moisture and increase the shelf life of fruits like oranges, apples and pears. Only peeling will remove this wax. Organically grown fruits only need to be rinsed under cold running water.

## How to Prevent Your Fruits from Discoloring

Browning occurs when certain fruits are cut and exposed to the air. To prevent browning of your fruit, place it in one cup of water mixed with one TBS of lemon, lime or orange juice. The vitamin C found in these fruit juices acts as an

antioxidant and slows down the activity of the enzymes that cause browning.

Once fruits have become brown, they should not be eaten as the brown color is an indication of oxidation and damage to some of the nutrients found in the fruit.

## No Bake Recipes

I often wonder why people settle for sugar and fat-laden desserts when they could be enjoying desserts made with delectable whole fruits. I have included many "No Bake" recipes to help you get the best flavor and most nutritional benefits from your fruit. Fruit is very delicate and cannot withstand the high temperatures used in baking. Its flavor and texture are so much better, and its nutritional content so much more preserved, when enjoyed raw rather than cooked. Another bonus of my "No Bake" recipes is how easily and quickly they can be prepared—much faster than recipes in which the fruit is cooked.

# glycemic index

## what is the glycemic index (GI) and how does it help find the best carbohydrates?

For many years, we have learned that carbohydrates fall into two categories: simple (including sugar and honey) and complex (including grains, starchy vegetables and legumes). We have been encouraged to eat plenty of complex carbohydrates and only moderate amounts of the simple carbohydrates. However, an increasing amount of evidence indicates that distinguishing which carbohydrates are good for you is more complicated than the simple-versus-complex paradigm suggests. What is important when differentiating between various types of carbohydrates is how rapidly a particular carbohydrate can be converted into sugar and raise levels of blood sugar (glucose), the body's source of energy for most activities. This can be measured by a food's glycemic index.

### What is Glycemic Index?

The glycemic index (GI) is a numerical scale used to indicate how fast and how high a particular food raises blood sugar levels. Glucose, the body's source of energy for many activities, is delivered to cells throughout our bodies via our bloodstream and is primarily derived from the carbohydrates in the foods we eat. A food with a low GI causes just a small rise in blood glucose, whereas a food with a high GI can cause blood glucose levels to spike.

When we look at the GI figures associated with various carbohydrates, we find that some of the foods classified as complex carbohydrates in the old system can actually increase blood glucose levels faster than some simple carbohydrates. Because the glycemic index provides a more accurate description of how quickly different carbohydrates are absorbed by the body than their classification as simple or complex carbohydrates, it has become an important tool for helping to select the right foods to help stabilize blood sugar levels and supply the energy our bodies need to promote both short-term and long-term health.

### How Awareness of Food's Glycemic Index Can Promote Optimal Health

An awareness of foods' GI can help you control your blood sugar levels. By doing so may help you improve cholesterol levels; prevent heart disease, insulin resistance and type-2 diabetes; prevent certain cancers; and achieve or maintain a healthy weight. Since substantial amount of research suggests a low GI diet provides these significant health benefits, it's worth taking a look at the basic principles of a low GI way of eating.

### Eating the Low Glycemic Way

The GI is somewhat counter-intuitive as some of the foods you would expect to have a high GI have a low GI, while others you might expect to have a low GI have a high GI. To get the most precise idea of whether your typical meals are high or low on the GI scale, it's best to look over a glycemic index list of foods (check the GI listing of the World's Healthiest Foods on the next page) and see where your favorite foods fit. Additionally, here are some basic principles that can help you estimate a food's GI and eat healthfully:

- Foods that are white tend to have a high GI. These include processed foods made with white sugar and white flour, as well as white potatoes.

- Concentrate on eating foods that are high in fiber. In general, high-fiber foods take longer to digest and therefore produce a slower rise in blood glucose levels.

- Protein foods, while not high in fiber, are typically low in GI.

- Fats do not raise glucose levels—but stick with healthy fats such as those found in extra virgin olive oil, fish, nuts and seeds.

- A person's glycemic response to a food also depends on the other foods eaten along with it. For a person without blood sugar problems, combining a food with a high GI with one with a low GI will balance the overall effect of the foods on blood sugar levels.

- Eating an array of nutrient-rich foods each day will naturally ensure that you maintain a healthy GI. Since your glycemic response to a food not only depends upon the other foods you eat along with it at that meal or snack, but also on the GI of foods eaten at your most recent meals, using GI as a guideline to help you control your blood sugar means eating healthfully day-by-day, week-by-week.

### More Practical Tips

A food is generally considered to have a high GI if it is

rated above 60. Individuals who have problems with maintaining proper blood sugar levels should restrict their selection to foods with a GI of 40 or less. These individual include those who have low blood sugar (hypoglycemia) or high blood sugar (hyperglycemia), as well as those who have a high sensitivity to sugar. Sugar includes not just refined sugars, honey and maple syrup, but also fruits, fruit juices, starchy vegetables and grain products or other foods with a high GI.

For a healthy person without any problems with blood sugar levels, all of the foods in a meal do not have to have a low GI. For example, consider a bean-and-cheese filled tortilla. The corn tortilla has a high GI (78) as do the pinto beans (GI of 63), but the tomatoes (GI of 15), onions (GI of 15), lettuce (GI of 15) and cheese (GI so low it is not recorded) balance out the overall GI effect. The result is a healthy meal that will not destabilize blood sugar levels.

When planning your healthy GI meals, keep the following simple guidelines in mind:

- Main components should have a GI of no more than 70
- Half of all components should have a GI below 50

### GLYCEMIC INDEX OF WORLD'S HEALTHIEST FOODS

In the table below, I've listed the glycemic index values primarily for the World's Healthiest Foods that are high in carbohydrates plus a few comparative foods. If a World's Healthiest Food is not on this list, it is because it does not have a high carbohydrate value and therefore, even if eaten alone, will not cause blood sugar levels to spike.

The values in the table are based on the more reliable white bread (starch) index rather than the glucose index. Should you compare these values to a GI table based on the glucose index, divide those values by 1.4.

| FOOD ITEMS | GLYCEMIC INDEX |
|---|---|
| **VEGETABLES\*** | |
| Spinach | 15 |
| Turnip Greens | 15 |
| Lettuce | 15 |
| Water Cress | 15 |
| Zucchini | 15 |
| Asparagus | 15 |
| Artichokes | 15 |
| Okra | 15 |
| Cabbage | 15 |
| Celery | 15 |
| Cucumbers | 15 |
| Dill Pickles | 15 |
| Radishes | 15 |
| Broccoli | 15 |
| Brussels Sprouts | 15 |
| Eggplant | 15 |
| Onions | 15 |
| Tomatoes | 15 |
| Cauliflower | 30 |
| Bell Peppers | 40 |
| Green Peas | 40 |
| Squash | 50 |
| Hearts of Palm | 50 |

\* I cannot find published research studies to confirm the GI of vegetables. Some consider them so low that they are not detectable, while most place their value between 15–50, and I suspect that this range is right on target based on their low carbohydrate and high-fiber content.

| FOOD ITEMS | GLYCEMIC INDEX |
|---|---|
| **GRAINS** | |
| **Barley** | |
| Pearled barley, cooked (average of 5 samples) | 35 |
| | |
| Barley kernel bread (50% kernels) | 64 |
| Barley flour bread (80% barley, 20% white white flour) | 94 |
| Whole meal barley porridge | 95 |
| | |
| **Buckwheat** | |
| Buckwheat bread (50% dehusked buckwheat groats, 50% white flour) | 66 |
| Buckwheat, cooked (average of 3 samples) | 76 |
| | |
| **Corn** | |
| Corn, yellow | 78 |
| Corn tortillas | 78 |
| Cornmeal, boiled in salted water 2 minutes | 95 |
| Taco shells | 97 |
| | |
| **Millet** | |
| Millet, boiled | 99 |
| | |
| **Multi-grains** | |
| Multi-grain bread | 60 |
| | |
| **Oats** | |
| Oat bran bread (45% oat bran, 50% white wheat flour) | 66 |
| Oatmeal (thick, dehulled oat flakes) | 77 |
| Oat bran cereal | 78 |
| Muesli | 80 |
| Oatmeal (rolled oats), cooked | 81 |

(Continued on Page 409)

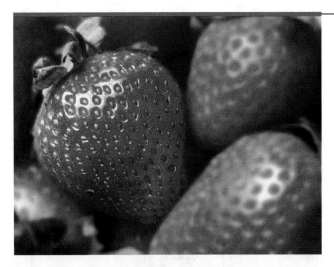

# strawberries

## highlights

| | |
|---|---|
| AVAILABILITY: | Year-round |
| REFRIGERATE: | Yes |
| SHELF LIFE: | 3 days refrigerated |
| PREPARATION: | Minimal |
| BEST WAY TO ENJOY: | Enjoy them raw |

## nutrient-richness chart

Total Nutrient-Richness: **24**    GI: **56**

One cup (144 grams) of fresh Strawberries contains 43 calories

| NUTRIENT | AMOUNT | %DV | DENSITY | QUALITY |
|---|---|---|---|---|
| Vitamin C | 81.7 mg | 136.1 | 56.7 | excellent |
| Manganese | 0.4 mg | 21.0 | 8.8 | excellent |
| Dietary Fiber | 3.3 g | 13.2 | 5.5 | very good |
| Iodine | 13.0 mcg | 8.6 | 3.6 | very good |
| Potassium | 239.0 mg | 6.8 | 2.8 | good |
| Folate | 25.5 mcg | 6.4 | 2.7 | good |
| B2 Riboflavin | 0.1 mg | 5.9 | 2.5 | good |
| B5 Pantothenic Acid | 0.5 mg | 4.9 | 2.0 | good |
| Omega-3 Fatty Acids | 0.1 g | 4.4 | 1.8 | good |
| B6 Pyridoxine | 0.1 mg | 4.0 | 1.7 | good |
| Vitamin K | 3.17 mcg | 4.0 | 1.7 | good |
| Magnesium | 14.4 mg | 3.6 | 1.5 | good |
| Copper | 0.1 mg | 3.5 | 1.5 | good |
| **CAROTENOIDS:** | | | | |
| Beta-Carotene | 10.1 mcg | | | |
| Lutein+Zeaxanthin | 37.4 mcg | | | |
| **FLAVONOIDS:** | | | | |
| (+)-Catechin | 6.4 mg | | | |
| Kaempferol | 1.1 mg | | | |
| Quercetin | 0.9 mg | | | |
| **PHYTOSTEROLS:** | | | | |
| Phytosterols - Total | 17.3 mg | | | |

Daily values for these nutrients have not yet been established.

For more on "Total Nutrient-Richness," "%DV," "Density," and The World's Healthiest Foods "Quality" Rating System, see page 805.

For more on GI, see page 342.

Strawberries were as popular during the times of the Pilgrims as they are today. They described Strawberries to be "the wonder of all fruits growing naturally" in the New World and found them in abundance as they had been planted by the Native Americans. Today, fragrantly sweet Strawberries are the most popular berries in the U.S. and for good reason. They are great enjoyed as a snack or as an addition to a summer salad or your favorite morning cereal. Once enjoyed only by the wealthy because they were so perishable and difficult to transport, Strawberries are now readily available and affordable enough for everyone to enjoy them almost any time of the year.

## why strawberries should be part of your healthiest way of eating

Strawberries are rich in antioxidants. They are an excellent source of vitamin C and also contain phenolic phytonutrients including ellagitannins and anthocyanins, which provide Strawberries with their rich red color. These heart-healthy nutrients provide powerful antioxidant and anti-inflammatory protection. Strawberries are an ideal food to add to your "Healthiest Way of Eating" not only because they are nutritious and taste great but also because they are low in calories: one cup of fresh Strawberries contains only 43 calories! (For more on the *Health Benefits of Strawberries* and a complete analysis of their content of over 60 nutrients, see page 346.)

## varieties of strawberries

Strawberries have grown wild for millennia in temperate regions throughout the world. There are more than 600 varieties of Strawberries that differ in flavor, size and texture, with 70 varieties grown in the United States. In addition to Strawberries that are cultivated, there are also varieties that grow wild. The most common scientific names for Strawberries are *Fragaria virginiana* and *Fragaria chilioensis*.

## the peak season

Although grown in all 50 states, most commercially grown

Strawberries come from California and Florida. They are available year-round, but the peak of the season runs from April through July. These are the months when their concentration of nutrients and flavor are highest, and their cost is at its lowest.

## biochemical considerations

Strawberries are a concentrated source of oxalates and goitrogens, which might be of concern to certain individuals. They are one of the foods most commonly associated with allergic reactions and also one of the 12 foods on which pesticide residues have been most frequently found. (For more on *Oxalates*, see page 725; *Goitrogens*, see page 751; *Food Allergies* see page 719; and *Pesticide Residues*, see page 726.)

## 3 steps for the best tasting and most nutritious strawberries

Enjoying the best tasting Strawberries with the most nutrients is simple if you just follow my 3 easy steps:

1. The Best Way to Select
2. The Best Way to Store
3. The Best Way to Prepare

# 1. the best way to select strawberries

Since Strawberries do not ripen after they have been picked, look for ones that are fully ripe. Fully ripe Strawberries will not only have the peak flavor and texture, but will also have more nutrients, including vitamins, antioxidants and enzymes. They have a beautiful aroma and are moderately soft and plump; they should have a shiny, deep red color and well-attached bright green caps. Medium-size Strawberries are often more flavorful than those that are excessively large. Since Strawberries are one of the foods on which pesticides residues are frequently found, I recommend selecting organically grown varieties whenever possible. (For more on *Organic Foods*, see page 113.)

Avoid Strawberries that are dull in color or have green or yellow patches since they are likely to be sour and of lesser quality. Their flavor will be inferior since they did not have time to ripen, and they will also have less nutrients. Avoid overripe Strawberries that are very soft, mushy or moldy. If you are buying Strawberries prepackaged in a container, make sure that they are not packed too tightly and that there are no signs of stains or moisture present. These are indications that the berries may be crushed, damaged or spoiled.

I have found that it is best to purchase Strawberries no more than 3 days prior to use as they are highly perishable and do not store well.

### How Do You Know Which Strawberries are Ready to Eat?

Strawberries that have a beautiful aroma, are moderately soft and plump, and have a shiny, deep red color and bright green well-attached caps are ready to eat.

# 2. the best way to store strawberries

Proper storage is an important step in keeping Strawberries fresh and preserving their nutrients, texture and unique flavor.

### Fresh Ripe Strawberries Can Last for Up to 3 Days When Properly Stored and Refrigerated

Strawberries continue to respire even after they have been harvested. The faster they respire, the more the Strawberries interact with air to produce carbon dioxide. The more carbon dioxide produced, the more quickly they will spoil. Strawberries kept at a room temperature of approximately 68°F (20°C) give off carbon dioxide at a rate of 150 mg per kilogram every hour. (For a *Comparison of Respiration Rates* for different fruits, see page 341.) Refrigerate Strawberries as soon as you bring them home. Since water encourages spoilage, do not wash Strawberries before refrigeration. While Strawberries that are stored properly will remain fresh for up to 3 days, if they are not stored properly, they will only last about 1–2 days.

### Handle with Care

Before storing in the refrigerator, remove any Strawberries that are moldy or damaged so that they will not contaminate others. Return unwashed, whole berries (with stems still attached) to their original container or spread them out on a plate. Cover with a paper towel, and then cover with plastic wrap.

# 3. the best way to prepare strawberries

Properly preparing Strawberries helps ensure that they will have the best flavor and retain the greatest number of nutrients.

*(Continued on Page 347)*

# health benefits of strawberries

### Provide Powerful Antioxidant Protection

Strawberries are a concentrated source of phenol phytonutrients, notably the anthocyanins and the ellagitannins. The anthocyanins in Strawberries not only provide them with their red color, but they also serve as potent antioxidants that have repeatedly been shown to help protect cell struc-

tures in the body and to prevent oxygen damage in all of the body's organ systems. Strawberries' unique phenol content makes them not only a heart-protective fruit, but an anti-inflammatory one as well. The anti-inflammatory properties of Strawberries include the ability of their phenols to lessen activity of the enzyme *cyclo-oxygenase* (COX). Non-steroidal anti-inflammatory drugs like aspirin or ibuprofen thwart pain by blocking the COX enzyme, whose overactivity has been shown to contribute to unwanted inflammation, such as that which is involved in arthritis, asthma, atherosclerosis and cancer.

### Promote Optimal Health

The ellagitannin content of Strawberries has actually been associated with decreased rates of cancer death. In one study, Strawberries topped a list of eight foods most linked to lower rates of cancer deaths among a group of elderly people. Recent test tube research found that all eight cultivars of Strawberries tested were able to significantly inhibit the proliferation of human liver cancer cells.

### Promote Brain Health

In animal studies, researchers have found that Strawberries help protect the brain from oxidative stress and may reduce the effects of age-related declines in brain function. Researchers found that feeding aging laboratory animals Strawberry-rich diets significantly improved both their learning capacity and motor skills.

### Promote Joint Health

While a study found that high doses of vitamin C dietary supplements made osteoarthritis worse in laboratory animals, another indicates that vitamin C-rich foods, such as Strawberries, provide humans with protection against inflammatory polyarthritis, a form of rheumatoid arthritis involving two or more joints. Vitamin C may promote joint health not only because it is a powerful antioxidant, and therefore can protect joints from the damaging effects of free-radicals, but also because it is necessary for an enzyme that promotes the production of collagen.

### Additional Health-Promoting Benefits of Strawberries

Strawberries are also a concentrated source of many other nutrients providing additional health-promoting benefits. These nutrients include bone-building vitamin K, magnesium, manganese and copper; heart-healthy omega-3 fatty acids, dietary fiber, folate, vitamin B6 and potassium; thyroid hormone-promoting iodine; and energy-producing vitamins B2 and B5. Since one cup of Strawberries contains only 43 calories, they are an ideal food for healthy weight control.

## Nutritional Analysis of 1 cup fresh Strawberries:

| NUTRIENT | AMOUNT | % DAILY VALUE |
|---|---|---|
| Calories | 43.20 | |
| Calories from Fat | 4.80 | |
| Calories from Saturated Fat | 0.26 | |
| Protein | 0.88 g | |
| Carbohydrates | 10.11 g | |
| Dietary Fiber | 3.31 g | 13.24 |
| Soluble Fiber | 1.20 g | |
| Insoluble Fiber | 2.12 g | |
| Sugar – Total | 6.80 g | |
| Monosaccharides | 5.50 g | |
| Disaccharides | 1.30 g | |
| Other Carbs | 0.00 g | |
| Fat – Total | 0.53 g | |
| Saturated Fat | 0.03 g | |
| Mono Fat | 0.07 g | |
| Poly Fat | 0.27 g | |
| Omega-3 Fatty Acids | 0.11 g | 4.40 |
| Omega-6 Fatty Acids | 0.16 g | |
| Trans Fatty Acids | 0.00 g | |
| Cholesterol | 0.00 mg | |
| Water | 131.86 g | |
| Ash | 0.62 g | |

**Vitamins**

| NUTRIENT | AMOUNT | % DAILY VALUE |
|---|---|---|
| Vitamin A IU | 38.88 IU | 0.78 |
| Vitamin A RE | 4.32 RE | |
| A - Carotenoid | 4.32 RE | 0.06 |
| A - Retinol | 0.00 RE | |
| B1 Thiamin | 0.03 mg | 2.00 |
| B2 Riboflavin | 0.10 mg | 5.88 |
| B3 Niacin | 0.33 mg | 1.65 |
| Niacin Equiv | 0.50 mg | |
| Vitamin B6 | 0.08 mg | 4.00 |
| Vitamin B12 | 0.00 mcg | 0.00 |
| Biotin | 1.58 mcg | 0.53 |
| Vitamin C | 81.65 mg | 136.08 |
| Vitamin D IU | 0.00 IU | 0.00 |
| Vitamin D mcg | 0.00 mcg | |
| Vitamin E Alpha Equiv | 0.20 mg | 1.00 |
| Vitamin E IU | 0.30 IU | |
| Vitamin E mg | 0.37 mg | |
| Folate | 25.49 mcg | 6.37 |
| Vitamin K | 3.17 mcg | 3.96 |

| NUTRIENT | AMOUNT | % DAILY VALUE |
|---|---|---|
| Pantothenic Acid | 0.49 mg | 4.90 |

**Minerals**

| NUTRIENT | AMOUNT | % DAILY VALUE |
|---|---|---|
| Boron | — mcg | |
| Calcium | 20.16 mg | 2.02 |
| Chloride | 25.92 mg | |
| Chromium | — mcg | |
| Copper | 0.07 mg | 3.50 |
| Fluoride | — mg | — |
| Iodine | 12.96 mcg | 8.64 |
| Iron | 0.55 mg | 3.06 |
| Magnesium | 14.40 mg | 3.60 |
| Manganese | 0.42 mg | 21.00 |
| Molybdenum | — mcg | — |
| Phosphorus | 27.36 mg | 2.74 |
| Potassium | 239.04 mg | |
| Selenium | 1.01 mcg | 1.44 |
| Sodium | 1.44 mg | |
| Zinc | 0.19 mg | 1.27 |

**Amino Acids**

| NUTRIENT | AMOUNT | % DAILY VALUE |
|---|---|---|
| Alanine | 0.04 g | |
| Arginine | 0.04 g | |
| Aspartate | 0.20 g | |
| Cystine | 0.01 g | 2.44 |
| Glutamate | 0.13 g | |
| Glycine | 0.03 g | |
| Histidine | 0.02 g | 1.55 |
| Isoleucine | 0.02 g | 1.74 |
| Leucine | 0.04 g | 1.58 |
| Lysine | 0.04 g | 1.70 |
| Methionine | 0.00 g | 0.00 |
| Phenylalanine | 0.03 g | 2.52 |
| Proline | 0.03 g | |
| Serine | 0.03 g | |
| Threonine | 0.03 g | 2.42 |
| Tryptophan | 0.01 g | 3.13 |
| Tyrosine | 0.03 g | 3.09 |
| Valine | 0.03 g | 2.04 |

(Note: "–" indicates data is unavailable. For more information, please see page 806.)

**STEP-BY-STEP**
## No Bake Recipes

# 10-Minute Strawberries with Chocolate Créme

*A delicious way to serve Strawberries!*

**3 TBS low-fat vanilla or soy yogurt**
**3 TBS organic cocoa**
**3 TBS maple syrup**
**1 pint Strawberries**

1. Whisk yogurt, cocoa and maple syrup in a small bowl. If your cocoa has lumps, sift it through a strainer before mixing with the other ingredients.

2. Place mixture in 2 small sauce cups on a plate and arrange the Strawberries around the cups.

3. Dip Strawberries into the chocolate créme and enjoy!

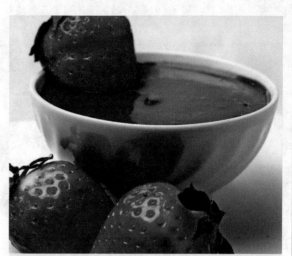

Strawberries with Chocolate Créme

**Preparation Hint**: The taste of this recipe will vary depending upon the brand of yogurt used. A creamy, custard-type yogurt works best. **SERVES 2**

Please write (address on back cover flap) or e-mail me at info@whfoods.org with your personal ideas for preparing Strawberries, and I will share them with others through our website at www.whfoods.org.

### 10 QUICK SERVING IDEAS for STRAWBERRIES:

1. Strawberries combine well with oranges, grapefruit, kiwifruit and other berries.

2. Add sliced Strawberries to mixed green salad.

3. **Strawberries and Mint:** Combine 1 cup sliced Strawberries with 1 TBS chopped fresh mint and 1 TBS creamy honey.

4. **Strawberry Parfait:** Layer sliced Strawberries, whole blueberries and plain yogurt in a wine glass for a colorful parfait dessert.

5. **Strawberry Smoothie:** Blend Strawberries with banana, papaya or grapefruit sections and orange juice for a great smoothie.

6. **High Energy Breakfast Shake:** In a blender combine 1 banana, 1/2 cup Strawberries (fresh or frozen), 1$^1$/2 cups orange juice, 1/2 cup water and your favorite protein addition, such as almond butter, spirulina or protein powder.

7. **Strawberries with Orange Sauce:** Grate 1/2 tsp orange zest. Combine the zest, 1/3 cup orange juice and 2 TBS creamy honey. Drizzle over fresh Strawberries.

8. **Waffle Topping:** Mix chopped Strawberries with cinnamon, lemon juice and maple syrup, and serve as a topping for waffles and pancakes.

9. **Strawberries and Balsamic Vinegar:** Combine 1 tsp good quality balsamic vinegar and 1/2 tsp honey and drizzle over 1 pint fresh, sliced Strawberries. Add a few grinds of black pepper for a kick. Serve at room temperature for dessert.

10. **Strawberries with Cashew Créme:** For Cashew Créme, see page 550. Pour over sliced Strawberries and chill 1 hour.

*(Continued from Page 345)*

## Cleaning Strawberries

Strawberries are very perishable and should not be washed until right before eating or using in a recipe. Do not remove their caps and stems until after you have gently washed the berries under cold running water and patted them dry. This will prevent them from absorbing excess water, which can degrade Strawberries' texture and flavor. To remove the stems, caps and white hulls, simply pinch these off with your fingers or use a paring knife. (For more on *Washing Fruit*, see page 341.)

## No Bake Recipes

I have discovered that Strawberries retain their maximum amount of nutrients and their best taste when they are fresh and not prepared in a cooked recipe. That is because their nutrients—including vitamins, antioxidants and enzymes—are unable to withstand the temperature (350°F/175°C) used in baking. So that you can get the most enjoyment and benefit from fruit, I created quick and easy recipes that require no cooking. I call them "No Bake Recipes."

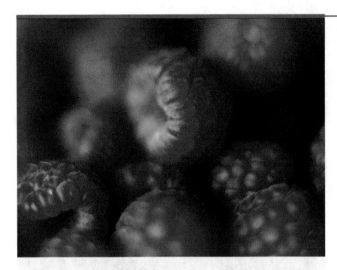

# raspberries

## highlights

| | |
|---|---|
| AVAILABILITY: | June through October |
| REFRIGERATE: | Yes |
| SHELF LIFE: | 3 days refrigerated |
| PREPARATION: | Minimal |
| BEST WAY TO ENJOY: | Enjoy them raw |

## nutrient-richness chart

Total Nutrient-Richness: **18**  GI: **n/a**

One cup (123 grams) of fresh Raspberries contains 60 calories

| NUTRIENT | AMOUNT | %DV | DENSITY | QUALITY |
|---|---|---|---|---|
| Manganese | 1.2 mg | 62.0 | 18.5 | excellent |
| Vitamin C | 30.8 mg | 51.3 | 15.3 | excellent |
| Dietary Fiber | 8.3 g | 33.4 | 10.0 | excellent |
| Folate | 32.0 mcg | 8.0 | 2.4 | good |
| B2 Riboflavin | 0.1 mg | 7.1 | 2.1 | good |
| Magnesium | 22.1 mg | 5.5 | 1.7 | good |
| B3 Niacin | 1.1 mg | 5.5 | 1.6 | good |
| Potassium | 187.0 mg | 5.3 | 1.6 | good |
| Copper | 0.1 mg | 5.0 | 1.5 | good |
| **CAROTENOIDS:** | | | | |
| Alpha-Carotene | 19.9 mcg | | | |
| Beta-Carotene | 14.8 mcg | | | |
| Lutein+Zeaxanthin | 167.3 mcg | | | |
| **FLAVONOIDS:** | | | | |
| (+)-Catechin | 1.2 mg | | | |
| (-)-Epicatechin | 10.2 mg | | | |
| Cyanidin | 51.9 mg | | | |
| Delphidin | 0.6 mg | | | |
| Pelargonidin | 4.6 mg | | | |
| Quercetin | 1.0 mg | | | |

Daily values for these nutrients have not yet been established.

For more on "Total Nutrient-Richness," "%DV," "Density," and The World's Healthiest Foods "Quality" Rating System, see page 805.

For more on GI, see page 342.

According to the ancient myths, Raspberries were originally white until the nymph Ida pricked her finger while collecting berries for baby Jupiter. The blood from her fingers caused the berries to turn their deep red color and from this came the botanical name for Raspberries, *Rubus idaeus,* with *Rubus* meaning "red" and *idaeus* meaning "belonging to Ida." Although Raspberries have been around since prehistoric times, it has only been within the past several hundred years that they have been cultivated. Sweet and subtly tart, fresh Raspberries are a great addition to your breakfast cereal or favorite dessert. And because they have a short growing season, remember to enjoy these delicately structured berries while they are in season since they are not available year-round.

## why raspberries should be part of your healthiest way of eating

Raspberries are unusually rich in health-promoting nutrients that provide powerful antioxidant protection from free-radicals that can damage cellular structures, including DNA. These include ellagic acid and flavonoids such as quercetin, kaempferol and the anthocyanins, which give red raspberries their deep red color. Like many berries, Raspberries are also exceptionally rich in dietary fiber. Raspberries are an ideal food to add to your "Healthiest Way of Eating" not only because they are nutritious and delicious, but also because they are low in calories: one cup of fresh Raspberries contains only 60 calories! (For more on the *Health Benefits of Raspberries* and a complete analysis of their content of over 60 nutrients, see page 350.)

## varieties of raspberries

Wild Raspberries are thought to have originated in eastern Asia, but there are also varieties that are native to the Western Hemisphere. Raspberries are known as "aggregate fruits" since they are a compendium of smaller seed-containing fruits, called drupelets, which are arranged around a hollow central cavity. Most Raspberries are red, but there are also yellow, amber, apricot, purple and black varieties. Although they may differ in color, they all are similar in texture and flavor.

## the peak season

Most cultivated varieties of Raspberries are grown in California from June through October and are only available during this time of the year.

## biochemical considerations

Raspberries are a concentrated source of oxalates, which might be of concern to certain individuals. (For more on *Oxalates*, see page 725.

## 3 steps for the best tasting and most nutritious raspberries

Enjoying the best tasting Raspberries with the most nutrients is simple if you just follow my 3 easy steps:
1. The Best Way to Select
2. The Best Way to Store
3. The Best Way to Prepare

# 1. the best way to select raspberries

When you select Raspberries, look for ones that are fully ripe because they will not ripen after they are picked. Fully ripe Raspberries are slightly soft, plump and deep in color. Vitamins and health-promoting phytonutrients, many of which can act as powerful antioxidants, are at their peak when Raspberries are ripe; therefore, by selecting ripe Raspberries, you will also be enjoying Raspberries with the highest nutritional value as well as the best flavor. Since Raspberries are one of the foods on which pesticide residues are frequently found, I recommend selecting organically grown varieties whenever possible. (For more on *Organic Foods*, see page 113.)

Avoid overripe Raspberries that are very soft, mushy or moldy. Make sure that they are not packed too tightly in the container and show no signs of stains or moisture. These are indications that they may be crushed, damaged or spoiled.

I have found it is best to purchase Raspberries no more than 1 or 2 days prior to use as they are highly perishable and do not store well.

### How Do You Know Which Raspberries are Ready to Eat?

If they are deep in color, plump and slightly soft, they are ready to eat. They must be ready to eat when you purchase them as they will not ripen.

# 2. the best way to store raspberries

Proper storage is an important step in keeping Raspberries fresh and preserving their nutrients, texture and unique flavor.

### Fresh Ripe Raspberries Can Last for Up to 3 Days When Properly Stored and Refrigerated

Raspberries continue to respire even after they have been harvested. The faster they respire, the more the Raspberries interact with air to produce carbon dioxide. The more carbon dioxide produced, the more quickly they will spoil. Raspberries kept at a room temperature of approximately 68°F (20°C) give off carbon dioxide at a rate of 125 mg per kilogram every hour. (For a *Comparison of Respiration Rates* for different fruits, see page 341.) Refrigeration helps slow the respiration rate of ripe Raspberries, retain their

vitamin content and increase their storage life.

Refrigerate Raspberries as soon as you bring them home. Since water encourages spoilage, do not wash Raspberries before refrigeration. While Raspberries that are stored properly will remain fresh for up to 3 days, if they are not stored properly they will only last about 1–2 days.

### Handle with Care

Like all berries, Raspberries are very perishable, so great care should be taken in their handling and storage. Before storing in the refrigerator, remove any Raspberries that are moldy or damaged so that they will not contaminate others. Return unwashed, whole berries to their original container or spread them out on a plate, cover with a paper towel, and then cover with plastic wrap.

*(Continued on bottom of Page 351)*

# health benefits of raspberries

### Provide Powerful Antioxidant Protection

Raspberries are rich in ellagic acid, a phytonutrient that is viewed as being responsible for a good portion of the antioxidant activity of Raspberries (and other berries). Ellagic acid helps prevent unwanted damage to cell membranes and other structures in the body by neutralizing overly reactive oxygen-containing molecules called free-radicals.

## Nutritional Analysis of 1 cup fresh Raspberries:

| NUTRIENT | AMOUNT | % DAILY VALUE | NUTRIENT | AMOUNT | % DAILY VALUE |
|---|---|---|---|---|---|
| Calories | 60.28 | | Pantothenic Acid | 0.30 mg | 3.00 |
| Calories from Fat | 6.08 | | | | |
| Calories from Saturated Fat | 0.22 | | **Minerals** | | |
| Protein | 1.12 g | | Boron | — mcg | |
| Carbohydrates | 14.24 g | | Calcium | 27.06 mg | 2.71 |
| Dietary Fiber | 8.34 g | 33.36 | Chloride | 27.06 mg | |
| Soluble Fiber | 1.50 g | | Chromium | — mcg | — |
| Insoluble Fiber | 6.84 g | | Copper | 0.10 mg | 5.00 |
| Sugar – Total | 5.90 g | | Fluoride | — mg | — |
| Monosaccharides | 8.24 g | | Iodine | — mcg | — |
| Disaccharides | 3.44 g | | Iron | 0.70 mg | 3.89 |
| Other Carbs | 0.00 g | | Magnesium | 22.14 mg | 5.54 |
| Fat – Total | 0.68 g | | Manganese | 1.24 mg | 62.00 |
| Saturated Fat | 0.02 g | | Molybdenum | — mcg | — |
| Mono Fat | 0.06 g | | Phosphorus | 14.76 mg | 1.48 |
| Poly Fat | 0.38 g | | Potassium | 186.96 mg | |
| Omega-3 Fatty Acids | 0.12 g | 4.80 | Selenium | 0.74 mcg | 1.06 |
| Omega-6 Fatty Acids | 0.26 g | | Sodium | 0.00 mg | |
| Trans Fatty Acids | 0.00 g | | Zinc | 0.56 mg | 3.73 |
| Cholesterol | 0.00 mg | | | | |
| Water | 106.48 g | | **Amino Acids** | | |
| Ash | 0.50 g | | Alanine | — g | |
| | | | Arginine | — g | |
| **Vitamins** | | | Aspartate | — g | |
| Vitamin A IU | 159.90 IU | 3.20 | Cystine | — g | — |
| Vitamin A RE | 16.00 RE | | Glutamate | — g | |
| A - Carotenoid | 16.00 RE | 0.21 | Glycine | — g | |
| A - Retinol | 0.00 RE | | Histidine | — g | — |
| B1 Thiamin | 0.04 mg | 2.67 | Isoleucine | — g | — |
| B2 Riboflavin | 0.12 mg | 7.06 | Leucine | — g | — |
| B3 Niacin | 1.10 mg | 5.50 | Lysine | — g | — |
| Niacin Equiv | 1.10 mg | | Methionine | — g | — |
| Vitamin B6 | 0.08 mg | 4.00 | Phenylalanine | — g | — |
| Vitamin B12 | 0.00 mcg | 0.00 | Proline | — g | |
| Biotin | 2.34 mcg | 0.78 | Serine | — g | |
| Vitamin C | 30.76 mg | 51.27 | Threonine | — g | — |
| Vitamin D IU | 0.00 IU | 0.00 | Tryptophan | — g | — |
| Vitamin D mcg | 0.00 mcg | | Tyrosine | — g | — |
| Vitamin E Alpha Equiv | 0.56 mg | 2.80 | Valine | — g | — |
| Vitamin E IU | 0.82 IU | | | | |
| Vitamin E mg | 0.56 mg | | | | |
| Folate | 31.98 mcg | 8.00 | | | |
| Vitamin K | — mcg | — | | | |

(Note: "–" indicates data is unavailable. For more information, please see page 806.)

However, ellagic acid is not the only well-researched phytonutrient component of Raspberries. They also contain flavonoids such as quercetin, kaempferol and anthocyanins. Anthocyanins give red Raspberries their rich red color as well as unique antioxidant and antimicrobial properties, including the ability to prevent overgrowth of certain bacteria and fungi (for example, the yeast *Candida albicans*, which is a frequent culprit in vaginal infections and can be a contributing cause in irritable bowel syndrome).

### Promote Heart Health

The antioxidant potential of Raspberries' ellagic acid, as well as their other phytonutrients, may help promote cardiovascular health since they reduce the oxidation of LDL ("bad" cholesterol) and help to safeguard the function of blood vessels. In addition to their phytonutrient concentrations, Raspberries' ability to support the heart also comes from the other nutrients that they provide. They are an excellent source of vitamin C and manganese and a good source of copper, three very powerful antioxidant nutrients that also help to protect the body from oxygen-related damage. Raspberries are also an excellent source of health-promoting dietary fiber, which can help to reduce elevated cholesterol levels. Additionally, Raspberries are a good source of folic acid, which reduces heart disease risk by lowering homocysteine levels, as well as a good source of potassium and magnesium, which help to regulate blood pressure.

### Promote Optimal Health

Research suggests that Raspberries may have cancer-preventive properties. Results from animal experiments suggest that Raspberries have the potential to inhibit cancer cell proliferation and tumor formation in various sites, including the colon and the mouth. In test tube experiments, Raspberries have been found to positively mediate cell signaling as well as inhibit an enzyme whose abnormal production has been linked to metastasis (invasion and spread of cancer cells). Deficiency of niacin, a B vitamin of which Raspberries are a good source, has been directly linked to genetic (DNA) damage.

### Additional Health-Promoting Benefits of Raspberries

Since Raspberries contain only 60 calories per one cup serving, they are an ideal food for healthy weight control.

## No Bake Recipes

# 5-Minute Raspberry Almond Parfait

*The combination of Raspberries and almonds makes a delicious dessert.*

8 oz (1 cup) low-fat vanilla or soy yogurt
1/2 tsp almond extract
2 TBS honey
1 pint Raspberries
1 TBS sliced almonds
Optional: grated dark chocolate

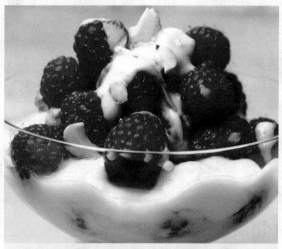
Raspberry Almond Parfait

1. Blend yogurt, honey and almond extract in a small mixing bowl with a whisk until the honey is incorporated and the mixture is smooth.

2. Divide the yogurt mixture into two dessert dishes. Place the Raspberries in one layer on top and garnish with the sliced almonds and, if desired, dark chocolate.

As an alternative to yogurt, make a sauce with 1 cup cashews and 1/2 cup of water, blended until smooth.

**Preparation Hint:** Taste the yogurt mixture for sweetness. You may want more honey depending upon the brand of yogurt. **SERVES 2**

Please write (address on back cover flap) or e-mail me at info@whfoods.org with your personal ideas for preparing Raspberries, and I will share them with others through our website at www.whfoods.org.

## 6 QUICK SERVING IDEAS for RASPBERRIES:

1. **Raspberries with Balsamic Vinegar:** Combine 1 tsp good quality balsamic vinegar and 1/2 tsp honey, and drizzle over 1 pint fresh Raspberries. Add a few grinds of black pepper for a little kick. Serve for dessert.

2. **Raspberries with Lemon Sauce:** For a zesty sauce, drizzle Quick Lemon Sauce (see page 431) over fresh Raspberries.

3. **Raspberries with Yogurt and Chocolate:** Top Fresh Raspberries with low-fat Raspberry or chocolate yogurt and grated dark chocolate.

4. **Porridge with Raspberries:** Mix fresh Raspberries in with cooked oatmeal (or other grain porridge) for a sweet morning breakfast treat.

5. **Raspberry Yogurt Topping:** Plain yogurt mixed with Raspberries, honey and freshly chopped mint is delicious eaten as is or used as a topping for waffles.

6. **Raspberry Sauce:** Blend a pint of Raspberries with 2 TBS honey on medium speed for 1 minute in a blender. Strain. Use the sauce over Raspberries that have been combined with chopped dark chocolate and sliced almonds or as a sauce for other desserts.

*(Continued from Page 349)*

# 3. the best way to prepare raspberries

Properly preparing Raspberries helps ensure that they will have the best flavor and retain the greatest number of nutrients.

## Cleaning Raspberries

As Raspberries are very delicate, wash them very gently, using the light pressure of the sink sprayer if possible, and then pat them dry. To prevent Raspberries from becoming waterlogged, wash them right before eating or using in a recipe. (For more on *Washing Fruit*, see page 341.)

## No Bake Recipes

I have discovered that Raspberries retain their maximum amount of nutrients and their best taste when they are fresh and not prepared in a cooked recipe. That is because their nutrients—including vitamins, antioxidants and enzymes—are unable to withstand the temperature (350°F/175°C) used in baking. So that you can get the most enjoyment and benefit from fruit, I created quick and easy recipes, which require no cooking. I call them "No Bake Recipes."

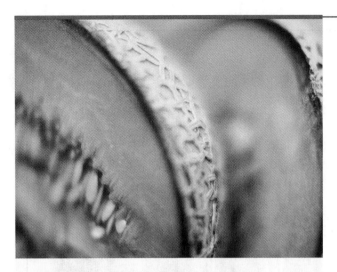

# cantaloupe

## highlights

| | |
|---|---|
| AVAILABILITY: | Year-round |
| REFRIGERATE: | Yes |
| SHELF LIFE: | 5 days refrigerated |
| PREPARATION: | Minimal |
| BEST WAY TO PREPARE: | Enjoy it raw |

## nutrient-richness chart

| Total Nutrient-Richness: | **14** | | | GI: **91** |
|---|---|---|---|---|

One cup (160 grams) of fresh Cantaloupe contains 56 calories

| NUTRIENT | AMOUNT | %DV | DENSITY | QUALITY |
|---|---|---|---|---|
| Vitamin C | 67.5 mg | 112.5 | 36.2 | excellent |
| Vitamin A | 5158.4 IU | 103.2 | 33.2 | excellent |
| Potassium | 494.4 mg | 14.1 | 4.5 | very good |
| B6 Pyridoxine | 0.2 mg | 9.0 | 2.9 | good |
| Folate | 27.2 mcg | 6.8 | 2.2 | good |
| Dietary Fiber | 1.3 g | 5.1 | 1.6 | good |
| B3 Niacin | 0.9 mg | 4.6 | 1.5 | good |
| **CAROTENOIDS:** | | | | |
| Alpha-Carotene | 25.6 mcg | | | |
| Beta-Carotene | 3232.0 mcg | | | |
| Beta-Cryptoxanthin | 1.6 mcg | | | |
| Lutein+Zeaxanthin | 41.6 mcg | | | |
| **PHYTOSTEROLS:** | | | | |
| Phytosterols - Total | 16.0 mg | | | |

Daily values for these nutrients have not yet been established.

For more on "Total Nutrient Richness," "%DV," "Density," and
The World's Healthiest Foods "Quality" Rating System, see page 805.

For more on GI, see page 342.

The popularity of Cantaloupe, with its refreshingly rich flavor and aroma, dates back to ancient Greece and Rome. It is believed that it was named for a former Papal garden near Rome called Cantalou where this variety of melon was developed. Cantaloupes were introduced to the U.S. during colonial times but not grown commercially until the late 19th century. Today, they are renowned for their wonderful flavor and minimal number of calories, making them a favorite snack, dessert or salad, especially among those watching their weight. As with most fruits, Cantaloupe requires little preparation and is ready to serve and eat in a matter of minutes.

## why cantaloupe should be part of your healthiest way of eating

Cantaloupe is an excellent source of vitamins A and C, powerful antioxidants that protect against damage to cellular structures and DNA. The distinctive orange color of Cantaloupe is provided by its wealth of beta-carotene, a carotenoid phytonutrient that is a precursor to vitamin A. Cantaloupe is an ideal food to add to your "Healthiest Way of Eating" not only because it is nutritious and tastes great but also because it is low in calories: one cup of Cantaloupe contains only 56 calories! (For more on the *Health Benefits of Cantaloupe* and a complete analysis of its content of over 60 nutrients, see page 354.)

## varieties of cantaloupe

The fruit that we call Cantaloupe is, in actuality, really a muskmelon. The true Cantaloupe is a different species of melon, which is mostly grown in France and rarely found in the United States. Cantaloupe is a melon that belongs to the same family as the cucumber, squash, pumpkin and gourd. Like many of its relatives, it grows on the ground on a trailing vine. The botanical name for Cantaloupe is *Cucumis melo*. Other popular melon varieties include the honeydew, casaba and crenshaw melon.

Cantaloupes range in color from orange-yellow to salmon and have a soft and juicy texture with a sweet, musky aroma that you can smell when they are ripe.

## the peak season

While Cantaloupe may be available throughout the year, the peak of the season runs from June through August.

These are the months when its concentration of nutrients and flavor are highest, and its cost is at its lowest.

## biochemical considerations

Cantaloupe is one of the foods most commonly associated with allergic reactions in individuals with latex allergies. (For more on *Latex Food Allergies*, see page 722.)

## 3 steps for the best tasting and most nutritious cantaloupe

Enjoying the best tasting Cantaloupe with the most nutrients is simple if you just follow my 3 easy steps:
1. The Best Way to Select
2. The Best Way to Store
3. The Best Way to Prepare

# 1. the best way to select cantaloupe

You can select the best tasting Cantaloupe by looking for one that is fully ripe with a sweet aroma. Ripe Cantaloupe will not only have the best flavor and texture but will also feature the highest level of vitamins, antioxidants and enzymes. Cantaloupe will not ripen after it has been picked. I have discovered some clues that will help you find a ripe Cantaloupe: (1) tap the melon with the palm of your hand and listen for a hollow sound, (2) look for one that seems heavy for its size, (3) look for rind underneath the netting that is yellow- or cream-colored, (4) look for a "full slip" (the area where the stem was attached) that is smooth and slightly indented, (5) look for one whose end opposite the full slip is slightly soft and (6) you should be able to smell the fruit's sweetness subtly coming through.

Cantaloupe is so fragrant that you can check for its aroma even when it has been pre-cut and packaged in a plastic container. As with all fruits, I recommend selecting organically grown Cantaloupe whenever possible. (For more on *Organic Foods*, see page 113.)

Avoid Cantaloupe that has no aroma or has green undertones since both indicate it is not ripe. Not only will it not have a good flavor, but it will provide less nutrients. Do not purchase Cantaloupe that is bruised or has spots that are overly soft, two signs of an overripe melon. Be careful not to select a Cantaloupe with an overly strong odor as this also indicates an overripe or fermented melon.

### How Do You Know Which Cantaloupe is Ready to Eat?

If the Cantaloupe is ripe with a rich, sweet melon aroma, and the end opposite the full slip is slightly soft, it is ready to eat. Cantaloupe tastes best at room temperature.

# 2. the best way to store cantaloupe

Proper storage is an important step in keeping Cantaloupe fresh and preserving its nutrients, texture and unique flavor.

### Fresh Ripe Cantaloupe Can Last for Up to 5 Days When Properly Stored and Refrigerated

Cantaloupe continues to respire even after it has been harvested. The faster it respires, the more the Cantaloupe interacts with air to produce carbon dioxide. The more carbon dioxide produced, the more quickly it will spoil. Refrigeration helps slow the respiration rate of a ripe Cantaloupe, retain its vitamin content and increase its storage life.

While refrigerating Cantaloupe will increase storage time and the coolness will make it more refreshing, it may also blunt its flavor. Cantaloupe that is stored properly will remain fresh for up to 5 days; if it is not stored properly, it will only last about 2 days.

### How to Store Cut Cantaloupe

Cantaloupe that has been cut should be refrigerated in a tightly sealed container to ensure that the ethylene gas that it emits does not affect the taste or texture of other fruits and vegetables.

# 3. the best way to prepare cantaloupe

Properly preparing Cantaloupe helps ensure it will have the best flavor and retain the greatest number of nutrients.

*(Continued on bottom of Page 355)*

*Q I was told that it is better to not eat fruits, such as Cantaloupe, right before a meal. Is this true?*

*A* Whether to wait a certain time before or after a meal to eat fruit is one of the most common questions I get asked regarding food combining. Although there appears to be no research evidence about when it is best to eat fruits in

relation to the rest of your meal, many people report better overall digestion when they follow the practice of waiting about one half hour or so before or after a meal to enjoy their fruit. A number of healthcare practitioners also advocate fruit consumption separate from meals.

# health benefits of cantaloupe

## Promotes Vision Health

As a result of its concentration of beta-carotene, Cantaloupe is an excellent source of vitamin A. Both vitamin A and beta-carotene are important vision nutrients. One large-scale research study found that those who had the highest dietary intake of vitamin A had a 39% reduced risk of developing cataracts. A study investigating the relationship between the need for cataract surgery and diet revealed that those who ate diets that included Cantaloupe were half as likely to need cataract surgery. Additionally, another study showed that eating 3 servings of fruit per day may reduce the risk of macular degeneration by 36% compared to eating 1.5 servings per day.

## Promotes Immune Health

In addition to its antioxidant activity, Cantaloupe's vitamin C is critical for good immune function. Vitamin C stimulates white cells to fight infection, directly kills many bacteria and viruses, and regenerates vitamin E back into its active form.

## Promotes Heart Health

Cantaloupe contains many nutrients that promote cardiovascular health. It is a very good source of potassium, which enhances healthy muscle contractions and is therefore important for maintaining healthy blood pressure levels and heart function. Its folate and vitamin B6 help keep levels of homocysteine in check; elevated levels of homocysteine can damage artery walls, contributing to the development of cardiovascular disease. Intake of vitamin C is also associated with a reduced risk of heart disease. Additionally, Cantaloupe is a good addition to a fiber-rich diet, which has been found to be beneficial for heart health.

## Promotes Healthy Cells

Melons have been found to be one of the best sources of myoinositol, a building block of cell membranes. This nutrient has been the focus of recent studies on treating depression, panic disorder, diabetic nerve damage and liver disease as well as preventing some cancers. Although findings are preliminary, it is certainly an exciting new area of research. Cantaloupe is also a good source of niacin, a B vitamin whose deficiency has been directly linked to genetic (DNA) damage.

## Additional Health-Promoting Benefits of Cantaloupe

Since Cantaloupe contains only 56 calories per one cup serving, it is an ideal food for healthy weight control.

## Nutritional Analysis of 1 cup of fresh Cantaloupe:

| NUTRIENT | AMOUNT | % DAILY VALUE |
|---|---|---|
| Calories | 56.00 | |
| Calories from Fat | 4.03 | |
| Calories from Saturated Fat | 1.02 | |
| Protein | 1.41 g | |
| Carbohydrates | 13.38 g | |
| Dietary Fiber | 1.28 g | 5.12 |
| Soluble Fiber | 0.38 g | |
| Insoluble Fiber | 0.90 g | |
| Sugar – Total | 12.10 g | |
| Monosaccharides | 4.37 g | |
| Disaccharides | 7.73 g | |
| Other Carbs | 0.00 g | |
| Fat – Total | 0.45 g | |
| Saturated Fat | 0.11 g | |
| Mono Fat | 0.01 g | |
| Poly Fat | 0.18 g | |
| Omega-3 Fatty Acids | 0.10 g | 4.00 |
| Omega-6 Fatty Acids | 0.08 g | |
| Trans Fatty Acids | 0.00 g | |
| Cholesterol | 0.00 mg | |
| Water | 143.65 g | |
| Ash | 1.14 g | |

| Vitamins | | |
|---|---|---|
| Vitamin A IU | 5158.40 IU | 103.17 |
| Vitamin A RE | 515.20 RE | |
| A - Carotenoid | 515.20 RE | 6.87 |
| A - Retinol | 0.00 RE | |
| B1 Thiamin | 0.06 mg | 4.00 |
| B2 Riboflavin | 0.03 mg | 1.76 |
| B3 Niacin | 0.92 mg | 4.60 |
| Niacin Equiv | 1.13 mg | |
| Vitamin B6 | 0.18 mg | 9.00 |
| Vitamin B12 | 0.00 mcg | 0.00 |
| Biotin | — mcg | — |
| Vitamin C | 67.52 mg | 112.53 |
| Vitamin D IU | 0.00 IU | 0.00 |
| Vitamin D mcg | 0.00 mcg | |
| Vitamin E Alpha Equiv | 0.24 mg | 1.20 |
| Vitamin E IU | 0.36 IU | |
| Vitamin E mg | 0.50 mg | |
| Folate | 27.20 mcg | 6.80 |
| Vitamin K | — mcg | — |

| NUTRIENT | AMOUNT | % DAILY VALUE |
|---|---|---|
| Pantothenic Acid | 0.20 mg | 2.00 |

| Minerals | | |
|---|---|---|
| Boron | — mcg | |
| Calcium | 17.60 mg | 1.76 |
| Chloride | 70.40 mg | |
| Chromium | — mcg | — |
| Copper | 0.07 mg | 3.50 |
| Fluoride | — mg | — |
| Iodine | 6.40 mcg | 4.27 |
| Iron | 0.34 mg | 1.89 |
| Magnesium | 17.60 mg | 4.40 |
| Manganese | 0.08 mg | 4.00 |
| Molybdenum | — mcg | — |
| Phosphorus | 27.20 mg | 2.72 |
| Potassium | 494.40 mg | |
| Selenium | 0.64 mcg | 0.91 |
| Sodium | 14.40 mg | |
| Zinc | 0.26 mg | 1.73 |

| Amino Acids | | |
|---|---|---|
| Alanine | — g | |
| Arginine | — g | |
| Aspartate | — g | |
| Cystine | — g | — |
| Glutamate | — g | |
| Glycine | — g | |
| Histidine | — g | — |
| Isoleucine | 0.03 g | 2.61 |
| Leucine | 0.05 g | 1.98 |
| Lysine | 0.07 g | 2.98 |
| Methionine | — g | — |
| Phenylalanine | 0.04 g | 3.36 |
| Proline | — g | |
| Serine | — g | |
| Threonine | — g | — |
| Tryptophan | 0.01 g | 3.13 |
| Tyrosine | — g | — |
| Valine | 0.04 g | 2.72 |

(Note: "–" indicates data is unavailable. For more information, please see page 806.)

## No Bake Recipes

# Cantaloupe with Lime and Mint

*For the best flavor, enjoy Cantaloupe with lime and mint.*

**1 Cantaloupe**
**2 TBS fresh lime juice**
**4 mint leaves**

1. Cut Cantaloupe in half and scoop out the seeds.
2. Sprinkle each half with 1 TBS lime juice.
3. Tear mint leaves by hand and sprinkle over cantaloupe.

**SERVES 2**

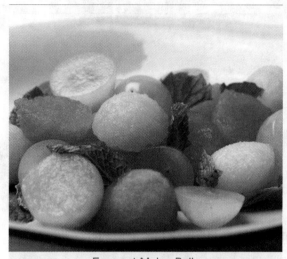
Fragrant Melon Balls

Please write (address on back cover flap) or e-mail me at info@whfoods.org with your personal ideas for preparing Cantaloupe, and I will share them with others through our website at www.whfoods.org.

## 12 QUICK SERVING IDEAS for CANTALOUPE:

1. Enhance the flavor of Cantaloupe with lime juice and freshly grated ginger.
2. Fill with cottage cheese or yogurt.
3. Serve with feta cheese or cottage cheese.
4. Add diced Cantaloupe to your favorite chicken salad recipe.
5. Add chopped Cantaloupe to chutneys and fruit salsas.
6. **Cantaloupe-Blueberry Frozen Yogurt:** Blend cubed Cantaloupe with blueberries and low-fat frozen yogurt for a cool and refreshing summer treat.
7. **Cantaloupe Sorbet:** Whip Cantaloupe in a blender or food processor and freeze.
8. **Whole Cantaloupe Shake:** For a creamy, refreshing shake, blend fruit and seeds of a whole, skinned Cantaloupe for 2–3 minutes at high speed.
9. **Sparkling Cantaloupe Cooler:** Purée Cantaloupe and add cold sparkling water for a delightfully refreshing drink that can be enjoyed throughout the year.
10. **Refreshing Cantaloupe Soup:** Purée Cantaloupe in blender and mix in orange or other fruit juices for a cold refreshing soup.
11. **Cantaloupe Fruit Salad:** Combine diced Cantaloupe and watermelon, berries, oranges and bananas.
12. **Fragrant Melon Balls:** Slice 1 Cantaloupe in half and scoop out seeds. Starting at the outside edge, scoop out balls with a melon baller, working your way towards the center. Toss the melon balls with the leaves of one cup of fresh mint or basil. Add 1 TBS lemon or lime juice and refrigerate at least 4 hours, stirring occasionally to infuse the flavor of the herbs. (Pictured above.) *Optional:* Use a combination of Cantaloupe, honeydew and watermelon in this recipe.

*(Continued from Page 353)*

## Cleaning Cantaloupe

It is important to scrub Cantaloupe under running water before cutting it. This helps to remove any bacteria on the surface and prevents it from being transferred to the flesh when you cut into the melon. (For more on *Washing Fruit*, see page 341.)

## Cutting Cantaloupe

After washing, cut the Cantaloupe in half, remove the seeds and netting, and cut it into pieces of desired thickness. Alternatively, you can scoop out the flesh with a melon baller.

## No Bake Recipes

I have discovered that Cantaloupe retains its maximum amount of nutrients and its best taste when it is enjoyed raw and not prepared in a cooked recipe. That is because its nutrients—including vitamins, antioxidants and enzymes—are unable to withstand the temperature (350°F/175°C) used in baking. So that you can get the most enjoyment and benefit from fruit, I created quick and easy recipes, which require no cooking. I call them "No Bake Recipes."

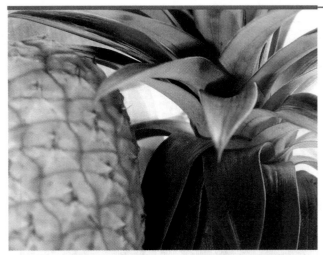

# pineapple

## highlights

| | |
|---|---|
| AVAILABILITY: | Year-round |
| REFRIGERATE: | No |
| SHELF LIFE: | 5 days |
| PREPARATION: | Peel |
| BEST WAY TO ENJOY: | Enjoy them raw |

## nutrient-richness chart

| Total Nutrient-Richness: | **12** | | | GI: **83** |
|---|---|---|---|---|

One cup (155 grams) of fresh Pineapple contains 76 calories

| NUTRIENT | AMOUNT | %DV | DENSITY | QUALITY |
|---|---|---|---|---|
| Manganese | 2.6 mg | 128.0 | 30.3 | excellent |
| Vitamin C | 23.9 mg | 39.8 | 9.4 | excellent |
| B1 Thiamin | 0.1 mg | 9.3 | 2.2 | good |
| Copper | 0.8 mg | 8.5 | 2.0 | good |
| Dietary Fiber | 1.9 g | 7.4 | 1.8 | good |
| B6 Pyridoxine | 0.1 mg | 6.5 | 1.5 | good |
| **CAROTENOIDS:** | | | Daily values for this nutrient have not yet been established. | |
| Beta-Carotene | 52.7 mcg | | | |

For more on "Total Nutrient-Richness," "%DV," "Density," and
The World's Healthiest Foods "Quality" Rating System, see page 805.

For more on GI, see page 342.

Pineapples were named by European explorers who believed they looked like pinecones with the flesh of an apple. Fresh Pineapples were once reserved for the elite, who served them as a sign of prestige since they were very expensive, owing to the costs of transporting them stateside from the Caribbean Islands. Today, since they are more affordable and easily found at most local markets, Pineapples have become second only to bananas as America's favorite tropical fruit. Exceptionally sweet and juicy with a wonderful flavor, Pineapples are a great way to add a little taste of the tropics to your meal. Friends have asked me why the same batch of Pineapples that taste great in Hawaii don't taste as good when transported to the Mainland. A Pineapple farmer told me that the reason Pineapples taste best in Hawaii is because they are served or canned the same day they are picked. Pineapples develop an acidic taste after 24 hours.

## why pineapple should be part of your healthiest way of eating

Pineapple contains a special group of enzymes called *bromelain*, which function both as a digestive aid and anti-inflammatory compound. Pineapple is also an excellent source of the trace mineral manganese—an essential cofactor in a number of enzymes important in energy production and antioxidant defenses—as well as vitamin C, a powerful antioxidant that protects against oxidative damage to cell structures. Pineapples are an ideal food to add to your "Healthiest Way of Eating" not only because they are nutritious and taste great, but also because they are low in calories: one cup of Pineapple contains only 76 calories! (For more on the *Health Benefits of Pineapple* and a complete analysis of its content of over 60 nutrients, see page 360.)

## varieties of pineapple

While Pineapples are thought to have originated in South America, they were first discovered on the Caribbean island of Guadeloupe by Christopher Columbus in 1493. Pineapple (*Ananas comosus*) belongs to the *Bromeliaceae* family, from which the name of one of its most important health-promoting compounds, the enzyme *bromelain*, was derived. Pineapples are a composite of many flowers whose individual fruitlets fuse together around a central core. Each fruitlet can be identified by an "eye," the rough spiny marking on the Pineapple's surface.

### SMOOTH CAYENNE

This is the most popular, and often considered the best tasting, of the varieties most commonly found in markets. It is a Pineapple grown in Hawaii with a cone-like shape and weighs from 3 to 5 pounds.

**MAUI GOLD**

A hybrid variety that is exceptionally sweet and has a longer storage life than the Smooth Cayenne.

**QUEEN**

Small with firmer, less acidic flesh. Drier than the Smooth Cayenne and not quite as sweet.

**RED SPANISH**

Grown in the Caribbean, they are similar to the Smooth Cayenne but have a "squarish" shape and tough outer shell.

**SUGAR LOAF**

Grown in Mexico, these larger Pineapples weigh from 5 to 10 pounds.

## the peak season

Although Pineapples are available year-round, the peak of the Pineapple season runs from March through June. These are the months when their concentration of nutrients and flavor are highest, and their cost is at its lowest.

## 3 steps for the best tasting and most nutritious pineapple

Enjoying the best tasting Pineapples with the most nutrients is simple if you just follow my 3 easy steps:

1. The Best Way to Select
2. The Best Way to Store
3. The Best Way to Prepare

# 1. the best way to select pineapple

When you select Pineapples, look for ones that are fully ripe. Pineapples will not ripen after they are picked. Fully ripened Pineapples will have a well developed flavor as well as the most developed concentration of nutrients, including vitamins, minerals and antioxidants. It is best to smell the aroma of a Pineapple before you purchase it. Fully ripe Pineapples have the sweet fragrant aroma of Pineapple and give slightly to pressure. While larger Pineapples will have a greater proportion of edible flesh, there is usually no difference in quality between those that are small or large. Leaves should look fresh and green. Vitamins and antioxidants are at their peak when Pineapples are ripe, so by selecting ripe Pineapples, you will also be enjoying Pineapples with the highest nutritional value. Pineapples will soften and become juicier after they are picked, but they will not get sweeter because their starches will not turn to sugar. As with all fruits, I recommend selecting organically grown varieties when-

ever possible. (For more on *Organic Foods*, see page 113.)

Avoid Pineapples that are too soft or have a sour or fermented smell. If they are green, they will be fibrous, lack sweetness and not contain their optimal concentration of nutrients. They should be free of soft spots, bruises and darkened "eyes," all of which may indicate that the Pineapple is past its prime. Avoid Pineapples with dry brown leaves because they will have a very sour taste. The flesh of the Pineapple darkens in color as it becomes overripe, an indication of the formation of free-radicals. Overripe Pineapples should not be eaten.

### How Do You Know
### Which Pineapples are Ready to Eat?

If Pineapples are heavy for their size and have the sweet aroma of Pineapple, they are ready to eat. Since Pineapples do not ripen after they have been picked, be sure to select a ripe one.

# 2. the best way to store pineapple

Proper storage is an important step in keeping Pineapples fresh and preserving their nutrients, texture and unique flavor.

### Fresh Ripe Pineapples
### Can Last for Up to 5 Days

Pineapples continue to respire even after they have been harvested. The faster they respire, the more the Pineapples interact with air to produce carbon dioxide. The more carbon dioxide produced, the more quickly they will spoil.

Pineapples kept at a room temperature of approximately 68°F (20°C) give off carbon dioxide at a rate of 24 mg per kilogram every hour. (For a *Comparison of Respiration Rates* for different fruits, see page 341.)

Pineapples are most flavorful when served at room temperature. Although refrigeration may enhance the freshness of Pineapples, it will also cause them to get "chill injury" and lose some of their flavor compounds. If you do refrigerate your Pineapple, place it on the top shelf, which is the warmest part of the refrigerator (over 50°F/10°C).

Avoid storing Pineapples in sealed plastic bags. The combination of limited oxygen exchange and the excessive amounts of ethylene gas that the Pineapples naturally produce under these conditions will cause them to rot.

While Pineapples that are stored at room temperature will have more flavor than those stored in the refrigerator, they will have a shorter shelf life. They will remain fresh for 3 days, while those stored in the refrigerator can last for up to 5 days.

## Handle with Care

Pineapples can bruise easily, so handle them with care.

# 3. the best way to prepare pineapple

Properly preparing Pineapples helps ensure that they will have the best flavor and retain the greatest number of nutrients.

## Cutting Pineapples

Pineapples can be cut and peeled in a variety of ways. Regardless of how you proceed, the first step is always to remove the crown and the base of the fruit with a knife.

### PINEAPPLE CHUNKS

Cut off and discard both ends of the Pineapple. Stand Pineapple up on one end on the cutting board and cut off peel by going around Pineapple. If the Pineapple has deep eyes, remove them with the tip of a knife. Cut Pineapple into fourths lengthwise and cut out core from each section. Slice each section lengthwise in half or into thirds. Cut across slices into desired size.

### USING PINEAPPLE CORERS

You can also use Pineapple corers that are available in kitchen-supply stores. While they provide a quick and convenient method for peeling and coring Pineapples, they can result in a large amount of wasted fruit since they often cannot be adjusted for different size fruit. Some markets offer devices that will peel and core the Pineapple, but this process may waste a lot of fruit.

## No Bake Recipes

I have discovered that Pineapples retain their maximum amount of nutrients and their best taste when they are fresh and not prepared in a cooked recipe. That is because their nutrients—including vitamins, antioxidants and enzymes—are unable to withstand the temperature (350°F/175°C) used in baking. So that you can get the most enjoyment and benefit from fruit, I created quick and easy recipes, which require no cooking. I call them "No Bake Recipes."

---

**BROMELAIN FROM PINEAPPLES AS A DIGESTIVE AID**

*Bromelain* is a unique group of enzymes found in fresh Pineapples that breaks down protein and aids digestion; it can also be purchased in powder form. Canned or cooked Pineapples contain no *bromelain* because the Pineapples are heated to the boiling point, which inactivates the enzyme. Pineapples' ability to break down proteins is the reason that they should not be combined with yogurt or cottage cheese until immediately before serving as the *bromelain* will break down the proteins in these foods, altering their flavor and texture. On the other hand, adding Pineapple to a marinade for meat or poultry will not only add extra flavor to these foods, but will also help tenderize them.

---

Here are questions that I received from readers of the whfoods.org website about Pineapple:

**Q** *If I wanted to take advantage of bromelain's enzyme activity, how much before or after eating a meal should I eat Pineapple?*

**A** The time frame for digestion of our food varies greatly. Pure proteins typically move through our stomach and small intestine in the two to five hour range. Bromelain is a protein-digesting enzyme, so one to two hours before or after eating (so that it's not sitting in our stomach or small intestine right next to the proteins in our food) would be the best way to make use of its anti-inflammatory benefits.

*(Continued on bottom of adjacent Page)*

**STEP-BY-STEP**
## No Bake Recipes

# 5-Minute Ginger Pineapple

*Ginger adds a zing to Pineapple for a great dessert.*

**1/2 medium Pineapple**
**1 tsp finely minced fresh ginger**

1. Cut Pineapple into 1-inch chunks.
2. Combine Pineapple and minced ginger in a bowl and refrigerate for 1/2 hour.

   Best if eaten within an hour.

**SERVES 2**

*Variation...* Substitute chopped mint for the ginger.

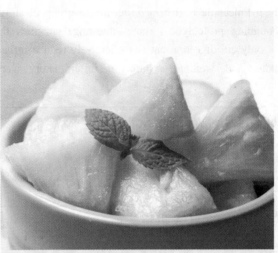

Ginger Pineapple

Please write (address on back cover flap) or e-mail me at info@whfoods.org with your personal ideas for preparing Pineapple, and I will share them with others through our website at www.whfoods.org.

## 7 QUICK SERVING IDEAS for PINEAPPLE:

1. Add Pineapple to your favorite smoothie.
2. **Pineapple Fruit Salad:** Combine Pineapple with other tropical fruits, such as papaya, kiwi and mango.
3. **Pineapple Chutney:** Combine 1 medium diced Pineapple, 2 TBS raisins, 1 medium minced onion, 1 TBS minced mint and a pinch of red pepper flakes. Serve with meat and fish.
4. **Pineapple Salsa:** Mix 1 medium diced Pineapple and 1 medium deseeded and minced hot chili pepper (jalapeño or serrano). Add juice of one lime and sea salt to taste. This is an easy-to-prepare salsa that's an exceptional complement to fish such as halibut, tuna and salmon.
5. **Pineapple Shish-Ka-Bobs:** Skewer Pineapple chunks with shrimp or chicken and bell peppers. Brush with tamari (soy sauce) and grill.
6. **Pineapple Shrimp Salad:** Combine 1 medium diced Pineapple with 1 lb of cooked shrimp, 1 TBS grated ginger and 3 TBS olive oil. Season to taste with sea salt and black pepper, and serve this fragrant shrimp salad on a bed of romaine lettuce.
7. **Pineapple Chicken Salad:** Combine 1 medium diced Pineapple, 1 small grated fennel bulb, 2 TBS chopped cashews and 1 cup diced cooked chicken. Toss with your favorite vinaigrette.

Q *Does the high heat involved in canning destroy the beneficial enzymes in Pineapple? If so, is canned Pineapple not one of the World's Healthiest Foods?*

A That's a great question you ask since it brings up the definition of a healthy food in general as compared more specifically to a World's Healthiest Food.

It is true that the canning process does destroy the activity of the *bromelain* enzyme and reduces the content of other nutrients as well. The nutrient loss that occurs with canning is why I prefer fresh fruit to canned fruit. Fresh fruit is more of a whole food if we include as part of the definition of a whole food one that has the least amount of processing. (It is rare that no processing would occur to a food, as you could even

say that the very act of picking the Pineapple is actually processing and takes away from its wholeness—but that's a whole other philosophical conversation.)

But should the loss of some nutrients disqualify the canned Pineapple from being a World's Healthiest Food? I don't think so. If I apply the standard that processing affects the nutrient content of a food and therefore disqualifies it, then I would have to apply that to all of the World's Healthiest Foods and object to cooking, even light cooking of vegetables, which I think is appropriate. Canned Pineapple is still rich in nutrients, and I would rather see people eat canned Pineapple than not enjoy this food at all. In my view, choosing canned Pineapple that is organic and not packed with sugar water would also make it closer to a whole food.

# health benefits of pineapple

## Promotes Inflammatory Balance

Fresh Pineapple is rich in *bromelain*, a group of sulfur-containing proteolytic (protein-digesting) enzymes that not only aid digestion but can effectively reduce inflammation and swelling. A variety of inflammatory agents are inhibited by the action of *bromelain*. In clinical human trials, *bromelain* has demonstrated significant anti-inflammatory effects, reducing swelling in inflammatory conditions such as acute sinusitis, sore throat, arthritis and gout, and speeding recovery from injuries and surgery. To maximize *bromelain*'s anti-inflammatory effects, Pineapple should be eaten alone between meals or its enzymes will be used up digesting food.

## Provides Powerful Antioxidant Protection

Pineapple is an excellent source of vitamin C, the body's primary water-soluble antioxidant, which defends all aqueous areas of the body against free-radicals that attack and damage cells. Free radicals have been shown to promote the artery plaque build-up of atherosclerosis and diabetic heart disease, cause the airway spasm that leads to asthma attacks, damage the cells of the colon so that they become colon cancer cells and contribute to the joint pain and disability seen in osteoarthritis and rheumatoid arthritis. This would explain why diets rich in vitamin C have been shown to be useful for preventing or reducing the severity of all of these conditions. In addition, vitamin C is vital for the proper function of the immune system, making it a nutrient helpful for the prevention of recurrent ear infections, colds and flu.

## Promotes Energy Production

Pineapple is an excellent source of the trace mineral manganese, which is an essential cofactor in a number of enzymes important in energy production and antioxidant defenses. For example, the key oxidative enzyme, *superoxide dismutase,* which disarms free-radicals produced within the mitochondria (the energy production factories within our cells), requires manganese. In addition to manganese, Pineapple is a good source of thiamin, a B vitamin that acts as a cofactor in enzymatic reactions central to energy production.

## Additional Health-Promoting Benefits of Pineapple

Pineapple is also a concentrated source of many other nutrients providing additional health-promoting benefits. These nutrients include heart-healthy dietary fiber and vitamin B6 and free-radical-scavenging copper. Since one cup of Pineapple contains only 76 calories, it is an ideal food for healthy weight control.

### Nutritional Analysis of 1 cup of fresh Pineapple:

| NUTRIENT | AMOUNT | % DAILY VALUE |
|---|---|---|
| Calories | 75.95 | |
| Calories from Fat | 6.00 | |
| Calories from Saturated Fat | 0.45 | |
| Protein | 0.60 g | |
| Carbohydrates | 19.20 g | |
| Dietary Fiber | 1.86 g | 7.44 |
| Soluble Fiber | 0.16 g | |
| Insoluble Fiber | 1.71 g | |
| Sugar – Total | 17.34 g | |
| Monosaccharides | 7.75 g | |
| Disaccharides | 4.81 g | |
| Other Carbs | 0.00 g | |
| Fat – Total | 0.67 g | |
| Saturated Fat | 0.05 g | |
| Mono Fat | 0.07 g | |
| Poly Fat | 0.23 g | |
| Omega-3 Fatty Acids | 0.10 g | 4.00 |
| Omega-6 Fatty Acids | 0.13 g | |
| Trans Fatty Acids | 0.00 g | |
| Cholesterol | 0.00 mg | |
| Water | 134.07 g | |
| Ash | 0.45 g | |
| **Vitamins** | | |
| Vitamin A IU | 35.65 IU | 0.71 |
| Vitamin A RE | 3.10 RE | |
| A - Carotenoid | 3.10 RE | 0.04 |
| A - Retinol | 0.00 RE | |
| B1 Thiamin | 0.14 mg | 9.33 |
| B2 Riboflavin | 0.06 mg | 3.53 |
| B3 Niacin | 0.65 mg | 3.25 |
| Niacin Equiv | 0.78 mg | |
| Vitamin B6 | 0.13 mg | 6.50 |
| Vitamin B12 | 0.00 mcg | 0.00 |
| Biotin | 0.47 mcg | 0.16 |
| Vitamin C | 23.87 mg | 39.78 |
| Vitamin D IU | 0.00 IU | 0.00 |
| Vitamin D mcg | 0.00 mcg | |
| Vitamin E Alpha Equiv | 0.16 mg | 0.80 |
| Vitamin E IU | 0.23 IU | |
| Vitamin E mg | 0.16 mg | |
| Folate | 16.43 mcg | 4.11 |
| Vitamin K | 1.09 mcg | 1.36 |

| NUTRIENT | AMOUNT | % DAILY VALUE |
|---|---|---|
| Pantothenic Acid | 0.25 mg | 2.50 |
| **Minerals** | | |
| Boron | — mcg | |
| Calcium | 10.85 mg | 1.08 |
| Chloride | — mg | |
| Chromium | — mcg | — |
| Copper | 0.17 mg | 8.50 |
| Fluoride | — mg | — |
| Iodine | — mcg | — |
| Iron | 0.57 mg | 3.17 |
| Magnesium | 21.70 mg | 5.42 |
| Manganese | 2.56 mg | 128.00 |
| Molybdenum | — mcg | — |
| Phosphorus | 10.85 mg | 1.08 |
| Potassium | 175.15 mg | |
| Selenium | 0.93 mcg | 1.33 |
| Sodium | 1.55 mg | |
| Zinc | 0.12 mg | 0.80 |
| **Amino Acids** | | |
| Alanine | 0.03 g | |
| Arginine | 0.03 g | |
| Aspartate | 0.09 g | |
| Cystine | 0.00 g | 0.00 |
| Glutamate | 0.07 g | |
| Glycine | 0.03 g | |
| Histidine | 0.01 g | 0.78 |
| Isoleucine | 0.02 g | 1.74 |
| Leucine | 0.03 g | 1.19 |
| Lysine | 0.04 g | 1.70 |
| Methionine | 0.02 g | 2.70 |
| Phenylalanine | 0.02 g | 1.68 |
| Proline | 0.02 g | |
| Serine | 0.04 g | |
| Threonine | 0.02 g | 1.61 |
| Tryptophan | 0.01 g | 3.13 |
| Tyrosine | 0.02 g | 2.06 |
| Valine | 0.02 g | 1.36 |

(Note: "–" indicates data is unavailable. For more information, please see page 806.)

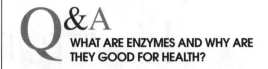

## OVERVIEW

Virtually all living things—including those we cook and eat—contain enzymes. Acting as the spark plugs for the vast majority of chemical reactions that make life possible, enzymes are a *sine qua non* for life.

Although most food eaten in the United States has been cooked, which inactivates the enzymes it contains, all the plant and animal foods in our meals are derived from once-living, enzyme-abundant things.

Over 2,500 different kinds of enzymes are found in living things. All enzymes are very special kinds of proteins that act as catalysts. Enzymes give our body chemistry its vitality, literally giving our metabolism a jumpstart. Plus, as molecules that enable the breaking down of our food, they also play a critically important role within our digestive system. Enzymes in our saliva allow us to break apart starches. Enzymes in our stomach help us break apart proteins. Enzymes in our intestines help us break apart fats, proteins and carbohydrates of all kinds.

When we eat fresh, uncooked foods, those foods can still contain active enzymes. When we chew a freshly picked leaf of lettuce, we break the cells in the leaf apart, releasing its nutrients, including enzymes. Enzymes are not automatically destroyed by the acids or temperatures in our digestive tract. Enzymes in the stomach—called gastric enzymes—are specially designed to function in the stomach's extremely acidic conditions and are critical to our health. Our bodies can overheat from fever, extreme exercise or summer weather but not to temperatures that will prevent the enzymes inside us from continuing to function.

Our digestive tract has specialized areas for absorbing large molecules, including enzymes, from food into our bloodstream. These areas house our M cells, specialized cells designed to selectively deliver large molecules from our intestines into our cells and bloodstream. The passing of enzymes from a mother to her nursing newborn is a good example of this M-cell function. A mother's milk contains the milk sugar, lactose. An enzyme called *lactase* is needed to digest *lactose*, but an infant's body is not yet capable of manufacturing this enzyme. So, the mother sends lactase along with her milk, enabling the baby to digest and absorb its lactose.

Ordinarily, we cook food at temperatures at least twice that of normal body temperature. For this reason, fresh, raw plant foods are our primary source of food enzymes. (Due to their high potential for bacterial contamination, most animal foods would be too risky for us to eat raw.) While there have been no large-scale, controlled studies to document the impact of enzyme-containing, fresh, raw plant foods on digestion and health, practitioners in the fields of complementary, natural and functional medicine have long advocated for the inclusion of fresh, organic, raw plant foods in the diet.

## TYPES OF ENZYMES
### Digestive Enzymes

Plant foods contain many of the same enzymes that humans use to metabolize different kinds of macronutrients. *Proteases* and *peptidases*, which help digest protein; *lipases*, which help digest fat; and *cellulases* and *saccharidases*, which help digest starches and sugars, are examples of the kind of digestive enzymes that would normally be secreted in our digestive tract or in nearby organs like the pancreas or liver. However, these same digestive enzymes can be found in the plant foods that we eat.

### Antioxidant Enzymes

Like humans, plants must protect themselves against oxygen-related damage, and they depend on enzymes to help them do so. A recently germinated sprout, for example, starts to generate many new oxidative enzymes in preparation for its journey up through the soil and into the open air. *Superoxide dismutase* and *catalase* are examples of oxidative enzymes that occur in higher concentrations in young plant sprouts than in the older, mature leaves. *Glutathione peroxidase* is another example of an important oxidative enzyme that is found in the human body and in the plants we eat.

## FUNCTIONS OF ENZYMES
### Necessary for Proper Digestion

Digestive enzymes play an integral role in the digestion of proteins, fats and carbohydrates since they catabolize these macronutrients into smaller molecules, which can be absorbed in the intestines. Our optimal physiological functioning depends upon the proper digestion and absorption of these nutrients.

### Confer Inflammatory and Oxidative Protection

Certain enzymes, such as *bromelain* (found in pineapple), have anti-inflammatory properties. *Bromelain* seems to confer anti-inflammatory protection through a variety of mechanisms. It is thought to inhibit intermediates of the clotting cascade, increase fibrinolysis (the dissolution of clots) and reduce the production of inflammatory molecules such as bradykinin.

### Support for the Immune System

Enzymes support the immune system in a few different ways. Since enzymes can work on substrates wherever the substrate is found, some of their targets include molecules other than the macronutrients associated with food. For example, *protease* enzymes can break apart the proteins that are found in unwanted bacteria and therefore reduce our risk of infection. In addition, the enzyme *bromelain* has been found to increase the production of a host of different immune system messenger molecules, including cytokines such as tumor necrosis factor-alpha, interleukin-1-beta and interleukin-6.

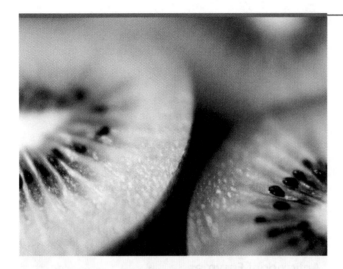

# kiwifruit

## nutrient-richness chart

Total Nutrient-Richness: **11**    GI: **74**
One (76 grams) fresh Kiwifruit contains 46 calories

| NUTRIENT | AMOUNT | %DV | DENSITY | QUALITY |
|---|---|---|---|---|
| Vitamin C | 57.0 mg | 95.0 | 36.9 | excellent |
| Dietary Fiber | 2.6 g | 10.3 | 4.0 | very good |
| Potassium | 252.3 mg | 7.2 | 2.8 | good |
| Copper | 0.1 mg | 6.0 | 2.3 | good |
| Magnesium | 22.8 mg | 5.7 | 2.2 | good |
| Vitamin E | 0.9 mg | 4.3 | 1.7 | good |
| Manganese | 0.1 mg | 4.0 | 1.6 | good |
| **CAROTENOIDS:** | | | | |
| Beta-Carotene | 39.5 mcg | | | |
| Lutein+Zeaxanthin | 92.7 mcg | | | |
| **FLAVONOIDS:** | | | | |
| (-)-Epicatechin | 0.3 mg | | | |

Daily values for these nutrients have not yet been established.

For more on "Total Nutrient-Richness," "%DV," "Density," and The World's Healthiest Foods "Quality" Rating System, see page 805.

For more on GI, see page 342.

While Kiwifruit are associated with New Zealand, they actually originated in China, where they have long been considered a delicacy. They were brought to New Zealand by missionaries in the early 20th century and known as Chinese Gooseberries. They were introduced into North America and other areas of the world in the 1960s when they also took on their new name in honor of the national bird of New Zealand, the kiwi. One of the traditional names for them in Chinese translates into "wonder fruit," which is definitely one way to describe these little fruits; underneath their brown fuzzy exterior you'll find bright emerald green or golden yellow flesh that has a creamy consistency and an invigorating, unique taste reminiscent of a combination of strawberries, pineapple and bananas.

## highlights

| | |
|---|---|
| AVAILABILITY: | Year-round |
| REFRIGERATE: | If desired |
| SHELF LIFE: | 5 days refrigerated |
| PREPARATION: | Peel before eating |
| BEST WAY TO ENJOY: | Enjoy them raw |

## why kiwifruit should be part of your healthiest way of eating

You may be surprised to learn that Kiwifruit actually contain more vitamin C than an equivalent amount of orange! Their rich concentration of vitamin C, combined with the health-promoting carotenoids and flavonoids found in Kiwifruit, provide powerful antioxidant protection against the oxidative damage caused by free-radicals. They are an ideal food to add to your "Healthiest Way of Eating" not only because they are nutritious and taste great, but also because they are low in calories: one Kiwifruit contains only 46 calories! (For more on the *Health Benefits of Kiwifruit* and a complete analysis of its content of over 60 nutrients, see page 366.)

## varieties of kiwifruit

The most common species of Kiwifruit is *Actinidia deliciosa*, also commonly known as Hayward. This is the type that you most often find in supermarkets, the ones with fuzzy brown skin and emerald green flesh.

With the growing interest in Kiwifruit, other species are beginning to appear in supermarket produce sections and farmer's markets. They include *Actinidia arguta* (Hardy Kiwi) and *Actinidia polygama* (Silvervine Kiwi), two smooth-skinned varieties that are the size of cherries and have a golden yellow-green hue.

## the peak season

Although Kiwifruit are commonly available throughout the year because they can be kept in cold storage for up to 10 months, the peak of their season in the United States runs from November through May. Kiwifruit from New Zealand are available from June through October. These are the months when their concentration of nutrients and flavor are highest, and their cost is at its lowest.

## biochemical considerations

Kiwifruit are one of the foods most commonly associated with allergic reactions in individuals with latex allergies. (For more on *Latex Food Allergies*, see page 722.)

## 3 steps for the best tasting and most nutritious kiwifruit

Enjoying the best tasting Kiwifruit with the most nutrients is simple if you just follow my 3 easy steps:
1. The Best Way to Select
2. The Best Way to Store
3. The Best Way to Prepare

# 1. the best way to select kiwifruit

For the best tasting Kiwifruit, look for ones that yield to gentle pressure, a sign that they are fully ripe. Fully ripened Kiwifruit not only taste best but are also highest in nutritional value. Concentrations of vitamins and health-promoting phytonutrients, many of which can act as powerful antioxidants, are at their peak when Kiwifruit are ripe. By selecting the best tasting Kiwifruit, you will also be enjoying ones with the highest nutritional value. As with all fruits, I recommend selecting organically grown Kiwifruit whenever possible. (For more on *Organic Foods*, see page 113.)

Avoid Kiwifruit that are shriveled or have bruised or damp spots. Overripe Kiwifruit will be very soft, may be brown in color and will have reduced nutritional value. Overripe Kiwifruit that have turned brown should not be eaten as they may contain free-radicals.

### How Do You Know Which Kiwifruit are Ready to Eat?

Kiwifruit that yield to gentle pressure will have reached the peak of their sweetness and are ripe and ready to eat.

# 2. the best way to store kiwifruit

Proper storage is an important step in keeping Kiwifruit fresh and preserving their nutrients, texture and unique flavor.

### Fresh Ripe Kiwifruit Can Last for Up to 5 Days When Properly Stored, Either Refrigerated or Kept at Room Temperature

Kiwifruit continue to respire even after they have been harvested. The faster they respire, the more the Kiwifruit interact with air to produce carbon dioxide. The more carbon dioxide produced, the more quickly they will spoil. Kiwifruit kept at a room temperature of approximately 68°F (20°C) give off carbon dioxide at a rate of 19 mg per kilogram every hour. (For a *Comparison of Respiration Rates* for different fruits, see page 341.) Kiwifruit can be either stored at room temperature or in the refrigerator, depending on your personal preference.

### How to Ripen Kiwifruit

Kiwifruit will become sweet and juicy (ripen) at home after they have been purchased, if they have not been picked too green. Kiwifruit can be ripened by leaving them at room temperature from 2 to 7 days. Be sure not to expose them to sunlight or heat. If you don't want them to ripen too quickly, store them away from all other fruits and vegetables since proximity to these foods will hasten the ripening process.

Another very natural way to ripen Kiwifruit is to place them in a paper bag for 2 to 3 days. The paper bag traps the ethylene gas produced by the Kiwifruit. The ethylene gas helps the Kiwifruit to ripen more quickly, while the paper bag allows for healthy oxygen exchange through the bag. Keep the paper bag in a dark, cool, ventilated place as excessive heat will cause the Kiwifruit to rot rather than ripen. To speed up the ripening, add a banana, apple or avocado to the bag.

Avoid storing Kiwifruit in sealed plastic bags or restricted spaces where they touch each other. Limited oxygen exchange and excessive amounts of ethylene gas naturally produced by the Kiwifruit will cause them to rot.

### Handle with Care

Kiwifruit are delicate and bruise easily, so handle them with care.

# 3. the best way to prepare kiwifruit

Properly preparing Kiwifruit helps ensure they will have the best flavor and retain the greatest number of nutrients.

## Peeling and Slicing Kiwifruit

Cut off the ends of the Kiwifruit, peel with a paring knife and then cut into pieces. Peeling is easier when ends are cut off first.

Alternatively, cut the Kiwifruit in half horizontally and scoop out the flesh with a spoon. Or you can wash off the brown fuzz before cutting and eat the Kiwifruit skin and all.

Kiwifruit should be eaten soon after cutting. Cutting activates enzymes (*actinic* and *bromic acids*) that act as food tenderizers and may result in the whole Kiwifruit becoming very soft soon after it has been cut.

If you are adding Kiwifruit to a fruit salad, you should do so at the last minute to prevent the other fruits from becoming too soggy from the enzymes found in Kiwifruit.

## No Bake Recipes

I have discovered that Kiwifruit retain their maximum amount of nutrients and their best taste when they are fresh and not prepared in a cooked recipe. That is because their nutrients—including vitamins, antioxidants and enzymes—are unable to withstand the temperature (350°F/175°C) used in baking. So that you can get the most enjoyment and benefit from fruit, I created quick and easy recipes, which require no cooking. I call them "No Bake Recipes."

---

Here are questions that I received from readers of the whfoods.org website about Kiwifruit:

### Q How does the small hardy Kiwifruit compare to the large fuzzy ones?

A Hardy Kiwifruit are becoming more and more popular. While it is difficult to find them in many markets because they are very delicate and don't hold up as readily to shipping as larger Kiwifruit, some specialty markets and farmer's markets offer them. In addition, more and more home gardeners are growing their own. While I haven't seen a nutritional comparison between hardy and larger-sized Kiwifruit, I assume that they are very similar and even offer a bit more fiber because their thin skin is readily edible, unlike the skin of larger Kiwifruit's skin.

### Q I don't like the texture of Kiwifruit. Since it is such a healthy fruit, can I juice it instead?

A Kiwifruit juice will not provide all of the nutrients that whole Kiwifruit does. No juice does. That's because the percentage of nutrients retained in a pulp-free juice is usually lower than the percentage retained in the pulp. Unless you take all of the pulp that is separated out from your juice and add it back into your juice before you drink it, you are not getting anywhere close to all of the nutrients that you would from eating the whole fruit. For example, virtually all of the fiber remains with the pulp and a signifi-

cant amount of beta-carotene does as well. Yet, if you want to enjoy Kiwifruit and don't like eating the whole fruit then by all means go ahead and make juice since you will still attain a wealth of nutrients. Try the Kiwi Cantaloupe Soup (page 365) as an alternative way to enjoy Kiwifruit.

### Q Can you freeze Kiwifruit?

A You can freeze almost any fruit, although it may not maintain the same taste and texture of the fresh fruit. But if you have more Kiwifruit than you can eat or if you want to freeze them for a recipe (smoothies, for example), by all means go ahead. I would probably suggest peeling them first (unless you enjoy the skin, as some people do) as it would be easier than peeling them once they have been frozen.

### Q I have a latex allergy and was recently told that Kiwifruit and latex are somewhat related. Can you clarify?

A Between 30–50% of individuals who have allergies to latex may also have allergic reactions to certain plant foods including Kiwifruit, avocados, bananas and chestnuts. Currently, the most conclusive evidence suggests that foods that cross-react with latex are those that contain enzymes called chitinases, which have similar protein structures to those found in latex. Consult your healthcare practitioner for more guidance on this topic.

STEP-BY-STEP
## No Bake Recipes

# 10-Minute
# Kiwi Mandala

*Make a mosaic of Kiwi and strawberries for a beautiful dessert.*

8 oz low-fat vanilla or soy yogurt
3 TBS fresh orange juice
1 TBS cream honey**
1/2 tsp grated orange rind*
1/4 tsp grated lemon rind*
1 Kiwifruit
4 strawberries
Optional: 2 TBS chopped walnuts or pecans

1. In a small bowl, whisk the yogurt, orange juice, honey, and grated orange and lemon rind, making sure the honey is completely blended into the yogurt.

2. Place in 2 shallow soup dishes.

3. Peel the Kiwifruit and slice into 1/8-inch rounds.

4. Take off the stems and cut strawberries lengthwise into 4 pieces.

5. Arrange the fruit in a beautiful pattern on top of the yogurt mixture and sprinkle with some grated orange rind and nuts if desired.

6. Refrigerate 1/2 hour so that the yogurt is well chilled. Enjoy immediately!

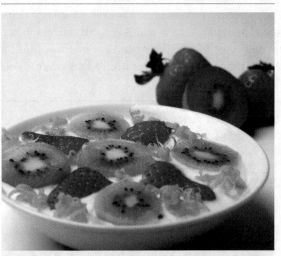

Kiwi Mandala

**Preparation Hint:** Some brands of yogurt are more acidic than others. This will determine how much honey you will use. Taste and adjust accordingly. The best honey to use is cream honey. This will keep your mixture thick.

\* Use an organic orange and lemon, if possible, to avoid wax coating.

\*\* Cream honey is whipped honey found in most health food stores.

**SERVES 2**

Please write (address on back cover flap) or e-mail me at info@whfoods.org with your personal ideas for preparing Kiwifruit, and I will share them with others through our website at www.whfoods.org.

## 5 QUICK SERVING IDEAS for KIWIFRUIT:

1. Add Kiwifruit to tossed green salads or fruit salads.

2. **Kiwi with Lemon Sauce:** Combine 3 TBS honey, 1 tsp lemon juice and 1/4 tsp lemon zest. Drizzle over sliced Kiwifruit.

3. **Kiwi Chutney:** Combine 4 chopped Kiwifruit, 1 small chopped orange and 1/2 cup chopped pineapple together to make chutney that can be served as an accompaniment to chicken or fish.

4. **Kiwi Cantaloupe Soup:** Blend equal amounts of Kiwifruit and cantaloupe in a blender to make a chilled soup. For a creamier consistency blend yogurt in with the fruit mixture. Add honey to sweeten.

5. **Marinade:** Include some Kiwifruit in a marinade or rub it on meat before cooking. The enzymes found in Kiwifruit act as a meat tenderizer.

# health benefits of kiwifruit

## Promote Respiratory Health

The protective properties of Kiwifruit have been demonstrated in a study with 6- and 7-year-old children in northern and central Italy. The more Kiwi or citrus fruit these children consumed, the less likely they were to have respiratory-related health problems including wheezing, shortness of breath or night coughing. The antioxidants found in these fruits may be involved in their health-promoting properties.

## Promote Heart Health

The small Kiwifruit may be a big friend to your heart. Kiwifruit are an excellent source of vitamin C, an antioxidant that helps to reduce oxidation of LDL cholesterol; LDL oxidation is one of the first steps in the development of atherosclerosis. Additionally, dietary fiber, a nutrient of which Kiwifruit are a very good source, has been shown to reduce high cholesterol levels, which may reduce the risk of heart disease and heart attack. Kiwifruit are also a good source of potassium and magnesium, two minerals important for regulating blood pressure. Yet, it may not be just their individual components that make Kiwifruit so heart-healthy but the synergy of the whole matrix of nutrients found in these fruits; recent research showed that individuals who ate two to three Kiwifruit per day reduced their platelet aggregation response (potential for blood clot formation) and triglyceride levels.

## Promote Optimal Health

Kiwifruit has fascinated researchers for its ability to protect DNA in human cells from oxygen-related damage. Researchers are not yet certain which compounds in Kiwi give it this protective antioxidant capacity, but they are sure that this healing property is not limited to those nutrients most commonly associated with Kiwifruit, including its vitamin C content. Since Kiwifruit contain a variety of flavonoids and carotenoids that have demonstrated antioxidant activity, these phytonutrients may be responsible for Kiwi's DNA protection.

## Promote Optimal Antioxidant Status

The vitamin C contained in Kiwifruit is the primary water-soluble antioxidant in the body, neutralizing free-radicals that can cause damage to cells and lead to inflammation. Kiwifruit is also a good source of copper and manganese, which are cofactors in the powerful antioxidant *superoxide dismutase*, as well as vitamin E, an important fat-soluble antioxidant. This combination of both fat- and water-soluble antioxidants makes Kiwi able to provide free-radical protection on all fronts.

## Additional Health-Promoting Benefit of Kiwifruit

Since each Kiwifruit contains only 46 calories, it is an ideal food for healthy weight control.

### Nutritional Analysis of 1 fresh Kiwifruit:

| NUTRIENT | AMOUNT | % DAILY VALUE | NUTRIENT | AMOUNT | % DAILY VALUE |
|---|---|---|---|---|---|
| Calories | 46.36 | | Pantothenic Acid | 0.14 mg | 1.40 |
| Calories from Fat | 3.01 | | | | |
| Calories from Saturated Fat | 0.20 | | **Minerals** | | |
| Protein | 0.75 g | | Boron | — mcg | |
| Carbohydrates | 11.31 g | | Calcium | 19.76 mg | 1.98 |
| Dietary Fiber | 2.58 g | 10.32 | Chloride | 29.64 mg | |
| Soluble Fiber | 0.86 g | | Chromium | — mcg | — |
| Insoluble Fiber | 1.73 g | | Copper | 0.12 mg | 6.00 |
| Sugar – Total | 8.51 g | | Fluoride | — mg | — |
| Monosaccharides | 7.14 g | | Iodine | — mcg | — |
| Disaccharides | 0.84 g | | Iron | 0.31 mg | 1.72 |
| Other Carbs | 0.21 g | | Magnesium | 22.80 mg | 5.70 |
| Fat – Total | 0.33 g | | Manganese | 0.08 mg | 4.00 |
| Saturated Fat | 0.02 g | | Molybdenum | — mcg | — |
| Mono Fat | 0.03 g | | Phosphorus | 30.40 mg | 3.04 |
| Poly Fat | 0.18 g | | Potassium | 252.32 mg | |
| Omega-3 Fatty Acids | 0.03 g | 1.20 | Selenium | 0.30 mcg | 0.43 |
| Omega-6 Fatty Acids | 0.16 g | | Sodium | 3.80 mg | |
| Trans Fatty Acids | 0.00 g | | Zinc | 0.13 mg | 0.87 |
| Cholesterol | 0.00 mg | | | | |
| Water | 63.12 g | | **Amino Acids** | | |
| Ash | 0.49 g | | Alanine | — g | |
| | | | Arginine | — g | |
| **Vitamins** | | | Aspartate | — g | |
| Vitamin A IU | 133.00 IU | 2.66 | Cystine | — g | — |
| Vitamin A RE | 13.68 RE | | Glutamate | — g | |
| A - Carotenoid | 13.68 RE | 0.18 | Glycine | — g | |
| A - Retinol | 0.00 RE | | Histidine | — g | — |
| B1 Thiamin | 0.02 mg | 1.33 | Isoleucine | — g | — |
| B2 Riboflavin | 0.04 mg | 2.35 | Leucine | — g | — |
| B3 Niacin | 0.38 mg | 1.90 | Lysine | — g | — |
| Niacin Equiv | 0.38 mg | | Methionine | — g | — |
| Vitamin B6 | 0.04 mg | 2.00 | Phenylalanine | — g | — |
| Vitamin B12 | 0.00 mcg | 0.00 | Proline | — g | |
| Biotin | — mcg | — | Serine | — g | |
| Vitamin C | 57.00 mg | 95.00 | Threonine | — g | |
| Vitamin D IU | 0.00 IU | 0.00 | Tryptophan | — g | — |
| Vitamin D mcg | 0.00 mcg | | Tyrosine | — g | — |
| Vitamin E Alpha Equiv | 0.85 mg | 4.25 | Valine | — g | — |
| Vitamin E IU | 1.27 IU | | | | |
| Vitamin E mg | 0.85 mg | | | | |
| Folate | 8.06 mcg | 2.02 | | | |
| Vitamin K | — mcg | — | | | |

(Note: "−" indicates data is unavailable. For more information, please see page 806.)

## Q&A
### WHAT ARE THE BENEFITS OF EATING FOODS IN SEASON?

Seasons form the natural backdrop for eating. All of the World's Healthiest Foods are seasonal. Imagine a vegetable garden in the dead of winter. Now imagine this same garden on a sunny, summer day. How different things are during these two seasons of the year! For ecologists, seasons are considered a source of natural diversity. Changes in growing conditions from spring to summer or fall to winter are considered essential for balancing the earth's resources and its life-forms. But today it's so easy for us to forget about seasons when we eat! Modern food processing and worldwide distribution of food make foods available year-round, and grocery stores shelves look much the same in December as they do in July.

### Research Supporting Seasonal Eating

In a research study conducted in 1997 by the Ministry of Agriculture, Fisheries and Food in London, England, significant differences were found in the nutrient content of pasteurized milk in summer versus winter. Iodine was higher in the winter; beta-carotene was higher in the summer. The ministry discovered that these differences in milk composition were primarily due to differences in the diets of the cows. With more salt-preserved foods in winter and more fresh plants in the summer, cows ended up producing nutritionally different milks during the two seasons. Similarly, researchers in Japan found three-fold differences in the vitamin C content of spinach harvested in summer versus winter.

### Guides for Eating Seasonally

What does this mean for you? Eat seasonally! To enjoy the full nourishment of food, you should make your menu a seasonal one. In different parts of the world, and even in different regions of one country, seasonal menus can vary. But here are some overriding principles you can follow to ensure optimal nourishment in every season:

- In spring, focus on tender, leafy vegetables that represent the fresh new growth of this season. The greening that occurs in springtime should be represented by greens on your plate, including Swiss chard, spinach, romaine lettuce, fresh parsley and basil.

- In summer, stick with light, cooling foods as defined in traditional Chinese medicine. These foods include fruits like strawberries, apples, pears, and plums; vegetables like summer squash, broccoli, cauliflower and corn; and spices and seasonings like peppermint and cilantro.

- In fall, turn toward the more warming, autumn harvest foods, including carrots, sweet potatoes, onions and garlic. Also emphasize the more warming spices and seasonings including ginger, peppercorns and mustard seeds.

- In winter, turn even more exclusively toward warming foods. Remember the principle that foods taking longer to grow are generally more warming than foods that grow quickly. All of the animal foods fall into the warming category including fish, chicken, beef, lamb and venison. So do most of the root vegetables, including carrots, potatoes, onions and garlic. Eggs also fit in here, as do corn and nuts.

In all seasons, be creative! Let the natural backdrop of spring, summer, fall and winter be your guide.

## Q&A
### HOW THE WORLD'S HEALTHIEST FOODS CAN HELP ADULTS OVER 50

As a general rule, it is true that our metabolism slows down somewhat as we age. For this reason, it is also generally true that we need fewer calories. For example, as Marion Nestle, PhD, MPH, and author of the book, "What to Eat," has noted, a woman in her 30s may need 2,400 daily calories, while at 50 she'll need about 2,100 and at 70, only 1,500 while a teenage boy may need 3,000 calories each day, but when he's 50 he'll only need 2,400 and when he's 70 he'll only need 2,200.

Calorie needs depend upon age but also upon activity level. One of the best ways to balance your calorie needs is to become more physically active. You definitely need to change your diet; you have to eat more nutrient-rich foods and less nutrient-poor foods.

Requirements for some nutrients increase for adults over 50. These include calcium for strong bones, vitamin D for calcium absorption, B vitamins such as B6 for a healthy heart and protection against the hardening of the arteries (by helping to keep homocysteine levels low) and antioxidant-rich foods to help prevent age-related cataracts and macular degeneration. For food sources of calcium, see page 738; for food sources of vitamin D, see page 796; for food sources of vitamin B6, see page 790; for food sources of antioxidants, see pages 735 and 804.

Research suggests that animals live 50% longer when they consume nutrient-rich foods without excess calories. Reducing caloric intake can lead to nutrient deficiencies if the food you eat is not highly nutrient-rich. By enjoying nutrient-rich World's Healthiest Foods, you not only won't ever feel hungry but you can eat large amounts of food at the same time that you are reducing your caloric intake. Enjoying nutrient-rich World's Healthiest Foods is a great way to meet your nutritional needs as you age while taking in fewer calories to accommodate a slowing metabolism, making it much easier to maintain a healthy weight.

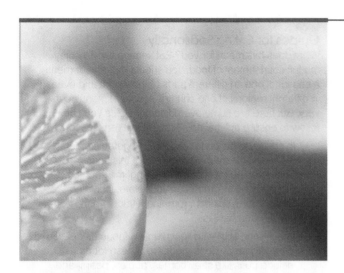

# oranges

| | |
|---|---|
| AVAILABILITY: | Year-round |
| REFRIGERATE | If desired |
| SHELF LIFE: | 10 days refrigerated |
| PREPARATION: | Peel |
| BEST WAY TO ENJOY: | Enjoy them raw |

## nutrient-richness chart

Total Nutrient-Richness: **11**          GI: **59**

One (131 grams) fresh Orange contains 62 calories

| NUTRIENT | AMOUNT | %DV | DENSITY | QUALITY |
|---|---|---|---|---|
| Vitamin C | 69.7 mg | 116.2 | 34.0 | excellent |
| Dietary Fiber | 3.1 g | 12.5 | 3.7 | very good |
| Folate | 39.7 mcg | 9.9 | 2.9 | good |
| B1 Thiamin | 0.1 mg | 7.3 | 2.1 | good |
| Potassium | 237.1 mg | 6.8 | 2.0 | good |
| Vitamin A | 268.6 IU | 5.4 | 1.6 | good |
| Calcium | 52.4 mg | 5.2 | 1.5 | good |

**CAROTENOIDS:**

| | | |
|---|---|---|
| Alpha-Carotene | 14.4 mcg | |
| Beta-Carotene | 93.0 mcg | Daily values for these nutrients have not yet been established. |
| Beta-Cryptoxanthin | 152.0mcg | |
| Lutein+Zeaxanthin | 169.0 mcg | |

For more on "Total Nutrient-Richness," "%DV," "Density," and
The World's Healthiest Foods "Quality" Rating System, see page 805.

For more on GI, see page 342.

Oranges were once reserved for special occasions. In medieval times, Oranges and their blossoms were used on a couple's wedding day, while in England, during the time of Queen Victoria, Oranges were presented as gifts during the Christmas holidays. Spanish explorers brought Oranges to Florida in the 16th century, while Spanish missionaries brought them to California in the 18th century, beginning their cultivation in the two states widely known for their Oranges. Historically, Oranges were also very expensive, but with advances in transportation and better means of utilizing their by-products, they are now affordable, available year-round and have become one of the world's most popular fruits. Delightful as a snack or as a recipe ingredient, these sweet juicy fruits are easy to pack and fun to eat.

## why oranges should be part of your healthiest way of eating

Oranges have been found to contain more than 60 flavonoids that provide powerful anti-inflammatory and antioxidant protection. These flavonoids work synergistically with vitamin C, of which Oranges are known to be a great source; vitamin C is the primary water-soluble antioxidant, providing protection against oxidative damage to cell structures, including DNA. These are just some of the reasons why Oranges can be an important part of your "Healthiest Way of Eating." Oranges are not only nutritious and delicious, but they are also low in calories: one Orange contains only 62 calories! (For more on the *Health Benefits of Oranges* and a complete analysis of their content of over 60 nutrients, see page 372.)

## varieties of oranges

Oranges originated thousands of years ago in Asia, in the region extending from southern China to Indonesia and spreading to India. They are classified into two general categories—bitter and sweet. Bitter Oranges (*Citrus aurantium*), such as Seville, are oftentimes used to make jam or marmalade, and their zest serves as the flavoring for liqueurs, such as Grand Marnier and Cointreau. Sweet Oranges are the ones most commonly found in the supermarket. Popular varieties of sweet Oranges (*Citrus sinensis*) include:

### VALENCIA

These medium- to large-size Oranges have smooth skin and a round or oval shape. They are the most commonly grown Oranges and can be peeled and eaten or squeezed for their juice. Florida Valencias are considered the best Oranges for juice.

### NAVEL
These thick-skinned Oranges are distinguished by a characteristic "belly button" scar on the blossom end. They are seedless, and the inner fruit is easily segmented, making them ideal for eating. Squeeze Navel Oranges for their juice as needed because the juice tends to turn bitter over time.

### JAFFA
Imported from Israel, they are similar to Valencias with a slightly sweeter flavor.

### BLOOD
As their name implies, these Oranges have blood-red flesh and juice. Imported from the Mediterranean area, they are small- to medium-size Oranges with smooth or pitted skin that sometimes has a reddish hue.

## the peak season

Oranges are available year-round, although their peak season runs from winter through summer with seasonal variations between varieties:

Valencia Oranges – March through June

Navel Oranges – November through April
Jaffa Oranges – December through February
Blood Oranges – March through May

These are the months when their concentration of nutrients and flavor are highest, and their cost is at its lowest.

## biochemical considerations

Oranges are one of the foods most commonly associated with allergic reactions. Conventionally grown Oranges often have a wax coating to help protect their surface and increase their shelf life. Avoiding the wax and the other compounds used on conventionally grown Oranges is one reason to choose organically grown Oranges whenever possible. (For more on *Food Allergies*, see page 719; and *Wax Coatings*, see page 732.)

## 3 steps for the best tasting and most nutritious oranges

Enjoying the best tasting Oranges with the most nutrients is simple if you just follow my 3 easy steps:

1. The Best Way to Select
2. The Best Way to Store
3. The Best Way to Prepare

# 1. the best way to select oranges

For the best tasting Oranges, look for ones that are fully ripe as Oranges will not ripen after they have been picked. Fully ripened Oranges will also have the greatest concentration of nutrients, including vitamins, antioxidants and enzymes. Ripe Oranges are heavy for their size. They will have higher juice content than ones that are spongy or lighter in weight. In general, smaller Oranges with thinner skins will be juicier than those that are larger in size. Oranges do not necessarily have to have a bright Orange skin to be good. Oranges that are partially green or have brown russeting may be just as ripe and tasty as those that are solid Orange in color. In fact, the uniform color of con-

ventionally grown Oranges may be due to the injection of Citrus Red Number 2 (an artificial dye) into their skins at the level of 2 parts per million. As with all fruits, I recommend selecting organically grown Oranges whenever possible. (For more on *Organic Foods*, see page 113.)

Avoid Oranges with soft spots or traces of mold.

### How Do You Know Which Oranges are Ready to Eat?
Almost all Oranges are picked ripe. The best Oranges are heavy for their size.

# 2. the best way to store oranges

Proper storage is an important step in keeping Oranges fresh and preserving their nutrients, texture and unique flavor.

### Fresh Ripe Oranges Can Last for Up to 10 Days When Properly Stored and Refrigerated
Oranges continue to respire even after they have been

harvested. The faster they respire, the more the Oranges interact with air to produce carbon dioxide. The more carbon dioxide produced, the more quickly they will spoil. Oranges kept at room temperature of approximately 68°F (20°C) give off carbon dioxide at a rate of 28 mg per kilogram every hour. (For a *Comparison of Respiration Rates* for different fruits, see page 341.)

Refrigeration helps slow the respiration rate of ripe Oranges, retain their vitamin content and increase their storage life. Oranges are juicier at room temperature where they will store for approximately 5 days. If you have more Oranges than you can enjoy within a week, it is best to place them in the refrigerator where they will last for about 10 days.

The best way to store Oranges is to keep them loose rather than in a plastic bag or restricted space where they touch each other. The combination of limited oxygen exchange and the excessive amounts of ethylene gas produced under these conditions will cause them to rot.

# 3. the best way to prepare oranges

Properly preparing Oranges helps ensure that they will have the best flavor and retain the greatest number of nutrients.

### Cleaning Oranges

Rinse Oranges under cold running water before peeling. (For more on *Washing Fruit*, see page 341.)

### Peeling Oranges

Thin-skinned Oranges can be easily peeled with your fingers. For easy peeling of the thicker-skinned varieties, first cut a small section of the peel from the top of the Orange. You can then either make four longitudinal cuts from the top to bottom and peel away these sections of skin, or starting at the top, peel the Orange in a spiral fashion.

### Juicing Oranges

Recipes often call for Orange juice. Oranges, like most citrus fruits, will produce more juice when they are not cold, so always juice them when they are at room temperature. To get the most juice out of an Orange, gently roll it on the counter top, applying soft pressure, before you cut and juice it.

Cut the Oranges in half and remove the visible seeds from the fruit before juicing or remove them from the juice after you are done juicing.

The juice can be extracted in a variety of ways. You can use a juicer or reamer or do it the old fashioned way, squeezing by hand.

### Grated Zest

Using a hand grater, grate the skin of the Orange; be careful to avoid the white membrane beneath the peel as it is bitter. Scrape the grated zest off the underside of the grater. Make sure that you use fruit that is organically grown since most conventionally grown fruits will have pesticide residues on their skin and are often coated with wax. If you use conventionally grown Oranges to make zest for your tea, you may find wax residues floating on top.

### Chopping Orange Rind

With a sharp knife, cut off thin pieces of Orange peel, getting as little of the white membrane as possible. Chop with a knife into desired size. Chopped Orange rind used to flavor sauces should be discarded once the sauce is done. Orange rind that is chopped very fine can be incorporated into a dish.

### Orange Segments

Cut the ends off a seedless Orange just far enough to expose the flesh. Place Orange cut end down and cut away as little of the peel as possible by following the Orange's shape. Using a sharp knife, cut along the inside of the membranes that separate the Orange segments. Continue around entire Orange cutting out each section.

### Cutting Oranges for Snacks

To eat as a snack, first wash the skin so that any dirt or bacteria residing on the surface will not be transferred to the fruit. Cut Oranges horizontally through the center. Cut the sections into halves or thirds, depending upon your personal preference.

### No Bake Recipes

I have discovered that Oranges retain their maximum amount of nutrients and their best taste when they are fresh and not prepared in a cooked recipe. That is because their nutrients—including vitamins, antioxidants and enzymes —are unable to withstand the temperature (350°F/175°C) used in baking. So that you can get the most enjoyment and benefit from fruit, I created quick and easy recipes, which require no cooking. I call them "No Bake Recipes."

STEP-BY-STEP
## No Bake Recipes

# 10-Minute Orange Treat

*Turn Oranges into a tangy dessert!*

**2 medium Oranges**
**1/2 tsp grated lemon rind***
**1¹/2 TBS fresh lemon juice**
**2 TBS cream honey****
**2¹/2 TBS low-fat vanilla yogurt**

1. In a small bowl, whisk lemon rind, lemon juice and honey until the honey is incorporated.
2. Add yogurt and whisk thoroughly.
3. Peel and separate the individual sections of the Orange. Be sure to remove the membrane covering from each section. Cut the sections in thirds crosswise. Place in 2 dessert bowls.
4. Spoon sauce over the Oranges.

**SERVES 2**

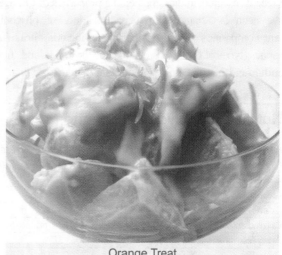

Orange Treat

\* Use an organic lemon for zest, if possible.
\*\* Cream honey is whipped honey found in most health food stores.

***Variations...*** • This sauce is delicious without the yogurt. • Substitute a banana for one of the Oranges.

Please write (address on back cover flap) or e-mail me at info@whfoods.org with your personal ideas for preparing Oranges, and I will share them with others through our website at www.whfoods.org.

## 6 QUICK SERVING IDEAS for ORANGES:

1. **Orange and Fennel Salad:** Combine segments from 2 medium Oranges, 1 medium thinly sliced fennel bulb and 2 TBS shaved Parmesan cheese for a delightfully refreshing salad. (Optional: top with chopped dill.)
2. **Orange and Avocado Salad:** Add extra flavor to a green salad by adding Orange sections and diced avocado.
3. **Orange Salsa:** Make a sweet salsa by combining 1 medium diced Orange, 1/2 medium finely diced jicama, 1 tsp lemon juice, 1 tsp minced fresh mint, 1 tsp Dijon mustard, red pepper flakes to taste and 2 TBS extra virgin olive oil.
4. **Orange Granita:** Freeze Orange juice in ice cube trays. When they are almost frozen, gently blend in a food processor to create a frozen granita dessert.
5. **Orange Cooler:** For a refreshing drink, blend Orange sections, strawberries, honey and ice in a blender.
6. **Orange French Toast:** Use Orange juice instead of milk when making French toast.

## Easy Way to Prepare Oranges, Step-by-Step

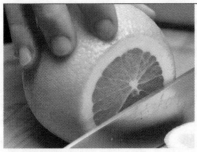
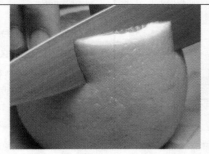
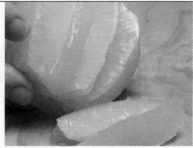

### ORANGE SEGMENTS

❶ Cut the ends off a seedless Orange. ❷ Place Orange cut end down and cut away the peel. ❸ Using a sharp knife, cut along the inside of the membranes that separate the Orange segments. Slice only down to the center of the Orange.

# health benefits of oranges

## Promote Optimal Health

In recent research studies, the healing properties of Oranges have been associated with a wide variety of phytonutrient compounds. These phytonutrients include citrus flavanones (types of flavonoids that include the compounds hesperidin and naringenin), anthocyanins, hydroxycinnamic acids and a variety of polyphenols. When these phytonutrients are studied in combination with Oranges' vitamin C, the significant antioxidant properties of this fruit are understandable. An increasing number of studies have also shown that nutrients such as vitamin C are more readily absorbed when consumed together with the other biologically active phytonutrients contained in citrus fruits than when taken singly as supplements.

The flavonoids in Oranges have been shown to have anti-inflammatory, anti-tumor and blood clot-inhibiting properties.

## Promote Heart Health

Oranges are a concentrated source of many heart-healthy nutrients including vitamin C, fiber, folate, potassium and flavonoids. The flavonoid hesperidin has been singled out in phytonutrient research on Oranges and shown to lower high blood pressure as well as cholesterol in animal studies. It has also been found to have strong anti-inflammatory properties. Importantly, most of this phytonutrient is found in the peel and inner white pulp of the Orange, rather than in the flesh used for juice, so it's important to eat the whole fruit rather than just drinking the juice.

Recent research has suggested that another class of compounds concentrated in citrus fruit peels, called polymethoxylated flavones (PMFs), has the potential to lower cholesterol more effectively than some prescription drugs, and without side effects. In this study, when animals with diet-induced high cholesterol were given the same diet containing PMFs, their blood levels of total cholesterol, VLDL and LDL (bad cholesterol) were reduced. Since these flavonoids are found in a much more concentrated amount in the peel, the best way to receive their benefits is by grating a tablespoon or so of the peel from a well-scrubbed organic Orange or tangerine each day and using it to flavor your meals.

## Additional Health-Promoting Benefits of Oranges

Oranges are also a concentrated source of other nutrients providing additional health-promoting benefits. These nutrients include free-radical-scavenging vitamin A, bone-building calcium and energy-producing vitamin B1. Since a medium-size Orange contains only 62 calories, it is an ideal food for healthy weight control.

### Nutritional Analysis of 1 Orange:

| NUTRIENT | AMOUNT | % DAILY VALUE | NUTRIENT | AMOUNT | % DAILY VALUE |
|---|---|---|---|---|---|
| Calories | 61.57 | | Pantothenic Acid | 0.33 mg | 3.30 |
| Calories from Fat | 1.41 | | | | |
| Calories from Saturated Fat 0.18 | | | **Minerals** | | |
| Protein | 1.23 g | | Boron | — mcg | |
| Carbohydrates | 15.39 g | | Calcium | 52.40 mg | 5.24 |
| Dietary Fiber | 3.13 g | 12.52 | Chloride | 3.93 mg | |
| Soluble Fiber | 2.06 g | | Chromium | — mcg | — |
| Insoluble Fiber | 1.07 g | | Copper | 0.06 mg | 3.00 |
| Sugar – Total | 12.26 g | | Fluoride | — mg | — |
| Monosaccharides | 6.16 g | | Iodine | — mcg | — |
| Disaccharides | 5.90 g | | Iron | 0.13 mg | 0.72 |
| Other Carbs | 0.00 g | | Magnesium | 13.10 mg | 3.27 |
| Fat – Total | 0.16 g | | Manganese | 0.03 mg | 1.50 |
| Saturated Fat | 0.02 g | | Molybdenum | — mcg | — |
| Mono Fat | 0.03 g | | Phosphorus | 18.34 mg | 1.83 |
| Poly Fat | 0.03 g | | Potassium | 237.11 mg | |
| Omega-3 Fatty Acids | 0.01 g | 0.40 | Selenium | 0.66 mcg | 0.94 |
| Omega-6 Fatty Acids | 0.02 g | | Sodium | 0.00 mg | |
| Trans Fatty Acids | 0.00 g | | Zinc | 0.09 mg | 0.60 |
| Cholesterol | 0.00 mg | | | | |
| Water | 113.64 g | | **Amino Acids** | | |
| Ash | 0.58 g | | Alanine | 0.07 g | |
| | | | Arginine | 0.09 g | |
| **Vitamins** | | | Aspartate | 0.15 g | |
| Vitamin A IU | 268.55 IU | 5.37 | Cystine | 0.01 g | 2.44 |
| Vitamin A RE | 27.51 RE | | Glutamate | 0.12 g | |
| A - Carotenoid | 27.51 RE | 0.37 | Glycine | 0.12 g | |
| A - Retinol | 0.00 RE | | Histidine | 0.02 g | 1.55 |
| B1 Thiamin | 0.11 mg | 7.33 | Isoleucine | 0.03 g | 2.61 |
| B2 Riboflavin | 0.05 mg | 2.94 | Leucine | 0.03 g | 1.19 |
| B3 Niacin | 0.37 mg | 1.85 | Lysine | 0.06 g | 2.55 |
| Niacin Equiv | 0.57 mg | | Methionine | 0.03 g | 4.05 |
| Vitamin B6 | 0.08 mg | 4.00 | Phenylalanine | 0.04 g | 3.36 |
| Vitamin B12 | 0.00 mcg | 0.00 | Proline | 0.06 g | |
| Biotin | 1.31 mcg | 0.44 | Serine | 0.04 g | |
| Vitamin C | 69.69 mg | 116.15 | Threonine | 0.02 g | 1.61 |
| Vitamin D IU | 0.00 IU | 0.00 | Tryptophan | 0.01 g | 3.13 |
| Vitamin D mcg | 0.00 mcg | | Tyrosine | 0.02 g | 2.06 |
| Vitamin E Alpha Equiv | 0.31 mg | 1.55 | Valine | 0.05 g | 3.40 |
| Vitamin E IU | 0.47 IU | | | | |
| Vitamin E mg | 0.31 mg | | | | |
| Folate | 39.69 mcg | 9.92 | | | |
| Vitamin K | 1.31 mcg | 1.64 | | | |

(Note: "–" indicates data is unavailable. For more information, please see page 806.)

# Q&A
## IS BREAKFAST REALLY THE MOST IMPORTANT MEAL?

Making time for a healthy breakfast sets the stage for healthy eating throughout the day. For most people, breakfast time comes at least eight hours after their previous meal. So, in essence, while sleeping you have also been "fasting." In fact, the word itself, when broken down, means to "break a fast." When you wake up in the morning, your blood sugar may be low, and you may feel hungry.

Eating a breakfast that contains a good source of both protein and complex carbohydrates will allow your blood sugar to rise at a steady pace throughout the morning and provide your cells with the energy they need to carry out your morning activities.

Oatmeal topped with fruit and soymilk, along with a generous helping of nuts and seeds, is one good way to start the day. Or, try a poached egg over whole grain toast. For a super-quick "meal on the run," spread some almond butter on a piece of whole grain toast and eat a piece of fruit along with it.

Try not to eat foods that are high in refined carbohydrates (for example, bagels, muffins or pastries made from white flour), first thing in the morning. These foods can cause a rapid spike in your blood sugar and may give you a short burst of energy but will cause you to "crash" a few hours later.

What happens if you skip breakfast? If you don't give your body some fuel first thing in the morning, your blood sugar will continue to drop. In addition, you will begin using your nutrient stores to hold you over until your next meal. Over the next few hours, you may begin to feel sleepy or fatigued. And, by the time lunch rolls around, you will probably be so hungry that you will eat anything in sight! At this point, it will be more difficult to select healthy foods, as you will be mostly interested in grabbing something quick to satisfy your body's need for fuel as soon as possible. These may be some of the reasons that studies have shown that eating breakfast regularly was a common characteristic of people who had lost weight. Researchers involved with the National Weight Control Registry say that there are several possible reasons that regular breakfast eating may be an essential behavior for weight loss maintenance:

- Eating breakfast may reduce the hunger experienced later in the day that leads to overeating.
- Breakfast eaters are able to better resist fatty and high-calorie foods throughout the day.
- Nutrients consumed at breakfast may give people a better ability to be more physically active.

Many people say that they are not hungry first thing in the morning, which makes it difficult to eat breakfast. Begin the habit of eating breakfast by starting with something very small, such as a half piece of whole grain toast with nut butter or a small bowl of whole grain cereal (with no added sugars!) with milk. As your body gets used to digesting food in the morning, you might notice you have a bigger appetite for breakfast.

# Q&A
## WHAT DO YOU THINK ABOUT FOOD COMBINING?

There's really no good research evidence to support the practice of food combining. However, many people have found food combining to be essential in their overall health, and many healthcare practitioners continue to support this practice despite the absence of research evidence. Sometimes proper food combining just means avoiding extremes. For example, some food combining advocates recommend eating protein alone or carbohydrates alone rather than protein and carbohydrates together. However, this goal is essentially impossible, since most vegetables, grains, nuts, seeds and legumes contain both proteins and carbohydrates. You would have to eliminate all of the above foods from your diet in order to avoid eating protein and carbohydrates together. However, large amounts of protein (like the 80+ grams of protein that would be found in a 12-ounce steak) together with large amounts of carbohydrates (like the 40+ grams of sugar found in a 16-ounce glass of orange juice) might be a taxing combination for your digestive tract, more difficult than either food alone. Nonetheless, I see the basic problem here as one of going to extremes (too much protein at once and too much sugar at once) rather than food combining.

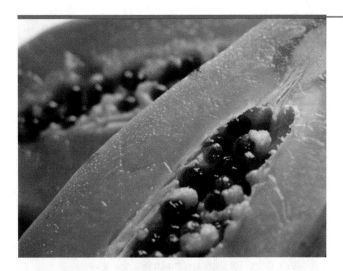

# papaya

## highlights

| | |
|---|---|
| AVAILABILITY: | Year-round |
| REFRIGERATE: | Yes, after ripening |
| SHELF LIFE: | 3 days |
| PREPARATION: | Peel |
| BEST WAY TO ENJOY: | Enjoy it raw |

## nutrient-richness chart

Total Nutrient-Richness: **11**   GI: **83**

One medium (304 grams) fresh Papaya contains 119 calories

| NUTRIENT | AMOUNT | %DV | DENSITY | QUALITY |
|---|---|---|---|---|
| Vitamin C | 187.9 mg | 313.1 | 47.5 | excellent |
| Folate | 115.5 mcg | 28.9 | 4.4 | very good |
| Potassium | 781.3 mg | 22.3 | 3.4 | very good |
| Dietary Fiber | 5.5 g | 21.9 | 3.3 | good |
| Vitamin A | 863.4 IU | 17.3 | 2.6 | good |
| Vitamin E | 3.4 mg | 17.0 | 2.6 | good |
| Vitamin K | 7.90 mcg | 9.9 | 1.5 | good |

| **CAROTENOIDS:** | | |
|---|---|---|
| Beta-Carotene | 839.0 mcg | Daily values for these nutrients have not yet been established. |
| Beta-Cryptoxanthin | 2389.5 mcg | |
| Lutein+Zeaxanthin | 228.0 mcg | |

For more on "Total Nutrient-Richness," "%DV," "Density," and The World's Healthiest Foods "Quality" Rating System, see page 805.

For more on GI, see page 342.

Bring the luscious taste and sunlit color of the tropics to your table by adding a ripe Papaya to your meal. Papaya trees are actually herbs that grow 10 to 12 feet high and produce the sweet, refreshing fruit, which you can now find in most local markets. Combining Papayas with other tropical fruits, like bananas and pineapples, is just one way you can enjoy them. And don't throw away those seeds. In some countries, they are used in place of black pepper; their peppery taste can be a great addition to salad dressings.

## why papaya should be part of your healthiest way of eating

Papayas' rich orange color reflects an abundance of beta-carotene and beta-cryptoxanthin, two carotenoid phytonutrients that not only get converted into vitamin A, but also provide powerful antioxidant protection against the oxidative damage free-radicals that inflict on cell structures. Green unripe Papayas are also rich in a unique enzyme called *papain*, which helps in the digestion of proteins. Papayas are an ideal food to add to your "Healthiest Way of Eating" because they are not only nutritious, but also truly delicious. (For more on the *Health Benefits of Papayas* and a complete analysis of their content of over 60 nutrients, see page 378.)

## varieties of papaya

Native to Central America, Papayas have a wonderfully soft, butter-like consistency and a deliciously sweet, musky taste. Botanically, they are known as *Carica papaya*. Inside the inner cavity of the fruit are black, round seeds encased in a gelatinous-like substance. Papayas' seeds are edible with a peppery flavor. The most popular varieties of Papaya include:

### HAWAIIAN VARIETIES

Hawaiian grown Papayas are the ones most commonly found in local markets. They are a pear-shaped fruit with a green-yellow outer skin—which turns yellow-orange when ripe—and bright orange-gold flesh. They range from six to eight inches in length and weigh about one pound. Sunrise Solo and Strawberry Sunrise are two Hawaiian varieties. All Papayas that are not organically grown on the Big Island in Hawaii are from genetically modified (GMO) seeds.

### MEXICAN VARIETIES

These are much larger than Hawaiian Papayas and reach upwards of two feet in length and ten pounds in weight. Their skin is also green in color, but they are not as sweet as Hawaiian Papayas.

## the peak season

Although there is a slight seasonal peak in early summer and fall, Papaya trees produce fruit throughout the year.

## biochemical considerations

Papayas are one of the foods most commonly associated with allergic reactions in individuals with latex allergies. Conventionally grown dried Papayas may be treated with sulfites, which may be problematic for some individuals. Papaya seeds are safe to eat in an amount proportional to the natural amount of fresh Papaya fruit being enjoyed. Problems with Papaya seeds discussed in the research have focused on high-dose, synthetic Papaya seed extracts; I don't believe that these studies on laboratory animals apply to direct consumption of Papaya seeds. (For more on *Latex Food Allergies*, see page 722; and *Sulfites*, see page 729.)

## 3 steps for the best tasting and most nutritious papaya

Enjoying the best tasting Papaya with the most nutrients is simple if you just follow my 3 easy steps:

1. The Best Way to Select
2. The Best Way to Store
3. The Best Way to Prepare

# 1. the best way to select papaya

The best tasting and most nutritious Papayas are those that are fully ripe. They have fully developed flavor and have the most concentrated amounts of nutrients. Unlike pineapples, you cannot use the smell of Papayas as a test for ripeness. Papayas that have patches of yellow color will take two to three more days to ripen. Fully ripe Papayas have yellow-orange skin and are slightly soft to the touch. Papayas with spotty coloring usually have more flavor. Since this is when their vitamins and powerful antioxidants are at their peak, by selecting ripe Papayas you will also be enjoying those with the highest nutritional value. Green (unripe) Papayas make a wonderful salad. They contain *papain* and are therefore good for digestion. As with all fruits, I recommend selecting organically grown varieties whenever possible. (For more on *Organic Foods*, see page 113.)

Avoid overripe Papayas, which become mushy, have more of an acidic taste and have begun to lose their nutritional value. Avoid those with black spots on the outside as they can penetrate the skin of the Papaya and negatively affect its taste. Also, avoid those that are bruised or overly soft. Do not purchase Papayas that are totally green or overly hard unless you are planning on making a green Papaya salad; they will not ripen when picked too green.

### How Do You Know Which Papayas are Ready to Eat?

Yellow-orange Papayas that are slightly soft to the touch are ready to eat.

# 2. the best way to store papaya

Proper storage is an important step in keeping Papayas fresh and preserving their nutrients, texture and unique flavor.

### Fresh Ripe Papaya Can Last for Up to 3 Days When Properly Stored and Refrigerated

Papayas continue to respire even after they have been harvested. The faster they respire, the more the Papayas interact with air to produce carbon dioxide. The more carbon dioxide produced, the more quickly they will spoil. Papayas kept at a room temperature of approximately 68°F (20°C) give off carbon dioxide at a rate of 80 mg per kilogram every hour. (For a *Comparison of Respiration Rates* for different fruits, see page 341.) Refrigeration helps slow the respiration rate of ripe Papayas, retain their vitamin content and increase their storage life.

Store fully ripened, but not unripened, Papayas in the refrigerator. While Papayas that are stored properly will remain fresh for up to 3 days, if they are not stored properly, they will only last about 1-2 days.

### How to Ripen Papaya

Papayas will become sweet and juicy at home if they have not been picked too green. Papayas are one of the few fruits that will ripen after they have been picked. Papayas are not ripe if they are hard and green. Unripe Papayas can be left at room temperature where they will ripen in 2–3 days. Don't refrigerate Papayas until they are ripe; they will not ripen in the refrigerator. Place Papayas on a flat surface with space between the fruit. It is best to turn them occasionally so that they will ripen evenly. Once their skin turns yellow-orange and they yield to gentle pressure, they are ripe and ready to eat. If you will not be consuming them immediately after they have ripened, place them in the refrigerator.

Another natural way to ripen Papayas is to place them in a paper bag for 2 to 3 days. The paper bag traps the ethylene gas produced by the Papayas. The ethylene gas helps them to ripen more quickly, while the paper bag allows for healthy oxygen exchange through the bag. Keep the paper bag in a dark, cool place as excessive heat will cause the Papayas to rot rather than ripen. Turn Papayas occasionally. Adding a banana, apple or avocado to the bag will speed up the ripening because they increase the amount of ethylene gas in the bag.

Avoid storing Papayas in sealed plastic bags or restricted spaces where they touch each other. The combination of limited oxygen exchange and the excessive amount of ethylene gas that the Papayas naturally produce under these conditions will cause them to rot.

## Do You Refrigerate Your Papayas After Ripening?

Yes, but they are very perishable and do not store well, so it is best to eat them as soon as possible.

## Handle with Care

Handle Papayas with care as they are a delicate fruit and bruise easily.

# 3. the best way to prepare papaya

Properly preparing Papaya helps ensure that it will have the best flavor and retain the greatest number of nutrients.

## Cleaning Papaya

Rinse Papaya under cold running water before cutting. (For more on *Washing Fruit*, see page 341.)

## Cutting Papaya

One of the easiest (and most delightful) ways to eat Papaya is to eat it just like a melon. After washing the fruit, cut it lengthwise, scoop out the seeds and eat the flesh with a spoon.

To cut Papaya into smaller pieces for fruit salad or recipes, first peel it with a paring knife and then cut into the desired size and shape. You can also use a melon baller to scoop out the fruit of a halved Papaya. If you are adding it to a fruit salad, you should

do so just before serving as it tends to cause the other fruits to become very soft.

Avoid the use of uncooked Papaya in gelatin recipes as the enzymes in Papaya prevent it from gelling.

## No Bake Recipes

I have discovered that Papaya retains its maximum amount of nutrients and its best taste when it is fresh and not prepared in a cooked recipe. That is because its nutrients—including vitamins, antioxidants and enzymes—are unable to withstand the temperature (350°F/175°C) used in baking. So that you can get the most enjoyment and benefit from fruit, I created quick and easy recipes, which require no cooking. I call them "No Bake Recipes."

### Easy Way to Prepare Papaya, Step-by-Step

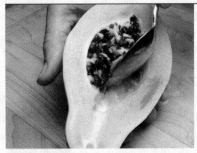 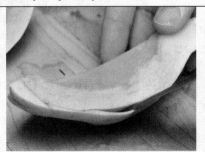 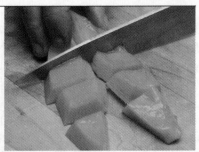

**PAPAYA CUBES**
❶ Cut Papaya in half and spoon out seeds from the center. ❷ Cut off peel with a sharp knife.
❸ Cut Papaya into quarters lengthwise. Cut across the width of each section into about 1- inch pieces.

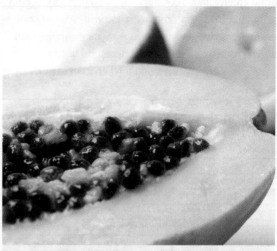

**STEP-BY-STEP**
## No Bake Recipes

# 5-Minute
# Papaya with Lime

*The best way to enjoy Papaya is to sprinkle it with lime.*

1 ripe Papaya
1 TBS lime juice
1/4 tsp lime zest*

1. Cut the Papaya in half and scoop out the seeds with a spoon. Place each half on a small dessert plate.

2. Squeeze lime over the Papaya, sprinkle with lime zest, and enjoy!

**SERVES 2**

## Variations...

- Drizzle with 1 TBS honey.
- Serve with 1/2 sliced banana and coconut flakes.

Papaya with Lime

\* Use an organic lime, if possible, to avoid wax coating.

# 10-Minute
# Papaya-Apricot Smoothie

*Enjoy this great tasting smoothie for breakfast or snack.*

1 small to medium Papaya
4 dried apricots soaked in 1¹/2 cups water
1 banana
2 TBS tahini (sesame seed butter)
1 TBS honey
1 tsp chopped fresh ginger
1/2 cup plain low-fat yogurt

1. Soak dried apricots in 1¹/2 cups of water for about 10–15 minutes.

2. Remove seeds from Papaya and scoop out fruit into blender.

3. Place rest of ingredients in blender, including soaking water for apricots, and blend until smooth.

**SERVES 2**

Please write (address on back cover flap) or e-mail me at info@whfoods.org with your personal ideas for preparing Papaya, and I will share them with others through our website at www.whfoods.org.

## 6 QUICK SERVING IDEAS for PAPAYAS:

1. **Tropical Papaya Smoothie:** Papaya adds thickness, tropical flavor and sweetness to a smoothie. For a refreshing treat blend fruit of 1 medium Papaya, 1 banana and enough orange juice to cover.

2. **Papaya Seeds:** While most people discard the black seeds, they are actually edible and have a delightful peppery flavor. They can be chewed whole or can be dried and then crushed and used like pepper.

3. **Papaya Fruit Cup:** Combine 1/2 medium diced Papaya, 1 sliced banana and 1/4 diced pineapple. Add juice of 1/2 an orange and mix well.

4. **Papaya Chicken Salad:** Combine 1 medium diced Papaya, 1 cup chopped chicken breast, 1/4 sliced sweet onion and 1/4 cup cashew nuts. Toss with Healthy Vinaigrette (see page 143).

5. **Ginger Papaya Salsa:** Combine 1 medium diced Papaya, 1 TBS minced cilantro, 1 tsp fresh grated ginger and 1 TBS lime juice to make a unique salsa that is a delicious accompaniment to shrimp, scallops and halibut.

6. **Green Papaya Salad:** You must use a totally green (unripe) Papaya for this recipe. Peel and deseed 1 medium green Papaya. Shred in food processor. Toss with 1/2 cup diced tomato, 2 TBS chopped cilantro, 1 clove pressed garlic, 2 TBS lime juice, 1 tsp sea salt, 1 tsp honey and 1/8 tsp cayenne. Sprinkle with 3 TBS chopped peanuts.

# health benefits of papaya

## Promotes Digestive Health

Unripe green Papaya contains *papain*, a proteolytic enzyme that is able to digest proteins; *papain* is well-known as a digestive enzyme and taken as a dietary supplement. Not only is it used to aid digestion, but natural healthcare practitioners sometimes recommend it when a person has allergic reactions to food since some of these reactions are thought to be caused by undigested protein. It may also be because of its *papain* that one of the traditional uses of Papaya in Central America is to eradicate dysentery infections caused by *Entamoeba histolytica*.

## Promotes Inflammatory Balance

In addition to *papain*, Papaya also contains *chymopapain*. This protein-digesting enzyme has been shown to help lower inflammation and improve healing from burns. In addition, the antioxidant nutrients found in Papaya, including vitamin C, vitamin E and beta-carotene, are very good at reducing inflammation. This may explain why people with diseases that get worse with inflammation—such as asthma, osteoarthritis and rheumatoid arthritis—find that the severity of their condition is reduced when they get more of these nutrients.

## Promotes Lung Health

Papaya is rich in the carotenoids beta-carotene and beta-cryptoxanthin. Not only are these carotenoids considered to be "pro-vitamin A" nutrients because they are converted into vitamin A in the body, but they have powerful antioxidant activity as well. Both of these functions make them important nutrients for promoting lung health.

While vitamin A has long been known to promote the health of the lungs since it is vital to the growth and development of epithelial tissues, such as those that line the lungs, recent research has suggested that vitamin A may also protect the lungs from the harmful effects of cigarette smoke. In laboratory animals exposed to cigarette smoke, levels of vitamin A dropped significantly in direct correlation with their development of emphysema. Another group of animals given a vitamin A-rich diet had less incidence of emphysema than those given a diet without extra amounts of this important nutrient. Yet, it may not only be Papaya's vitamin A content that has benefit; its beta-cryptoxanthin has also been found to promote lung health, potentially through its ability to scavenge free-radicals.

## Additional Health-Promoting Benefits of Papaya

Papaya is also a concentrated source of many other nutrients providing additional health-promoting benefits. These nutrients include heart-healthy folate, potassium and dietary fiber.

### Nutritional Analysis of 1 medium Papaya:

| NUTRIENT | AMOUNT | % DAILY VALUE | NUTRIENT | AMOUNT | % DAILY VALUE |
|---|---|---|---|---|---|
| Calories | 118.56 | | Pantothenic Acid | 0.66 mg | 6.60 |
| Calories from Fat | 3.83 | | | | |
| Calories from Saturated Fat | 1.18 | | **Minerals** | | |
| Protein | 1.85 g | | Boron | — mcg | |
| Carbohydrates | 29.82 g | | Calcium | 72.96 mg | 7.30 |
| Dietary Fiber | 5.47 g | 21.88 | Chloride | 33.44 mg | |
| Soluble Fiber | — g | | Chromium | — mcg | — |
| Insoluble Fiber | — g | | Copper | 0.05 mg | 2.50 |
| Sugar – Total | 17.94 g | | Fluoride | — mg | — |
| Monosaccharides | 12.46 g | | Iodine | — mcg | — |
| Disaccharides | 5.47 g | | Iron | 0.30 mg | 1.67 |
| Other Carbs | 6.41 g | | Magnesium | 30.40 mg | 7.60 |
| Fat – Total | 0.43 g | | Manganese | 0.03 mg | 1.50 |
| Saturated Fat | 0.13 g | | Molybdenum | — mcg | — |
| Mono Fat | 0.12 g | | Phosphorus | 15.20 mg | 1.52 |
| Poly Fat | 0.09 g | | Potassium | 781.28 mg | |
| Omega-3 Fatty Acids | 0.08 g | 3.20 | Selenium | 1.82 mcg | 2.60 |
| Omega-6 Fatty Acids | 0.02 g | | Sodium | 9.12 mg | |
| Trans Fatty Acids | 0.00 g | | Zinc | 0.21 mg | 1.40 |
| Cholesterol | 0.00 mg | | | | |
| Water | 270.04 g | | **Amino Acids** | | |
| Ash | 1.85 g | | Alanine | 0.04 g | |
| | | | Arginine | 0.03 g | |
| **Vitamins** | | | Aspartate | 0.15 g | |
| Vitamin A IU | 863.36 IU | 17.27 | Cystine | 0.00 g | 0.00 |
| Vitamin A RE | 85.12 RE | | Glutamate | 0.10 g | |
| A - Carotenoid | 85.12 RE | 1.13 | Glycine | 0.05 g | |
| A - Retinol | 0.00 RE | | Histidine | 0.02 g | 1.55 |
| B1 Thiamin | 0.08 mg | 5.33 | Isoleucine | 0.02 g | 1.74 |
| B2 Riboflavin | 0.10 mg | 5.88 | Leucine | 0.05 g | 1.98 |
| B3 Niacin | 1.03 mg | 5.15 | Lysine | 0.08 g | 3.40 |
| Niacin Equiv | 1.43 mg | | Methionine | 0.01 g | 1.35 |
| Vitamin B6 | 0.06 mg | 3.00 | Phenylalanine | 0.03 g | 2.52 |
| Vitamin B12 | 0.00 mcg | 0.00 | Proline | 0.03 g | |
| Biotin | — mcg | — | Serine | 0.05 g | |
| Vitamin C | 187.87 mg | 313.12 | Threonine | 0.03 g | 2.42 |
| Vitamin D IU | 0.00 IU | 0.00 | Tryptophan | 0.02 g | 6.25 |
| Vitamin D mcg | 0.00 mcg | | Tyrosine | 0.02 g | 2.06 |
| Vitamin E Alpha Equiv | 3.40 mg | 17.00 | Valine | 0.03 g | 2.04 |
| Vitamin E IU | 5.07 IU | | | | |
| Vitamin E mg | 3.40 mg | | | | |
| Folate | 115.52 mcg | 28.88 | | | |
| Vitamin K | 7.90 mcg | 9.88 | | | |

(Note: "—" indicates data is unavailable. For more information, please see page 806.)

# Q&A

## WHAT ARE THE KEYS TO SUPPORTING HEALTHY ENERGY PRODUCTION?

- **Support healthy digestion.** Healthy energy production begins with healthy digestion. Support healthy digestion by eating lightly and stopping as soon as you begin to feel satisfied. This places less burden on your digestion; you will feel lighter and more energetic. Eat slowly and deliberately. Include foods high in fiber in your meals. Enjoy herbs and spices that support digestion, such as ginger, pepper, cinnamon, fennel, rosemary, garlic, turmeric and chili spices.

- **Eat low-glycemic-index foods as much as possible.** Low-glycemic-index foods provide your body with sources of longer lasting energy and help you avoid the feeling of energy peaks and valleys. Good examples of low-glycemic-index foods include leafy green vegetables and legumes. Limit foods or drinks that have a high glycemic index.

- **Eat whole grains rather than refined grains.** Whole grains are one of the best sources of the full spectrum of the key vitamins needed for energy generation, especially the B-vitamins.

- **Include a good source of protein with each meal, especially during the first half of the day.** Good dietary sources of protein include fish, eggs and venison. Researchers have found that eating a varied diet featuring whole grains, legumes and vegetables provides all of the important amino acid building blocks to provide healthy proteins in the cells. In addition, some plant-based foods, such as soy, feature an essential amino acid protein profile similar to animal-based foods and can directly substitute for animal protein.

- **Provide a source of essential fatty acids or monounsaturated fats with each meal.** These fats support healthy cell membranes. Good sources for healthy fats include whole raw almonds, walnuts, pecans, flaxseeds, sesame seeds, sunflower seeds or pumpkin seeds or their oils; salmon, sardines, tuna, cod, halibut, sole, perch, turbot or orange roughy; and olive oil. In addition to these fats, inositol is a component of membrane phospholipids that are involved in various functions including cellular signaling. Increases in dietary inositol and choline have been found to significantly influence the concentration of membrane phospholipids and support healthy cell membranes. Good dietary sources of inositol include whole grains; choline is also present in high amounts in egg yolks.

- **Provide your body with foods rich in protective phytonutrients like the antioxidants.** The vitamin E family contains powerful antioxidants that are able to protect both the lipid and protein components in your cell membranes from damage caused by free-radicals and other oxidative compounds. Research has suggested that through their powerful antioxidant activity, vitamin E may be able to protect DNA from the damage caused by oxidative stress. It can also protect the mitochondria from the effects of the free-radicals produced during ATP manufacture. Good dietary sources of the vitamin E family include wheat germ and wheat germ oil.

- **Eat foods rich in antioxidants.** The body's premier water-soluble antioxidant, vitamin C, is critical to cellular membrane health since it plays an integral role in recycling vitamin E back to its active form. By regenerating vitamin E back to its active form, vitamin C also plays a role in protecting the mitochondria from potential damage by reactive oxygen species, like free-radicals. Excellent dietary sources of vitamin C include broccoli, bell pepper, strawberries, oranges, lemon juice, papaya, cauliflower, kale, mustard greens and Brussels sprouts.

- **Limit your alcohol intake and avoid foods or drinks to which you are sensitive or intolerant** and avoid the temptations of stimulants and sweet snacks, especially soft drinks, coffee and candy.

- **Select organic food whenever possible and avoid food cultivated with pesticides.** Several of the agricultural chemicals used in the conventional growing of foods have also been shown to have a negative effect upon mitochondrial function. These chemicals include paraquat, parathion, dinoseb and 2,4-D, all of which have been found to affect the mitochondria and cellular energy production in a variety of ways, including increasing membrane permeability (which exposes the mitochondria to damaging free-radicals) and inhibiting the protein that creates ATP, the energy currency of the body. Avoid foods containing preservatives, additives and colorants when possible, since many of these compounds have been associated with membrane damage, DNA mutations or altered energy production.

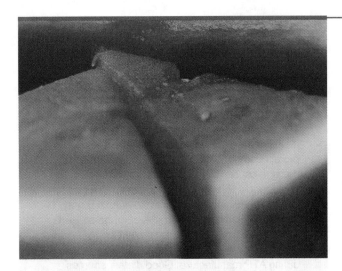

## nutrient-richness chart

Total Nutrient-Richness: **11**                    GI: **100**
One cup (152 grams) of fresh Watermelon contains 49 calories

| NUTRIENT | AMOUNT | %DV | DENSITY | QUALITY |
|---|---|---|---|---|
| Vitamin C | 14.6 mg | 24.3 | 9.0 | excellent |
| Vitamin A | 556.3 IU | 11.1 | 4.1 | very good |
| B6 Pyridoxine | 0.2 mg | 11.0 | 4.1 | very good |
| B1 Thiamin | 0.1 mg | 8.0 | 3.0 | good |
| Potassium | 176.3 mg | 5.0 | 1.9 | good |
| Magnesium | 16.7 mg | 4.2 | 1.5 | good |
| **CAROTENOIDS:** | | | | |
| Beta-Carotene | 466.6 mcg | | | |
| Beta-Cryptoxanthin | 120.1 mcg | | | |
| Lutein+Zeaxanthin | 12.3 mcg | | | |
| Lycopene | 6979.3 mcg | | | |
| **PHYTOSTEROLS:** | | | | |
| Phytosterols—Total | 3.1 mg | | | |

Daily values for these nutrients have not yet been established.

For more on "Total Nutrient Richness," "%DV," "Density," and
The World's Healthiest Foods "Quality" Rating System, see page 805.
For more on GI, see page 342.

Originating in Africa, Watermelons were first culti-vated in Egypt where testaments to their legacy were recorded in hieroglyphics painted on building walls. The fruit was held in such regard that it was even placed in the tombs of many Egyptian kings. Today, no other fruit is more enjoyable on a hot summer day than sweet, juicy Watermelon; it has an extremely high water content, approximately 92%, giving its flesh a crumbly and subtly crunchy texture and making it a favorite thirst-quenching fruit. It is so much a part of American food culture that it may come as a surprise to find that it is not the United States, but China, that is the top Watermelon-producing country in the world. Among its nutritional claim to frame, Watermelon is a rich source of lycopene; in fact, one cup of Watermelon contains more lycopene than one cup of raw tomatoes.

# watermelon

## highlights

## why watermelon should be part of your healthiest way of eating

Watermelon is a rich source of heart-healthy nutrients, such as vitamin C and the carotenoid phytonutrient, lycopene, which also provides reddish-pink Watermelon with its distinctive coloration. Lycopene, along with beta-carotene and vitamin A, provides powerful antioxidant protection from the oxidative damage to cellular structures caused by free-radicals. Watermelon is an ideal food to add to your "Healthiest Way of Eating" not only because it is nutritious and tastes great, but also because it is low in calories: one cup of Watermelon contains only 49 calories! (For more on the *Health Benefits of Watermelon* and a complete analysis of its content of over 60 nutrients, see page 382.)

## varieties of watermelon

Watermelon is a member of the *Cucurbitaceae* family and related to the squash and pumpkin. Its botanical name is *Citrullis lanatus*.

Watermelons are often associated with a deep red-pink color, but several varieties feature orange, yellow or white flesh. While most Watermelons have black, brown, white, green or yellow seeds, seedless varieties are also available. Watermelon's fifty different varieties are classified as:

### PICNIC
Round, oblong or oval, they weigh from 12 to 50 pounds.

### ICE BOX
Round or oval and designed to fit into a refrigerator, they weigh from 5 to 10 pounds.

### SEEDLESS WATERMELON
Hybrid Watermelon (not genetically modified) that contain small, edible white seeds.

## the peak season

Although Watermelon can now be found in markets throughout the year, the season for Watermelon is in the summer. This is the time of year when its concentration of nutrients and flavor are highest, and its cost is at its lowest.

## 3 steps for the best tasting and most nutritious watermelon

Enjoying the best tasting Watermelon with the most nutrients is simple if you just follow my 3 easy steps:

1. The Best Way to Select
2. The Best Way to Store
3. The Best Way to Prepare

# 1. the best way to select watermelon

Watermelons will not ripen after they are picked, so it is important to select a ripe Watermelon at the market. These will be the ones with the best flavor and peak concentration of nutrients, including vitamins, antioxidants and enzymes. Ripe Watermelons have a yellow or cream-yellow "ground spot," the place the melon rested on the soil. If this spot is green or white, the Watermelon is probably not ripe. If you thump a ripe Watermelon, it will sound like a dull thud rather than a tighter ringing or hollow sound. The rind should be relatively smooth and neither overly shiny nor overly dull. As with all fruits, I recommend selecting organic Watermelon whenever possible. (For more on *Organic Foods*, see page 113.)

Avoid Watermelons that do not have the "ground spot" markings on their underbelly as this may be an indication that they have been harvested prematurely. Unripe Watermelons will have less taste and contain less juice. Seedless Watermelons, however, are an exception to this rule; they often do not have this marking on their underbelly.

If you are purchasing Watermelons that are already cut, I would look for deeply colored flesh that is devoid of white streaks. The seeds should also be deep in color.

### How Do You Know Which Watermelon is Ready to Eat?

Watermelon is ready to eat if it has a yellow or cream-yellow "ground spot" (this does not apply to seedless Watermelons) and produces a dull thud sound when thumped.

# 2. the best way to store watermelon

Proper storage is an important step in keeping Watermelon fresh and preserving its nutrients, texture and unique flavor.

### Fresh Watermelon Can Last Up to 1 Week When Properly Stored

Watermelon continues to respire even after it has been harvested. The faster it respires, the more the Watermelon interacts with air to produce carbon dioxide. The more carbon dioxide produced, the more quickly it will spoil. Watermelon kept at a room temperature of approximately 68°F (20°C) gives off carbon dioxide at a rate of 21 milligrams per kilogram every hour. (For a *Comparison of Respiration Rates* for different fruits, see page 341.) Although refrigeration helps slow the respiration rate of Watermelon, retain its vitamin content and increase its storage life, most refrigerators are not large enough to store a Watermelon. It is fine to store the whole Watermelon at room temperature. Once the Watermelon has been cut, store the remaining portion by cutting into small pieces that can be stored in airtight containers in the refrigerator.

# 3. the best way to prepare watermelon

### Cleaning Watermelon

Wash the Watermelon before cutting it to remove any excess soil and bacteria. Due to its large size, you will probably not be able to run it under water in the sink. Instead, clean it thoroughly with a wet cloth or paper towel. (For more on *Washing Fruit,* see page 341.)

### No Bake Recipes

I have discovered that Watermelon retains its maximum amount of nutrients and its best taste when it is fresh. That is because its nutrients—including vitamins, antioxidants and enzymes—are unable to withstand the temperature (350°F/175°C) used in baking. So that you can get the most enjoyment and benefit from fruit, I created quick and easy recipes, which require no cooking. I call them "No Bake Recipes."

# health benefits of watermelon

## Promotes Heart Health

Watermelon is rich in many heart-healthy nutrients. It is a concentrated and bioavailable source of lycopene, a carotenoid phytonutrient that gives Watermelon, as well as other red and pink foods—such as tomatoes, pink grapefruits, papaya and guavas—their beautiful rosy hue.

Lycopene is a powerful antioxidant, and, in fact, is thought to be even more active than other well-known carotenoids, such as beta-carotene. Body levels of lycopene have been found to be inversely associated with both cardiovascular disease (such as atherosclerosis and heart attack) and cerebrovascular disease (such as stroke). One study even showed that women who had the highest plasma levels of lycopene demonstrated a 33% lower risk for developing cardiovascular disease.

Watermelon is also an excellent source of vitamin C as well as a very good source of vitamin A (since it is a rich source of the "pro-vitamin A" carotenoid, beta-carotene). High intake of vitamin C and beta-carotene have been shown in a number of scientific studies to reduce the risk of heart disease. In addition, Watermelon is a good source of magnesium and potassium, two minerals known for helping to balance blood pressure, as well as a very good source of vitamin B6, which helps to keep artery-damaging homocysteine in check.

## Provides Powerful Antioxidant Protection

In addition to providing heart-healthy benefits, the antioxidant nutrients offered by Watermelon promote health in numerous other ways since they can quench free-radicals that could otherwise cause damage. High intakes of vitamin C and beta-carotene have been shown in a number of scientific studies to reduce the airway spasm that occurs in asthma, reduce the risk of colon cancer and alleviate some of the symptoms of osteoarthritis and rheumatoid arthritis.

## Promotes Healthy Weight Control

Like many fruits, Watermelon is a great food for people interested in losing weight or maintaining a healthy weight. That's because it contains so many nutrients for so few calories—one cup has only 49 calories! It is high in water content, so it is refreshing as well as appetite satisfying. But, it is best to not eat Watermelon alone too frequently since it is rather high on the glycemic index (GI) scale and can lead to spikes of blood sugar. This effect can be blunted when it is consumed with foods that have a lower GI.

## Additional Health-Promoting Benefit of Watermelon

Watermelon is also a concentrated source of energy-producing vitamin B1.

### Nutritional Analysis of 1 cup fresh Watermelon:

| NUTRIENT | AMOUNT | % DAILY VALUE |
|---|---|---|
| Calories | 48.64 | |
| Calories from Fat | 5.88 | |
| Calories from Saturated Fat | 0.66 | |
| Protein | 0.94 g | |
| Carbohydrates | 10.91 g | |
| Dietary Fiber | 0.76 g | 3.04 |
| Soluble Fiber | 0.49 g | |
| Insoluble Fiber | 0.27 g | |
| Sugar – Total | 10.15 g | |
| Monosaccharides | 5.47 g | |
| Disaccharides | 4.68 g | |
| Other Carbs | 0.00 g | |
| Fat – Total | 0.65 g | |
| Saturated Fat | 0.07 g | |
| Mono Fat | 0.16 g | |
| Poly Fat | 0.22 g | |
| Omega-3 Fatty Acids | 0.00 g | 0.00 |
| Omega-6 Fatty Acids | 0.22 g | |
| Trans Fatty Acids | 0.00 g | |
| Cholesterol | 0.00 mg | |
| Water | 139.10 g | |
| Ash | 0.40 g | |

**Vitamins**

| NUTRIENT | AMOUNT | % DAILY VALUE |
|---|---|---|
| Vitamin A IU | 556.32 IU | 11.13 |
| Vitamin A RE | 56.24 RE | |
| A - Carotenoid | 56.24 RE | 0.75 |
| A - Retinol | 0.00 RE | |
| B1 Thiamin | 0.12 mg | 8.00 |
| B2 Riboflavin | 0.03 mg | 1.76 |
| B3 Niacin | 0.30 mg | 1.50 |
| Niacin Equiv | 0.48 mg | |
| Vitamin B6 | 0.22 mg | 11.00 |
| Vitamin B12 | 0.00 mcg | 0.00 |
| Biotin | 1.52 mcg | 0.51 |
| Vitamin C | 14.59 mg | 24.32 |
| Vitamin D IU | 0.00 IU | 0.00 |
| Vitamin D mcg | 0.00 mcg | |
| Vitamin E Alpha Equiv | 0.23 mg | 1.15 |
| Vitamin E IU | 0.34 IU | |
| Vitamin E mg | 0.23 mg | |
| Folate | 3.34 mcg | 0.83 |
| Vitamin K | — mcg | — |

| NUTRIENT | AMOUNT | % DAILY VALUE |
|---|---|---|
| Pantothenic Acid | 0.32 mg | 3.20 |

**Minerals**

| NUTRIENT | AMOUNT | % DAILY VALUE |
|---|---|---|
| Boron | — mcg | |
| Calcium | 12.16 mg | 1.22 |
| Chloride | — mg | |
| Chromium | — mcg | — |
| Copper | 0.05 mg | 2.50 |
| Fluoride | — mg | — |
| Iodine | — mcg | — |
| Iron | 0.26 mg | 1.44 |
| Magnesium | 16.72 mg | 4.18 |
| Manganese | 0.06 mg | 3.00 |
| Molybdenum | — mcg | — |
| Phosphorus | 13.68 mg | 1.37 |
| Potassium | 176.32 mg | |
| Selenium | 0.15 mcg | 0.21 |
| Sodium | 3.04 mg | |
| Zinc | 0.11 mg | 0.73 |

**Amino Acids**

| NUTRIENT | AMOUNT | % DAILY VALUE |
|---|---|---|
| Alanine | 0.03 g | |
| Arginine | 0.09 g | |
| Aspartate | 0.06 g | |
| Cystine | 0.00 g | 0.00 |
| Glutamate | 0.10 g | |
| Glycine | 0.02 g | |
| Histidine | 0.01 g | 0.78 |
| Isoleucine | 0.03 g | 2.61 |
| Leucine | 0.03 g | 1.19 |
| Lysine | 0.09 g | 3.83 |
| Methionine | 0.01 g | 1.35 |
| Phenylalanine | 0.02 g | 1.68 |
| Proline | 0.04 g | |
| Serine | 0.02 g | |
| Threonine | 0.04 g | 3.23 |
| Tryptophan | 0.01 g | 3.13 |
| Tyrosine | 0.02 g | 2.06 |
| Valine | 0.02 g | 1.36 |

(Note: "—" indicates data is unavailable. For more information, please see page 806.)

**STEP-BY-STEP**
## No Bake Recipes

# 5-Minute Watermelon Frappé

*A great alternative to Watermelon slices.*

**4 cups cold Watermelon chunks
8 mint leaves**

1. Run the blender at medium speed and drop chunks of Watermelon through the feed hole one at a time until they are well integrated.

2. Add the mint and run the blender at medium speed for 1 minute until the Watermelon has liquefied.

3. Strain into glasses, garnish with a sprig of mint and enjoy!

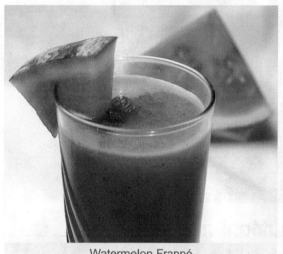

Watermelon Frappé

**Preparation Hint:** Selecting juicy red Watermelon will make the drink more flavorful. This is best served icy cold. If the Watermelon has been chilled first, it may not be necessary to chill it again. Serve it in chilled glasses to make a special presentation!

This recipe uses Watermelon with seeds. You may remove the seeds if you prefer.

**SERVES 2**

Please write (address on back cover flap) or e-mail me at info@whfoods.org with your personal ideas for preparing Watermelon, and I will share them with others through our website at www.whfoods.org.

## 6 QUICK SERVING IDEAS for WATERMELON:

1. Squeeze lime juice on cubed Watermelon.
2. Mix Watermelon chunks with minced mint.
3. Watermelon is a wonderful addition to any fruit salad.
4. **Watermelon and Jicama:** For a wonderful accompaniment to your favorite Mexican meals, toss 1/2-inch cubes of Watermelon with jicama, lime juice, cilantro, cayenne pepper, and sea salt and pepper to taste.
5. **Watermelon Granita:** Freeze puréed Watermelon in ice cube trays. Once frozen, gently blend in a food processor to create a frozen granita dessert treat.
6. **Watermelon-Kiwi Soup:** Purée 3 cups Watermelon, 1 cup cantaloupe and 1 cup kiwifruit together. Swirl in a little plain yogurt and serve as refreshing cold soup.

Here are questions that I received from readers of the whfoods.org website about Watermelons:

## Q *Are seedless Watermelons genetically engineered?*

A The seedless Watermelons that I know of are not genetically engineered. They are simple hybrids, the offspring of a cross between two varieties of Watermelon. It's actually fascinating, because seedless Watermelons are sterile and can only be grown through cross-pollination. Bees are used to accomplish this cross-pollination process.

## Q *Is there a benefit to eating Watermelon seeds?*

A Watermelon seeds contain a reasonable amount of magnesium, phosphorus, potassium and other minerals. There is also quite a health tradition involving Watermelon seeds, which are used in Asian medicine and other traditions for kidney cleansing and other medicinal purposes. In Nigeria, they use Watermelon seeds to make soup, while in China, they are eaten after removing their outer skin.

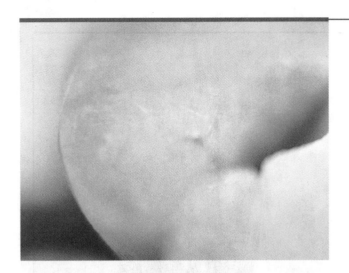

# apricots

| | |
|---|---|
| AVAILABILITY: | May through August |
| REFRIGERATE: | If desired |
| SHELF LIFE: | 3 days |
| PREPARATION: | Minimal |
| BEST WAY TO ENJOY: | Enjoy them raw |

## nutrient-richness chart

Total Nutrient-Richness: **9**     GI: **80**

One (35 grams) fresh Apricot contains 17 calories

| NUTRIENT | AMOUNT | %DV | DENSITY | QUALITY |
|---|---|---|---|---|
| Vitamin A | 914.2 IU | 18.3 | 19.6 | excellent |
| Vitamin C | 3.5 mg | 5.8 | 6.3 | very good |
| Dietary Fiber | 0.9 g | 3.4 | 3.6 | good |
| Tryptophan | 0.01 g | 3.1 | 3.3 | good |
| Potassium | 103.6 mg | 3.0 | 3.2 | good |
| **CAROTENOIDS:** | | | | |
| Alpha-Carotene | 6.7 mcg | | | |
| Beta-Carotene | 382.9 mcg | | | |
| Beta-Cryptoxanthin | 36.4 mcg | | | |
| Lutein+Zeaxanthin | 31.2 mcg | | | |
| **FLAVONOIDS:** | | | | |
| (+)-Catechin | 1.7 mg | | | |
| (-)-Epicatechin | 2.1 mg | | | |
| Quercetin | 0.9 mg | | | |
| **PHYTOSTEROLS:** | | | | |
| Phytosterols - Total | 6.3 mg | | | |

Daily values for these nutrients have not yet been established.

For more on "Total Nutrient-Richness," "%DV," "Density," and The World's Healthiest Foods "Quality" Rating System, see page 805.

For more on GI, see page 342.

Indigenous to the mountain slopes of China, Apricots have been cultivated for more than 4,000 years. In Latin, Apricot means "early matured fruit" because this close relative to the peach is one of the first fruits of summer. Although their flavor is often described as a cross between a peach and a plum, no words can adequately describe the uniquely delicious flavor of Apricots. I experienced the most exquisite tasting Apricots on the road to Istanbul in Eastern Turkey, which is renowned for having the best tasting Apricots in the world. I will never forget the experience of biting into a juicy, tree-ripened Apricot, which I purchased from a roadside stand that sat right next to the farm where the Apricots were picked. This is where I learned that you can only enjoy the delicious flavor of Apricots if they are truly ripe.

## why apricots should be part of your healthiest way of eating

Apricots may be little but they are large when it comes to nutritional benefits. Apricots are a rich source of carotenoid phytonutrients such as beta-carotene and beta-cryptoxanthin (both of which are precursors to vitamin A). They are also one of the few foods that are rich in the carotenoid lycopene. All of these antioxidant carotenoids not only provide Apricots with their red, orange and yellow hues, but also with the ability to defend cells against oxidative damage caused by free-radicals. Apricots are an ideal food to add to your "Healthiest Way of Eating" not only because they are nutritious and taste great, but also because they are low in calories: one Apricot contains only 17 calories! (For more on the *Health Benefits of Apricots* and a complete analysis of their content of over 60 nutrients, see page 388.)

## varieties of apricots

Apricots are cousins of peaches with golden-orange velvety skin and flesh that is not too juicy but definitely smooth and sweet. Their flavor is almost musky, with a faint tartness that is more pronounced when they are dried. Their botanical name is *Prunus armeniaca*.

The varieties of Apricots, including Sungold, Harglow and Goldcat, differ in size and color but are all similar in taste. Some hybrid varieties include:

### PLUMCOT

This cross between a plum and an Apricot is more like a plum.

**APRIUM**

This cross between a plumcot and Apricot is more like an Apricot than a plum.

**PLUOT**

A cross between a plumcot and a plum.

**PEACHCOT**

This is a cross between a peach and an Apricot.

## the peak season

One of the first fruits of the summer, Apricots are in season in the United States from May through August. These are the months when their concentration of nutrients and flavor are highest, and their cost is at its lowest. In the winter, Apricots are imported from South America and New Zealand.

Dried and canned Apricots are available year-round. Dried Apricots have less vitamin C than fresh, but they provide a concentrated supply of iron, potassium, beta-carotene and fiber. An equal amount of dried Apricots (by weight) will also contain more calories than the fresh fruit. Canned fruits are

less nutritious, and if packed in light syrup, they will contain double the calories.

## biochemical considerations

Conventionally dried Apricots may be treated with sulfite preservatives. (For more on *Sulfites*, see page 729.)

### Don't Eat the Pit Kernels

The inner pits of Apricots contain amygdalin, a naturally occurring compound that breaks down into prussic acid, or hydrogen cyanide, when digested. Cases of fatal poisoning from eating Apricot pits have been reported.

## 3 steps for the best tasting and most nutritious apricots

Enjoying the best tasting Apricots with the most nutrients is simple if you just follow my 3 easy steps:

1. The Best Way to Select
2. The Best Way to Store
3. The Best Way to Prepare

# 1. the best way to select apricots

For the best tasting Apricots, look for ones that are fully ripe and have a rich aroma. Smelling Apricots is one of the best ways to determine whether they are ripe. They should also be soft with an even orange color. Vitamins and health-promoting phytonutrients, many of which act as powerful antioxidants, are at their peak when Apricots are ripe; therefore, by selecting ripe Apricots you will also be enjoying Apricots with the highest nutritional value. As with all fruits, I recommend selecting organic varieties whenever possible. (For more on *Organic Foods*, see page 113.)

Avoid Apricots that are pale and yellow, an indication they have not been tree-ripened and therefore will not have much flavor. I have found that Apricots that still have a greenish tinge or are too firm have been picked too early and will never

ripen. They will just get softer (not juicier) and rot. Also avoid overripe Apricots that are soft and mushy since they will have lost much of their nutritional value. Overripe Apricots that have turned brown should not be eaten as the brown color is an indication of oxidation and the formation of harmful free-radicals.

### How Do You Know Which Apricots are Ready to Eat?

If Apricots have a rich aroma, a deep orange color and they yield to gentle pressure, they are ready to eat. They taste best at room temperature. If they are hard but have an orange color, you can ripen them (see next section).

# 2. the best way to store apricots

Proper storage is an important step in keeping Apricots fresh and preserving their nutrients, texture and unique flavor.

### Fresh Ripe Apricots Can Last for Up to 3 Days When Properly Stored and Refrigerated

Apricots continue to respire even after they have been har-

vested. The faster they respire, the more the Apricots interact with air to produce carbon dioxide. The more carbon dioxide produced, the more quickly they will spoil. Apricots kept at a room temperature of approximately 68°F (20°C) give off carbon dioxide at a rate of 40 mg per kilogram every hour. (For a *Comparison of Respiration Rates* for different fruits, see page 341.) Refrigeration helps slow the respiration rate of ripe Apricots, retain their vitamin content and increase their storage life.

Keep as many ripe Apricots at room temperature as you will be able to consume in a day or two. Store the rest in the refrigerator. While Apricots that are stored properly will remain fresh for up to 3 days, if they are not stored properly, they will only last about 1–2 days.

## How to Ripen Apricots

Apricots will become sweet and juicy at home if they have not been picked too green. Apricots that have been picked green or even have a slight tinge of green will not ripen. Unripe Apricots are hard and have no flavor.

Apricots that are orange, but still hard, will get softer and juicier. Don't refrigerate Apricots until they are ripe; they will not ripen in the refrigerator. Place Apricots on a flat surface with space between the fruit to ripen them at room temperature. It is best to turn them occasionally so that they will ripen evenly. Once they yield to gentle pressure, they are ripe and ready to eat. If you will not be consuming the Apricots immediately after they have ripened, place them in the refrigerator. Unlike tree-ripened Apricots, ones you have ripened this way will remain fresh for only 1 to 2 days.

Another very natural way to ripen Apricots is to place them in a paper bag for 2 to 3 days. The paper bag traps the ethylene gas produced by the Apricots. The ethylene gas helps the Apricots to ripen more quickly, while the paper bag allows for healthy oxygen exchange through the bag. Keep the paper bag in a dark cool place as excessive heat will cause the Apricots to rot rather than ripen.

Avoid storing Apricots in sealed plastic bags or restricted spaces where they touch each other. The combination of limited oxygen exchange and the excessive amounts of ethylene gas produced under these conditions will cause them to rot.

## How to Speed Up the Ripening of Apricots

Adding a banana, apple or avocado to the bag with the Apricots will increase the amount of ethylene gas trapped in the bag. The increased amount of gas will hasten the ripening process.

## Is It Best to Refrigerate Apricots After Ripening?

Yes, they will keep in the refrigerator for 1 to 2 days after ripening.

## Handle with Care

Apricots are a delicate fruit and bruise easily, so handle them with care.

# 3. the best way to prepare apricots

Properly preparing Apricots helps ensure that they will have the best flavor and retain the greatest number of nutrients.

## Peeling and Slicing Apricots

Peeling or slicing fresh Apricots tears their cell walls, which releases an enzyme that is easily oxidized, turning the cut portion of the Apricot brown when it is exposed to the air. You can slow down this browning process by dipping peeled or sliced Apricots into a mixture of 2 cups of water and 2 TBS of fresh lemon juice. Dipping Apricots into the lemon and water solution is unnecessary if the slices are being added to a fruit salad that contains any type of citrus fruit, as the juices from these fruits will provide the same protection against browning.

## No Bake Recipes

I have discovered that Apricots retain their maximum amount of nutrients and their best taste when they are fresh and not prepared in a cooked recipe. That is because their nutrients—including vitamins, antioxidants and enzymes— are unable to withstand the temperature (350°F/175°C)

used in baking. So that you can get the most enjoyment and benefit from fruit, I created quick and easy recipes, which require no cooking. I call them "No Bake Recipes."

Here is a question that I received from a reader of the whfoods.org website about Apricots:

**Q** *What can you tell me about the vitamin B17 found in Apricots?*

**A** Vitamin B17 is also known as laetrile as well as amygdalin. It is found in the kernels of Apricots (as well as in lesser amounts in the pits/kernels of other stone fruit). It is composed of two sugar molecules, a benzaldehyde molecule and a cyanide molecule. Vitamin B17 gained its reputation as an alternative cancer treatment, although there is currently inadequate clinical data to support this claim; additionally, concerns have been raised about the consumption of Apricot kernels since they contain cyanogenic compounds (compounds that may be metabolized into cyanide). For these reasons, while I enjoy eating delicious Apricots I don't eat the kernels.

STEP-BY-STEP
## No Bake Recipes

# 5-Minute Apricot Fruit Cup

*The taste of oranges and Apricots is a great combination!*

**4 Apricots
4 TBS fresh orange juice
1 tsp orange zest\*
2 TBS sliced almonds**

1. Cut Apricots in half, then in half twice more, so that Apricots are sliced into eighths.
2. Mix Apricots, orange juice and orange zest.
3. Top with sliced almonds.

**SERVES 2**

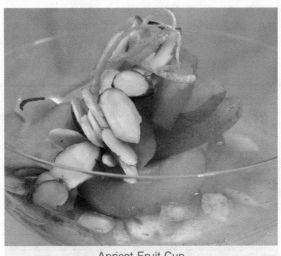

Apricot Fruit Cup

## Variations...

- Top Apricots with raspberry sauce (see pg 351) instead of orange juice.
- Use walnuts instead of Almonds.

\* Use an organic orange, if possible, to avoid wax coating.

# 10-Minute Apricot Bars

*Sweet fruit bars for a nutritious treat!*

**1 cup chopped dried Apricots
1/2 cup cream honey
1/2 cup almond butter**

**1¹/2 tsp almond extract
1/2 cup cinnamon granola
1/2 cup chopped almonds**

1. In a mixing bowl, blend honey, almond butter and almond extract with a spoon.
2. Mix together almond butter mixture, granola, almonds and Apricots. You can start mixing with a spoon, but it will require kneading with your hands to fully combine the ingredients.
3. Press into a loaf pan with slightly damp hands. Refrigerate for at least 1 hour.

4. Slice into 1-inch bars.

**MAKES 8 BARS**

**Preparation Hints:**

- If Apricots are hard, soak for 1 hour in warm water. They should still be firm. Drain well and pat dry with paper towels.
- Stir the almond butter in the jar before measuring.
- Cutting the Apricots with kitchen scissors is quicker, neater and requires no cutting board.

## Variations...

- Add 1/4 cup of chopped dark chocolate. Or melt the chocolate and dip 10-Minute Apricot bars half way into the melted chocolate. Refrigerate.
- Add grated coconut to the mixture.

- Make the recipe with peanut butter and chopped peanuts. Substitute vanilla for the almond extract.
- Try with different flavors of granola.
- Use walnuts instead of almonds.

Please write (address on back cover flap) or e-mail me at info@whfoods.org with your personal ideas for preparing Apricots, and I will share them with others through our website at www.whfoods.org.

## 5 QUICK SERVING IDEAS for APRICOTS:

1. Top Apricots with Quick Lemon Sauce (see page 431).
2. Add sliced Apricots to cereal.
3. Slice and add to yogurt.
4. Add fresh Apricots to fruit cups.
5. Apricots make a great addition to fruit salads and tossed green salads.

# health benefits of apricots

## Promote Optimal Antioxidant Status

Apricots are an excellent source of vitamin A, notably through their high concentration of carotenoid phytonutrients, including beta-carotene and beta-cryptoxanthin. Both of these carotenoids have been receiving attention for their antioxidant activity as well as for their anticancer and anti-aging potentials. Beta-carotene is also important for promoting healthy immune function as well as helping cells to communicate with each other.

Apricots also contain numerous flavonoid phytonutrients that have antioxidant activity. These include catechins (like those that give green tea many of its healthful properties) and quercetin. In addition, Apricots are a very good source of vitamin C. This antioxidant powerhouse helps to quench free-radicals in aqueous environments both inside and outside of the cell. Inside the cell, it plays an important role in protecting DNA, the cornerstone of our genetic material.

## Promote Vision Health

Apricots may help to protect eye health since they are a concentrated source of vitamin A, which can protect the lens of the eye from free-radical damage. This damage can lead to cataracts or macular degeneration since it inhibits proper blood supply to the eye. Researchers have found that women with the highest vitamin A intake have a 40% reduced risk of developing cataracts. Another recent study found that eating 3 or more servings of fruit per day reduced risk of developing macular degeneration.

Another way that vitamin A promotes vision health is through its participation in the synthesis of rhodopsin, a photopigment found in the eye. Rhodopsin plays a fundamental role in the adaptation of the eye to low-light conditions and night vision.

## Promote Digestive Health

Apricots are a good source of fiber. Eating three of these small fruits will give you about 10% of the Daily Value for this important nutrient. Dietary fiber has many health benefits. It helps to promote intestinal regularity and is suggested to help prevent colon cancer. Fiber may also benefit heart health since it helps to keep cholesterol levels balanced.

## Additional Health-Promoting Benefits of Apricots

Apricots are also a concentrated source of other nutrients providing additional health-promoting benefits. These nutrients include heart-healthy potassium and sleep-promoting tryptophan. Since each Apricot contains only 17 calories, it is an ideal food for healthy weight control.

### Nutritional Analysis of 1 fresh Apricot:

| NUTRIENT | AMOUNT | % DAILY VALUE | NUTRIENT | AMOUNT | % DAILY VALUE |
|---|---|---|---|---|---|
| Calories | 16.80 | | Pantothenic Acid | 0.08 mg | 0.80 |
| Calories from Fat | 1.23 | | | | |
| Calories from Saturated Fat | 0.09 | | **Minerals** | | |
| Protein | 0.49 g | | Boron | — mcg | |
| Carbohydrates | 3.89 g | | Calcium | 4.90 mg | 0.49 |
| Dietary Fiber | 0.84 g | 3.36 | Chloride | 1.05 mg | |
| Soluble Fiber | 0.47 g | | Chromium | — mcg | — |
| Insoluble Fiber | 0.37 g | | Copper | 0.03 mg | 1.50 |
| Sugar – Total | 3.05 g | | Fluoride | — mg | — |
| Monosaccharides | 0.81 g | | Iodine | — mcg | — |
| Disaccharides | 2.17 g | | Iron | 0.19 mg | 1.06 |
| Other Carbs | 0.01 g | | Magnesium | 2.80 mg | 0.70 |
| Fat – Total | 0.14 g | | Manganese | 0.03 mg | 1.50 |
| Saturated Fat | 0.01 g | | Molybdenum | — mcg | — |
| Mono Fat | 0.06 g | | Phosphorus | 6.65 mg | 0.67 |
| Poly Fat | 0.03 g | | Potassium | 103.60 mg | |
| Omega-3 Fatty Acids | 0.00 g | 0.00 | Selenium | 0.14 mcg | 0.20 |
| Omega-6 Fatty Acids | 0.03 g | | Sodium | 0.35 mg | |
| Trans Fatty Acids | 0.00 g | | Zinc | 0.09 mg | 0.60 |
| Cholesterol | 0.00 mg | | | | |
| Water | 30.22 g | | **Amino Acids** | | |
| Ash | 0.26 g | | Alanine | 0.02 g | |
| | | | Arginine | 0.02 g | |
| **Vitamins** | | | Aspartate | 0.11 g | |
| Vitamin A IU | 914.20 IU | 18.28 | Cystine | 0.00 g | 0.00 |
| Vitamin A RE | 91.35 RE | | Glutamate | 0.05 g | |
| A - Carotenoid | 91.35 RE | 1.22 | Glycine | 0.01 g | |
| A - Retinol | 0.00 RE | | Histidine | 0.01 g | 0.78 |
| B1 Thiamin | 0.01 mg | 0.67 | Isoleucine | 0.01 g | 0.87 |
| B2 Riboflavin | 0.01 mg | 0.59 | Leucine | 0.03 g | 1.19 |
| B3 Niacin | 0.21 mg | 1.05 | Lysine | 0.03 g | 1.28 |
| Niacin Equiv | 0.30 mg | | Methionine | 0.00 g | 0.00 |
| Vitamin B6 | 0.02 mg | 1.00 | Phenylalanine | 0.02 g | 1.68 |
| Vitamin B12 | 0.00 mcg | 0.00 | Proline | 0.04 g | |
| Biotin | — mcg | — | Serine | 0.03 g | |
| Vitamin C | 3.50 mg | 5.83 | Threonine | 0.02 g | 1.61 |
| Vitamin D IU | 0.00 IU | 0.00 | Tryptophan | 0.01 g | 3.13 |
| Vitamin D mcg | 0.00 mcg | | Tyrosine | 0.01 g | 1.03 |
| Vitamin E Alpha Equiv | 0.31 mg | 1.55 | Valine | 0.02 g | 1.36 |
| Vitamin E IU | 0.46 IU | | | | |
| Vitamin E mg | 0.31 mg | | | | |
| Folate | 3.01 mcg | 0.75 | | | |
| Vitamin K | 1.15 mcg | 1.44 | | | |

(Note: "–" indicates data is unavailable. For more information, please see page 806.)

# Q&A

## HOW CAN THE WORLD'S HEALTHIEST FOODS BENEFIT MY CHILDREN?

The World's Healthiest Foods feature numerous benefits that can nourish your children. These healthy foods provide an abundant supply of essential nutrients; when these healthy foods comprise the bulk of children's diets, it's easier for them to maintain a healthy weight and minimize their exposure to potentially harmful chemicals and additives.

## THE WORLD'S HEALTHIEST FOODS ARE PACKED WITH NUTRIENTS

Healthy foods provide a wealth of important nutrients vital to your child's well-being including:

### Vitamins and Minerals

Many children in the United States consume a diet that does not meet the RDA for most vitamins and minerals. For example, of children aged nine and under, only 71% meet the daily requirement for vitamin A. Often called the anti-infection vitamin since it is protects the integrity of the skin and all mucosal surfaces, vitamin A is also necessary for a healthy complexion, good eye-sight, bone development, growth and sexual develop-ment. The data for vitamin E, the body's primary antioxidant defender of our cells' membranes, is even more striking. Only 32% of American children meet the daily requirement for vitamin E. Minerals are also compromised in many children; for example, only 35% of our children receive the daily requirement of zinc, a critical mineral for good immune function, and 47% of children fall below the RDA for daily intake of calcium, a must-have for growing bones and healthy teeth. These vitamin and mineral deficiencies reflect the fact that most children do not consume the minimum recommendation of five servings of fruits and vegetables per day.

Fruits, vegetables, whole grains, legumes, nuts and seeds—foods that comprise a majority of the World's Healthiest Foods—are concentrated sources of vitamins and minerals. On the other hand, the majority of vitamins and minerals is removed from processed foods. Even when key vitamins and minerals are added back—and often the vitamins added back are synthetic rather than the natural forms—processed foods still contain a limited number of vitamins and minerals, not the full complement found in the World's Healthiest Foods.

### Dietary Fiber

It is estimated that between 55-90% of all children do not consume the recommended amount of dietary fiber.

Intake of dietary fiber is very important for children's health. Fiber is necessary to keep their digestion regular and reduce the incidence of constipation, maintain the health of their large intestines and increase the feeling of fullness they experience from eating, thus preventing overeating and excess weight gain. This is especially important in today's world as we are experiencing an explosion in the rate of childhood obesity. Good dietary sources of fiber include fruits (including their skin), vegetables, whole grains, nuts, seeds and legumes.

### Omega-3 Fatty Acids

Children (and adults) consuming the standard American diet receive a negligible amount of omega-3 essential fatty acids, making omega-3 deficiency the most widespread nutrient deficiency in the U.S. In addition, the typical American diet is quite high in omega-6 fats, which, when excessive, further promote functional deficiency of these critical omega-3s.

Omega-3 essential fatty acids provide a variety of important health benefits for children. Since they comprise a significant portion of the lipids in the brain, deficiencies of omega-3s in children are suggested to be linked to cognitive and psychosocial problems such as attention-deficit-hyperactivity disorder (ADHD), motor skill dysfunction, depression and, possibly, dyslexia. In addition, since these fatty acids have anti-inflammatory properties, foods rich in these "good fats" can help to reduce the incidence of allergen-induced asthma and dermatitis. Good dietary sources of omega-3 fats include wild-caught, cold-water fish, such as salmon, sardines, tuna and halibut; flaxseeds; and nuts, especially walnuts.

### The Benefits of Organically Grown Foods

One of the most important benefits organically grown foods provide for the health of our children lies in what they do not contain—the array of agricultural chemicals used in conventional methods of growing foods. Many of the foods that comprise a substantial portion of the diets of children, especially our youngest ones, are those that have been found to have the highest levels of pesticide residues. Reports by the government and some non-profit associations indicate that many children may be exposed to pesticides through their food at levels that surpass safe limits.

Pesticides in foods are of special concern for children for a variety of reasons. Since children have lower body weights than adults, even a small amount of these toxic chemicals can have a detrimental effect in their systems. Some of these pesticides have neurotoxic properties and are thought to cause damage to the developing brain and central nervous system. In addition, some researchers caution that the ill effects of pesticides may be more pronounced during times of growth and development.

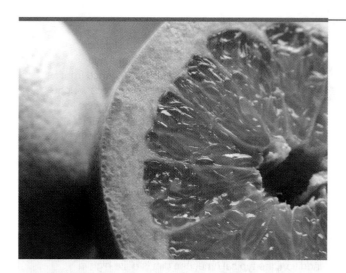

# grapefruit

## highlights

| | |
|---|---|
| AVAILABILITY: | Year-round |
| REFRIGERATE: | Yes |
| SHELF LIFE: | 10 days refrigerated |
| PREPARATION: | Minimal |
| BEST WAY TO ENJOY: | Enjoy them raw |

## nutrient-richness chart

Total Nutrient-Richness: **8**          GI: **35**

One-half (123 grams) fresh pink Grapefruit contains 37 calories

| NUTRIENT | AMOUNT | %DV | DENSITY | QUALITY |
|---|---|---|---|---|
| Vitamin C | 46.9 mg | 78.1 | 38.1 | excellent |
| Dietary Fiber | 1.7 g | 6.8 | 3.3 | good |
| Vitamin A | 318.6 IU | 6.4 | 3.1 | good |
| Potassium | 158.7 mg | 4.5 | 2.2 | good |
| Folate | 15.0 mcg | 3.8 | 1.8 | good |
| B5 Pantothenic Acid | 0.4 mg | 3.5 | 1.7 | good |

**CAROTENOIDS:**

| | |
|---|---|
| Alpha-Carotene | 5.1 mcg |
| Beta-Carotene | 706.6 mcg |
| Beta-Cryptoxanthin | 7.7 mcg |
| Lutein+Zeaxanthin | 7.7 mcg |
| Lycopene | 1452.8 mcg |

Daily values for these nutrients have not yet been established.

For more on "Total Nutrient-Richness," "%DV," "Density," and The World's Healthiest Foods "Quality" Rating System, see page 805.

For more on GI, see page 342.

The name Grapefruit reflects the way they grow in clusters, like Grapes, on the tree. This slightly larger cousin of the orange has a relatively short history dating back only to 18th century Barbados, with its Latin name *Citrus paradisi* reflecting its paradise-like origins. Many botanists believe the Grapefruit was actually the result of natural cross breeding between the orange and the pomelo, a citrus fruit that was brought from Indonesia to Barbados in the 17th century. Grapefruit are juicy, tart and tangy with an underlying sweetness that makes them a breakfast favorite. Both as the whole fruit and as juice, Grapefruit are a tasty addition to many recipes and a great between-meal snack.

## why grapefruit should be part of your healthiest way of eating

Pink Grapefruit contain lycopene, a carotenoid phytonutrient, that is responsible for its pink coloration and also provides protection against harmful free-radical activity. Grapefruit are also an excellent source of vitamin C and a good source of vitamin A, two vitamins that support the immune system and provide additional powerful antioxidant protection. Grapefruit are an ideal food to add to your "Healthiest Way of Eating" not only because they are nutritious and taste great, but also because they are low in calories: one-half Grapefruit contains only 37 calories! (For more on the *Health Benefits of Grapefruit* and a complete analysis of its content of over 60 nutrients, see page 394.)

## varieties of grapefruit

Grapefruit are designated as white, pink or ruby reflecting the color of their flesh rather than the color of their skin, which is usually yellow or pinkish-yellow. They range in size from four to six inches in diameter. Grapefruit are increasing in popularity with the development of sweeter, seedless varieties that are now easy to find in local markets.

### DUNCAN

A large Grapefruit with yellow skin that is primarily used to make juice.

### LAVENDER GEM

A Grapefruit-tangelo hybrid with a lemon-yellow rind or a pink blush. Its pinkish-blue flesh has a delicate flavor.

### MARSH SEEDLESS

The White Marsh is the most popular variety of Grapefruit.

There is also a pink and ruby red variety that is sweeter than the white variety.

Three varieties that resulted from a cross between a Grapefruit and a pomelo are: Melogold, Oroblanco and Sweeties.

White Grapefruit have negligible amounts of vitamin A, whereas the pink and red varieties contain more vitamin A and beta-carotene:

### COMPARISON BETWEEN PINK AND WHITE GRAPEFRUIT (1/2 FRUIT)

|  | VITAMIN A | DAILY VALUE | BETA-CAROTENE* |
|---|---|---|---|
| PINK AND RED GRAPEFRUIT | 319 IU | 6% | 192 mcg |
| WHITE GRAPEFRUIT | 12 IU | 1% | 7 mcg |

*There are currently no Daily Values for beta-carotene.

## the peak season

Although Grapefruit are available throughout the year, the peak of their season runs from winter through early spring. These are the months when their concentration of nutrients and flavor are highest, and their cost is at its lowest.

## biochemical considerations

### Drug Interactions

Taking certain pharmaceutical drugs with Grapefruit juice can make the drugs more bioavailable, so they have more powerful effects on the body. This is because compounds such as naringenin in Grapefruit juice may slow the normal detoxification and metabolic processes in the intestines and liver, hindering the breakdown of certain drugs.

Grapefruit interacts with drugs such as the immunosuppressant cyclosporine and calcium channel blocker drugs, such as felodipine, nifedipine and verapamil. Drugs enhanced by Grapefruit and Grapefruit juice include: the antihistamine, terfenadine; the hormone, estradiol; and the antiviral agent, saquinavir. Check with your healthcare practitioner if you are taking pharmaceutical drugs with Grapefruit or Grapefruit juice.

## 3 steps for the best tasting and most nutritious grapefruit

Enjoying the best tasting Grapefruit with the most nutrients is simple if you just follow my 3 easy steps:
1. The Best Way to Select
2. The Best Way to Store
3. The Best Way to Prepare

# 1. the best way to select grapefruit

You can select the best tasting Grapefruit by looking for ones that are heavy with smooth thin skin. I have found that these will have the best taste and most juice. Ripe Grapefruit are heavy and firm, yet slightly springy when gentle pressure is applied. They should have a sweet aroma when left at room temperature. Grapefruit do not ripen after they have been picked; however, most are picked after they have ripened. Selecting ripe Grapefruit will ensure that you are also enjoying Grapefruit with the highest nutritional value. I have found that Grapefruit don't have to be perfect in color to be good. Skin discoloration, scratches or scales may affect the appearance of Grapefruit but do not affect the taste. As with all fruits, I recommend selecting organically grown Grapefruit whenever possible. (For more on *Organic Foods*, see page 113.)

Avoid Grapefruit that show signs of decay or overly soft spots at the stem end of the fruit. These are usually signs that they will be less flavorful and more bitter than a good quality Grapefruit. Avoid fruit with overly rough or wrinkled skin, which also tends to be thick.

### How Do You Know Which Grapefruit is Ready to Eat?

If the Grapefruit is heavy and firm, but slightly springy when gentle pressure is applied, it is ready to eat.

---

**HEALTH BENEFITS OF GRAPEFRUIT PEELS**

The colored part of the Grapefruit rind contains d-limonene, a flavonoid phytonutrient that acts as a powerful antioxidant and helps prevent oxidative damage to cell structures and DNA. The white pithy portion under the skin also contains flavonoids that help lower LDL ("bad") cholesterol. If you ar going to enjoy Grapefruit rind, I'd suggest using organically grown Grapefruit, if possible.

# 2. the best way to store grapefruit

Proper storage is an important step in keeping Grapefruit fresh and preserving their nutrients, texture and unique flavor.

### Fresh Ripe Grapefruit Can Last for Up to 10 Days When Properly Stored and Refrigerated

Grapefruit continue to respire even after they have been harvested. The faster they respire, the more the Grapefruit interact with air to produce carbon dioxide. The more carbon dioxide produced, the more quickly they will spoil. Grapefruit kept at a room temperature of approximately 68°F (20°C) give off carbon dioxide at a rate of 10 mg per kilogram every hour. (For a *Comparison of Respiration Rates* for different fruits, see page 341.) Refrigeration helps slow the respiration rate of ripe Grapefruit, retain their vitamin content and increase their storage life.

Since Grapefruit are juicier when they are slightly warm, store them at room temperature where they will keep for approximately 5 days. If you have more Grapefruit than you can enjoy within a week, it is best to place them in the refrigerator where they will last for about 10 days.

Avoid storing Grapefruit in sealed plastic bags or restricted spaces where they are in too close proximity to each other. Limited oxygen exchange and excessive amounts of ethylene gas naturally produced by the Grapefruit will cause them to rot.

# 3. the best way to prepare grapefruit

Properly preparing Grapefruit helps ensure that they will have the best flavor and retain the greatest number of nutrients.

### Cleaning Grapefruit

Rinse Grapefruit under cold running water before eating.

### Cutting and Peeling Grapefruit

Grapefruit are usually eaten fresh by slicing the fruit horizontally and scooping out sections of the halves with a spoon. To separate the flesh from the membrane, you can first cut it with a sharp knife, a special Grapefruit knife with a curved blade or a serrated Grapefruit spoon.

Grapefruit can also be eaten like oranges. You can either peel them by hand or with a knife. If choosing the latter method, start at the top, make a vertical incision that runs downward and then back up to the top on the other side, and then repeat so that there will be four sections of similar size. Be careful to just cut through skin and not into the membrane. The skin can then be peeled back with your hands or with the knife. You can then separate the sections and enjoy them the same way you would an orange.

### No Bake Recipes

I have discovered that Grapefruit retain their maximum amount of nutrients and their best taste when they are f resh and not prepared in a cooked recipe. That is because their nutrients—including vitamins, antioxidants and enzymes—are unable to withstand the temperature (350°F/175°C) used in baking. So that you can get the most enjoyment and benefit from fruit, I created quick and easy recipes, which require no cooking. I call them "No Bake Recipes."

Here is a question that I received from a reader of the <u>whfoods.org</u> website about Grapefruit:

**Q** *I heard you should not eat Grapefruit if you are taking certain kinds of medication. Is that true?*

**A** Yes, grapefruit can have interactions with certain medications. That is because one of its flavonoids, naringenin, affects enzymes in the liver and large intestines that detoxify drugs and therefore affects the rate at which these drugs are metabolized in the body. These drugs include the immunosuppressent cyclosporine and calcium channel blocker drugs, such as felodipine, nifedipine and verapamil. Other drugs enhanced by grapefruit juice are the antihistamine terfenadine, the hormone estradiol and the antiviral agent saquinavir.

Research also indicates that individuals taking statin drugs should avoid grapefruit. Grapefruit increases the amount of statin drug that reaches the general circulation in two ways. First, Grapefruit's naringenin inactivates an enzyme (cytochrome P450 3A4) in the small intestine that metabolizes statin drugs. Secondly, Grapefruit also inhibits P-glycoprotein, a carrier molecule produced in the intestinal wall that would normally transport the statin drug back to the gut.

STEP-BY-STEP
## No Bake Recipes

# Grapefruit Sunrise

*Grapefruit, oranges and strawberries are a great combination for this refreshing, satisfying treat!*

Juice of 2 Grapefruit
Juice of 4 oranges
1 cup fresh or frozen strawberries
2 tsp honey

Sections from 1 Grapefruit
1/2 cup sliced strawberries

1. Place Grapefruit juice, orange juice, 1 cup strawberries and honey in blender, and blend until smooth.
2. Strain into 2 chilled glasses.
3. Top with Grapefruit sections and strawberries.

**Preparation Hint:** Chill the fruit first for cold juice or

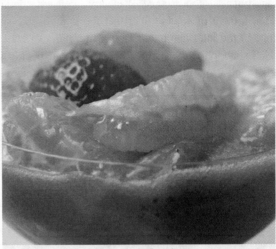
Grapefruit Sunrise

add some ice cubes while blending. Try adding your favorite protein powder to make a light breakfast or snack.

**SERVES 2**

# Grapefruit Arugula Salad

*The flavors of this fresh tasting Grapefruit salad complement each other nicely and are a wonderful addition to many meals.*

1 pink Grapefruit
1 large bunch arugula (about 4 cups)
1 bunch watercress (about 2 cups)
4 TBS coarsely chopped walnuts

DRESSING:
2 TBS fresh lemon juice
2 tsp honey
2 tsp prepared Dijon mustard
3 TBS extra virgin olive oil
Sea salt and pepper to taste

1. Peel Grapefruit and cut out each section, removing the membrane covering.
2. Prepare arugula by tearing into pieces, washing and drying. Remove stems of watercress, then wash it and dry along with the arugula. A salad spinner is the best way of doing this.
3. Mix together dressing ingredients, toss with salad greens and Grapefruit sections, and top with chopped walnuts.

**Preparation Hint:** Use young, tender arugula for this salad as older leaves can be too bitter for some people.

**SERVES 4**

Please write (address on back cover flap) or e-mail me at info@whfoods.org with your personal ideas for preparing Grapefruit, and I will share them with others through our website at www.whfoods.org.

## 4 QUICK SERVING IDEAS for GRAPEFRUIT:

1. Grapefruit sections add a tangy spark to green salads.
2. **Grapefruit Shrimp Salad:** Combine chopped Grapefruit pieces, cooked shrimp and avocados. Serve on a bed of romaine lettuce for a salad with a tropical flair.
3. **Grapefruit Salsa:** Combine diced Grapefruit with cilantro and chili peppers to make a unique salsa.
4. **Grapefruit Granita:** Freeze Grapefruit juice and honey to taste in ice cube trays and then purée in a food processor to make a simple and refreshing granita.

# health benefits of grapefruit

## Promotes Heart Health

Grapefruit is a good source of dietary fiber and contains pectin, a form of soluble fiber that forms a gel-like substance in the intestinal tract that can trap fats like cholesterol. In laboratory animal studies, Grapefruit pectin has been found to inhibit the development of atherosclerosis.

### Nutritional Analysis of 1/2 fresh Pink Grapefruit:

| NUTRIENT | AMOUNT | % DAILY VALUE | NUTRIENT | AMOUNT | % DAILY VALUE |
|---|---|---|---|---|---|
| Calories | 36.90 | | Pantothenic Acid | 0.35 mg | 3.50 |
| Calories from Fat | 1.11 | | | | |
| Calories from Saturated Fat | 0.15 | | **Minerals** | | |
| Protein | 0.68 g | | Boron | — mcg | |
| Carbohydrates | 9.45 g | | Calcium | 13.53 mg | 2.50 |
| Dietary Fiber | 1.69 g | 6.79 | Chloride | — mg | |
| Soluble Fiber | 1.05 g | | Chromium | — mcg | — |
| Insoluble Fiber | 0.64 g | | Copper | 0.05 mg | 2.50 |
| Sugar – Total | 7.76 g | | Fluoride | — mg | — |
| Monosaccharides | 3.08 g | | Iodine | — mcg | — |
| Disaccharides | 4.18 g | | Iron | 0.15 mg | 0.83 |
| Other Carbs | 0.00 g | | Magnesium | 9.84 mg | 2.46 |
| Fat – Total | 0.12 g | | Manganese | 0.01 mg | 0.50 |
| Saturated Fat | 0.02 g | | Molybdenum | — mcg | — |
| Mono Fat | 0.02 g | | Phosphorus | 11.07 mg | 1.11 |
| Poly Fat | 0.03 g | | Potassium | 158.67 mg | |
| Omega-3 Fatty Acids | 0.01 g | 0.40 | Selenium | 1.06 mcg | 1.51 |
| Omega-6 Fatty Acids | 0.02 g | | Sodium | 0.00 mg | |
| Trans Fatty Acids | 0.00 g | | Zinc | 0.09 mg | 0.60 |
| Cholesterol | 0.00 mg | | | | |
| Water | 112.40 g | | **Amino Acids** | | |
| Ash | 0.36 g | | Alanine | 0.02 g | |
| | | | Arginine | 0.05 g | |
| **Vitamins** | | | Aspartate | 0.13 g | |
| Vitamin A IU | 318.57 IU | 6.37 | Cystine | 0.00 g | 0.00 |
| Vitamin A RE | 31.98 RE | | Glutamate | 0.05 g | |
| A - Carotenoid | 31.98 RE | 0.43 | Glycine | 0.01 g | |
| A - Retinol | 0.00 RE | | Histidine | 0.01 g | 0.78 |
| B1 Thiamin | 0.04 mg | 2.67 | Isoleucine | 0.01 g | 0.87 |
| B2 Riboflavin | 0.02 mg | 1.18 | Leucine | 0.02 g | 0.79 |
| B3 Niacin | 0.23 mg | 1.15 | Lysine | 0.02 g | 0.85 |
| Niacin Equiv | 0.28 mg | | Methionine | 0.00 g | 0.00 |
| Vitamin B6 | 0.05 mg | 2.50 | Phenylalanine | 0.01 g | 0.84 |
| Vitamin B12 | 0.00 mcg | 0.00 | Proline | 0.06 g | |
| Biotin | 1.23 mcg | 0.41 | Serine | 0.03 g | |
| Vitamin C | 46.86 mg | 78.10 | Threonine | 0.01 g | 0.81 |
| Vitamin D IU | 0.00 IU | 0.00 | Tryptophan | 0.00 g | 0.00 |
| Vitamin D mcg | 0.00 mcg | | Tyrosine | 0.01 g | 1.03 |
| Vitamin E Alpha Equiv | 0.31 mg | 1.55 | Valine | 0.02 g | 1.36 |
| Vitamin E IU | 0.46 IU | | | | |
| Vitamin E mg | 0.32 mg | | (Note: "–" indicates data is unavailable. For more information, please see page 806.) | | |
| Folate | 15.01 mcg | 3.75 | | | |
| Vitamin K | — mcg | — | | | |

Animals fed a high cholesterol diet with added Grapefruit pectin had 24% narrowing of their arteries, while animals fed only the high-fat diet had 45% narrowing. Grapefruit is also a good source of the mineral potassium, which helps to regulate blood pressure. Additionally, red and pink Grapefruit contain lycopene, the powerful antioxidant carotenoid phytonutrient that has been found to inhibit free-radical damage to LDL cholesterol; body levels of lycopene (a reflection of dietary intake) have been associated with reduced risk of cardiovascular disease. The white pithy portion under the skin contains flavonoids that may help lower LDL cholesterol.

## Promotes Optimal Health

Pink Grapefruit is an excellent source of vitamin C and a good source of vitamin A (due to its concentration of pro-vitamin A beta-carotene). These nutrients help to support the immune system and protect cells from free-radical damage. Vitamin C-rich foods like Grapefruit may help reduce cold symptoms or severity of cold symptoms; over 20 scientific studies have supported that vitamin C is a cold-fighter.

Additionally, phytonutrients in Grapefruit called limonoids act as antioxidants and promote the formation of *glutathione-S-transferase*, a detoxifying enzyme. This enzyme sparks a reaction in the liver that helps to make toxic compounds more water-soluble for excretion from the body. The pulp of citrus fruits, such as Grapefruit, contain glucarates, compounds that may help to prevent breast cancer.

In humans, drinking three 6-ounce glasses of Grapefruit juice a day was shown to reduce the activity of an enzyme that activates cancer-causing chemicals found in tobacco smoke. In laboratory animals whose colons were injected with carcinogens, Grapefruit and its isolated active compounds (apigenin, hesperidin, limonin, naringin, naringenin, nobiletin) not only increased the suicide (apoptosis) of cancer cells, but also the production of normal colon cells.

## Promotes Energy Production

Grapefruit is a good source of pantothenic acid (vitamin B5), which plays an important role in the body's production of cellular energy.

## Additional Health-Promoting Benefit of Grapefruit

Since one-half Grapefruit contains only 37 calories, it is an ideal food for healthy weight control.

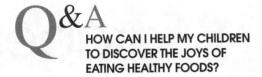

## Q&A

### HOW CAN I HELP MY CHILDREN TO DISCOVER THE JOYS OF EATING HEALTHY FOODS?

Understanding that a healthy foods diet can provide your children with good nutrition that will benefit their health is one thing. Getting them to eat and enjoy those foods is another. Here are some tips to help you inspire your children to eat healthy foods.

### Educate Your Children About the Benefits of the World's Healthiest Foods

We can probably all remember our parents telling us that eating healthy would help us to grow up big and strong, yet many parents did not tell us of the benefits we would experience while still being a child. Since kids are very "now-focused," explaining how eating healthy foods will help them feel good, look great, give them the kind of long-lasting energy that will make them stars in their school's sports program and help them to learn and think clearly so they can excel in the classroom, will motivate them.

Depending upon their age, explain to them the specific benefits they will notice and appreciate. For example, you could tell them how foods that contain fiber and complex carbohydrates will give them more energy for playing longer than foods made from refined carbohydrates and sugars, which, like firecrackers, quickly fizzle out after a brief burst of energy. Tell them how a complete spectrum of vitamins and minerals will increase their concentration and ability to learn and do well in their schoolwork. Talk to them about how omega-3 fatty acids not only support brain development, but are essential for clear skin and shiny hair and also help prevent or reduce itchy eyes, runny noses and other allergic reactions.

### Introduce Them to a New World's Healthiest Food Every Week

Most young children are fascinated by new things, and the colors, shapes, textures and tastes of different foods are no exception. And since foods have a rich history of tradition and heritage that kids can enjoy, learning about and eating new foods can be a lot of fun—and it's easy to do. There are lots of interesting facts about the World's Healthiest Foods in this book and on the whfoods.org website that children will find fascinating.

### Make Grocery Shopping Fun for Your Little Ones

Take your kids with you to the market and make it an educational and participatory experience for them. Explore the colorful produce department together. If you purchase food items from bulk bins, let your children help you scoop them into the bags. If they are old enough to read, play the "food label game" with them by having them read the labels, trying to determine by looking at the ingredients which foods are the most healthy.

### Visit a Local Farm, Explore a Farmer's Market or Talk to Your Greengrocer

Nature, living things and the process of how things work captivate children. By seeing where food comes from, how it is grown and meeting the people who work with the food, such as local farmers who grow the food or the produce manager at your local grocery who knows the farms in your area, your children will develop a real appreciation and more intimate relationship with the food they eat.

### Involve Your Children With Growing Foods Themselves

Children love to be productive and creative and accomplish something on their own. You can help them create their own mini-"farm" right at home by simply growing a pot or two of herbs or sprouting some seeds or grains. Once your children have experienced the miracle of a tender green shoot emerging from the soil you have watered together, they will understand through personal experience that food is a miraculous gift from the earth—not from a factory.

### Let Your Children "Help" You Cook

All children can participate in cooking (even toddlers can "help" with your assistance). Design their involvement depending upon their age. Small children can help measure and mix ingredients. Older children can cut and cook food and choose new recipes to try. Involving your children in the cooking process will award them with a sense of achievement, a pride in eating what they helped to prepare and cooking skills that they can rely on as adults. Make your kitchen the heart of your home, a warm and friendly place where healthy food prepared with love makes memories that will nourish your children throughout their lives. Remember, the more colorful the meal, the greater the range of phytonutrients it contains, so let your children be creative with colorful vegetables and fruits and help choose a vivid palette for your meals.

### Buy or Make Special Decorative Containers for School Meals and Snacks

Packing the foods your children take to school in bright and decorative containers can help them feel special and loved. Let them select containers they like at the store or decorate any of the new, inexpensive, reusable containers with their favorite stickers. A healthy meal is a present for your child's body; gift wrapping adds to the fun.

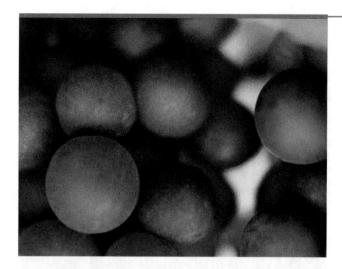

# grapes

## highlights

| | |
|---|---|
| AVAILABILITY: | Year-round |
| REFRIGERATE: | Yes |
| SHELF LIFE: | 5 days refrigerated |
| PREPARATION: | Minimal |
| BEST WAY TO ENJOY: | Enjoy them raw |

## nutrient-richness chart

Total Nutrient-Richness: **8**      GI: **64**

One cup (92 grams) of fresh Grapes contains 62 calories

| NUTRIENT | AMOUNT | %DV | DENSITY | QUALITY |
|---|---|---|---|---|
| Manganese | 0.7 mg | 33.0 | 9.6 | excellent |
| Vitamin C | 3.7 mg | 6.1 | 1.8 | good |
| B1 Thiamin | 0.2 mg | 5.3 | 1.6 | good |
| Potassium | 175.7 mg | 5.0 | 1.5 | good |
| B6 Pyridoxine | 0.1 mg | 5.0 | 1.5 | good |

| CAROTENOIDS: | | |
|---|---|---|
| Alpha-Carotene | 0.9 mcg | Daily values for these nutrients have not yet been established. |
| Beta-Carotene | 54.3 mcg | |
| Lutein+Zeaxanthin | 66.2 mcg | |

For more on "Total Nutrient-Richness," "%DV," "Density," and The World's Healthiest Foods "Quality" Rating System, see page 805.

For more on GI, see page 342.

Grapes were once considered to be the "food of the gods" and were closely associated with Dionysus, the Greek god of wine, agriculture and fertility. They are one of the oldest foods to be cultivated, dating as far back as biblical times. Fresh Grapes are the original high-energy food. Nature has conveniently packaged their natural sweetness so that they are easy to carry and easy to eat, making them a great between-meal snack or addition to any meal.

## why grapes should be part of your healthiest way of eating

Grapes (particularly black Grapes) contain quercetin and resveratrol, two phytonutrients that have been credited with providing an explanation to what has become known as the French Paradox: the interesting phenomenon that low rates of heart disease are present in France, a culture that has a diet high in fats. Increasing evidence suggests that the phytonutrients found in Grapes, Grape juice and red wine might be the key to their heart health. Grapes are also an excellent source of manganese, which facilitates protein and carbohydrate metabolism and activates the enzymes responsible for the utilization of key nutrients, such as the energy-producing B vitamins, biotin and thiamin. Grapes are an ideal food to add to your "Healthiest Way of Eating" not only because they are nutritious and taste great, but also because they are low in calories so are good for healthy weight control: one cup of Grapes contains only 62 calories! (For more on the *Health Benefits of Grapes* and a complete analysis of their content of over 60 nutrients, see page 400.)

## varieties of grapes

Grapes fall into three classifications: table Grapes, wine Grapes and raisin Grapes. As their names suggest, table Grapes are those that we enjoy raw in our favorite salads or desserts, while wine Grapes are used in viniculture to produce wine and raisin Grapes are used to make the dried fruit. Grapes are known botanically as *Vitis vinifera*.

While there are thousands of varieties of Grapes, only about 20 constitute the majority of table Grapes consumed; they differ in color (green, amber, red, blue-black and purple), size, taste and other characteristics.

Grapes are available in three main varieties:

### EUROPEAN GRAPES

These include Thompson (seedless and amber-green in color), Emperor (seeded and purple in color) and Champagne Black Corinth (tiny in size and purple in color). European varieties feature skins that adhere closely to their flesh.

**NORTH AMERICAN GRAPES**

These include Concord (large in size, blue-black in color), Delaware (pink-red in color with a tender skin) and Niagara (amber colored and less sweet than other varieties). A characteristic feature of North American varieties is that their skins slip easily away from their flesh.

**FRENCH HYBRIDS**

These include varieties that were developed from the *vinifera* Grapes after the majority of these Grape varietals were destroyed in Europe in the 19th century.

## the peak season

European Grape varieties are available throughout most of the year, while North American varieties are available only in September and October. These are the months when their concentration of nutrients and flavor are highest, and their cost is at its lowest.

## biochemical considerations

Grapes are a concentrated source of oxalates, which might be of concern to certain individuals. Imported Grapes are among the 12 foods on which pesticide residues have been most frequently found. Wine may contain sulfite preservatives. (For more on *Oxalates*, see page 725; *Pesticide Residues*, see page 726; and *Sulfites*, see page 729.)

## 3 steps for the best tasting and most nutritious grapes

Enjoying the best tasting Grapes with the most nutrients is simple if you just follow my 3 easy steps:

1. The Best Way to Select
2. The Best Way to Store
3. The Best Way to Prepare

# 1. the best way to select grapes

For the best tasting Grapes, look for ones that are fully ripe. Fully ripened Grapes are firm, plump and wrinkle-free. The stem should be firmly attached to the Grape, and the area around the attachment should have the same color as the rest of the Grape. It is best to taste them to determine their flavor and ripeness. Most Grapes are picked ripe; they will not ripen after they have been picked. Fully ripened Grapes are also highest in nutritional value because this is when the concentration of vitamins and health-promoting phytonutrients are at their peak. Since imported Grapes are one of the foods on which pesticide residues are most commonly found, I highly recommend selecting organically grown Grapes whenever possible. (For more on *Organic Foods*, see page 113.)

Avoid Grapes that are overripe or damaged. Overripe Grapes are shriveled and mushy; they will have lost much of their nutritional value.

### How Do You Know Which Grapes are Ready to Eat?

Green Grapes are ready to eat when they have a slightly yellowish hue. Red Grapes should be mostly red, while blue-black Grapes should have a deep color. All varieties should be plump, firm, free of wrinkles and firmly attached to the stem.

# 2. the best way to store grapes

Proper storage is an important step in keeping Grapes fresh and preserving their nutrients, texture and unique flavor.

### Fresh Ripe Grapes Can Last for Up to 5 Days When Properly Stored and Refrigerated

Grapes continue to respire even after they have been harvested. The faster they respire, the more the Grapes interact with air to produce carbon dioxide. The more carbon dioxide produced, the more quickly they will spoil. Grapes kept at a room temperature of approximately 68°F (20°C) give off carbon dioxide at a rate of 27 mg per kilogram every hour. (For a *Comparison of Respiration Rates* for differ-

ent fruits, see page 341.) Refrigeration helps slow the respiration rate of ripe Grapes, retain their vitamin content and increase their storage life.

Store Grapes in the refrigerator to reduce their respiration rate and increase their storage life. While Grapes that are stored properly will remain fresh for up to 5 days, if they are not stored properly they will only last about 2–3 days.

### Handle with Care

Grapes are a delicate fruit and bruise easily, so handle them with care.

# 3. the best way to prepare grapes

Properly preparing Grapes helps ensure that they will have the best flavor and retain the greatest number of nutrients.

## Cleaning Grapes

Grapes should be rinsed under cold running water right before consuming or using in a recipe. After rinsing, drain the Grapes in a colander or gently pat them dry. (For more on *Washing Fruit*, see page 341.)

## Peeling Grapes

Select American varieties of Grapes if you want to peel them because their skins come off more easily. You can blanch other varieties by dropping them in boiling water for a few seconds and then into a bowl of ice water to help loosen the skin from the flesh so that you can peel them more easily.

## Separating Grape Clusters

If you are not going to consume the whole bunch of Grapes at one time, use scissors to separate small clusters of Grapes from the stem instead of removing individual Grapes. This will prevent the stem from drying out and will keep the remaining Grapes fresher.

## No Bake Recipes

I have discovered that Grapes retain their maximum amount of nutrients and their best taste when they are fresh and not prepared in a cooked recipe. That is because their nutrients—including vitamins, antioxidants and enzymes—are unable to withstand the temperature (350°F/175°C) used in baking. So that you can get the most enjoyment and benefit from fruit, I created quick and easy recipes, which require no cooking. I call them "No Bake Recipes."

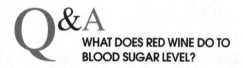

Q&A

**WHAT DOES RED WINE DO TO BLOOD SUGAR LEVEL?**

### Health Properties of Red Wine

Red wine contains health-supportive polyphenols, including resveratrol and other phytonutrients, called saponins. These phytonutrients, which are powerful antioxidants, appear to be heart protective and cancer preventive; they may even have anti-aging properties. Red wine also contains tannins that can help prevent blood cells from clumping together and causing a heart attack. Studies have also indicated that alcohol consumption in general helps raise the level of HDL (heart-protective cholesterol) and prevent the clumping of blood cells. In the Copenhagen City Heart Study, one to seven glasses of red wine per week were sufficient to provide some of these heart-protective benefits.

### Misinformation About Red Wine: blood sugar control

With more and more folks on the red wine bandwagon, I'm also starting to see some misinformation about red wine, including claims that red wine is helpful for blood sugar control. I don't think the research supports this conclusion. In fact, I think the research points in the opposite direction.

Some of the popular press writing points out that red wine is actually low in carbohydrates and sugar. They are correct. An 8-ounce glass of red wine only has 2–4 grams of carbohydrates, mostly in the form of sugar. An 8-ounce glass of grape juice has about 38 grams—all sugar. So it's true that a glass of wine is easier on your blood sugar than a glass of grape juice when it comes to the sugar and carbohydrate content.

However, the sugar content doesn't tell the whole story when it comes to blood sugar balance. The reason? Alcohol affects insulin production. Our bodies make less insulin when we drink alcohol-containing beverages, and so our ability to clear sugar from our blood decreases when we drink. It does appear that food consumption alongside of alcohol can lessen this effect, but it doesn't eliminate it entirely. The bottom line? Alcohol from red wine decreases, in varying degrees, our ability to keep blood sugar stable.

Consumption of healthy foods—meaning whole natural foods with some protein and fiber—appears to lessen the impact of alcohol on insulin production. For this reason, having your red wine alongside of a meal with some tuna or salmon, for example, would be a plus. If you overdo it on the red wine, you will definitely increase the likelihood of insufficient insulin production.

If you keep your red wine to some moderate level, you'll minimize that risk, while still preserving the possible benefits of the red wine polyphenols and saponins. As with everything, moderation is the key. Excessive amounts of any type of alcohol are harmful to your liver and wines often contain sulfites, additives which can be detrimental to your health.

STEP-BY-STEP
## No Bake Recipes

### 5-Minute Grapes in Honey-Lemon Sauce

*A quick flavorful way to serve Grapes for dessert.*

1/2 cup green Grapes
1/2 cup red Grapes
2 tsp lemon juice
1 tsp lemon zest*
2 TBS honey

1. Remove Grapes from stem and place in two dessert dishes.
2. Mix honey with lemon juice and lemon zest in a small bowl.
3. Spoon over the Grapes and serve.

**SERVES 2**

\* Use an organic lemon, if possible, to avoid wax coating.

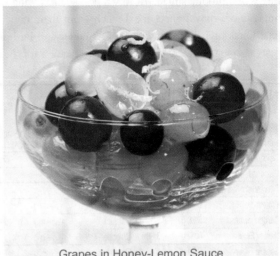

Grapes in Honey-Lemon Sauce

### 10-Minute Grape Arugula Salad

*This easy salad recipe makes a wonderful accompaniment to almost any meal.*

1 cup seedless green Grapes
1 bunch arugula (4 cups)
1/2 cup thinly sliced fresh fennel
3 TBS extra virgin olive oil
1 TBS fresh lemon juice
Sea salt and pepper to taste
3 oz crumbled gorgonzola cheese

1. Wash and dry Grapes, arugula and fennel to prevent the dressing from becoming diluted. Dry in a salad spinner, if you have one, or pat dry with paper towels.
2. Combine olive oil, lemon juice, and salt and pepper to taste.
3. Arrange Grapes, arugula and fennel on a plate with cheese. Drizzle with dressing.

**Preparation Hint:** Use young, tender arugula for this salad. Older leaves can be too bitter for some people.

**SERVES 4**

Please write (address on back cover flap) or e-mail me at info@whfoods.org with your personal ideas for preparing Grapes, and I will share them with others through our website at www.whfoods.org.

### 7 QUICK SERVING IDEAS for GRAPES:

1. For a healthy "sundae," serve a bowl of Grapes topped with yogurt and granola.
2. Grapes add flavor, texture and color to green or fruit salads.
3. Include Grapes in a curry recipe for a delicious fruity punch.
4. Serve a simple snack of Grapes and low-fat cheese.
5. **Grapes with Yogurt Sauce:** Combine 1 TBS honey, 1/2 tsp chopped mint, 1/4 tsp lemon zest and 1 cup yogurt. Spoon over green Grapes.
6. **Curried Waldorf Salad with Grapes:** Mix together 1 cup Grapes, 1 medium diced apple, 3 stalks diced celery, 1 medium diced avocado and 1 TBS chopped walnuts. In a small bowl combine 1 TBS cider vinegar, 2 tsp cream honey, 3 TBS extra virgin olive oil, 1 tsp curry powder and 1/4 tsp tamari (soy sauce). Drizzle this dressing over the diced fruit and vegetables.
7. **Frozen Grapes:** Freeze Grapes for a delicious snack.

# health benefits of grapes

## Promote Heart Health

Grapes and products made from Grapes, such as wine and Grape juice, may protect the French from their high-fat diets. Diets high in saturated fats like butter and lard and lifestyle habits like smoking are risk factors for heart

disease. Yet, French people with these habits have a lower risk of heart attack than Americans do. One clue that may help to explain this "French paradox" is their frequent consumption of Grapes and red wines.

Featured among the many health-promoting nutrients that Grapes contain are beneficial compounds called flavonoids, which are phytonutrients that give their vibrant color to purple Grapes, Grape juice and red wine; the richer the color, the higher the concentration of flavonoids.

These flavonoid compounds include catechins, epicatechins and quercetin as well as a second flavonoid-type compound called resveratrol. These compounds appear to decrease the risk of heart disease by reducing platelet clumping and harmful blood clots and protecting LDL cholesterol from the free-radical damage that initiates LDL's artery-damaging actions.

In a study in which blood samples were drawn from 20 healthy volunteers both before and after they drank Grape juice, researchers found several beneficial effects from their juice consumption. First, an increase occurred in levels of nitric oxide, a compound produced in the body that helps relax blood vessels, which in turn can reduce blood pressure. Second, a decrease occurred in platelet aggregation, reducing the risk of blood clot formation. Lastly, researchers saw an increase in levels of alpha-tocopherol, a form of vitamin E, and this increase was accompanied by a 50% increase in plasma antioxidant activity.

Resveratrol has recently been found to promote heart health through numerous unique mechanisms. It has been found to inhibit the production of both a molecule that constricts blood vessels as well as one that causes the production of excessive collagen, which leads to the stiffening of the heart muscle.

As interest in the heart-health-promoting properties of Grapes grows, so do researchers' findings as to other phytonutrient compounds, in addition to flavonoids, found in Grapes that may help protect cardiovascular health. These include saponins and pterostilbene.

## Promote Women's Health

Red Grape skins and seeds contain isolated compounds, called procyanidin B dimers, which a recent test tube study has suggested are able to reduce the size of estrogen-dependent breast cancer tumors. Another study found that resveratrol can inhibit the growth, and even trigger programmed cell death, of highly invasive and metastatic breast cancer cells.

## Nutritional Analysis of 1 cup of fresh Grapes:

| NUTRIENT | AMOUNT | % DAILY VALUE | NUTRIENT | AMOUNT | % DAILY VALUE |
|---|---|---|---|---|---|
| Calories | 61.64 | | Pantothenic Acid | 0.02 mg | 0.20 |
| Calories from Fat | 2.90 | | | | |
| Calories from Saturated Fat | 0.94 | | **Minerals** | | |
| Protein | 0.58 g | | Boron | — mcg | |
| Carbohydrates | 15.78 g | | Calcium | 12.88 mg | 1.29 |
| Dietary Fiber | 0.92 g | 3.68 | Chloride | — mg | |
| Soluble Fiber | 0.24 g | | Chromium | — mcg | — |
| Insoluble Fiber | 0.70 g | | Copper | 0.04 mg | 2.00 |
| Sugar – Total | 14.72 g | | Fluoride | — mg | — |
| Monosaccharides | 12.42 g | | Iodine | 0.92 mcg | 0.61 |
| Disaccharides | 2.66 g | | Iron | 0.26 mg | 1.44 |
| Other Carbs | 0.14 g | | Magnesium | 4.60 mg | 1.15 |
| Fat – Total | 0.32 g | | Manganese | 0.66 mg | 33.00 |
| Saturated Fat | 0.10 g | | Molybdenum | — mcg | — |
| Mono Fat | 0.02 g | | Phosphorus | 9.20 mg | 0.92 |
| Poly Fat | 0.10 g | | Potassium | 175.72 mg | |
| Omega-3 Fatty Acids | 0.02 g | 0.80 | Selenium | 0.18 mcg | 0.26 |
| Omega-6 Fatty Acids | 0.08 g | | Sodium | 1.84 mg | |
| Trans Fatty Acids | 0.00 g | | Zinc | 0.04 mg | 0.27 |
| Cholesterol | 0.00 mg | | | | |
| Water | 74.80 g | | **Amino Acids** | | |
| Ash | 0.52 g | | Alanine | 0.02 g | |
| | | | Arginine | 0.04 g | |
| **Vitamins** | | | Aspartate | 0.08 g | |
| Vitamin A IU | 92.00 IU | 1.84 | Cystine | 0.00 g | 0.00 |
| Vitamin A RE | 9.20 RE | | Glutamate | 0.12 g | |
| A - Carotenoid | 9.20 RE | 0.12 | Glycine | 0.02 g | |
| A - Retinol | 0.00 RE | | Histidine | 0.02 g | 1.55 |
| B1 Thiamin | 0.08 mg | 5.33 | Isoleucine | 0.00 g | 0.00 |
| B2 Riboflavin | 0.06 mg | 3.53 | Leucine | 0.02 g | 0.79 |
| B3 Niacin | 0.28 mg | 1.40 | Lysine | 0.02 g | 0.85 |
| Niacin Equiv | 0.32 mg | | Methionine | 0.02 g | 2.70 |
| Vitamin B6 | 0.10 mg | 5.00 | Phenylalanine | 0.02 g | 1.68 |
| Vitamin B12 | 0.00 mcg | 0.00 | Proline | 0.02 g | |
| Biotin | 0.28 mcg | 0.09 | Serine | 0.02 g | |
| Vitamin C | 3.68 mg | 6.13 | Threonine | 0.02 g | 1.61 |
| Vitamin D IU | 0.00 IU | 0.00 | Tryptophan | 0.00 g | 0.00 |
| Vitamin D mcg | 0.00 mcg | | Tyrosine | 0.02 g | 2.06 |
| Vitamin E Alpha Equiv | 0.32 mg | 1.60 | Valine | 0.02 g | 1.36 |
| Vitamin E IU | 0.46 IU | | | | |
| Vitamin E mg | 0.32 mg | | | | |
| Folate | 3.58 mcg | 0.89 | | | |
| Vitamin K | — mcg | — | | | |

(Note: "—" indicates data is unavailable. For more information, please see page 806.)

## Additional Health-Promoting Benefits of Grapes

Grapes are also a concentrated source of many other nutrients, providing additional health-promoting benefits. These nutrients include free-radical-scavenging vitamin C and manganese, heart-healthy vitamin B6 and potassium, and energy-producing vitamin B1. Since one cup of Grapes contains only 62 calories, they are an ideal food for healthy weight control.

Here are questions that I received from readers of the whfoods.org website about Grapes:

**Q** *Does red wine help lower cholesterol levels?*

**A** Research presented at the 226th national meeting of the American Chemical Society provided another explanation for red wine's cardio-protective effects. Saponins, a plant protective agent found in Grapes' waxy skin, which dissolves into the wine during its fermentation process, are believed to bind to and prevent the absorption of cholesterol. They are also known to settle down inflammation pathways, an effect that could have implications in not only heart disease, but also in cancer prevention. The research team thinks that alcohol may make the saponins more soluble and thus more available in wine.

**Q** *I was just wondering which types of Grapes are more beneficial— red Grapes or green Grapes?*

**A** The deeper red color of red and purple Grapes as compared to green Grapes reflects a higher concentration of flavonoid phytonutrients. These phytonutrients have powerful antioxidant activity, which can be a great asset to promoting overall health. Therefore, although I also like green Grapes, I would say that to get the most benefit from flavonoids, you may want to choose darker colored red or purple Grapes instead.

**Q** *I have heard that the seeds of Grapes contain proanthocyanins. Are these antioxidant phytonutrients contained in Grapes themselves?*

**A** Although research does suggest that Grape seeds are a more concentrated source of proanthocyanins, according to the USDA Database for the Proanthocyanidin Content of Selected Foods–August 2004, Grapes also contain these phytonutrients. For example, 100 grams of green Grapes contains 59 mg of proanthocyanidin polymers while 100 grams of red Grapes contains 45 mg. This is more than contained in many fruits, such as pears, pineapples and peaches. How does this compare to some proanthocyanidin-rich foods? One hundred grams of cacao beans (from which cocoa is extracted) contains 1,568 mg, fresh cranberries contain 233 mg and hazelnuts contain 322 mg.

**Q** *I heard that sour (unripe) Grapes offer a variety of health benefits. Can you tell me anything about the chemical composition of an unripe Grape that supports this?*

**A** In comparison to fully ripened Grapes, unripe Grapes are a fairly concentrated source of glycolic acid. Glycolic acid is a member of the alpha-hydroxy family of acids that you may be familiar with from their listing on many facial products, especially exfoliants. Research studies suggest that glycolic acid may be able to help stimulate collagen production and may help repair skin from UV light damage. I haven't seen any research studies linking unripe Grapes to health benefits, however. In some non-Western medical traditions, I've also heard about unripe Grapes being used to treat sore throats, although I've never seen any research studies that support this use.

**Q** *Is it harmful to eat seedless Grapes? Are they a genetically modified food?*

**A** I haven't seen any research showing problems with consumption of either seeded or seedless organic Grapes. The "organic" factor here is important, because I've seen numerous studies that show pesticide residues on conventionally grown Grapes, and imported Grapes usually make the "top 12" list for unwanted levels of pesticides. Seedless Grapes began as hybrids, not as genetically modified foods. In other words, it's possible to create seedless Grapes without the use of genetic engineering. However, there are genetically modified (GM) seeded and seedless Grapes out in the marketplace. Since GM foods have no labeling requirement in the U.S., it can be difficult to determine whether any food has been genetically modified. However, since organic foods cannot be certified if they are GM, organic Grapes are the safe option here.

## Q Are there health benefits to eating Grape seeds? If so, should I chew them or simply swallow them?

A Unique phytonutrients found in Grapes are located in both the skins and the seeds. But the types of phytonutrients found in these two parts of the fruit can be very different. I've looked, but have been unable to find any research raising safety issues with the consumption of Grape seeds, provided that the Grapes are organically grown. Best absorption of nutrients from nuts and seeds (including Grape seeds) would usually require chewing of the seeds. In order for nutrients to be absorbed from food, our body has to break the food down either by mechanical or chemical means. Our body must work harder chemically to break down any food that we swallow without chewing. Small seeds can often pass through the digestive tract unchanged if they are not subjected to some chewing.

## Q Do Grapes and Grape juice provide the same health benefit as red wine?

A Red wine is recognized as an integral part of the "French paradox," the fact that when compared to Americans, French people eat more saturated fat-rich foods and smoke more cigarettes yet have a lower risk of heart attacks. Eating Grapes or drinking Grape juice may provide similar health benefits.

While wine has far greater concentrations of resveratrol, the antioxidant phytonutrient thought to play an important role in explaining the "French paradox," than Grapes, Grapes do contain concentrated amounts of other phytonutrients; these include flavonoids such as catechins, epicatechins and pterostilbene, all of which are thought to have important heart-healthy benefits.

Resveratrol has also been the focus of recent cancer research. Cancer researchers have shown that resveratrol has the ability to selectively target and destroy cancer cells.

Other studies have shown that resveratrol helps prevent cancer during all three phases of the cancer process: initiation, promotion and progression.

Although resveratrol has been identified in over 70 species of plants, including eucalyptus, spruce, lily, mulberries and peanuts, resveratrol's most abundant natural food source is Grapes, especially the varieties used to make wine. According to the website of The Linus Pauling Institute, one cup of red grapes contains 0.24–1.25 mg of resveratrol while 5 oz of red wine contains 0.29–1.89 mg.

Resveratrol belongs to a group of compounds called phytoalexins that plants produce in self-defense against environmental stressors like adverse weather or attack by insects or pathogenic microbes. Since Grapes produce resveratrol as a defensive agent against fungal infection, this cancer-fighting phytonutrient is found at higher levels in organically grown Grapes, which have not been artificially protected by treatment with man-made fungicides.

Like red wine, Grape juice has been found to have numerous cardiovascular benefits such as reducing blood pressure, inhibiting platelet aggregation and protecting LDL cholesterol from oxidation (one of the primary processes involved in the development of atherosclerosis).

While studies show red wine offers numerous protective benefits, Grapes and Grape juice also provide the majority of these effects without the risks of alcohol consumption, which, if excessive, can lead to accidents, liver problems, higher blood pressure, heart arrhythmias, fetal alcohol syndrome and alcoholism.

To receive comparable benefits as those gained from drinking a glass of red wine, you need to drink more Grape juice. A recent study found that six glasses of Grape juice produced the same beneficial effect as two glasses of red wine in reducing platelet aggregation (the clumping that leads to blood clots), heart attacks and strokes. Another option is to drink dealcoholized red wine. A study published in the January 2004 issue of the *American Journal of Clinical Nutrition* suggests that the alcohol-free alternative provides comparable cardioprotective benefit. Therefore, if you want to avoid alcohol and protect your heart, toast your health with at least three daily glasses of red or purple Grape juice or dealcoholized red wine.

So, if you prefer not to consume alcoholic beverages, take heart—Grapes may still provide many of the cardioprotective benefits attributed to red wine.

# raisins

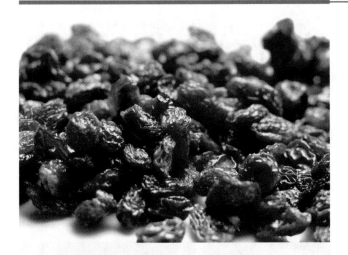

## nutrient-richness chart

1/4 cup (36.25 grams) of seedless Raisins contains 109 calories

| NUTRIENT | AMOUNT | |
|---|---|---|
| **FLAVONOIDS:** | | Daily values for these nutrients have not yet been established. |
| (+)-Catechin (mg) | 1.1 | |
| (-)-Epicatechin (mg) | 0.3 | |

Raisins are easy to pack, easy to eat and almost never go bad. It is no wonder that they are a favorite for school lunches, backpackers and hikers. Raisins do contain fewer phenols than grapes since many of grape's phenols are largely lost in the conversion of grapes to Raisins. The drying of grapes into Raisins has been practiced since ancient times. They were produced in Persia and Egypt as early as 2,000 BC. Raisins are grapes that have been dehydrated under the heat of the sun or through a mechanical oven-drying process.

## varieties of raisins

Some of the most popular varieties of Raisins include:

### CURRANTS

Approximately one-fourth the size of other Raisins, they are made from Black Corinth grapes that are seedless and very dark in color.

### GOLDEN SEEDLESS

Made from Thompson seedless grapes that have been oven dried, which prevents them from darkening. Non-organic varieties are treated with sulfur dioxide to help preserve their golden color.

### NATURAL SEEDLESS

The most popular variety of Raisins, they are made from sun-dried Thompson seedless grapes.

### MONUKKA

From the grape by the same name, they are large, dark, seedless Raisins with limited availability.

### highlights

| | |
|---|---|
| AVAILABILTY: | Year-round |
| REFRIGERATE: | Yes |
| SHELF LIFE: | 1 year refrigerated |
| PREPARATION: | Minimal |
| BEST WAY TO ENJOY: | Enjoy as a snack |

### MUSCAT

Large, brown, fruity tasting Raisins made from Muscat grapes. Since these grapes contain seeds, unless the seeds are mechanically removed, these Raisins will contain seeds. Most commonly used in fruit cakes, they are considered a specialty item.

### SULTANAS

Made from large yellow-green grapes. This variety is popular in Europe.

## biochemical considerations

Conventionally dried Raisins may be treated with sulfites, which might be of concern to certain individuals. (For more on *Sulfites*, see page 729.)

## 6 quick serving ideas for raisins:

1. **RAISINS FOR BREAKFAST:** Raisins are a great addition to homemade granola or can be sprinkled over any breakfast cereal, hot or cold.
2. **FRUIT COMPOTE:** Soak Raisins and other dried fruits in hot water to soften for easy-to-make compote. Use in a dessert parfait layered with yogurt or serve on top of grilled chicken.
3. **RAISINS AND RICE:** Add Raisins and almonds to brown rice to make a tasty side dish.
4. **TRAIL MIX:** Mix Raisins with your favorite nuts for a high energy, fiber-packed homemade snack.
5. **5-MINUTE RYE RAISIN SNACKS:** Spread 1 TBS peanut or almond butter on 4 rye crackers. Sprinkle cinnamon and 1 TBS Raisins on each cracker.
6. **RAISIN BUTTER:** Soak 1/2 cup each of Raisins and dates in 3/4 cup orange juice with the zest of one orange for at least 2 hours and as long as overnight. Blend together with 1 tsp cinnamon until it is thick and creamy.

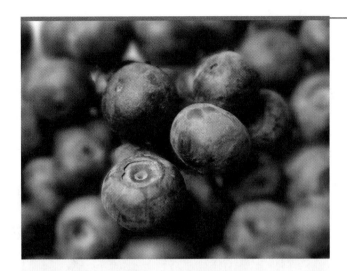

# blueberries

## highlights

| | |
|---|---|
| AVAILABILITY: | May through October |
| REFRIGERATE: | Yes |
| SHELF LIFE: | 3 days refrigerated |
| PREPARATION: | Minimal |
| BEST WAY TO ENJOY: | Enjoy them raw |

## nutrient-richness chart

Total Nutrient-Richness: **7**    GI: **n/a**

One cup (145 grams) of fresh Blueberries contains 81 calories

| NUTRIENT | AMOUNT | %DV | DENSITY | QUALITY |
|---|---|---|---|---|
| Vitamin C | 18.9 mg | 31.4 | 7.0 | very good |
| Manganese | 0.4 mg | 20.0 | 4.4 | very good |
| Dietary Fiber | 3.92 g | 15.7 | 3.5 | very good |
| Vitamin E | 1.5 mg | 7.3 | 1.6 | good |
| **CAROTENOIDS:** | | | | |
| Beta-Carotene | 46.4 mcg | | | |
| Lutein+Zeaxanthin | 116.0 mcg | | | |
| **FLAVONOIDS:** | | | | |
| (-)-Epicatechin | 1.6 mg | | | |
| Cyanidin | 21.8 mg | | | |
| Delphidin | 42.8 mg | | | |
| Malvidin | 71.4 mg | | | |
| Myricitin | 1.1 mg | | | |
| Peonidin | 10.2 mg | | | |
| Petunidin | 17.0 mg | | | |
| Quercetin | 4.5 mg | | | |

Daily values for these nutrients have not yet been established.

For more on "Total Nutrient-Richness," "%DV," "Density," and
The World's Healthiest Foods "Quality" Rating System, see page 805.

For more on GI, see page 342.

When it comes to berries, Blueberries are second only to strawberries in popularity. They are bursting with flavor, low in calories and make a quick-and-easy addition to your favorite breakfast or dessert. They can also serve as a nutritious and tasty between-meal snack. Blueberries played an important role in the food culture of the Native Americans, but the early settlers did not appreciate the tart flavor of the wild berries. It was not until the 20th century that Blueberries gained general popularity with the development of the sweet, plump, juicy varieties that we enjoy today. Modern means of transportation have also helped to make them widely available.

## why blueberries should be part of your healthiest way of eating

Blueberries have consistently been ranked among the top fruits and vegetables tested for antioxidant activity. They feature nutrients known as anthocyanidins; these flavonoids not only provide Blueberries with their dark blue color, but, along with other nutrients such as vitamin C, resveratrol, and ellagic acid, they deliver powerful antioxidant protection from the cellular damage caused by free-radicals. Blueberries are an ideal food to add to your "Healthiest Way of Eating" because they are nutritious, taste great and are low in calories: one cup of fresh Blueberries contains only 81 calories! (For more on the *Health Benefits of Blueberries* and a complete analysis of their content of over 60 nutrients, see page 408.)

## varieties of blueberries

Blueberries grow in the woods and mountainous regions throughout the U.S. and Canada. This fruit is rarely found growing in Europe (although its cousin, the bilberry grows there) and has only been recently introduced to Australia. Blueberries are the fruits of a shrub that belong to the heath family (*Ericaceae*), which includes the cranberry and bilberry as well as the azalea, mountain laurel and rhododendron. Like their other berry cousins, they are often referred to by their genus name of *Vaccinium*.

Cultivated Blueberries have a delicious taste that is mildly sweet with a slight tang. Wild Blueberries have a more tart, tangy and intense flavor than cultivated Blueberries and are about one-third the size.

Approximately 30 different species of Blueberries are now cultivated, many of which are indigenous to specific regions of North America:

**HIGHBUSH**

This variety can be found throughout the Eastern seaboard from Maine to Florida.

**LOWBUSH**

They grow throughout the Northeast U.S. and Eastern Canada.

**EVERGREEN**

This variety grows throughout the Pacific Northwest.

**DRIED BLUEBERRIES**

Dried Blueberries may be healthful but remember that dried fruit does not have the same nutrient profile as fresh or frozen fruit. For example, flavonoids—like peonidin, petunidin, malvidin and many other—found in Blueberries are susceptible to damage from heat, light and oxygen, factors that may be involved in the drying process.

## the peak season

Blueberries cultivated in the U.S. are available from May through October. These are the months when their concentration of nutrients and flavor are highest, and their cost is at its lowest. Imported Blueberries may be found at other times of the year.

## biochemical considerations

Blueberries are a concentrated source of oxalates, which might be of concern to certain individuals. (For more on *Oxalates*, see page 725.)

## 3 steps for the best tasting and most nutritious blueberries

Enjoying the best tasting Blueberries with the most nutrients is simple if you just follow my 3 easy steps:

1. The Best Way to Select
2. The Best Way to Store
3. The Best Way to Prepare

# 1. the best way to select blueberries

When you select Blueberries, look for ones that are fully ripe. Fully ripe Blueberries are ones that have a deep blue color with a whitish bloom and are firm to the touch. Shake the container to make sure that the Blueberries move freely and that they are free of moisture as the presence of water will cause them to spoil. Fully ripened Blueberries are highest in nutritional value, bursting with vitamins, antioxidants and enzymes. As with all fruits, I recommend selecting organically grown varieties whenever possible. (For more on *Organic Foods*, see page 113.)

Avoid Blueberries with a reddish tinge, an indication that they are not ripe and therefore will not have developed either their wonderful taste or the extent of their nutritional bene-fits. Also avoid Blueberries that are overripe. If you shake the container and the berries don't move freely, it is an indication that they may be soft, overripe or damaged and will have decreased in nutritional value. Overripe Blueberries are dull in color, soft and tend to fall apart; they are likely to get mushy and moldy. Alternatively, they may have lost their moisture and be very dry. Discard Blueberries that are soft and moldy. Overripe Blueberries should not be eaten.

### How Do You Know Which Blueberries are Ready to Eat?

If Blueberries are firm and have a uniform blue color, they are ready to eat. If they have a slight reddish coloration, they can be ripened (see next section).

# 2. the best way to store blueberries

Proper storage is an important step in keeping Blueberries fresh and preserving their nutrients, texture and unique flavor.

### Fresh Ripe Blueberries Can Last for Up to 3 Days When Properly Stored and Refrigerated

Blueberries continue to respire even after they have been harvested. The faster they respire, the more the Blueberries interact with air to produce carbon dioxide. The more carbon dioxide that is produced, the more quickly they will spoil. Blueberries kept at a room temperature of approximately 68°F (20°C) give off carbon dioxide at a rate of 70 mg per kilogram every hour. (For a *Comparison of Respiration Rates* for different fruits, see page 341.) Refrigeration helps slow the respiration rate of ripe Blueberries, retain their vitamin content and increase their storage life.

When you bring your Blueberries home, remove any crushed or moldy berries to prevent the rest from spoiling, and then place them in the refrigerator. While Blueberries that are stored properly will remain fresh for up to 3 days, if they are not stored properly, they will only last about 1–2 days.

## How to Ripen Blueberries

Blueberries will become sweet and juicy at home if they have not been picked too green. Blueberries are best if they are ripe before they are picked, but if they are tart and have a slight reddish coloration when you purchase them (signaling that they are not ripe), you can ripen them at home.

The natural way to ripen Blueberries is to place them in their container in a paper bag until they get softer and juicier. The paper bag traps the ethylene gas produced by the Blueberries. The ethylene gas helps them to ripen more quickly, while the paper bag allows for healthy oxygen exchange through the bag. (Don't use a plastic bag as it provides for limited oxygen exchange and will lead to the rotting of your Blueberries.) Keep the paper bag in a dark cool place as excessive heat will also cause the Blueberries to rot rather than ripen.

Do not refrigerate Blueberries until they are ripe; they will not ripen in the refrigerator.

## How to Speed Up the Ripening of Blueberries

Adding a banana, apple or avocado to the bag with the Blueberries will increase the amount of ethylene gas trapped in the bag. The increased amount of gas hastens the ripening process. They should ripen in 2 to 3 days.

## Is It Best to Refrigerate Your Blueberries After Ripening?

Yes, but because fully ripened blueberries do not store well and are very perishable, it is best to eat them as soon as possible.

## Handle with Care

Blueberries are a delicate fruit and bruise easily, so handle them with care.

# 3. the best way to prepare blueberries

Properly preparing Blueberries helps ensure that they will have the best flavor and retain the greatest number of nutrients.

## Cleaning Blueberries

Blueberries are very delicate, so wash them very gently. Use the light pressure of the sink sprayer, if you have one, and pat them dry. Do not wash until right before using your Blueberries to prevent them from becoming waterlogged. Do not use any Blueberries that are overly soft and mushy unless you will be puréeing them for a sauce or coulis. (For more on *Washing Fruit*, see page 341.)

## No Bake Recipes

I have discovered that Blueberries retain their maximum amount of nutrients and their best taste when they are fresh and not prepared in a cooked recipe. That is because their nutrients—including vitamins, antioxidants and enzymes —are unable to withstand the temperature (350°F/175°C) used in baking. So that you can get the most enjoyment and benefit from fruit, I created quick and easy recipes, which require no cooking. I call them "No Bake Recipes."

Q *What are bilberries?*

A Bilberries are closely related to Blueberries. They belong to the same genus of plants (*Vaccinium*). The Blueberries native to North America include the species *corymbosum, ashei,* and *angustifolium; Vaccinum angustifolium* are also called "lowbush" or "wild" blueberries. The *myrtillus* species grown in Europe are what we commonly call "bilberries."

The anthocyanin flavonoids, for which Blueberries are highly regarded, are also found in high concentrations in bilberries. The antioxidant activity of these flavonoids has many benefits including the suggested ability to promote eye health. In fact, there is some specialized research in the area of macular degeneration and eye health that shows bilberry extract to be effective in improving visual function under specific circumstances. Modern day research into bilberry's benefits on vision has interesting roots of inspiration: during World War II, British Royal Air Force pilots who consumed jam made from bilberries during nighttime raids reported that they had better nocturnal vision.

## No Bake Recipes

# 5-Minute Fresh Blueberries with Yogurt

*The vanilla yogurt sets off the flavor of Blueberries in this quick and easy dessert.*

**1 pint of fresh Blueberries**
**4 oz vanilla or soy yogurt, stirred**
**1 TBS chopped walnuts**
**Optional: Add 2 tsp grated chocolate**

1. Place Blueberries into two bowls. Top with yogurt, walnuts and chocolate.

**SERVES 2**

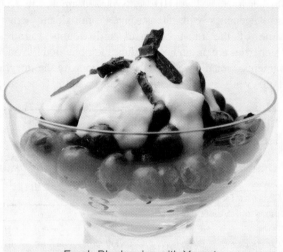

Fresh Blueberries with Yogurt

## Variation...

- For a delicious dessert, layer vanilla yogurt and Blueberries in wine glasses and top with crystallized ginger.

Please write (address on back cover flap) or e-mail me at info@whfoods.org with your personal ideas for preparing Blueberries, and I will share them with others through our website at www.whfoods.org.

### 4 QUICK SERVING IDEAS for BLUEBERRIES

1. Fresh or dried Blueberries add a colorful punch to cold breakfast cereals.
2. **Blueberry Shake:** Add Blueberries to your breakfast shake. If the blender is plastic, and you are using frozen berries, allow them a few minutes to soften, so they will not damage the blender.
3. **Blueberry-Peach Yogurt:** Combine fresh Blueberries and sliced peaches. Top with vanilla yogurt.
4. **Blueberries with Cashew-Almond Sauce:** Divide 1 pint of fresh Blueberries into 2 bowls. For sauce, make Cashew Cream (page 550), adding almond extract. Pour over Blueberries and chill 1 hour. Top with sliced almonds.

Here are questions that I received from readers of the whfoods.org website about Blueberries:

**Q** *Are there seeds in Blueberries? I am unable to eat any foods with seeds.*

**A** Blueberries do have very tiny seeds found suspended within their flesh.

**Q** *Do Blueberries have tannic acid?*

**A** Tannic acid and tannins are a classification of chemicals, all of which share certain chemical characteristics including having a phenolic structure. Some phytonutrients, chemicals found in plant foods that promote health, are tannins. Blueberries (as well as cranberries) do contain special phytonutrients that are classified as tannins. These tannins have been found to act as astringents in the digestive tract and reduce inflammation.

**Q** *Does freezing and thawing cause any loss in Blueberries' antioxidant value?*

**A** Freezing Blueberries results in minimal loss of nutrients, including its nutrients that have powerful antioxidant activity. While they may lose a little bit of their vitamin C content during freezing and thawing, their manganese content should remain pretty consistent since this mineral is found in its more stable, chelated form in Blueberries. Although their anthocyanin flavonoids are considered rather delicate, a recent study showed that there was no significant decrease in Blueberries' anthocyanin level after three months of freezing. If you are going to eat your Blueberries within a few days of purchase, I think it's still better to eat them fresh. Yet, if you buy a lot of fresh berries and you want to save them for a later date when they are less likely to be readily available, by all means, go ahead and freeze them.

# health benefits of blueberries

## Provide Powerful Antioxidant Protection

Blueberries have been repeatedly ranked among the fruits and vegetables with the strongest antioxidant activity. Some of the most powerful antioxidants found in Blueberries are the anthocyanidins, their blue-red flavonoid pigments, which have been shown to improve the integrity of the veins and the entire vascular system. Blueberries work their protective magic by preventing free-radical damage and supporting the stability of the collagen matrix. Since collagen damage can lead to cataracts, glaucoma, varicose veins, hemorrhoids, peptic ulcers, heart disease and cancer, adequate anthocyanidin intake may be inextricably linked to optimal health. Anthocyanidins have also been shown to enhance the effects of vitamin C, an antioxidant nutrient of which Blueberries are a very good source.

In addition, Blueberries are an important source of resveratrol, a phytonutrient found in red wine and to which many of its benefits have been assigned. The resveratrol in Blueberries is found mostly in their skin, and research studies support its effectiveness in preventing different types of heart disease and cancer. (Cooking Blueberries has been found to degrade their resveratrol concentration, so don't just enjoy Blueberry pies and cobblers, but some fresh berries as well.)

In addition to their antioxidant phytonutrients and vitamin C, Blueberries are a very good source of the antioxidant manganese and a good source of vitamin E.

## Promote Brain Health

In animal studies, researchers have found that Blueberries help protect the brain from oxidative stress and may reduce the effects of age-related conditions such as dementia. Researchers found that diets rich in Blueberries significantly improved both the learning capacity and motor skills of aging laboratory animals, making them mentally equivalent to those that were much younger.

## Promote Healthy Elimination

Blueberries are a very good source of dietary fiber, which promotes more regular elimination. In addition, Blueberries contain tannins, which act as astringents in the digestive system to reduce the inflammation that oftentimes causes loose bowel movements. Blueberries also promote urinary tract health. They contain the same compounds found in cranberries that help prevent or eliminate urinary tract infections by reducing the ability of E. coli, the bacteria that is the most common cause of urinary tract infections, to adhere.

## Promote Optimal Health

In addition to their powerful anthocyanidins and resveratrol, Blueberries contain another antioxidant compound called ellagic acid that blocks metabolic pathways that can lead to cancer. Blueberries are also high in the soluble fiber pectin, which has been shown to prevent bile acid from being transformed into a potentially cancer-causing compound.

## Additional Health-Promoting Benefits of Blueberries

Since Blueberries contain only 81 calories per one cup serving, they are an ideal food for healthy weight control.

### Nutritional Analysis of 1 cup of fresh Blueberries

| NUTRIENT | AMOUNT | % DAILY VALUE | NUTRIENT | AMOUNT | % DAILY VALUE |
|---|---|---|---|---|---|
| Calories | 81.20 | | Pantothenic Acid | 0.14 mg | 1.40 |
| Calories from Fat | 4.96 | | | | |
| Calories from Saturated Fat | 0.42 | | **Minerals** | | |
| Protein | 0.98 g | | Boron | — mcg | |
| Carbohydrates | 20.48 g | | Calcium | 8.70 mg | 0.87 |
| Dietary Fiber | 3.92 g | 15.68 | Chloride | — mg | |
| Soluble Fiber | 1.16 g | | Chromium | — mcg | — |
| Insoluble Fiber | 2.76 g | | Copper | 0.08 mg | 4.00 |
| Sugar – Total | 16.54 g | | Fluoride | — mg | — |
| Monosaccharides | 10.30 g | | Iodine | — mcg | — |
| Disaccharides | 0.28 g | | Iron | 0.24 mg | 1.33 |
| Other Carbs | 0.04 g | | Magnesium | 7.26 mg | 1.81 |
| Fat – Total | 0.56 g | | Manganese | 0.40 mg | 20.00 |
| Saturated Fat | 0.04 g | | Molybdenum | — mcg | — |
| Mono Fat | 0.08 g | | Phosphorus | 14.50 mg | 1.45 |
| Poly Fat | 0.24 g | | Potassium | 129.06 mg | |
| Omega-3 Fatty Acids | 0.10 g | 4.00 | Selenium | 0.88 mcg | 1.26 |
| Omega-6 Fatty Acids | 0.14 g | | Sodium | 8.70 mg | |
| Trans Fatty Acids | 0.00 g | | Zinc | 0.16 mg | 1.07 |
| Cholesterol | 0.00 mg | | | | |
| Water | 122.68 g | | **Amino Acids** | | |
| Ash | 0.30 g | | Alanine | 0.04 g | |
| | | | Arginine | 0.04 g | |
| **Vitamins** | | | Aspartate | 0.08 g | |
| Vitamin A IU | 145.00 IU | 2.90 | Cystine | 0.02 g | 4.88 |
| Vitamin A RE | 14.50 RE | | Glutamate | 0.12 g | |
| A - Carotenoid | 14.50 RE | 0.19 | Glycine | 0.04 g | |
| A - Retinol | 0.00 RE | | Histidine | 0.02 g | 1.55 |
| B1 Thiamin | 0.06 mg | 4.00 | Isoleucine | 0.04 g | 3.48 |
| B2 riboflavin | 0.08 mg | 4.71 | Leucine | 0.06 g | 2.37 |
| B3 Niacin | 0.52 mg | 2.60 | Lysine | 0.02 g | 0.85 |
| Niacin Equiv | 0.60 mg | | Methionine | 0.02 g | 2.70 |
| Vitamin B6 | 0.06 mg | 3.00 | Phenylalanine | 0.04 g | 3.36 |
| Vitamin B12 | 0.00 mcg | 0.00 | Proline | 0.04 g | |
| Biotin | — mcg | — | Serine | 0.02 g | |
| Vitamin C | 18.86 mg | 31.43 | Threonine | 0.02 g | 1.61 |
| Vitamin D IU | 0.00 IU | 0.00 | Tryptophan | 0.00 g | 0.00 |
| Vitamin D mcg | 0.00 mcg | | Tyrosine | 0.02 g | 2.06 |
| Vitamin E Alpha Equiv | 1.46 mg | 7.30 | Valine | 0.04 g | 2.72 |
| Vitamin E IU | 2.16 IU | | | | |
| Vitamin E mg | 2.72 mg | | | | |
| Folate | 9.28 mcg | 2.32 | | | |
| Vitamin K | — mcg | — | | | |

(Note: "—" indicates data is unavailable. For more information, please see page 806.)

(Continued from Page 343)

| FOOD ITEMS | GLYCEMIC INDEX |
|---|---|
| **GRAINS (Continued)** | |
| Oat bread (80% intact oat kernels, 20% white wheat flour) | 91 |
| Oatmeal (one-minute oats) | 92 |
| **Rice** | |
| Wild rice | 81 |
| Rice cakes | 81 |
| Rice noodles, cooked | 85 |
| White, boiled (average of 12 samples) | 90 |
| Parboiled rice | 100 |
| Rice bread | 100 |
| **Rye** | |
| Whole kernels, cooked (average of 3 samples) | 48 |
| Rye kernel bread (80% rye 20% white wheat flour) (average of 6 samples) | 70 |
| Whole meal rye bread (average of 4 samples) | 81 |
| **Spelt** | |
| Whole meal spelt bread | 88 |
| **Wheat** | |
| Spaghetti, whole meal (average of 2 samples) | 52 |
| Whole wheat kernels, cooked 10–15 minutes (average of 7 samples) | 62 |
| Cracked wheat, bulgur, boiled (average of 4 samples) | 67 |
| Wheat kernel bread (80% intact kernels, 20% white wheat flour) | 73 |
| Couscous, boiled 5 minutes (from semolina-durham wheat) | 91 |
| Whole wheat bread (average of 13 samples) | 95 |
| White flour bread (average of 6 samples) | 100 |
| Gluten-free | 129 |
| **FRUITS** | |
| Grapefruit | 35 |
| Apples, dried (average of 2 samples) | 40 |
| Prunes | 41 |
| Apricots, dried (average of 2 samples) | 43 |
| Apples, raw (average of 6 samples) | 53 |
| Pears (average of 4 samples) | 53 |
| Plums (average of 2 samples) | 55 |
| Strawberries | 56 |
| Oranges (average of 6 samples) | 59 |

| FOOD ITEMS | GLYCEMIC INDEX |
|---|---|
| Pineapple juice | 64 |
| Grapes (average of 2 samples) | 64 |
| Orange juice (average of 3 samples) | 73 |
| Bananas (average of 10 samples) | 73 |
| Kiwifruit (average of 2 samples) | 74 |
| Apricots, raw | 80 |
| Papaya (average 3 samples) | 83 |
| Pineapple (average of 2 samples) | 83 |
| Figs | 85 |
| Raisins | 90 |
| Cantaloupe | 91 |
| Watermelon | 100 |
| **STARCHY VEGETABLES** | |
| Yams (average of 3 samples) | 52 |
| Carrots (average 4 samples) | 66 |
| Potatoes, boiled 15 minutes, cubed, peeled | 81 |
| Sweet potatoes (average of 5 samples) | 85 |
| Beets | 90 |
| Mashed potatoes (average of 3 samples) | 104 |
| Potatoes, baked (average of 4 samples) | 119 |
| **LEGUMES** | |
| Soybeans, cooked (average of 2 samples) | 25 |
| Lentils, red, cooked (average of 4 samples) | 36 |
| Garbanzo beans, soaked, boiled 35 minutes (average of 4 samples) | 39 |
| Kidney beans (average of 8 samples) | 39 |
| Lentils, green, cooked (average of 3 samples) | 42 |
| Split peas, yellow, cooked | 45 |
| Soymilk, full fat, with maltodextrin, calcium-fortified | 50 |
| Navy beans, cooked (average of 5 samples) | 53 |
| Pinto beans, cooked | 55 |
| Pinto beans, canned | 63 |
| **DAIRY** | |
| Yogurt, low-fat, plain | 20 |
| Whole fat milk | 39 |
| Skim milk | 46 |
| Yogurt, low-fat, with fruit | 47 |
| **SWEETENERS** | |
| Honey (average of 11 samples) | 77 |
| Sucrose (white sugar) | 95 |

*For more information go to www.mendosa.com.*

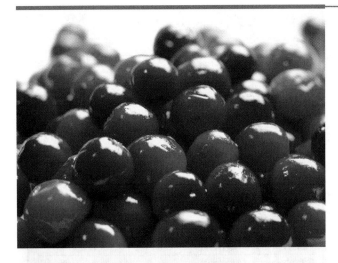

# cranberries

| | |
|---|---|
| AVAILABILITY: | October through December |
| REFRIGERATE: | Yes |
| SHELF LIFE: | 20 days refrigerated |
| PREPARATION: | Minimal |
| BEST WAY TO ENJOY: | Cooked with natural sweetener or dried |

## nutrient-richness chart

Total Nutrient-Richness: 7     GI: **n/a**
One-half cup (47.5 grams) of fresh Cranberries contains 23 calories

| NUTRIENT | AMOUNT | %DV | DENSITY | QUALITY |
|---|---|---|---|---|
| Vitamin C | 6.41 mg | 10.7 | 8.3 | excellent |
| Dietary Fiber | 1.99 g | 8.0 | 6.2 | very good |
| Manganese | 0.07 mg | 3.5 | 2.7 | good |
| Vitamin K | 2.42 mcg | 3.0 | 2.3 | good |
| **CAROTENOIDS:** | | | | |
| Beta-Carotene | 17.1 mcg | | | |
| Lutein+Zeaxanthin | 43.2 mcg | | | |
| **FLAVONOIDS:** | | | | |
| (-)-Epicatechin | 2.0 mg | | | |
| Malvidin | 2.2 mg | | | |
| Quercetin | 6.7 mg | | | |

Daily values for these nutrients have not yet been established.

For more on "Total Nutrient-Richness," "%DV," "Density," and The World's Healthiest Foods "Quality" Rating System, see page 805.
For more on GI, see page 342.

Cranberries have also been called "bounceberries," because ripe ones bounce, and "craneberries," a poetic allusion to the fact that their pale pink blossoms look a bit like the heads of the cranes that frequent Cranberry bogs. American Indians enjoyed Cranberries cooked and sweetened with honey or maple syrup—a Cranberry sauce recipe that was likely a treat at early New England Thanksgiving feasts. Cranberries were also used by the Indians as a source of red dye. They were also used medicinally as a poultice for wounds since the berries' astringent tannins contract tissues and help stop bleeding. In the 18th century, American sailors carried vitamin C-rich Cranberries on their voyages to help prevent scurvy. If that were not enough benefits to boast of, compounds in Cranberries have also been found to have antibiotic effects.

## why cranberries should be part of your healthiest way of eating

Cranberries are not just for Thanksgiving anymore. These little red jewels are so full of nutrients and flavor that they can help make everyday a holiday of well-being. They are an incredible source of antioxidants. In fact, one study conducted at Cornell University found Cranberries to have the highest antioxidant levels compared to 19 other commonly eaten fruits. These antioxidants include proanthocyanidins that help to prevent urinary tract infections by blocking the infection-causing bacteria from attaching to the urinary tract lining. Cranberries are also an excellent source of vitamin C, the body's primary water-soluble antioxidant. Nutrient-rich Cranberries can be prepared so many delicious ways that you should give thanks everyday and include them as part of your "Healthiest Way of Eating." Not only are they rich in nutrients but they are also low in calories: one half-cup contains only 23 calories. (For more on the *Health Benefits of Cranberries* and a complete analysis of their content of over 60 nutrients, see page 414.)

## varieties of cranberries

A glossy, scarlet red, very tart berry, the Cranberry belongs to the same *Vaccinium* genus as the blueberry. The three most common varieties of Cranberries are American, Mountain and European.

### AMERICAN

A bright red berry, it is the most commonly cultivated variety in the northern United States and southern Canada. The U.S. Department of Agriculture categorizes the

American as its standard variety. It is known botanically as *Vaccinium macrocarpon*.

### MOUNTAIN

A mostly uncultivated variety that can be occasionally found in markets, these are the fruits that are bright red to dark red in color and better known as lingonberry or cowberry. Botanically, they are known as *Vaccinium vitis-idaea*.

### EUROPEAN

This variety is much smaller than the popular American variety. It is eaten less often than other varieties and primarily used as an ornamental. It is known as *Vaccinium oxycoccos*.

### HIGHBUSH CRANBERRY

Primarily used for jams, jellies and sauces, this variety belongs to a different plant family *(Viburnum)* than the other three Cranberries.

### DRIED CRANBERRIES

Since Cranberries are inherently tart, the sweetness of dried Cranberries comes from added sugar (either in the form of refined sugar, cane sugar, honey or fruit juice concentrate). With their increased popularity, dried Cranberries are becoming easier to find at the local market.

## the peak season

Fresh Cranberries, which contain the highest levels of beneficial nutrients, are at their peak from October through December. These are the months when their concentration of nutrients and flavor are highest, and their cost is at its lowest.

## biochemical considerations

Cranberries are a concentrated source of oxalates, which might be of concern for certain individuals. (For more on *Oxalates*, see page 725.)

### Cranberries and Warfarin

Since 1999, the United Kingdom's Committee on the Safety of Medicines has had 12 reports of cases (one fatal) that suggest that Cranberry juice (from *Vaccinium macrocarpon*) enhances the effect of the anticoagulant drug warfarin (Coumadin). Until this possible interaction between warfarin and Cranberry juice has been investigated further, individuals taking warfarin are advised to avoid Cranberry juice.

## 3 steps for the best tasting and most nutritious cranberries

Enjoying the best tasting Cranberries with the most nutrients is simple if you just follow my 3 easy steps:

1. The Best Way to Select
2. The Best Way to Store
3. The Best Way to Prepare

# 1. the best way to select cranberries

Fresh Cranberries that are firm, plump, deep red in color and firm to the touch are the most flavorful.

Firmness is a primary indicator of quality. In fact, during harvesting, high quality Cranberries are often sorted from lesser quality fruits by bouncing the berries against barriers made of slanted boards. The best berries bounce over the barriers, while the inferior ones collect in the reject pile.

The deeper red their color, the more highly concentrated are Cranberries' beneficial anthocyanin compounds. Fresh Cranberries contain the most antioxidants, and dried Cranberries are second to fresh in their concentration of antioxidants. Bottled Cranberry drinks and Cranberry cocktails with added sugars or low-calorie sweeteners contain the least.

Avoid fresh Cranberries that are soft, mushy and pale in color as they will be sour or lack flavor.

Although typically packed in 12-ounce plastic bags, fresh Cranberries, especially if organic, may be available in pint containers. Frozen Cranberries keep well and are available throughout the year. Dried Cranberries are sold in many groceries and may be found with other dried fruits. Look for those that are sweetened with cane juice, fruit juice concentrate or honey rather than refined sugar. As with all fruits, I recommend selecting organically grown Cranberries whenever possible. (For more on *Organic Foods*, see page 113.)

### How Do You Know Which Cranberries are Ready to Use?

Fresh Cranberries that are firm with deep red color are ripe and ready to use.

# 2. the best way to store cranberries

Proper storage is an important step in keeping Cranberries fresh and preserving their nutrients, texture and unique flavor.

### Fresh Ripe Cranberries Can Last for Up to 20 Days When Properly Stored and Refrigerated

Cranberries continue to respire even after they have been harvested. The faster they respire, the more the Cranberries interact with air to produce carbon dioxide. The more carbon dioxide produced, the more quickly they will spoil. Cranberries kept at a room temperature of approximately 68°F (20°C) give off carbon dioxide at a rate of 16 mg per kilogram every hour. (For a *Comparison of Respiration Rates* for different fruits, see page 341.) Refrigeration helps slow down the respiration rate of ripe Cranberries, retain their vitamin content and increase their storage life.

Before storing Cranberries in the refrigerator, discard any that are soft, discolored, pitted or shriveled. Water encourages spoilage, so do not wash Cranberries before refrigeration. While Cranberries that are stored properly will remain fresh for up to 20 days, if they are not stored properly, they will only last about 10 days.

### Cranberries Store Well in the Freezer

Wash and dry Cranberries before freezing. To freeze, spread fresh Cranberries out on a cookie sheet and place in the freezer. In a couple of hours, the fully frozen berries will be ready to transfer to a freezer bag. Don't forget to date the bag before returning to the freezer. Once frozen, Cranberries may be kept for one year. Once thawed, frozen berries will be quite soft and should be used immediately.

### Storing Dried Cranberries

Dried Cranberries stored in a well-sealed container in a cool dark place will keep fresh for several weeks. They can also be kept in the refrigerator. Frozen dried cranberries will keep for at least one year.

# 3. the best way to prepare cranberries

Properly preparing Cranberries helps ensure that they will have the best flavor and retain the greatest number of nutrients. When removed from the refrigerator, Cranberries may look damp, but such moistness does not indicate spoilage, unless the Cranberries are discolored or feel sticky, leathery or tough.

### Cleaning Cranberries

While not as fragile as blueberries, fresh Cranberries should be treated with care. Just prior to use, place Cranberries in bowl of cold water. Discard berries that float to the surface as they are not ripe.

### Frozen Cranberries

When using frozen Cranberries in recipes that do not require cooking, thaw them well and then drain them prior to using. For cooked recipes, use unthawed berries since this will ensure maximum flavor and provide you with berries that best hold their shape. Extend the cooking time a few minutes to accommodate the frozen berries.

### No Bake Recipes

I have discovered that Cranberries retain their maximum amount of nutrients and their best taste when they are enjoyed fresh and not prepared in a cooked recipe. That is because their nutrients—including vitamins, antioxidants and enzymes—are unable to withstand the temperature (350°F/175°C) used in baking. So that you can get the most enjoyment and benefit from fruit, I created quick and easy recipes, which require no cooking. I call them "No Bake Recipes."

STEP-BY-STEP
**No Bake Recipes**

# Cranberry and Fresh Pear Cobbler

*A fresh and delicious dessert.*

1 medium orange*
1/2 cup dried Cranberries
2 tsp honey
1/2 ripe pear (Bosc or other firm variety)
1/2 cup + 2 TBS lightly roasted walnuts (for light roasting walnuts, see Walnut chapter)

1. Grate enough orange rind to make 1 tsp zest and place in a mixing bowl.

2. Cut the orange in half and juice both halves into the same bowl as the rind.

3. Add the Cranberries and honey. Mix until the honey is dissolved. Let sit for 1/2 hour to allow Cranberries to soften.

4. After the Cranberries have softened, cut the pear into 1/4-inch cubes and add to the bowl. Add 1/2 cup lightly roasted walnuts.

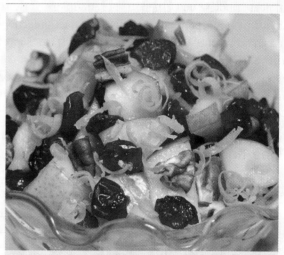

Cranberry and Fresh Pear Cobbler

5. Divide the mixture into 2 dessert dishes and sprinkle each with 1 TBS of the chopped walnuts.

**Preparation Hint:** Enjoy this dish right away, before the pear starts to brown.

* Use organic oranges, if possible, to avoid wax coating.

**SERVES 2**

## Variations...

- In summer, make the cobbler with fresh strawberries, blueberries and blackberries.
- Serve the cobbler with low-fat yogurt.
- Apples may be substituted for the pears.
- Top the mixture with granola.

# Cranberry Relish

*One of the best ways to enjoy fresh raw Cranberries is to make relish, which goes well with cooked chicken and turkey.*

12 oz fresh or frozen Cranberries
1 medium apple, chopped
1 medium pear, chopped
1/2 cup honey
1 TBS horseradish

1. Chop Cranberries very fine. A food processor may be used.

2. Chop the apple and pear into 1/2-inch cubes.

3. Combine all ingredients and mix well.

Please write (address on back cover flap) or e-mail me at info@whfoods.org with your personal ideas for preparing Cranberries, and I will share them with others through our website at www.whfoods.org.

## 7 QUICK SERVING IDEAS for CRANBERRIES:

1. Add Cranberries to rice pudding, quick breads or muffins for variety and color.
2. Use dried Cranberries instead of raisins in any recipe.
3. Add to chicken or turkey salad.
4. **Oatmeal with Cranberries:** Sprinkle a handful of dried Cranberries over a bowl of hot oatmeal (or any hot or cold cereal).
5. **Green Salad with Cranberries:** Add chopped fresh or dried Cranberries to your favorite green salad. Their tartness will add a zing, replacing the need for the vinegar or lemon used in the dressing.
6. **Cranberry Trail Mix:** Mix dried Cranberries with lightly roasted and salted nuts for a delicious snack.
7. **Cranberry Spritzer:** Combine unsweetened Cranberry juice in equal parts with your favorite fruit juice and sparkling mineral water.

# health benefits of cranberries

## Prevent Urinary Tract Infections

Clinical studies now support the traditional use of Cranberries for prevention of urinary tract infections. Researchers believe that Cranberries' ability to support urinary tract health is multifold: it acidifies the urine, contains an antibacterial agent called hippuric acid and also contains other compounds that reduce the ability of *E. coli*

### Nutritional Analysis of One-half cup fresh Cranberries:

| NUTRIENT | AMOUNT | % DAILY VALUE | NUTRIENT | AMOUNT | % DAILY VALUE |
|---|---|---|---|---|---|
| Calories | 23.27 | | Pantothenic Acid | 0.10 mg | 1.00 |
| Calories from Fat | 0.85 | | | | |
| Calories from Saturated Fat | 0.07 | | **Minerals** | | |
| Protein | 0.19 g | | Boron | — mcg | |
| Carbohydrates | 6.02 g | | Calcium | 3.33 mg | 0.33 |
| Dietary Fiber | 1.99 g | 7.96 | Chloride | — mg | |
| Soluble Fiber | 0.66 g | | Chromium | — mcg | — |
| Insoluble Fiber | 1.33 g | | Copper | 0.03 mg | 1.50 |
| Sugar – Total | 4.03 g | | Fluoride | — mg | — |
| Monosaccharides | — g | | Iodine | — mcg | — |
| Disaccharides | — g | | Iron | 0.10 mg | 0.56 |
| Other Carbs | 0.00 g | | Magnesium | 2.38 mg | 0.59 |
| Fat – Total | 0.10 g | | Manganese | 0.07 mg | 3.50 |
| Saturated Fat | 0.01 g | | Molybdenum | — mcg | — |
| Mono Fat | 0.01 g | | Phosphorus | 4.28 mg | 0.43 |
| Poly Fat | 0.04 g | | Potassium | 33.73 mg | |
| Omega-3 Fatty Acids | 0.02 g | 0.80 | Selenium | 0.28 mcg | 0.40 |
| Omega-6 Fatty Acids | 0.03 g | | Sodium | 0.47 mg | |
| Trans Fatty Acids | 0.00 g | | Zinc | 0.06 mg | 0.40 |
| Water | 41.11 g | | | | |
| Ash | 0.09 g | | **Amino Acids** | | |
| | | | Alanine | — g | |
| **Vitamins** | | | Arginine | — g | |
| Vitamin A IU | 21.85 IU | 0.44 | Aspartate | — g | |
| Vitamin A RE | 2.38 RE | | Cystine | — g | — |
| A - Carotenoid | 2.38 RE | 0.03 | Glutamate | — g | |
| A - Retinol | 0.00 RE | | Glycine | — g | |
| B1 Thiamin | 0.01 mg | 0.67 | Histidine | — g | — |
| B2 Riboflavin | 0.01 mg | 0.59 | Isoleucine | — g | — |
| B3 Niacin | 0.05 mg | 0.25 | Leucine | — g | — |
| Niacin Equiv | 0.05 mg | | Lysine | — g | — |
| Vitamin B6 | 0.03 mg | 1.50 | Methionine | — g | — |
| Vitamin B12 | 0.00 mcg | 0.00 | Phenylalanine | — g | — |
| Biotin | — mcg | — | Proline | — g | |
| Vitamin C | 6.41 mg | 10.68 | Serine | — g | |
| Vitamin D IU | 0.00 IU | 0.00 | Threonine | — g | — |
| Vitamin D mcg | 0.00 mcg | | Tryptophan | — g | — |
| Vitamin E Alpha Equiv | 0.05 mg | 0.25 | Tyrosine | — g | — |
| Vitamin E IU | 0.07 IU | | Valine | — g | — |
| Vitamin E mg | 0.47 mg | | | | |
| Folate | 0.81 mcg | 0.20 | (Note: "–" indicates data is unavailable. For more information, please see page 806.) | | |
| Vitamin K | 2.42 mcg | 3.02 | | | |

bacteria, the pathogen responsible for 80–90% of urinary tract infections, to adhere to the walls of the urinary tract. Cranberries may have such potential to protect urinary tract health that even consumption of a single serving of 1.5 ounces of dried Cranberries had the ability to reduce the adhesion of bacteria to the urinary tract walls.

Researchers suggest that some of Cranberries' beneficial properties come from the unique proanthocyanidin phytonutrients that they contain. A recent small scale study suggests that Cranberries' benefits are dose dependent; for example, eight ounces of Cranberry juice may be twice as effective as four ounces in preventing the adherence of bacteria.

In a manner similar to the way the tannins in Cranberries protect against bladder infection by preventing bacteria from adhering to the bladder wall, Cranberries' antiviral compound, proanthocyanidin A-1, has recently been found in test tube research to inhibit the attachment and penetration of the herpes type 2 virus.

## Prevent Kidney Stone Formation

Cranberries also contain quinic acid, which slightly acidifies the urine, preventing calcium and phosphate ions from joining to form insoluble stones. In patients who have had recurrent kidney stones, Cranberry juice has been shown to reduce the amount of ionized calcium in their urine by more than 50%—a highly protective effect since in the U.S., 75–85% of kidney stones are composed of calcium salts. Findings from another study led researchers to suggest that Cranberry juice may be useful in the treatment of brushite (calcium) and struvite (non-calcium) stones.

## Promote Gastrointestinal Health

Research suggests that Cranberries may be able to inhibit the growth of common foodborne pathogens, including *Listeria monocytogenes* and *E. coli* 0157:H7, and to decrease the salivary levels of *Streptococcus mutans*, the major cause of tooth decay. It may also enhance the growth of the beneficial bacterium *Lactobacillus fermentum*. Cranberry juice has also been found to prevent the bacterium responsible for most gastric ulcers, *Helicobacter pylori*, from adhering to stomach lining cells.

## Promote Heart Health

Cranberries may have heart health benefits not limited to their being a very good source of dietary fiber. After test tube research demonstrated that Cranberries' antioxidants could protect LDL cholesterol from oxidation, and animal research at three universities provided evidence that Cranberries can decrease levels of total cholesterol and

LDL (low density or "bad" cholesterol), a human study has also corroborated these positive results. In this study, drinking three glasses of cranberry juice for three months was associated with increased HDL levels. The increase was 10%; based upon known epidemiological data on heart disease, this corresponds to approximately a 40% reduction in heart disease risk.

Similarly, subjects' plasma antioxidant capacity, a measure of the total amount of antioxidants available in the body, was significantly increased—by as much as 121% after two or three servings of juice per day. Increased antioxidant levels are also associated with a decreased risk of heart disease. While the mechanism by which Cranberry juice changes cholesterol levels has not been clearly established, the researchers have theorized that the effect is due to the fruit's high levels of polyphenols, a type of potent antioxidant.

One of the interesting things about the study is that they used juice with only 27% Cranberry juice by volume, which raises the question of whether juice with higher levels of real fruit may have even more benefit.

## Provide Powerful Antioxidant Protection

In addition to being an excellent source of vitamin C and a good source of manganese, Cranberries are loaded with other antioxidants—phenolic phytonutrients. One study found that Cranberries are packed with five times the antioxidant content of broccoli; another found that they had the highest phenolic content of numerous commonly eaten fruits, while a third looked at 20 different fruit juices and found that Cranberry juice had the most phenols and the highest free-radical scavenging capacity of all of them.

## Additional Health-Promoting Benefits of Cranberries

Since one-half cup of Cranberries contains only 23 calories, they are an ideal food for healthy weight control.

Here are questions that I received from readers of the whfoods.org website about Cranberries:

### Q Since Cranberries lose nutritional value when dried, does that mean that their heart health benefits are greatly reduced?

A While the drying process can reduce the amount of nutrients in fruit, I wouldn't worry that much about its heart-health benefits being greatly reduced. That is because while there is a reduction in vitamin C and beta-carotene, the amount that regular Cranberries initially had is so small that it is not likely to have been a contributing factor to this benefit.

It seems that other phytonutrients such as polyphenolics may, in fact, be responsible for the great antioxidant activity attributed to Cranberries. Not only are polyphenolics usually conserved during the drying process, but many seem to actually increase.

### Q In the research studies that showed the health benefits of Cranberry juice, how much did the participants consume?

A In published research on Cranberries and kidney stone prevention, subjects consumed 2 cups of Cranberry juice per day, and these 2 cups were diluted with 6 cups of water. In one cholesterol-lowering study, subjects drank only 1 cup of Cranberry juice per day, while in another, they drank 3 glasses per day. The juice in these studies was the store-bought variety, not the concentrated variety. Store-bought, pre-diluted Cranberry juices are usually diluted at a ratio of about 3 cups of water per 1 cup of juice (therefore if someone wanted to mix their own using concentrate, a 3 to 1 ratio would reflect what was used in the studies). In studies on Cranberry juice used in prevention of urinary tract infection, however, Cranberry juice concentrate is often used. For example, in a well-known study from Finland in 2001, a small amount of concentrate (about 50 milliliters, or 1.6 ounces) was consumed.

### Q Are raw Cranberries good for you?

A Yes, raw Cranberries—especially if they are high quality and organically grown—are good for you. The reason that most people don't eat Cranberries raw is because they are very tart. (Some people might experience a stomachache from this amount of tartness, but from a nutritional standpoint, I would still describe raw Cranberries as being a highly nutritious food and a food without natural toxicity risks). One of my favorite ways to incorporate raw Cranberries into my diet is to slice them very thin and add them to salads or cooked vegetables. By slicing them very thin, you won't have to worry about an overload of tartness; you'll get just enough zing to brighten the taste of the dish to which you add them.

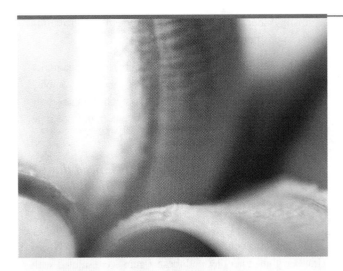

# bananas

## highlights

| | |
|---|---|
| AVAILABILITY: | Year-round |
| REFRIGERATE: | No |
| SHELF LIFE: | 5 days |
| PREPARATION: | Peel |
| BEST WAY TO ENJOY: | Enjoy them raw |

## nutrient-richness chart

Total Nutrient-Richness: **6**     GI: **73**

One (118 grams) medium fresh Banana contains 109 calories

| NUTRIENT | AMOUNT | %DV | DENSITY | QUALITY |
|---|---|---|---|---|
| B6 Pyridoxine | 0.7 mg | 34.0 | 5.6 | very good |
| Vitamin C | 10.7 mg | 17.9 | 3.0 | good |
| Potassium | 467.3 mg | 13.4 | 2.2 | good |
| Dietary Fiber | 2.8 g | 11.3 | 1.9 | good |
| Manganese | 0.2 mg | 9.0 | 1.5 | good |

**CAROTENOIDS:**

| | | |
|---|---|---|
| Alpha-Carotene | 29.5 mcg | |
| Beta-Carotene | 30.7 mcg | Daily values for these nutrients have not yet been established. |
| Lutein+Zeaxanthin | 26.0 mcg | |

**PHYTOSTEROLS:**

| | |
|---|---|
| Phytosterols - Total | 18.88 mg |

For more on "Total Nutrient-Richness," "%DV," "Density," and The World's Healthiest Foods "Quality" Rating System, see page 805.

For more on GI, see page 342.

B ananas were first mentioned in Buddhist texts in 600 BC. According to Indian legend, a Banana, not an apple, was the fruit offered to Adam in the Garden of Eden; this is why Bananas were once known in India as the "fruit of paradise." Bananas were introduced to Africa by Arabian traders and discovered there by Portuguese explorers who took them to the Americas, the place where the majority of Bananas are now grown. Today, Bananas are the most popular fruit in the United States and a dietary staple in many countries around the world. Wonderfully sweet with firm and creamy flesh, Bananas come prepackaged in their own yellow jackets and are available for harvest throughout the year. They can be enjoyed as a part of a "Healthiest Way of Eating" by everyone, from infants to the elderly.

## why bananas should be part of your healthiest way of eating

Sports enthusiasts and those on-the-go especially appreciate the portability and high energy delivered by Bananas. Bananas are one of the best sources of potassium as well as vitamin B6. And the vitamin C and manganese found in Bananas provide antioxidant protection against free-radical damage to cellular structures. (For more on the *Health Benefits of Bananas* and a complete analysis of their content of over 60 nutrients, see page 420.)

## varieties of bananas

The hundreds of varieties of edible Bananas fall under two distinct categories—sweet and plantain. Sweet Bananas are generally referred to botanically as *Musa sapienta* and *Musa nana* while the plantain Banana is known as *Musa paradisiacal.*

### SWEET BANANAS

Sweet Bananas vary in size and color. While we are accustomed to thinking of sweet Bananas having yellow skins, some varieties feature red, pink, purple and black tones when ripe. Bananas also have a wide range of flavors and textures with some varieties being very sweet, while others have much starchier characteristics.

In the United States, the most familiar varieties are Big Michael, Martinique and Cavendish. The yellow fruit available in most U.S. stores is usually the Cavendish variety.

### PLANTAIN BANANAS

Usually cooked and considered more like a vegetable due to their starchier qualities, Plantain Bananas are often used as a substitute for starchy vegetables such as potatoes in soups, stews or as a side dish. Unlike sweet Bananas, Plantain Bananas contain significant amounts of beta-carotene.

### EXOTIC VARIETIES

These include Manzano (apple or finger) Bananas, Saba Bananas and Brazilian Red Bananas, which are sometimes available in Hawaiian, Hispanic and specialty stores.

## the peak season

Bananas are available throughout the year.

## biochemical considerations

Bananas are one of the foods most commonly associated with allergic reactions in individuals with latex allergies. (For more on *Latex Food Allergies*, see page 722.)

## 3 steps for the best tasting and most nutritious bananas

Enjoying the best tasting Bananas with the most nutrients is simple if you just follow my 3 easy steps:

1. The Best Way to Select
2. The Best Way to Store
3. The Best Way to Prepare

# 1. the best way to select bananas

You can select the best tasting Bananas by looking for ones that are fully ripe. Ripe Bananas are plump and evenly colored with few brown spots. They have intact stems. Fully ripened Bananas are highest in nutritional value. Vitamins, enzymes and health-promoting phytonutrients are at their peak when Bananas are ripe. Since Bananas are always picked green and do not begin to ripen until after they have been picked, most of the Bananas you find at the market will not be ripe. Base your selection of Bananas on when you will want to use them. The greener the fruit, the longer it will take them to ripen. The size of the Banana does not affect its quality. As with all fruits, I recommend selecting organically grown varieties whenever possible. (For more on *Organic Foods*, see page 113.)

Avoid Bananas that have bruises or other injuries. Even a slightly green color indicates they are not ripe, while a brown color means they are overripe. Do not purchase overripe Bananas as they will be soft and mushy, turn brown easily and have lost some of their nutritional value. The brown coloration is an indication of the formation of free-radicals.

### How Do You Know Which Bananas are Ready to Eat?

If Bananas are plump and evenly colored with few brown spots, they are ready to eat.

# 2. the best way to store bananas

Proper storage is an important step in keeping Bananas fresh and preserving their nutrients, texture and unique flavor.

### Fresh Ripe Bananas Can Last for Up to 5 Days When Properly Stored

Bananas continue to respire even after they have been harvested. The faster they respire, the more the Bananas interact with air to produce carbon dioxide. The more carbon dioxide produced, the more quickly they will spoil. Bananas kept at a room temperature of approximately 68°F (20°C) give off carbon dioxide at a rate of 280 mg per kilogram every hour. (For a *Comparison of Respiration Rates* for different fruits, see page 341.) Refrigeration helps slow the respiration rate of ripe Bananas, retain their vitamin content and increase their storage life.

If you are not going to use ripened Bananas right away, you can refrigerate them to help retain their vitamin content. Do not be alarmed when their peels turn a very dark brown; the flesh will not be affected. Bananas taste best when they are at room temperature, so take them out of the refrigerator and allow them to return to room temperature before using. This will maximize their flavor.

If you have a large number of ripe Bananas, they can be kept frozen for up to 6 months and used to make Banana bread, Banana pudding, waffles, smoothies or other fruit drinks. I recommend peeling them before freezing.

While Bananas that are stored properly will remain fresh for up to 5 days, if they are not stored properly, they will only last about 3 days.

### How to Ripen Bananas

Bananas will become sweet at home. Bananas are a fruit that will fully ripen after they have been picked green. You will know if your Bananas are not ripe if they are hard, green and have little flavor.

A very natural way to ripen Bananas is to place them in a paper bag until they yield to gentle pressure, an indication that they are ripe, flavorful and ready to eat. The paper bag traps the ethylene gas produced by the Bananas. The ethylene gas helps them to ripen more quickly, while the paper bag allows for healthy oxygen exchange through the bag. Keep the paper bag in a dark, cool place as excessive heat will cause the Bananas to rot rather than ripen.

### How to Speed Up the Ripening of Bananas

Adding an apple or avocado to the bag with the Bananas will increase the amount of ethylene gas trapped in the bag. The increased amount of gas will hasten the ripening process.

Do not refrigerate Bananas until they are ripe. Placing unripe Bananas in the refrigerator will cause chill injury and disrupt their ripening process; they will not ripen even if they are returned to room temperature.

Avoid storing Bananas in sealed plastic bags or restricted spaces where they touch each other. The combination of limited oxygen exchange and the excessive amounts of ethylene gas produced under these conditions will cause them to rot.

### Handle with Care

Bananas are a delicate fruit and bruise easily, so handle them with care.

# 3. the best way to prepare bananas

Properly preparing Bananas helps ensure that they will have the best flavor and retain the greatest number of nutrients.

### Peeling and Slicing Bananas

Don't peel or slice Bananas until you are ready to use them because exposing peeled Bananas to the air causes oxidation of enzymes that will turn them brown. You can slow down this process by dipping peeled Bananas into a mixture of 2 cups of water and 2 TBS of fresh lemon juice. Dipping Bananas into the lemon and water solution is unnecessary if the slices are being added to a fruit salad that contains any type of citrus fruit, as the juices from these fruits will provide the same protection against browning.

### No Bake Recipes

I have discovered that Bananas retain their maximum amount of nutrients and their best taste when they are enjoyed fresh and not prepared in a cooked recipe. That is because their nutrients—including vitamins, antioxidants and enzymes—are unable to withstand the temperature (350°F/175°C) used in baking. So that you can get the most enjoyment and benefit from fruit, I created quick and easy recipes, which require no cooking. I call them "No Bake Recipes."

---

### An Easy Way to Prepare Bananas, Step-by-Step

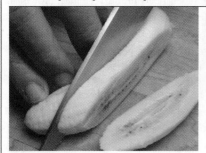 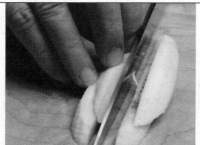 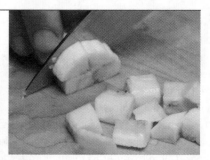

**DICED BANANA**

❶ Peel the Banana and cut lengthwise in slices about 1/4-inch wide. ❷ Take the slices one at a time, or 2 stacked on top of each other, and cut again lengthwise into 1/4-inch slices. ❸ Cut across the slices, ending up with small cubes.

STEP-BY-STEP
## No Bake Recipes

# 5-Minute Tropical Banana Treats

*A great nutritious snack, as easy as 1-2-3!*

**2 Bananas**
**4 tsp cashew, almond or peanut butter**
**1/4 cup grated coconut**
**Optional: 2 TBS dark chocolate chips**

1. Peel the Banana and cut in half crosswise then lengthwise, trimming the ends.

2. Spread 1 tsp of nut butter on each flat side.

3. Place the coconut in a saucer and dip the slices into the coconut covering the nut butter completely.

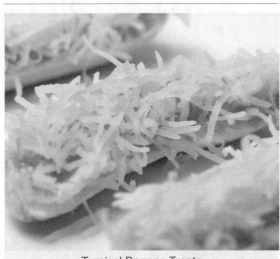

Tropical Banana Treats

4. Press chocolate chips into the nut butter (optional).

**SERVES 2**

## Variations...

- Try different thicknesses of grated coconut to find the texture you like.
- Use granola instead of coconut.
- Use raisins in place of the coconut.
- Spread Bananas with peanut butter and chopped peanuts.

Please write (address on back cover flap) or e-mail me at info@whfoods.org with your personal ideas for preparing Bananas, and I will share them with others through our website at www.whfoods.org.

## 10 QUICK SERVING IDEAS for BANANAS:

1. **Most Popular: Breakfast Power Smoothie.** Blend 2 TBS almond butter, 1 medium Banana, 1/2 cup strawberries, 2 cups soymilk or orange juice, 2 TBS flaxseeds, and 1 TBS molasses.

2. Add sliced Bananas, sunflower seeds, raisins and cinnamon to your oatmeal for a long-lasting breakfast.

3. Add chopped Bananas, walnuts and maple syrup to rice pudding.

4. Squeeze lime juice on sliced Bananas and garnish with coconut.

5. Bananas are packaged so perfectly that they make a great, take-along snack all on their own.

6. A peanut butter and Bananas sandwich drizzled with honey is an all-time favorite comfort food for children and adults alike.

7. Add Bananas to fruit salad.

8. Bananas and grated chocolate go great with vanilla ice cream.

9. **Rich Chocolate Banana Smoothie:** In blender combine 2 Bananas (frozen are better), 1 TBS cocoa powder, 1–2 tsp maple syrup or honey, and soy or rice milk to cover. Blend until smooth. *Optional:* for mocha flavor, add 1 tsp instant coffee or granulated coffee substitute (grain beverage).

10. **Frozen Banana Treat:** Place popsicle stick in one end of peeled Banana. Place on a tray lined with wax paper and freeze. When frozen, dip in melted chocolate until most of the Banana is well covered. For extra flavor, you can then roll in chopped nuts, coconut flakes or granola. Place on lined tray and return to freezer. Enjoy when chocolate becomes firm, about 2–3 hours.

# health benefits of bananas

## Promote Heart Health

Bananas are one of the best sources of potassium, a mineral essential for maintaining normal blood pressure and heart function. The effectiveness of potassium-rich foods in lowering blood pressure has been demonstrated by a number of studies. These delicious fruits are also rich in heart-healthy fiber; in a recent study, individuals who ate the most fiber had 12% less coronary heart disease and 11% less cardiovascular disease than those eating the least amount of fiber. Additionally, Bananas are a very good source of vitamin B6, which helps to keep levels of the cardiovascular disease risk factor, homocysteine, in balance. Bananas also contain phytosterols, which may promote heart health through their ability to inhibit cholesterol absorption.

## Promote Stomach Health

Bananas have long been recognized for their antacid effects, protecting the stomach against ulcers and ulcerative damage. In one study, a mixture of Banana and milk significantly suppressed acid secretion. Researchers have also found fewer stomach wounds in animals that consumed fresh Bananas.

Bananas work their protective magic in two ways. First, substances in Bananas help activate stomach lining cells to produce a thicker protective mucus barrier against stomach acids. Second, compounds in Bananas called protease inhibitors help eliminate *H. pylori*, the bacteria in the stomach that has been recognized as a primary cause of ulcers.

## Promote Proper Elimination

Bananas can be an important addition to the diet for those suffering from elimination problems. A bout of diarrhea can quickly deplete the body of important electrolytes. Bananas can replenish stores of potassium, one of the most important electrolytes, which helps regulate heart function as well as fluid balance.

In addition, Bananas are a good source of pectin, a soluble fiber that absorbs fluid, thus helping to normalize movement of food through the digestive tract and ease constipation. In Bananas, pectin is combined with a good supply of starch, supplying complex carbohydrate for slow-burning energy.

## Promote Optimal Antioxidant Status

Bananas are also a good source of vitamin C and manganese. These nutrients help to promote optimal health through their potent antioxidant activity; therefore they protect cells from free-radical oxidative damage. Vitamin C plays an important role in protecting DNA from oxidative damage. Manganese is a component of *superoxide dismutase*, an enzyme that guards the cells' energy production factories, the mitochondria, from free-radicals generated during energy production. Uncontrolled free-radical production has been linked to increased risk of diseases including cardiovascular disease, arthritis and certain forms of cancer.

### Nutritional Analysis of 1 medium fresh Banana:

| NUTRIENT | AMOUNT | % DAILY VALUE | NUTRIENT | AMOUNT | % DAILY VALUE |
|---|---|---|---|---|---|
| Calories | 108.56 | | Pantothenic Acid | 0.31 mg | 3.10 |
| Calories from Fat | 5.10 | | | | |
| Calories from Saturated Fat | 1.96 | | **Minerals** | | |
| Protein | 1.22 g | | Boron | — mcg | |
| Carbohydrates | 27.65 g | | Calcium | 7.08 mg | 0.71 |
| Dietary Fiber | 2.83 g | 11.32 | Chloride | 93.22 mg | |
| Soluble Fiber | 0.91 g | | Chromium | — mcg | — |
| Insoluble Fiber | 1.92 g | | Copper | 0.12 mg | 6.00 |
| Sugar – Total | 21.82 g | | Fluoride | — mg | — |
| Monosaccharides | 8.97 g | | Iodine | 9.44 mcg | 6.29 |
| Disaccharides | 12.27 g | | Iron | 0.37 mg | 2.06 |
| Other Carbs | 3.00 g | | Magnesium | 34.22 mg | 8.55 |
| Fat – Total | 0.57 g | | Manganese | 0.18 mg | 9.00 |
| Saturated Fat | 0.22 g | | Molybdenum | — mcg | — |
| Mono Fat | 0.05 g | | Phosphorus | 23.60 mg | 2.36 |
| Poly Fat | 0.11 g | | Potassium | 467.28 mg | |
| Omega-3 Fatty Acids | 0.04 g | 1.00 | Selenium | 1.30 mcg | 1.86 |
| Omega-6 Fatty Acids | 0.07 g | | Sodium | 1.18 mg | |
| Trans Fatty Acids | 0.00 g | | Zinc | 0.19 mg | 1.27 |
| Cholesterol | 0.00 mg | | | | |
| Water | 87.63 g | | **Amino Acids** | | |
| Ash | 0.94 g | | Alanine | 0.05 g | |
| | | | Arginine | 0.06 g | |
| **Vitamins** | | | Aspartate | 0.13 g | |
| Vitamin A IU | 95.58 IU | 1.91 | Cystine | 0.02 g | 4.88 |
| Vitamin A RE | 9.44 RE | | Glutamate | 0.13 g | |
| A - Carotenoid | 9.44 RE | 0.13 | Glycine | 0.04 g | |
| A - Retinol | 0.00 RE | | Histidine | 0.10 g | 7.75 |
| B1 Thiamin | 0.05 mg | 3.33 | Isoleucine | 0.04 g | 3.48 |
| B2 Riboflavin | 0.12 mg | 7.06 | Leucine | 0.08 g | 3.16 |
| B3 Niacin | 0.64 mg | 3.20 | Lysine | 0.06 g | 2.55 |
| Niacin Equiv | 0.87 mg | | Methionine | 0.01 g | 1.35 |
| Vitamin B6 | 0.68 mg | 34.00 | Phenylalanine | 0.04 g | 3.36 |
| Vitamin B12 | 0.00 mcg | 0.00 | Proline | 0.05 g | |
| Biotin | 3.07 mcg | 1.02 | Serine | 0.06 g | |
| Vitamin C | 10.74 mg | 17.90 | Threonine | 0.04 g | 3.23 |
| Vitamin D IU | 0.00 IU | 0.00 | Tryptophan | 0.01 g | 3.13 |
| Vitamin D mcg | 0.00 mcg | | Tyrosine | 0.03 g | 3.09 |
| Vitamin E Alpha Equiv | 0.32 mg | 1.60 | Valine | 0.06 g | 4.08 |
| Vitamin E IU | 0.47 IU | | | | |
| Vitamin E mg | 0.38 mg | | | | |
| Folate | 22.54 mcg | 5.63 | | | |
| Vitamin K | 0.59 mcg | 0.74 | | | |

(Note: "–" indicates data is unavailable. For more information, please see page 806.)

Here are questions that I received from readers of the whfoods.org website about Bananas:

## Q I am allergic to Bananas. Does this mean I can't eat plaintains either?

A Many people have adverse reactions to Bananas because they have a latex allergy, and they react to Bananas since Bananas contain enzymes that exhibit cross-reactivity to latex. If this is what causes your Banana allergy, then you should also avoid plaintains since they are also known to have a cross reactivity with latex. Even if your reaction to Bananas is not related to latex allergy, you may want to be careful when trying plantains as these two fruits belong to the same botanical family, and some people who react to one food in a family are often sensitive to other family members.

## Q I have read that green Bananas aid nutrient absorption. Yet, eating them is not fun since they are bitter and chalky. Any suggestions?

A Green Bananas do contain indigestible short chain fatty acids, such as butyric acid, that help to nourish the cells that line the intestines. When these cells are well nourished, nutrient absorption is enhanced.

Yet, green Bananas are not the only food that contains short chain fatty acids. For example, whole grains such as brown rice, barley, whole wheat and buckwheat also contain compounds called resistant starches that promote short chain fatty acid development. Therefore, eating a diet that is rich in whole foods, including whole grains, can provide you with a well balanced supply of these nutrients that promote both the health of the cells that line the intestines and nutrient absorption. This way, you can limit your consumption of green Bananas to the amount that you find pleasing.

## Q If I make Banana shakes in a blender will I still benefit from all of the nutrients that this fruit has to offer?

A When fruits are juiced, and the process separates out the pulp from the juice, some of the nutrients are lost (unless, of course, the pulp is completely mixed back with the juice). Yet, if you are adding the Banana to the blender, all of it will remain in the blender and will become part of your shake. There may be a little bit of loss from exposure to air and from the mechanical processing, but since you are not heating the Banana or discarding any of its components, you are losing very little here—especially in comparison with juicing—so I think that making the Banana shake in a blender is fine from a nutritional perspective.

## Q I read on your website that "In Bananas, pectin is combined with a good supply of starch, supplying complex carbohydrate for slow-burning energy." You also say they are favored by athletes. I assume this is because they provide fast-burning energy. I have always understood that Bananas are fast-burning, instant energy—not slow-burning with a high GI. So what's correct?

A Thank you for taking the time to write to me with your comments about the Banana text. Bananas are a fascinating food from the standpoint of digestion and metabolism, because their degree of ripeness is so influential in determining the results. When consumed during their less ripe stages, Bananas not only contain starch at a level of about 20% total calories, but this starch is typically classified as "resistant starch," meaning that it is resistant to digestion in the stomach and small intestine. In addition to this starch, Bananas contain the water-soluble hydrocolloids called pectins. The combination of resistant starch and pectin in less ripe Bananas is partly responsible for the unusually low end glycemic index (GI) and glycemic load (GL) numbers that can be associated with Bananas. GIs as low as 30 and GLs as low as 6 have been found in research on less ripe Bananas. Since a GI under 50 is usually considered low, as is a GL under 10, Bananas would be classified as low GI and GL foods in their early (less ripe) stages.

As they increase in ripeness, the GI of Bananas will increase to a maximum value ranging from 60–70, and a GL between 15–17. These values would qualify Bananas as medium GI and GL foods. GI values aren't usually described as high until they are above 70 and GL values when they are above 20.

The speed with which Bananas provide energy depends on many factors. Whether they should be called fast-burning or slow-burning depends on the foods they're being compared to. In general, we agree with you that they are better described as "fast-burning" than "slow-burning," since that term ("slow-burning") is usually used to describe foods that are higher in fat and, to a lesser extent, protein. I have made some changes in our website text to try and clarify some of these issues.

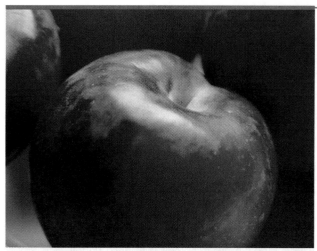

# plums

| | |
|---|---|
| AVAILABILITY: | May through October |
| REFRIGERATE: | Yes, after ripening |
| SHELF LIFE: | 10 days refrigerated |
| PREPARATION: | Minimal |
| BEST WAY TO ENJOY: | Enjoy them raw |

## nutrient-richness chart

Total Nutrient-Richness: **6**          GI: **55**

One (66 grams) fresh Plum contains 36 calories

| NUTRIENT | AMOUNT | %DV | DENSITY | QUALITY |
|---|---|---|---|---|
| Vitamin C | 6.3 mg | 10.4 | 5.2 | very good |
| Vitamin A | 213.2 IU | 4.3 | 2.1 | good |
| Dietary Fiber | 1.0 g | 4.0 | 2.0 | good |
| B2 Riboflavin | 0.1 mg | 3.5 | 1.8 | good |
| Potassium | 113.5 mg | 3.2 | 1.6 | good |
| **CAROTENOIDS:** | | | | |
| Beta-Carotene | 125.4 mcg | | | |
| Beta-Cryptoxanthin | 23.1 mcg | | | |
| Lutein+Zeaxanthin | 48.2 mcg | | | |
| **FLAVONOIDS:** | | | | |
| (+)-Catechin | 2.2mg | | | |
| (-)-Epicatechin | 1.9 mg | | | |
| Quercetin | 0.8mg | | | |
| **PHYTOSTEROLS:** | | | | |
| Phytosterols–Total | 4.6 mg | | | |

Daily values for these nutrients have not yet been established.

For more on "Total Nutrient-Richness," "%DV," "Density," and
The World's Healthiest Foods "Quality" Rating System, see page 805.
For more on GI, see page 342.

Plums have been cultivated since ancient times. European Plums are believed to have originated from fruits from Damascus, Syria and Persia, while Japanese Plums originated in China. One of the unique things about Plums is that there are so many varieties available; even in ancient Roman times, there were already over 300 varieties of European Plums. Today, thousands of varieties of these colorful fruits can be found of which over 100 are available in the United States alone! There are few fruits that come in such a wide range of sizes and colors, including red, yellow, green and purple.

## why plums should be part of your healthiest way of eating

Plums are richly endowed with antioxidants, containing unique flavonoid and phenolic phytonutrients including neochlorogenic acid, chlorogenic acid and catechins. These phytonutrients, along with the vitamin C of which Plums are a very good source, provide powerful antioxidant protection from the oxidative damage caused by free-radicals. Plums are an ideal food to add to your "Healthiest Way of Eating" because they are highly nutritious and taste great while being quite low in calories: one Plum contains only 36 calories! (For more on the *Health Benefits of Plums* and a complete analysis of their content of over 60 nutrients, see page 424.)

## varieties of plums

Plums belong to the genus *Prunus* and are related to peaches, nectarines and almonds. They are all considered "drupes," fruits that have a hard stone pit surrounding their seeds. When Plums are dried, they are also known as prunes. The scientific name for Plums is *Prunus domestica*.

Plums are classified into six general categories: Japanese, American, Damson, Ornamental, Wild and European/Garden. The Plums in each category vary by size, shape and color. Most of the Plums found in the market in the United States are either Japanese or European Plums.

### JAPANESE

Japanese Plums are known as clingstones because their flesh clings to the pit. The skins of Japanese Plums range from crimson to black-red (but never purple). They are juicy with yellow or reddish flesh.

**EUROPEAN**

Characterized by their blue- or purple-colored skins, they are smaller, more dense and less juicy than their Japanese counterparts. They are also considered freestone because their flesh is easily separated from their pits. European Plums are most often used to make prunes.

## the peak season

The Plum season extends from May through October with the Japanese varieties first on the market from May and peaking in August, followed by the European varieties in the fall. These are the months when their concentration of nutrients and flavor are highest, and their cost is at its lowest.

## biochemical considerations

Plums are a concentrated source of oxalates, which might be of concern to certain individuals. (For more on *Oxalates*, see page 725.)

## 3 steps for the best tasting and most nutritious plums

Enjoying the best tasting Plums with the most nutrients is simple if you just follow my 3 easy steps:

1. The Best Way to Select
2. The Best Way to Store
3. The Best Way to Prepare

# 1. the best way to select plums

When you select Plums, look for ones that are fully ripe. Fully ripened Plums will yield to gentle pressure and are slightly soft at their tip. I have also found that good quality Plums will feature a rich color and may still have a slight whitish "bloom," indicating that they have not been over-handled. Vitamins and health-promoting phytonutrients, many of which can act as powerful antioxidants, are at their peak when Plums are ripe, so by selecting ripe Plums, you will also be enjoying Plums with the highest nutritional value as well as the best flavor. As with all fruits, I recommend selecting organically grown varieties whenever possible. (For more on *Organic Foods*, see page 113.)

Avoid Plums with soft spots, an indication that they are overripe. Overripe Plums with brown-colored flesh should not be eaten. Plums should be free of punctures, bruises or any signs of decay. Also avoid Plums that are excessively hard because they have probably been picked too green and will never develop their full taste, texture or nutritional benefits.

### How Do You Know Which Plums are Ready to Eat?

Plums that yield to gentle pressure and have a deep rich color are ready to eat. Plums that have not been picked too green can be ripened at room temperature.

# 2. the best way to store plums

Proper storage is an important step in keeping Plums fresh and preserving their nutrients, texture and unique flavor.

### Fresh Ripe Plums Can Last for Up to 10 Days When Properly Stored and Refrigerated

Plums continue to respire even after they have been harvested. The faster they respire, the more the Plums interact with air to produce carbon dioxide. The more carbon dioxide produced, the more quickly they will spoil. Plums kept at a room temperature of approximately 68°F (20°C) give off carbon dioxide at a rate of 20 mg per kilogram every hour. (For a *Comparison of Respiration Rates* for different fruits, see page 341.) Refrigeration helps slow the respiration rate of ripe Plums, retain their vitamin content and increase their storage life.

Keep as many ripe Plums at room temperature as you will be able to consume in a day or two. Store the rest in the refrigerator. You will enjoy maximum juiciness and sweetness from refrigerated Plums if you allow them to approach room tem-

perature before eating. While Plums that are stored properly will remain fresh for up to 10 days, if they are not stored properly, they will only last 5 days.

### How to Ripen Plums

Plums will become sweet and juicy at home if they have not been picked too green. Plums that are not yet ripe can be left at room temperature to ripen. Place Plums on a flat surface with space between the fruit to ripen them. It is best to turn them occasionally so that they will ripen evenly. Once they yield to gentle pressure, they are ripe and ready to eat. Don't refrigerate Plums until they are ripe; they will not ripen in the refrigerator.

Another natural way to ripen Plums is to place them in a paper bag for 2 to 3 days. The paper bag traps the ethylene gas produced by the Plums, which helps the Plums to ripen more quickly. Do not use plastic bags as they deprive Plums of oxygen and cause them to rot. Keep the paper bag in a dark cool place as excessive heat will also cause the Plums to rot rather than ripen.

*(Continued on bottom of Page 424)*

# health benefits of plums

## Provide Powerful Antioxidant Protection

Plums in both their fresh and dried version (prunes) have been the subject of repeated health research for their high content of unique phytonutrients called neochlorogenic acid and chlorogenic acid. These substances are classified as phenols, and their function as antioxidants has been well documented. These damage-preventing substances are effective in neutralizing a particularly destructive oxygen radical called superoxide anion radical. These antioxidants have also been shown to help prevent oxygen-based damage to fats, such as the fats that comprise a substantial portion of our brain cells (neurons), the cholesterol and triglycerides circulating in our bloodstream and the fats that make up our cell membranes.

## Promote Heart Health

Plums also contain catechins, flavonoid phytonutrients that have brought so much attention to the benefits of green tea. Catechins are powerful antioxidants that have many benefits including protecting LDL ("bad") cholesterol from oxidation; LDL oxidation is a primary step in the development of atherosclerosis. Cholesterol is afforded additional protection by Plums since they are a very good source of vitamin C, which also safeguards LDL from oxidation. In addition, Plums are also a good source of other heart-healthy nutrients, such as vitamin A, potassium and dietary fiber.

## Promote Vision Health

Research has found that fruit may be one of your eyes' best friends. A recent study found that those who eat 3 or more servings of fruit per day have a 36% lower risk of developing age-related macular degeneration (ARM), the primary cause of vision loss in older adults, compared to those who consume less than 1.5 servings daily.

*(Continued from Page 423)*
Adding a banana, apple or avocado to the bag with the Plums will increase the amount of ethylene gas trapped in the paper bag, which will hasten the ripening process. Storing Plums in sealed plastic bags or restricted spaces where they are in too close proximity to each other will cause them to rot.

## Handle with Care

Plums are a delicate fruit and bruise easily, so handle them with care.

## Nutritional Analysis of 1 fresh Plum:

| NUTRIENT | AMOUNT | % DAILY VALUE | NUTRIENT | AMOUNT | % DAILY VALUE |
|---|---|---|---|---|---|
| Calories | 75.95 | | Pantothenic Acid | 0.25 mg | 2.50 |
| Calories from Fat | 6.00 | | | | |
| Calories from Saturated Fat | 0.45 | | **Minerals** | | |
| Protein | 0.60 g | | Boron | — mcg | |
| Carbohydrates | 19.20 g | | Calcium | 10.85 mg | 1.08 |
| Dietary Fiber | 1.86 g | 7.44 | Chloride | — mg | |
| Soluble Fiber | 0.16 g | | Chromium | — mcg | — |
| Insoluble Fiber | 1.71 g | | Copper | 0.17 mg | 8.50 |
| Sugar – Total | 17.34 g | | Fluoride | — mg | — |
| Monosaccharides | 7.75 g | | Iodine | — mcg | — |
| Disaccharides | 4.81 g | | Iron | 0.57 mg | 3.17 |
| Other Carbs | 0.00 g | | Magnesium | 21.70 mg | 5.42 |
| Fat – Total | 0.67 g | | Manganese | 2.56 mg | 128.00 |
| Saturated Fat | 0.05 g | | Molybdenum | — mcg | — |
| Mono Fat | 0.07 g | | Phosphorus | 10.85 mg | 1.08 |
| Poly Fat | 0.23 g | | Potassium | 175.15 mg | |
| Omega-3 Fatty Acids | 0.10 g | 4.00 | Selenium | 0.93 mcg | 1.33 |
| Omega-6 Fatty Acids | 0.13 g | | Sodium | 1.55 mg | |
| Trans Fatty Acids | 0.00 g | | Zinc | 0.12 mg | 0.80 |
| Cholesterol | 0.00 mg | | | | |
| Water | 134.07 g | | **Amino Acids** | | |
| Ash | 0.45 g | | Alanine | 0.03 g | |
| | | | Arginine | 0.03 g | |
| **Vitamins** | | | Aspartate | 0.09 g | |
| Vitamin A IU | 35.65 IU | 0.71 | Cystine | 0.00 g | 0.00 |
| Vitamin A RE | 3.10 RE | | Glutamate | 0.07 g | |
| A - Carotenoid | 3.10 RE | 0.04 | Glycine | 0.03 g | |
| A - Retinol | 0.00 RE | | Histidine | 0.01 g | 0.78 |
| B1 Thiamin | 0.14 mg | 9.33 | Isoleucine | 0.02 g | 1.74 |
| B2 Riboflavin | 0.06 mg | 3.53 | Leucine | 0.03 g | 1.19 |
| B3 Niacin | 0.65 mg | 3.25 | Lysine | 0.04 g | 1.70 |
| Niacin Equiv | 0.78 mg | | Methionine | 0.02 g | 2.70 |
| Vitamin B6 | 0.13 mg | 6.50 | Phenylalanine | 0.02 g | 1.68 |
| Vitamin B12 | 0.00 mcg | 0.00 | Proline | 0.02 g | |
| Biotin | 0.47 mcg | 0.16 | Serine | 0.04 g | |
| Vitamin C | 23.87 mg | 39.78 | Threonine | 0.02 g | 1.61 |
| Vitamin D IU | 0.00 IU | 0.00 | Tryptophan | 0.01 g | 3.13 |
| Vitamin D mcg | 0.00 mcg | | Tyrosine | 0.02 g | 2.06 |
| Vitamin E Alpha Equiv | 0.16 mg | 0.80 | Valine | 0.02 g | 1.36 |
| Vitamin E IU | 0.23 IU | | | | |
| Vitamin E mg | 0.16 mg | | | | |
| Folate | 16.43 mcg | 4.11 | | | |
| Vitamin K | — mcg | — | | | |

(Note: "—" indicates data is unavailable. For more information, please see page 806.)

STEP-BY-STEP
## No Bake Recipes

# 5-Minute Fresh Plums in Sweet Sauce

*Try this great dessert recipe when Plums are in season.*

**3 Plums**
**1 TBS apple juice**
**1 TBS cream honey***
**1/8 tsp cinnamon**
**1/4 tsp almond extract**
**1 TBS chopped almonds**

1. Slice Plums lengthwise into eighths.
2. In a small bowl, stir together the apple juice, honey, cinnamon and almond extract.
3. Spoon mixture over the Plums.
4. Top Plums with chopped almonds. **SERVES 2**

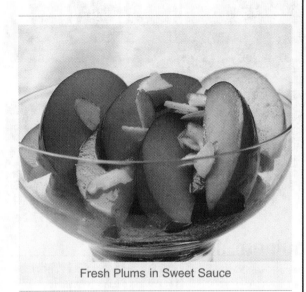

Fresh Plums in Sweet Sauce

## Variations...
* Top with your favorite granola.
* Combine the Plums with sliced peaches or nectarines.
* Substitute the cinnamon and almond extract with 1 tsp

\* Cream honey is whipped honey found in most health food stores.

of lemon juice and 1/2 tsp lemon zest.
* Use walnuts instead of almonds.
* Substitute the almond extract, cinnamon and apple juice with 1 TBS orange juice and 1/2 tsp orange zest.

Please write (address on back cover flap) or e-mail me at info@whfoods.org with your personal ideas for preparing Plums, and I will share them with others through our website at www.whfoods.org.

### 4 QUICK SERVING IDEAS for PLUMS:
1. Add Plum slices to your cold cereal.
2. Mash peeled Plums and mix them into your oatmeal.
3. Combine Plums, low-fat yogurt and crystallized ginger for a delicious breakfast or snack.
4. For a sandwich with a sweet twist, combine goat cheese, walnuts, fresh sage and Plum slices in a whole wheat pita bread.

# 3. the best way to prepare plums

Properly preparing Plums helps ensure that they will have the best flavor and retain the greatest number of nutrients.

## Cleaning Plums
Rinse Plums under cold running water before eating. (For more on *Washing Fruit*, see page 341.)

## Removing the Pit
If you want to remove the pit before eating, cut the Plum in half lengthwise, gently twist the halves in opposite directions, then carefully take out the pit.

## No Bake Recipes
I have discovered that Plums retain their maximum amount of nutrients and their best taste when they are enjoyed fresh and not prepared in a cooked recipe. That is because their nutrients—including vitamins, antioxidants and enzymes—are unable to withstand the temperature (350°F/175°C) used in baking. So that you can get the most enjoyment and benefit from fruit, I created quick and easy recipes, which require no cooking. I call them "No Bake Recipes."

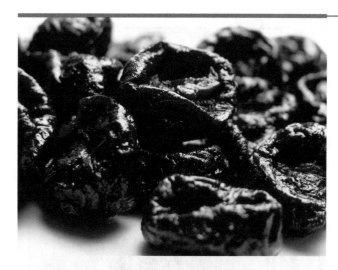

# prunes

## highlights

| | |
|---|---|
| AVAILABILITY: | Year-round |
| REFRIGERATE: | Yes |
| SHELF LIFE: | Up to 6 months in the refrigerator |
| PREPARATION: | Minimal |
| BEST WAY TO ENJOY: | Enjoy them as a snack |

## nutrient-richness chart

Total Nutrient-Richness: **4**    GI: **41**
One-quarter cup (42.50 grams) of Prunes contains 102 calories

| NUTRIENT | AMOUNT | %DV | DENSITY | QUALITY |
|---|---|---|---|---|
| Vitamin A | 844.5 IU | 16.9 | 3.0 | good |
| Dietary Fiber | 3.0 g | 12.1 | 2.1 | good |
| Potassium | 316.6 mg | 9.0 | 1.6 | good |
| Copper | 0.2 mg | 9.0 | 1.6 | good |
| **CAROTENOIDS:** | | | | |
| Alpha-Carotene | 24.2 mcg | | | |
| Beta-Carotene | 167.5 mcg | | | |
| Beta-Cryptoxanthin | 39.5 mcg | | | |
| Lutein+Zeaxanthin | 62.9 mcg | | | |

Daily values for these nutrients have not yet been established.

For more on "Total Nutrient-Richness," "%DV," "Density," and The World's Healthiest Foods "Quality" Rating System, see page 805.
For more on GI, see page 342.

Prunes have recently officially been renamed "dried plums," a very appropriate name for the dried version of the European plum.

## why prunes should be part of your healthiest way of eating

In a study conducted by Tufts University, Prunes outranked all other fruits and vegetables tested for their antioxidant values. Phenolic and carotenoid phytonutrients found in Prunes, such as chlorogenic acid and neochlorogenic acid, beta-carotene, alpha-carotene and beta-cryptoxanthin, provide powerful antioxidant protection against the oxidative damage caused by free-radicals. Prunes also are a good source of vitamin A because of their concentration of "provitamin A" carotenoids.

## varieties of prunes

Prunes are the dried version of the European plum. Most of

Prunes come from the California French Prune plum. A few other varieties of Prunes that are available include:

**DRIED MIRABELLES**
This fleshy variety is smaller than the average Prune.

**SOUR PRUNES**
A staple in Middle Eastern and Greek cuisines, they are orange or red in color and have a taste that is a combination of tart and sweet.

## the peak season available year-round.

## biochemical consideration

Prunes are a concentrated source of oxalates, and conventially grown Prunes may also contain sulfites, which might be of concern to certain individuals. (For more on *Oxalates*, see page 725; and *Sulfites*, see page 729.)

## the best way to prepare prunes

### Soaking Prunes
If you have Prunes that are extremely dry, soaking them in hot water for a few minutes will help to refresh them. If you are planning on cooking the Prunes, soak them in water or juice beforehand to reduce the cooking time.

### Reconstituting Prunes
Pour hot water over Prunes and let sit overnight. Avoid boiling the Prunes as it will cause their skins to split.

**Q** *Is it true that Prunes have very high antioxidant activity?*

**A** Phenolic phytonutrients in Prunes are especially effective at neutralizing the superoxide anion radical, which is a very dangerous oxygen radical that can damage cells.

**STEP-BY-STEP**
## No Bake Recipes

### *15-Minute Dark Chocolate Truffles*

*Chocolate and Prunes—a winning combination!*

1/2 cup pitted Prunes
1/4 cup pitted dates
3 TBS almond butter
1 TBS maple syrup
3 TBS unsweetened cocoa
1/2 cup finely grated unsweetened coconut

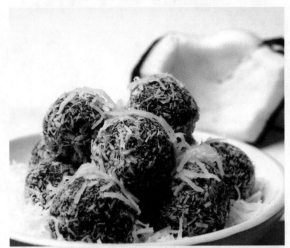

Dark Chocolate Truffles

1.  In a food processor, drop the Prunes and dates through the feed hole one by one. Scrape the processor bowl and run until the Prunes and dates are smooth.

2.  Add remaining ingredients except for the coconut. Run until smooth and scrape the bowl as needed.

3.  Roll the mixture into 12 one-inch balls and roll in coconut to coat. Refrigerate for at least 1/2 hour.

    **Preparation Hint:** If you don't have a food processor, this recipe may be done by hand, which, of course, will take longer (but well worth it). Cut dates and

Prunes in quarters. Toss with 1 TBS of the cocoa and chop the mixture until minced. Chopping with the cocoa keeps the mixture from sticking together. Place the chopped mixture in a mixing bowl and combine with remaining cocoa, almond butter and maple syrup. Knead the mixture on your cutting board until well combined. This version will be chunkier than those prepared in the food processor. Continue with the recipe as described in Step 3. **MAKES 12 PIECES**

Please write (address on back cover flap) or e-mail me at info@whfoods.org with your personal ideas for preparing Prunes, and I will share them with others through our website at www.whfoods.org.

### 5 SERVING IDEAS for PRUNES:

1.  **Prunes for Breakfast:** For a nourishing breakfast, soak 1 cup diced Prunes in 1/2 cup orange juice overnight in the refrigerator. Serve with chopped almonds or as a topping for pancakes or waffles.
2.  **Spiced Prunes with Yogurt:** Soak 1 cup Prunes in 1/2 cup orange juice, 1/4 tsp cinnamon, 1/4 tsp ground coriander and 2 tsp honey overnight in the refrigerator. Serve with plain yogurt.
3.  **Prunes with Lemon Sauce:** Soak Prunes in warm water until rehydrated. Drain, place in a dessert dish and serve with Quick Lemon Sauce (see page 431).
4.  **Trail Mix:** Combine diced Prunes with other dried fruits and nuts to make homemade trail mix.
5.  **Prunes and Almond Treat:** Slice open a moist Prune and put in a teaspoon of almond butter or a whole almond.

# health benefits of prunes

### Promote Digestive Health

Prunes are well known for their ability to prevent constipation. In addition to providing bulk and decreasing the transit time of fecal matter (thereby reducing the risk of colon cancer and hemorrhoids), Prunes' insoluble fiber also provides food for the "friendly" bacteria in the large intestine. When these helpful bacteria ferment Prunes' insoluble fiber, they produce a short-chain fatty acid called butyric acid, which serves as the primary fuel for the cells of the large intestine and helps maintain a healthy colon. These helpful bacteria also create two other short-chain fatty acids, propionic and acetic acid, which are used as fuel by the cells of the liver and muscles.

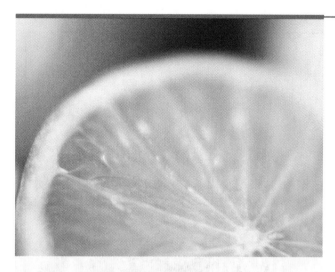

## nutrient-richness chart

Total Nutrient-Richness: **4**          GI: **n/a**

One-quarter cup (61 grams) of Lemon juice* contains 15 calories

| NUTRIENT | AMOUNT | %DV | DENSITY | QUALITY |
|----------|--------|-----|---------|---------|
| Vitamin C | 28.1 mg | 46.8 | 55.2 | excellent |
| **CAROTENOIDS:** | | | | |
| Beta-Carotene | 1.8 mcg | | | |
| Beta-Cryptoxanthin | 10.4 mcg | | | |
| Lutein+Zeaxanthin | 5.5 mcg | | Daily values for these | |
| **FLAVONOIDS:** | | | nutrients have not yet been | |
| Hesperitin | 7.3 mg | | established. | |
| Naringenin | 0.9 mg | | | |
| Quercetin | 0.2 mg | | | |

For more on "Total Nutrient-Richness," "%DV," "Density," and
The World's Healthiest Foods "Quality" Rating System, see page 805.
* Lime juice is comparable to Lemon juice.

For more on GI, see page 342.

L emons were so highly prized during the California Gold Rush for preventing scurvy that people were willing to pay up to $1 per Lemon, a price considered costly today and extremely expensive back in 1849. It wasn't until vitamin C was discovered in 1932 that researchers found it was not the fruits themselves, but the vitamin, that provided protection against the disease. Limes are native to the East Indies and can be found in tropical and subtropical areas around the world. Lemons are a cross between a Lime and a citron, native to either China or India, and have been cultivated for over 2,500 years. In the 18th century, the British navy ordered ships to carry Limes to prevent scurvy, and British sailors became known as "limeys." Both Lemons and Limes are powerhouses in their ability to enhance the flavor of other foods, so I encourage you use Lemons and Limes to enrich the flavor of your favorite "Healthiest Way of Cooking" recipes.

# lemons and limes

## highlights

| | |
|---|---|
| AVAILABILITY: | Year-round |
| REFRIGERATE: | Yes |
| SHELF LIFE: | 10 days refrigerated |
| PREPARATION: | Minimal |
| BEST WAY TO ENJOY: | As a flavor enhancer |

## why lemons and limes should be part of your healthiest way of eating

Lemons and Limes contain unique flavonoid phytonutrients, such as hesperitin and naringenin, which have been found to have powerful antioxidant properties and promote a healthy heart. They are also renowned as excellent sources of vitamin C, the primary water-soluble antioxidant in the body, which helps protect against the oxidative damage caused by free-radicals. Lemons and Limes are an ideal food to add to your "Healthiest Way of Eating" not only because they are nutritious and add great flavor to many dishes, but also because they are low in calories: 1/4 cup of fresh Lemon juice contains only 15 calories! (For more on the *Health Benefits of Lemons and Limes* and a complete analysis of their content of over 60 nutrients, see page 432.)

## varieties of lemons and limes

### Lemons

Lemons are scientifically known as *Citrus limon*. While most Lemons are tart, acidic and astringent, they are also surprisingly refreshing. Lemons are classified as either sour or sweet.

### SOUR LEMONS

Sour Lemons include: Eureka Lemons, which have textured skin, a short neck at one end and few seeds; and Lisbon Lemons, which have smoother skin, no neck and are generally seedless.

### SWEET LEMONS

Sweet Lemons include Meyer Lemons, a cross between a

Lemon and either an orange or mandarin. They have orange-yellow flesh and thin, smooth skin.

## Limes

Limes *(Citrus aurantifolia)* are a small citrus fruit and also come in sour and sweet varieties. Sour Limes contain citric acid, giving them an acidic, tart taste, while sweet Limes lack citric acid and are sweet in flavor. Sweet Limes are not readily available in the United States.

### SOUR LIMES

The sour Limes most commonly found in markets, Tahitian Limes, come in two varieties: Persian Limes, which are grown in Florida and are oval, egg-sized fruits, and Bearss Limes, which are grown in California, are smaller than Persian Limes and are seedless.

Key Limes or Mexican Limes are also sour Limes. They are rounder and more yellow than Tahitian Limes. They have a higher acid content and are most renowned as an ingredient for Key Lime pie.

### SWEET LIMES

They have lower sugar content than sour Limes but no acidity.

## the peak season

Lemons are available year-round with seasonal peaks around May, June and August. Limes are also available year-round but are in peak season from May through October. These are the months when their concentration of nutrients and flavor are highest, and their cost is at its lowest.

## biochemical considerations

Lemon and Lime peels are a concentrated source of oxalates, which may be of concern to some individuals. Commercially available Lemon and Lime juice may contain sulfite preservatives. Conventionally grown Lemons and Limes often have a wax coating to help protect their surface and increase their shelf life. Avoiding the wax and the other compounds used on Lemons and Limes is just one of the reasons to choose organically grown Lemons and Limes. (For more on *Oxalates*, see page 725; *Sulfites*, see page 729; and *Wax Coatings*, see page 732.)

## 3 steps for the best tasting and most nutritious lemons and limes

Enjoying the best tasting Lemons and Limes with the most nutrients is simple if you just follow my 3 easy steps:
1. The Best Way to Select
2. The Best Way to Store
3. The Best Way to Prepare

# 1. the best way to select lemons and limes

As with all fruits, I recommend selecting organically grown varieties of Lemons and Limes whenever possible. (For more on *Organic Foods*, see page 113.)

## Lemons

You can select the best quality Lemons by looking for ones that are fully ripe and heavy for their size with smooth, thin skin. Lemons that give slightly under gentle pressure are usually juicier. Fully ripe Lemons are yellow in color with no green tinge to their skin. An unripe Lemon with a green tinge will be more acidic in flavor. Lemons with thicker peels have less flesh and less juice. Avoid overly mature Lemons that are wrinkled, have soft or hard patches, or are dull in color.

## Limes

The best way to select Limes is to look for ones that are heavy for their size, give slightly to gentle pressure and are free of decay and mold. They should have a glossy skin that is deep green in color. Although Limes turn more yellow as they ripen, they are at the height of their lively, tart flavor when they are green. While a few brown spots on the skin will not affect their taste, it is best to avoid Limes that are primarily brown in color as this is an indication of "scald," which may give them an undesirable moldy taste.

### How Do You Know Which Lemons and Limes are Ready to Use?

Lemons that are heavy for their size with smooth skins that are fully yellow in color will have the most juice and best flavor. Limes are best when they are heavy for their size, give slightly to gentle pressure and are deep green in color.

# 2. the best way to store lemons and limes

### Fresh Lemons Can Last Up to 10 Days and Fresh Limes Can Last Up to 7 Days When Properly Stored and Refrigerated

Lemons and Limes continue to respire even after they have been harvested. The faster they respire, the more the Lemons and Limes interact with air to produce carbon dioxide. The more carbon dioxide produced, the more quickly they will spoil. Lemons kept at a room temperature of approximately 68°F (20°C) give off carbon dioxide at a rate of 24 mg per kilogram every hour, while Limes kept at this temperature give off carbon dioxide at a rate over 24 mg per kilogram every hour. (For a *Comparison of Respiration Rates* for different fruits, see page 341.) Refrigeration helps slow the respiration rate of ripe Lemons and Limes, retain their vitamin content and increase their storage life.

Avoid storing Lemons and Limes in sealed plastic bags or restricted spaces where they are in too close proximity to each other. The resulting limited oxygen exchange and trapping of excessive amounts of ethylene gas naturally produced by the Lemons and Limes will cause them to rot.

Fresh Lemons are juicier when kept at room temperature and will keep for 5 days if not refrigerated. If you are not going to use your Lemons within a few days after purchase, it is best to refrigerate them where they will store for up to 10 days. Even when refrigerated, Meyer Lemons will keep for only 5 days. It is best to refrigerate any Limes that you are not going to use the day you purchase them as they will spoil quickly at room temperature. While Limes that are stored properly will remain fresh for up to 7 days, if they are not stored properly they will only last about 3 days.

### How to Ripen Lemons and Limes

Lemons and Limes will not get sweet and juicy after they have been picked. They can get softer at home, but never sweeter or juicer. Lemons and Limes must be picked or purchased ripe.

### How to Store Lemon and Lime Juice and Zest

Lemon and Lime juice and zest can also be stored for later use. Place freshly squeezed Lemon or Lime juice in ice cube trays until frozen and then store the cubes in plastic bags in the freezer. Dried Lemon or Lime zest should be stored in a cool and dry place in an airtight glass container.

# 3. the best way to prepare lemons and limes

Properly preparing Lemons and Limes helps ensure that they will have the best flavor and retain the greatest number of nutrients.

### Cleaning Lemons and Limes

Rinse Lemons and Limes under cold running water before cutting. (For more on *Washing Fruit*, see page 341.)

### Cutting and Juicing Lemons and Limes

Lemons and Limes, like most citrus fruits, will produce more juice when they are not cold, so always juice them

*(Continued on Page 433)*

---

### An Easy Way to Prepare Lemons and Limes, Step-by-Step

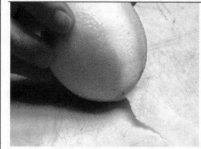 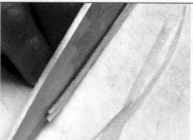 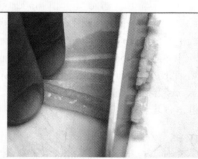

CHOPPED LEMON RIND

❶ With a sharp knife cut between the Lemon peel and white membrane of the Lemon. You will have thin pieces of Lemon peel. ❷ Cut Lemon peel lengthwise into thin strips. ❸ Cut across strips for chopped rind.

STEP-BY-STEP
**No Bake Recipes**

# 10-Minute Lime Coconut Cooler

*This creamy refreshing beverage is wonderful with any of your favorite Asian recipes.*

1 cup canned coconut milk (not non-fat)
1/4 cup Lime juice (1-2 Limes)
1/3 cup mint leaves plus mint leaves
   for garnish
4 TBS honey
2 cups cracked or crushed ice

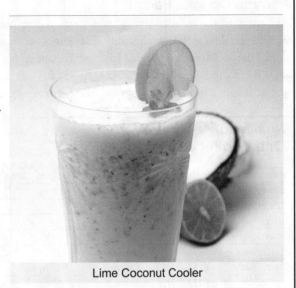

Lime Coconut Cooler

1. Place all ingredients, except the ice, in a blender and run on medium speed until the honey is dissolved and the liquid is well blended (about 1 minute).

2. Add ice and blend on medium speed for about 5 seconds, until it has the consistency of shaved ice.

3. Pour into two chilled glasses and serve garnished with mint.

**Preparation Hint:** To crack ice for easier blending, wrap ice cubes in a tea towel and cover them well. Hit with a mallet or the back of a heavy knife until all the cubes are in small pieces.

**SERVES 2**

## Variations...

• Add sliced banana for a richer beverage.

• Try substituting Lemon juice for the Lime juice.

# Quick Lemon Sauce*

*A versatile sauce that is quick and easy to prepare and complements many types of fruits!*

3 TBS cream honey**
2 tsp Lemon juice
1 tsp Lemon zest***

1. Mix all ingredients in a small mixing bowl.

2. Spoon over fresh fruit or low-fat yogurt.

3. Squeeze Lime or Lemon juice and a few drops of tamari (soy sauce) onto avocado slices and enjoy.

* Quick Lemon Sauce may also be made with lime.

** Cream honey is whipped honey found in most health food stores.

*** Use organic Lemons, if possible, to avoid wax coating.

Please write (address on back cover flap) or e-mail me at info@whfoods.org with your personal ideas for preparing Lemons and Limes, and I will share them with others through our website at www.whfoods.org.

## 5 QUICK SERVING IDEAS for LEMONS AND LIMES:

1. Sprinkle Lemon juice over spinach and other iron-rich vegetables since its vitamin C will help to make the iron more absorbable.

2. If you are watching your salt intake (and even if you are not), serve Lemon or Lime wedges with meals as their tartness makes a great salt substitute.

3. Squeeze some Lime juice and a few drops of tamari (soy sauce) onto avocado slices and enjoy.

4. **Brown Rice with a Zing:** Add an easy-to-prepare zing to dinner tonight by tossing seasoned cooked brown rice with garden peas, chicken pieces, scallions, pumpkin seeds, Lime juice and Lime zest.

5. **Refreshing Lemonade:** Stir together 2 TBS fresh Lemon juice and 2 TBS maple syrup in a glass. Fill glass with 6 oz of water, add ice cubes, and garnish with mint and a Lemon slice.

# health benefits of lemons and limes

## Promote Optimal Health

Like many of the fruits and vegetables found among the World's Healthiest Foods, Lemons and Limes contain unique flavonoid compounds that have antioxidant properties. The antibiotic effects of these flavonoids are of special interest. In several villages in West Africa where cholera epidemics had occurred, the inclusion of Lime juice during the main meal of the day was found to have been protective against the contraction of cholera, a disease triggered by *Vibrio cholera* bacteria.

Additionally, Lemons and Limes are also excellent sources of vitamin C, which is vital to the function of a strong immune system. The immune system's main goal is to protect you from illness, so a little extra vitamin C may be useful in conditions like colds, flus and recurrent ear infections.

## Promote Heart Health

Vitamin C is one of the main antioxidants found in food and the primary water-soluble antioxidant in the body. Vitamin C travels through the body neutralizing any free-radicals with which it comes into contact in the aqueous environments in the body, both inside and outside cells. Since free-radicals can damage blood vessels and can change cholesterol to make it more likely to build up in artery walls, vitamin C can be helpful for preventing the development and progression of atherosclerosis and diabetic heart disease. Lemons and Limes may also provide protection from cerebrovascular diseases (such as strokes) because they contain flavonoid phytonutrients, such as hesperitin and naringenin, whose intake has been associated with lower incidence of these diseases.

## Promote Respiratory Health

Lemons and Limes may help support lung health since they are a concentrated source of both vitamin C and flavonoids. Since free-radicals are responsible for causing smooth muscle contraction and airway constriction in asthma, having extra supplies of vitamin C, with its antioxidant ability, on hand can be helpful. Vitamin C also helps breakdown histamine, an inflammatory chemical produced by overly reactive immune cells. Studies have shown that people with low levels of vitamin C in their diets are at a much greater risk—as much as five times greater—of reacting to pollutants in the air. Research also suggests that higher intake of the flavonoids naringenin, hesperitin and quercetin is related to a lower incidence of asthma.

## Additional Health-Promoting Benefits of Lemons and Limes

Since Lemons and Limes can be used to add flavor to many dishes yet are low in calories (one quarter cup of Lemon and Lime juice contains only 15 calories), they are ideal foods for healthy weight control.

### Nutritional Analysis of One-quarter cup Lemon Juice:

| NUTRIENT | AMOUNT | % DAILY VALUE | NUTRIENT | AMOUNT | % DAILY VALUE |
|---|---|---|---|---|---|
| Calories | 15.25 | | Pantothenic Acid | 0.07 mg | 0.70 |
| Calories from Fat | 0.00 | | | | |
| Calories from Saturated Fat | 0.00 | | **Minerals** | | |
| Protein | 0.23 g | | Boron | — mcg | |
| Carbohydrates | 5.27 g | | Calcium | 4.27 mg | 0.43 |
| Dietary Fiber | 0.25 g | 1.00 | Chloride | — mg | |
| Soluble Fiber | 0.12 g | | Chromium | — mcg | — |
| Insoluble Fiber | 0.13 g | | Copper | 0.02 mg | 1.00 |
| Sugar - Total | 2.08 g | | Fluoride | — mg | — |
| Monosaccharides | 1.28 g | | Iodine | — mcg | — |
| Disaccharides | 0.19 g | | Iron | 0.02 mg | 0.11 |
| Other Carbs | 2.95 g | | Magnesium | 3.66 mg | 0.92 |
| Fat - Total | 0.00 g | | Manganese | 0.01 mg | 0.50 |
| Saturated Fat | 0.00 g | | Molybdenum | — mcg | — |
| Mono Fat | 0.00 g | | Phosphorus | 3.66 mg | 0.37 |
| Poly Fat | 0.00 g | | Potassium | 75.64 mg | |
| Omega-3 Fatty Acids | 0.00 g | 0.00 | Selenium | 0.06 mcg | 0.09 |
| Omega-6 Fatty Acids | 0.00 g | | Sodium | 0.61 mg | |
| Trans Fatty Acids | 0.00 g | | Zinc | 0.03 mg | 0.20 |
| Cholesterol | 0.00 mg | | | | |
| Water | 55.35 g | | **Amino Acids** | | |
| Ash | 0.16 g | | Alanine | 0.02 g | |
| | | | Arginine | 0.02 g | |
| **Vitamins** | | | Aspartate | 0.03 g | |
| Vitamin A IU | 12.20 IU | 0.24 | Cystine | 0.01 g | 2.44 |
| Vitamin A RE | 1.22 RE | | Glutamate | 0.03 g | |
| A - Carotenoid | 1.22 RE | 0.02 | Glycine | 0.02 g | |
| A - Retinol | 0.00 RE | | Histidine | 0.01 g | 0.78 |
| B1 Thiamin | 0.02 mg | 1.33 | Isoleucine | 0.01 g | 0.87 |
| B2 Riboflavin | 0.01 mg | 0.59 | Leucine | 0.01 g | 0.40 |
| B3 Niacin | 0.06 mg | 0.30 | Lysine | 0.01 g | 0.43 |
| Niacin Equiv | 0.08 mg | | Methionine | 0.01 g | 1.35 |
| Vitamin B6 | 0.03 mg | 1.50 | Phenylalanine | 0.01 g | 0.84 |
| Vitamin B12 | 0.00 mcg | 0.00 | Proline | 0.01 g | |
| Biotin | 0.19 mcg | 0.06 | Serine | 0.01 g | |
| Vitamin C | 28.06 mg | 46.77 | Threonine | 0.01 g | 0.81 |
| Vitamin D IU | 0.00 IU | 0.00 | Tryptophan | 0.00 g | 0.00 |
| Vitamin D mcg | 0.00 mcg | | Tyrosine | 0.01 g | 1.03 |
| Vitamin E Alpha Equiv | 0.06 mg | 0.30 | Valine | 0.01 g | 0.68 |
| Vitamin E IU | 0.08 IU | | | | |
| Vitamin E mg | 0.14 mg | | | | |
| Folate | 7.87 mcg | 1.97 | | | |
| Vitamin K | 0.00 mcg | 0.00 | | | |

(Note: "–" indicates data is unavailable. For more information, please see page 806.)

*(Continued from Page 430)*

when they are at room temperature. Rolling Lemons and Limes under the palm of your hand on a flat surface will also help to extract more juice.

Cut the Lemons and Limes in half and remove the visible seeds from the fruit before juicing or remove them from the juice after you are done juicing.

The juice can be extracted in a variety of ways. You can use a juicer or reamer. Or you can do it the old fashioned way, squeezing by hand.

## Grated Zest

Using a hand grater, grate the skin of the Lemon or Lime, being careful to avoid the white membrane beneath the peel as it is bitter. Scrape the grated zest off the underside of the grater. If the recipe calls for Lemon or Lime zest (or rind), make sure that you use fruit that is organically grown since most conventionally grown fruits will have pesticide residues on their skin and Lemons and Limes are often coated with wax. If you use conventionally grown Lemon or Lime to make zest for your tea, you may find wax residues floating on top.

## Chopped Rind

With a sharp knife, cut thin strips of peel from the Lemon or Lime, avoiding as much of the white membrane beneath the peel as possible as it is bitter. Use a rocking motion with a chef's knife and chop peel.

## Minced Rind

Use the same method as in chopped rind, but chop peel very fine.

## No Bake Recipes

I have discovered that Lemons and Limes retain their maximum amount of nutrients and their best taste when they are enjoyed fresh and not prepared in a cooked recipe. That is because their nutrients—including vitamins, anti-oxidants and enzymes—are unable to withstand the temperature (350°F/175°C) used in baking. So that you can get the most enjoyment and benefit from fruit, I created quick and easy recipes, which require no cooking. I call them "No Bake Recipes."

---

### HEALTH BENEFITS OF LEMON/LIME PEELS

The colored part of Lemons and Limes contain d-limonene, a flavonoid phytonutrient that acts as a powerful antioxidant and helps prevent oxidative damage to cell structures and DNA. The white pithy portion under the skin also contains flavonoids that help lower LDL ("bad") cholesterol. Be sure to use organically grown Lemons or Limes to make zest to avoid wax and pesticide residues. While zest adds great flavor to recipes, it can be a stomach irritant for some individuals if consumed in large quantities.

---

Here are questions that I received from readers of the whfoods.org website about Lemons:

## Q *Are Lemons considered acidic?*

A The idea of acidic foods is confusing because it doesn't necessarily mean that the food itself is acidic (i.e., has a low chemical pH level), but that the food decreases the pH levels in our digestive tract when we eat it. Lemons are a good example of this. They are an acidic food (have a low pH of about 2) that makes the body more alkaline. In other words, they have the effect of increasing the pH in the body when we eat them. In general, animal foods are viewed as more acid-forming and less alkalizing than plant foods. Fruits and vegetables are considered alkalizing in comparison with other foods groups (rutabagas and cranberries are exceptions).

## Q *Is there anything special I need to do if I want to freeze fresh Lemon juice?*

A There is nothing special you need to do to freeze fresh-squeezed Lemon juice, although I have found that it is very convenient to freeze it in ice cube trays so that I can have easy access to small amounts of the juice. After the cubes have frozen, place them in plastic freezer bags. The juice will retain its flavor for about 3 months when frozen.

## Q *Does Lemon help in reducing body weight?*

A No, Lemon or its juice does not help reduce body weight. Lemon can act as a diuretic and increase elimination of water from the body, but the water balance in our body is constantly shifting and is supposed to shift according to our physiological needs. It's the excess fat stored on our body that we want to get rid of when we lose weight—not the body water that usually accounts for about 60% of our total body weight and that keeps our cells and organ systems healthy.

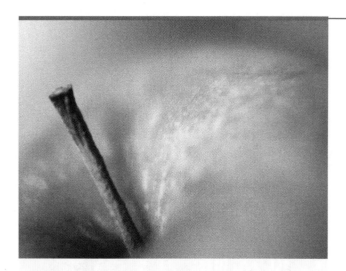

# apples

| | |
|---|---|
| AVAILABILITY: | Year-round |
| REFRIGERATE: | Yes |
| SHELF LIFE: | 1 week refrigerated |
| PREPARATION: | Minimal |
| BEST WAY TO ENJOY: | Enjoy them raw |

## nutrient-richness chart

Total Nutrient-Richness: **3**          GI: **53**
One (138 grams) fresh Apple contains 81 calories

| NUTRIENT | AMOUNT | %DV | DENSITY | QUALITY |
|---|---|---|---|---|
| Dietary Fiber | 3.7 g | 14.9 | 3.3 | good |
| Vitamin C | 7.9 mg | 13.1 | 2.9 | good |
| **CAROTENOIDS:** | | | | |
| Beta-Carotene | 37.3 mcg | | | |
| Beta-Cryptoxanthin | 15.2 mcg | | | |
| **FLAVONOIDS:** | | | | |
| (+)-Catechin | 1.3 mg | | | |
| (-)-Epicatechin | 11.2 mg | | | |
| Quercetin | 6.1 mg | | | |
| **PHYTOSTEROLS:** | | | | |
| Phytosterols—Total | 16.6 mg | | | |

Daily values for these nutrients have not yet been established.

For more on "Total Nutrient-Richness" "%DV," "Density," and
The World's Healthiest Foods "Quality" Rating System, see page 805.

For more on GI, see page 342.

Apples were the favorite fruit of the ancient Greeks and Romans, and their popularity has not diminished—the average American consumes 65 fresh Apples each year! Historically, they have been called the "forbidden fruit," the "fruit of knowledge" and in Norse mythology, "the fruit that promised everlasting youth." Today, "An Apple a day keeps the doctor away" is a popular adage that reflects their valuable contribution to our "Healthiest Way of Eating." The original colonists who migrated to North America planted the first Apples here in the early 1600s. Yet, it was Johnny Appleseed, a real person named John Chapman—who walked barefoot across an area of 100,000 square miles in the 1800s planting Apple trees—to whom we often give credit for ensuring that subsequent generations had plenty of these delicious fruits to enjoy.

## why apples should be part of your healthiest way of eating

Apples are especially rich in antioxidant nutrients, including flavonoid and phenolic antioxidants and vitamin C. They also contain plenty of soluble and insoluble fiber. Apples are not only fun to eat, but are also easy to pack, making them a quick, convenient snack addition to your "Healthiest Way of Eating." They are also low in calories: one medium Apple contains 81 calories. (For more on the *Health Benefits of Apples* and a complete analysis of their content of over 60 nutrients, see page 439.)

## varieties of apples

The Apple is actually a member of the rose family (*Rosaceae*), with a compartmentalized core that classifies it as a pome fruit. In Latin "pome" means "Apple." Apples are crisp, white-fleshed fruits with red, yellow or green skin. Depending on the variety, they can be moderately sweet and refreshing or have a pleasant degree of tartness. Over 7,500 varieties of Apples are grown throughout the world, but only a small percentage of them are of commercial importance. Eight varieties represent 80% of the current market in the United States. The following are a few of the most popular varieties in the United States.

### Varieties Best Eaten Raw Include:

#### RED DELICIOUS
This bright red Apple is available year-round and is the most popular variety in the United States. It has thin, tough skin with flesh that is crisp, juicy and sweet. It is best eaten raw. Its flavor and texture do not hold up well when cooked.

### FUJI

Crisp and sweet, these large, green-red Apples are usually eaten raw. They are available year-round.

### GALA

Sweet, orange-yellow colored Apples that are great addition to salads. They are available year-round.

## Varieties Enjoyed Both Raw and Cooked:

### GOLDEN DELICIOUS

A variety distinct from the Red Delicious, this golden yellow, freckled fruit is great eaten raw, makes delicious Applesauce and is also suitable for baking a delicious Apple pie. Because Golden Delicious Apples are slower to brown than other varieties when sliced, they are a welcome addition to salads. This Apple is a favorite in Europe and is available year-round.

### GRANNY SMITH

Originally from Australia, they are green Apples that are now widely grown on the West Coast of the United States. Notably brisk and tart, they are often the preferred variety for cooked desserts like Apple pie because they retain their shape and texture. They are available year-round. This is the variety featured in the photograph on the first page of this chapter.

### MCINTOSH

Grown in the East and Midwest, these green-red Apples are very juicy and slightly tart. They can be enjoyed raw or cooked. They are in season from September through March.

### JONATHAN

Jonathans are smaller Apples that have a vibrant red color with yellow undertones. They can be enjoyed raw, cooked in pies or made into Applesauce. They are in season September through March.

### PIPPIN

Large greenish-yellow Apples with a red blush. They are great for making Apple butter, jelly and cider.

### BRAEBURN

With a red hue layered over a yellow skin tone, Braeburn Apples have a flavor that blends both sweet and tart. They are an excellent choice for salads, pies and sauces.

## Varieties Used Primarily for Cooking:

### ROME BEAUTY

These red Apples are prized for baking because they hold their shape and retain their flavor well when baked but are rather bland and mealy when eaten raw. They are in season from October through July.

### CRAB APPLES

This tiny variety of Apple (about the size of a large cherry tomato) is rarely eaten fresh. They are, however, popular for making jellies and Apple butter because of their high pectin content.

# the peak season

In the Northern Hemisphere, Apple season begins at the end of summer and lasts until early winter. These are the months when their concentration of nutrients and flavor are highest, and their cost is at its lowest. Apples available at other times have been in cold storage or are imported from the Southern Hemisphere.

# biochemical considerations

Apples are one of the 12 foods on which pesticide residues have been most frequently found. Conventionally grown varieties also usually have a wax coating to help protect their surface and increase shelf life. To avoid both pesticide residues and the wax coating on Apples, purchase organically grown varieties whenever possible. Dried Apples may be treated with sulfites, which may be problematic for some individuals.

## NEW SCIENTIFIC FINDINGS

### ANTIOXIDANTS FOUND IN APPLE SKINS

The health benefits of Apples do not just come from the fiber, vitamins and minerals they provide but also from their flavonoid phytonutrients, which act as powerful antioxidants. These include quercetin and other polyphenolic compounds that contribute significantly to the total antioxidant activity of Apples, with the peel of the Apple providing greater concentrations of quercetin than the flesh. The concentration of polyphenols in Apples varies between the different varieties with Red Delicious and Northern Spy having the higher concentration and Empire having lower concentrations. One special flavonoid, cyanidin 3-galactoside, is found only in red Apple peels; it has strong antioxidant activity, with laboratory research showing its ability to inhibit the oxidation of LDL cholesterol.

The benefits derived from Apples are attributed to the complex mixture of phytonutrients in the whole fruit, which work together synergistically to provide potent antioxidant protection.

Apples are also one of the foods most commonly associated with allergic reactions in individuals with latex allergies. (For more on *Pesticide Residues*, see page 726; *Wax Coatings*, see page 732; *Sulfites*, see page 729; and *Latex Food Allergies*, see page 722.)

### Poisonous Seeds

Apple seeds, like many fruit seeds, contain compounds called cyanogenic glycosides; when broken down, these compounds can release small amounts of cyanide. While Apple seeds have lower levels than other fruits (like prune and peach pits), they could still pose problems in terms of stomachache or food poisoning. A few seeds chewed by small child could result in poisoning. While the severity of this problem would depend upon many factors, including the person's health, I don't think that the potential risk of eating the seeds is worth taking.

## 3 steps for the best tasting and most nutritious apples

Enjoying the best tasting Apples with the most nutrients is simple if you just follow my 3 easy steps:
1. The Best Way to Select
2. The Best Way to Store
3. The Best Way to Prepare

# 1. the best way to select apples

For the best tasting Apples and those that feature the maximal concentration of vitamins, antioxidants and enzymes, look for ones that are fully ripe. Fully ripe Apples are heavy and firm; they have vibrant color and a fresh aroma. Smelling Apples when you purchase them is a good way to find ones that are fresh and ripe. I have found that yellow and green Apples are best with a slight blush, and heavier Apples have more moisture and therefore are less likely to have a mealy texture. By selecting the best tasting Apples, you will also be getting Apples with the highest nutritional value. As with all fruits, I recommend selecting organically grown Apples at the peak of their season whenever possible. (For more on *Organic Foods*, see page 113.)

Avoid overripe Apples and ones that are bruised. Overripe Apples are usually very light and will have a mealy texture.

### How Do You Know Which Apples are Ready to Eat?

If Apples are heavy and firm with a vibrant color and fresh aroma they are ready to eat.

# 2. the best way to store apples

Proper storage is an important step in keeping Apples fresh and preserving their nutrients, texture and unique flavor.

### Fresh Ripe Apples Can Last for Up to 7 Days When Properly Stored and Refrigerated

Apples continue to respire even after they have been harvested. The faster they respire, the more the Apples interact with air to produce carbon dioxide. The more carbon dioxide produced, the more quickly they will spoil. Apples kept at a room temperature of approximately 68°F (20°C) give off carbon dioxide at a rate of 20 mg per kilogram every hour. (For a *Comparison of Respiration Rates* for different fruits, see page 341.) Refrigeration helps slow the respiration rate of ripe Apples, retain their vitamin content and increase their storage life.

Keep as many ripe Apples at room temperature as you will be able to consume in a day or two. Store the rest in the refrigerator. While Apples that are stored properly will remain fresh for up to 7 days, if they are not stored properly, they will only last about 3 days.

### How to Ripen Apples

Apples will become sweet and juicy at home if they have not been picked too green. Apples are best if they are ripe before they are picked, but if the apples you purchase are tart (or are red and yellow Apples, but have green tints to them), you can ripen them by placing them in a paper bag. This is a very natural way to ripen Apples. The paper bag traps the ethylene gas produced by the Apples. The ethylene gas helps the Apples to ripen more quickly, while the paper bag allows for healthy oxygen exchange through the bag. Keep the bag in a dark, cool, well-ventilated place, and the Apples will get sweeter and more flavorful in a few days; excessive heat, however, will cause the Apples to rot rather than ripen. Avoid storing Apples in sealed plastic bags or restricted spaces where they touch each other. The combination of limited oxygen exchange

*(Continued on Page 438)*

STEP-BY-STEP
## No Bake Recipes

# 5-Minute Apple Treats

*Fresh, crisp Apples are a perfect snack any time of day.*

**1 Apple, sliced 1/2-inch thick, unpeeled**
**4 TBS almond butter**
**Cinnamon to taste**
**1/4 cup granola**

1. Spread one side of sliced Apple with almond butter and sprinkle with cinnamon.

2. Dip the Apple slices into granola to cover the almond butter.

   Use sweet Delicious, tart Granny Smith, tangy Fuji or your favorite variety of Apple; in seconds, you'll have a satisfying snack or dessert.

**SERVES 2**

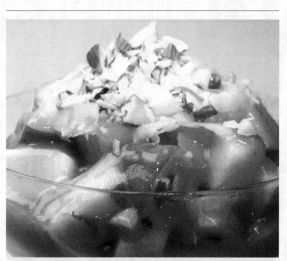

Apple Sundae

# 10-Minute Apple Sundae

*This is a wonderful way to start the day or end a meal.*

**2 Apples**
**2 TBS almond butter**
**1/4 cup maple syrup**
**1½ tsp almond extract**
**2 TBS chopped almonds**
**2 TBS grated coconut**

1. Coarsely chop almonds and set aside for topping.

2. In a small mixing bowl, blend the almond butter, maple syrup and almond extract until smooth. It should be the consistency of caramel sauce.

3. Cut the Apples into quarters and core. Then cut the quarters into 3 pieces lengthwise and 1/4-inch pieces crosswise. Place in two serving bowls.

4. Drizzle the sauce over the two bowls of Apples and top with almonds and coconut.

**SERVES 2**

## Variations...

- Use different varieties of Apples such as Golden Delicious, Granny Smith and Braeburn for a mixture of taste and color.
- Use the sauce on other fresh fruit such as apricots or pears.
- For breakfast, top Apples with ground flaxseeds before adding the sauce.

Please write (address on back cover flap) or e-mail me at info@whfoods.org with your personal ideas for preparing Apples, and I will share them with others through our website at www.whfoods.org.

## 6 QUICK SERVING IDEAS for APPLES:

1. Apples make great on-the-go snacks. They are easy to carry and refreshing to eat.
2. Sliced Apples (either alone or with other fruit) and cheese are a European favorite when it comes to dessert.
3. Add diced Apples to fruit or green salads.
4. Combine diced Apple, low-fat yogurt, chopped walnuts, raisins and honey for breakfast or a snack.
5. Tart Apples combine well with dark greens (spinach, arugula, kale) and sharp cheeses in salads.
6. **Apple-Carrot Salad:** Combine 1 diced medium Apple, 1 shredded medium carrot, 1/2 cup diced pineapple and 1/4 cup raisins for a great tasting salad.

*(Continued from Page 436)*

and the excessive amounts of ethylene gas produced under these conditions will cause them to rot. Don't refrigerate your Apples until they are ripe; they will not ripen in the refrigerator.

### How to Speed Up the Ripening of Apples

Adding a banana or avocado to the bag with the Apples will increase the amount of ethylene gas trapped in the bag. The increased amount of gas will hasten the ripening process.

### Is It Best to Refrigerate Your Apples After Ripening?

Yes. They will keep in the refrigerator for up to 7 days.

### Handle with Care

Be careful not to bruise Apples as this will result in loss of some of their nutritional value.

# 3. the best way to prepare apples

Properly preparing Apples helps ensure that they will have the best flavor and retain the greatest number of nutrients.

### Cleaning Apples

Rinse your Apples under cold running water. (For more on *Washing Fruit*, see page 341.)

### How to Keep Apples from Turning Brown

Once Apples are cut, the enzymes in the flesh will oxidize, causing them to turn brown. To prevent Apples from turning brown, prepare a bowl of water large enough to hold the quantity of Apples you will be slicing. For every 2 cups of water, add 2 TBS of fresh lemon juice. Add Apple slices to the lemon and water solution as you cut them. When you are done slicing, use a colander to strain the Apples.

### Cooking Apples

Some Apples are best used for cooking. If you are going to cook Apples, good choices include Granny Smith, McIntosh, Jonathan and Rome Apples. Apples can be poached, baked or made into a sauce. Vanilla, cinnamon, clove and almond flavoring complement the flavor of Apples.

### No Bake Recipes

I have discovered that Apples retain their maximum amount of nutrients and their best taste when they are fresh and not prepared in a cooked recipe. That is because their nutrients—including vitamins, antioxidants and enzymes—are unable to withstand the temperature (350°F/175°C) used in baking. So that you can get the most enjoyment and benefit from fruit, I created quick and easy recipes, which require no cooking. I call them "No Bake Recipes."

**Q** *Does Apple juice provide the same nutritional benefits as Apples?*

**A** Unfortunately, Apple juice does not provide the same range of nutritional benefits as do Apples. Not only does it contain none of the fiber in which Apples are so rich, but processing Apples into juice greatly lowers their phytonutrient content. A review article in the May 2004 edition of *Nutrition Journal* reported that Apple juice obtained from Jonagold Apples by pulping and straight pressing had only 10% of the antioxidant activity of fresh Apples, while juice obtained after pulp enzyming had only 3% of fresh Apples' antioxidant activity.

### An Easy Way to Prepare Apples, Step-By-Step

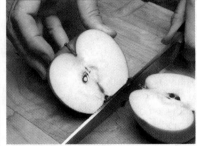 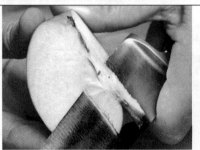 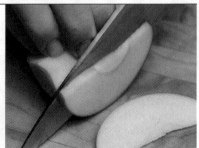

**SLICING APPLES**
❶ Cut Apples in half. ❷ Cut each half in half again and cut out core. ❸ Slice each quarter the thickness desired. Place in the bowl of lemon water as you slice.

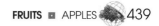

# health benefits of apples

## Provide Powerful Antioxidant Protection

Apples are a very important source of flavonoids and phenolic antioxidants. For example, in the United States, 22% of the phenolic compounds consumed from fruits come from Apples, making them the largest source of phenols in the American diet.

Apples are also a rich source of other antioxidants; when compared to many other commonly consumed fruits in the United States, they have been found to have the second highest level of antioxidant activity. Many of the antioxidants found in Apples, including quercetin, catechin, phloridzin and chlorogenic acid, have very powerful activity. In a study that measured the total antioxidant activity of Apples, 100 grams (about $3^1/2$ ounces) of whole Apple with peel was found to be equivalent in antioxidant effect to about 1,500 mg of vitamin C. Since the amount of vitamin C in 100 grams of Apples is only about 5.7 mg, this suggests that nearly all of Apples' antioxidant activity comes from a variety of other compounds, such as these flavonoid phytonutrients.

## Promote Heart Health

Apples' two types of fiber pack a double punch that can knock down cholesterol levels, reducing your risk of hardening of the arteries, heart attack, and stroke. Apples' insoluble fiber works like bran, latching onto LDL cholesterol in the digestive tract and removing it from the body, while Apples' soluble fiber, pectin, reduces the amount of LDL cholesterol produced in the liver. Adding just one large Apple (about 2/3 of a pound) to the daily diet has been shown to decrease serum cholesterol by 8–11%. Eating two large Apples a day has been found to lower cholesterol levels by up to 16%! A large-scale study confirmed that eating high-fiber foods, such as Apples, helps prevent heart disease. People eating the most fiber, 21 grams per day, had 12% less CHD (coronary heart disease) and 11% less CVD (cardiovascular disease) compared to those eating the least, 5 grams daily. Those eating the most water-soluble dietary fiber fared even better with a 15% reduction in risk of CHD and a 10% risk reduction in CVD.

Apples' flavonoids have been extensively researched and found to help prevent heart disease. A recent meta-analysis of seven prospective studies found that individuals whose diets most frequently included Apples, tea, onions, and broccoli—the richest sources of flavonoids—gained a 20% reduction in their risk of heart disease.

When it comes to heart health, one of the Apple flavonoids of greatest benefit is thought to be quercetin. Quercetin is a potent antioxidant, especially when it teams up with another antioxidant also found in Apples, vitamin C, to bolster the body's immune defenses. This dynamic antioxidant duo helps prevent the free-radical damage to LDL cholesterol that promotes heart disease. *(Continued on Page 440)*

## Nutritional Analysis of 1 Apple:

| NUTRIENT | AMOUNT | % DAILY VALUE | NUTRIENT | AMOUNT | % DAILY VALUE |
|---|---|---|---|---|---|
| Calories | 81.42 | | Pantothenic Acid | 0.08 mg | 0.80 |
| Calories from Fat | 4.47 | | | | |
| Calories from Saturated Fat | 0.72 | | **Minerals** | | |
| Protein | 0.26 g | | Boron | — mcg | |
| Carbohydrates | 21.05 g | | Calcium | 9.66 mg | 0.97 |
| Dietary Fiber | 3.73 g | 14.92 | Chloride | — mg | |
| Soluble Fiber | 1.42 g | | Chromium | — mcg | — |
| Insoluble Fiber | 2.30 g | | Copper | 0.06 mg | 3.00 |
| Sugar – Total | 16.56 g | | Fluoride | — mg | — |
| Monosaccharides | 11.45 g | | Iodine | — mcg | — |
| Disaccharides | 3.59 g | | Iron | 0.25 mg | 1.39 |
| Other Carbs | 0.76 g | | Magnesium | 6.90 mg | 1.73 |
| Fat – Total | 0.50 g | | Manganese | 0.06 mg | 3.00 |
| Saturated Fat | 0.08 g | | Molybdenum | — mcg | — |
| Mono Fat | 0.02 g | | Phosphorus | 9.66 mg | 0.97 |
| Poly Fat | 0.14 g | | Potassium | 158.70 mg | |
| Omega-3 Fatty Acids | 0.02 g | 0.80 | Selenium | 0.41 mcg | 0.59 |
| Omega-6 Fatty Acids | 0.12 g | | Sodium | 0.00 mg | |
| Trans Fatty Acids | 0.00 g | | Zinc | 0.06 mg | 0.40 |
| Cholesterol | 0.00 mg | | | | |
| Water | 115.82 g | | **Amino Acids** | | |
| Ash | 0.36 g | | Alanine | 0.01 g | |
| | | | Arginine | 0.01 g | |
| **Vitamins** | | | Aspartate | 0.05 g | |
| Vitamin A IU | 73.14 IU | 1.46 | Cystine | 0.00 g | 0.00 |
| Vitamin A RE | 6.90 RE | | Glutamate | 0.03 g | |
| A - Carotenoid | 6.90 RE | 0.09 | Glycine | 0.01 g | |
| A - Retinol | 0.00 RE | | Histidine | 0.00 g | 0.00 |
| B1 Thiamin | 0.02 mg | 1.33 | Isoleucine | 0.01 g | 0.87 |
| B2 Riboflavin | 0.02 mg | 1.18 | Leucine | 0.02 g | 0.79 |
| B3 Niacin | 0.11 mg | 0.55 | Lysine | 0.02 g | 0.85 |
| Niacin Equiv | 0.15 mg | | Methionine | 0.00 g | 0.00 |
| Vitamin B6 | 0.07 mg | 3.50 | Phenylalanine | 0.01 g | 0.84 |
| Vitamin B12 | 0.00 mcg | 0.00 | Proline | 0.01 g | |
| Biotin | 1.73 mcg | 0.58 | Serine | 0.01 g | |
| Vitamin C | 7.87 mg | 13.12 | Threonine | 0.01 g | 0.81 |
| Vitamin D IU | 0.00 IU | 0.00 | Tryptophan | 0.00 g | 0.00 |
| Vitamin D mcg | 0.00 mcg | | Tyrosine | 0.01 g | 1.03 |
| Vitamin E Alpha Equiv | 0.44 mg | 2.20 | Valine | 0.01 g | 0.68 |
| Vitamin E IU | 0.66 IU | | | | |
| Vitamin E mg | 0.91 mg | | | | |
| Folate | 3.86 mcg | 0.97 | | | |
| Vitamin K | 3.00 mcg | 3.75 | | | |

(Note: "—" indicates data is unavailable. For more information, please see page 806.)

*(Continued from Page 439)*

Apples' protective effects against free-radical damage to cholesterol have been found to reach their peak at three hours following Apple consumption and drop off after 24 hours, providing yet another good reason to eat a whole fresh Apple a day. As the research shows that both the flesh (which contains the pectin) and the skin (where the flavonoids, including quercetin, are concentrated) have health-promoting benefits, it is best to eat the whole fruit, skin and all.

## Promote Digestive Health

When it comes to bowel regularity, Apples' two types of fiber tackle the job—no matter what it is. Both the insoluble fiber in Apples and their soluble fiber pectin help relieve constipation. The insoluble fiber works like roughage, while the pectin, which is found primarily in the skin, acts as a stool softener by drawing water into the stool and increasing stool bulk. On the other hand, because pectin firms up an excessively loose stool, it's also used to treat diarrhea.

## Promote Lung Health

In several large epidemiological (population) studies conducted in the United Kingdom, Finland and the Netherlands, Apple consumption (a minimum of 2 Apples per week) was found to be inversely linked with asthma (as well as type 2 diabetes), and positively associated with general lung health. Researchers attribute Apples' protective effects in these conditions to Apples' high concentration of anti-inflammatory flavonoids, such as quercetin and catechins.

## Promote Optimal Health

New research suggests an innovative way that Apples may be able to promote optimal health—by regulating cell-to-cell communication. Researchers at the University of California, Davis, found that Apple extracts were able to protect cells from the effects of tumor necrosis factor—a compound that triggers cell death and promotes inflammation—by inhibiting the signals in its pathway that would otherwise damage or kill cells.

---

Here are questions that I received from readers of the whfoods.org website about Apples:

Q *Can you tell me a little bit about Apple cider vinegar. I was told that it is rich in minerals. Is that true?*

A The quality of a vinegar depends on how it was made and upon the ingredients used to make it. The highest-quality vinegars are made from fresh, organically grown fruits, including Apples. The sugars in these fruits make them good candidates for fermentation, and a bacterium called *Acetobacter* is usually used for the fermentation. (If you notice cloudy strands and translucent shapes floating in your vinegar, this is the *Acetobacter.*) Potassium, magnesium, phosphorus and calcium are some of the minerals that remain in the vinegar when it is produced in this way.

It would be wrong, however, to overemphasize the value of fermented cider vinegar when it comes to minerals alone. For example, there are less than 2 mg of calcium in a full ounce of fermented Apple cider vinegar. But there may be other benefits to high-quality vinegars. There is preliminary evidence in animals that vinegar may help calcium be better absorbed by rendering it more soluble. In humans, there is initial evidence that vinegar may help slow down the rate at which our stomachs pass food along to our intestines. This slowing down process may mean better control of our blood sugar when we are eating high-carbohydrate meals.

I prefer to purchase organically grown Apple cider vinegar that was made through a traditional fermentation process and that is unfiltered as it retains more nutrients when it is produced that way.

Q *What is the benefit of eating a whole Apple compared with one that has been peeled?*

A The peel of fruit provides special nutritional benefits, and Apples are no exception. Apple peel is a concentrated source of dietary fiber; in fact, Apples with peel have almost double the amount of fiber compared to ones that are peeled. The peel features most of the Apple's concentration of pectin, a type of insoluble fiber that helps to regulate proper digestion. In addition, Apple's flavonoid and phenolic antioxidants are found in much greater amounts in the peel than in the flesh; for example, the peel is rich in rutin, catechin and quercetin, the phytonutrient for which Apples have gained such great recent acclaim. Their benefits must be synergistic since when quercetin was tested by itself in laboratory animals, it had no protective effect. And when Apple flesh and Apple juice were tested, they provided less than a tenth the benefit of whole Apple. Try to buy organically grown Apples so that you can enjoy the whole Apple without having to worry about the pesticide residues and waxes found on the skin of their conventionally grown counterparts.

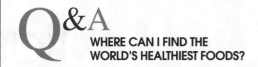

## Q&A

### WHERE CAN I FIND THE WORLD'S HEALTHIEST FOODS?

One of the great things about the World's Healthiest Foods is that they are not hard-to-find foods but ones that are widely available in a many different retail outlets. The abundance of shopping alternatives provides something for everyone as the different options also provide their own unique benefits and experiences. Here is an overview of some of the places where you can purchase the World's Healthiest Foods.

### Community supported agriculture (CSAs)

Community supported agriculture (CSAs) are a good resource for organically grown fruits, vegetables, herbs and dairy foods. CSAs are a partnership between food growers and consumers with consumers becoming members of a local farm. Membership money supports the operation of the farm and, in return, members receive a portion of the farm's food production on a continual basis (usually weekly) throughout the growing season. Since most CSA farmers use organic farming methods, joining a CSA is one way to ensure yourself access to delicious, fresh and nutritionally rich foods that can be enjoyed at the height of their growing season and the apex of their freshness and vitality. Plus, you will be supporting local farmers in their commitment to ecologically sound management of the land and the sustainable production of organically grown foods.

### Ethnic food stores

Since some of the World's Healthiest Foods have Asian, Indian and Latin American origins, ethnic food stores are a great place to shop for these foods. While many of these foods—tofu, lentils and certain herbs and spices—are commonly offered in supermarkets and natural foods stores, going to an ethnic food store still provides an enchanting experience for many people. Buying the World's Healthiest Foods at ethnic stores will provide you with the opportunity to explore other indigenous foods and spices and learn more about the traditional ways of preparing these healthy foods, expanding your repertoire of ingredients and recipes.

### Farmer's markets

While many people think of farmer's markets as a novelty place to shop, in fact they are one of the oldest and most traditional ways of buying food. Before the advent of roads, refrigeration and large-scale transportation that contributed to the establishment of supermarkets, most people bought their foods at community markets where farmers would gather to sell their fresh-from-the-field foods. Today, with the interest in fresh and natural foods, farmer's markets are booming, bringing together small family farmers with health-conscious consumers. Farmer's markets not only provide you with the opportunity to purchase the World's Healthiest Foods that are fresh and in season but also provide you with a way to connect with the people who are actually growing the foods that you enjoy eating. In addition, strolling through a farmer's market and exploring the ripe produce, handmade cheeses, local handicrafts and more is a fun and rewarding activity that can be shared together by friends and family alike.

### Home delivery service

In several regions of the country, entrepreneurial businesses have sprung up that cater to people who are not only health conscious but for whom convenience is key. These companies not only offer a wide selection of organic produce and dry goods but also deliver these foods right to your doorstep. And because these businesses don't have the overhead that stores do, oftentimes they are not only a more convenient way to get your organic produce but a more cost-effective way as well.

### Natural food stores

Natural food stores have always been the bastion of healthy foods, supporting the community in attaining the "Healthiest Way of Eating." With a longstanding commitment to organic foods, natural foods stores offer an extensive selection of foods grown in this sustainable manner. Natural foods stores are a great resource for buying foods such as grains, beans, legumes, nuts and seeds since these stores oftentimes have extensive bulk bin sections where these foods can be purchased at lower costs than offered when they are prepackaged. In addition to small, locally owned stores, natural foods supermarket chains are opening in more and more cities around the country. These stores offer a broad selection of natural and organic foods, including meats, fish and dairy products, while providing an extensive array of organically grown fruits and vegetables.

### Supermarkets

As consumers become more interested in whole and organic foods, many supermarkets are responding to this demand and becoming a valuable resource where many of the World's Healthiest Foods can be purchased. While traditionally you could always find certain varieties of the World's Healthiest Foods (notably fruits and vegetables) at supermarkets, as more and more foods are produced that are organically grown or additive-free, these healthier versions are now also being offered in many supermarkets. For example, while you could always buy oats in your local supermarket, it is now becoming more and more common to find oats that are organically grown and free of synthetic preservatives on the supermarket shelf. What is also exciting is that organic produce offerings are becoming more and more common as well.

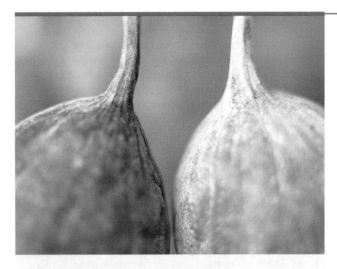

# figs

| | |
|---|---|
| AVAILABILITY: | May through October |
| REFRIGERATE: | Yes |
| SHELF LIFE: | 3 days |
| PREPARATION: | Minimal |
| BEST WAY TO ENJOY: | Enjoy them raw |

## nutrient-richness chart

Total Nutrient-Richness: **3**  GI: **85**

8 oz (226.80 grams) of fresh Figs contains 167 calories

| NUTRIENT | AMOUNT | %DV | DENSITY | QUALITY |
|---|---|---|---|---|
| Dietary Fiber | 7.5 g | 29.9 | 3.2 | good |
| Potassium | 526.2 mg | 15.0 | 1.6 | good |
| Manganese | 0.3 mg | 14.5 | 1.6 | good |
| **CAROTENOIDS:** | | | | |
| Beta-Carotene | 193.0 mcg | | | |
| Lutein+Zeaxanthin | 20.4 mcg | | | |
| **PHYTOSTEROLS:** | | | | |
| Phytosterols - Total | 70.4 mg | | | |

Daily values for these nutrients have not yet been established.

For more on "Total Nutrient-Richness," "%DV," "Density," and The World's Healthiest Foods "Quality" Rating System, see page 805.

For more on GI, see page 342.

Figs can trace their history back to the earliest of times with mentions in the Bible and other ancient texts. According to Greek mythology, the luscious, sweet-tasting Fig was presented by the Goddess Demeter as the autumn fruit. Considering their great taste and unique texture, it is no surprise that they have been revered throughout history. Figs are believed to have originated in western Asia and were then brought to the Mediterranean region where they are held in high esteem. There is nothing like the unique taste and texture of fresh Figs; they are deliciously sweet with a texture that combines the chewiness of their flesh, the smoothness of their skin and the crunchiness of their seeds. I enjoyed the truly fresh taste of Figs just outside of Athens, where farmers picked the Figs just before taking them to the market. Figs have a very short growing season and are extremely perishable. So, be sure to enjoy Figs when they are in season. Although fresh Figs are only available a few months out of the year, you can enjoy dried Figs throughout the year.

## why figs should be part of your healthiest way of eating

Like bananas, Figs provide easy-to-pack, convenient potassium power, which is especially important for athletes and those on-the-go. Their rich supply of dietary fiber is important for general health as well as in helping to control weight. Figs are one of the richest sources of phytosterols of all of the World's Healthiest Foods; phytosterols are plant nutrients that can help reduce cholesterol levels. Figs are an ideal food to add to your "Healthiest Way of Eating" because they are nutritious and taste great. (For more on the *Health Benefits of Figs* and a complete analysis of their content of over 60 nutrients, see page 446.)

## varieties of figs

Figs grow on the Ficus tree (*Ficus carica*), which is a member of the Mulberry family. There are more than 150 varieties of Figs, which range dramatically in color and subtly in texture. Some of the most popular varieties are:

**BLACK MISSION**
Blackish-purple skin with pink-colored flesh. This is the variety featured in the photographs in this chapter.

**KADOTA**
Green skin with purple flesh.

**CALIMYRNA**
Greenish-yellow skin with amber flesh.

**BROWN TURKEY**
Purple skin with red flesh.

**ADRIATIC**
This variety is most often used to make Fig bars; it has light green skin with pink-tan flesh.

**DRIED FIGS**

Black Mission and Calimyrna are the varieties of Figs that are the most commonly dried. Conventionally grown Figs that are dried usually contain sulfites.

## the peak season

Figs are available from May through October (depending on the variety). These are the months when their concentration of nutrients and flavor are highest, and their cost is at its lowest. Dried Figs are available throughout the year.

## biochemical considerations

Figs are a concentrated source of oxalates, which might be of concern to certain individuals. Conventionally grown Figs that are dried may contain sulfite preservatives. (For more on *Oxalates*, see page 725; and on *Sulfites*, see page 729.)

## 3 steps for the best tasting and most nutritious figs

Enjoying the best tasting Figs with the most nutrients is simple if you just follow my 3 easy steps:

1. The Best Way to Select
2. The Best Way to Store
3. The Best Way to Prepare

# 1. the best way to select figs

To select the best tasting Figs, look for ones that are fully ripe. These Figs will not only have the best flavor and texture, but fully ripe Figs also feature the most nutrients, including vitamins, antioxidants and enzymes. Fully ripe Figs are plump, have a rich deep color and yield to gentle pressure. They are soft, but not mushy, and exude syrupy nectar from the side opposite the stem. They should have firm stems and be free of bruises. As with all fruits, I recommend selecting organically grown varieties whenever possible. (For more on *Organic Foods*, see page 113.)

Avoid Figs that are overripe. Overripe Figs are soft and mushy, have a sour odor and will have begun to lose their nutritional value. Overripe Figs should not be eaten as they will have formed free-radicals. Make sure Figs are free of mold.

Since fresh ripe Figs are one of the most perishable fruits, be sure to purchase them only a day or two in advance of when you are planning on eating them.

### How Do You Know Which Figs are Ready to Eat?

If fresh Figs are plump and give slightly under gentle pressure, they are ready to eat.

# 2. the best way to store figs

Proper storage is an important step in keeping Figs fresh and preserving their nutrients, texture and unique flavor.

### Fresh Ripe Figs Can Last for Up to 3 Days When Properly Stored and Refrigerated

Figs continue to respire even after they have been harvested. The faster they respire, the more the Figs interact with air to produce carbon dioxide. The more carbon dioxide produced, the more quickly they will spoil. Figs kept at room temperature of approximately 68°F (20°C) give off carbon dioxide at a rate of 50 mg per kilogram every hour. (For a *Comparison of Respiration Rates* for different fruits, see page 341.) While refrigeration helps slow the respiration rate of ripe Figs, retain their vitamin content and increase their storage life, they will cause Figs to lose some of their flavor. While Figs that are stored properly and refrigerated will remain fresh for 3 days, if they are not stored properly, they will last only 1–2 days.

Dried Figs will stay fresh for several months and can either be kept in a cool, dark, ventilated place or stored in the refrigerator. They should be well wrapped so that they are not overexposed to air, which may cause them to become hard or dry.

### How to Ripen Figs

Figs will become sweet and juicy at home after they have been picked or purchased, if they have not been picked too green. Place Figs on a flat surface with space between the fruit to ripen them at room temperature for a day or two. It is best to turn them occasionally so that they will ripen evenly. Once they yield to gentle pressure, they are ripe and ready to eat. If you will not be consuming the Figs immediately after they have ripened, place them in the refrigerator. Don't refrigerate Figs until they are ripe; they will not ripen in the refrigerator.

## Handle with Care

Figs are a delicate fruit and bruise easily, so handle them with care.

# 3. the best way to prepare figs

Properly preparing Figs helps ensure that they will have the best flavor and retain the greatest number of nutrients.

## Cleaning Figs

Rinse fresh Figs under cold running water before serving and gently remove stem. (For more on *Washing Fruit*, see page 341.)

## Cutting and Peeling Figs

Fresh Figs can be consumed either peeled or unpeeled, depending upon the thickness of the skin (which differs with variety) as well as personal preference. The soft and sticky inner portion of the Fig makes them difficult to cut. To simplify this process, place them in the freezer for up to an hour before cutting to make them firm and easier to handle. Dip the knife in hot water as you are cutting the Figs to prevent them from sticking to the knife.

## Reconstituting Dried Figs

To reconstitute dried Figs, simmer them in boiling water or fruit juice for two minutes.

## No Bake Recipes

I have discovered that Figs retain their maximum amount of nutrients and their best taste when they are enjoyed fresh and not prepared in a cooked recipe. That is because their nutrients—including vitamins, antioxidants and enzymes—are unable to withstand the temperature (350°F/175°C) used in baking. So that you can get the most enjoyment and benefit from fruit, I created quick and easy recipes, which require no cooking. I call them "No Bake Recipes."

---

Here is a question that I received from a reader of the whfoods.org website about Figs:

**Q** *I've seen websites that note that dried Figs contain omega-3 essential fatty acids. Is that true, and if so how much omega-3s do Figs contain?*

**A** I have also found several website references to research at various universities revealing the omega-3 content of Figs. However, I can find no published research showing any omega-3 fatty acids in raw or dried Figs. The U.S. Department of Agriculture's most recent food data-base, as well as the Food Processor software (ESHA Research, Salem Oregon) we used in the construction of our website, show 0.0 grams of omega-3s in both raw and dried Figs.

In addition, it wouldn't make sense to me that Figs would be a good source of omega-3 fatty acids. There is less than one gram of total fat in 8 ounces of raw Figs, and over 1/3 of that fat occurs in either monounsaturated or saturated. About 1/2 occurs as linoleic acid, an omega-6 fatty acid. Not much room would be left here for omega-3s. Until I see research evidence to the contrary, I will continue to assume that dried Figs are not a source of omega-3 fatty acids.

STEP-BY-STEP
## No Bake Recipes

# 10-Minute Fig and Fresh Apple Cobbler

*Fresh and flavorful, this Fig and apple cobbler is quick and easy to make any time of the year. Choose your favorite type of apple for a treat the family can enjoy for dessert or even for breakfast.*

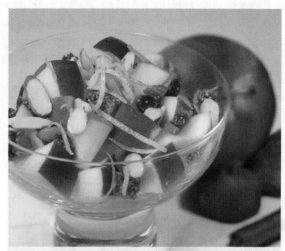
Fig and Fresh Apple Cobbler

**2 small apples**
**1/4 tsp lemon juice**
**1 TBS apple juice**
**4 dried Figs (or fresh when in season)**
**4 TBS chopped almonds**
**2 tsp honey**
**1/2 tsp lemon zest***
**1/4 tsp cinnamon**
**Pinch of cloves**
**Pinch of allspice**

1. Cut apples into quarters. Cut out core and slice fruit into 1/4-inch thick slices. Turn apples and cut across slices for diced apples. In a mixing bowl, toss with lemon and apple juice.

2. Cut the stem off the Figs. Cut Figs into quarters and chop to produce pieces 1/4-inch in size or smaller. Add to the apples.

3. Add the remaining ingredients and toss until well combined. For best nutrition, eat immediately. To chill, cover well and place in the refrigerator for up to 8 hours.

### SERVES 2

## Variations...

* Top with your favorite granola.
* Top with vanilla yogurt.

* Use organic lemon for zest, if possible.

# 5-Minute Fig Energy Bars

*If you are looking for a true Fig bar, here it is. Almonds and Figs make a great combination.*

**1/2 cup cream honey**
**1/2 cup almond butter**
**1/2 cup dried Figs**
**1/4 cup dried cranberries**
**1/4 cup chopped almonds**
**1 cup granola**

1. In a mixing bowl, mix the honey and almond butter.
2. Cut the dried Figs into 1/8-inch pieces.
3. Add Figs, cranberries, almonds and granola to the honey and almond butter mixture. Press into a loaf pan. Refrigerate for at least 1 hour. Slice into 1-inch bars.

### MAKES 8 BARS

Please write (address on back cover flap) or e-mail me at info@whfoods.org with your personal ideas for preparing Figs, and I will share them with others through our website at www.whfoods.org.

## 4 QUICK SERVING IDEAS for FIGS:

1. When preparing oatmeal or any other whole grain breakfast porridge, add some dried or fresh Figs.
2. Fresh Figs and dried Figs are great in salads, fruit cups, cobblers and with cereal.
3. **Stuffed Figs with Cheese:** Stuff fresh Figs with goat cheese and chopped almonds for a great hors d'oeuvre or dessert. Alternatively, place Figs with cheese under the broiler for a minute or two to melt the cheese. Broiling exposes the Figs to heat for such a short time that it does not really affect their nutrient content.
4. **Figs and Almond Treat:** Pierce a hole in the Figs and stuff each with 1 whole almond.

# health benefits of figs

## Promote Blood Sugar Balance

You probably do not think about the leaves of the Fig tree as one of Fig's edible parts. But in some cultures, Fig leaves are a common part of the menu and for good reason. The leaves of the Fig have been shown to have anti-dia-

betic properties and can actually reduce the amount of insulin needed by persons with diabetes who require insulin injections. In one study, a liquid extract made from Fig leaves was simply added to the breakfast of insulin-dependent diabetic subjects in order to produce this insulin-lowering effect.

## Promote Heart Health

Serving for serving, Figs are one of the most concentrated sources of phytosterols of all of the World's Healthiest Foods. Phytosterols can block cholesterol absorption in the body and therefore reduce cholesterol levels.

Figs are also a good source of potassium, a mineral that helps to control blood pressure. Since many people have an inadequate intake of fruits and vegetables, they may be deficient in potassium. Low intake of potassium-rich foods can lead to hypertension.

In the Dietary Approaches to Stop Hypertension (DASH) study, one group ate servings of fruits and vegetables in place of snacks and sweets and also ate low-fat dairy foods. This diet delivered more potassium, magnesium and calcium. Another group ate a "usual" diet low in fruits and vegetables with a fat content similar to the average American Diet. After eight weeks, the group that ate the enhanced diet lowered their blood pressure by an average of 5.5 points (systolic) over 3.0 points (diastolic).

## Promote Optimal Weight

Figs are a good source of dietary fiber, especially soluble fiber. Fiber and fiber-rich foods may have a positive effect on weight management. In one study, women who increased their fiber intake with supplements significantly decreased their energy intake, yet their hunger and satiety scores did not change.

## Promote Optimal Health

In addition to their blood sugar-stabilizing properties, in *in vitro* (test tube) studies, Fig leaves have been shown to inhibit the growth of certain types of cancer cells. Researchers have not yet determined exactly which substances in Fig leaves are responsible for these remarkable healing effects.

The Fig fruit is also a good source of manganese, a cofactor of the *superoxide dismutase* (SOD) enzyme. Manganese-containing SOD protects the mitochondria, the energy producing parts of our cells, from free-radical damage.

### Nutritional Analysis of 8 oz of fresh Figs:

| NUTRIENT | AMOUNT | % DAILY VALUE | NUTRIENT | AMOUNT | % DAILY VALUE |
|---|---|---|---|---|---|
| Calories | 167.83 | | Pantothenic Acid | 0.68 mg | 6.80 |
| Calories from Fat | 6.12 | | | | |
| Calories from Saturated Fat | 1.22 | | **Minerals** | | |
| Protein | 1.70 g | | Boron | — mcg | |
| Carbohydrates | 43.50 g | | Calcium | 79.38 mg | 7.94 |
| Dietary Fiber | 7.48 g | 29.92 | Chloride | 40.82 mg | |
| Soluble Fiber | 1.47 g | | Chromium | — mcg | — |
| Insoluble Fiber | 6.01 g | | Copper | 0.16 mg | 8.00 |
| Sugar – Total | 36.02 g | | Fluoride | — mg | — |
| Monosaccharides | — g | | Iodine | — mcg | — |
| Disaccharides | — g | | Iron | 0.84 mg | 4.67 |
| Other Carbs | 0.00 g | | Magnesium | 38.56 mg | 9.64 |
| Fat – Total | 0.68 g | | Manganese | 0.29 mg | 14.50 |
| Saturated Fat | 0.14 g | | Molybdenum | — mcg | — |
| Mono Fat | 0.15 g | | Phosphorus | 31.75 mg | 3.17 |
| Poly Fat | 0.33 g | | Potassium | 526.18 mg | |
| Omega-3 Fatty Acids | 0.00 g | 0.00 | Selenium | 1.36 mcg | 1.94 |
| Omega-6 Fatty Acids | 0.33 g | | Sodium | 2.27 mg | |
| Trans Fatty Acids | 0.00 g | | Zinc | 0.34 mg | 2.27 |
| Cholesterol | 0.00 mg | | | | |
| Water | 179.42 g | | **Amino Acids** | | |
| Ash | 1.50 g | | Alanine | 0.10 g | |
| | | | Arginine | 0.04 g | |
| **Vitamins** | | | Aspartate | 0.40 g | |
| Vitamin A IU | 322.06 IU | 6.44 | Cystine | 0.03 g | 7.32 |
| Vitamin A RE | 31.75 RE | | Glutamate | 0.16 g | |
| A - Carotenoid | 31.75 RE | 0.42 | Glycine | 0.06 g | |
| A - Retinol | 0.00 RE | | Histidine | 0.02 g | 1.55 |
| B1 Thiamin | 0.14 mg | 9.33 | Isoleucine | 0.05 g | 4.35 |
| B2 Riboflavin | 0.11 mg | 6.47 | Leucine | 0.07 g | 2.77 |
| B3 Niacin | 0.91 mg | 4.55 | Lysine | 0.07 g | 2.98 |
| Niacin Equiv | 1.13 mg | | Methionine | 0.01 g | 1.35 |
| Vitamin B6 | 0.26 mg | 13.00 | Phenylalanine | 0.04 g | 3.36 |
| Vitamin B12 | 0.00 mcg | 0.00 | Proline | 0.11 g | |
| Biotin | — mcg | — | Serine | 0.08 g | |
| Vitamin C | 4.54 mg | 7.57 | Threonine | 0.05 g | 4.03 |
| Vitamin D IU | 0.00 IU | 0.00 | Tryptophan | 0.01 g | 3.13 |
| Vitamin D mcg | 0.00 mcg | | Tyrosine | 0.07 g | 7.22 |
| Vitamin E Alpha Equiv | 2.02 mg | 10.10 | Valine | 0.06 g | 4.08 |
| Vitamin E IU | 3.01 IU | | | | |
| Vitamin E mg | 2.02 mg | | | | |
| Folate | 13.61 mcg | 3.40 | | | |
| Vitamin K | 10.66 mcg | 13.32 | | | |

(Note: "–" indicates data is unavailable. For more information, please see page 806.)

# Q&A

## WHAT DOES "GMO" MEAN?

If you've shopped in a natural foods store in recent months, you've probably seen products bearing the label "GMO-free" or "contains only non-GMO ingredients." The acronym "GMO" stands for Genetically Modified Organism, which refers to any food product that has been altered at the gene level. Genetically modified foods are also frequently described as "genetically engineered," "genetically altered" or "genetically manipulated."

It can be said that modification of plants is not a new phenomenon. For centuries, gardeners and farmers have been crossbreeding different species of plants to create plants that produce heartier, better tasting or more beautiful crops. However, the type of genetic engineering of foods that has caused a groundswell of concern around the world is vastly different from these traditional plant-breeding practices. With modern genetic engineering, genes from an animal, plant, bacterium or virus are inserted into a different organism (most often a plant), thereby irreversibly altering the genetic code— the "blueprint" that determines all of an organism's physical characteristics—of the organism that received the gene. Through this technology, scientists have created tomatoes with a longer shelf life by adding flounder genes, soybeans that are resistant to weed killers, potatoes that produce their own pesticides and potatoes with jellyfish genes that glow in the dark when they need water. Genetic engineers are also working to develop fruits, vegetables and grains with higher levels of vitamins and foods that contain vaccines against diseases like malaria, cholera and hepatitis.

While proponents of genetic engineering believe that this technology will make it possible to produce enough food to ensure that everyone in the world has enough to eat, farmers, scientists, environmentalists, health professionals and consumers throughout the world are outraged by the growing number of genetically altered foods in our food supply and are very skeptical about the purported benefits of this technology. Since 1996, when the first large-scale commercial harvest of genetically engineered crops occurred in the United States, the percentage of genetically engineered crops grown in the United States has increased to 25%, including 35% of all corn, 55% of all soybeans and nearly half of all cotton. In addition, much of the canola oil produced in Canada comes from genetically manipulated rapeseed. It has been estimated that as many as two-thirds of all food products in grocery stores contain genetically engineered ingredients. In fact, unless you buy exclusively organic, you will likely bring home foods that contain genetically modified ingredients, especially if you purchase foods that contain soybeans, corn or their derivatives (soy oil, soy flour, soy protein isolates, corn oil, corn starch, corn flour and high-fructose corn syrup).

At this point in time, the health risks of consuming genetically altered foods have not been clearly identified, since few studies have been conducted to evaluate the impact of these foods on human health. However, many scientists have speculated that it is likely that these foods will trigger allergic reactions in some people, create new toxins that produce disease and lead to antibiotic resistance and a subsequent resurgence of infectious disease. The impact on the environment may be even more devastating. Many farmers are concerned that it will be impossible to prevent genetically engineered crops from "polluting" organic farms, as the wind and bees will naturally carry pollen from the genetically engineered crops to nearby organic farms. In addition, farmers and environmentalists fear that foods that are genetically engineered to be resistant to herbicides, such as Roundup Ready soybeans, will result in heavier herbicide use, further polluting the groundwater, lakes and rivers. Heavy use of herbicides may also encourage the development of "superweeds" that are resistant to herbicides, which could threaten crops throughout the country. The results of a 1999 study conducted by researchers at Cornell University suggest that genetically engineered crops also endanger wildlife, specifically the Monarch butterfly. These researchers found that nearly half of the Monarch caterpillars that ate milkweed leaves dusted with pollen from genetically engineered corn died within four days. A study conducted one year later at Iowa State University found that plants that neighbor farms of genetically engineered corn are dusted with enough corn pollen to kill Monarch caterpillars.

As more is learned about the environmental and health risks of genetically engineered foods, people around the world are demanding that food producers eliminate these so-called "Frankenfoods" from their products. While the law in the United States does not mandate that foods containing genetically modified ingredients be labeled, many proactive food producers have stopped using these ingredients and are now labeling their products as "GMO-free." For more information about genetically modified foods, please visit the official website of The Campaign to Label Genetically Engineered Foods at www.thecampaign.org and Earthsave's webpage at www.earthsave.org.

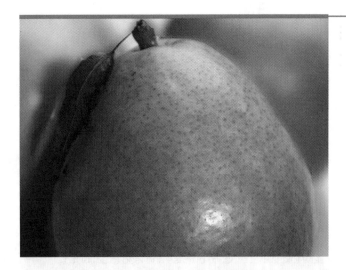

# pears

## highlights

| | |
|---|---|
| AVAILABILITY: | Year-round |
| REFRIGERATE: | Yes, after ripening |
| SHELF LIFE: | 3 days refrigerated |
| PREPARATION: | Minimal |
| BEST WAY TO ENJOY: | Enjoy them raw |

## nutrient-richness chart

Total Nutrient-Richness: **3**          GI: **53**
One (166 grams) fresh Pear contains 98 calories

| NUTRIENT | AMOUNT | %DV | DENSITY | QUALITY |
|---|---|---|---|---|
| Dietary Fiber | 4.0 g | 15.9 | 2.9 | good |
| Vitamin C | 6.6 mg | 11.1 | 2.0 | good |
| Copper | 0.2 mg | 9.5 | 1.7 | good |
| Vitamin K | 7.47 mcg | 9.3 | 1.7 | good |
| **CAROTENOIDS:** | | | | |
| Beta-Carotene | 21.6 mcg | | | |
| Beta-Cryptoxanthin | 3.3 mcg | | | |
| Lutein+Zeaxanthin | 74.7 mcg | | | |
| **FLAVONOIDS:** | | | | |
| (+)-Catechin | 0.4 mg | | | |
| (-)-Epicatechin | 5.3 mg | | | |
| Isorhamnetin | 0.5 mg | | | |
| Quercetin | 0.7 mg | | | |
| **PHYTOSTEROLS:** | | | | |
| Phytosterols—Total | 13.3 mg | | | |

Daily values for these nutrients have not yet been established.

For more on "Total Nutrient-Richness," "%DV," "Density," and
The World's Healthiest Foods "Quality" Rating System, see page 805.
For more on GI, see page 342.

Originating in Central Asia, Pears have been cultivated for more than 3,000 years. I tasted the best Pears from a local fruit stand when I was trekking in Africa on my way to Nairobi, Kenya. They were just the right combination of crisp and juicy. I knew then why Homer referred to Pears as the "gift of the gods" in his epic poem, *The Odyssey*. Considered an item of luxury in the French court of Louis XIV, Pears were brought by the early colonists to America, where the first Pear tree was planted in 1620. Easy to pack and fun to eat, the buttery sweetness of Pears makes them a great between-meal snack, and they can be easily added to your favorite salad or dessert or enjoyed as an appetizer.

## why pears should be part of your healthiest way of eating

A good source of dietary fiber, Pears contain flavonoid phytonutrients, including catechins and quercetin, as well as phytosterols, which have been found to be important for a healthy heart. Pears are an ideal food to add to your "Healthiest Way of Eating" not only because they are nutritious and taste great, but also because they are low in calories making them a good choice for weight control: one Pear contains only 98 calories! (For more on the *Health Benefits of Pears* and a complete analysis of their content of over 60 nutrients, see page 450.)

## varieties of pears

There are thousands of varieties of Pears *(Pyrus communis),* each differing in size, shape, color, flavor and shelf life. Varieties such as Conference, Passe Crassane and Packham, which are popular in other countries, are becoming more widely available in the United States, where the most popular varieties currently include:

### ANJOU
These slightly stubby, oval-shaped Pears with smooth, yellow-green skin and creamy flesh are the most abundant of the winter Pears.

### BARTLETT
These large, juicy summer Pears turn from dark green to golden yellow when ripe. They are the variety primarily used for canning and exclusively used for drying.

### BOSC
These Pears are characterized by their long tapering neck and rough reddish-brown skin. They have a firm, crunchy texture, which makes them perfect for baking and poaching.

**COMICE**

This squat-shaped, dull green Pear is often considered the sweetest and most flavorful of the common varieties of Pears.

## the peak season

Because Pear season varies depending on variety, Pears are available year-round. However, the peak of their season runs from August through October.

## biochemical considerations

Pears are one of the 12 foods on which pesticide residues have been most frequently found. Conventionally grown dried Pears may be treated with sulfites, which may be problematic for some individuals. (For more on *Pesticide Residues*, see page 726; and *Sulfites*, see page 729.)

## 3 steps for the best tasting and most nutritious pears

Enjoying the best tasting Pears with the most nutrients is simple if you just follow my 3 easy steps:

1. The Best Way to Select
2. The Best Way to Store
3. The Best Way to Prepare

# 1. the best way to select pears

You will often find that the Pears in the market are not soft. Pears are picked hard because they are very perishable once they have ripened. So, plan to allow a few days for Pears to soften after you purchase them.

When you're selecting Pears, look for ones that are firm but not too hard, and free from bruises and mold. Don't feel you have to look for Pears with uniform color because several varieties feature russeting or brown-speckled patches on the skin. Russeting is an acceptable characteristic and may even reflect a more intense flavor. Fully ripened Pears have a delightfully sweet taste and the highest nutritional value since their content of vitamins, antioxidants and enzymes is at its peak. Pears will be juicy, flavorful and ready to eat once they yield to gentle pressure. They have the best taste when they are enjoyed at room temperature. As with all fruits, I recommend selecting organically grown Pears whenever possible. (For more on *Organic Foods,* see page, 113.)

Avoid overripe Pears, which should not be eaten because they have lost nutritional value and have formed free-radicals. You can recognize overripe Pears because they are soft and brown.

# 2. the best way to store pears

You can eat Pears crisp or soft depending upon your preference. If you like them crisp purchase them that way at the store and then you won't need to ripen them. But if you like them soft, either purchase ripe ones or ripen them at home. Proper storage is an important step in keeping Pears fresh and preserving their nutrients, texture and unique flavor.

### Fresh Tree-Ripened Pears Can Last for Up to 3 Days When Properly Stored and Refrigerated

Pears continue to respire even after they have been harvested. The faster they respire, the more the Pears interact with air to produce carbon dioxide. The more carbon dioxide produced, the more quickly they will spoil. Placing ripe pears in the refrigerator will help to slow down their respiration rate and keep them fresh for longer.

### How to Ripen Pears

To ripen them at room temperature, place Pears standing upright on a flat surface with space between the fruit. Once they yield to gentle pressure, they will be soft and ready to eat. This will usually take from 3 to 5 days.

Another natural way to ripen Pears is to place them in a paper bag for 2 to 3 days. The paper bag traps the ethylene gas produced by the Pears. The ethylene gas helps the Pears to soften more quickly, while the paper bag allows for healthy oxygen exchange through the bag. To speed up ripening, add an apple, banana or avocado to the bag. Keep the paper bag in a dark, cool, ventilated place as excessive heat will cause the Pears to rot rather than ripen. Avoid storing Pears in sealed plastic bags or restricted spaces where they touch each other as this will cause them to deteriorate prematurely.

### Is it Best to Refrigerate Your Pears After Ripening?

I suggest refrigerating ripened pears (whether tree-ripened or ripened at home), but I would eat them soon after you ripen them since they get overripe very quickly.

### Handle with Care

Pears are a delicate fruit and bruise easily, so handle them with care. *(Continued on bottom of Page 451)*

# health benefits of pears

## Promote Heart Health

In addition to being a good source of vitamin C, Pears also contain a spectrum of flavonoids. Vitamin C and flavonoids have a synergistic relationship, each helping to improve the antioxidant potential of the other. Vitamin C helps to protect cells from oxygen-related damage due to free-radicals; for example, vitamin C protects LDL ("bad") cholesterol from oxidation, which is one of the ways in which this vitamin protects against heart disease. The flavonoids contained in Pears—including catechins and quercetin—are antioxidants that have also been linked with cardiovascular disease prevention.

Additionally, Pears are packed with phytosterols. These phytonutrients have been shown to be able to inhibit cholesterol absorption and therefore potentially help to lower cholesterol levels. Yet, Pears' benefits in relation to cholesterol don't stop there since they are a good source of dietary fiber, which numerous studies have shown helps reduce cholesterol.

## A Hypoallergenic Fruit

Although their hypoallergenicity is not well-documented in scientific research, Pears are often recommended by healthcare practitioners as a fruit less likely to produce an allergic response than other fruits. Particularly in the introduction of first fruits to infants, Pear is often recommended as a safe way to start.

## Promote Optimal Antioxidant Status

In addition to the antioxidant vitamin C and flavonoids that Pears contain, they are also a good source of copper. An important trace mineral, copper helps protect the body from free-radical damage via its role as a necessary component of *superoxide dismutase* (SOD), a copper-dependent enzyme that eliminates superoxide radicals. Superoxide radicals are a type of free-radical generated during normal metabolism as well as when white blood cells attack invading bacteria and viruses. If not eliminated quickly, superoxide radicals damage cell membranes.

## Promote Digestive Health

Pear's fiber does a lot more than just help prevent constipation and ensure regularity. Fiber also binds to cancer-causing chemicals in the colon, preventing them from damaging colon cells. This may be one reason why diets high in fiber-rich foods, such as Pears, are associated with a reduced risk of colon cancer. Additionally, the fact that low dietary intake of copper seems to also be associated with risk factors for colon cancer serves as yet another reason in support of why this delicious fruit may be very beneficial for digestive health.

## Nutritional Analysis of 1 Pear:

| NUTRIENT | AMOUNT | % DAILY VALUE | NUTRIENT | AMOUNT | % DAILY VALUE |
|---|---|---|---|---|---|
| Calories | 97.94 | | Pantothenic Acid | 0.12 mg | 1.20 |
| Calories from Fat | 5.98 | | | | |
| Calories from Saturated Fat | 0.33 | | **Minerals** | | |
| Protein | 0.65 g | | Boron | — mcg | |
| Carbohydrates | 25.08 g | | Calcium | 18.26 mg | 1.83 |
| Dietary Fiber | 3.98 g | 15.92 | Chloride | 1.66 mg | |
| Soluble Fiber | 0.83 g | | Chromium | — mcg | — |
| Insoluble Fiber | 3.15 g | | Copper | 0.19 mg | 9.50 |
| Sugar – Total | 17.50 g | | Fluoride | — mg | — |
| Monosaccharides | 13.78 g | | Iodine | — mcg | — |
| Disaccharides | 3.65 g | | Iron | 0.42 mg | 2.33 |
| Other Carbs | 3.60 g | | Magnesium | 9.96 mg | 2.49 |
| Fat – Total | 0.66 g | | Manganese | 0.13 mg | 6.50 |
| Saturated Fat | 0.04 g | | Molybdenum | — mcg | — |
| Mono Fat | 0.14 g | | Phosphorus | 18.26 mg | 1.83 |
| Poly Fat | 0.16 g | | Potassium | 207.50 mg | |
| Omega-3 Fatty Acids | 0.00 g | 0.00 | Selenium | 1.66 mcg | 2.37 |
| Omega-6 Fatty Acids | 0.15 g | | Sodium | 0.00 mg | |
| Trans Fatty Acids | 0.00 g | | Zinc | 0.20 mg | 1.33 |
| Cholesterol | 0.00 mg | | | | |
| Water | 139.13 g | | **Amino Acids** | | |
| Ash | 0.46 g | | Alanine | 0.02 g | |
| | | | Arginine | 0.01 g | |
| **Vitamins** | | | Aspartate | 0.13 g | |
| Vitamin A IU | 33.20 IU | 0.66 | Cystine | 0.01 g | 2.44 |
| Vitamin A RE | 3.32 RE | | Glutamate | 0.05 g | |
| A - Carotenoid | 3.32 RE | 0.04 | Glycine | 0.02 g | |
| A - Retinol | 0.00 RE | | Histidine | 0.01 g | 0.78 |
| B1 Thiamin | 0.03 mg | 2.00 | Isoleucine | 0.02 g | 1.74 |
| B2 Riboflavin | 0.07 mg | 4.12 | Leucine | 0.03 g | 1.19 |
| B3 Niacin | 0.17 mg | 0.85 | Lysine | 0.02 g | 0.85 |
| Niacin Equiv | 0.17 mg | | Methionine | 0.01 g | 1.35 |
| Vitamin B6 | 0.03 mg | 1.50 | Phenylalanine | 0.02 g | 1.68 |
| Vitamin B12 | 0.00 mcg | 0.00 | Proline | 0.02 g | |
| Biotin | 0.33 mcg | 0.11 | Serine | 0.02 g | |
| Vitamin C | 6.64 mg | 11.07 | Threonine | 0.02 g | 1.61 |
| Vitamin D IU | 0.00 IU | 0.00 | Tryptophan | 0.00 g | 0.00 |
| Vitamin D mcg | 0.00 mcg | | Tyrosine | 0.00 g | 0.00 |
| Vitamin E Alpha Equiv | 0.83 mg | 4.15 | Valine | 0.02 g | 1.36 |
| Vitamin E IU | 1.24 IU | | | | |
| Vitamin E mg | 0.83 mg | | | | |
| Folate | 12.12 mcg | 3.03 | | | |
| Vitamin K | 7.47 mcg | 9.34 | | | |

(Note: "—" indicates data is unavailable. For more information, please see page 806.)

**STEP-BY-STEP**
## No Bake Recipes

# 10-Minute Pears with Orange Ginger Topping

*Ginger adds a zing to Pears for a savory dessert.*

6 oz low-fat vanilla or soy yogurt
3 TBS undiluted frozen orange juice
    concentrate
1/4 tsp grated fresh ginger
2 TBS honey
2 fresh Pears                    **SERVES 2**

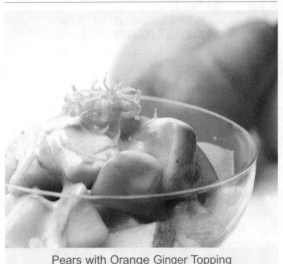

Pears with Orange Ginger Topping

1. Whisk orange juice concentrate, ginger and honey into yogurt until the honey is well incorporated and the mixture is smooth.

2. Cut Pear in quarters and core. Dice into 1/4-inch pieces and divide into 2 dessert dishes.

3. Spoon the yogurt sauce over Pears.

   **Preparation Hint:** If you do not have fresh ginger, 1/2 tsp powdered ginger may be used.

Please write (address on back cover flap) or e-mail me at info@whfoods.org with your personal ideas for preparing Pears, and I will share them with others through our website at www.whfoods.org.

## 5 QUICK SERVING IDEAS for PEARS:

1. Serve sliced Pears with gorgonzola, goat or blue cheese for a delightful dessert.

2. **Pear and Watercress Salad:** Combine Pear slices with watercress, thinly sliced leeks, mustard greens and walnuts for a delicious salad. Serve with Healthy Vinaigrette (page 143).

3. **Pear and Millet Porridge** (see page 660): Add 1 medium chopped Pear, 1 tsp grated fresh ginger and 1 TBS honey to millet porridge for a pungently sweet breakfast treat.

4. **Pears with Lemon Sauce:** Drizzle sliced Pears with Quick Lemon Sauce (see page 431).

5. **Pears with Almond Cashew Cream:** Make cashew cream (page 550) using almond extract. Slice 1–2 Pears and sprinkle with lemon juice. Dip Pear slices in sauce. Optional: sprinkle with cinnamon.

*(Continued from Page 449*

# 3. the best way to prepare pears

Properly preparing Pears helps ensure that they will have the best flavor and retain the greatest number of nutrients.

## Cleaning Pears

Rinse Pears gently under cold running water. (For more on *Washing Fruit*, see page 341.)

## Cutting and Peeling Pears

It is best not to peel Pears as the skin contains many of their nutrients and dietary fiber. This is another reason to select organically grown Pears whenever possible as you will not have the concern over pesticide residues on the skin.

## How to Keep Pears from Turning Brown

Once Pears are cut, the enzymes in the flesh will oxidize causing them to turn brown. To prevent Pears from turning brown, prepare a bowl of water large enough to hold the quantity of Pears you will be slicing. For each 2 cups of water, add 2 TBS of fresh lemon juice. Add cut Pears to the lemon and water solution as you cut them. When you are done slicing, use a colander to strain the Pears.

## No Bake Recipes

I have discovered that Pears retain their maximum amount of nutrients and their best taste when they are enjoyed fresh and not prepared in a cooked recipe. That is because their nutrients—including vitamins, antioxidants and enzymes—are unable to withstand the temperature (350°F/175°C) used in baking. So that you can get the most enjoyment and benefit from fruit, I created quick and easy recipes, which require no cooking. I call them "No Bake Recipes."

# Q&A

### HOW DO YOU SELECT FRUITS AND VEGETABLES BY COLOR?

The rainbow hues of fruits and vegetables don't just make these healthy foods attractive to our eyes—they are actually part of the reason that these foods are so healthy in the first place.

That's because these foods contain nutrients, called phytonutrients, which are unique to plants (*phyto* = plant) and endow them with their beautiful pigments. Phytonutrients actually provide a lot of benefit to the plant as well as to those whose diets are rich in these plant foods. For example, many of them have powerful antioxidant activity, able to quench free-radicals that could otherwise do harm to our cells and genetic material. Darker colored fruits and vegetables reflect higher concentrations of nutrients and more flavor than those that are pale in color.

## Color and nutrients in food

Let's travel through the spectrum of colors to further explore how eating color-rich foods can also mean eating nutrient-rich foods.

**Red**-colored foods such as tomatoes, watermelon and grapefruits feature a phytonutrient known as lycopene. This member of the carotenoid phytonutrient family has powerful antioxidant activity, more effective actually than its well-known carotenoid cousin, beta-carotene. Lycopene is especially effective at thwarting a free-radical called singlet oxygen and as such is important for protecting the lipid-containing parts of cell membranes from the damage usually caused by that free-radical.

**Yellow**- and **orange**-colored foods such as papaya, apricots, carrots and sweet potatoes are rich in the carotenoids, alpha-carotene, beta-carotene and beta-cryptoxanthin, which lend them their sunshine-colored hues. Not only do these carotenoids fight free-radicals but they are also converted in the body to retinol, the active form of vitamin A.

**Green**-colored foods such as spinach, kale, asparagus and other leafy green vegetables are rich in phytonutrients such as chlorophyll and lutein. Chlorophyll is structurally similar to the hemoglobin molecule in our bodies that transports oxygen, although instead of containing iron at its center it contains magnesium. Lutein is a carotenoid antioxidant that has been found to be especially beneficial to vision health since it is concentrated in the eyes.

**Blue**- and **purple**-colored foods such as grapes, blueberries, eggplant, black beans and purple potatoes get their royal colors from phytonutrients such as anthocyanins. These flavonoid phytonutrients have many important functions in the body; they improve the integrity of support structures in the veins and the entire vascular system, enhance the effects of vitamin C, improve capillary integrity and stabilize the collagen matrix (the ground substance of all body tissues).

## Variation among the same food

Yet, it's not just different foods that feature different colors. There are certain fruits and vegetables that can be found in an array of colors and therefore offer you an array of nutritional benefits. Green, red or yellow apples? Yellow, white or blue corn? Purple, green or white asparagus? Depending upon which one you choose you will receive different nutritional benefits.

For example, different colored onions contain different levels of nutrients. Of the storage onions, white ones have the least amount overall. Not surprisingly, red and yellow onions contain more quercetin, a flavonoid phytonutrient pigment, than white onions. Red onions also contain more anthocyanin flavonoid phytonutrients than white or yellow ones, which is reflected in their red coloring.

## Deeper in color, richer in nutrients

When given the choice I like to eat deeply colored foods. If choosing between two heads of lettuce, I choose the one that has a deeper, richer green color. When choosing between red apples, I usually opt for the one with the more brilliant scarlet color. Not only do deeper, darker colors enrich my sensory experience of a food, but I also feel that they enrich my health as well.

That's because their deeper colors are often a reflection of their having a greater concentration of phytonutrient pigments. For example, pink grapefruit contains about 27 times more beta-carotene than white grapefruit while red bell peppers contain about 18 times more beta-carotene than yellow ones and 6 times more than green ones! So, remember that it's not just color in general that's important but the intensity of color that can also make a big difference when it comes to the nutritional benefits that you'll receive from fruits and vegetables.

## See color, see better health

To benefit most from these wonderful phytonutrients that nature has provided for us, I think it is important to eat a diet that features a range of colors. Create a salad with vegetables from all parts of the rainbow. Make your dinner plate a spectrum of many deeply colored foods. This way you can help ensure that you are receiving the unique benefits that different phytonutrients have to offer.

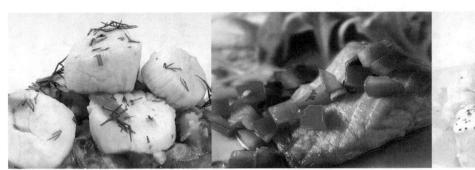
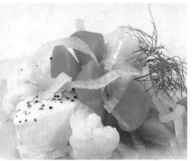

# fish & shellfish

The numbers beside each food indicate their Total Nutrient-Richness. (For more details, see page 805.)

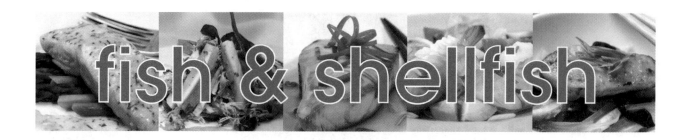

# fish & shellfish

With the increased wave of interest in foods that provide great nutrition, it is not surprising that the demand for fish and shellfish has doubled within the last ten years. Nutrition experts encourage eating more fish and shellfish because they are excellent sources of protein and rich in omega-3 fatty acids, and their consumption has been linked to a reduced risk of many diseases. Many research studies have shown that cultures in which seafood plays a prominent role in the diet not only have more abundant health but live longer. Not surprisingly, seafood are sometimes referred to as the "perfect food."

Yet, it's not just their health benefits that can make fish and shellfish such wonderful additions to your "Healthiest Way of Eating." They can also be delicious and offer a wide range of tastes and textures. Some are light and flaky, while others are sweet and meaty. Some lend just the right depth to make a summer salad a filling meal, while others are a perfect addition to a hearty winter stew. There are fish and shellfish to meet everyone's individual preferences, and since a little goes a long way, they are certain to not only please your taste buds but your wallet as well.

Recently, attention has been drawn to some concerns about consuming seafood. Because of environmental contamination, some fish are laden with mercury and may pose a problem for certain people. Additionally, practices of indiscriminate fishing are depleting some fish and shellfish species, while processes involved in fish farming are endangering the environment. The bottom line is that when you purchase fish and shellfish, you need to be an educated consumer in order to protect both your health and the health of the environment. Because I believe this is so important, this chapter features a Fish & Shellfish Guide that can help you easily decipher which fish and shellfish are the best options.

## Fish and Shellfish: Definition

When I refer to fish, I am referring to the flesh of aquatic vertebrate animals (usually having scales and fins) that are consumed as food. Examples of fish include salmon, tuna, cod, sardines, tilapia and striped bass. Shellfish refers to the flesh of aquatic invertebrate animals that have a hard shell. Examples of shellfish include shrimp and scallops.

## How Fish and Shellfish Can Help You Stay Slim, Energized and Healthy

Fish and shellfish can play a very important role in a health-promoting diet. So many important nutrients—protein, selenium, magnesium, vitamin B12, vitamin B6, niacin and omega-3 fatty acids to name just a few—are concentrated in these foods that it is no wonder they are referred to as treasures of the sea. Just 4 ounces (cooked) of most fish and shellfish can supply 50% of your daily value for protein, vitamin B12 and selenium for relatively very few calories. Now that's what I call nutrient-rich!

The healthfulness of fish and shellfish is a reflection of the compounds which they concentrate, but also the compounds they do not. In addition to the low caloric content of many fish, most also have less saturated fat and cholesterol than their land animal counterparts (an exception would be shrimp, which are noted sources of cholesterol).

Additionally, for those who are focused on attaining or maintaining their ideal body weight, these foods can be instrumental in helping them achieve their goal. For example, a 6-ounce serving of shrimp provides almost 36 grams of protein for a mere 168 calories. Compare this to a 6-ounce serving of beef that contains 48 grams of protein at a caloric cost of 360 calories or a 6-ounce serving of chicken containing 51 grams of protein for 335 calories and you can see how seafood will fill you up without filling out your waistline. Featuring fish and shellfish as the centerpiece of your meals will keep your taste buds satisfied and your appetite satiated, while providing so many of the nutrients vital to optimal physiological functioning. And since all of the benefits of these foods cost you very little in terms of calories, they can also help you attain your ideal weight goals.

# fish & shellfish guide

Since there are thousands of different types of fish and shellfish, making a seafood selection is sometimes difficult and confusing. I have developed a Fish & Shellfish Guide (The Guide) to help you make informed decisions about which fish and shellfish are best for you and decide which ones to purchase.

There are three things to consider when purchasing fish and shellfish.

1. Which fish have the lowest mercury content?

2. Which fish and shellfish provide the highest concentration of those hard-to-find omega-3 fatty acids?

3. What is the environmental impact of different fishing and farming methods used to catch and raise fish and shellfish? What is their effect on the sustainability of wild stocks of fish and shellfish?

## How to Avoid Mercury in Fish and Shellfish

You can select fish and shellfish that are safe to eat by simply following The Guide included in this chapter. Some fish and shellfish contain higher mercury levels than others, but you will be surprised that there are many types of fish and shellfish with low levels of mercury.

Mercury is a heavy metal that has contaminated many of our seas and oceans. Mercury toxicity can cause birth defects, damage to the nervous system, premature aging, vision loss and the onset of certain diseases. The U.S. Food and Drug Administration (FDA) has urged individuals, notably children and women who are pregnant, lactating or of childbearing age, to avoid certain fish because of their high mercury concentrations. These fish include swordfish, tuna, king

mackerel (ono or wahoo), shark and tilefish. Most fish that grow slowly and become very large tend to have higher mercury levels. The Guide helps you to select the fish and shellfish lowest in mercury levels. (For more on *Mercury in Fish*, see page 463.)

The U.S. FDA standard considers fish safe if it contains less than 1 ppm of methyl mercury. Canada's recommendation is that 0.5 ppm is considered safe.

## How to Select Fish and Shellfish that Provide the Richest Source of Omega-3 Fatty Acids

Most people in the U.S. are deficient in omega-3 fatty acids. One of the qualities for which many fish and shellfish have gained such great acclaim is that many of their fats are "good fats," which includes omega-3 fatty acids in the form of eicosapentaenoic acid (EPA) and docosahexaenoic acid (DHA). Fish and shellfish can directly provide your body with these important essential fatty acids.

Many species of fish and shellfish—including salmon, sardines, trout, halibut and scallops—contain rich concentrations of omega-3 fatty acids while others—such as lobsters, crabs, crayfish, oysters, squid and mahi mahi—are low in omega-3 fatty acids.

Omega-3 fatty acids have many health benefits, and cultures whose diets feature these important nutrients have been found to have reduced incidence of many different diseases as well as increased longevity. The Guide is designed to help you select the fish that will provide you with all of the beneficial omega-3 fatty acids you need. It includes ratings of high, medium, low and very low concentrations of omega-3 fatty acids, which are defined as follows: high (2.0+ g), medium (1.0-2.0 g), low (0.3-1.0 g) and very low (below 0.2). These amounts are based on a 6-ounce serving. (For more on *Omega-3 Fatty Acids*, see page 770.)

## How to Choose Fish and Shellfish that are Environmentally Sustainable

When deciding which fish or shellfish to purchase, it is very important to consider the environmental impact that these decisions may produce if you are concerned with the health and safety of our oceans and waterways. You can help protect fish and shellfish and the sustainability of the oceans, lakes and rivers by making environmentally aware choices.

Due to overfishing and depleted stocks of fish and shellfish, the 1996 Sustainable Fisheries Act was created to address the necessity of better management of both fish and shellfish. Size of the fish caught, overall catch size, seasonal fishing and how fish are harvested are now being more commonly considered in fisheries' management practices. If you are concerned about conservation, there are many types of fish and shellfish that you can enjoy that are considered sustainable and whose consumption does not greatly impact the environment. The Guide will provide you with information about how you can be an aqua-environmentally responsible citizen.

Fortunately, a growing number of resources, such as Seafood Watch provided by the non-profit Monterey Bay Aquarium (http://www.mbayaq.org/cr/seafoodwatch.asp), provide online information about how to support the fisheries and fish farms that maintain practices that are healthier for both the fish and the environment. The Monterey Bay Aquarium provides you with three lists (Best Choices, Good Alternatives and Avoid) to help you select fish and shellfish whose consumption will least impact the environment. I have used their sustainability ratings in The Guide.

At the time of this writing, wild-caught Alaskan salmon and Pacific cod are on the Monterey Bay Aquarium's list of Best Choices, while monkfish, Atlantic cod, Chilean sea bass and orange roughy are on the list of fish and shellfish to Avoid. Fish like Chilean sea bass and orange roughy mature very slowly, and heavy fishing pressure on slow growing fish results in depletion of their population. However, fish like mahi mahi that grow and reproduce quickly are considered to be less affected by fishing pressures and therefore more ecologically sound. They can grow up to 20 pounds in one year, reproduce at a young age and live only four to five years, so their consumption does not generally pose a problem for sustainability. Salmon also have very a short lifespan ranging from two to five years, depending on the species, after which they return to the rivers where they were hatched to spawn and die.

Most tilapia and striped bass now found in markets are farm-raised, using methods that have little environmental impact, and are therefore considered environmentally sustainable. Information regarding sustainability can change; updated information will be posted on the World's Healthiest Foods website, www.whfoods.org.

The Fish & Shellfish Guide is divided into separate categories: Wild Fish & Shellfish Safe to Eat, Farm-Raised Fish & Shellfish Safe to Eat, Fish & Shellfish OK to Eat One Meal Per Week and Fish & Shellfish OK to Eat One Meal Per Month. In The Guide you will also find information on Fish & Shellfish to Avoid.

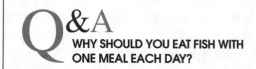

## Q&A
### WHY SHOULD YOU EAT FISH WITH ONE MEAL EACH DAY?

For years we have been told to eat fish a couple of times a week for optimal health, however, a recent research study shows why it is important to eat fish with one meal every day. Researchers in Japan found that daily consumption of omega-3-rich fish results in a significantly greater reduction in the risk of coronary heart disease compared to eating fish just a couple of times a week.

When participants who consumed fish eight times per week were compared with those whose intake was just once per week, it was found that those eating the most fish had a 37% lower risk of developing coronary heart disease and a 56% percent lower risk of heart attack. None of the participants had cardiovascular disease or cancer when the study began.

When the effect of omega-3 fatty acid intake on cardiovascular risk was analyzed, coronary heart disease risk was lowered by 42% among those whose intake was the highest, at 2.1 grams per day or more, compared to those whose intake was the lowest at 300 milligrams (0.3 grams) per day. Those whose intake of Omega-3s was in the top tier received a 65% reduction in the risk of heart attack compared to those whose omega-3 intake was lowest.

The authors theorize that daily fish consumption is highly protective largely due to the resulting daily supply of omega-3 fatty acids, which not only reduce platelet aggregation, but also decrease the production of pro-inflammatory leukotrienes. Lowering leukotrienes reduces damage to the endothelium (the lining of the blood vessels), a key factor in the development of atherosclerosis.

"Our results suggest that a high fish intake may add a further beneficial effect for the prevention of coronary heart disease among middle-aged persons," note the study's authors.

Iso H, Kobayashi M, Ishihara J, etal; JPHC Study Group. Intake of fish and n3 fatty acids and risk of coronary heart disease among Japanese: the Japan Public Health Center-Based (JPHC) Study Cohort I. Circulation. 2006 Jan 17;113(2):195-202. Epub 2006 Jan 9.

# fish & shellfish guide

## Wild Fish & Shellfish
## Several Meals Per Week

| | MERCURY LEVEL (PPM)* | OMEGA-3 FATTY ACIDS PER 6-OZ SERVING | ENVIRONMENTAL IMPACT/ SUSTAINABILITY RATINGS** |
|---|---|---|---|
| † Salmon, king | Very Low | 3.1 g High | Best Choice |
| † Salmon, sockeye | Very Low | 2.4 g High | Best Choice |
| † Salmon, coho | Very Low | 1.8 g Medium | Best Choice |
| † Salmon pink, canned, wild | Very Low | 2.8 g High | Best Choice |
| † Salmon king, smoked | Very Low | 0.8 g Low | Best Choice |
| Flounder, Pacific | Very Low | 0.9 g Low | Good Alternative |
| Sole, Pacific | Very Low | 0.9 g Low | Good Alternative |
| Sardines, canned | Very Low | 1.6 g Medium | Best Choice |
| Anchovies | Very Low | 2.4 g High | Best Choice |
| Squid (calamari) | Very Low | 1.0 g Medium | Good Alternative |
| Shrimp (domestic) | Very Low | 0.6 g Low | Good Alternative |
| Scallops (except from U.S. Mid-Atlantic) | Very Low | 0.6 g Low | Good Alternative |
| Oysters | Very Low | 0.6 g Low | Good Alternative |

## Farm-Raised Fish & Shellfish
## Several Meals Per Week

| | MERCURY LEVEL (PPM)* | OMEGA-3 FATTY ACIDS PER 6-OZ SERVING | ENVIRONMENTAL IMPACT/ SUSTAINABILITY RATINGS** |
|---|---|---|---|
| Striped bass | Very Low | 1.4 g Medium | Best Choice |
| Rainbow trout | Very Low | 2.0 g Medium | Best Choice |
| Char (small salmon) | Very Low | 2.0 g Medium | N/A |
| Shrimp (domestic) | Very Low | 0.6 g Low | Good Alternative |
| Catfish (domestic) | Very Low | 0.6 g Low | Best Choice |
| Crayfish (domestic) | Very Low | 0.2 g Very Low | N/A |
| Tilapia | Very Low | 1.8 g Medium | Best Choice |
| Scallops | Very Low | 0.6 g Low | N/A |
| Oysters | Very Low | 0.6 g Low | Best Choice |
| Clams | Very Low | 0.4 g Low | Best Choice |
| Mussels | Very Low | 1.4 g Medium | Best Choice |

† Best Choice = Alaskan wild-caught salmon, Good Alternative = California, Oregon and Washington wild-caught salmon,
      Avoid = Atlantic salmon

*(Fish and Shellfish Guide continued on next Page)*

## fish & shellfish guide (continued)

### Fish & Shellfish
### One Meal Per Week

| | MERCURY LEVEL (PPM)* | OMEGA-3 FATTY ACIDS PER 6-OZ SERVING | ENVIRONMENTAL IMPACT/ SUSTAINABILITY RATINGS** |
|---|---|---|---|
| Tuna (canned light) | Low | 0.2 g Very Low | Good Alternative |
| Mahi mahi | Low | 0.2 g Very Low | Good Alternative |
| Cod, Atlantic | Low | 0.4 g Low | Avoid |
| Cod, Pacific | Low | 0.4 g Low | Good Alternative |
| Haddock | Low | 0.4 g Low | Good Alternative (hook-and-line) |
| Herring | Low | 3.4 g High | Best Choice |
| Crabs, Dungeness | Low | 0.6 g Low | Best Choice |
| Lobsters (spiny and rock) | Low | 0.2 g Very Low | Best Choice |
| Whitefish | Low | 2.8 g High | N/A |
| Crab, Alaskan king | Low | 0.8 g Low | Good Alternative |
| Pollack | Low | 1.0 g Medium | N/A |
| Mackerel, canned (except king mackerel) | Low | 2.2 g High | Best Choice |

### Fish & Shellfish
### One Meal Per Month

| | MERCURY LEVEL (PPM)* | OMEGA-3 FATTY ACIDS PER 6-OZ SERVING | ENVIRONMENTAL IMPACT/ SUSTAINABILITY RATINGS** |
|---|---|---|---|
| Halibut, Pacific | Medium | 0.8 g Low | Best Choice |
| Halibut, Atlantic | Medium | 0.8 g Low | Avoid |
| Sea Bass, wild | Medium | 1.2 g Medium | N/A |
| Grouper, wild | Medium | 1.2 g Medium | Good Alternative |
| Tuna, albacore/yellowfin, troll/pole caught | Medium | 0.8 g Low | Best Choice |
| Bluefish | Medium | 1.6 g Medium | Good Alternative |
| Lobster, Maine | Medium | 0.2 g Very Low | Good Alternative |

### Fish & Shellfish
### One Meal on Very Rare Occasions
### (but avoid if pregnant or a child under 44 lbs/20 kg)

| | MERCURY LEVEL (PPM)* | OMEGA-3 FATTY ACIDS PER 6-OZ SERVING | ENVIRONMENTAL IMPACT/ SUSTAINABILITY RATINGS** |
|---|---|---|---|
| Swordfish (domestic) | High | 1.4 g Medium | Good Alternative |
| Tilefish | High | 2.0 g Medium | Good Alternative (U.S. Mid-Atlantic) |
| Marlin | High | N/A | Good Alternative |
| Shark | High | 0.8 g Low | Avoid |
| Tuna, bluefin | High | 2.6 g High | Avoid |
| King Mackerel, ono or wahoo | High | 0.6 g Low | Best Choice |

### Farm-Raised Fish & Shellfish
### NOT Recommended

| | |
|---|---|
| Salmon | Avoid for now because they have been found to contain PCs and artificial coloring. Farmed salmon are sold under the name of Atlantic salmon and Norwegian salmon. |
| Shrimp, imported | Avoid because of use of preservatives and antibiotics. |
| Scallops, imported | Avoid because of use of preservatives. |

# Wild Fish & Shellfish To Avoid
## Not Sustainable/Overfished

| | |
|---|---|
| Chilean Sea Bass and Orange Roughy | Fish like Chilean sea bass and orange roughy live over 100 years, mature very slowly and will not reproduce until they are approximately 30 years of age. |
| Pacific Snapper (Pacific Rock Cod, Rock Fish, Red Snapper) | Overfished. Snapper matures very slowly and will not reproduce until approximately 20 years of age. |
| Monkfish, wild | Overfished |
| Catfish, wild | Overfished |
| King Crab, wild | Overfished |
| Caviar, wild | Overfished |
| Flounder, Atlantic, wild | Overfished |
| Sturgeon, wild | Overfished |

## Fish & Shellfish Guide Legend

### Mercury Level
*Sources of Information:

Sunderland EM. (2007). Mercury Exposure from Domestic and Imported Estuarine and Marine Fish in the U.S. Seafood Market Environmental Health Perspectives Volume 115, Number 2, February 2007.

U.S. Food and Drug Administration. (1978) and (2000). "National Marine Fisheries Service Survey of Trace Elements in the Fishery Resource" Report 1978; "The Occurrence of Mercury in the Fishery Resources of the Gulf of Mexico" Report 2000. This data was published by the U.S. Department of Health and Human Services (HHS) and the U.S. Environmental Protection Agency (EPA) in 2001 under the title, "Mercury Levels in Commercial Fish and Shellfish" and then updated in 2006.

Consumer's Union of U.S., Inc. (2003). Statement by Consumers Union of U.S., Inc. Regarding Federal Dietary Advice on Methyl Mercury in Fish and Seafood. FDA/EPA Stakeholders Meeting, College Park, Maryland, July 30, 2003.

The mercury content of all fish and shellfish can vary substantially. Region of catch, species of fish, exact age of fish, exact size of fish, and other factors can all influence mercury accumulation. The safety of fish consumption depends not only on mercury content, but also on the health status of the individual who is eating the fish. In general, individuals who have special health needs (for example, pregnant women or children) or individuals who have poor health status should talk to their healthcare provider about the role of fish and shellfish in their overall meal plan.

### Mercury Level rating system:

**Very Low** = less than .1 ppm
This level is 1/10th of the U.S. Food and Drug Administration (FDA) Action Level for mercury in fish and seafood.

**Low** = greater than .1 ppm but less than .25 ppm
This level is always below the U.S. Food and Drug Administration (FDA) Action Level for mercury in fish and seafood. In addition, it is also below the amount of mercury that would be present in 6 ounces of fish and still prevent a woman weighing 132 lbs. (60 kg) from going over the EPA's Reference Dose (RfD) level for mercury.

**Medium** = greater than .25 ppm but less than .5 ppm
This level is always below the U.S. Food and Drug Administration (FDA) Action Level for mercury in fish and seafood. In addition, it is also below the amount of mercury that would be present in 3 ounces of fish and still prevent a woman weighing 132 lbs. (60 kg) from going over the EPA's Reference Dose (RfD) level for mercury.

**High** = greater than .5 ppm
While this level is still below the U.S. Food and Drug Administration (FDA) Action Level for mercury, it is sufficiently high to cause a woman weighing 132 lbs. (60 kg) to exceed the EPA's Reference Dose (RfD) level for mercury when only 3 ounces of fish are consumed.

**PPM** = parts per million.
PPM is the gold standard of measurement in scientific research on mercury levels in fish and shellfish.

### Environmental Impact / Sustainability Ratings

**Sustainability ratings from Monterey Bay Aquarium Seafood Watch, http://www.mbayaq.org/cr/seafoodwatch.asp

**Best Choice:** These rank well against all their criteria for sustainability. The wild population is abundant and well managed, and there are low levels of wasted catch (bycatch). The fish are not caught or farmed in ways that harm the environment.

**Good Alternative:** There are some concerns with how they are fished or farmed or with the health of their habitats. Yet, they are good alternatives to the Best Choices seafood and are better than those on the Avoid List.

**Avoid:** These fish are not sustainable and should, at least for now, be avoided. They rank poorly on many of their criteria. For example, the wild population may be threatened and need time to multiply or the management of these fish needs improvement. Additionally, the fish may be caught or farmed in ways that negatively impact other fish species or the environment in general.

## Who to Call for Information on What Fish and Shellfish are Safe to Eat

If you, your family or friends have caught local freshwater fish and want to know whether they are safe to eat, call the Environmental Protection Agency at 1-888-SEAFOOD.

## Is Farmed Fish Safe to Eat?

Many fish and seafood are now farmed. If they are farmed in clean waters using environmentally sound production practices, they do not provide much of an environmental problem. Shellfish such as scallops, clams, mussels and oysters are filter feeders (they filter the surrounding water for the food they eat) and therefore can easily accumulate pollutants if they are farmed in unclean waters. Striped bass, rainbow trout, tilapia and white sturgeon are grown in inland farms and have not been found to present an environmental problem.

Atlantic salmon and shrimp are produced in coastal operations, which have often been found to be environmentally unfriendly. While shrimp farming is well regulated in the United States, operations in foreign countries are not.

## Fish or Fish Oil Supplements?

Fresh fish is best. Not only does fresh fish supply you with important omega-3 fatty acids but like all whole foods they provide an entire range of protein, vitamins and minerals that work together to promote optimal health. If you decide to purchase fish oil capsules to supplement your diet with omega-3 fatty acids, you'll want to select a product from a very high-quality manufacturer to make sure that the omega-3 fat content is what it's supposed to be and that these fragile oils are not rancid.

Some fish oil products go through a refining process that removes contaminants that may be found in the fish itself. To be sure that your supplements are free of such contaminants, such as PCBs and dioxins, purchase a brand that has undergone "molecular distillation," which removes contaminants; this will be stated on the product label.

Mercury in fish oil capsules does not seem to be a general problem. According to www.consumerlab.com's 2004 testing of 20 fish oil products currently available in the marketplace, none of the products contained detectable mercury levels. Most mercury has been found to be in the flesh rather than the oil.

## The Easy Way to Eat Three to Four Servings of Fish Each Week

The American Heart Association recommends that healthy individuals eat at least 2 servings per week of fish or shellfish. But to get an optimal amount of omega-3 fatty acids, I recommend 3–4 servings per week of fish or shellfish that are low in mercury content, rich in omega-3 fats and considered environmentally sustainable.

This goal should not be too difficult because you can enjoy many varieties of fish that fit these criteria. Salmon, shrimp, cod and scallops are just a few to choose from. And with the numerous recipes that I have included for each of the World's Healthiest Fish and Shellfish, you'll have a cornucopia of different preparation options. Because these recipes are so quick and easy to prepare, they will not only help satisfy the needs of your taste buds but of your busy schedule as well.

## What is a Serving Size of Fish or Shellfish?

The American Heart Association's recommended serving size for seafood is 6 ounces raw or 4 ounces cooked.

## How to Use the Individual Fish and Shellfish Chapters

Each fish and shellfish chapter is dedicated to one of the World's Healthiest Fish and Shellfish and contains everything you need to know to enjoy and maximize its flavor and nutritional benefits. Each chapter is organized into two parts:

1. **FISH AND SHELLFISH FACTS** describes each fish and shellfish, their different varieties and peak season. It also addresses biochemical considerations of each fish and shellfish by describing any unique compounds they contain that may be potentially problematic to individuals with specific health problems. Detailed information of the health benefits of each fish and shellfish can be found at the end of the chapter, as can a complete nutritional profile.

2. **THE 4 STEPS TO THE BEST TASTING AND MOST NUTRITIOUS FISH AND SHELLFISH** includes information to help you select, store, prepare and cook each one of the World's Healthiest Fish and Shellfish. This section also features Step-by-Step Recipes and Flavor Tips. While specific information for individual fish and shellfish is given in each of the specific chapters, here are the 4 Steps that can be applied to seafood in general, including those not on the list of the World's Healthiest Foods.

# 1. the best way to select fish and shellfish —

It is important to buy the freshest fish and shellfish possible as the differences in taste and nutritional value are greatly affected by how long they have been "out of the sea." By talking to the people that work in the seafood departments of your local markets (often known as fishmongers) and asking them about where and how often their market gets its fish, you can ascertain which stores have the freshest selection. Ask questions about the fish's origin, whether it is farm-raised or wild and whether it contains artificial coloring. Using the Fish & Shellfish Guide, determine whether the fish is on the Best Choice, Good Alternative or Avoid list for sustainability. While each individual chapter will provide you with tips on how to make the best selection for individual fish or shellfish, a general rule of thumb follows:

You can tell a lot by how the fish looks: the older the fish, the duller the appearance. Generally speaking, thicker cuts of fish (1" to 2" thick) work better in most recipes as they are more moist and hold together better when cooked. These cuts come from the part of the fish that is closest to the head.

The U.S. Food and Drug Administration suggests looking for the following qualities to ensure that you are purchasing fresh fish:

"• Be sure that the fish has been refrigerated or properly iced.
• Fresh fish smells fresh and mild, not "fishy" or ammonia-like.
• The flesh should spring back when pressed.
• The flesh should be firm and shiny (whether it is whole or filleted).
• There should be no darkening around the edges of the fish or brown or yellowish discoloration.
• The eyes should be clear and bulge slightly.
• The gills should be bright red and free from slime.
• Don't purchase frozen seafood if the packages are open, torn or crushed on the edges.
• Don't purchase cooked seafood, such as shrimp, crab or smoked fish if it is displayed in the same case as raw fish, since cross-contamination can occur."

# 2. the best way to store fish and shellfish —

Most fish come from cold waters and require colder temperatures than fruits and vegetables to stay fresh. Fish and shellfish are very perishable and, in contrast to fruits and vegetables, normal refrigerator temperatures of 36°–40°F (2°–4°C) do not inhibit the enzymatic activity that causes them to spoil. Fish and shellfish are best when stored at 28°–32°F (-2°–0°C). I have tried the traditional method of packing fish with ice before placing it in the refrigerator to decrease the temperature. What I discovered was that when the ice melts, the fish ends up sitting in a pool of water losing much of its flavor.

## The Way I Store My Fish

I have since refined the method above, and I want to share with you the best way I found to keep your fish and shellfish fresh. This method is the most effective when you have a large amount of fish.

Place your fish in a zip-lock plastic storage bag, place the bag in a bowl and cover with ice. The benefit to this method is that you don't have to worry about the fish ending up in a pool of water and losing flavor, so there is less concern about remembering to drain the water away from the fish as the ice melts. However, the down side to this method is that the fish will end up sitting in some of its own juices as they collect inside the bag. Fish stored using this method will last an extra day.

You can use ice packs in place of the ice in both methods. Remember to replace the ice packs as necessary. Although the fish will keep for two to three days using these methods, I recommend using it the day of purchase or within one or two days.

It is interesting what proper storage can do. Many times when my fish has a little fishy odor, I cover it for three to four hours with ice, which I have found to remove the odor. This will not work if the fish has already developed a strong odor.

# 3. the best way to prepare fish and shellfish —

Minimal preparation is required for many varieties of fish. You don't need to start with whole fish because they are usually already filleted or cut into steaks for your convenience when you purchase them at your local market. Yet, some shellfish, like shrimp, scallops and oysters, may require some preparation. In the individual chapters, I will present you with the best ways to prepare specific varieties of fish and shellfish.

# 4. the healthiest way of cooking fish and shellfish

Although the recipes in the book include the best cooking methods for each individual fish and shellfish, here is some general information on the best ways to cook these foods:

## Healthy Cooking Times

Traditionally, it has been suggested that you cook your fish for approximately 7 minutes for every inch of thickness. Some fish can take a little longer, up to 10 minutes. In the individual chapters, I will provide you with more specific instructions on how to cook your fish. The length of cooking time recommended for each of the recipes is based on the type of fish or shellfish that is to be prepared and the cooking method used for that particular recipe.

Cooking time is also dependent on the desired doneness of the fish or shellfish. For example, tuna is preferably cooked rare to medium-rare while white fish, like striped bass and halibut, can be cooked through and still retain their moistness and flavor. It is very important to pay close attention to the cooking time of fish and shellfish because if it is overcooked, it will be dry and lose much of its flavor.

## Healthy Cooking Methods

The variety of tastes and textures of fish and shellfish can be adapted to different cooking techniques, recipes and seasons. With the wide variety of fish and shellfish available, your taste is certain to always be satisfied, while your sense of well-being is enhanced. Unhealthy cooking methods include frying battered fish as well as topping fish with rich sauces. Once you have started with fresh fish and shellfish, it is then important to choose the most appropriate "Healthiest Way of Cooking" methods (listed below) for the type of fish and shellfish you are preparing. Detailed descriptions on these methods are given in each of the individual fish and shellfish chapters.

### QUICK BROIL

This is a good cooking method to use when you want to quickly cook a fish fillet or steak and seal in its moisture and flavor. It cooks the fish simultaneously on both sides and is a good way to prepare fish if you want to serve it lightly seasoned or with a sauce that you can prepare on the side. (For more on "Quick Broil," see page 61.)

### POACHING

Poaching is a great way of cooking fish to retain its moisture. To get the most flavor, I like to poach fish with a simple homemade fish and shellfish broth whose essence infuses itself into the fish during cooking. (For more on Poaching, see page 61.)

### HEALTHY STEAMING

Many types of fish take well to steaming. You can steam fillets as well as bite-sized pieces of fish, either by themselves or placed on top of vegetables. (For more on "Healthy Steaming," see page 58.)

### HEALTHY SAUTÉ

If your recipe calls for fish or shellfish cut in bite-size pieces and cooked with other ingredients (such as vegetables or other fish and shellfish), you may want to use this cooking method. It cooks the fish quickly, requires no fat and makes a simmering sauce that can be served with the fish. (For more on "Healthy Sauté," see page 57.)

### HEALTHY STOVETOP SEARING

A great cooking method if you want to quickly cook a fillet of fish. Because the skillet is hot, it immediately seals the fish and keeps the moisture from escaping. It is a great way to prepare fish during the warmer weather since it does not require you to turn on the oven or broiler, so your kitchen won't heat up too much. This method is also good when you want to make a sauce to pour over the fish because you can use the same pan to prepare the sauce. The pan will already be hot, plus it will contain a lot of flavor from the fish that will enhance the flavor of your sauce. Stovetop searing is best for oily fish such as tuna or salmon; this method does not work as well on drier varieties of fish.

---

**Q** *I heard that shrimp, although high in cholesterol, have been found to have more of the "good" (HDL) than the "bad" (LDL). Is this true?*

**A** HDL and LDL aren't types of cholesterol. HDL stands for "high-density lipoprotein," and it's the form in which cholesterol (and other substances) gets transported in the bloodstream back toward the liver from other locations in the human body. LDL, which stands for "low-density lipoprotein," is the form in which cholesterol (and other substances) gets transported in the bloodstream out from the liver toward other locations in the body. Since shrimp are arthropods, they don't have a bloodstream like humans with veins, capillaries and arteries, and their cholesterol does not get transported around in the same way. Therefore, shrimp won't provide you with HDL or LDL.

Shrimp do contain cholesterol, however. Four ounces of shrimp contain about 220 mg of cholesterol. (By comparison, one whole egg contains about 187 mg). Most public health organizations allow at least 200 mg daily.

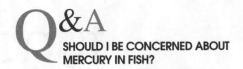

## Q&A

### SHOULD I BE CONCERNED ABOUT MERCURY IN FISH?

Yes, mercury contamination of fish is a definite concern for all individuals, particularly for pregnant women, women considering pregnancy and children. Here is a brief exploration of the causes of mercury contamination, whether the health benefits of fish outweigh the mercury risks and how much mercury exposure is considered safe.

### Sources of Mercury Contamination

Mercury finds its way into the environment from a variety of sources including industrial practices, the incineration of medical and municipal wastes, coal-fired power plants, and the presence in the landfills of mercury-containing products such as fluorescent light bulbs and thermometers. Once it has found its way into the air or the soil, it can move through naturally occurring ecological channels into lakes, streams, rivers and oceans where it becomes a toxic contaminant for fish.

### The Problems of a Global Food Supply

Globalization of the food supply is another reason all individuals need to be concerned about fish and mercury. In certain parts of the world, like the Mediterranean Sea, naturally occurring ore deposits serve as an ongoing source of mercury contamination. A February 2007 report by the U.S. Environmental Protection Agency (EPA) has shown that the geographical origin of different fish (i.e., their original habitat) can play a more important role in degree of mercury contamination than many other factors, including the size of the fish or the length of its lifespan. For example, this 2007 EPA report found Atlantic herring (a very small fish) to contain three times the mercury level of Pacific herring, or even many larger fish like cod.

### Do the Health Benefits Outweigh the Mercury Risks?

Fish has always been recognized to be an excellent source of protein. In more recent years, cold-water fish have also been recognized as excellent sources of omega-3 fatty acids, including EPA (eicosapentaenoic acid) and DHA (docosahexaenoic acid). Risk of mercury contamination has thrown some of these nutritional benefits into question, and the benefits-versus-risks of fish have become a matter of widespread debate. Do the nutritional benefits of fish, including their rich omega-3 fatty acid content, outweigh the risk of mercury exposure?

I believe the answer to this question is "yes"—but a conditional yes, rather than an unconditional one. Yes, the nutritional benefits of fish outweigh the risk of

mercury exposure, provided that (1) lower mercury fish are chosen for consumption and (2) total weekly intake of fish stays fairly restricted. Here's a closer look at the details involved in this risk-benefit analysis.

### Risk-Benefit Analysis of Fish in the Bristol, United Kingdom Study

A study published in the February 17, 2007 issue of The Lancet answers this question with a definite "yes" based on questionnaire data obtained from more than 10,000 women living in Bristol, United Kingdom in the early 1990s. Researchers found that women consuming over 12 ounces (340 grams) of fish per week during their pregnancy had children with higher IQs and better nervous system development than women who consumed less than this amount. While I respect the quality of the research presented in this study, I do not totally agree with the interpretation of its findings, nor do I believe that the findings are necessarily applicable to U.S. women who are trying to evaluate the advantages and disadvantages of fish. My reasoning is fairly simple.

In this 1991–1992 study, women who ate more than 12 ounces of fish per week during their pregnancy were also women who smoked less, had greater amounts of income, were better educated, owned homes and sustained marriages and a family environment in the home. Even though these factors were analyzed statistically by the researchers, I believe that they influenced many aspects of the children's upbringing that were not adequately analyzed by the research team. (There are many reasons I would expect children from these households to do better on IQ tests). In addition, I am concerned about the fact that no daily food records were ever kept by pregnant women in the study, and no food contents—either nutritional or toxicity-related—were ever subjected to laboratory analysis. The fact that all of the women in the study lived in one town in the United Kingdom 15–16 years ago is also of concern, given the increasingly dynamic nature of the global food supply and geographical origins of fish in the U.S. marketplace.

### Risk-Benefit Approach to Fish by the U.S. Food and Drug Administration (FDA)

My own conclusion about the risk-benefit profile of fish is much closer to the position taken by the U.S. Food and Drug Administration (FDA) in its March 19, 2004 advisory on mercury and fish. Like the FDA, I believe that a restriction on fish intake is prudent for all individuals. While setting a 12-ounce guideline for maximum weekly intake of all fish, the FDA also recommended that this 12-ounce intake be restricted to fish and shellfish that are lower in mercury. I support this type of approach, and I like the idea of a dividing line between lower mercury

*(Continued on Page 498)*

# tuna

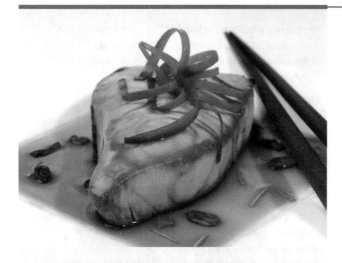

| | |
|---|---|
| AVAILABILITY: | Year-round |
| REFRIGERATE: | Yes |
| SHELF LIFE: | Up to 4 days refrigerated |
| PREPARATION: | Minimal |
| BEST WAY TO COOK: | "Quick Broil" in just 2 minutes |

## nutrient-richness chart

Total Nutrient-Richness: **24**
4 ounces (113 grams) of baked/broiled Tuna contains 158 calories

| NUTRIENT | AMOUNT | %DV | DENSITY | QUALITY |
|---|---|---|---|---|
| Tryptophan | 0.4 g | 118.8 | 13.6 | excellent |
| Selenium | 53.1 mcg | 75.8 | 8.7 | excellent |
| Protein | 34.0 g | 68.0 | 7.8 | excellent |
| B3 Niacin | 13.5 mg | 67.7 | 7.7 | excellent |
| Pyroxidine B6 | 1.2 mg | 59.0 | 6.7 | very good |
| B1 Thiamin | 0.6 mg | 38.0 | 4.3 | very good |
| Phosphorus | 277.8 mg | 27.8 | 3.2 | good |
| Potassium | 645.3 mg | 18.4 | 2.1 | good |
| Magnesium | 72.6 mg | 18.1 | 2.1 | good |
| Omega-3 Fatty Acids | 0.3 g | 13.2 | 1.5 | good |

For more on "Total Nutrient-Richness," "%DV," "Density," and
The World's Healthiest Foods "Quality" Rating System, see page 805.

Tuna is second only to shrimp in popularity largely due to the demand for canned Tuna. While canned Tuna may be convenient, it does not compare to the wonderful taste treat provided by fresh Tuna. Fresh Tuna has been enjoyed by coastal populations throughout history, while smoked and pickled Tuna have been widely consumed since ancient times. The firm, dense flesh of Tuna gives it one of the meatiest flavors and textures of any fish. Because the moisture content of Tuna can be easily lost through cooking, making it tough and dry, I want to share with you how the "Healthiest Way of Cooking" methods can not only keep Tuna moist, but also bring out its wonderful flavor.

## why tuna should be part of your healthiest way of eating

Like other varieties of fish, Tuna is a rich source of protein.

Its omega-3 fatty acids are important for cardiovascular health and reducing inflammation, while its selenium, potassium and magnesium also support a healthy heart. Tuna is an ideal food to add to your "Healthiest Way of Eating" because not only is it high in protein but it is also low in fat. (For more on the *Health Benefits of Tuna* and a complete analysis of its content of over 60 nutrients, see page 468.)

## varieties of tuna

Tuna are found in the warm water areas of the Pacific, Atlantic and Indian Oceans as well as the Mediterranean Sea. The meat is a reddish color because Tuna are hydrodynamically designed to swim more than other species of fish, resulting in greater oxygenation of their muscle mass. Tuna are not farm-raised. Popular varieties include:

### ALBACORE OR WHITE TUNA

Weighing up to 130 pounds, it has pinkish flesh, which turns white when cooked, and a delicate taste. In Hawaii, it is called tombo. Most Albacore Tuna is canned and sold as Albacore, white Tuna or white chunk. Although it is sometimes sold in markets and served in restaurants, it is not as flavorful or as popular as Yellowfin or Ahi.

### YELLOWFIN OR AHI

True to its name, the fins and tail of this variety are a distinctive yellow color. The meat is pale, fatty, firm and dense; it is usually canned as "light" Tuna. It is called Ahi in Hawaii. It is sold fresh as steaks.

### BLUEFIN

It is the largest member of the Tuna family, weighing up to 400 pounds. It is difficult to find, has reddish brown flesh and is fattier than other varieties. Bluefin is very tasty and used for sashimi.

**BONITO OR SKIPJACK**

This small (up to 5 pounds) and most frequently caught variety of Tuna has dark red flesh and is usually canned with Yellowfin Tuna and sold as "light" Tuna. The Japanese often use dried bonito for seasoning and garnish.

## the peak season

Canned and fresh Tuna are available throughout the year.

## biochemical considerations

In the spring of 2004, due to concerns about mercury levels in certain fish, the FDA issued recommendations that children, pregnant and nursing women, and women of childbearing age should limit their consumption of canned Albacore Tuna and Tuna steaks to no more than 6 ounces per week and light Tuna to no more than 12 ounces per week. (For more on *Mercury in Fish*, see page 463.)

## 4 steps for the best tasting and most nutritious tuna

Turning Tuna into a flavorful dish with the most nutrients is simple if you just follow my 4 easy steps:

1. The Best Way to Select
2. The Best Way to Store
3. The Best Way to Prepare
4. The Healthiest Way of Cooking

---

### POLE-CAUGHT YELLOWFIN, SKIPJACK AND ALBACORE TUNA ARE THE BEST CHOICE* AS ECOLOGICALLY SUSTAINABLE SPECIES

Sustainable species of Tuna are those that can be sustained long-term without compromising their survival or the integrity of the ecosystem in which they live. Yellowfin and Skipjack Tuna are abundant in number because they reproduce quickly. Albacore Tuna have healthy and stable populations; however, fishing methods can affect their level of sustainability.

Pole and troll caught Albacore, Yellowfin and Skipjack Tuna are the best choices for sustainability because this method results in the least amount of bycatch (unintended catch of other species such as dolphins due to the method of fishing). You should use "caution" when selecting Tuna (Albacore, Yellowfin or canned Tuna) that was caught using a long-line or purse seines; these methods of fishing result in more undesirable bycatch.

Bluefin Tuna are severely overfished and are on the list of fish to "avoid" eating because they are not considered a sustainable resource at the present time.

*\* Information from Monterey Bay Aquarium Seafood Watch*

---

# 1. the best way to select tuna

Fresh Tuna such as Yellowfin Tuna (also called Ahi) is the most flavorful and the best type of Tuna to cook. Tuna is sold in many different forms. It is available fresh as steaks, fillets or pieces, but is most popular in its canned form. (See *The Guide* for mercury content, page 457.)

Just as with any seafood, it is best to purchase fresh Tuna from a store that has a good reputation for having a frequent turnover of their fresh fish. Get to know a fishmonger (the person who sells the fish) at the store, so you have someone from whom you can purchase your fish with confidence.

Fresh whole Tuna should be displayed buried in ice, while fillets and steaks should be placed on top of the ice. The flesh should be firm to the touch. Try to avoid purchasing Tuna that has dry or brown spots.

Smell is a good indicator of freshness. Since a slightly "off" smell cannot be detected through plastic, if you have the option, it is preferable to purchase displayed fish as opposed to pieces that are prepackaged. Once the fishmonger wraps and hands you the fish that you have selected, smell it through the paper wrapping and return it if it has a very strong fishy odor.

If you are going to have a full day of errands after you purchase your Tuna, be sure to keep a cooler in the car to ensure it stays cold and does not spoil.

**CANNED TUNA** is available either solid or in chunks and is packaged in oil, broth or water. Although the Tuna packed in oil usually has the greatest amount of moisture, it also has the highest fat content, and the oils in which it is packed are high in omega-6 fats. Since omega-6 fatty acids and omega-3 fatty acids compete for the same enzymes that activate them for use in the body, and most Americans already consume too many omega-6 fats in comparison to omega-3s, it is best to purchase Tuna packed in water or broth (for more on *Omega-3 Fatty Acids*, see page 770). Oftentimes, cans of Tuna do not specify the species of Tuna that was canned except to indicate that it is either light Tuna (Skipjack and/or Yellowfin) or white Tuna (usually Albacore).

**LIGHT CANNED TUNA** contains less mercury than white or albacore Tuna. You can find canned specialty Tuna, which is pole-caught with no bycatch and therefore ecologically sustainable. The specialty Tunas claim to have higher concentration of omega-3 fatty acids and lower concentrations of mercury and can be found online and in specialty and natural food stores.

## 2. the best way to store tuna

Fresh Tuna, like other fish, is very perishable, and normal refrigerator temperatures of 36°–40°F (2°–4°C) do not inhibit the enzymatic activity that causes it to spoil; it is best when stored at 28°–32°F (-2°–0°C). I have tried various methods to find the best way to store Tuna including packing the Tuna with ice before placing it in the refrigerator to decrease the temperature. Although this method kept the Tuna cool, once the ice melted, the Tuna ended up sitting in a pool of water, causing it to lose much of its flavor.

I have refined this method and want to share with you the best way to keep your Tuna fresh. Remove Tuna from store packaging, rinse and place in a plastic storage bag as soon as you bring it home from the market. Place Tuna in a large bowl and cover with ice cubes or ice packs to reduce the temperature of the Tuna. Although fresh Tuna will keep for a few days using this method, I recommend using it within a day or two of purchase. Remember to drain off the melted ice water and replenish the ice or replace the ice packs as necessary.

If you have more Tuna than you can use, freezing will increase its shelf life to 3 – 6 months.

## 3. the best way to prepare tuna

Fresh Tuna is usually bought precut in steaks and requires very little preparation. Make sure it is very fresh. The skin of Tuna is inedible and bitter, so you rarely see Tuna sold with skin on.

Rinse and wipe Tuna dry. Rub with a little fresh lemon juice and season with salt and pepper before cooking. Tuna is excellent if given the chance to marinate for 24 hours before cooking. There are many marinades that are suitable for fresh Tuna.

Canned Tuna requires no preparation and can be used in a variety of different ways.

## 4. the healthiest way of cooking tuna

Searing Tuna is the best for keeping it moist and tender. Tuna cooks very quickly and can be prepared in 2–3 minutes as it is best cooked rare. If you want your Tuna cooked through, cook for 7–10 minutes for each inch of thickness; this is the general rule for cooking fish. It can be easily overcooked and become dry, so be sure to watch your cooking times. "Quick Broil" is the method I found best to sear Tuna. (Cooking times are based on 1-inch thickness. Fish that is 1/2-inch thick will take half the amount of time.)

### How to Avoid Overcooking Tuna

To prevent overcooking Tuna, I highly recommend using a timer. And since Tuna cooks in only 2–3 minutes, it is important to begin timing as soon as you place it onto the skillet. Remove Tuna from the heat and transfer it to a plate after the allocated time because it will continue to cook if left in the pan. Overcooked Tuna will become dry and tough.

### Methods Not Recommended for Tuna

#### COOKING WITH OIL

I don't recommend cooking Tuna in oil because high temperature heat can damage delicate oils and potentially create harmful free radicals. (For more on *Why it is Important to Cook without Heated Oils*, see page 52.)

Here are questions that I received from readers of the whfoods.org website about Tuna:

**Q** *I often order Tuna in restaurants and wanted to know what the best way is for me to have it prepared (i.e., rare, medium, etc.)? Does it make a difference in terms of its nutritional value?*

**A** There are slight nutritional differences between fish that is cooked medium rare or medium, and in many nutrient categories these differences would not be great enough to rule out either choice as a healthy option. In fact, using Tuna as an example, there are only very slight differences between the vitamin E, vitamin A and omega-3 fatty acid content of raw Tuna in comparison to medium broiled Tuna. The protein content of fish will not change significantly even if the fish is overcooked. However, an overcooked fish is usually dry, more rubbery in texture, non-flaky and lacking in flavor. In terms of nutrition, you're also going to want to look for restaurants that pay close attention to the overall freshness of the fish (length of time since it was caught). Of course, the more recent the catch, the better the nutritional value.

## Q How do you know when fresh Tuna has gone bad?

**A** Use smell as your guide. Does the Tuna have a funny, fishy, strong, "off" odor? If so, it has probably gone bad. Also, how long has it been stored? Unless the Tuna was caught the day before you purchased it, I wouldn't recommend storing it in the refrigerator for more than one or two days. Especially with fish and meat, I like to follow the old kitchen adage—when in doubt, throw it out! So if you are unsure of whether it is bad, I would suggest not using it.

## Q How does vacuum cooking work?

**A** Vacuum cooking typically involves the use of a plastic pouch to surround a food and provide a small, enclosed space in which a combination of steam and heated air can cook the food. I've usually seen this process applied to meats and fish. These foods are vacuum-sealed together with spices and seasonings, and the flavor of these seasonings can be very effectively retained through the use of vacuum packing. However, I don't recommend this technique due to the possible risk of plastic migration from the pouch into the food. Such migration of plastic has been clearly demonstrated in research with the use of plastic bags in microwave ovens. So yes, vacuum cooking works, but I do not recommend vacuum cooking due to the toxicity risk I've described.

## Q I don't care for any type of seafood, but I still want the benefits that seafood provides. Are there other foods that can provide me the same benefits?

**A** No food will have the same exact benefits in totality that another food provides. Yet, you can look for other foods that also contain the nutrients concentrated in the original food.

For example, seafood has gained a lot of recent acclaim because it is rich in omega-3 fatty acids, a group of nutrients with anti-inflammatory properties that have shown benefit for overall health. The omega-3 fatty acids that are concentrated in seafood are the longer chain varieties, notably eicosapentaenoic acid (EPA) and docosahexaenoic acid (DHA).

---

## Tuna Salad without Mayo

*Enjoy a great tuna salad or sandwich without using mayonnaise.*

**2 6.5-oz cans of light Tuna, drained**

**Dressing:**
**3 medium cloves garlic, pressed**
**1 TBS prepared Dijon mustard**
**1 tsp honey**
**4 TBS fresh lemon juice**
**1/4 cup sunflower seeds**
**4 oz silken tofu**
**1/2 tsp Italian herbs**
**2 TBS extra virgin olive oil**
**Sea salt and pepper to taste**
**\*a little water to thin if necessary**

Combine all dressing ingredients in blender and blend until smooth. Mix by hand with Tuna in a mixing bowl. Serve on a bed of salad greens or use in a sandwich.

### Flavor Tips: 9 Ways to Enjoy Tuna Salad

1. Add diced celery.
2. Add chopped walnuts.
3. Add chopped fresh parsley.
4. Add finely minced onions.
5. Add chopped tomatoes with excess seeds removed.
6. Add capers.
7. Add anchovy paste.
8. Add olives.
9. Add 1/2 cup tahini instead of tofu.

---

Unfortunately, no other food is as concentrated in these long-chain fatty acids as seafood. Yet, certain foods are rich in the omega-3 fatty acid, alpha-linolenic acid (ALA), which is the precursor to EPA and DHA. ALA is found in some vegetables and is especially concentrated in flaxseeds and walnuts. About 10% of ALA gets converted to these longer-chain fatty acids, yet most of it seems to be converted to EPA, with less being converted to DHA. Many vegetarians concerned about their omega-3 intake often include nuts and seeds in their diet and then may take an algae supplement rich in DHA to make sure that they get adequate amounts of this important nutrient. For more information about omega-3 fatty acids, see page 770.

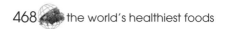
# health benefits of tuna

## Promotes Heart Health

Tuna is a good source of the omega-3 fatty acids, notably EPA and DHA, which provide a broad array of cardiovascular benefits. Omega-3s benefit the cardiovascular system by helping to prevent erratic heart rhythms, making blood less likely to clot inside arteries (which is the ultimate cause of most heart attacks) and reducing triglyceride levels. Because inflammation is a key component in converting cholesterol into artery-clogging plaques, the ability of omega-3s to reduce inflammation helps prevent atherosclerosis; therefore, it further reduces the risk of heart disease. Omega-3 fatty acids may be partially responsible for a recent study's finding that eating fish lowers the risk of certain types of strokes. Tuna is also a concentrated source of other heart-health-promoting nutrients including selenium, vitamin B6, potassium and magnesium.

## Helps Reduce Stress

Eating fish rich in omega-3 fatty acids, such as Tuna, may help to reduce stress. A recent study found a relationship between consuming fish rich in omega-3 fats and a lower hostility rate in young adults. Other studies have suggested that DHA supplementation can reduce levels of aggression and enhance the stress response. In addition, plasma levels of omega-3 fatty acids have been found to be reduced in people who express more aggressive behavior.

## Promotes Vision Health

Eating fish may protect against age-related macular degeneration (ARMD), a currently untreatable disease that causes fuzziness, shadows or other distortions in the center of vision. In a recently published study, investigators found that those who ate the greatest amount of fat overall increased their risk of ARMD, while those who ate fish reduced their risk of developing the eye disease. One of the reasons that fish like Tuna may benefit eye health is that they provide DHA, which is actually concentrated in the retina of the eye and may help protect and promote healthy retinal function.

## Promotes Optimal Health

Tuna is rich in selenium, a necessary component of one of the body's most important antioxidants, *glutathione peroxidase*, which is critical for the liver to detoxify and clear potentially harmful compounds such as pesticides, drugs and heavy metals from the body. Selenium also helps prevent cancer and heart disease.

## Additional Health-Promoting Benefits of Tuna

Tuna is also a concentrated source of many nutrients providing additional health benefits. These nutrients include muscle-building protein, energy-producing vitamin B1 and phosphorus, and sleep-promoting tryptophan.

### Nutritional Analysis of 4 ounces of baked/broiled Tuna:

| NUTRIENT | AMOUNT | % DAILY VALUE | NUTRIENT | AMOUNT | % DAILY VALUE |
|---|---|---|---|---|---|
| Calories | 157.63 | | Pantothenic Acid | 0.98 mg | 9.80 |
| Calories from Fat | 12.45 | | | | |
| Calories from Saturated Fat | 3.07 | | **Minerals** | | |
| Protein | 33.99 g | | Boron | — mcg | |
| Carbohydrates | 0.00 g | | Calcium | 23.81 mg | 2.38 |
| Dietary Fiber | 0.00 g | 0.00 | Chloride | — mg | |
| Soluble Fiber | 0.00 g | | Chromium | — mcg | — |
| Insoluble Fiber | 0.00 g | | Copper | 0.09 mg | 4.50 |
| Sugar – Total | 0.00 g | | Fluoride | — mg | — |
| Monosaccharides | 0.00 g | | Iodine | — mcg | — |
| Disaccharides | 0.00 g | | Iron | 1.07 mg | 5.94 |
| Other Carbs | 0.00 g | | Magnesium | 72.58 mg | 18.14 |
| Fat –Total | 1.38 g | | Manganese | 0.02 mg | 1.00 |
| Saturated Fat | 0.34 g | | Molybdenum | 3.86 mcg | 5.15 |
| Mono Fat | 0.22 g | | Phosphorus | 277.83 mg | 27.78 |
| Poly Fat | 0.41 g | | Potassium | 645.25 mg | |
| Omega-3 Fatty Acids | 0.33 g | 13.20 | Selenium | 53.07 mcg | 75.81 |
| Omega-6 Fatty Acids | 0.05 g | | Sodium | 53.30 mg | |
| Trans Fatty Acids | 0.00 g | | Zinc | 0.76 mg | 5.07 |
| Cholesterol | 65.77 mg | | | | |
| Water | 71.23 g | | **Amino Acids** | | |
| Ash | 1.95 g | | Alanine | 2.06 g | |
| | | | Arginine | 2.03 g | |
| **Vitamins** | | | Aspartate | 3.48 g | |
| Vitamin A IU | 77.11 IU | 1.54 | Cystine | 0.36 g | 87.80 |
| Vitamin A RE | 22.68 RE | | Glutamate | 5.07 g | |
| A - Carotenoid | 0.00 RE | 0.00 | Glycine | 1.63 g | |
| A - Retinol | 22.68 RE | | Histidine | 1.00 g | 77.52 |
| B1 Thiamin | 0.57 mg | 38.00 | Isoleucine | 1.57 g | 136.52 |
| B2 Riboflavin | 0.06 mg | 3.53 | Leucine | 2.76 g | 109.09 |
| B3 Niacin | 13.54 mg | 67.70 | Lysine | 3.12 g | 132.77 |
| Niacin Equiv | 19.89 mg | | Methionine | 1.01 g | 136.49 |
| Vitamin B6 | 1.18 mg | 59.00 | Phenylalanine | 1.33 g | 111.76 |
| Vitamin B12 | 0.68 mcg | 11.33 | Proline | 1.20 g | |
| Biotin | — mcg | — | Serine | 1.39 g | |
| Vitamin C | 1.13 mg | 1.88 | Threonine | 1.49 g | 120.16 |
| Vitamin D IU | — IU | — | Tryptophan | 0.38 g | 118.75 |
| Vitamin D mcg | — mcg | | Tyrosine | 1.15 g | 118.56 |
| Vitamin E Alpha Equiv | 0.71 mg | 3.55 | Valine | 1.75 g | 119.05 |
| Vitamin E IU | 1.06 IU | | | | |
| Vitamin E mg | 0.71 mg | | (Note: "–" indicates data is unavailable. For more information, please see page 806.) | | |
| Folate | 2.27 mcg | 0.57 | | | |
| Vitamin K | — mcg | — | | | |

STEP-BY-STEP RECIPE
## The Healthiest Way of Cooking Tuna

# 2-Minute "Quick Broiled" Tuna Steaks

*"Quick Broil" seals in Tuna's natural flavor and moisture, and the Tuna is ready in a matter of minutes!*

3/4 lb Tuna steaks (2 steaks each 1" thick)
2 TBS + 1 tsp fresh lemon juice
Sea salt and black pepper to taste
2 TBS extra virgin olive oil
1 medium clove garlic

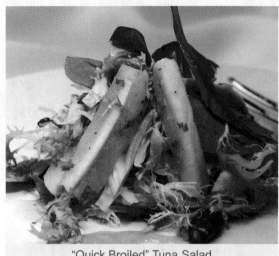

"Quick Broiled" Tuna Salad

1. Chop or press garlic and let sit for 5 minutes (Why?, see page 261.)

2. Preheat the broiler on high and place an all stainless steel skillet (be sure the handle is also stainless steel) or cast iron pan under the heat for about 10 minutes to get it very hot. The pan should be 5–7 inches from the heat source.

3. While pan is heating, prepare Tuna by rubbing steaks with 2 TBS fresh lemon juice and salt and pepper. The pan requires no oil as the lemon from the fish sufficiently coats the pan.

4. Using a hot pad, remove pan from heat, place Tuna on hot pan and return pan to broiler. Keep in mind that it is cooking rapidly on both sides, so it is done very quickly, usually in 2–3 minutes, depending on thickness.

5. Dress with olive oil, 1 tsp lemon juice and garlic.

**SERVES 2**

## Flavor Tips: Try these 7 great serving suggestions with the recipe above. ✱

1. **Most Popular: "Quick Broiled" Tuna Salad.** In a small bowl, whisk together: 3 TBS extra virgin olive oil, 1 TBS lemon juice, 2 tsp Dijon mustard, 1 tsp rinsed capers and 2 TBS minced parsley. Prepare 2-Minute "Quick Broiled" Tuna, omitting dressing. Cut Tuna into slices and toss with the mustard mixture. Serve on a bed of fresh greens.

2. Coat with Olive Tapenade (page 325) after broiling. Omit salt from above recipe.

3. Spread Tuna steaks with Dijon mustard and fresh chopped rosemary before "Quick Broiling."

4. Add Tuna to a Niçoise salad (see page 144).

5. For an Asian flavor, add tamari (soy sauce), ginger and rice vinegar. Replace black pepper with white pepper and omit salt.

6. Tamari, lime juice, and sesame seeds are natural complements to Tuna.

7. Make a sauce of wasabi horseradish and tamari. Drizzle over cooked Tuna. Tuna can take a lot of heat, so go as spicy as you like!

Please write (address on back cover flap) or e-mail me at info@whfoods.org with your personal ideas for preparing Tuna, and I will share them with others through our website at www.whfoods.org.

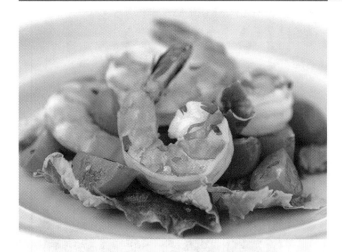

# shrimp

| | |
|---|---|
| AVAILABILITY: | Year-round |
| REFRIGERATE: | Yes |
| SHELF LIFE: | Up to 2 days refrigerated |
| PREPARATION: | Shell and devein |
| BEST WAY TO COOK: | "Healthy Sauté" in just 3 minutes |

## nutrient-richness chart

Total Nutrient-Richness: **23**
4 ounces (113 grams) of boiled Shrimp contain 112 calories

| NUTRIENT | AMOUNT | %DV | DENSITY | QUALITY |
|---|---|---|---|---|
| Tryptophan | 0.3 g | 103.1 | 16.5 | excellent |
| Selenium | 44.9 mcg | 64.2 | 10.3 | excellent |
| Protein | 23.7 g | 47.4 | 7.6 | excellent |
| Vitamin D | 162.4 IU | 40.6 | 6.5 | very good |
| Vitamin B12 | 1.7 mcg | 28.2 | 4.5 | very good |
| Iron | 3.5 mg | 19.4 | 3.1 | good |
| Phosphorus | 155.4 mg | 15.5 | 2.5 | good |
| Omega-3 Fatty Acids | 0.4 g | 14.8 | 2.4 | good |
| B3 Niacin | 2.9 mg | 14.7 | 2.4 | good |
| Zinc | 1.8 mg | 11.8 | 1.9 | good |
| Copper | 0.2 mg | 11.0 | 1.8 | good |
| Magnesium | 38.6 mg | 9.6 | 1.5 | good |

For more on "Total Nutrient-Richness," "%DV," "Density," and
The World's Healthiest Foods "Quality" Rating System, see page 805.

Shrimp may be small in size, but they are huge in nutritional value and taste appeal. Close relatives to lobster and crayfish, Shrimp's delicious taste and ease of preparation make them the most popular seafood in the United States; they are consumed more than salmon or tuna. The English name for Shrimp is prawns. Shrimp prepared with garlic is called *scampi* in Italy. Shrimp can be served hot or cold and offer a great alternative to meat protein. I want to share with you how using the "Healthiest Way of Cooking" Shrimp can enhance their flavor in just a matter of minutes!

## why shrimp should be part of your healthiest way of eating

Shrimp are an excellent source of protein and a good source of those hard-to-find, health-promoting omega-3 fatty acids, which are not only important for heart health, but also for reducing inflammation. They are a rich source of minerals, including copper, selenium and zinc, which provide powerful antioxidant protection against the oxidative damage to cellular structures caused by free radicals. Shrimp are an ideal food to add to your "Healthiest Way of Eating" not only because they are high in nutrients and low in fat, but also because they are low in calories making them a good choice for healthy weight control: 4 ounces of Shrimp contain only 112 calories! (For more on the *Health Benefits of Shrimp* and a complete analysis of their content of over 60 nutrients, see page 474.)

## varieties of shrimp

Although farm-raised Shrimp are now sold in the United States, most Shrimp are still caught in the wild. Over 300 different species of Shrimp are harvested worldwide, and within these 300 species are thousands of different varieties. Shrimp freeze well, and most Shrimp in the market have been frozen.

Saltwater Shrimp are classified as either warm-water or cold-water Shrimp. Warm-water shrimp are caught off the coast of North Carolina, Texas, California and Mexico; they include White, Brown, Rock and Pink Shrimp. Pink Shrimp are three to four inches in length, reddish-pink in color and the most popular variety in the United States. Cold-water Shrimp are caught in the north Atlantic and north Pacific; they have firmer meat than warm-water varieties and a sweeter flavor. Some common varieties of Shrimp include:

### PINK SHRIMP
The most popular variety is northern Pink Shrimp or Maine Shrimp.

### SPOTTED PRAWNS

Also known as Alaskan prawns, these are caught in the Pacific Ocean off the West Coast of the United States.

### GIANT TIGER PRAWNS

These large Shrimp measure six to twelve inches in length.

### FARM-RAISED SHRIMP

They are raised both domestically or can be imported. The farm raising of Shrimp in the U.S. is well regulated, and farmers must adhere to laws limiting environmental impact. Imported Shrimp production is not well regulated.

## the peak season

Fresh and frozen Shrimp are available throughout the year.

## biochemical considerations

Shrimp may be considered a high cholesterol food for individuals watching their cholesterol intake (221 mg in a 4-ounce serving). Shrimp also contain purines, which may be problematic for certain individuals. (For more on *Purines*, see page 727.)

## 4 steps for the best tasting and most nutritious shrimp

Turning Shrimp into a flavorful dish with the most nutrients is simple if you just follow my 4 easy steps:

1. The Best Way to Select
2. The Best Way to Store
3. The Best Way to Prepare
4. The Healthiest Way of Cooking

# 1. the best way to select shrimp

Pink Shrimp from Oregon and spotted Shrimp from British Columbia are the best Shrimp to purchase. However, they may be difficult to find, so U.S. farmed or trawl-caught Shrimp or wild Shrimp from the Canadian Atlantic are your next best alternatives. Avoid other imported Shrimp whenever possible. (For more on *Sustainability*, see page 473.)

The first step in selecting the best Shrimp is to find a store with a good reputation for having a fresh supply of fish and shellfish. Get to know a fishmonger (person who sells the seafood) at the store so you can have a trusted person from whom you can purchase your Shrimp.

Fresh Shrimp should have firm bodies that are still attached to their shells, which should be free of black spots since this indicates that the flesh has begun to break down. In addition, the shells should not appear yellow or gritty as this may reflect the use of sodium bisulfate or another chemical to bleach the shells. Whenever possible, purchase displayed Shrimp rather than prepackaged Shrimp. Smell is a good indicator of freshness, and it is difficult to detect smells through the plastic of prepackaged seafood. I have found that fresh Shrimp never smells fishy but more like seawater. Once the fishmonger wraps and hands you the Shrimp, smell it through the paper

wrapping and return it if it does not smell right.

Since Shrimp freeze well, it is best to buy Shrimp while still frozen. This will ensure you are getting the freshest Shrimp possible because they are usually frozen as soon as they are caught. One pound of frozen Shrimp with shells on will yield about a half pound of cooked shelled Shrimp. Frozen Shrimp have the longest shelf life and can be kept for several weeks, whereas fresh Shrimp will only keep for a day or two.

The number of Shrimp you get per pound will depend on their size:

- Small Shrimp: 40–50 per pound
- Medium Shrimp: 31–40 per pound
- Large Shrimp: 26–30 per pound
- Extra Large Shrimp: 21–25 per pound
- Jumbo Shrimp: 16–20 per pound

Shrimp that come over 40 per pound are usually precooked and used for salads and Shrimp cocktail.

If you are going to have a full day of errands after you purchase your Shrimp, be sure to keep a cooler in the car to ensure they stay cold and do not spoil.

# 2. the best way to store shrimp

Like most seafood, Shrimp are very perishable and normal refrigerator temperatures of 36°–40°F (2°–4°C) do not inhibit the enzymatic activity that causes them to spoil; they are best when stored at 28°–32°F (-2°–0°C). I have tried various methods to find the best way to store Shrimp, including

packing the Shrimp with ice before placing it in the refrigerator to decrease the temperature. Although this method kept the Shrimp cool, once the ice melted, the Shrimp ended up sitting in a pool of water, causing them to lose much of their flavor.

I have refined this method and want to share with you the

best way to keep Shrimp fresh. Remove Shrimp from store packaging, rinse and place in a plastic zip-lock bag as soon as you bring them home from the market. Place in a large bowl and cover with ice cubes or ice packs to reduce the temperature of the Shrimp. Although fresh Shrimp will keep for a few days using this method, I recommend using your Shrimp within a day or two of purchase. Remember to drain off the melted ice water and replenish the ice or replace the ice packs as necessary. Frozen Shrimp can be kept for several weeks. Cooked shrimp should be consumed within 24 hours.

# 3. the best way to prepare shrimp

Properly preparing Shrimp helps to ensure that the Shrimp you serve will have the best flavor and retain the greatest number of nutrients.

### Defrosting Shrimp
Defrost frozen Shrimp in the refrigerator. Do not thaw Shrimp at room temperature or in a microwave.

### Peeling and Deveining Shrimp
Remove the shell by pulling it away from the Shrimp meat starting at the legs on the underside of the Shrimp. The tail can be removed, if desired. With a sharp paring knife, make a slit down the back of the Shrimp about 1/8 inch deep. You may see a dark string (the intestines of the shrimp) that runs the length of the Shrimp. Rinse under cold water to remove.

If you are not going to remove the shells, rinse Shrimp under cold running water and pat dry before cooking.

# 4. the healthiest way of cooking shrimp

The best way to cook Shrimp is by using methods that will keep them moist and tender. Shrimp can be easily over-cooked and become dry, so be sure to watch your cooking times. Shrimp are delicate, and I have found that they can be best prepared by using the "Healthy Sauté" method. (For more on *Healthy Sauté,* see page 57.)

While grilled Shrimp tastes great, make sure that they do not burn. It is best to grill Shrimp on an area without a direct flame as the temperatures directly above or below the flame can reach as high as 500°F to 1000°F (260°C to 578°C). Extra care should be taken when grilling as burning can damage nutrients and create free radicals that can be harmful to your health. (For more on *Grilling*, see page 61.)

### How to Avoid Overcooking Shrimp
Shrimp cook quickly and are easily overcooked. To prevent overcooking Shrimp, I highly recommend using a timer. And since Shrimp cook in only 3–4 minutes, it is important to begin timing as soon as you place them into the skillet. Shrimp will become tough and lose their flavor when overcooked.

### Methods Not Recommended for Cooking Shrimp
#### COOKING WITH OIL
I don't recommend cooking Shrimp in oil because high temperature heat can damage delicate oils and potentially create harmful free radicals. (For more on *Why it is Important to Cook without Heated Oils*, see page 52.)

## An Easy Way to Prepare Shrimp, Step-by-Step

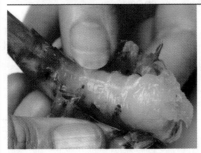 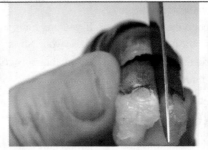 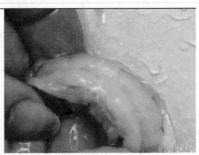

### PEELING AND DEVEINING SHRIMP
❶ Pull shell away from Shrimp meat starting at the legs on the underside of Shrimp. Remove tail if the recipe calls for it. ❷ With a sharp paring knife make a slit down the back of the Shrimp about 1/8 inch deep. ❸ You may see a dark string the length of the Shrimp. Rinse under cold water to remove this.

Here is a question that I received from a reader of the whfoods.org website about Shrimp:

## Q *Should I devein my Shrimp, and what is the "vein" that gets removed?*

A Some people prefer to devein their Shrimp while others don't (I actually prefer shrimp deveined). The reason is not just from an appearance perspective, but because the "vein" is actually the intestines of the Shrimp and any material that may be in it.

---

### OREGON PINK SHRIMP AND B.C. SPOTTED PRAWNS ARE THE BEST CHOICE* AS ECOLOGICALLY SUSTAINABLE SPECIES

Sustainable species of Shrimp are those that can be sustained long-term without compromising their survival or the integrity of the ecosystem in which they live. Pink Shrimp from Oregon and spotted Shrimp from British Columbia are your best choices for sustainability. U.S. farmed or trawl-caught Shrimp or wild Canadian Atlantic Shrimp are your next best alternative. Farm-raised Shrimp operations in the United States are well regulated with the use of the antibiotic chloramphenicol strictly prohibited; the Shrimp are also never treated with iodine. U.S. trawling methods are also more ecologically sound than methods used by foreign fishing fleets as boats are outfitted with devices to let turtles and fish escape from their nets.

Imported foreign Shrimp should be "avoided." Fishing methods used to catch them may be very detrimental to Shrimp habitat and the surrounding ecological environment, and there are high levels of bycatch using these methods. Shrimp from the Gulf of Thailand can have 14 pounds of bycatch per pound of Shrimp! They are oftentimes not frozen immediately after being harvested. Shrimp from foreign Shrimp farms are also treated with iodine as well as antibiotic chloramphenicol to keep them white.

*\* Information from Monterey Bay Aquarium Seafood Watch*

---

## 5-Minute Boiled Large Shrimp

*Boiling Shrimp is quick and easy, and you can use boiled Shrimp in a variety of different recipes.*

**1/2 lb large Shrimp
3 TBS + 1 tsp fresh lemon juice
3 TBS extra virgin olive oil
Sea salt and pepper to taste**

1. Chop or press garlic and let sit for 5 minutes. (Why?, see page 261.)

2. Use a 3-quart saucepan filled halfway with water. Add salt to taste and 3 TBS lemon juice to the water and bring to a boil.

3. Peel and devein Shrimp as directed under *The Best Way to Prepare*.

4. When water is at a full boil, place Shrimp into the pot. Stir briefly, remove the pot from the heat and **cover**. Steep small Shrimp for 1 minute, medium Shrimp for 2 minutes and large Shrimp for 5 minutes. Cooked Shrimp look pink and are firm and opaque in the center. If the center is still translucent, steep for an additional 30 seconds **covered**. Be extremely careful to avoid burning yourself when adding Shrimp to the boiling water.

5. Dress with extra virgin olive oil, remaining lemon juice, garlic and salt and pepper to taste.

**SERVES 2**

### HOW TO ENJOY BOILED SHRIMP:

- Add chilled, small cooked Shrimp to Tangy Gazpacho recipe (page 288) for a great twist with added nutrition and flavor.
- **Asian Dipping Sauce:** In a small bowl, combine 4 TBS tamari (soy sauce), 1 tsp minced ginger, 2 tsp sesame seeds, 1 tsp honey and a pinch of red pepper flakes. Place in individual bowls. Dip cooked hot or cold Shrimp into the sauce.
- **Shrimp Cocktail:** In a medium bowl, combine 1 cup organic ketchup, 1–2 TBS horseradish, 1 tsp chili powder, 2 tsp lemon juice, 1 tsp Worcestershire Sauce, and sea salt and black pepper to taste. Dip boiled Shrimp into sauce.

---

### WHY COOKED SHRIMP TURNS PINK

When you cook Shrimp, the color of its shell and flesh change from gray-white to bright red, orange and pink. The reason for this colorful transformation is related to a carotenoid—astaxanthin—that is present not only in Shrimp but also in other seafood such as salmon, lobster, crabs and crawfish, and which gives these foods their reddish-pink tone. Yet, unlike in other seafood, the astaxanthin found in Shrimp is bound to a protein that conceals its natural color, making the Shrimp appear gray-white. When heat is applied in the process of cooking, the bond between the astaxanthin and the protein dissolves, so its red-pink tone can naturally appear.

The benefits of astaxanthin are not limited to the beautiful color that it provides. It is also a powerful antioxidant and plays an important role in the function of the immune and reproductive systems of sea animals.

# health benefits of shrimp

## Promote Heart Health

Many people are confused about the fat and cholesterol content of Shrimp. Shrimp is very low in total fat, yet it has a high cholesterol content (about 220 mg in 4 ounces, or 13 large boiled Shrimp), which has caused some people to avoid eating it. However, based on research involving Shrimp and blood cholesterol levels, avoidance of Shrimp for this reason may not be justified.

In a peer-reviewed scientific study, researchers reviewed the effect of a diet containing Shrimp or eggs on the cholesterol levels of subjects with normal lipid levels. The results of this randomized crossover trial showed that while LDL levels ("bad" cholesterol) increased by 7% in those eating the Shrimp diet, HDL levels ("good" cholesterol) increased by 12%. In contrast, subjects eating the egg diet had a 10% increase in LDL levels and only a 7% increase in HDL levels. The results indicated that the Shrimp diet produced significantly lower ratios of total to HDL cholesterol and lower ratios of LDL to HDL cholesterol than the egg diet. In addition, subjects who ate the Shrimp diet lowered their levels of triglycerides by 13%.

Shrimp are a very good source of vitamin B12, an important nutrient for a healthy heart since this B vitamin is necessary for keeping levels of homocysteine low. Homocysteine is a molecule that can directly damage blood vessel walls and is considered a significant risk factor for cardiovascular disease. Shrimp is also a good source of cardioprotective omega-3 fatty acids, noted for their anti-inflammatory effects and suggested ability to prevent the formation of blood clots. They are also a concentrated source of other heart-healthy nutrients including niacin and magnesium.

## Promote Optimal Health

Shrimp are a concentrated source of many antioxidants, including selenium, copper and zinc. Selenium is a co-factor of *glutathione peroxidase*, which is used by the liver to detoxify a wide range of potentially harmful molecules. Accumulated evidence from prospective studies, intervention trials and studies on animal models of cancer has suggested a strong inverse correlation between selenium intake and cancer incidence. Copper is a component of *superoxide dismutase*, an antioxidant enzyme that scavenges free radicals in the lungs and the red blood cells. Zinc is necessary for keeping the immune system functioning properly.

## Additional Health-Promoting Benefits of Shrimp

Shrimp are also a concentrated source of many other nutrients providing additional health benefits. These nutrients include muscle-building protein, energy-producing iron, bone-building vitamin D and phosphorus, and sleep-promoting tryptophan.

### Nutritional Analysis of 4 ounces of boiled Shrimp:

| NUTRIENT | AMOUNT | % DAILY VALUE | NUTRIENT | AMOUNT | % DAILY VALUE |
|---|---|---|---|---|---|
| Calories | 112.27 | | Pantothenic Acid | 0.39 mg | 3.90 |
| Calories from Fat | 11.02 | | | | |
| Calories from Saturated Fat | 2.95 | | **Minerals** | | |
| Protein | 23.71 g | | Boron | — mcg | |
| Carbohydrates | 0.00 g | | Calcium | 44.23 mg | 4.42 |
| Dietary Fiber | 0.00 g | 0.00 | Chloride | — mg | |
| Soluble Fiber | 0.00 g | | Chromium | — mcg | — |
| Insoluble Fiber | 0.00 g | | Copper | 0.22 mg | 11.00 |
| Sugar – Total | 0.00 g | | Fluoride | — mg | — |
| Monosaccharides | 0.00 g | | Iodine | — mcg | — |
| Disaccharides | 0.00 g | | Iron | 3.50 mg | 19.44 |
| Other Carbs | 0.00 g | | Magnesium | 38.56 mg | 9.64 |
| Fat – Total | 1.22 g | | Manganese | 0.04 mg | 2.00 |
| Saturated Fat | 0.33 g | | Molybdenum | — mcg | — |
| Mono Fat | 0.22 g | | Phosphorus | 155.36 mg | 15.54 |
| Poly Fat | 0.50 g | | Potassium | 206.39 mg | |
| Omega-3 Fatty Acids | 0.37 g | 14.80 | Selenium | 44.91 mcg | 64.16 |
| Omega-6 Fatty Acids | 0.10 g | | Sodium | 254.02 mg | |
| Trans Fatty Acids | 0.00 g | | Zinc | 1.77 mg | 11.80 |
| Cholesterol | 221.13 mg | | | | |
| Water | 87.64 g | | **Amino Acids** | | |
| Ash | 1.78 g | | Alanine | 1.34 g | |
| | | | Arginine | 2.07 g | |
| **Vitamins** | | | Aspartate | 2.45 g | |
| Vitamin A IU | 248.35 IU | 4.97 | Cystine | 0.27 g | 65.85 |
| Vitamin A RE | 74.84 RE | | Glutamate | 4.04 g | |
| A - Carotenoid | 0.00 RE | 0.00 | Glycine | 1.43 g | |
| A - Retinol | 74.84 RE | | Histidine | 0.48 g | 37.21 |
| B1 Thiamin | 0.04 mg | 2.67 | Isoleucine | 1.15 g | 100.00 |
| B2 Riboflavin | 0.04 mg | 2.35 | Leucine | 1.88 g | 74.31 |
| B3 Niacin | 2.94 mg | 14.70 | Lysine | 2.06 g | 87.66 |
| Niacin Equiv | 8.41 mg | | Methionine | 0.67 g | 90.54 |
| Vitamin B6 | 0.14 mg | 7.00 | Phenylalanine | 1.00 g | 84.03 |
| Vitamin B12 | 1.69 mcg | 28.17 | Proline | 0.78 g | |
| Biotin | — mcg | — | Serine | 0.93 g | |
| Vitamin C | 2.49 mg | 4.15 | Threonine | 0.96 g | 77.42 |
| Vitamin D IU | 162.39 IU | 40.60 | Tryptophan | 0.33 g | 103.13 |
| Vitamin D mcg | 4.06 mcg | | Tyrosine | 0.79 g | 81.44 |
| Vitamin E Alpha Equiv | 0.58 mg | 2.90 | Valine | 1.11 g | 75.51 |
| Vitamin E IU | 0.86 IU\ | | | | |
| Vitamin E mg | 0.85 mg | | | | |
| Folate | 3.97 mcg | 0.99 | | | |
| Vitamin K | 0.02 mcg | 0.03 | | | |

(Note: "—" indicates data is unavailable. For more information, please see page 806.)

STEP-BY-STEP RECIPE
## The Healthiest Ways of Cooking Shrimp

# 3-Minute "Healthy Sautéed" Shrimp

*"Healthy Sautéed" Shrimp has a rich flavor and can easily be combined with a variety of vegetables for a complete meal.*

1/2 lb medium size Shrimp,
    peeled and deveined
2 TBS + 1 TBS fresh lemon juice
Sea salt and pepper to taste
3 TBS low-sodium chicken or vegetable broth
2 medium garlic cloves
2 TBS extra virgin olive oil

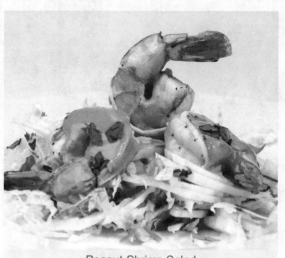

Peanut Shrimp Salad

1. Chop garlic and let sit for 5 minutes. (Why?, see page 261.)

2. Peel and devein Shrimp as directed under *The Best Way to Prepare.*

3. Rub Shrimp with 2 TBS lemon juice, and salt and pepper to taste.

4. Heat 3 TBS broth over medium-low heat in a stainless steel skillet.

5. When broth begins to steam, add Shrimp and sauté.

Stir frequently. After 2 minutes, turn the Shrimp over and add garlic. Sauté until Shrimp are pink and opaque throughout (approximately 3 minutes). Cook 4–5 minutes for large Shrimp. Shrimp cook quickly, so watch your cooking time. They become tough if overcooked.

6. Dress with extra virgin olive oil and the remaining 1 TBS lemon juice.

### SERVES 2

## Flavor Tips: Try these 9 great serving suggestions with the recipe above. ✳

1. **Most Popular: Peanut Shrimp Salad.** Toss Napa Cabbage with tamari (soy sauce) and rice vinegar. Top with "Healthy Sautéed Shrimp (omit dressing) and your favorite bottled peanut sauce (pictured above).

2. In addition to the dressing, toss Shrimp with pesto, chopped tomatoes and capers after cooking.

3 Fresh dill weed is delicious with Shrimp.

4. Hot or cold Shrimp combine well with your favorite chili hot sauce.

5. **Spicy Asian Shrimp:** Add 1/8 tsp red pepper flakes, 1/4 cup orange juice and 1 TBS minced fresh ginger while sautéing. Serve over hot rice.

6. **Shrimp Nicosia:** "Healthy Sauté" finely chopped onion and mushrooms for 1 minute. Add diced tomatoes and large Shrimp. Cook for 2 minutes. Stir. Add rinsed capers and chopped black olives,

and cook for 2 more minutes. Toss with dressing.

7. **Asian Sauté:** "Healthy Sauté" sliced onions and snap peas. Combine with 3-Minute "Healthy Sautéed Shrimp recipe, 1 chopped tomato and grated ginger. Replace salt with tamari (soy sauce). Serve with noodles or rice.

8. **Shrimp Salad:** Combine 3-Minute "Healthy Sautéed" Shrimp, one small diced avocado, 3 diced celery stalks and 2 TBS Mediterranean Dressing (see page 331) mixed with 1 TBS of Dijon mustard. Serve in a lettuce leaf or cored tomato.

9. **Classic Shrimp Scampi:** "Healthy Sauté" 1/2 lb large Shrimp using 1 TBS lemon juice and 1/2 cup of white wine in place of the broth for 4 minutes. Add 3 minced garlic cloves and sea salt to taste. Cook for 1 minute. Remove from heat, drizzle with olive oil and sprinkle with parsley.

Please write (address on back cover flap) or e-mail me at info@whfoods.org with your personal ideas for preparing Shrimp, and I will share them with others through our website at www.whfoods.org.

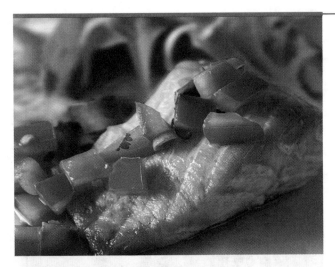

# salmon

| | |
|---|---|
| AVAILABILITY: | Year-round |
| REFRIGERATE: | Yes |
| SHELF LIFE: | Up to 4 days refrigerated |
| PREPARATION: | Minimal |
| BEST WAY TO COOK: | "Quick Broil" in just 7 minutes |

## nutrient-richness chart

Total Nutrient-Richness: **21**
4 ounces (113 grams) of broiled Chinook Salmon contains 262 calories

| NUTRIENT | AMOUNT | %DV | DENSITY | QUALITY |
|---|---|---|---|---|
| Tryptophan | 0.3 g | 103.1 | 7.1 | excellent |
| Omega-3 Fatty Acids | 2.1 g | 83.6 | 5.7 | excellent |
| Selenium | 53.2 mcg | 75.8 | 5.2 | excellent |
| Protein | 29.1 g | 58.3 | 4.0 | very good |
| B3 Niacin | 11.3 mg | 56.7 | 3.9 | very good |
| Vitamin B12 | 3.3 mcg | 54.2 | 3.7 | very good |
| Phosphorus | 420.7 mg | 42.1 | 2.9 | good |
| Magnesium | 138.4 mg | 34.6 | 2.4 | good |
| B6 Pyroxidine | 0.5 mg | 26.0 | 1.8 | good |

For more on "Total Nutrient-Richness," "%DV," "Density," and
The World's Healthiest Foods "Quality" Rating System, see page 805.

S almon is an incredible food providing exceptional flavor and nutrition. The story of Salmon before it reaches your table is just as remarkable. As a family of fish, Salmon have an amazing life cycle. Born in fresh water, they travel to saltwater oceans, returning not only to fresh water, but to the very place where they were spawned! As with other types of fish, it is important to cook Salmon properly to enhance its flavor and maintain its moisture. I want to share with you how to prepare Salmon using the "Healthiest Way of Cooking" methods for a dish that only takes minutes to prepare but one you will want to share with your favorite guests.

## why salmon should be part of your healthiest way of eating

Low in calories and saturated fats and high in protein, wild-caught Salmon is one of the best sources of those hard-to-find, health-promoting fats known as the omega-3 fatty acids, specifically eicosapentaenoic acid (EPA) and docosahexaenoic acid (DHA). These fatty acids play an important role as anti-inflammatory agents and are also sorely deficient in the American diet. Add the benefit of Salmon's EPA and DHA to its being a rich source of protein, vitamins and minerals, many of which act as powerful antioxidants, and you have some of the many reasons why Salmon is included among the World's Healthiest Foods and is a valuable addition to your "Healthiest Way of Eating." (For more on the *Health Benefits of Salmon* and a complete analysis of its content of over 60 nutrients, see page 480.)

## varieties of salmon

The life cycles of the different species of Salmon range from two to five years, and the diet they consume during that time accounts for their wide variation in color (from pink to red to orange) and the differences in their fat content and flavor. Salmon can be either caught wild or are farm-raised. They are sold as fillets, steaks and whole fish.

### Wild-Caught Salmon

All of the wild-caught Salmon we find in the market are from the Pacific coast and are labeled as "Wild Salmon." They have a deeper, more complex and fuller flavor than farm-raised Salmon. Given the concerns that have been raised about farm-raised fish (see Farm-Raised Salmon Section), I recommend choosing wild-caught Salmon whenever possible.

### WILD CHINOOK (King Salmon)

The largest of all of the Pacific Salmon, they remain out to sea for 4 to 5 years before they spawn and die. The flesh of Chinook or King Salmon can range from deep red to almost white. It is higher in fat content and has a better flavor than other species of Salmon. One 4-ounce serving contains 2.1 grams of omega-3 fatty acids. King Salmon comes fresh, frozen and smoked.

### WILD SOCKEYE (Red Salmon)

It has deep red-colored flesh and is considered the finest of the canned Salmon. It is also sold fresh in season and has the second highest fat content with a 4-ounce serving containing 1.5 grams of omega-3 fatty acids. Sockeye Salmon are out to sea for three to four years before they spawn and die.

### WILD HUMPBACK (Pink Salmon)

One 4-ounce serving of Humpback Salmon contains 1.5 grams of omega-3 fatty acids. It has soft, pale-pink flesh and bland flavor and is usually canned. Pink Salmon are out to sea for two years before they spawn and die.

### WILD COHO (Silver Salmon)

This species ranges in size from 5 to 15 pounds, has red colored flesh and a lower fat content than Chinook or Sockeye; a 4-ounce serving contains 1.3 grams of omega-3 fatty acids. It is sold fresh. Coho Salmon are out to sea for three to four years before they spawn and die.

### WILD CHUM (Dog Salmon)

Lower in omega-3 fatty acids with only 1.0 grams per 4-ounce serving, this species of Salmon has firm, coarse flesh that is pale in color. It is oftentimes used for smoked Salmon. Chum Salmon are out to sea for three to four years before they spawn and die.

## Farm-Raised Salmon

Salmon raised in pens and fed fish pellets for nourishment results in an omega-3 fatty acid to omega-6 fatty acid ratio that is different than found in wild Salmon; farmed Salmon have far more omega-6 fatty acids in relation to omega-3 fatty acids. Because the pellets do not give them their natural pink color, their feed must include an artificial coloring for their flesh to have a pink hue.

In addition, a number of concerns have been noted about Salmon farming. Crowded pens result in a large amount of waste discharge in the water that disrupts the ecological balance of the environment where the pens are located. Because these feed lot rearing conditions are also very conducive to the development of disease, farmed Salmon are protected with the use of antibiotics. As noted above, they are fed artificial coloring to achieve the peach-colored flesh naturally present in wild Salmon (a result of their consumption of carotenoid-rich krill). Farm-raised Salmon may also cause problems in the wild since some do escape from their pens and end up competing with wild stocks for resources or interbreeding with wild stocks and changing their genetic make-up.

Farmed Salmon are lower in protein (because they do not swim long distances) and fattier and higher in saturated fats than their wild counterparts. While they contain omega-3 fatty acids, they also contain significantly higher amounts of pro-inflammatory omega-6 fatty acids, making the ratio between these two types of fats less desirable than those found in wild stocks of Salmon.

FDA statistics on the nutritional content (protein and fat ratios) of farmed versus wild-caught Salmon detail many findings. They show that the fat content of farmed Salmon is excessively high (30–35% by weight) and that wild Salmon have a 20% higher protein content. And while wild Salmon have a 20% lower overall fat content than farm-raised Salmon, they have 33% more omega-3 fatty acids.

When you purchase Atlantic Salmon, you are purchasing farm-raised Salmon. Farm-raised Salmon comes from Norway, Chili and New Zealand as well as the United States. One thing to remember that is not well-known is that not only Atlantic but Norwegian Salmon are now almost always generic terms for farm-raised Salmon.

---

### WILD-CAUGHT SALMON FROM ALASKA ARE THE BEST CHOICES* FOR SUSTAINABILITY

Sustainable species of Salmon are those that can be sustained long-term without compromising their survival or the integrity of the ecosystem in which they live. Three species of wild-caught Alaskan Salmon including Coho, Sockeye and King Salmon are rated as Best Choice for sustainability by the Monterey Bay Aquarium Seafood Watch. Wild-caught Salmon from Washington, Oregon and California are considered Good Alternatives by that organization.

Farm-raised Salmon are rated "Avoid" because raising them in pens produces waste products and damages the ecosystem of the area in which they are raised; the process of farm raising Salmon can also spread disease and parasites to wild stocks of fish. If the Salmon escape they will also compete for the natural resources used by wild stocks and interbeed with them, changing their genetics.

*Rating information from Monterey Bay Aquarium Seafood Watch*

New labeling regulations now specify that farm-raised Salmon must be labeled as "Farm-Raised" and indicate that artificial colorings were used in processing. Wild-caught Salmon must be labeled as "Wild Salmon." These new labeling regulations make distinguishing farm-raised from wild Salmon at the market easy and clear.

(For more on wild-caught versus farm-raised Salmon see *"What are the Nutritional Differences between Wild-Caught and Farm-Raised Fish?"* page 495.)

### Canned Salmon

Canned Salmon used to always be wild-caught, but not anymore. Some companies have started to can farmed Salmon, so be sure to read the label. Remember that when the label on the can reads Atlantic or Norwegian Salmon, the Salmon was farm-raised.

## the peak season

It's always best to enjoy any fish during its peak season. These are the months when its concentration of nutrients and flavor are highest, and its cost is at its lowest. The different species of wild Salmon are available during different times of the year with the peak of their respective seasons running between February and November. Although farm-raised Salmon is available year-round, I recommend eating wild Salmon whenever possible.

## biochemical considerations

Salmon contains purines, which may be problematic for some individuals. Recent studies have shown that farm-raised Salmon have high levels of PCBs and dioxins. Synthetic dyes are also used to give them a pink coloration. It is recommend that farm-raised Salmon not be eaten more than once a month. (For more on *Purines*, see page 727.)

## 4 steps for the best tasting and most nutritious salmon

Turning Salmon into a flavorful dish with the most nutrients is simple if you just follow my 4 easy steps:

1. The Best Way to Select
2. The Best Way to Store
3. The Best Way to Prepare
4. The Healthiest Way of Cooking

## 1. the best way to select salmon

All species of wild-caught Salmon from Alaska, Washington, Oregon and California are sustainable choices. King Salmon, Sockeye and Coho Salmon are the best for flavor.

The first step in selecting the best Salmon, like all other fish, is to find a store with a good reputation for having a fresh supply of seafood and get to know a fishmonger (person who sells the seafood) at the store, so you can have a trusted person from whom you can purchase your fish.

Fresh whole Salmon should be displayed buried in ice, while fillets should be placed on top of the ice. Whenever possible, purchase displayed fish rather than prepackaged fish. Smell is a good indicator of freshness, and it is difficult to detect smells through the plastic of prepackaged fish. I have found that fresh fish never smells fishy; instead, it smells like seawater. Once the fishmonger wraps and hands you the fish, smell it through the paper wrapping and return it if it does not smell right.

If you are going to have a full day of errands after you purchase your Salmon, be sure to keep a cooler in the car to ensure it stays cold and does not spoil.

## 2. the best way to store salmon

Like most fish, Salmon is very perishable, and normal refrigerator temperatures of 36°–40°F (2°–4°C) do not inhibit the enzymatic activity that causes it to spoil; it is best when stored at 28°–32°F (-2°–0°C). I have tried various methods to find the best way to store Salmon including packing the Salmon with ice before placing it in the refrigerator to decrease the temperature. Although this method kept the Salmon cool, once the ice melted the Salmon ended up sitting in a pool of water, causing it to lose much of its flavor.

I have refined this method and want to share with you the best way to keep your Salmon fresh. Remove Salmon from store packaging, rinse and place in a plastic storage bag as soon as you bring it home from the market. Place in a large bowl and cover with ice cubes or ice packs to reduce the temperature of the fish. Although fresh Salmon will keep for a few days using this method, I recommend using your Salmon as soon as possible, within a day or two. Remember to drain off the melted water and replenish the ice water or ice packs as necessary.

Remember that fish not only starts to smell but will dry out or become slimy if it is not stored correctly.

# 3. the best way to prepare salmon

Salmon comes in the form of steaks, fillets or whole fish.

Rinse under cold running water and pat dry before cooking.

# 4. the healthiest way of cooking salmon

The best way to cook Salmon is by using methods that will keep it moist and tender. Salmon can be easily overcooked and become dry, so be sure to watch your cooking times.

Salmon is a delicate fish, and I have found that it can be most easily prepared by using the "Quick Broil" method. You do not have to skin Salmon before cooking. As a general rule, each inch of thickness requires 7–10 minutes of cooking; fish that is 1/2-inch thick will take half the amount of time. (For more on "*Quick Broil*," see page 60.)

While grilled Salmon tastes great, make sure it does not burn. It is best to grill Salmon on an area without a direct flame as the temperatures directly above or below the flame can reach as high as 500°F to 1000°F (260°C to 538°C). Extra care should be taken when grilling, as burning can damage nutrients and create free radicals that can be harmful to your health. (For more on *Grilling*, see page 61.)

## How to Avoid Overcooking Salmon

Salmon cooks quickly and is easily overcooked. To prevent overcooking Salmon, I highly recommend using a timer. And since Salmon cooks in only 7–10 minutes, it is important to begin timing as soon as you place it into the skillet. Salmon cooks quickly and will become tough and lose its flavor when overcooked. You can also use a thermometer to determine doneness; remove from the heat when the internal temperature reads 135°F (57°C) to prevent overcooking. The internal temperature will continue to rise to 140°–145°F (60°–63°C) once the fish is removed from the heat. You will know when Salmon is done when it flakes easily with a fork. Cooking times are based on Salmon that is less than 1-inch thick. Never cook longer than 10 minutes per inch of thickness as the fish will become tough. Previously frozen Salmon fillets cook 25% more quickly than fresh Salmon, so adjust your cooking time appropriately. It is best to follow the recipe directions.

## Remove Salmon Skin After Cooking

I usually like to remove the skin from fish, such as Salmon, after it is cooked because the skin is a source of potential contaminants. For example, I've seen one study on Salmon harvested from the Great Lakes that showed 50% fewer pesticide residues (including DDT residues) in skinned versus unskinned salmon. In fish obtained from uncontaminated waters, I would consider the skin to be a nutrient-rich portion of the fish (containing important concentrations of omega-3 fatty acids). While the skin of Salmon and other fish is definitely considered edible, and even considered a valued food in some cuisines and some restaurants, it is the risk of potential toxins that I am trying to avoid when I remove the skin.

## Methods Not Recommended for Cooking Salmon

### COOKING WITH OIL

I don't recommend cooking Salmon in oil because high temperature heat can damage delicate oils and potentially create harmful free radicals. (For more on *Why it is Important to Cook Without Heated Oils*, see page 52.)

---

## Preparing Salmon, Step-by-Step

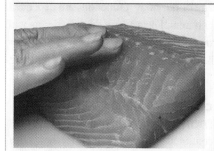 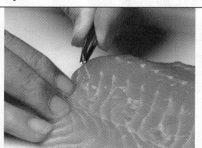 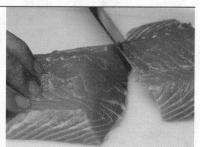

### REMOVING BONES FROM SALMON FILLETS

❶ Lay Salmon fillet skin side down and run your fingers along the flesh in both directions until you locate the line of bones. ❷ Pull them out one at a time with your fingers or tweezers. ❸ Cut into desired size.

# health benefits of salmon

## Promotes Brain Health

Salmon is well known as an excellent source of omega-3 fatty acids, notably EPA and DHA. Cold-water fatty fish like Salmon have often been thought of as a "brain food" because of their high concentration of these omega-3 fats.

### Nutritional Analysis of 4 ounces of broiled Chinook Salmon:

| NUTRIENT | AMOUNT | % DAILY VALUE | NUTRIENT | AMOUNT | % DAILY VALUE |
|---|---|---|---|---|---|
| Calories | 261.95 | | Pantothenic Acid | 0.98 mg | 9.80 |
| Calories from Fat | 136.76 | | | | |
| Calories from Saturated Fat | 32.76 | | **Minerals** | | |
| Protein | 29.14 g | | Boron | — mcg | |
| Carbohydrates | 0.00 g | | Calcium | 31.75 mg | 3.17 |
| Dietary Fiber | 0.00 g | 0.00 | Chloride | — mg | |
| Soluble Fiber | 0.00 g | | Chromium | — mcg | — |
| Insoluble Fiber | 0.00 g | | Copper | 0.06 mg | 3.00 |
| Sugar – Total | 0.00 g | | Fluoride | — mg | — |
| Monosaccharides | 0.00 g | | Iodine | — mcg | — |
| Disaccharides | 0.00 g | | Iron | 1.03 mg | 5.72 |
| Other Carbs | 0.00 g | | Magnesium | 138.35 mg | 34.59 |
| Fat – Total | 15.20 g | | Manganese | 0.02 mg | 1.00 |
| Saturated Fat | 3.64 g | | Molybdenum | 3.86 mcg | 5.15 |
| Mono Fat | 6.51 g | | Phosphorus | 420.71 mg | 42.07 |
| Poly Fat | 3.02 g | | Potassium | 572.67 mg | |
| Omega-3 Fatty Acids | 2.09 g | 83.60 | Selenium | 53.07 mcg | 75.81 |
| Omega-6 Fatty Acids | 0.38 g | | Sodium | 68.04 mg | |
| Trans Fatty Acids | 0.00 g | | Zinc | 0.64 mg | 4.27 |
| Cholesterol | 96.39 mg | | | | |
| Water | 74.39 g | | **Amino Acids** | | |
| Ash | 2.00 g | | Alanine | 1.77 g | |
| | | | Arginine | 1.75 g | |
| **Vitamins** | | | Aspartate | 2.98 g | |
| Vitamin A IU | 562.46 IU | 11.25 | Cystine | 0.31 g | 75.61 |
| Vitamin A RE | 168.97 RE | | Glutamate | 4.35 g | |
| A - Carotenoid | 0.00 RE | 0.00 | Glycine | 1.39 g | |
| A - Retinol | 168.97 RE | | Histidine | 0.86 g | 66.67 |
| B1 Thiamin | 0.05 mg | 3.33 | Isoleucine | 1.35 g | 117.39 |
| B2 Riboflavin | 0.17 mg | 10.00 | Leucine | 2.37 g | 93.68 |
| B3 Niacin | 11.34 mg | 56.70 | Lysine | 2.68 g | 114.04 |
| Niacin Equiv | 16.78 mg | | Methionine | 0.86 g | 116.22 |
| Vitamin B6 | 0.52 mg | 26.00 | Phenylalanine | 1.13 g | 94.96 |
| Vitamin B12 | 3.25 mcg | 54.17 | Proline | 1.03 g | |
| Biotin | 4.54 mcg | 1.51 | Serine | 1.19 g | |
| Vitamin C | 4.65 mg | 7.75 | Threonine | 1.28 g | 103.23 |
| Vitamin D IU | — IU | — | Tryptophan | 0.33 g | 103.13 |
| Vitamin D mcg | — mcg | | Tyrosine | 0.98 g | 101.03 |
| Vitamin E Alpha Equiv | 1.94 mg | 9.70 | Valine | 1.51 g | 102.72 |
| Vitamin E IU | 2.89 IU | | | | |
| Vitamin E mg | 1.94 mg | | | | |
| Folate | 39.69 mcg | 9.92 | | | |
| Vitamin K | 0.00 mcg | 0.00 | | | |

(Note: "−" indicates data is unavailable. For more information, please see page 806.)

The human brain is more than 60% structural fat and for brain cells to function properly, this structural fat needs to be primarily omega-3 fats such as the EPA and DHA found in Salmon. There has been a lot of research into the relationship between "brain health" and omega-3 fatty acids. Epidemiological studies in various countries including the U.S. suggest a connection between increased rates of depression and decreased omega-3 consumption. A recent study showed that kids deficient in omega-3 essential fatty acids are significantly more likely to be hyperactive, have learning disorders and display behavioral problems. And if preventing these problems weren't enough benefits, here are two more—one recent study found eating omega-3-rich fish several times each week reduced the risk of developing impaired cognitive function, while another one found that those who consumed fish at least once per week had a lower risk of developing Alzheimer's disease.

## Promotes Heart Health

The benefits upon cardiovascular health of the omega-3 fatty acids found in Salmon have been well documented in the scientific literature. They have been found to reduce hypertension (high blood pressure), protect against coronary heart disease, improve blood flow, prevent against erratic heart rhythm and lower triglyceride levels. In addition, a recent meta-analysis review of eight studies suggests that eating fish, such as Salmon, as little as one to three times per month may protect against the occurrence of ischemic stroke. Salmon's heart-health benefits are not limited to its omega-3 fats; it is also an excellent source of selenium, a very good source of vitamin B12 and niacin, and a good source of vitamin B6 and magnesium, all of which are intricately tied to cardiovascular health.

## A Concentrated Source of Protein

Salmon is a very good source of protein. Not only does protein provide us with long-lasting energy to help us feel our very best, but so many of our body's functions are dependent upon this important nutrient. Dietary protein provides us with the amino acids from which our body makes our muscles, tissues, enzymes, health-protective antibodies and nutrient-carrying proteins.

## Additional Health-Promoting Benefits of Salmon

Salmon is a concentrated source of many other nutrients providing numerous health benefits. These nutrients include energy-producing phosphorus and sleep-promoting tryptophan.

STEP-BY-STEP RECIPE
## The Healthiest Ways of Cooking Salmon

# 7-Minute "Quick Broiled" Salmon

*This is a great way to prepare Salmon that seals in its wonderful juices, brings out its best flavor and retains its moisture. It is not necessary to turn the Salmon over as it cooks on both sides simultaneously.*

**1 lb Salmon fillet, cut in half**
**2 tsp + 1 TBS fresh lemon juice**
**Sea salt and black pepper to taste**
**2 TBS extra virgin olive oil**
**1 medium clove garlic**

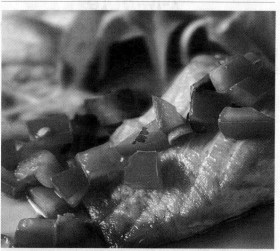
"Quick Broiled" Salmon with Ginger Mint Salsa

1. Preheat the broiler on high and place an all stainless steel skillet (be sure the handle is also stainless steel) or cast iron pan under the heat for about 10 minutes to get it very hot. The pan should be 5 to 7 inches from the heat source.

2. While pan is heating, chop or press garlic and let it sit for 5 minutes. (Why?, see page 261.)

3. Rub Salmon with 2 tsp fresh lemon juice, salt and pepper. (You can "Quick Broil" with the skin on, it just takes a minute or two longer. The skin will peel right off after cooking.)

4. Using a hot pad, pull pan away from heat and place Salmon on hot pan, skin side down. Return to broiler. Keep in mind that it is cooking rapidly on both sides, so it will be done very quickly, usually in 7 minutes, depending on thickness. Test with a fork for doneness. It will flake easily when it is cooked. Salmon is best when it is still pink inside.

5. Dress with olive oil, 1 TBS lemon juice, garlic, and salt and pepper to taste.

**SERVES 2**

## Flavor Tips: Try these 10 great serving suggestions with the recipe above. ✱

1. **Most Popular: Salmon with Ginger Mint Salsa.** Prepare 1 recipe of "Quick Broiled" Salmon. Combine 1 ripe diced tomato, 1/2 cup finely minced green onion, 1 tsp finely chopped ginger, 2 tsp finely minced fresh mint, 1 tsp lime juice, and sea salt and pepper to taste. Spoon salsa over cooked Salmon. Garnish with mint leaves and a sprinkle of extra virgin olive oil.

2. Mint, cilantro, ginger, mustard and tamari (soy sauce) also complement the taste of Salmon.

3. Spread Dijon mustard on Salmon before broiling. Garnish with capers and dill weed.

4. Top Salmon with pesto (see page 508) or Olive Tapenade (page 325).

5. Add shredded Salmon to a frittata (see next page).

6. Top your green salad with "Quick Broiled" Salmon for a light meal. Drizzle with your favorite dressing.

7. **Miso Salmon:** Prepare the 7-Minute "Quick Broiled" Salmon. While it cooks, whisk together 1 TBS miso, 3 tsp mirin (rice cooking wine), 1 tsp rice vinegar, 1 tsp water and 1 tsp fresh grated ginger. Spread on cooked Salmon and garnish with green onions.

8. **Salmon in Dill Sauce:** Combine 1 cup low-fat plain yogurt, a medium-size diced seeded cucumber, 1 TBS dill weed, 1 tsp minced fresh mint and black pepper to taste. Serve on chilled 7-Minute "Quick Broiled" Salmon.

9. **Asian Marinade:** Marinate Salmon before "Quick Broiling." In a plastic storage bag, combine 1/2 cup tamari, 1/4 cup mirin, and 1/4 cup water. Place Salmon fillets in the bag and let marinate in the refrigerator 1 hour to overnight. Add scallions, minced ginger and red pepper flakes to marinade for more flavor.

10. **Egg-Salmon Salad:** Combine 1 cup cold cooked Salmon (flaked), 1 diced boiled egg, 1/2 small finely chopped sweet onion, minced dill pickle, 3 TBS olive oil and sea salt and pepper. Scoop onto a bed of dressed greens.

Please write (address on back cover flap) or e-mail me at info@whfoods.org with your personal ideas for preparing Salmon, and I will share them with others through our website at www.whfoods.org.

# 7-Minute "Healthy Sautéed" Salmon

*When you "Healthy Sauté" Salmon, you will be pleasantly surprised by its rich flavor.*

**3/4 lb Salmon fillet, cut in half**
**3 TBS low-sodium chicken broth**
**2 tsp + 1 TBS fresh lemon juice**
**Sea salt and pepper to taste**
**2 TBS extra virgin olive oil**
**1 medium clove garlic**
**Optional: 1 TBS chopped fresh dill**

**SERVES 2**

1. Press or chop garlic and let it sit for 5 minutes. (Why?, see page 261.)
2. Rub Salmon with 2 tsp fresh lemon juice, salt and pepper.
3. Heat broth on medium heat in a stainless steel skillet.
4. When broth begins to steam, add Salmon fillets and sauté for about 3-4 minutes.
5. Turn Salmon and sauté for another 3 to 4 minutes depending on thickness. Salmon is done when it flakes easily with a fork.
6. Dress with 1 TBS lemon juice, olive oil and garlic. (For more flavor, add 1 TBS basil.)

   OPTIONAL: For more mellow garlic flavor, add chopped garlic to Salmon for the last minute of sautéing.

# 7-Minute "Healthy Steamed" Salmon

*"Healthy Steaming" is a moist gentle way to prepare Salmon on your stovetop. It is one of the best ways to preserve the delicate flavor and texture of Salmon.*

**3/4 lb Salmon fillet, cut in half**
**2 tsp + 1 TBS fresh lemon juice**
**Sea salt and pepper to taste**
**2 TBS extra virgin olive oil**
**1 medium clove garlic**
**Optional: 1 TBS fresh ginger**

**SERVES 2**

1. Press or chop garlic and let it sit for 5 minutes. (Why?, see page 261.)
2. While steam is building up in steamer, prepare Salmon. Rub fillets with 2 tsp lemon juice and season with salt and pepper to taste.
3. Place Salmon in steamer basket, **cover** and steam for about 7 minutes. To avoid burning yourself, be sure to open the steamer lid away from you and let the steam dissipate for a few seconds before fully removing the lid. Salmon is done when it flakes easily with a fork. Remove the skin after cooking.
4. Dress with olive oil, remaining lemon juice and garlic. (For more flavor, add 1 TBS fresh chopped ginger.)

# 7-Minute Poached Salmon

*If you would like to poach your fish, here is a quick and easy way. Your fish will come out moist, tender and flavorful because it is cooked in broth.*

**4 cups cold water or low-sodium chicken broth**
**1 medium onion**
**3 ribs celery, sliced**
**3 sprigs parsley**
**3/4 lb Salmon fillet, cut in half**
**1 tsp fresh lemon juice**
**2 TBS extra virgin olive oil**
**1 medium clove garlic**
**Sea salt and pepper to taste**

**SERVES 2**

1. Chop onions and chop or press garlic and let sit for 5 minutes. (Why?, see page 261.)
2. Place onion, celery, parsley and water or broth into a 2-quart pan. Optional: 2 TBS dry white wine. (If using water, add 1/2 tsp salt.) **Cover** and bring to a boil.
3. Place halved Salmon fillets in the boiling liquid. **Be sure that the Salmon is covered with the liquid.** A few drops of sherry will further enhance the flavor. Lower the heat to medium, **cover** and cook for 7 minutes. Remove Salmon with a slotted spoon.
4. Dress with olive oil, 1 tsp lemon juice, garlic, and salt and pepper to taste. For Mediterranean flavor, add fresh basil, thyme or parsley. Save broth for soups.

# Salmon Frittata

*This quick, protein-rich breakfast makes use of precooked Salmon.*

**2 TBS + 2 TBS vegetable or chicken broth**
**1/4 medium red bell pepper, diced**
**1/4 medium red onion, diced**
**1/2 medium zucchini, diced**
**3 eggs**
**1/2 cup cooked Salmon, shredded**
**Sea salt and pepper to taste**
**1–2 TBS extra virgin olive oil**
**Optional: 1 TBS chopped fresh basil or dill**

**SERVES 2**

1. Heat 2 TBS broth in a stainless steel skillet on medium-high. When broth begins to steam, add the bell pepper and onions. **Cover** and sauté 3 minutes.
2. Add zucchini and sauté 1 minute.
3. While vegetables are cooking, whisk together eggs, Salmon, salt and pepper.
4. Add remaining 2 TBS broth to vegetables and pour the egg mixture over them. Add basil or dill if desired. **Cover**, reduce heat to medium and cook 2–3 minutes or until the eggs are done on top.
5. Slice frittata in half in the pan and remove each half carefully with a spatula.
6. Sprinkle each serving with olive oil and serve.

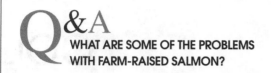

# Q&A
### WHAT ARE SOME OF THE PROBLEMS WITH FARM-RAISED SALMON?

## Synthetic Pigment Used to Color Flesh of Farm-Raised Salmon Pink

In the wild, Salmon absorb carotenoids from eating pink krill. On the aquafarm, their rich pink hue is supplied by canthaxanthin, a synthetic pigment. Fish farmers can choose just what shade of pink their fish will display from a pharmaceutical company's trademarked SalmoFan™, a color swatch similar to those you'd find in a paint store. Without help from synthetic pigments, the flesh of farmed Salmon would be a pale gray. To date, no government has banned canthaxanthin from animal feed. Cantha-xanthin was linked to retinal damage in people when taken as a sunless tanning pill, leading the British to ban its use as a tanning agent. (In the U.S., it's still available.) Consumed in high amounts, canthaxanthin can produce an accumulation of pigments in the retina of the eye and adversely affect sight.

## Antibiotic and Pesticide Use in Farm-Raised Salmon

Disease and parasites, which would normally exist in rela-tively low levels in fish scattered around the oceans, can run rampant in densely packed oceanic feedlots. To sur-vive, farmed fish are vaccinated when they are small. Later, they are given antibiotics or pesticides to ward off infection.

Sea lice, in particular, are a problem. In a recent L.A. Times story, Alexandra Morton, an independent biologist and critic of Salmon farms, is quoted as beginning to see sea lice in 2001 when a fisherman brought her two baby pink Salmon covered with them. Examining more than 700 baby pink Salmon around farms, she found that 78% were covered with a fatal load of sea lice while juvenile Salmon she netted farther from the farms were largely lice-free.

While Salmon farmers have discounted Morton's concerns, saying that sea lice are also found in the wild, at the first sign of an outbreak, they add the pesticide emamectin benzoate to the feed. According to officials, the use of pesticides should pose no problem for consumers.

## Toxic Compounds Found in Farm-Raised Salmon

Scientists in the U.S. are far more concerned about two preliminary studies—one in British Columbia and one in Great Britain—both of which showed farmed Salmon accumulate more cancer-causing polychlorinated biphenyls (PCBs) and toxic dioxins than wild-caught Salmon. The reason for this pesticide concentration is the Salmon feed. Pesticides, including those now outlawed in the United States, have circulated into the ocean where they are absorbed by marine life and accumulate in their fat, which is distilled into the concentrated fish oil that is a major ingredient in Salmon feed. Salmon feed contains higher concentrations of fish oil—extracted from sardines, anchovies and other ground-up fish—than wild-caught Salmon normally consume. Scientists in the U.S. are currently trying to determine the extent of the pesticide contamination in farmed Salmon and what levels are safe for human consumption.

Research on this issue published July 30, 2003, by the Environmental Working Group, indicates that levels of carcinogenic chemicals called PCBs found in farmed Salmon purchased from U.S. grocery stores are so much higher than levels of PCBs found in wild-caught Salmon that they pose an increased risk for cancer. PCBs have been banned in the U.S. for use in all but completely closed areas since 1979, but they persist in the environment and end up in animal fat. When farmed Salmon from U.S. grocery stores was tested, the farmed Salmon, which contains up to twice the fat of wild-caught Salmon, was found to contain 16 times the PCBs found in wild-caught Salmon, 4 times the levels in beef and 3.4 times the levels found in other seafood. Other studies done in Canada, Ireland and Britain have produced similar findings.

Flame-retardant additives used widely in electronics and furniture are also appearing in increasing amounts in fish, and farmed Salmon contain significantly higher levels of these polybrominated diphenyl ether (PBDE) compounds than wild-caught Salmon, according to research published in the August 11, 2004, issue of *Environmental Science and Technology*.

## New Labeling Regulations

Since September 2004, U.S. supermarkets have been required to label Salmon as farmed or wild-caught. Ask for line-caught Alaskan fish first. The healthiest populations and habitats exist in Alaska.

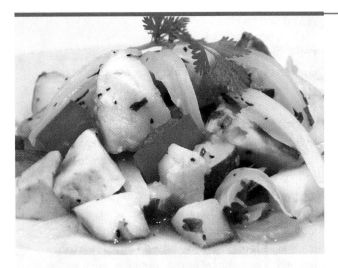

# cod

## highlights

| | |
|---|---|
| AVAILABILITY: | Year-round |
| REFRIGERATE: | Yes |
| SHELF LIFE: | Up to 4 days refrigerated |
| PREPARATION: | Minimal |
| BEST WAY TO COOK: | "Quick Broil" in just 5 minutes |

## nutrient-richness chart

Total Nutrient-Richness: **21**
4 ounces (113 grams) of baked/broiled Pacific Cod contains 119 calories

| NUTRIENT | AMOUNT | %DV | DENSITY | QUALITY |
|---|---|---|---|---|
| Tryptophan | 0.3 g | 90.6 | 13.7 | excellent |
| Selenium | 53.1 mcg | 75.8 | 11.5 | excellent |
| Protein | 26.0 g | 52.1 | 7.9 | excellent |
| B6 Pyridoxine | 0.5 mg | 26.0 | 3.9 | very good |
| Phosphorus | 252.9 mg | 25.3 | 3.8 | very good |
| Vitamin B12 | 1.2 mcg | 19.7 | 3.0 | good |
| Potassium | 586.3 mg | 16.8 | 2.5 | good |
| Vitamin D | 63.5 IU | 15.9 | 2.4 | good |
| B3 Niacin | 2.8 mg | 14.1 | 2.1 | good |
| Omega-3 Fatty Acids | 0.3 g | 12.8 | 1.9 | good |

For more on "Total Nutrient-Richness," "%DV," "Density," and
The World's Healthiest Foods "Quality" Rating System, see page 805.

People have been enjoying Cod as a subsistence food since time immemorial. Cod has historically been enjoyed not only fresh but salted, smoked and dried. The Massachusetts town of Cape Cod derived its name from the Cod that was once abundant in the coastal waters of this seaside town and along the eastern seaboard of the United States and Canada. Cod has a wonderfully mild flavor, and its versatility makes it easily adaptable to different types of recipes. I want to share with you how using the "Healthiest Way of Cooking" methods helps retain Cod's moisture, bring out its best flavor and maximize its nutritional benefits in a matter of minutes.

## why cod should be part of your healthiest way of eating

Cod is a great low-fat source of protein and contains hard-to-find, heart-healthy omega-3 fatty acids, which help reduce inflammation. Cod is an ideal food to add to your "Healthiest Way of Eating" because it is not only rich in nutrients but low in calories so it is a great choice for healthy weight control: 4 ounces of Pacific Cod contains only 119 calories! (For more on the *Health Benefits of Cod* and a complete analysis of its content of over 60 nutrients, see page 486.)

## varieties of cod

All Cod in the market is wild-caught. There are some varieties of fish known as Cod, such as rock Cod and ling Cod, which do not actually belong to the Cod family. The different types of Cod fall under two classifications:

### PACIFIC COD

There are many varieties of Pacific Cod that are still considered abundant. These include Alaskan pollack, Pacific whiting, hake, grenadier and opah (known more commonly as monkfish).

### ATLANTIC COD OR HADDOCK

This is the most well-known variety of Cod. It has a light color and a rich taste. Once very abundant, Atlantic Cod is, unfortunately, now rarely available at the market.

## the peak season

Cod is available year-round.

## 4 steps for the best tasting and most nutritious cod

Turning Cod into a flavorful dish with the most nutrients is simple if you just follow my 4 easy steps:
1. The Best Way to Select
2. The Best Way to Store
3. The Best Way to Prepare
4. The Healthiest Way of Cooking

# 1. the best way to select cod

The first step in selecting the best Cod, and all varieties of fish, is to find a store with a good reputation for having a fresh supply of seafood. Get to know a fishmonger (person who sells the fish) at the store, so you can have a trusted person from whom you can purchase your fish.

The flesh of the Cod fillets should glisten white with no signs of browning or gaping. Fresh whole Cod should be displayed buried in ice, while fillets should be placed on top of the ice. Whenever possible, purchase displayed fish rather than pre-packaged fish. Smell is a good indicator of freshness, and it is difficult to detect smells through the plastic of prepackaged fish. I have found that fresh fish never smells fishy but more like seawater. Once the fishmonger wraps and hands you the Cod, smell it through the paper wrapping and return it if it does not smell right.

If you are going to have a full day of errands after you purchase your fish, be sure to keep a cooler in the car to ensure it stays cold and does not spoil.

# 2. the best way to store cod

Like most fish, Cod is very perishable, and normal refrigerator temperatures of 36°–40°F (2°–4°C) do not inhibit the enzymatic activity that causes it to spoil; it is best when stored at 28°–32°F (-2°–0°C). I have tried various methods to find the best way to store Cod including packing the Cod with ice before placing it in the refrigerator to decrease the temperature. Although this method kept the Cod cool, once the ice melted, the Cod ended up sitting in a pool of water causing it to lose much of its flavor.

I have refined this method and want to share with you the way I have found that keeps Cod fresh. Remove Cod from store packaging, rinse it, and place it in a plastic storage bag as soon as you bring it home from the market. Place in a large bowl and cover with ice cubes or ice packs to reduce the temperature of the fish. Although fresh Cod will keep for a few days using this method, I recommend using your Cod within a day or two of purchase. Remember to drain off the melted water and replenish the ice or replace the ice packs as necessary.

# 3. the best way to prepare cod

Cod is usually purchased as fillets. It is best to rinse the fillets and pat dry before cooking.

# 4. the healthiest way of cooking cod

The best way to cook Cod is by using methods that will keep it moist and tender. Cod can be easily overcooked and become dry, so be sure to watch your cooking times.

Cod is a delicate fish, and I have found that it can be best prepared by using the "Quick Broil" method. Most Cod fillets do not come with skin on, but if the skin has not been removed, you can cook it with skin on. As a general rule, each inch of thickness requires 7–10 minutes of cooking; fish that is 1/2-inch thick will take half the amount of time. (For more on "Quick Broil," see page 60.)

## How to Avoid Overcooking Cod

Cod cooks quickly and is easily overcooked. To prevent overcooking Cod, I highly recommend using a timer. And since Cod cooks in only 7–10 minutes, it is important to begin timing as soon as you place it into the skillet. Cod cooks quickly and will become tough and lose its flavor when overcooked. You can also use a thermometer to determine doneness; remove Cod from the heat when the internal temperature reads 135°F (57°C) to prevent overcooking. The internal temperature will continue to rise to 140°–145°F (60°–63°C) once the fish is removed from the heat. You will know when Cod is done when it flakes easily with a fork. The recommended cooking time is based on Cod that is less than 1-inch thick. Never cook longer than 10 minutes per inch of thickness as the fish will become tough. Previously frozen Cod fillets cook 25% more quickly than fresh Cod, so adjust your cooking time appropriately. It is best to follow the recipe directions.

## Methods Not Recommended for Cooking Cod

### GRILLING OR COOKING WITH OIL

I don't recommend grilling Cod because it is so delicate and is easily burned.

*(Continued on Page 488)*

# health benefits of cod

## Promotes Heart Health

Fish, particularly cold-water fish like Cod, have been shown to be a protein-rich food very beneficial for people looking to support cardiovascular health. Studies show that people who eat fish regularly have a much lower risk of heart disease and heart attack than people who don't consume fish. Additionally, a recent meta-analysis (study that compiles data from many studies) suggests that eating fish, such as Cod, as little as one to three times per month may protect against ischemic stroke. Risk was reduced by as much as 31% in those who ate fish 5 times a week.

Cod, specifically, promotes cardiovascular health because it is not only a good source of omega-3 fatty acids, which have beneficial effects on blood lipid levels and reduce platelet aggregation, but is also a good source of vitamin B12 and a very good source of vitamin B6; both are needed to keep homocysteine levels low. This is important because homocysteine is a dangerous molecule that is directly damaging to blood vessel walls, and high homocysteine levels are associated with an increased risk of heart attack and stroke. Cod is also a good source of both niacin and potassium, two other nutrients noted to be important for heart health.

## Promotes Protection Against Inflammation

The selenium, vitamin D and omega-3 fats found in Cod have anti-inflammatory actions that reduce the inflammation that may lead to asthma attacks, rheumatoid arthritis, osteoarthritis and even migraines. Studies have shown that children who eat fish several times a week are at a much lower risk of developing asthma than children who don't eat fish. In societies where fish is eaten regularly, the rate of rheumatoid arthritis is much lower than in areas where fish is not commonly eaten.

## Promotes Optimal Health

Fish consumption is correlated with a reduced incidence of colon cancer—the more fish people eat, the less likely they are to develop this condition. The selenium, vitamin B12 and vitamin D concentrated in Cod have all been shown to reduce the risk of the development of colon cancer by protecting colon cells from the damage caused by toxic substances found in certain foods and cancer-causing chemicals produced by certain intestinal bacteria.

## Additional Health-Promoting Benefits from Cod

Cod is also a concentrated source of other nutrients providing additional health benefits. These nutrients include energy-producing phosphorus and sleep-promoting tryptophan.

### Nutritional Analysis of 4 ounces of baked/broiled Pacific Cod:

| NUTRIENT | AMOUNT | % DAILY VALUE | NUTRIENT | AMOUNT | % DAILY VALUE |
|---|---|---|---|---|---|
| Calories | 119.07 | | Pantothenic Acid | 0.18 mg | 1.80 |
| Calories from Fat | 8.27 | | | | |
| Calories from Saturated Fat | 1.06 | | **Minerals** | | |
| Protein | 26.03 g | | Boron | — mcg | |
| Carbohydrates | 0.00 g | | Calcium | 10.21 mg | 1.02 |
| Dietary Fiber | 0.00 g | 0.00 | Chloride | — mg | |
| Soluble Fiber | 0.00 g | | Chromium | — mcg | — |
| Insoluble Fiber | 0.00 g | | Copper | 0.04 mg | 2.00 |
| Sugar - Total | 0.00 g | | Fluoride | — mg | — |
| Monosaccharides | 0.00 g | | Iodine | — mcg | — |
| Disaccharides | 0.00 g | | Iron | 0.37 mg | 2.06 |
| Other Carbs | 0.00 g | | Magnesium | 35.15 mg | 8.79 |
| Fat - Total | 0.92 g | | Manganese | 0.02 mg | 1.00 |
| Saturated Fat | 0.12 g | | Molybdenum | 3.86 mcg | 5.15 |
| Mono Fat | 0.12 g | | Phosphorus | 252.88 mg | 25.29 |
| Poly Fat | 0.35 g | | Potassium | 586.28 mg | |
| Omega-3 Fatty Acids | 0.32 g | 12.80 | Selenium | 53.07 mcg | 75.81 |
| Omega-6 Fatty Acids | 0.03 g | | Sodium | 103.19 mg | |
| Trans Fatty Acids | 0.00 g | | Zinc | 0.58 mg | 3.87 |
| Cholesterol | 53.30 mg | | | | |
| Water | 86.18 g | | **Amino Acids** | | |
| Ash | 1.75 g | | Alanine | 1.57 g | |
| | | | Arginine | 1.56 g | |
| **Vitamins** | | | Aspartate | 2.66 g | |
| Vitamin A IU | 36.29 IU | 0.73 | Cystine | 0.28 g | 68.29 |
| Vitamin A RE | 11.34 RE | | Glutamate | 3.89 g | |
| A - Carotenoid | 0.00 RE | 0.00 | Glycine | 1.25 g | |
| A - Retinol | 11.34 RE | | Histidine | 0.77 g | 59.69 |
| B1 Thiamin | 0.03 mg | 2.00 | Isoleucine | 1.20 g | 104.35 |
| B2 Riboflavin | 0.06 mg | 3.53 | Leucine | 2.11 g | 83.40 |
| B3 Niacin | 2.82 mg | 14.10 | Lysine | 2.39 g | 101.70 |
| Niacin Equiv | 7.67 mg | | Methionine | 0.77 g | 104.05 |
| Vitamin B6 | 0.52 mg | 26.00 | Phenylalanine | 1.02 g | 85.71 |
| Vitamin B12 | 1.18 mcg | 19.67 | Proline | 0.92 g | |
| Biotin | — mcg | — | Serine | 1.06 g | |
| Vitamin C | 3.40 mg | 5.67 | Threonine | 1.14 g | 91.94 |
| Vitamin D IU | 63.50 IU | 15.88 | Tryptophan | 0.29 g | 90.62 |
| Vitamin D mcg | 1.59 mcg | | Tyrosine | 0.88 g | 90.72 |
| Vitamin E Alpha Equiv | 0.39 mg | 1.95 | Valine | 1.34 g | 91.16 |
| Vitamin E IU | 0.59 IU | | | | |
| Vitamin E mg | 0.39 mg | | | | |
| Folate | 9.07 mcg | 2.27 | | | |
| Vitamin K | — mcg | — | | | |

(Note: "—" indicates data is unavailable. For more information, please see page 806.)

STEP-BY-STEP RECIPE
## The Healthiest Ways of Cooking Cod

# 5-Minute "Quick Broiled" Cod

*The "Quick Broil" method seals in Cod's delicious juices, brings out is best flavor and retains its moisture. It is not necessary to turn the Cod over as it cooks on both sides simultaneously.*

> 3/4 lb Cod fillets, cut in half
> 2 TBS + 1 TBS fresh lemon juice
> 2 TBS extra virgin olive oil
> 1 medium clove garlic
> Sea salt and pepper to taste

1. Chop or press garlic and let sit for 5 minutes. (Why?, see page 261.)

2. Preheat the broiler on high and place an all stainless steel skillet (be sure the handle is also stainless steel) or cast iron pan under the heat for about 10 minutes to get it very hot. The pan should be 5 to 7 inches from the heat source.

3. Rub Cod fillets with 2 TBS lemon juice and salt and pepper to taste. If Cod comes with its skin on, cook it skin side down.

4. Using a hot pad, remove pan from heat, place Cod

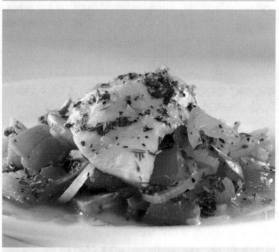

Mediterranean Cod

on hot pan and return to broiler. Keep in mind that it is cooking rapidly on both sides, so it is done very quickly, usually in 3–5 minutes, depending on thickness. (Most Cod fillets are less than 1-inch thick.) Test with a fork for doneness. Cod will flake easily when it is done. Make sure it is not overcooked and dry.

5. Dress with extra virgin olive oil, 1 TBS lemon juice and garlic.

**SERVES 2**

## Flavor Tips: Try these 7 great serving suggestions for Cod. ✳

If you would like to "Healthy Sauté," "Healthy Steam" or poach Cod, see instructions in the salmon chapter, page 482. Because it is thinner, the Cod will cook more quickly than the salmon.

1. **Most Popular: Mediterranean Cod.** Combine 2 TBS honey, 2 TBS sherry wine and 2 diced tomatoes in a mixing bowl. "Healthy Sauté" 1 thinly sliced onion and 1 diced red bell pepper for 2 minutes. Add 1/2 cup chicken or vegetable broth, 2 medium Cod fillets and tomato mixture. **Cover** and cook over medium heat for 3–5 minutes or until fish is cooked. Add minced basil and parsley and sea salt and pepper to taste. Serve over brown rice or quinoa (pictured above).

2. Marjoram and thyme combine well with Cod.

3. Top Cod with pesto (see page 508) or Olive Tapenade (see page 325) after broiling.

4. For an Asian flavor add tamari (soy sauce), ginger, and rice vinegar and replace black pepper with white pepper.

5. **Cod Tacos:** Combine "Healthy Sautéed" Cod with chopped romaine lettuce, tomatoes, avocados and cheese in a corn tortilla. Top with your favorite salsa.

6. **Sweet and Spicy Cod:** "Healthy Sauté" diced onion, add Cod fillets and cook for 2 minutes. Add 1/2 cup diced tomatoes, 1/3 cup diced pineapple, 1 TBS honey, 2 TBS lemon juice and red pepper flakes to taste. Cook for 3 minutes. Add minced parsley and sea salt to taste. Serve with brown rice.

7. **Cod with Herbs:** Combine minced fresh rosemary, ground cumin and fennel seeds in a small bowl. Press the herbs and spices into the Cod fillets. "Healthy Sauté" the fillets and drizzle with olive oil, sea salt and pepper to taste.

Please write (address on back cover flap) or e-mail me at info@whfoods.org with your personal ideas for preparing Cod, and I will share them with others through our website at www.whfoods.org.

*(Continued from Page 485)*

I also don't recommend cooking Cod in oil because high temperature heat can damage delicate fats and potentially create harmful free radicals. (For more on *Why it is Important to Cook Without Heated Oils*, see page 52.)

---

### PACIFIC COD ARE THE BEST CHOICE* AS AN ECOLOGICALLY SUSTAINABLE SPECIES

Sustainable species of Cod are those that can be sustained long-term without compromising their survival or the integrity of the ecosystem in which they live. Pacific Cod are not overfished, and fish managers currently believe that they are a sustainable resource. There are no immediate conservation concerns regarding stocks of Cod harvested off the coast of Alaska. Alaskan Cod is being considered by the Marine Stewardship Council for one of its coveted eco-labels for sustainability and sound management.

Atlantic Cod is rated "avoid." Due to heavy overfishing and destruction of their seafloor habitat by the trawling methods used to catch them, Atlantic Cod stocks are very low. It is estimated it will take decades for stocks to recover. While not as common, you can sometimes find Atlantic Cod caught with sustainable fishing methods (hook and line), making them a relatively eco-friendly choice.

*\* Rating information from Monterey Bay Aquarium Seafood Watch*

---

## Q *Is there such a thing as organic fish and shellfish?*

A The labeling of fish and shellfish as "organic" is controversial since the United States Department of Agriculture (USDA) has not yet allowed for its organic seal to be used on seafood. As of early 2007, it has not even come up with a standard that could be used as a basis for certification of seafood as organic. Precisely because there is no USDA organics standard for seafood, it is also impossible for the USDA to regulate organic labeling claims on seafood imported into the U.S. from other countries.

At present, all seafood purchased in the U.S. that is labeled as organic is imported from other countries. In other countries, organic standards may be significantly different than U.S. standards. For example, fish labeled organic in other countries may carry residues of compounds and drugs that are prohibited in existing U.S. standards for other (non-seafood) foods.

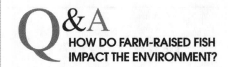

## Q&A HOW DO FARM-RAISED FISH IMPACT THE ENVIRONMENT?

### A Threat to Small Commercial Fisheries

Salmon farmed in open pen nets are now the source of 50% of the world's salmon. (Hatchery fish account for about 30%, and wild-caught fish provide the remaining 20%.) Flooding the market with fish—farm salmon has resulted in a drop in the fisherman's asking price for wild-caught salmon—a price decrease that has forced many small fishing boats off the water.

### Polluting the Immediate Environment

Aquafarms, called "floating pig farms," by Daniel Pauly, professor of fisheries at the University of British Columbia in Vancouver, put a significant strain upon their surrounding environment. According to Pauly, "They consume a tremendous amount of highly concentrated protein pellets and they make a terrific mess." Uneaten feed and fish waste blankets the sea floor beneath these farms, a breeding ground for bacteria that consume oxygen vital to shellfish and other bottom-dwelling sea creatures. A good sized salmon farm produces an amount of excrement equivalent to the sewage of a city of 10,000 people.

### Polluting the Food Chain

Sulfa drugs and tetracycline used to prevent infectious disease epidemics in the dense aquafarm populations are added to food pellet mixes along with, in farm-raised salmon, the orange dye canthaxanthin, to color their otherwise grey flesh. These food additives drift to the ocean bottom below the open net pens where they are invariably recycled into our food chain.

### A Threat to Wild Fish

Pesticides fed to the fish and toxic copper sulfate used to keep nets free of algae are building up in seafloor sediments. Antibiotic use has resulted in the development of resistant strains that can infect not only farm-raised but wild fish as they swim past. Sea lice that infest captive fish beset wild salmon as they swim past on their migration to the ocean. *(Continued on Page 489.)*

## HOW DO FARM-RAISED FISH IMPACT THE ENVIRONMENT?

*(Continued from Page 488.)*

Perhaps the most serious concern is a problem fish farms were meant to alleviate: the depletion of marine life from overfishing. Salmon aquafarming increases the depletion because captive salmon, unlike vegetarian catfish which thrive on grains, are carnivores and must be fed fish during the two to four year period when they are raised to a marketable size. To produce one pound of farmed salmon, approximately two to four pounds of wild sardines, anchovies, mackerel, herring and other fish must be ground up to render the oil and meal that is compressed into pellets of salmon chow.

Similar to the raising of cattle, farming fish creates a problematic redistribution of protein in the food system. Removing such immense amounts of small prey fish from an ecosystem can significantly upset its balance. According to Rosamond L. Naylor, an agricultural economist at Stanford's Center for Environmental Science and Policy, "We are not taking strain off wild fisheries. We are adding to it. This cannot be sustained forever."

### A Threat to Other Marine Life

Other reported environmental impacts from salmon aquaculture include seabirds ensnared in protective netting and sea lions shot for preying on penned fish. Penned salmon also directly threaten their wild counterparts, preying on migrating smolts (immature wild salmon) as they journey to the sea and competing for the krill and herring that nourish wild fish before their final journey home to their spawning grounds. Escapees of farm fish also create problems by competing with wild fish for habitat, spawning grounds and food sources. (About 1 million Atlantic salmon have escaped through holes in nets from storm-wracked farms in the Pacific Northwest's Puget Sound.)

### A Threat to Biodiversity

The interbreeding of wild and farm stocks also poses a threat of dilution to the wild salmon gene pool. Biologists fear these invaders will outcompete Pacific salmon and trout for food and territory, hastening the demise of the native fish. An Atlantic salmon takeover could knock nature's balance out of whack and turn a healthy, diverse marine habitat into one dominated by a single invasive species.

Recently, Aqua Bounty Farms Inc., of Waltham, Mass., has begun seeking U.S. and Canadian approval to alter genes to produce a growth hormone that could shave a year off the usual two and one-half to three years it takes to raise a market-size fish. The prospect of genetically modified salmon that can grow six times faster than normal fish has heightened anxiety that these "Frankenfish" will escape and pose an even greater danger to native species than do the Atlantic salmon.

### A Possible Contributor to Antibiotic Resistance

Rearing fish in such high densities presents problems. Infectious disease outbreaks pose financial threats to operators, so vaccines and antibiotics are often used to prevent potential epidemics. Sulfa drugs and tetracycline are often added to food pellet mixes as well as canthaxanthin (a synthetic dye) to impart a rich pink color to an otherwise pale gray flesh. Antibiotics are also given to speed growth and increase profits.

In some of the more progressive salmon-rearing operations, fish farmers are raising their Chinook and other species in closed, floating pens so that antibiotics and other wastes can be filtered from the water before it's released back into the environment.

In the majority of aquafarms, however, these drugs and additives, which quickly build up in the sediment, will invariably find their way into our food stream. In a paper published in 2002, Bent Halling-Sørensen and his colleagues at the Royal Danish School of Pharmacy noted that one such growth-promoting antibiotic—oxytetracycline—has been found in the sediment of fish-farming sites at concentrations of up to 4.9 milligrams per kilogram. These scientists are concerned that "Antibiotic resistance in sediment bacteria is often found in locations with fish farms"—and may play a growing role in the development of antibiotic-resistant germs. Should their fears be true, aquafarming may be eroding the efficacy of life-saving drugs, argues Stuart Levy, the director of the Center for Adaptation Genetics and Drug Resistance at the Tufts Medical School in Boston.

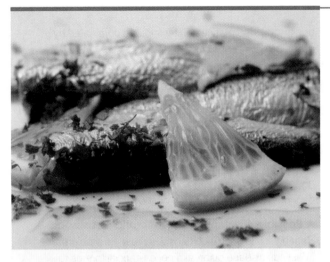

# sardines

| | |
|---|---|
| AVAILABILITY: | Year-round |
| REFRIGERATE: | No |
| PREPARATION: | Minimal |
| BEST WAY TO COOK: | Needs no cooking |

## nutrient-richness chart

Total Nutrient-Richness: **20**
3.25 ounce can (93 grams) of Sardines in oil contains 191 calories

| NUTRIENT | AMOUNT | %DV | DENSITY | QUALITY |
|---|---|---|---|---|
| Vitamin B12 | 8.22 mcg | 137.0 | 12.9 | excellent |
| Tryptophan | 0.25 g | 78.1 | 7.3 | excellent |
| Selenium | 48.4 g | 69.3 | 6.5 | very good |
| Vitamin D | 250.2 IU | 62.6 | 5.9 | very good |
| Omega-3 Fatty Acids | 1.36 g | 54.4 | 5.1 | very good |
| Protein | 22.7 g | 45.3 | 4.3 | very good |
| Phosphorus | 450.8 mg | 45.1 | 4.2 | very good |
| Calcium | 351.4 | 35.1 | 3.3 | good |
| B3 Niacin | 4.8 mg | 24.1 | 2.3 | good |

For more on "Total Nutrient-Richness," "%DV," "Density," and
The World's Healthiest Foods "Quality" Rating System, see page 805.

Sardines are named after Sardinia, the Italian island where large schools of these fish were once found. While Sardines are delightful enjoyed fresh, they are most commonly found canned, since they are so perishable. Sardines date back to time immemorial, but it was the emperor Napoleon Bonaparte who helped to popularize these little fish by initiating the canning of Sardines, the first fish to ever be canned, in order to feed his people. Extremely popular in the United States in the beginning of the 20th century, Sardines are now making a comeback as people realize that they are an incredibly rich source of omega-3 fatty acids. With concern over the health of the seas, people are also turning to Sardines since they are at the bottom of the aquatic food chain, feeding solely on plankton, and therefore do not concentrate heavy metals, such as mercury, and contaminants as do some other fish. Although they are small, Sardines will make a large contribution to your "Healthiest

Way of Eating." The information in this chapter is mostly about canned Sardines, as fresh Sardines are not readily available in most parts of the country.

## why sardines should be part of your healthiest way of eating

The adage "big things come in small packages" could not be truer than for Sardines. These little fish, which can grow to up to 14 inches but generally range from 6–8 inches in length, are packed with health-promoting nutrients. They are rich in heart-healthy omega-3 fatty acids and bone-building calcium and vitamin D. They are the second most concentrated source of vitamin B12 of all of the World's Healthiest Foods. (For more on the *Health Benefits of Sardines* and a complete analysis of their content of over 60 nutrients, see page 494.)

## varieties of sardines

Sardines are classified in a group known as cold-water fish, which also includes mackerel, herring, smelt, salmon and halibut, which are rich in omega-3 fatty acids.

While there are six different species of Sardines belonging to the *Clupeidae* family, more than 20 varieties of fish are sold as Sardines throughout the world. What these fish share is that they are all small, saltwater, oil-rich, silvery fish that are soft-boned. In the United States, Sardine actually refers to a small herring, and adult Sardines are known as "pilchards," a name that is commonly used in other parts of the world. Sardines are abundant in the seas of the Atlantic, Pacific and Mediterranean with Spain, Portugal, France and Norway being the leading producers of canned sardines.

### FRESH SARDINES

Since they are very perishable, fresh Sardines are more

difficult to find in many fish markets. If you can find them they are a treat and are delicious grilled or broiled.

### CANNED SARDINES

Canned Sardines are widely available. Before canning, their heads are removed and they are gutted and steamed. They are not deboned, as their bones become soft and edible after steaming. To retain their moisture, Sardines are canned in liquid mediums including oil, water, tomato sauce and mustard sauce. Smoked Sardines are also available canned.

## the peak season

Fresh Sardines are in season during the summer months. Canned Sardines are available throughout the year.

## biochemical considerations

Sardines contain purines, which might be of concern to certain individuals. (For more on *Purines*, see page 727.)

## 4 steps to the best tasting and most nutritious sardines

Turning Sardines into a flavorful dish with the most nutrients is simple if you just follow my 4 easy steps:

1. The Best Way to Select
2. The Best Way to Store
3. The Best Way to Prepare
4. The Healthiest Way of Cooking

---

### SARDINES ARE BEST CHOICE* AS AN ECOLOGICALLY SUSTAINABLE SPECIES

The name "Sardine" is applied to many small fishes of the herring family. These fish reproduce rapidly and travel in gigantic schools, but their success depends strongly on a favorable marine environment. Warmer weather is more favorable for Sardines. Pacific Sardines, which once supported the largest and most profitable U.S. fishery, nearly disappeared in the 1940s. Although overfishing may have sped up this decline, the population dip was part of a natural Sardine "boom and bust" cycle. Sardines have made a comeback on both coasts — good news for people who enjoy these tasty little fish, and for the many kinds of sea birds, sea mammals and large fish that feed on Sardines.

The wild population is abundant and well managed with low levels of wasted catch (bycatch), and the fish are not caught or farmed in ways that harm the environment.

*Rating information from Monterey Bay Aquarium Seafood Watch*

---

# 1. the best way to select sardines

Canned Sardines packed in olive oil are preferable to those in soybean oil. Those concerned about their intake of fat may want to choose Sardines packed in water. Look at the expiration date stamped on the package to ensure that they are still fresh.

Fresh Sardines are not often available, but if you are purchasing fresh Sardines, look for ones that smell fresh, are firm to the touch, and have bright eyes and shiny skin.

# 2. the best way to store sardines

Canned Sardines can be stored in the kitchen cupboard, ideally one that is cool and not exposed to excess heat. They have a long storage life; check the package for the expiration date, so you know by when you should use it. Turn the can every now and then to ensure that all parts of the Sardines are exposed to the oil or liquid in which they are packed; this will keep them well-moistened. Unused portions of opened canned Sardines should be refrigerated.

Fresh Sardines are very perishable, and normal refrigerator temperatures of 36°–40°F (2°–4°C) do not inhibit the enzymatic activity that causes them to spoil; they are best when stored at 28°–32°F (-2°–0°/C). I have tried various methods to find the best way to store Sardines including packing the Sardines with ice before placing them in the refrigerator to decrease the temperature. Although this method kept the Sardines cool, once the ice melted, the Sardines ended up sitting in a pool of water causing them to lose much of their flavor.

I have refined this method and want to share with you the best way to keep your Sardines fresh. Remove Sardines from store packaging, rinse and place in a plastic storage bag as soon as you bring them home from the market. Place in a large bowl and cover with ice cubes or ice packs to reduce the temperature of the fish. Although fresh Sardines will keep for a few days using this method, I recommend using your Sardines as soon as possible, within a day or two. Remember to drain off the melted water and replenish the ice or ice packs as necessary. Remember that fish not only starts to smell but will dry out or become slimy if it is not stored correctly.

# 3. the best way to prepare sardines

Canned Sardines require minimal preparation. For canned Sardines packed in oil, gently rinse them under water to remove excess oil before eating.

Fresh Sardines need to be gutted and rinsed under cold running water.

# 4. the healthiest way of cooking sardines

**CANNED SARDINES**

Canned Sardines require no cooking.

**FRESH SARDINES**

Fresh Sardines can be grilled or broiled. Sardines cook quickly and are easily overcooked. To prevent overcooking Sardines, I highly recommend using a timer. And since Sardines cook in only 7–10 minutes (3 to 5 minutes on each side), it is important to begin timing as soon as you place them in the broiler. Sardines cook quickly and will become tough and lose flavor when overcooked. You will know when Sardines are done when they flake easily with a fork. Cooking times are based on Sardines that are about 6–7 inches in length.

---

**Q** *What are your thoughts on canned Sardines and tuna as I eat these foods as way of getting my fish oils?*

**A** Canned fish can be a great addition to a "Healthiest Way of Eating." Sardines are one of the best sources of omega-3 fatty acids (as well as other nutrients such as vitamin D). They are very delicate and seasonal, so canned Sardines are the best way to really enjoy this great fish throughout the year. If you eat a lot of canned tuna and you are concerned about mercury, you may want to consume light tuna versus albacore tuna. The FDA recently advised women who are pregnant, lactating or of childbearing age as well as young children to limit the amount of canned tuna they consume; since albacore tuna is more prone to mercury contamination, they advised that these groups limit their consumption to 6 ounces per week of albacore tuna and to no more than 12 ounces per week of light tuna. If possible, I think that it is best to purchase canned fish that is packaged in water as opposed to packaged in oil to avoid excess calories.

**Q** *Is a metallic taste in the mouth a sign of mercury toxicity?*

**A** There are many symptoms of chronic mercury over-exposure with a metallic taste in the mouth being one of them. Other potential symptoms include shakiness, slurred speech, impaired memory, joint pain and headaches. But, because these symptoms—including the metallic taste—have a wide variety of possible causes, they aren't particularly helpful in singling out mercury as the main culprit. There are blood tests and hair tests available for measuring mercury toxicity. If you are considering mercury testing, we recommend that you do so in consultation with your healthcare provider.

**Q** *I'm in charge of facilitating group process at the company where I work. Are there any foods that we can serve at our meetings to help decision making and affect our mood?*

**A** Although food can affect our mood, the connection between eating and behaving in a particular way is much less direct than you ask about. All of our organ systems need nutrients to function properly, including our brain and nervous systems. When we are poorly nourished, we may start to think less clearly. All of us have experienced that phenomenon where we are very tired, have gotten too little sleep and are much quicker to become irritated or impatient. Sometimes one good night's sleep will fix our mood—sometimes not. But food seldom works that quickly. We become nourished over time, over days and weeks and months of eating well. The food eaten at a meeting isn't even absorbed until hours after that meeting has already ended. In addition, it isn't food that decides how we treat our fellow human beings. That takes place in our heart and in our conscience, and even when we are poorly nourished, we can usually be decent people if we want to be. I believe that the World's Healthiest Foods are the best long-term way of maintaining optimal health, including healthy organ systems that aid good listening skills and decision making.

## The Healthiest Ways to Prepare Sardines

# 3-Minute Sardine Spread

*Great as an appetizer served on crackers or as a dip.*

1 can (3.25 ounces) of sardines packed
    in olive oil or water
4 ounces Parmesan cheese, grated
1 TBS fresh lemon juice
2 TBS parsley, chopped
1 tsp capers
1/2 tsp paprika
3 TBS extra virgin olive oil

1. Drain the oil or water from the can of Sardines.
2. Combine all ingredients in a food processor or blender. Process or blend until smooth. Serve with crackers or vegetables.

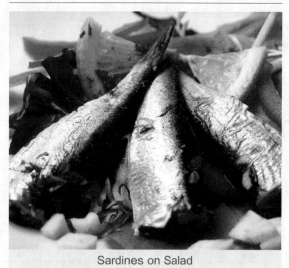

Sardines on Salad

**SERVES 2–4**

## Flavor Tips: 7 Ways to Enjoy Sardines and Canned Sardines. ✳

1. **Sardines with Dijon Caper Sauce:** In a bowl whisk together 3 TBS extra virgin olive oil, 2 tsp lemon juice, 1 clove pressed garlic, 1 TBS Dijon mustard, 1 tsp capers, and 2 tsp minced basil or parsley. Pour over Sardines.
2. Drain and sprinkle with lemon and olive oil.
3. Sprinkle with basil, oregano or rosemary and combine with chopped tomatoes.
4. Balsamic vinegar gives Sardines a nice zing.
5. Combine with chopped onion, olives or fennel.
6. **Sardine Wrap:** Wrap Sardines, tomatoes, chopped onions, chopped olives, chopped avocados, fresh basil and goat cheese in a leaf of romaine lettuce.
7. **Sardines on Salad:** For added protein, top a salad with canned Sardines and your favorite "Healthy Vinaigrette" (see page 143) (pictured above).

# Fresh Broiled Sardines

*Tasty, quick and easy.*

6 fresh Sardines
2 TBS + 1 tsp fresh lemon juice
Sea salt and pepper to taste
3 cloves garlic
3 TBS extra virgin olive oil
2 TBS fresh basil, chopped

1. Chop garlic and let sit for 5 minutes. (Why?, see page 261.)

2. Preheat broiler.
3. While broiler is heating, gut and clean Sardines. Brush Sardines with lemon juice and salt and pepper to taste.
4. Place them in the broiler 7 inches from the heating element, and cook 5 minutes on each side or until brown. Dress with olive oil, basil and garlic.

**SERVES 2**

Please write (address on back cover flap) or e-mail me at info@whfoods.org with your personal ideas for preparing Sardines, and I will share them with others through our website at www.whfoods.org.

# health benefits of sardines

## Promote Heart Health

Sardines are rich in numerous nutrients that have been found to support cardiovascular health. They are one of the most concentrated sources of the omega-3 fatty acids EPA and DHA, which have been found to lower triglyceride and cholesterol levels; one serving of Sardines actually contains over 50% of the daily value for these important nutri-ents. Sardines are also an excellent source of vitamin B12, second only to calf's liver as the World's Healthiest Food most concentrated in this nutrient. Vitamin B12 promotes cardiovascular well-being since it is intricately tied to keeping levels of homocysteine in balance; homocysteine can damage artery walls, with elevated levels being a risk factor for atherosclerosis.

## Promote Bone Health

If you don't think of fish as being a bone-building food, Sardines will make you think again. Not only are Sardines a good source of calcium, but they are also incredibly rich in vitamin D, a nutrient not so readily available in the diet and one that is most often associated with fortified dairy products. Vitamin D plays an essential role in bone health since it helps to increase the absorption of calcium. Sardines are also a very good source of phosphorus, a mineral that is important to strengthening the bone matrix. Additionally, as high levels of homocysteine are also related to osteoporosis, Sardines' vitamin B12 rounds out their repertoire of nutrients that support bone health.

## Promote Optimal Health

For many years, researchers have known that vitamin D, in the form of calcitriol, participates in the regulation of cell activity. Because cell cycles play such a key role in the development of cancer, optimal vitamin D intake may turn out to play an important role in the prevention of various cancers. Selenium, of which Sardines are also a very good source, is a mineral with powerful antioxidant activity, whose dietary intake has been associated with reduced risk of cancer.

## Packed with Protein

Sardines are rich in protein, which provides us with amino acids. Our bodies use amino acids to create new proteins, which serve as the basis for most of the body's cells and structures. Proteins form the basis of muscles and connective tissues, antibodies that keep our immune system strong and transport proteins that deliver oxygen and nutrients throughout the body.

## Additional Health-Promoting Benefits of Sardines

Sardines are also a concentrated source of other nutrients providing additional health benefits. These nutrients include energy-producing niacin and sleep-promoting tryptophan.

### Nutritional Analysis of 3.25 ounce can of Sardines in oil:

| NUTRIENT | AMOUNT | % DAILY VALUE | NUTRIENT | AMOUNT | % DAILY VALUE |
|---|---|---|---|---|---|
| Calories | 191.36 | | Pantothenic Acid | 0.59 mg | 5.90 |
| Calories from Fat | 94.81 | | | | |
| Calories from Saturated Fat | 12.65 | | **Minerals** | | |
| Protein | 22.65 g | | Boron | — mcg | |
| Carbohydrates | 0.00 g | | Calcium | 351.44 mg | 35.14 |
| Dietary Fiber | 0.00 g | 0.00 | Chloride | — mg | |
| Soluble Fiber | 0.00 g | | Chromium | — mcg | — |
| Insoluble Fiber | 0.00 g | | Copper | 0.17 mg | 8.50 |
| Sugar – Total | 0.00 g | | Fluoride | — mg | — |
| Monosaccharides | 0.00 g | | Iodine | — mcg | — |
| Disaccharides | 0.00 g | | Iron | 2.69 mg | 14.94 |
| Other Carbs | 0.00 g | | Magnesium | 35.88 mg | 8.97 |
| Fat – Total | 10.53 g | | Manganese | 0.10 mg | 5.00 |
| Saturated Fat | 1.41 g | | Molybdenum | 3.13 mcg | 4.17 |
| Mono Fat | 3.56 g | | Phosphorus | 450.80 mg | 45.08 |
| Poly Fat | 4.74 g | | Potassium | 365.24 mg | |
| Omega-3 Fatty Acids | 1.36 g | 54.40 | Selenium | 48.48 mcg | 69.26 |
| Omega-6 Fatty Acids | 3.26 g | | Sodium | 464.60 mg | |
| Water | 54.84 g | | Zinc | 1.21 mg | 8.07 |
| Ash | 3.11 g | | | | |
| | | | **Amino Acids** | | |
| **Vitamins** | | | Alanine | 1.37 g | |
| Vitamin A IU | 206.08 IU | 4.12 | Arginine | 1.36 g | |
| Vitamin A RE | 61.64 RE | | Aspartate | 2.32 g | |
| A - Carotenoid | 0.00 RE | 0.00 | Cystine | 0.24 g | 58.54 |
| A - Retinol | 61.64 RE | | Glutamate | 3.38 g | |
| B1 Thiamin | 0.07 mg | 4.67 | Glycine | 1.09 g | |
| B2 Riboflavin | 0.21 mg | 12.35 | Histidine | 0.67 g | 51.94 |
| B3 Niacin | 4.83 mg | 24.15 | Isoleucine | 1.04 g | 90.43 |
| Niacin Equiv | 9.06 mg | | Leucine | 1.84 g | 72.73 |
| Vitamin B6 | 0.15 mg | 7.50 | Lysine | 2.08 g | 88.51 |
| Vitamin B12 | 8.22 mcg | 137.00 | Methionine | 0.67 g | 90.54 |
| Biotin | — mcg | — | Phenylalanine | 0.88 g | 73.95 |
| Vitamin C | 0.00 mg | 0.00 | Proline | 0.80 g | |
| Vitamin D IU | 250.24 IU | 62.56 | Serine | 0.92 g | |
| Vitamin D mcg | 6.26 mcg | | Threonine | 0.99 g | 79.84 |
| Vitamin E Alpha Equiv | 0.28 mg | 1.40 | Tryptophan | 0.25 g | 78.13 |
| Vitamin E IU | 0.41 IU | | Tyrosine | 0.76 g | 78.35 |
| Vitamin E mg | 0.28 mg | | Valine | 1.17 g | 79.59 |
| Folate | 10.86 mcg | 2.71 | | | |
| Vitamin K | 0.07 mcg | 0.09 | | | |

(Note: "—" indicates data is unavailable. For more information, please see page 806.)

# Q&A

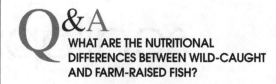

**WHAT ARE THE NUTRITIONAL DIFFERENCES BETWEEN WILD-CAUGHT AND FARM-RAISED FISH?**

### Farm-raised Fish are Fattier

The fat content of farmed salmon is excessively high—30–35% by weight. Wild salmon have a 20% higher protein content and a 20% lower fat content than farm-raised salmon. According to a USDA study, farm-raised catfish, rainbow trout and coho salmon were fattier compared to wild stocks of the same species. This is not surprising since farm-raised fish do not spend their lives vigorously swimming through cold ocean waters or leaping up rocky streams. Marine couch potatoes, they circle lazily in crowded pens fattening up on pellets of fish chow.

In each of the species evaluated by the USDA, the farm-raised fish were found to contain more total fat than their wild counterparts. For rainbow trout, the difference in total fat (4.6 g/100 g in wild trout vs. 5.4 g/100 g in cultivated trout) was the smallest, while cultivated catfish had nearly five times as much fat as wild catfish (11.3 g/100 g in cultivated vs. 2.3 g/100 g in wild). Farm-raised coho salmon had approximately 2.7 times the total fat as wild samples.

### Farm-raised Fish Provide Less Usable Omega-3 Fats

Although the farm-raised catfish, rainbow trout and coho salmon contained similar amounts of omega-3 fatty acids as their wild equivalents, in proportion to the amount of omega-6 fats they also contained, they actually provided less usable omega-3s.

The reason for this apparent discrepancy is that both omega-3 and omega-6 fats use the same enzymes for conversion into the forms in which they are active in the body. The same *elongase* and *desaturase* enzymes that convert omega-3 fats into their beneficial anti-inflammatory forms (the series-3 prostaglandins and the less inflammatory thromboxanes and leukotrienes) also convert omega-6 fats into their pro-inflammatory forms (the series-2 prostaglandins and the pro-inflammatory thromboxanes and leukotrienes). So, when a food is eaten that contains high amounts of omega-6s in proportion to its content of omega-3s, the omega-6 fats use up the available conversion enzymes to produce pro-inflammatory compounds while preventing the manufacture of anti-inflammatory substances from omega-3s, even when these beneficial fats are present.

### Farm-raised Fish Contain More Pro-inflammatory Omega-6 Fats

In all three types of fish, the amount of omega-6 fats was substantially higher in farm-raised compared to wild fish. Cultivated trout, in particular, had much higher levels of one type of omega-6 fat called linoleic acid than wild trout (14% in farm-raised compared to 5% in wild samples). The total of all types of omega-6 fats found in cultivated fish was twice the level found in the wild samples (14% vs 7%, respectively).

### Wild Fish Provide More Omega-3 Fats

In all three species evaluated, the wild fish were found to have a higher proportion of omega-3 fats in comparison to omega-6 fats than the cultivated fish. The wild coho were not only much lower in overall fat content but also were found to have 33% more omega-3 fatty acids than their farm-raised counterparts. Omega-3s accounted for 29% of the fats in wild coho versus 19% of the fats in cultivated coho. Rainbow trout showed similar proportions in fatty acid content; wild trout contained approximately 33% more omega-3s than cultivated trout; however, both cultivated and wild trout did have much lower amounts of omega-6 fats than the other types of fish.

---

**Q** *I typically eat 1/4 cup of walnuts a day, 4–5 times a week. I am considering adding an omega-3 supplement (cold-water fish oil capsules), but I'm having trouble evaluating whether the supplement offers me anything additional over the walnut omega-3 source?*

**A** In general, it makes no sense to compare a food to a supplement. Whenever you can obtain nutrients from food rather than supplements, you should do so. Unless you need a therapeutic dose of a nutrient, are unable to obtain foods that contain the nutrients you need or are unable to consume certain foods for allergy or other physical reasons, you should always be sticking with foods versus supplements. The omega-3 fatty acids in fish include alpha-linolenic acid (ALA), eicosapentaenoic acid (EPA) and docosahexaenoic acid (DHA). Walnuts have ALA, but they do not have EPA or DHA. The amount of EPA and DHA contained in one fish oil capsule is approximately the same as you could find in one ounce of salmon. Our bodies, when healthy, make EPA and DHA from ALA. For this reason, only ALA is considered an essential omega-3 fatty acid. The only reason you would want to turn to a processed supplemental oil is if you needed larger doses of EPA and DHA for some personal health reason, if you suspected your body could not make enough EPA and DHA from ALA, of if you were having trouble incorporating enough ALA-containing foods into your meal plan.

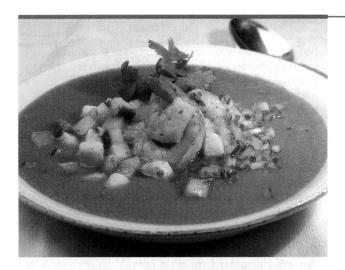

# scallops

## highlights

| | |
|---|---|
| AVAILABILITY: | Year-round |
| REFRIGERATE: | Yes |
| SHELF LIFE: | Up to 1-2 days refrigerated |
| PREPARATION: | Minimal |
| BEST WAY TO COOK: | "Healthy Sauté" in just 3 minutes |

## nutrient-richness chart

Total Nutrient-Richness: **14**
4 ounces (113 grams) of broiled/baked Scallops contain 152 calories

| NUTRIENT | AMOUNT | %DV | DENSITY | QUALITY |
|---|---|---|---|---|
| Tryptophan | 0.3 g | 81.3 | 9.6 | excellent |
| Protein | 23.1 g | 46.2 | 5.5 | very good |
| Omega-3 Fatty Acids | 1.1 g | 44.0 | 5.2 | very good |
| Vitamin B12 | 2.0 mcg | 33.3 | 4.0 | very good |
| Phosphorus | 302.1 mg | 30.2 | 3.6 | very good |
| Magnesium | 77.1 mg | 19.3 | 2.3 | good |
| Potassium | 444.5 mg | 12.7 | 1.5 | good |

For more on "Total Nutrient-Richness," "%DV," "Density," and
The World's Healthiest Foods "Quality" Rating System, see page 805.

People have been enjoying Scallops as a food since antiquity, ever since this beautiful mollusk appeared in the Earth's waters. The soft, fleshy texture and delicious mild flavor of Scallops make them a seafood favorite even among those who are not particularly fond of other types of fish or shellfish. The great Scallop gained prestige during medieval times when pilgrims visiting the shrine of St. James in Spain began to use empty Scallop shells for both eating and begging. Scallops are quick and easy to prepare. They are almost always shucked and trimmed when you purchase them, and they take only minutes to cook. I would like to share with you how using the "Healthiest Way of Cooking" methods can help enhance the flavor and texture of your Scallops.

## why scallops should be part of your healthiest way of eating

Scallops are exceptionally rich in vitamin B12, an important vitamin for cardiovascular health, as well as those hard-to-find omega-3 fatty acids, which help reduce inflammation in the body. Scallops are an ideal food to add to your "Healthiest Way of Eating" not only because they are high in nutrients, but also because they are low in calories: 4 ounces of Scallops contain only 152 calories! (For more on the *Health Benefits of Scallops* and a complete analysis of their content of over 60 nutrients, see page 500.)

## varieties of scallops

There are several hundred species of Scallops found in shallow saltwater areas throughout the world. In the United States, the most widely available types of Scallops include the Atlantic Sea Scallop and the Bay Scallop. Scallops can be either wild-caught or farm-raised.

### SEA SCALLOPS

These are large Scallops from the North Atlantic that can be up to two inches in diameter. Their flesh is ivory-colored and translucent. They have a chewier texture and a less delicate flavor than Bay Scallops. Most Sea Scallops are wild-caught; only small quantities are farm-raised.

### BAY SCALLOPS

Sweet and delicate in flavor, the Bay Scallop is tiny, averaging only about one-half of an inch in diameter. Wild Bay Scallops are harvested from protected bays and shallow waters from New England to North Carolina. Bay Scallop stocks in the U.S. are largely depleted with most of the Bay Scallops currently farmed. Most farmed Bay Scallops found in the U.S. market are imported from China; small quantities are still farmed in New England and Nova Scotia.

### CALICO SCALLOPS

Small Sea Scallops from the coast of Florida, they are often sold as Bay Scallops. These are the least expensive of the

Scallops and often considered inferior by Scallop lovers. They are partially cooked by the time they reach the consumer because they must be steamed to open the shells.

### GREAT SCALLOPS

The most popular type of Scallop consumed in Europe, they are more commonly known as Coquille St. Jacques.

# the peak season

The peak season for fresh Sea Scallops and Bay Scallops is from October through March, although Sea Scallops are available year-round; fresh Calico Scallops are available from December through May. It is during the peak of their respective seasons that they are the most flavorful and least expensive. Frozen Scallops are available throughout the year.

# biochemical considerations

Scallops contain purines, which might be of concern to certain individuals. (For more on *Purines*, see page 727.)

# 4 steps for the best tasting and most nutritious scallops

Turning Scallops into a flavorful dish with the most nutrients is simple if you just follow my 4 easy steps:

1. The Best Way to Select
2. The Best Way to Store
3. The Best Way to Prepare
4. The Healthiest Way of Cooking

---

**WILD-CAUGHT SEA SCALLOPS FROM NORTHEAST U.S. AND CANADA AND BAY SCALLOPS WORLDWIDE ARE GOOD ALTERNATIVES**

Sustainable species of Scallops are those that can be sustained long-term without compromising their survival or the integrity of the ecosystem in which they live. Wild-caught Sea Scallops from Northeast U.S. and Canada and wild-caught Bay Scallops worldwide are the most likely to be ecologically sound and chemical free.

Sea Scallops are most commonly caught by dredging. Sea Scallops caught using this method are rated "Caution" because it causes damage to the seafloor. Most Bay Scallops in the United States are imported from China. Imported Scallops may be treated with sodium triphosphate. This preservative causes the Scallops to absorb 25% more water, increasing their apparent weight and freshness. Because there is little information regarding the environmental impact of this industry, they are rated as "Caution."

*\* Rating information from Monterey Bay Aquarium Seafood Watch.*

---

# 1. the best way to select scallops

Wild-caught Sea Scallops from the North Atlantic and wild-caught Bay Scallops are your best choices for Scallops. These methods of production are environmentally sound, and the Scallops are typically not chemically treated. Avoid Scallops which have been "soaked" with sodium triphosphate to increase their shelf life and water absorption. They will have a "soapy" feel to them and not have the rich, sweet taste of untreated Scallops.

The first step in selecting the best Scallops is to find a store with a good reputation for having a fresh supply of seafood. Get to know a fishmonger (person who sells the fish) at the store, so you can have a trusted person from whom you can purchase your fish.

Since Scallops are extremely perishable, they are usually shelled, washed and frozen, or packed in ice, as soon as they are caught. Fresh Scallops should be white, firm and show no evidence of browning. I have found that frozen Scallops are best when they are solid and shiny and the inside of their packaging is free of frost. If you are planning on freezing the Scallops, make sure to ask the fishmonger whether they are fresh or defrosted (if it is not clearly marked) since you will need to cook previously frozen Scallops before refreezing.

It is best to purchase displayed Scallops, whenever possible, rather than those that are already prepackaged. Smell is a good indicator of freshness, and it is difficult to detect smells through the plastic of prepackaged seafood. Once the fishmonger wraps and hands you the Scallops, smell them through the paper wrapping and return them if they do not smell right.

The number of Scallops you get per pound will depend on their size:

> Sea Scallops: 20–30 per pound
> Bay Scallops: 60–100 per pound

If you are going to have a full day of errands after you purchase your Scallops, be sure to keep a cooler in the car to ensure they stay cold and do not spoil.

## 2. the best way to store scallops

Like most shellfish, Scallops are very perishable and normal refrigerator temperatures of 36°–40°F (2°–4°C) do not inhibit the enzymatic activity that causes them to spoil; they are best when stored at 28°–32°F (-2°–0°C). I have tried various methods to find the best way to store Scallops, including packing the Scallops with ice before placing them in the refrigerator to decrease the temperature. Although this method kept the Scallops cool, once the ice melted the Scallops ended up sitting in a pool of water, causing them to lose much of their flavor.

I have refined this method and want to share with you the best way to keep your Scallops fresh. Remove Scallops from store packaging, rinse and place in a plastic storage bag as soon as you bring them home from the market. Place in a large bowl and cover with ice cubes or ice packs to reduce the temperature of the fish. Although fresh Scallops will keep for a few days using this method, I recommend using your Scallops within a day or two of purchase. Remember to drain off the melted ice water and replenish the ice or replace the ice packs as necessary.

## 3. the best way to prepare scallops

There is little preparation necessary before cooking Scallops. Just rinse the Scallops under cold running water and pat dry. Do not excessively rinse them or some of the flavor will also rinse away.

## 4. the healthiest way of cooking scallops

The best way to cook Scallops is by using methods that will keep them moist and tender. Scallops can be easily overcooked and become dry, so be sure to watch your cooking times. Scallops are a delicate shellfish, and I have found that they can be best prepared by using the "Healthy Sauté" method. (For more on "*Healthy Sauté*," see page 57.)

### How to Avoid Overcooking Scallops

Scallops cook quickly and are easily overcooked. To prevent overcooking Scallops, I highly recommend using a timer. And since Scallops cook in only 3 to 5 minutes (depending on size), it is important to begin timing as soon as you place them into the skillet. Scallops cook quickly and will become tough and lose their flavor when overcooked.

### Methods Not Recommended for Cooking Scallops

#### GRILLING AND COOKING WITH OIL

I don't recommend grilling Scallops because they are so delicate and will burn easily.

I don't recommend cooking Scallops in oil because high temperature heat can damage delicate oils and potentially create harmful free radicals. (For more on *Why it is Important to Cook Without Heated Oils*, see page 52.)

---

*(Continued from Page 463)*

and higher mercury fish—especially when it comes to tuna. (For more on where different fish rate in terms of mercury levels, please see page 457.)

**2007 EPA Update on Current Levels of Mercury in Fish**

According to a February 2007 EPA report, 39% of all mercury exposure from fish in the U.S. comes from tuna. Of this 39%, 18% comes from canned light tuna, 10% from canned albacore or white tuna and 11% from fresh or frozen tuna. (Swordfish, pollack, shrimp and cod account for another 25% of all mercury exposure from fish.) Even though canned light tuna accounts for almost double the total mercury exposure as canned albacore or white tuna, albacore/white tuna are actually much higher in mercury content. (As a nation, we just eat much more canned light tuna because of the lower price). In the EPA update report, both Pacific and Atlantic albacore tuna (all forms, including canned and fresh) contained about triple the mercury content of both Pacific and Atlantic light (yellowfin) tuna (all forms, including canned and fresh). But it should also be noted that Atlantic tuna was always higher in mercury content than Pacific tuna. The average numbers for Atlantic tuna in this 2007 EPA study were: 0.47 milligrams/kilogram for albacore and 0.31 milligrams/kilogram for yellowfin (light). By comparison, Pacific albacore only contained an average of 0.17 milligrams/kilogram of mercury and Pacific yellowfin (light) only 0.06 milligrams per kilogram. *(Continued on Page 783)*

STEP-BY-STEP RECIPES
## The Healthiest Ways of Cooking Scallops

# 3-Minute "Healthy Sautéed" Scallops

*For great flavor without the use of heated fats or oils, "Healthy Sauté" your Scallops.*

**1/2 lb Bay Scallops or Sea Scallops**
**1 TBS low-sodium chicken or**
  **vegetable broth**
**2 medium cloves garlic**
**2 TBS extra virgin olive oil**
**1 TBS fresh lemon juice**
**Sea salt and pepper to taste**

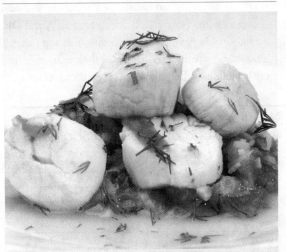

"Healthy Sautéed" Scallops on Bed of Vegetables

1. Chop garlic and let sit for 5 minutes. (Why?, see page 261.)

2. Heat 1 TBS broth over medium heat in a stainless steel skillet.

3. When broth begins to steam, add Scallops and garlic and sauté for 2 minutes stirring frequently. After 2 minutes, turn Scallops over and let cook on the other side for 1 minute. Scallops cook very quickly, so watch your cooking time. Overcooked Scallops become tough (if you are using larger Sea Scallops, you will need to cook for 1–2 minutes longer.

4. Dress with extra virgin olive oil, lemon juice, garlic, and salt and pepper to taste.

**SERVES 2**

## Flavor Tips: Try these 8 great serving suggestions with the recipe above. ✳

1. Serve with salsa made with diced papaya, cilantro, jalapeño peppers and ginger.

2. For an Asian flavor add ginger, rice vinegar and tamari (soy sauce). Replace the black pepper with white pepper.

3. Combine cooked Scallops with "Healthy Sautéed" shiitake mushrooms. Serve on a bed of chopped romaine lettuce and Swiss chard, and top with the dressing of your choice.

4. Toss Scallops with pesto (page 508) or top with Olive Tapenade (page 325) after cooking.

5. Serve on a bed of hot spinach and garnish with toasted almonds.

6. Sprinkle Scallops with Cajun spice before sautéing.

7. Tarragon pairs beautifully with Scallops.

8. In a small mixing bowl, combine mashed anchovies, minced garlic and minced fresh thyme. Pour over hot sautéed Scallops to coat.

**ADDITIONAL RECIPE:**

**Mediterranean Scallops:** Combine 2 TBS honey, 2 TBS white wine, 2 diced tomatoes and 1 tsp sweet paprika in a mixing bowl. "Healthy Sauté" diced onion and 1-inch pieces of asparagus for 1 minute. Add Scallops and tomato mixture. Cook for 5 minutes.

# 4-Minute Scallops Poached in Orange Juice

**2 TBS fresh orange juice**
**1 TBS white wine**
**1 tsp tarragon**
**1/2 lb Sea Scallops**
**Extra virgin olive oil to taste**
**Sea salt and pepper to taste**

1. Heat orange juice and wine in a stainless steel skillet until boiling.

2. Add tarragon and Sea Scallops, and stir constantly while cooking. After 2 minutes, turn Scallops over to cook 2 minutes more on the other side.

3. When Scallops are opaque, remove form heat and drizzle with extra virgin olive oil. Add salt and pepper to taste.

**SERVES 2**

Please write (address on back cover flap) or e-mail me at info@whfoods.org with your personal ideas for preparing Scallops, and I will share them with others through our website at www.whfoods.org.

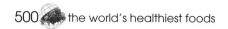

# health benefits of scallops

## Promote Heart Health

Scallops are a very good source of omega-3 fatty acids, providing us with concentrated amounts of EPA and DHA. These fatty acids have emerged as nutrition stars over the last few years as researchers discover their extensive health benefits, including the promotion of cardiovascular health.

### Nutritional Analysis of 4 ounces of broiled/baked Scallops:

| NUTRIENT | AMOUNT | % DAILY VALUE | NUTRIENT | AMOUNT | % DAILY VALUE |
|---|---|---|---|---|---|
| Calories | 151.70 | | Pantothenic Acid | 0.16 mg | 1.60 |
| Calories from Fat | 40.36 | | | | |
| Calories from Saturated Fat | 6.95 | | **Minerals** | | |
| Protein | 23.11 g | | Boron | — mcg | |
| Carbohydrates | — g | | Calcium | 34.28 mg | 3.43 |
| Dietary Fiber | 0.00 g | 0.00 | Chloride | — mg | |
| Soluble Fiber | 0.00 g | | Chromium | — mcg | — |
| Insoluble Fiber | 0.00 g | | Copper | 0.07 mg | 3.50 |
| Sugar - Total | — g | | Fluoride | — mg | — |
| Monosaccharides | — g | | Iodine | — mcg | — |
| Disaccharides | — g | | Iron | 0.40 mg | 2.22 |
| Other Carbs | — g | | Magnesium | 77.12 mg | 19.28 |
| Fat - Total | 4.48 g | | Manganese | 0.10 mg | 5.00 |
| Saturated Fat | 0.77 g | | Molybdenum | — mcg | — |
| Mono Fat | 1.72 g | | Phosphorus | 302.05 mg | 30.20 |
| Poly Fat | 1.31 g | | Potassium | 444.46 mg | |
| Omega-3 Fatty Acids | 1.10 g | 44.00 | Selenium | — mcg | — |
| Omega-6 Fatty Acids | 0.15 g | | Sodium | 261.63 mg | |
| Trans Fatty Acids | 0.00 g | | Zinc | 1.31 mg | 8.73 |
| Cholesterol | 45.37 mg | | | | |
| Water | 80.34 g | | **Amino Acids** | | |
| Ash | 3.01 g | | Alanine | 1.39 g | |
| | | | Arginine | 1.68 g | |
| **Vitamins** | | | Aspartate | 2.22 g | |
| Vitamin A IU | 211.03 IU | 4.22 | Cystine | 3.03 g | 739.02 |
| Vitamin A RE | 51.67 RE | | Glutamate | 3.14 g | |
| A - Carotenoid | 5.85 RE | 0.08 | Glycine | 1.44 g | |
| A - Retinol | 45.82 RE | | Histidine | 0.44 g | 34.11 |
| B1 Thiamin | 0.01 mg | 0.67 | Isoleucine | 1.00 g | 86.96 |
| B2 Riboflavin | 0.07 mg | 4.12 | Leucine | 1.62 g | 64.03 |
| B3 Niacin | 1.50 mg | 7.50 | Lysine | 1.72 g | 73.19 |
| Niacin Equiv | 5.81 mg | | Methionine | 0.52 g | 70.27 |
| Vitamin B6 | 0.20 mg | 10.00 | Phenylalanine | 0.83 g | 69.75 |
| Vitamin B12 | 2.00 mcg | 33.33 | Proline | 0.94 g | |
| Biotin | — mcg | — | Serine | 1.03 g | |
| Vitamin C | 3.93 mg | 6.55 | Threonine | 0.99 g | 79.84 |
| Vitamin D IU | 4.54 IU | 1.14 | Tryptophan | 0.26 g | 81.25 |
| Vitamin D mcg | 0.11 mcg | | Tyrosine | 0.74 g | 76.29 |
| Vitamin E Alpha Equiv | 1.89 mg | 9.45 | Valine | 1.01 g | 68.71 |
| Vitamin E IU | 2.81 IU | | | | |
| Vitamin E mg | 1.89 mg | | | | |
| Folate | 20.94 mcg | 5.24 | | | |
| Vitamin K | — mcg | — | | | |

(Note: "—" indicates data is unavailable. For more information, please see page 806.)

Omega-3 fatty acids keep your blood flowing smoothly by preventing the formation of blood clots and by lowering triglyceride levels.

Additionally, Scallops are a very good source of vitamin B12, another very important nutrient for cardiovascular health. Vitamin B12 is needed by the body to convert homocysteine, a chemical that can directly damage blood vessel walls, into other benign chemicals. Since high levels of homocysteine are associated with an increased risk for atherosclerosis, diabetic heart disease, heart attack and stroke, it's a good idea to be sure that your diet contains plenty of vitamin B12 to help keep homocysteine levels low. Homocysteine is also associated with osteoporosis, and a recent study found that osteoporosis occurred more frequently among women whose vitamin B12 status was deficient or marginal compared with those who had normal B12 status.

In addition to their omega-3 fatty acids and vitamin B12 concentrations, Scallops are a good source of magnesium and potassium, two other nutrients that provide significant benefits for the cardiovascular system. Magnesium helps out by causing blood vessels to relax, thus helping to lower blood pressure while improving blood flow. Potassium helps to maintain normal blood pressure levels.

## A Concentrated Source of Protein

Scallops are a very good source of low-calorie, high-quality protein, with about 60% of their calories derived from this very important macronutrient. It is vital that our diets provide us with ample amounts of protein since we rely upon it to supply us with amino acids, which our bodies use for a variety of different functions. Our muscles and tissues are made from amino acids as are enzymes and some important immune-system compounds.

## Promote Optimal Health

A high intake of vitamin B12 has also been shown to be protective against colon cancer. Vitamin B12 helps protect the cells of the colon from mutations as a result of exposure to cancer-causing chemicals—another good reason to eat plenty of vitamin B12-rich foods. So, add Scallops, a very good source of protein and vitamin B12, to your list of healthy seafood and enjoy.

## Additional Health-Promoting Benefits of Scallops

Scallops are a concentrated source of other nutrients providing additional health benefits. These nutrients include energy-producing phosphorus and sleep-promoting tryptophan.

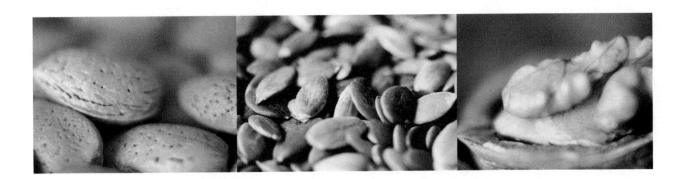

# nuts & seeds

The numbers beside each food indicate their Total Nutrient-Richness. (For more details, see page 805.)

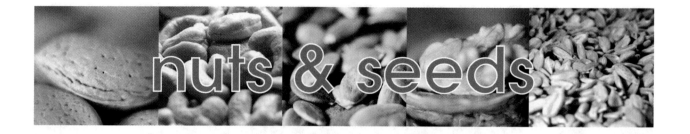

# nuts & seeds

When it comes to the "Healthiest Way of Eating," remember that nuts and seeds may be small in size, but they are big when it comes to nutrition! Not only are they rich sources of many vitamins and minerals and serve as a good plant-based protein source, but many of them contain monounsaturated fats, essential omega-3 fatty acids and phytosterol phytonutrients that do wonders for promoting overall health.

Throughout history, people have thrived on nuts and seeds. Abundant in the wild and not requiring any preparation (they are best eaten raw), nuts and seeds even made a significant contribution to the diets of the early hunter-gatherers. And their popularity continues today in numerous cultures around the world. That is not surprising when you recognize that they are not only delicious and nutritious, but also highly portable, providing good nutrition to those on-the-go, whether that be a tribal nomad or a soccer mom. Used in breakfast cereals, salads, grain dishes, desserts and "Healthy Sautéed" vegetables, the complex tastes and unique textures of nuts and seeds complement many dishes.

## Definition: Nuts and Seeds

Nuts are actually fruits that have a hard outer shell that encloses a kernel; the kernel is the meaty part we call the "nut."

Seeds are structures contained in fruits that can produce a new plant if returned back to the earth. If you think about how they are the essence of creating new life, it becomes more apparent why they are such a vitally concentrated source of nutrients.

### Why We Need to Eat Nuts Every Day

In March of 2004, three of the World's Healthiest Nuts—walnuts, peanuts and almonds—were awarded a qualified health claim (QHC) by the U.S. Food and Drug Administration. The quality health claim permits labels on packages of walnuts, peanuts and almonds (as well as other approved nuts) to state that eating 1.5 ounces of these nuts every day may reduce the risk of heart disease. This claim is qualified with the statement that the scientific evidence of their protective effect is supportive but not conclusive and a diet low in saturated fat and cholesterol without increased overall calorie intake is necessary in order for these nuts to benefit health.

## How Nuts and Seeds Can Keep You Healthy

Nuts and seeds are incredibly rich in nutrients. Many are a concentrated source of "good fats" such as the omega-3 essential fatty acid, alpha-linolenic acid (ALA), as well as heart-healthy monounsaturated fats, such as oleic acid.

Nuts and seeds are also filled with vitamins and minerals. Looking for vitamin E, copper, manganese, magnesium and zinc? Nuts and seeds should be one of the first foods to consider adding to your menu. Additionally, some of these foods can be a concentrated source of lignans, which have been found to have heart-health benefits; these include secoisolariciresinol diglycoside in flaxseeds, and sesamin and sesamolin in sesame seeds. They also contain other phytonutrients; for example, walnuts are a rich source of ellagic acid.

Nuts and seeds have a high satiety factor, which means that they are great for satisfying your appetite. Whether you eat them as a snack, sprinkle a few on a salad or cereal or add nut butter or seed butter to a smoothie, these foods can really fill you up. They also provide long lasting energy that can carry you through the day while maintaining stable blood sugar levels. Although nuts and seeds have a reputation for being high in calories, a small amount will go a long way in satisfying your hunger. Therefore you may actually end up consuming fewer calories than when you eat other foods that may have less calories but will not sustain you for as long a period of time.

## Nuts and Seeds Contain Healthy Fats

Many people are concerned about eating nuts and seeds because they view them as high-fat foods. Yet, for optimal health, you need fat. In fact, about 25–30% of your daily calories should come from fat. Nuts and seeds are good examples of looking at our diets in a more modern, discriminating way; they serve to remind us that not all fats are bad. A good proportion of fats in these foods is actually comprised of health-promoting "good fats," such as omega-3 essential fatty acids and monounsaturated fats.

Many nuts and seeds are a concentrated source of alpha-linolenic acid (ALA), the omega-3 fatty acid whose intake has been linked to a reduction of inflammatory markers, and therefore a healthy heart. ALA is also the precursor to eicosapentaenoic acid (EPA) and docosahexaenoic acid (DHA), the forms of omega-3 fatty acids that are found in cold-water fish and which have been found to be highly beneficial in supporting heart health, brain health and respiratory health. Flaxseeds and walnuts are good examples of nuts and seeds rich in ALA. Based on a decade of evidence supporting the health benefits of walnuts, researchers have found that eating $1^{1/2}$ ounces per day as part of a diet low in saturated fats and cholesterol may help reduce the risk of heart disease and stroke. The standard American diet does not regularly provide adequate amounts of these important fats, so adding nuts and seeds to your diet can do wonders for your health.

In addition to their omega-3 fatty acid content, the fat content of many nuts and seeds is also composed of a large percentage of monounsaturated fats such as oleic acid. Studies show that these fats promote good cardiovascular health, even in individuals with diabetes.

## The Easy Way to Eat 5 Servings of Nuts and Seeds Each Week

Leading health organizations recommend we eat 5 servings of nuts and seeds each week. To derive the optimal health benefits from nuts and seeds, I recommend including 1 to $1^{1/2}$ ounces of nuts or seeds per day in your "Healthiest Way of Eating."

Some of my favorite ways to include nuts and seeds in my diet are adding them to breakfast cereals and to blended smoothie drinks or sprinkling them on top of vegetables, fruit salads, fish and seafood dishes.

Here are some easy ways to incorporate nuts and seeds into your meals:

**NUTS**

| | |
|---|---|
| **BREAKFAST:** | Add chopped cashews to your cereal |
| **LUNCH:** | Top your salad with walnuts instead of croutons |
| **DINNER:** | Top broccoli, or any other vegetable, with walnuts or almonds |
| **SNACK:** | Walnuts, cashews or almonds combined with fruits make a great snack any time of day |

**SEEDS**

| | |
|---|---|
| **BREAKFAST:** | Sprinkle 2 TBS of ground flaxseeds on your cereal or smoothie |
| **LUNCH:** | Sprinkle sunflower seeds on top of your salad |
| **DINNER:** | Serve crudités with tahini (sesame seed spread) as an appetizer, and serve vegetables topped with sesame seeds or chopped pumpkin seeds |
| **SNACK:** | Sunflower and pumpkin seeds make a great snack any time of day |

## How to Use the Individual Nuts and Seeds Chapters

Each chapter is dedicated to one of the World's Healthiest Nuts and Seeds and contains everything you need to know to enjoy and maximize its flavor and nutritional benefits. Each chapter is organized into two parts:

1. **NUTS AND SEEDS FACTS** describes each of the nuts and seeds, its different varieties and its peak season. It also addresses the biochemical considerations of each nut and seed by describing any of its unique compounds that may be potentially problematic to individuals with specific health problems. Detailed information about the health benefits of each of the nuts and seeds can be found at the end of each chapter, as can a complete nutritional profile.

2. **THE 3 STEPS TO THE BEST TASTING AND MOST NUTRITIOUS NUTS AND SEEDS** includes information about how to best select, store and prepare each one of the World's Healthiest Nuts and Seeds. This section also features recipes and quick serving ideas. While specific information for individual nuts and seeds is given in each of the specific chapters, here are the 3 Steps that can be applied to nuts and seeds in general, including those not on the list of the World's Healthiest Foods.

# 1. the best way to select nuts and seeds

Selection is the first step in adding the freshest and most nutritious nuts and seeds to your "Healthiest Way of Eating." Here are some tips that apply to nuts and seeds:

Heat, air and light damage the fragile omega-3 fatty acids found in nuts and seeds. As rancidity sets in long before you can taste or smell the "off" flavor, it's important to buy nuts and seeds that are as fresh as possible. Buy them in their shell if you can, as the shell protects them from these environmental "hazards." If that is not possible, purchase them in vacuum-sealed opaque packaging that protects them from air and light.

If you buy nuts and seeds in bulk, go to a busy store that has a high turnover rate so the nuts and seeds you bring home will not have been sitting in the bins and exposed to room temperature, air and light for too long. Some natural food stores keep their nuts and seeds in a refrigerated section, which is an ideal way to protect their omega-3 fatty acids.

Avoid nuts and seeds that are overly salted or have been roasted using oil. They go rancid more quickly than whole, raw nuts and seeds. The damaged fats and high sodium content of these processed nuts may harm, not help, your heart.

I also highly recommend selecting organically grown nuts and seeds whenever possible.

# 2. the best way to store nuts and seeds

Proper storage maximizes the shelf life and retains the nutritional value of your nuts and seeds. After purchasing, do not let these foods sit in a hot car. When you get home, store nuts and seeds in airtight containers in the refrigerator or freezer.

# 3. the best way to prepare nuts and seeds

One way that I have found to add versatility to nuts and seeds is to finely grind them and put a couple of tablespoons on top of vegetables or add them to sauces, soups or salad dressings. Finely ground nuts can also be used in place of flour as a flavorful thickening agent. For added convenience, you can grind a small amount and store it in your freezer. For certain seeds, notably flaxseeds, grinding not only changes their texture but can also increase the bioavailability of their nutrients. Grinding flaxseeds cracks open their hard outer shell, which allows greater absorption of their essential fatty acids.

Roasting brings out the flavor of nuts and seeds, and develops their sweetness. It is safe to roast nuts and seeds if done at low temperatures—no higher than 170°F (77°C). Research has shown that roasting at high temperatures damages the delicate fats that they contain. Certain systems of healthcare, like Ayurveda, recommend always soaking nuts to help increase their digestibility; yet, while there may be certain advantages to doing so, I have not seen these advantages substantiated in any peer-reviewed, published research.

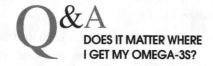
### Q&A
**DOES IT MATTER WHERE I GET MY OMEGA-3S?**

While there is universal agreement about the need for increased omega-3 fatty acids in our food, there is almost equally universal confusion about where these omega-3s should come from. Should we focus more on animal foods or plant foods? Are nuts better than seeds? Is there really enough total omega-3 fat in any diet, or do we absolutely need supplements to make ends meet?

### Two Key Starting Points: LA and ALA
Fatty acids are relatively easy to understand in terms of their chemical relationship. There are basic "starting point" fatty acids from which all other fatty acids are made. Even more important, there are only two key "starting point" fatty acids. One is called linoleic acid, or LA. This fatty acid is the starting point for all omega-6 fatty acids. In other words, every omega-6 fatty acid found in the body must either be directly obtained from food or produced in the body from LA. The other key starting point is alpha-linolenic acid, or ALA. ALA is the starting point for all omega-3s. Again, to repeat this most

*(Continued on Page 505)*

*(Continued from Page 504)*

important relationship, every omega-3 fat found in the body must either be consumed directly from food or be manufactured in the body from ALA.

## Except for ALA, All Omega-3s are Complicated

It's not particularly easy for the body to turn ALA into other omega-3s. In fact, it's pretty demanding in terms of nutrition. It's demanding because the enzymes that process ALA require a long list of nutrients in order to function. For example, the first enzyme required for processing ALA is called *delta-6 desaturase*. In order to function properly, this enzyme requires the presence of vitamins B3, B6 and C and the minerals, zinc and magnesium. A person who is deficient in any of these vitamins or minerals might not be able to start processing ALA and might become deficient in all other omega-3 fats (if they rely upon it as their only dietary source of omega-3s), since all of them are made from ALA.

Multiple processing steps are involved in turning ALA into the best-researched omega-3s in terms of disease prevention: EPA (eicosapentaenoic acid) and DHA (docosahexaenoic acid). Both of these omega-3 fats are critical for prevention of virtually all major chronic diseases, and they can only be made in the body from ALA if a person is reasonably well-nourished because their production is demanding in terms of nutrient metabolism.

## Plants Do Not Naturally Produce EPA or DHA

In general, there is virtually no preformed EPA or DHA in plants. We know that genetic engineering is being done on some plants like thale cress to encourage production of EPA and DHA in the leaves, and we know that some non-engineered, hybridized plants, like the rapeseed used to produce canola oil, can result in very small percentages of EPA or DHA (less than 3%) becoming present in the oil. But as a rule, you simply cannot get the EPA or DHA you need from plant foods. To get your EPA and DHA, you will need to either (1) consume animal foods (or supplements) that contain preformed EPA and DHA or (2) depend on your body to make EPA and DHA from the ALA found in plant foods.

## Should I Depend on My Body To Make EPA and DHA from Plant Foods?

While I would love to give a single "yes" or "no" answer to this question, it just doesn't have a "yes" or "no" answer. But I can give you three categories and let you decide into which one you fit. The three categories are:

(1) If you know you are generally malnourished, you should not depend on your body to make EPA and DHA from plant foods. If you fit into this category, it is simply too likely that you won't have the nutritional support

needed to convert ALA into EPA and DHA. You'll need to either (a) consume animal foods that contain preformed EPA and DHA or (b) take dietary supplements containing these omega-3s.

(2) If, at the other end of the spectrum, you are well-nourished and enjoy what you would describe as excellent health, you are very likely to make the EPA and DHA you need from plant foods. In fact, many alternative health practitioners like the idea of relying on a healthy body to make EPA and DHA from ALA, rather than supplementing with preformed EPA or DHA. The reason is simple. Our body, when healthy, is in the best position to decide on the omega-3 balance we need. (Our body, when healthy, is in the best position to decide on all nutritional balances, for that matter.) Our body will decide when to keep ALA and use it directly for health purposes or when to convert ALA into the more complicated EPA and DHA omega-3s.

(3) If you find yourself somewhere in the middle—not well-nourished and in excellent health, but not malnourished either—you will need to take a much closer look at the details of your health to decide about your optimal food choices. Why are you not well-nourished, and what is below excellent when it comes to your health? Is fat quality a problem in your diet overall? Is fat intake related to the health risks you face? These kinds of questions are important to answer if you fall into this middle category. Often, a licensed healthcare practitioner is needed to help you sort through all of the health details.

## If I Do Turn to Animal Foods, Which Ones are Best for EPA and DHA?

Virtually all fish, both finfish and shellfish, contain some amount of both EPA and DHA. Salmon, cod, mackerel and herring would be standouts here. Unfortunately, the pollution of our environment has made the benefits of eating these fish contingent on their being free of common toxins like dioxins and mercury. Across the board, the research shows that you are safer consuming wild-caught fish than farmed fish. In addition, the research shows that you are safer eating wild-caught salmon and tuna than wild-caught mackerel in terms of mercury risk. The unusually high EPA and DHA content of these "cold water" fish is also the reason that cod liver oil is one of the most concentrated sources of EPA and DHA in the dietary supplement world.

## How Are Omega-3s Related to Inflammation?

Our immune system uses a family of molecules called eicosanoids to increase or decrease our body's inflammatory response. Eicosanoids that increase the

*(Continued on Page 550)*

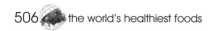

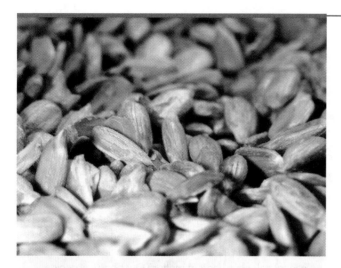

## nutrient-richness chart

Total Nutrient-Richness: **18**
One-quarter cup (36 grams) of Sunflower Seeds contains 205 calories

| NUTRIENT | AMOUNT | %DV | DENSITY | QUALITY |
|---|---|---|---|---|
| Vitamin E | 18.1 mg | 90.5 | 7.9 | excellent |
| B1 Thiamin | 0.8 mg | 54.7 | 4.8 | very good |
| Manganese | 0.7 mg | 36.5 | 3.2 | good |
| Magnesium | 127.4 mg | 31.9 | 2.8 | good |
| Copper | 0.6 mg | 31.5 | 2.8 | good |
| Tryptophan | 0.1 g | 31.3 | 2.7 | good |
| Selenium | 21.4 mcg | 30.6 | 2.7 | good |
| Phosphorus | 253.8 mg | 25.4 | 2.2 | good |
| B5 Pantothenic Acid | 2.4 mg | 24.3 | 2.1 | good |
| Folate | 81.9 mcg | 20.5 | 1.8 | good |

For more on "Total Nutrient-Richness," "%DV," "Density," and
The World's Healthiest Foods "Quality" Rating System, see page 805.

Looking for a health-promoting snack? A handful of mild, nutty-tasting Sunflower Seeds will take the edge off your hunger while providing you with a wealth of health-promoting nutrients to add to your "Healthiest Way of Eating." Sunflowers are thought to have originated in Mexico and Peru and are one of the first plants to ever be cultivated in the United States. They have been used for more than 5,000 years by Native Americans, who not only used the seeds as a food and a source of oil, but also used the flowers, roots and stems for various purposes including dye pigment.

## why sunflower seeds should be part of your healthiest way of eating

Sunflower Seeds are an excellent source of vitamin E, a nutrient essential for cardiovascular health because it provides

# sunflower seeds

## highlights

| | |
|---|---|
| AVAILABILITY: | Year-round |
| REFRIGERATE: | Yes |
| SHELF LIFE: | 3 months in the refrigerator; 6 months in the freezer |
| PREPARATION: | Minimal |

antioxidant protection from the oxidative damage to cells caused by free radicals. Sunflower Seeds are so rich in nutrients that they have the highest Total Nutrient-Richness of any of the World's Healthiest Nuts or Seeds. (For more on the *Health Benefits of Sunflower Seeds* and a complete analysis of their content of over 60 nutrients, see page 510.)

## varieties of sunflower seeds

The sunflower's Latin scientific name, *Helianthus annuus*, reflects its solar appearance since *helios* is the Greek word for sun, and *anthos* is the Greek word for flower. The sunflower produces grayish-green or black seeds encased in teardrop-shaped gray or black shells that oftentimes feature black and white stripes. Sunflower Seeds' very high oil content makes them one of the primary sources of polyunsaturated oil. Their taste is oftentimes compared with the Jerusalem artichoke (not to be confused with the bulb artichoke), another member of the *Helianthus* family. Sunflower Seeds used for consumption are called "confectionary seeds" and are a different variety from those used to make oil. They come in several forms:

**HULLED**

The kernels can be raw, roasted, dry roasted or oil roasted and are often salted.

**UNHULLED**

Whole seeds that do not have the outer hull removed, so more nutrients are still intact. They are dried on the flower and brined (put in saltwater) once they are harvested.

**the peak season** available year-round.

## 3 steps for the best tasting and most nutritious sunflower seeds

Enjoying the best tasting Sunflower Seeds with the most nutrients is simple if you just follow my 3 easy steps:

1. The Best Way to Select
2. The Best Way to Store
3. The Best Way to Prepare

# 1. the best way to select sunflower seeds

Sunflower Seeds are generally available in prepackaged containers as well as bulk bins. It is best to check and make sure that the store where you buy Sunflower Seeds in bulk has a quick turnover of inventory and that the bulk containers are well sealed in order to ensure maximum freshness. The Sunflower Seeds should be uniform in color and not shriveled. They should also smell sweet and nutty; be sure they do not smell rancid or musty. When purchasing unshelled seeds, I make sure that the shells are firm, not broken, dirty or limp. Avoid shelled seeds that appear yellowish in color as they have most likely gone rancid. As with all seeds, I recommend selecting organically grown Sunflower Seeds whenever possible. (For more on *Organic Foods*, see page 113.)

If you want Sunflower Seeds with a roasted flavor and texture, choose ones that have been "dry roasted" as they are not cooked in oil. The commercial roasting process of nuts is often a form of deep-frying, usually in saturated fat, such as coconut or palm kernel oil. Consumption of deep-fried foods has been linked to high levels of LDL (the "bad" form of cholesterol) and to thickening of larger artery walls. Even "dry roasted" Sunflower Seeds may be cooked at high temperatures that damage their natural oils. It is also important to read the label to be sure that no additional ingredients such as sugar, corn syrup or preservatives have been added. For the highest quality, least expensive "dry roasted" Sunflower Seeds, it's best to just roast them yourself using "The Healthiest Way to Dry Roast Sunflower Seeds" (see page 508).

# 2. the best way to store sunflower seeds

Since Sunflower Seeds have a high fat content and are prone to rancidity, it is best to store them in an airtight container in the refrigerator. They can also be stored in the freezer since the cold temperature will not greatly affect their texture or flavor. They will keep for 3 months in the refrigerator and 6 months in the freezer.

# 3. the best way to prepare sunflower seeds

The best way to prepare Sunflower Seeds is to dry roast them. For details, see page 508.

Q *Is it harmful to eat the shells of Sunflower Seeds?*

A The shells of Sunflower Seeds contain approximately 40% digestible and 60% nondigestible components. Of the nondigestible components, the majority are types of fiber. While it isn't necessarily bad to consume nondigestible parts of food, including non-digestible fibers, it isn't clear why a person would want to do so. I haven't seen research showing intestinal problems following consumption of the hulls and shells of seeds and nuts, but I can imagine a person's digestive tract having trouble processing these components under certain circumstances. Because the pieces of the shells could have sharp ends, it would obviously be important to chew them extremely well. The hulls of conventionally grown Sunflower Seeds would contain a higher level of certain pesticides in comparison to the seeds since they are at higher risk of exposure. It would be important to select organically grown Sunflower Seeds for this reason.

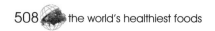
# Sunflower Seed Pesto

*Sunflower Seeds make an amazing pesto!*

2 TBS Sunflower Seeds, roasted
1/2 cup extra virgin olive oil
2 cloves medium garlic, pressed
2 cups basil leaves (discard stems)
Sea salt and pepper to taste
1/2 cup grated Parmesan cheese

1. Begin blending the Sunflower Seeds, garlic, basil, salt, pepper and 1/4 cup of extra virgin olive oil, scraping the sides of the blender as necessary.

2. Gradually add the remaining 1/4 cup of olive oil through the blender's feed hole until it is well integrated. Stir in Parmesan cheese before serving.

## The Healthiest Way to Dry Roast Sunflower Seeds

**Dry Roasting Sunflower Seeds the healthiest way gives them a lightly roasted flavor and develops their sweetness. It is safe to dry roast seeds if done at a low temperature.**

2 cups Sunflower Seeds

1. Preheat oven to 160–170°F (70–75°C).
2. Place a thin layer of seeds on a cookie sheet.
3. Roast for 15–20 minutes.

To enhance the "roasted" flavor, try putting a little liquid aminos seasoning or tamari (soy sauce) into a spray bottle and misting the seeds before roasting.

Roasting Sunflower Seeds at a temperature higher than 170°F (75°C) will cause a breakdown of their fats and the production of free radicals. Commercially roasted Sunflower Seeds have been heated to high temperatures (over 350°F or 175°C) that damage their delicate oils, resulting in the formation of free radicals and causing lipid peroxidation—the oxidizing of fats in your bloodstream that can trigger tiny injuries in artery walls—a first step in the buildup of plaque and cardiovascular disease.

Roasted Sunflower Seeds have a shorter shelf life and spoil more quickly than raw Sunflower Seeds because the unsaturated oils found in seeds oxidize more quickly after exposure to the heat of the roasting process.

Although some find raw seeds more difficult to digest than roasted seeds, this appears to vary greatly between individuals. For more information, see page 69.

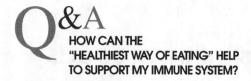

## Q&A

**HOW CAN THE "HEALTHIEST WAY OF EATING" HELP TO SUPPORT MY IMMUNE SYSTEM?**

### Nutrient-Rich Foods and the Immune System

Your ability to interact with the world around you and remain healthy is dependent to a large extent on the healthy functioning of your immune system. Your immune system is responsible for fighting foreign invaders to your body, like pathogenic bacteria and viruses responsible for colds and flu, and also for destroying cells within your body when they become cancerous. Poor nutrition has been shown to result in increased infections, to slow healing from injury and infections and to increase susceptibility to symptoms and complications from immune system dysfunction. Science has shown that immune function often decreases as we age, and recent research suggests this decrease is also related to nutrition and may be slowed or even stopped by maintaining healthy nutrition.

Medical science has established that one of the most important factors in supporting a healthy, balanced immune system is good nutrition. Research studies show that healthy eating can help in keeping your immune system ready and capable of functioning properly when necessary. The World's Healthiest Foods provide the kind of nutrition that supports your immune functions to its fullest, while minimizing the agents that may induce or activate your immune response when it should not be active.

The role of the World's Healthiest Foods in supporting your immune system is so vital that it is one of the reasons that I emphasized this benefit in the "Healthiest Way of Eating" Plan on page 34. While all nutrient-rich foods play a role in helping to keep an immune system running strong, let's take a look at some of the World's Healthiest Foods most well-known for their ability to support optimal immune function. As you will see, enhancing your immune system may be as simple as enjoying a delicious meal

*(Continued on Page 511)*

STEP-BY-STEP RECIPE

## The Healthiest Ways of Preparing Sunflower Seeds

# Creamy Sunflower Seed Dressing

*This non-dairy, creamy dressing will keep in your refrigerator for up to 2-3 weeks.*

1/4 cup Sunflower Seeds
3 TBS chopped fresh basil
3 medium cloves garlic
1 TBS prepared Dijon mustard
1 TBS honey
4 TBS fresh lemon juice
4 oz silken tofu
2 TBS extra virgin olive oil
Sea salt and pepper to taste
*a little water for thinning if needed

1. Press garlic and let sit for 5 minutes (Why?, see page 261).

2. Blend all ingredients in blender until smooth, adding oil a little at a time at end.

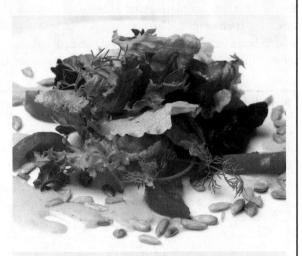

Creamy Sunflower Seed Dressing

**Preparation Hint:** This dressing can also be made without the tofu. It is not quite as creamy, but still has a nice consistency. Blend well, so it becomes smooth in texture.

### YIELDS ABOUT 1 1/2 CUPS

Please write (address on back cover flap) or e-mail me at info@whfoods.org with your personal ideas for preparing Sunflower Seeds, and I will share them with others through our website at www.whfoods.org.

## 12 QUICK SERVING IDEAS for SUNFLOWER SEEDS:

1. Add Sunflower Seeds to your favorite breakfast cereal.
2. Mix some ground Sunflower Seeds into your pancake batter.
3. Sprinkle Sunflower Seeds on top of low-fat yogurt.
4. Add Sunflower Seeds to scrambled eggs for a unique taste and texture.
5. Add Sunflower Seeds to your favorite tuna, chicken or turkey salad recipe.
6. Garnish mixed green salads with dry roasted Sunflower Seeds in place of croutons.
7. Dry roasted Sunflower Seeds complement green vegetables such as broccoli and kale.
8. Keep a bag of Sunflower Seeds handy for a between-meal snack.
9. **Energizing Snack:** Combine Sunflower Seeds, diced dried apricots and almonds to make a great snack to carry with you in your car.
10. **Sunflower Seed Porridge:** Soak 1/2 cup Sunflower Seeds in water overnight. In the morning, rinse the seeds. Place in a blender with an apple cut in 1-inch pieces, 1/2 tsp ground cinnamon and 1/2 cup water. Blend for 1 minute on medium speed. Drizzle with honey for extra sweetness.
11. **Sunflower Seed Butter:** Grind Sunflower Seeds in a food processor until pasty. Add sea salt or tamari (soy sauce) to taste. Use to fill celery stalks or serve on toast or crackers.
12. **Sunny Salad Dressing:** Blend 1 cup of your favorite vinaigrette with 1/2 cup of Sunflower Seeds for 1 minute at medium speed. Add water if the mixture needs to be thinned. Add 2 TBS ground flaxseeds, fresh basil, fresh cilantro or chopped tomatoes for added flavor. Using lightly roasted Sunflower Seeds will also add extra flavor.

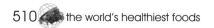 

# health benefits of sunflower seeds

## Promote Brain Health

Sunflower Seeds are an excellent source of vitamin E, which has been suggested to play an important role in promoting brain health. A multi-year population-based study showed that people with the highest intake of vitamin E from foods had a 32% reduction in their rate of mental decline compared to those with the least vitamin E in their diets. Previous research had suggested that people who consume more vitamin E retain mental function and are less likely to develop Alzheimer's disease. Sunflower Seeds are also a very good source of vitamin B1, which is necessary for the production of acetylcholine, a neurotransmitter molecule essential for memory.

## Promote Heart Health

Vitamin E also plays an important role in the prevention of cardiovascular disease. It helps prevent free radicals from oxidizing cholesterol, curbing the process of atherosclerosis, which can lead to blocked arteries, heart attack or stroke. In fact, studies show that people who get a good amount of vitamin E in their diet are at a much lower risk of dying of a heart attack than people whose intake of vitamin E is marginal or inadequate. Additionally, a recently published study showed that women whose diets provided them with the highest blood levels of vitamin E had the lowest risk of high cholesterol and atherosclerosis. Sunflower Seeds are also a good source of other nutrients that promote heart health. Their magnesium helps to maintain balanced blood pressure, while their folate keeps homocysteine levels in check. Additionally, in many cases of heart disease, when oxidative damage has been found to be the cause of blood vessel damage, low intake of selenium, a mineral concentrated in Sunflower Seeds, has been identified as a contributing factor to the disease.

## Promote Optimal Health

Vitamin E, the body's primary fat-soluble antioxidant, travels throughout the body neutralizing free radicals that would otherwise damage fat-containing structures and molecules, such as cell membranes, brain cells and cholesterol. By protecting these cellular and molecular components, vitamin E has significant anti-inflammatory effects that can contribute to the reduction of symptoms of asthma, osteoarthritis and rheumatoid arthritis, conditions where free-radicals and inflammation play a big role.

## Additional Health-Promoting Benefits of Sunflower Seeds

Sunflower Seeds are a concentrated source of many other nutrients providing additional health-promoting benefits. These nutrients include free-radical-scavenging manganese and copper, energy-producing vitamin B5 and phosphorus, and sleep-promoting tryptophan.

### Nutritional Analysis of 1/4 cup of Sunflower Seeds:

| NUTRIENT | AMOUNT | % DAILY VALUE | NUTRIENT | AMOUNT | % DAILY VALUE |
|---|---|---|---|---|---|
| Calories | 205.20 | | Pantothenic Acid | 2.43 mg | 24.30 |
| Calories from Fat | 160.61 | | | | |
| Calories from Saturated Fat | 16.83 | | **Minerals** | | |
| Protein | 8.20 g | | Boron | — mcg | |
| Carbohydrates | 6.75 g | | Calcium | 41.76 mg | 4.18 |
| Dietary Fiber | 3.78 g | 15.12 | Chloride | — mg | |
| Soluble Fiber | 1.21 g | | Chromium | — mcg | — |
| Insoluble Fiber | 2.57 g | | Copper | 0.63 mg | 31.50 |
| Sugar – Total | 1.19 g | | Fluoride | — mg | — |
| Monosaccharides | 0.00 g | | Iodine | — mcg | — |
| Disaccharides | 0.90 g | | Iron | 2.44 mg | 13.56 |
| Other Carbs | 1.79 g | | Magnesium | 127.44 mg | 31.86 |
| Fat – Total | 17.85 g | | Manganese | 0.73 mg | 36.50 |
| Saturated Fat | 1.87 g | | Molybdenum | — mcg | — |
| Mono Fat | 3.41 g | | Phosphorus | 253.80 mg | 25.38 |
| Poly Fat | 11.78 g | | Potassium | 248.04 mg | |
| Omega-3 Fatty Acids | 0.02 g | 0.80 | Selenium | 21.42 mcg | 30.60 |
| Omega-6 Fatty Acids | 11.75 g | | Sodium | 1.08 mg | |
| Trans Fatty Acids | 0.00 g | | Zinc | 1.82 mg | 12.13 |
| Cholesterol | 0.00 mg | | | | |
| Water | 1.93 g | | **Amino Acids** | | |
| Ash | 1.27 g | | Alanine | 0.37 g | |
| | | | Arginine | 0.79 g | |
| **Vitamins** | | | Aspartate | 0.80 g | |
| Vitamin A IU | 18.00 IU | 0.36 | Cystine | 0.15 g | 36.59 |
| Vitamin A RE | 1.80 RE | | Glutamate | 1.83 g | |
| A - Carotenoid | 1.80 RE | 0.02 | Glycine | 0.48 g | |
| A - Retinol | 0.00 RE | | Histidine | 0.21 g | 16.28 |
| B1 Thiamin | 0.82 mg | 54.67 | Isoleucine | 0.37 g | 32.17 |
| B2 Riboflavin | 0.09 mg | 5.29 | Leucine | 0.54 g | 21.34 |
| B3 Niacin | 1.62 mg | 8.10 | Lysine | 0.31 g | 13.19 |
| Niacin Equiv | 3.36 mg | | Methionine | 0.16 g | 21.62 |
| Vitamin B6 | 0.28 mg | 14.00 | Phenylalanine | 0.38 g | 31.93 |
| Vitamin B12 | 0.00 mcg | 0.00 | Proline | 0.39 g | |
| Biotin | — mcg | — | Serine | 0.35 g | |
| Vitamin C | 0.50 mg | 0.83 | Threonine | 0.30 g | 24.19 |
| Vitamin D IU | 0.00 IU | 0.00 | Tryptophan | 0.10 g | 31.25 |
| Vitamin D mcg | 0.00 mcg | | Tyrosine | 0.22 g | 22.68 |
| Vitamin E Alpha Equiv | 18.10 mg | 90.50 | Valine | 0.43 g | 29.25 |
| Vitamin E IU | 26.96 IU | | | | |
| Vitamin E mg | 18.11 mg | | | | |
| Folate | 81.86 mcg | 20.46 | | | |
| Vitamin K | 0.97 mcg | 1.21 | | | |

(Note: "—" indicates data is unavailable. For more information, please see page 806.)

(Continued from Page 508)
filled with fruits, vegetables, nuts, seeds and other World's Healthiest Foods.

## Organically Grown Fruits and Vegetables

From vitamin A to zinc, fruits and vegetables contain a virtual A-Z of vitamins and minerals that can support healthy immune system functioning. They are incredibly rich sources of the powerful antioxidants, vitamin C and pro-vitamin A carotenoids. One of the important roles that these nutrients fulfill is supporting the integrity of our body's tissues, bolstering their defenses so that they can serve as a fortress to protect against the invasion of bacteria and other microbes. Vitamin C is also concentrated in immune system cells; when these cells are under stress, their vitamin C levels decrease.

Fruits and vegetables are also rich in nutrients such as vitamin B6, folic acid, iron and zinc, whose deficiency has been linked to a reduction in cell-mediated immune response. They also contain abundant amounts of flavonoid phytonutrients (plant nutrients), antioxidants that can protect cells of the body, including those of the immune system, from the havoc caused by too many free radicals.

### GARLIC, ONIONS AND LEEKS

Garlic, onions and leeks are members of the *Allium* family; in addition to their vast array of vitamins and minerals, *Allium* family vegetables are especially renowned as being a source of sulfur-containing phytonutrients that have shown promise when it comes to supporting the immune system. For example, the sulfur-containing compound allicin is a powerful antibacterial and antiviral agent that joins forces with vitamin C to help kill harmful microbes (garlic and onions are very good sources of vitamin C while leeks are a good source). Allicin has been shown to be effective not only against common infections like colds and flu but a host of other pathogenic microbes. In addition, quercetin and other flavonoids concentrated in onions work with vitamin C to help kill harmful bacteria, making onions an especially good addition to soups and stews during cold and flu season.

### SHIITAKE MUSHROOMS

Long a staple in Asian diets, shiitake mushrooms are making their way to markets and restaurants in the U.S., a wonderful thing for people interested not only in a great tasting food, but foods that can offer great support to the immune system. While their ability to promote vibrant health is a result of their concentration of numerous nutrients, a lot of the research has focused on their unique polysaccharides, including lentinan. These phytonutrients have been found to power up the immune system, enhancing its ability to fight infection and disease.

## Nuts and Seeds

Nuts and seeds are rich in many minerals important for immune system support, including selenium and zinc. Selenium is a component of one of the body's most powerful antioxidant enzymes, *glutathione peroxidase*,

which is used in the liver to detoxify a wide range of potentially harmful molecules, reducing their impact on our immune system. Many types of immune cells appear to depend upon zinc for optimal function with its deficiency shown to compromise the number of white blood cells and immune response.

## Dietary Factors That Can Compromise the Immune System

To best support your immune system, it's not just what you eat, but what you don't eat, that's important. That's because while nutrients can help strengthen the immune system, other dietary factors may cause it stress, reducing its ability to perform at its optimal level.

### Food Intolerances

Your immune system is not just involved in fighting invaders like bacteria but also becomes activated when you eat foods to which you are intolerant or allergic. Food sensitivity reactions are an important consideration when planning a "Healthiest Way of Eating" that best supports your immune system. For more details on this subject, see Food Sensitivity, page 719.

### Chemical Additives

Processed foods and foods produced with pesticides or not grown organically may also be problematic for your immune function. Toxic metals such as cadmium, lead and mercury are immunosuppressive. Some pesticides and preservatives can negatively affect the gastrointestinal lining. Food additives can also have untoward effects on the nutrient content of the food. For example, sulfites destroy thiamin (vitamin B1) in foods to which they have been added.

### Other Dietary Factors

Cooking oils that are exposed to high heat can produce substances that are damaging to the immune system. The "Healthiest Way of Cooking" methods give you great alternatives to cooking with heated oils, such as "Healthy Sauté" (page 57).

Excessive consumption of calories and fat can weaken your immune system strength. The "Healthiest Way of Eating" emphasizes delicious, satiating foods that deliver a concentration of nutrients and do not contain excess fat or calories; this will help you to enjoy a diet that meets your caloric and fat intake goals for optimal health and weight management.

The "Healthiest Way of Eating" further supports your immune system since it avoids refined grain products, refined sugar and processed foods that deplete the body of vitamins and minerals necessary for promoting immunity. Specifically, sugar reduces the responsiveness of your immune cells and lowers your immune defenses; some studies have found that the infection-protective ability of white blood cells may be reduced by as much as 50% after ingestion of only four ounces of sugar-containing substances!

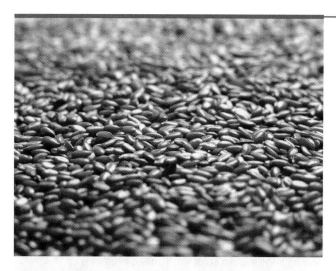

# flaxseeds

## highlights

| | |
|---|---|
| AVAILABILITY: | Year-round |
| REFRIGERATE: | Yes |
| SHELF LIFE: | 3 months in the refrigerator; 6 months in the freezer |
| PREPARATION: | Minimal |

## nutrient-richness chart

Total Nutrient-Richness: **13**

Two TBS (19 grams) of Flaxseeds contain 95 calories

| NUTRIENT | AMOUNT | %DV | DENSITY | QUALITY |
|---|---|---|---|---|
| Omega-3 Fatty Acids | 3.5 g | 140.4 | 26.5 | excellent |
| Manganese | 0.6 mg | 32.0 | 6.0 | very good |
| Dietary Fiber | 5.4 g | 21.6 | 4.1 | very good |
| Magnesium | 70.1 mg | 17.5 | 3.3 | good |
| Folate | 53.9 mcg | 13.5 | 2.5 | good |
| Copper | 0.2 mg | 10.0 | 1.9 | good |
| Phosphorus | 96.5 mg | 9.6 | 1.8 | good |
| B6 Pyridoxine | 0.2 mg | 9.0 | 1.7 | good |

**PHYTOESTROGEN LIGNANS:**

| | | |
|---|---|---|
| Secoisolariciresinol diglycoside | 136-368 mg | Daily values for this nutrient have not yet been established. |

For more on "Total Nutrient-Richness," "%DV," "Density," and The World's Healthiest Foods "Quality" Rating System, see page 805.

Charlemagne, the famous emperor who helped reshape European history, was also instrumental in the rise in popularity of Flaxseeds. He was so impressed with the versatility of Flax (as a food, medicine and as the source of fiber to make linen) that he passed laws requiring not only its cultivation, but also its consumption. Today, adding the warmly earthy and slightly nutty flavor of Flaxseeds to cereals, baked goods and other recipes is a great way to enjoy them as part of your "Healthiest Way of Eating."

## why flaxseeds should be part of your healthiest way of eating

Flaxseeds are the most concentrated plant source of the omega-3 fatty acid, alpha-linolenic acid (ALA), a precursor to the omega-3s found in cold-water fish. Omega-3 fatty acids are heart-healthy nutrients that also have anti-inflammatory properties. (For more on plant-based versus fish-based *Omega-3 Fatty Acids*, see page 770.) Flaxseeds also contain phytoestrogens, estrogen precursors found in plants, known as lignans, which help to balance estrogen levels in the body and also have antioxidant properties. (For more on the *Health Benefits of Flaxseeds* and a complete analysis of their content of over 60 nutrients, see page 513.)

## varieties of flaxseeds

The botanical name for the Flax plant, *Linum usitatissimum*, means "most useful." This aptly describes the versatility of Flax, with its ability to be used as a food, medicine and cloth material. Originating in Mesopotamia, it has been used since the Stone Age. One of the first records of the culinary use of Flaxseeds dates back to ancient Greece. Flaxseeds are slightly larger than sesame seeds and have a hard shell, which is smooth and shiny. Their color ranges from deep amber to reddish brown, depending upon whether the Flax is of the golden or brown variety. Flaxseeds can be purchased whole, as Flaxseed meal or as Flaxseed oil.

## the peak season available year-round.

## biochemical considerations

### GLYCOSIDE COMPOUNDS

While Flaxseeds contain cyanogenic glycoside compounds, at normal intake levels and without protein malnutrition, researchers currently maintain that this is not of concern and should cause no adverse effects (they consider 50 grams, which is more than 2 TBS, to be a safe amount for most people). The heat employed by cooking has been found to eliminate the presence of these compounds.

## 3 steps for the best tasting and most nutritious flaxseeds

Enjoying the best tasting Flaxseeds with the most nutrients is simple if you just follow my 3 easy steps:

1. The Best Way to Select
2. The Best Way to Store
3. The Best Way to Prepare

# 1. the best way to select flaxseeds

Flaxseeds are generally available in prepackaged containers as well as bulk bins. It is best to check and make sure that the store where you buy bulk Flaxseeds has a quick turnover of inventory and that the bulk containers are sealed well in order to ensure maximum freshness.

Whether purchasing Flaxseeds in bulk or in a packaged container, make sure that no evidence of moisture is present. While Flaxseeds can be purchased preground, I always prefer to buy whole Flaxseeds and grind them at home whenever I need them. Whole Flaxseeds have a longer shelf life than preground seeds. As with all seeds, I recommend selecting organically grown Flaxseeds whenever possible. (For more on *Organic Foods*, see page 113.)

Flaxseed oil should be expeller cold pressed and organic. It should be in an opaque bottle and kept in the refrigerator case at the grocery. Filtered Flaxseed oil is processed to remove many of the contaminants.

# 2. the best way to store flaxseeds

Whole Flaxseeds should be stored in an airtight container in a dark, dry and cool place (ideally, the refrigerator) where they will keep fresh for 3 months. To extend the shelf life of Flaxseeds, you can store them in the freezer where they will keep for 6 months.

Flaxseed oil should always be refrigerated. Since the most delicate part of the chemistry of Flaxseed oil is the portion containing the omega-3 fatty acids, refrigeration is important to help protect it from oxidative rancidity.

# 3. the best way to prepare flaxseeds

Always grind Flaxseeds before serving. In order to derive benefit from Flaxseeds, they need to be ground to break their hard shells and allow for the digestion and absorption of their nutrients. Whole shelled Flaxseeds can be ground in a coffee grinder. Be sure to clean the grinder well both before and after grinding seeds.

Flaxseeds are stabilized (at 110°F/43°C) before they are sold to help prevent them from going rancid, which allows the addition of Flaxseeds to baked items without damaging their delicate oils.

# health benefits of flaxseeds

### Promote Optimal Health

Flaxseeds are one of the most concentrated food source of alpha-linolenic acid (ALA), an omega-3 fatty acid, . ALA has numerous benefits including being a readily used form of energy and a fatty acid essential for proper skin function; it also inhibits inflammatory compounds made from linoleic acid. Additionally, ALA is the precursor to eicosapentaenoic acid (EPA) and docosahexaenoic acid (DHA), the acclaimed fatty acids found in fish. Omega-3 fatty acids are well-known for their anti-inflammatory properties.

### Promote Heart Health

While small in size, Flaxseeds have big benefits for heart health. Studies have found that diets rich in ALA are associated with a lower risk of atherosclerotic plaques and of dying from heart disease or sudden cardiac death. Individuals who followed ALA-rich diets have been found to have lower total cholesterol, LDL cholesterol and triglycerides, with recent studies also finding that individuals who consume Flaxseed oil have reduced levels of inflammatory markers, including C-reactive protein. Additionally, EPA and DHA have been found to be associated with reduced plasma triglycerides and VLDL (very low density cholesterol, the most dangerous form of LDL), protection against coronary heart disease and reduction of hypertension. Flaxseeds are also a good source of folate, vitamin B6 and magnesium, three other nutrients vital for heart health. (For more on plant-based *Omega-3 Fats*, see page 770.)

## Nutritional Analysis of 2 TBS of Flaxseeds:

| NUTRIENT | AMOUNT | % DAILY VALUE | NUTRIENT | AMOUNT | % DAILY VALUE |
|---|---|---|---|---|---|
| Calories | 95.33 | | Pantothenic Acid | 0.30 mg | 3.00 |
| Calories from Fat | 59.29 | | | | |
| Calories from Saturated Fat | 5.57 | | **Minerals** | | |
| Protein | 3.78 g | | Boron | — mcg | |
| Carbohydrates | 6.64 g | | Calcium | 38.56 mg | 3.86 |
| Dietary Fiber | 5.41 g | 21.64 | Chloride | — mg | |
| Soluble Fiber | — g | | Chromium | — mcg | — |
| Insoluble Fiber | — g | | Copper | 0.20 mg | 10.00 |
| Sugar – Total | — g | | Fluoride | — mg | — |
| Monosaccharides | — g | | Iodine | — mcg | — |
| Disaccharides | — g | | Iron | 1.21 mg | 6.72 |
| Other Carbs | — g | | Magnesium | 70.14 mg | 17.54 |
| Fat –Total | 6.59 g | | Manganese | 0.64 mg | 32.00 |
| Saturated Fat | 0.62 g | | Molybdenum | — mcg | — |
| Mono Fat | 1.33 g | | Phosphorus | 96.49 mg | 9.65 |
| Poly Fat | 4.35 g | | Potassium | 131.94 mg | |
| Omega-3 Fatty Acids | 3.51 g | 140.40 | Selenium | 1.07 mcg | 1.53 |
| Omega-6 Fatty Acids | 0.84 g | | Sodium | 6.59 mg | |
| Trans Fatty Acids | 0.00 g | | Zinc | 0.81 mg | 5.40 |
| Cholesterol | 0.00 mg | | | | |
| Water | 1.70 g | | **Amino Acids** | | |
| Ash | 0.68 g | | Alanine | — g | |
| | | | Arginine | — g | |
| **Vitamins** | | | Aspartate | — g | |
| Vitamin A IU | 0.00 IU | 0.00 | Cystine | — g | — |
| Vitamin A RE | 0.00 RE | | Glutamate | — g | |
| A - Carotenoid | 0.00 RE | 0.00 | Glycine | — g | |
| A - Retinol | 0.00 RE | | Histidine | — g | — |
| B1 Thiamin | 0.03 mg | 2.00 | Isoleucine | — g | — |
| B2 Riboflavin | 0.03 mg | 1.76 | Leucine | — g | — |
| B3 Niacin | 0.27 mg | 1.35 | Lysine | — g | — |
| Niacin Equiv | 0.27 mg | | Methionine | — g | — |
| Vitamin B6 | 0.18 mg | 9.00 | Phenylalanine | — g | — |
| Vitamin B12 | 0.00 mcg | 0.00 | Proline | — g | |
| Biotin | — mcg | — | Serine | — g | |
| Vitamin C | 0.25 mg | 0.42 | Threonine | — g | — |
| Vitamin D IU | — IU | — | Tryptophan | — g | — |
| Vitamin D mcg | — mcg | | Tyrosine | — g | — |
| Vitamin E Alpha Equiv | 0.97 mg | 4.85 | Valine | — g | — |
| Vitamin E IU | 1.44 IU | | | | |
| Vitamin E mg | 0.97 mg | | | | |
| Folate | 53.86 mcg | 13.46 | | | |
| Vitamin K | 0.00 mcg | 0.00 | | | |

(Note: "−" indicates data is unavailable. For more information, please see page 806.)

## Promote Women's Health

Of more than 60 foods tested, Flaxseeds were found to be the most concentrated source of special lignan phytoestrogens, phytonutrients that are converted by beneficial intestinal flora into two hormone-like substances called enterolactone and enterodiol. These hormone-like agents demonstrate a number of protective effects against breast cancer and are believed to be one reason that a vegetarian diet is associated with a lower risk for breast cancer. Studies show that women with breast cancer and women who eat meat typically excrete much lower levels of lignans in their urine than female vegetarians without breast cancer. In animal studies conducted to evaluate the beneficial effects of lignans, supplementing a high-fat diet with Flaxseed flour reduced early markers for mammary cancer in laboratory animals by more than 55%. (For more on *Phytoestrogens*, see page 774.)

## Promote Digestive Health

Flaxseeds are a very good source of dietary fiber, containing insoluble and soluble fiber in a ratio of 2 to 1. Flaxseeds have been found to have a laxative effect, decreasing symptoms of constipation and increasing frequency of bowel movements in both young and old subjects. The fiber in Flaxseeds is suggested to have a cholesterol-lowering effect by preventing the reabsorption of cholesterol from the colon.

## Additional Health-Promoting Benefits of Flaxseeds

Flaxseeds are a concentrated source of many other nutrients providing additional health-promoting benefits. These nutrients include free-radical-scavenging manganese and copper and bone-building phosphorus.

Here are questions that I have received from readers of the whfoods.org website about Flaxseeds:

**Q** *Can you bake with Flaxseeds or are the omega-3 fatty acids damaged by heat?*

**A** While it is not recommended to heat Flaxseed oil because it is very delicate and can oxidize, research shows that the combination of healthy omega-3 oils and lignan phytonutrients in Flaxseeds are surprisingly heat stable. Not only is it safe to leave whole Flaxseeds at room temperature, but you can also use them in baking.

Using ground or whole Flaxseeds in baking does not significantly impact their omega-3 fats. Numerous studies testing the amount of omega-3 fat in baked goods indicate no significant breakdown or loss of beneficial fats occurs in baking. In one study, women who ate raw, ground Flaxseeds daily for

*(Continued on bottom of next Page)*

**STEP-BY-STEP RECIPE**
## The Healthiest Ways of Preparing Flaxseeds

# *Flaxseed Dressing*

*Try this quick and easy dressing on your favorite salad.*

**4 TBS whole Flaxseeds**
**1/3 cup lemon juice**
**1 TBS Dijon mustard**
**1 clove garlic**
**1/2 cup extra virgin olive oil**
**Sea salt and pepper to taste**

1. Press garlic and let sit for 5 minutes. (Why?, see page 261.)
2. Grind Flaxseeds in a blender on medium speed until well ground.
3. Add the remaining ingredients and blend for 2 minutes.

### MAKES 1 CUP

**Preparation Hint:** This dressing should be used right away because the Flaxseeds will swell in liquid, making the dressing too thick.

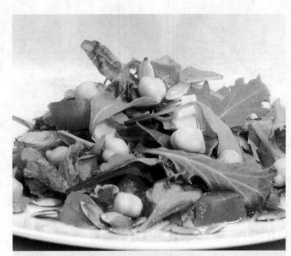

Salad with Flaxseed Dressing

## *Variations...*

- Add 1 tsp of curry powder.
- Add 1 TBS minced basil or rosemary.
- Add 1 TBS of honey.
- Add 2 pinches of cayenne.

Please write (address on back cover flap) or e-mail me at info@whfoods.org with your personal ideas for preparing Flaxseeds, and I will share them with others through our website at www.whfoods.org.

### 10 QUICK SERVING IDEAS for FLAXSEEDS:

1. Sprinkle ground Flaxseeds on your morning fruit or cereal and eat immediately.
2. Add ground Flaxseeds to a morning smoothie and drink immediately.
3. Add 1 TBS ground Flaxseed to green salads.
4. Sprinkle ground Flaxseeds on top of cooked vegetables for a nutty flavor.
5. Spread peanut butter on apple slices and dip in ground Flaxseeds.
6. Fill celery ribs with peanut butter and dip into ground Flaxseeds.
7. Make a fruit "sundae." Top a bowl of your favorite fruit salad with cottage cheese, ground Flaxseeds, maple syrup and a sprinkling of cinnamon.
8. Make your favorite dressing with Flaxseed oil.
9. Add ground Flaxseeds to Sesame Bars (page 519), Peanut Bars (page 543) and Apricot Bars (page 387).
10. Add ground Flaxseeds to granola.

*(Continued from previous Page)*

four weeks had similar plasma fatty acid profiles as those who ate milled Flaxseeds that had been baked in bread. Both groups of women showed a lowering of total cholesterol and "bad" LDL cholesterol.

Researchers speculate that the omega-3 fats in Flaxseeds are resistant to heat because of the presence of plant lignans (like secoisolariciresinol) in Flaxseeds; these phytonutrients are transformed into mammalian lignans (like enterodiol and enterolactone) in the body. So, enjoy this World's Healthiest Food in baked goods as well as raw—either way, you'll receive plenty of healthy benefits.

**Q** *I know that Flaxseeds are rich in dietary fiber. What is the breakdown of their insoluble and soluble fiber?*

**A** The ratio of insoluble fiber to soluble fiber in Flaxseed is 2:1. In other words, two-thirds of the fiber is insoluble and one-third is soluble. The insoluble fiber is mostly lignin (not to be confused with phytoestrogenic lignans), which has benefits on gastrointestinal health. The soluble fiber is mostly mucilage, and it's this type of fiber that benefits cholesterol levels and blood sugar balance and promotes the growth of intestinal "good flora."

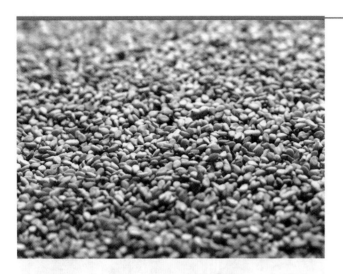

# sesame seeds

| | |
|---|---|
| AVAILABILITY: | Year-round |
| REFRIGERATE: | Yes |
| SHELF LIFE: | 6 months in the refrigerator; 1 year in the freezer |
| PREPARATION: | Minimal |

## nutrient-richness chart

Total Nutrient-Richness: **12**
One-quarter cup (36 grams) of Sesame Seeds contains 206 calories

| NUTRIENT | AMOUNT | %DV | DENSITY | QUALITY |
|---|---|---|---|---|
| Copper | 1.5 mg | 74.0 | 6.5 | very good |
| Manganese | 0.9 mg | 44.0 | 3.8 | very good |
| Tryptophan | 0.1 g | 37.5 | 3.3 | good |
| Calcium | 351.0 mg | 35.1 | 3.1 | good |
| Magnesium | 126.4 mg | 31.6 | 2.8 | good |
| Iron | 5.2 mg | 29.1 | 2.5 | good |
| Phosphorus | 226.4 mg | 22.6 | 2.0 | good |
| Zinc | 2.8 mg | 18.7 | 1.6 | good |
| B1 Thiamin | 0.3 mg | 18.7 | 1.6 | good |
| Dietary Fiber | 4.2 g | 17.0 | 1.5 | good |
| **PHYTOSTEROLS:** | | | Daily values for these nutrients have not yet been established. | |
| Phytosterols-Total | 257 mg | | | |

For more on "Total Nutrient-Richness," "%DV," "Density," and
The World's Healthiest Foods "Quality" Rating System, see page 805.

## why sesame seeds should be part of your healthiest way of eating

Sesame Seeds are a good source of copper, a trace mineral important in a number of anti-inflammatory and antioxidant enzyme systems. They are rich in unique lignan phytonutrients, sesamin and sesamolin, which have been found to have antioxidant and anti-inflammatory properties. (For more on the *Health Benefits of Sesame Seeds* and a complete analysis of their content of over 60 nutrients, see page 520.)

## varieties of sesame seeds

Sesame Seeds are the main ingredient in the Middle Eastern sweet dessert called halvah. "Open Sesame," the famous phrase from the Arabian Nights, reflects the distinguishing feature of the Sesame Seed pod, which bursts open when it reaches maturity. The scientific name for Sesame Seeds is *Sesamun indicum*. Sesame Seeds come in two forms and a variety of different colors, including white, yellow, black and red:

**UNHULLED**

These seeds are darker in color and have their bran intact. They are more nutritious than the hulled variety. One-hundred grams of unhulled Sesame Seeds contain 989 mg of calcium while the same amount of unhulled seeds contains 131 mg.

**HULLED**

These seeds are very light in color and have had their bran portion removed. They come both roasted and unroasted.

Sesame Seeds were believed to have originated in India where they are mentioned in early Hindu legends as a symbol of immortality. Sesame Seeds may be the oldest condiment known to man, dating back to as early as 1,600 BC. According to ancient Assyrian legends, wine made from Sesame Seeds was drunk by the gods when they created the world. Sesame Seeds are tiny, flat, oval seeds with a nutty taste and a delicate, almost invisible crunch that will make a tasty addition to your "Healthiest Way of Eating," especially for those dishes with an Asian flair.

**TAHINI**

Middle Eastern Sesame paste made from Sesame Seeds. Raw tahini is more nutrient-rich than roasted tahini.

**ASIAN SESAME PASTE**

Paste made from toasted Sesame Seeds.

**the peak season** available year-round.

## 3 steps for the best tasting and most nutritious sesame seeds

Enjoying the best tasting Sesame Seeds with the most nutrients is simple if you just follow my 3 easy steps:
1. The Best Way to Select
2. The Best Way to Store
3. The Best Way to Prepare

# 1. the best way to select sesame seeds

Sesame Seeds are generally available in prepackaged containers and can also be found in bulk bins. It is best to check and make sure that the store where you buy Sesame Seeds in bulk has a quick turnover of inventory and that the bulk containers are sealed well in order to ensure maximum freshness. Whether purchasing Sesame Seeds in bulk or in a packaged container, make sure no evidence of moisture is present. Additionally, since Sesame Seeds have high oil content and can become rancid, it is good to smell those from bulk bins to ensure that they smell sweet and fresh, not bitter or rancid. As with all seeds, I recommend selecting organically grown Sesame Seeds whenever possible. (For more on *Organic Foods*, see page 113.)

# 2. the best way to store sesame seeds

Unhulled Sesame Seeds are best stored in an airtight container in a cool, dry, dark place. They will last for 6 months in the refrigerator and 1 year in the freezer. Once the seeds are hulled, they are much more prone to rancidity; hulled Sesame Seeds should be stored in the refrigerator, where they will last for about 3 months, or in the freezer, where they should remain fresh for up to a year. Opened containers of tahini and Asian Sesame paste should be refrigerated.

# 3. the best way to prepare sesame seeds

The best way to prepare Sesame Seeds is to dry roast them. For details, see below.

### The Healthiest Way to Dry Roast Sesame Seeds

**Dry Roasting Sesame Seeds the healthiest way brings out their flavor and develops their sweetness. It is safe to dry roast seeds if done at a low temperature.**

2 cups Sesame Seeds
1. Preheat oven to 160–170°F (70–75°C).
2. Place a thin layer of seeds on a cookie sheet.
3. Roast for 15–20 minutes.

To enhance the "roasted" flavor, try putting a little liquid aminos seasoning or tamari (soy sauce) into a spray bottle and misting the seeds before roasting.

Commercially roasted Sesame Seeds have been heated to high temperatures (over 350°F or 175°C) that damage their delicate oils, resulting in the formation of free radicals and causing lipid peroxidation—the oxidizing of fats in your bloodstream, which can trigger tiny injuries in artery walls—a first step in the buildup of plaque and cardiovascular disease.

Roasted Sesame Seeds have a shorter shelf life and spoil more quickly than raw Sesame Seeds because the unsaturated oils found in seeds oxidize more quickly after exposure to the heat of the roasting process.

Although some find raw seeds more difficult to digest than roasted seeds, this appears to vary greatly between individuals.

For more information, see page 69.

## Sesame Tahini Sauce

*Adds great flavor to vegetables and legumes.*

2 TBS Sesame tahini
1 TBS fresh lemon juice
3 TBS water
Sea salt and cayenne pepper to taste
Optional: Add one minced garlic clove

Mix all ingredients in a small bowl until smooth.

**SERVES 2**

**4 WAYS TO ENJOY THE SESAME TAHINI SAUCE:**

1. Drizzle over cooked vegetables and sprinkle with Sesame Seeds.
2. Use as a dressing for green salad.
3. Use as a sauce for a sandwich wrap.
4. Pour over garbanzo beans and brown rice.

**Q** *I have been told that Sesame oil is good for reducing high blood pressure. Is this true?*

**A** While Sesame oil is not as nutrient-rich as Sesame Seeds, it has been researched for a variety of cardiovascular benefits, including blood pressure reduction. Most of the beneficial effects are thought to come from the special lignan phytonutrients that they contain. What is interesting is that while there are some naturally occurring lignans found in Sesame Seeds (sesamin and sesamolin), some of the lignans that are being studied for their health benefits (episesamin and sesaminol) are actually created during the process of making Sesame oil and don't exist in the seeds themselves.

There have been several animal studies that investigated the effect of dietary Sesame lignans on blood pressure and found that it caused reductions in blood pressure and the physiological damage usually associated with elevated blood pressure. Just recently, results of a human clinical trial supported these earlier animal study findings. Individuals who were on calcium-channel blocker medicine and given 35 grams of Sesame oil per day for 60 days were found to have not only a reduction in blood pressure but also a reduction of triglycerides and LDL (the "bad" cholesterol) and an elevation in HDL (the "good" cholesterol). Additionally, markers of antioxidant activity significantly increased in the Sesame oil supplemented individuals.

**Q** *Can you cook with Sesame oil?*

**A** Like with many other oils, I would rather use Sesame oil in either dressings or drizzled on foods as opposed to heating it in order to prevent oxidation from occurring. Yet, low temperature cooking, such as that involved with making sauces, may be okay for Sesame oil.

**Q** *Are Sesame Seeds OK for children to eat?*

**A** While Sesame Seeds are incredibly rich in nutrients, it is a food to which some people have adverse reactions. It seems that children are becoming increasingly sensitive to Sesame Seeds; sensitivity is growing in terms of its prevalence of allergenicity, especially among infants and children if there is a family history of allergies, asthma or eczema.

**Q** *Given the high calcium content of Sesame Seeds, is tahini a good source to use as I look to incorporate more non-dairy calcium sources into my diet?*

**A** Sesame Seeds are a rich source of calcium. One tablespoon of tahini contains 63 mg of calcium. Therefore, calcium intake is another good reason to incorporate tahini into your "Healthiest Way of Eating" (in addition to its other nutritional benefits including its lignan phytonutrients as well as its great taste and texture).

Yet, I wouldn't just focus on tahini as a non-dairy source of calcium as that 63 mg of calcium will "cost" you 86 calories. Therefore, if you were wanting to get a substantial amount of calcium, say 25% of your daily calcium needs (250 mg) from tahini, it would "cost you" over 340 calories.

A little known nutrition fact (although it should be a widely known one) is that there are actually many non-dairy foods that are rich in calcium. For example, one cup of boiled spinach has over 244 mg of calcium, yet only 41 calories, while one cup of cooked collard greens offers about 226 mg of calcium for less than 50 calories. Therefore, these and other plant-based foods can serve as great sources of calcium but "cost" you less calories.

*(Continued on bottom of next Page)*

**STEP-BY-STEP RECIPE**
## The Healthiest Ways of Preparing Sesame Seeds

# Sesame Bars

*A great dessert or energy bar—just mix ingredients and chill!*

1/2 cup Sesame Seeds, roasted or raw
1 cup walnuts
1½ cups pitted dates
1½ cups raisins
1/8 tsp salt

1. Pulse all ingredients in food processor just until mixture holds together when pressed. Avoid overprocessing which will turn the mixture into a paste.

2. Press mixture into 9-inch square pan, and chill for approximately 1 hour in the refrigerator.

3. Cut into 1½-inch squares to serve.

## MAKES 30 BARS

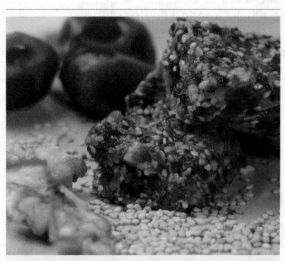

Sesame Bars

Please write (address on back cover flap) or e-mail me at info@whfoods.org with your personal ideas for preparing Sesame Seeds, and I will share them with others through our website at www.whfoods.org.

## 10 QUICK SERVING IDEAS for SESAME SEEDS:

1. Add toasted Sesame Seeds to your morning granola.

2. Sprinkle toasted Sesame Seeds over cooked grains, seafood or Asian vegetable dishes.

3. Add Sesame Seeds to Asian-flavored cabbage salad.

4. **Sesame Spread:** Spread Sesame tahini on toasted bread and either drizzle with honey for a sweet treat or combine with miso for a savory snack.

5. **Sesame Milk:** Blend 1/2 cup of Sesame tahini, 3 pitted dates, a pinch of sea salt and 2½ cups of water on high for 2 minutes. Strain through fine cheesecloth into a bowl or a quart measuring pitcher. Use on cereal or over sliced bananas. Sesame milk may be stored in a glass jar in the refrigerator for up to 3 days.

6. **Cool Cucumber Salad:** Place 2 thinly sliced cucumbers in a medium-size bowl and toss with 1 tsp tamari (soy sauce), 1 TBS lemon juice, 1 TBS extra virgin olive oil, 2 TBS toasted Sesame Seeds and 1 TBS honey.

7. **Sesame Spinach:** Combine cooked spinach with 1 TBS tamari (soy sauce), 1 TBS honey, 2 TBS extra virgin olive oil, 2 TBS Sesame Seeds and hot sauce to taste.

8. **Gomasio:** A traditional macrobiotic seasoning made from crushed Sesame Seeds and sea salt. Sprinkle on vegetables and grains. You can either purchase gomasio at a natural food store or make your own by using a mortar and pestle. Simply mix together one part sea salt with twelve parts dry roasted Sesame Seeds.

9. **Sesame Dressing:** Combine 2 TBS dry roasted Sesame Seeds with 2 TBS rice vinegar, 1 tsp tamari, 3 cloves crushed garlic and 3 TBS extra virgin olive oil. Use as a dressing for salads, vegetables and noodles.

10. **Sesame Chicken:** "Healthy Sauté" chicken pieces with 1 TBS Sesame Seeds, 1 tsp tamari, 2 cloves minced garlic, 1 TBS fresh grated ginger and your favorite vegetables for a healthy, but quick, Asian-inspired meal.

*(Continued from previous Page)*

This is not to dissuade you from eating tahini. It is a wonderful food and one of my favorites. I use it in a lot of recipes. But if you enjoy the other plant-based foods that are rich in calcium, I would not suggest that you make tahini your primary source for this important mineral.

# health benefits of sesame seeds

### Rich in Unique Health-Promoting Phytonutrients

Sesame Seeds contain the unique lignan phytonutrients, sesamin and sesamolin. Once in the body, sesamolin gets converted to sesamol, another lignan with health-promoting effects. Research on these compounds has yielded very exciting findings. In animals, Sesame Seed lignans have been found to have cholesterol- lipoprotein- and blood-pressure-lowering effects. They have been found to have antioxidant activity, to increase vitamin E supplies and to protect the liver from oxidative damage. In addition, preliminary research suggests that sesamin and sesamol may have anti-inflammatory properties since they have been found to inhibit the *delta-5-desaturase* enzyme, which converts omega-6 fatty acids into arachidonic acid; the latter fatty acid is known to be a precursor for molecules that promote inflammation. Sesame Seeds are also a highly concentrated source of phytosterols, plant nutrients that may help to reduce cholesterol.

### Promote Joint and Skin Health

Sesame Seeds are a very good source of copper, a trace mineral that is important in a number of anti-inflammatory and antioxidant enzyme systems. Copper plays an important role in the activity of *lysyl oxidase*, an enzyme needed for the cross-linking of collagen and elastin—the ground substances that provide structure, strength and elasticity to blood vessels, bones, joints and skin.

### Promote Bone Health

Calcium's most highly recognized role has been to prevent the bone loss that can occur as a result of menopause or other conditions, such as rheumatoid arthritis. Sesame Seeds are also rich in other bone-supportive nutrients. They are a good source of magnesium and phosphorus, minerals which serve as "scaffolding" to support the integrity of bone. They are also a very good source of copper and manganese and a good source of zinc, three trace minerals that are cofactors in enzymes that help to promote the construction of the bone matrix. In fact, a recent study found low dietary intake of zinc to be correlated with both low blood levels of this trace mineral and osteoporosis of the hip and spine in middle to older age men.

### Additional Health-Promoting Benefits of Sesame Seeds

Sesame Seeds are also a concentrated source of many other nutrients providing additional health-promoting benefits. These nutrients include energy-producing iron and vitamin B1, digestive-health-supporting dietary fiber, and sleep-promoting tryptophan.

## Nutritional Analysis of 1/4 cup of Sesame Seeds:

| NUTRIENT | AMOUNT | % DAILY VALUE |
|---|---|---|
| Calories | 206.28 | |
| Calories from Fat | 160.92 | |
| Calories from Saturated Fat | 22.56 | |
| Protein | 6.40 g | |
| Carbohydrates | 8.44 g | |
| Dietary Fiber | 4.24 g | 16.96 |
| Soluble Fiber | 0.88 g | |
| Insoluble Fiber | 3.36 g | |
| Sugar – Total | 0.40 g | |
| Monosaccharides | — g | |
| Disaccharides | 0.32 g | |
| Other Carbs | 3.80 g | |
| Fat – Total | 17.88 g | |
| Saturated Fat | 2.52 g | |
| Mono Fat | 6.76 g | |
| Poly Fat | 7.84 g | |
| Omega-3 Fatty Acids | 0.12 g | 4.80 |
| Omega-6 Fatty Acids | 7.72 g | |
| Trans Fatty Acids | 0.00 g | |
| Cholesterol | 0.00 mg | |
| Water | 1.68 g | |
| Ash | 1.60 g | |
| **Vitamins** | | |
| Vitamin A IU | 3.24 IU | 0.06 |
| Vitamin A RE | 0.36 RE | |
| A - Carotenoid | 0.36 RE | 0.00 |
| A - Retinol | 0.00 RE | |
| B1 Thiamin | 0.28 mg | 18.67 |
| B2 Riboflavin | 0.08 mg | 4.71 |
| B3 Niacin | 1.64 mg | 8.20 |
| Niacin Equiv | 3.44 mg | |
| Vitamin B6 | 0.28 mg | 14.00 |
| Vitamin B12 | 0.00 mcg | 0.00 |
| Biotin | 3.96 mcg | 1.32 |
| Vitamin C | 0.00 mg | 0.00 |
| Vitamin D IU | 0.00 IU | 0.00 |
| Vitamin D mcg | 0.00 mcg | |
| Vitamin E Alpha Equiv | 0.80 mg | 4.00 |
| Vitamin E IU | 1.20 IU | |
| Vitamin E mg | 0.80 mg | |
| Folate | 34.80 mcg | 8.70 |
| Vitamin K | 0.00 mcg | 0.00 |

| NUTRIENT | AMOUNT | % DAILY VALUE |
|---|---|---|
| Pantothenic Acid | 0.00 mg | 0.00 |
| **Minerals** | | |
| Boron | — mcg | |
| Calcium | 351.00 mg | 35.10 |
| Chloride | 3.60 mg | |
| Chromium | — mcg | |
| Copper | 1.48 mg | 74.00 |
| Fluoride | — mg | — |
| Iodine | — mcg | — |
| Iron | 5.24 mg | 29.11 |
| Magnesium | 126.36 mg | 31.59 |
| Manganese | 0.88 mg | 44.00 |
| Molybdenum | 10.64 mcg | 14.19 |
| Phosphorus | 226.44 mg | 22.64 |
| Potassium | 168.48 mg | |
| Selenium | 2.04 mcg | 2.91 |
| Sodium | 3.96 mg | |
| Zinc | 2.80 mg | 18.67 |
| **Amino Acids** | | |
| Alanine | 0.28 g | |
| Arginine | 0.84 g | |
| Aspartate | 0.52 g | |
| Cystine | 0.12 g | 29.27 |
| Glutamate | 1.24 g | |
| Glycine | 0.40 g | |
| Histidine | 0.16 g | 12.40 |
| Isoleucine | 0.24 g | 20.87 |
| Leucine | 0.44 g | 17.39 |
| Lysine | 0.20 g | 8.51 |
| Methionine | 0.20 g | 27.03 |
| Phenylalanine | 0.28 g | 23.53 |
| Proline | 0.24 g | |
| Serine | 0.32 g | |
| Threonine | 0.24 g | 19.35 |
| Tryptophan | 0.12 g | 37.50 |
| Tyrosine | 0.24 g | 24.74 |
| Valine | 0.32 g | 21.77 |

(Note: "–" indicates data is unavailable. For more information, please see page 806.)

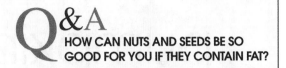

# Q&A

## HOW CAN NUTS AND SEEDS BE SO GOOD FOR YOU IF THEY CONTAIN FAT?

**A Serving of Nuts and Seeds Won't Make You Fat**

Yes, it's true that nuts and seeds do contain a good amount of fat and therefore calories. But, eaten in small quantities—a serving is just two to four tablespoons—these highly nutritious members of the World's Healthiest Foods deliver not only delicious flavor but also nutritional benefits that can help protect you against cardiovascular disease. A handful of almonds, pumpkin seeds or walnuts, eaten as a healthy snack or used as a flavorful addition to a tossed green salad, will not make you fat. Too many bowls full of salty nuts washed down with several beers may.

**Nuts' and Seeds' Healthy Fats**

Not only will reasonable amounts of nuts and seeds not make you fat but the fat found in nuts and seeds is the primary reason eating them promotes a healthy heart. The fats that nuts and seeds contain is mostly polyunsaturated, although they also contain a little monounsaturated and a very small amount of saturated fat. The proper balance between these types of fats is important, and many people do not get enough of certain types, especially one type of polyunsaturated fat called omega-3. Nuts and seeds are rich sources of a type of omega-3 fat called alpha-linolenic acid (ALA), which belongs to the same family of omega-3 fats as the heart-healthy fats you may have heard about in cold-water fish.

The omega-3 fatty acids found in nuts and seeds may help prevent heart disease and repeat heart attacks in several ways. Omega-3 fatty acids, including ALA, EPA and DHA, are protective fats that have been found to:

- *Lower blood cholesterol and triglyceride levels,* which, when elevated, are both risk factors for heart disease.
- *Decrease platelet aggregation, which when excessive can cause "sticky" blood.* Like aspirin, omega-3s "thin" the blood. The blood doesn't actually become thinner; what happens is that the red blood cells no longer clump together, so the blood flows more freely through the blood vessels, which is especially helpful in vessels that may be partially clogged with cholesterol build-up. If the blood is "sticky," clumps of red blood cells may form a clot that blocks a narrowed artery, triggering a heart attack if the blood vessel feeds the heart, or a stroke if the blood vessel is in the brain.

- *Reduce the formation of artery-clogging atherosclerotic plaque.* Once platelets aggregate or stick together, they release a substance that contributes to the process through which cholesterol is used to form atherosclerotic plaque. When atherosclerotic plaque builds up in the blood vessels, blood flow is decreased to a minimum or stopped altogether, precipitating a heart attack or stroke. By reducing platelet aggregation, omega-3s may help short-circuit this whole process.
- *Reduce inflammation of the blood vessels.* If blood vessels are inflamed, blood flow is reduced. Omega-3s are used within the body to produce anti-inflammatory chemical messengers called the series E3 prostaglandins, which by lessening blood vessel inflammation can improve blood flow.
- *Lower blood pressure, another major risk factor for heart attacks and strokes.* All the ways in which omega-3 fats promote blood vessel health contribute to maintenance of clear, open vessels through which blood flows easily.

**More Healthy Reasons to Eat Nuts and Seeds**

Nuts and seeds are a rich source of plant protein, which is needed not only to build and maintain all body tissues, but for a healthy immune system as well. A handful of nuts or seeds will also provide you with fiber. The fiber in nuts and seeds helps keep your digestive tract, specifically your colon, in good health and also promotes the health of your blood vessels since the soluble portion of their fiber helps lower blood cholesterol—another boon to heart health.

Nuts and seeds may even help those who wish to lose weight. The combination of protein, fiber and healthy fats provided by nuts and seeds helps keep blood sugar levels stable, which helps keep us from getting hungry too soon after eating.

In addition to the cardioprotective fats, plant protein and dietary fiber nuts provide, new research indicates that nuts and seeds are rich sources of other bioactive molecules that support cardiovascular health. These include plant sterols, antioxidant phenolics and numerous other phytonutrients—natural substances in plants that are beneficial to our health—that may be protective against chronic diseases.

Many phytonutrients act as powerful antioxidants, which can improve cardiovascular health because they destroy free radicals that can harm the lining of the blood vessels. Tiny micro-injuries in the lining of the vessel are a precursor to plaque development, which can eventually clog the artery. Yet another cardioprotective effect from a few nuts and seeds!

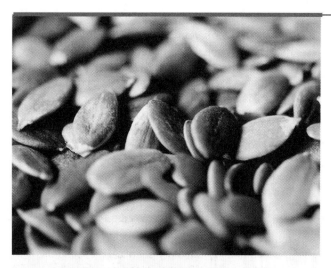

## nutrient-richness chart

Total Nutrient-Richness: **11**

One-quarter cup (35 grams) of dried Pumpkin Seeds contains 187 calories

| NUTRIENT | AMOUNT | %DV | DENSITY | QUALITY |
|---|---|---|---|---|
| Manganese | 1.0 mg | 52.0 | 5.0 | very good |
| Magnesium | 184.6 mg | 46.1 | 4.5 | very good |
| Phosphorus | 405.0 mg | 40.5 | 3.9 | very good |
| Tryptophan | 0.1 g | 34.4 | 3.3 | good |
| Iron | 5.2 mg | 28.7 | 2.8 | good |
| Copper | 0.5 mg | 24.0 | 2.3 | good |
| Vitamin K | 17.7 mcg | 22.2 | 2.1 | good |
| Zinc | 2.6 mg | 17.1 | 1.7 | good |
| Protein | 8.5 g | 16.9 | 1.6 | good |

For more on "Total Nutrient-Richness," "%DV," "Density," and
The World's Healthiest Foods "Quality" Rating System, see page 805.

Pumpkin Seeds were a celebrated food of the Native Americans, who treasured them for their dietary and medicinal properties. They are also a special hallmark of traditional Mexican cuisine and a popular snack in Mexico. So, don't toss away the seeds you scrape out of your Halloween pumpkin; they can be toasted and eaten as a delicious snack or added to your favorite salad, soup or fish dish. Of course, you don't have to wait for Halloween to enjoy Pumpkin Seeds. They are readily available in bulk or prepackaged at your local natural food store any time of year. Chewy, subtly sweet and nutty, Pumpkin Seeds make a great addition to your "Healthiest Way of Eating."

# pumpkin seeds

## highlights

| | |
|---|---|
| AVAILABILITY: | Year-round |
| REFRIGERATE: | Yes |
| SHELF LIFE: | 6 months in the refrigerator; 1 year in the freezer |
| PREPARATION: | Minimal |

## why pumpkin seeds should be part of your healthiest way of eating

Pumpkin Seeds are a good source of zinc, a hard-to-find mineral important for a healthy immune system. They are becoming increasingly popular not only because of their overall nutrient-richness, but because scientific research is finding their unique nutritional substances called cucurbitacins to have many health-promoting benefits. (For more on the *Health Benefits of Pumpkin Seeds* and a complete analysis of their content of over 60 nutrients, see page 526.)

## varieties of pumpkin seeds

Some varieties of Pumpkin Seeds are encased in a yellow-white husk, although some varieties of pumpkins produce seeds without shells. Pumpkin Seeds, also known as pepitas, are flat, dark green seeds. Like cantaloupe, cucumber and squash, pumpkins belong to the gourd or *Cucurbitaceae* family. The most common genus and species name for pumpkin is *Cucurbita maxima*.

## the peak season available year-round.

## 3 steps for the best tasting and most nutritious pumpkin seeds

Enjoying the best tasting Pumpkin Seeds with the most nutrients is simple if you just follow my 3 easy steps:

1. The Best Way to Select
2. The Best Way to Store
3. The Best Way to Prepare

# 1. the best way to select pumpkin seeds

Pumpkin Seeds are generally available in prepackaged containers as well as bulk bins. It is best to check and make sure that the store where you buy Pumpkin Seeds in bulk has a quick turnover of inventory and that the bulk containers are sealed well in order to ensure maximum freshness. The Pumpkin Seeds should be uniform in color and not limp or shriveled. They should also smell sweet and nutty; be sure they do not smell rancid or musty. As with all seeds, I recommend selecting organically grown Pumpkin Seeds whenever possible. (For more *Organic Foods*, see page 113.)

If you want Pumpkin Seeds with a roasted flavor and texture, choose ones that have been "dry roasted" as they are not cooked in oil. The commercial roasting process of seeds is often a form of deep-frying, usually in saturated fat, such as coconut oil or palm kernel oil. Consumption of deep-fried foods has been linked to high levels of LDL (the "bad" form of cholesterol) and to thickening of larger artery walls.

Even "dry roasted" Pumpkin Seeds may be cooked at high temperatures that damage their natural oils. It is important to read the label to be sure that no additional ingredients such as sugar, corn syrup or preservatives have been added. For the highest quality, least expensive "dry roasted" Pumpkin Seeds, it's best to just roast them yourself using "The Healthiest Way to Dry Roast Pumpkin Seeds." (See below.)

You can now also find Pumpkin Seed butter in some natural food stores. It is a delicious addition to a squash soup or can be used as a spread, like peanut butter.

# 2. the best way to store pumpkin seeds

Pumpkin Seeds should be stored in an airtight container in the refrigerator. While they may stay edible for about 6 months, they seem to lose their peak freshness after about 1–2 months. Pumpkin Seeds can be stored in an airtight container in the freezer where they will keep for 1 year.

# 3. the best way to prepare pumpkin seeds

The best way to prepare Pumpkin Seeds is to dry roast them. For details, see below.

---

### The Healthiest Way to Dry Roast Pumpkin Seeds

**Dry Roasting Pumpkin Seeds the healthiest way gives them a lightly roasted flavor and develops their sweetness. It is safe to dry roast seeds if done at a low temperature.**

2 cups Pumpkin Seeds

1. Preheat oven to 160–170°F (70–75°C).
2. Place a thin layer of seeds on a cookie sheet.
3. Roast for 15–20 minutes.

To enhance the "roasted" flavor, try putting a little liquid aminos seasoning or tamari (soy sauce) into a spray bottle and misting the seeds before roasting.

Roasting seeds at a temperature higher than 170°F (75°C) will cause a breakdown of their fats and the production of free radicals. Commercially roasted Pumpkin Seeds have been heated to high temperatures (over 350°F or 175°C) that damage their delicate oils resulting in the formation of free radicals and causing lipid peroxidation—the oxidizing of fats in your bloodstream that can trigger tiny injuries in artery walls—a first step in the buildup of plaque and cardiovascular disease.

Roasted Pumpkin Seeds have a shorter shelf life and spoil more quickly than raw Pumpkin Seeds because the unsaturated oils found in seeds oxidize more quickly after exposure to the heat of the roasting process.

Although some find raw seeds more difficult to digest than roasted seeds, this appears to vary greatly between individuals.

## Q *What is the difference between green and white Pumpkin Seeds?*

A Like all plants, there are different species and varieties of Pumpkins, even though they all belong to the same family of plants (*Cucurbitaceae*). Green hulled Pumpkin Seeds are a variety usually referred to as pepitas. This variety of Pumpkin Seeds is especially popular in the southwestern United States and in Mexico. The hulls of Pumpkin Seeds are edible and high in fiber, but typically not eaten. (They may also be different in color than the inner seed.) White seeds and white or whitish-yellow hulls are very common to other pumpkin varieties. There is even a variety of pumpkin (the *Lumina* variety) that not only contains white seeds, but has a white outer skin.

I haven't seen research documenting the nutritional differences between green and white varieties of Pumpkin Seeds. There can be a pretty wide range of values in the zinc and vitamin E content of Pumpkin Seeds, but I haven't seen any studies that showed these differences to be associated with the color of the inner seed or the hull.

## Q *Do I need to separate Pumpkin Seeds from the outside husk, or is the whole seed edible?*

A The hulls of Pumpkin Seeds are high in fiber, and although typically not eaten, they are edible, and you will find individuals who enjoy eating the hull.

## 8 QUICK SERVING IDEAS for PUMPKIN SEEDS:

1. Add Pumpkin Seeds to your morning cereal.
2. Add chopped Pumpkin Seeds to green salads.
3. Top broiled Salmon with chopped Pumpkin Seeds.
4. Sprinkle chopped Pumpkin Seeds on steamed broccoli or any healthy sautéed vegetable.
5. Add chopped Pumpkin Seeds to your favorite vegetable burger recipe.
6. Keep a bag of Pumpkin Seeds handy for a snack.

7. **High Energy Snack to Go:** Combine 1 cup each of Pumpkin Seeds, whole raw cashews, dried cranberries or blueberries, and diced dried apple.
8. **Diced Vegetable Salad:** Combine 1/2 cup chopped Pumpkin Seeds, 1 medium diced carrot, 1 medium diced tomato, 1 stalk diced celery, 1/2 cup quartered broccoli florets, 1/2 medium chopped sweet onion and your favorite vinaigrette.

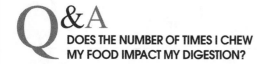

## Q&A
### DOES THE NUMBER OF TIMES I CHEW MY FOOD IMPACT MY DIGESTION?

Chewing is an extremely important, yet oftentimes overlooked, part of healthy digestion. Most people put food in their mouth, chew a few times and swallow their food, as if their sole focus was how quickly they could get their food to their stomach.

While our mothers might have repeatedly told us to "chew your food," most people do not do this well, probably out of habit, conditioning and attitude towards food. When the idea of sitting down for a relaxing meal that focuses truly on the enjoyment and nutritional benefits of food takes second fiddle to the pressures and stress of our modern-day, on-the-go lifestyles, it is no surprise that many people do not slow down when they eat and take the time to chew their food.

Yet, in reality it doesn't really take much time and effort to chew your food, and what you get in return is well worth it, with better health and a greater enjoyment of food being some of the rewards.

### Digestion begins in the mouth
Most people think that digestion begins in the stomach. Yet, with proper, health-promoting digestion, this process actually begins in the mouth. The process of chewing is a vital component of the digestive activities that occur in the mouth, inextricably linked to good digestion and, therefore, to good health.

### The mechanical process of digestion begins with chewing
The action of chewing mechanically breaks down very large aggregates of food molecules into smaller particles. This results in the food having increased surface area, an important contributing factor to good digestion. In addition to the obvious benefit of reduced esophageal stress that accompanies swallowing smaller, rather than larger, pieces of food, there is another very important benefit to chewing your food well that comes with its ability to be exposed to saliva for a longer period of time.

*(Continued on Page 527)*

**The Healthiest Ways of Preparing Pumpkin Seeds**

# Pumpkin Seed and Cilantro Pesto

*A quick, easy and exciting way to enjoy the many nutritional benefits of Pumpkin Seeds. This pesto goes well with pasta, chicken or fish.*

1/4 cup Pumpkin Seeds
1 cup chopped cilantro
1/2 cup coarsely chopped parsley
2 TBS coarsely chopped scallion
3 medium cloves garlic, chopped
2 TBS water
2 TBS fresh lemon juice
3 TBS extra virgin olive oil
Sea salt and white pepper to taste

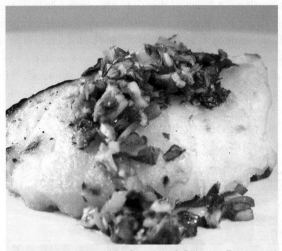

Cod with Pumpkin Seed and Cilantro Pesto

Blend all ingredients in a food processor, adding olive oil a little at a time at end. Do not overprocess. You may need to scrape down the sides of the bowl. Make sure that the mixture does not become too smooth; small pieces of Pumpkin Seeds should still be visible. This can be done by pulsing the food processor rather than leaving it running. The pesto is best served at room temperature. Do not heat it. It will keep in the refrigerator for about 5 days.

## Flavor Tips: Try these 4 great serving suggestions with the recipe above.

1. Serve over broccoli, cauliflower, summer squash, potatoes or your favorite healthy sautéed vegetable.
2. Spread on crackers or vegetable chips and top with cottage cheese.
3. Make a wrap with lettuce, sprouts, carrots and tomato in a whole wheat tortilla and spread with pesto.
4. Toss with cooked grains and vegetables.

# Spicy Pumpkin Seed Snack Mix

*Here's a great way to add extra zing to Pumpkin Seeds.*

1 cup Pumpkin Seeds
1 TBS tamari (soy sauce)
1 tsp curry powder
1/4 tsp hot chili sauce
Optional: Substitute chili powder
for curry powder

1. Combine all ingredients in a mixing bowl.
2. Place on a baking sheet and bake at 160°F (60°C) for 15–20 minutes. Let cool before serving or storing. Keep in a glass jar with a tightly fitting lid.

## Flavor Tips: Try these 4 great serving suggestions with the recipe above.

1. Sprinkle on green salads.
2. Garnish kale or Swiss chard with the Spicy Pumpkin Seed Snack Mix.
3. Coat a slice of goat cheese with Spicy Pumpkin Seed Snack Mix.
4. Blend it with your favorite vinaigrette.

Please write (address on back cover cover flap) or e-mail me at info@whfoods.org with your personal ideas for preparing Pumpkin Seeds, and I will share them with others through our website at www.whfoods.org.

# health benefits of pumpkin seeds

## Promote Prostate Health

Increasing incidence of prostate enlargement in U.S. men has catapulted Pumpkin Seeds into the health spotlight. These seeds contain phytonutrients called cucurbitacins that can prevent the body from converting testosterone into a much more potent form called dihydrotestosterone. This makes it more difficult for the body to produce more prostate cells and therefore more difficult for the prostate to keep enlarging.

## Promote Men's Health

Pumpkin Seeds are a good source of zinc, a mineral long renowned for promoting men's health. Now there may be yet another reason for men to concentrate on getting an adequate daily supply of zinc—bone mineral density. Although osteoporosis is often thought to be a disease for which postmenopausal women are at highest risk, it is also a potential problem for older men. Almost 30% of hip fractures occur in men, and one in eight men over age 50 will have an osteoporotic fracture. A recent study focusing on men over 45 years old found a clear correlation between low dietary intake of zinc, low blood levels of this trace mineral and osteoporosis at the hip and spine.

## Promote Joint Health

The healing properties of Pumpkin Seeds have also been recently investigated with respect to arthritis. In animal studies, the addition of Pumpkin Seeds to the diet has compared favorably with the use of the non-steroidal anti-inflammatory drug indomethacin in reducing inflammatory symptoms. Additionally, Pumpkin Seeds did not have one extremely undesirable effect of indomethacin: unlike the drug, Pumpkin Seeds do not increase the level of damaged fats in the linings of the joints, a side effect that actually contributes to the progression of arthritis. Some of Pumpkin Seeds' joint health benefits may come from their concentration of copper, which plays a role in promoting flexibility in bones and joints.

## Important Protein Source

Pumpkin Seeds are such a concentrated source of protein that they are one of only two World's Healthiest Nuts and Seeds that are rated as a good source of this important nutrient (the other one is peanuts). Our body uses dietary protein to create its structure, using it to build muscles and tissues. In addition, compounds vital to our health—such as enzymes and nutrient-transport proteins—are synthesized from dietary protein. And protein gives us slow burning energy that helps us to feel our best.

## Additional Health-Promoting Benefits of Pumpkin Seeds

Pumpkin Seeds are also a concentrated source of other nutrients providing additional health-promoting benefits. These nutrients include free-radical-scavenging manganese, muscle-relaxing magnesium, energy-promoting iron and phosphorus, and sleep-promoting tryptophan.

### Nutritional Analysis of 1/4 cup of Pumpkin Seeds:

| NUTRIENT | AMOUNT | % DAILY VALUE |
|---|---|---|
| Calories | 186.65 | |
| Calories from Fat | 142.36 | |
| Calories from Saturated Fat | 26.93 | |
| Protein | 8.47 g | |
| Carbohydrates | 6.14 g | |
| Dietary Fiber | 1.35 g | 5.40 |
| Soluble Fiber | 0.19 g | |
| Insoluble Fiber | 1.16 g | |
| Sugar – Total | 0.35 g | |
| Monosaccharides | 0.00 g | |
| Disaccharides | 0.35 g | |
| Other Carbs | 4.45 g | |
| Fat – Total | 15.82 g | |
| Saturated Fat | 2.99 g | |
| Mono Fat | 4.92 g | |
| Poly Fat | 7.21 g | |
| Omega-3 Fatty Acids | 0.06 g | 2.40 |
| Omega-6 Fatty Acids | 7.14 g | |
| Trans Fatty Acids | 0.00 g | |
| Cholesterol | 0.00 mg | |
| Water | 2.39 g | |
| Ash | 1.68 g | |

**Vitamins**

| NUTRIENT | AMOUNT | % DAILY VALUE |
|---|---|---|
| Vitamin A IU | 131.10 IU | 2.62 |
| Vitamin A RE | 13.11 RE | |
| A - Carotenoid | 13.11 RE | 0.17 |
| A - Retinol | 0.00 RE | |
| B1 Thiamin | 0.07 mg | 4.67 |
| B2 Riboflavin | 0.11 mg | 6.47 |
| B3 Niacin | 0.60 mg | 3.00 |
| Niacin Equiv | 2.48 mg | |
| Vitamin B6 | 0.08 mg | 4.00 |
| Vitamin B12 | 0.00 mcg | 0.00 |
| Biotin | — mcg | — |
| Vitamin C | 0.66 mg | 1.10 |
| Vitamin D IU | 0.00 IU | 0.00 |
| Vitamin D mcg | 0.00 mcg | |
| Vitamin E Alpha Equiv | 0.35 mg | 1.75 |
| Vitamin E IU | 0.51 IU | |
| Vitamin E mg | 3.76 mg | |
| Folate | 19.84 mcg | 4.96 |
| Vitamin K | 17.73 mcg | 22.16 |

| NUTRIENT | AMOUNT | % DAILY VALUE |
|---|---|---|
| Pantothenic Acid | 0.12 mg | 1.20 |

**Minerals**

| NUTRIENT | AMOUNT | % DAILY VALUE |
|---|---|---|
| Boron | — mcg | |
| Calcium | 14.84 mg | 1.48 |
| Chloride | — mg | |
| Chromium | — mcg | — |
| Copper | 0.48 mg | 24.00 |
| Fluoride | — mg | — |
| Iodine | — mcg | — |
| Iron | 5.16 mg | 28.67 |
| Magnesium | 184.58 mg | 46.15 |
| Manganese | 1.04 mg | 52.00 |
| Molybdenum | — mcg | — |
| Phosphorus | 405.03 mg | 40.50 |
| Potassium | 278.42 mg | |
| Selenium | 1.93 mcg | 2.76 |
| Sodium | 6.21 mg | |
| Zinc | 2.57 mg | 17.13 |

**Amino Acids**

| NUTRIENT | AMOUNT | % DAILY VALUE |
|---|---|---|
| Alanine | 0.35 g | |
| Arginine | 1.21 g | |
| Aspartate | 0.75 g | |
| Cystine | 0.09 g | 21.95 |
| Glutamate | 1.30 g | |
| Glycine | 0.54 g | |
| Histidine | 0.20 g | 15.50 |
| Isoleucine | 0.38 g | 33.04 |
| Leucine | 0.63 g | 24.90 |
| Lysine | 0.55 g | 23.40 |
| Methionine | 0.17 g | 22.97 |
| Phenylalanine | 0.37 g | 31.09 |
| Proline | 0.30 g | |
| Serine | 0.35 g | |
| Threonine | 0.27 g | 21.77 |
| Tryptophan | 0.11 g | 34.38 |
| Tyrosine | 0.31 g | 31.96 |
| Valine | 0.59 g | 40.14 |

(Note: "—" indicates data is unavailable. For more information, please see page 806.)

*(Continued from Page 524)*

## The chemical process of digestion begins with chewing

Food's contact with saliva is important because it helps to lubricate the food, making it easier for foods (notably dried ones) to pass more easily through the esophagus and because saliva contains enzymes that contribute to the chemical process of digestion. Carbohydrate digestion begins with salivary *alpha-amylase* as it breaks down some of the chemical bonds that connect the simple sugars that comprise starches. Additionally, the first stage of fat digestion also occurs in the mouth with the secretion of the enzyme, *lingual lipase,* by glands that are located under the tongue.

## Incomplete digestion can lead to bacterial overgrowth

When food is not well chewed, and the food fragments are too big to be properly broken down, incomplete digestion occurs. Not only do nutrients not get extracted from the food but undigested food becomes fodder for bacteria in the colon that can lead to bacterial overgrowth, flatulence and other symptoms of indigestion.

## Chewing relaxes the lower stomach muscle

Chewing is directly connected with the movement of food through your digestive tract and, in particular, with the movement of your food from your stomach into your small intestine. At the lower end of your stomach, there is a muscle called the pylorus. This muscle must relax in order for food to leave your stomach and pass into your small intestine. Sufficient saliva from optimal chewing helps relax the pylorus and, in this way, helps your food move through your digestive tract in a healthy fashion.

## Chewing triggers the rest of the digestive process

Yet, the contribution of chewing to good digestion does not even stop there. The process of chewing also activates signaling messages to the rest of the gastrointestinal system that triggers it to begin the entire digestive process. This is because when chewing is a well-paced, thorough process, it can actually be said to belong to the "cephalic stage of digestion," the phase in which you first see, smell and taste your food. The length of time spent chewing the food is related to the length of the cephalic stage of digestion since with more extensive chewing, the longer the food gets to be seen, tasted and smelled.

Cephalic phase responses have been extensively analyzed in the research literature. The release of small messaging molecules critical for digestion, such as cholecystokinin, somatostatin and neurotensin, has been found to increase by over 50% just by the mere sight and smell of food. Additionally, research has shown how chewing and the activation of taste receptors in the mouth can prompt the nervous system that, in turn, relays information to the gastrointestinal system that expedites the process of digestion. For example, stimulation of the taste receptors can signal the stomach lining to produce hydrochloric acid that helps in the breakdown of protein. Additionally, chewing signals the pancreas to prepare to secrete enzymes and bicarbonate into the lumen of the small intestine.

## Practical tips

For healthy digestion to occur, it is important to thoroughly chew your food. While various health professionals advocate distinct numbers of times you should chew food, I recommend more personal guidelines. I feel that instead of prescribing a set number of chews for each biteful people should get a sense of their own eating, and develop more of a relationship with their food, enhancing their own knowingness about what is best for their health.

My suggestion is that you chew your food completely until it is small enough and dissolved enough to be swallowed with ease. A good rule of thumb is as follows: if you can tell what kind of food you are eating from the texture of the food in your mouth (not the taste), then you haven't chewed it enough. For example, if you are chewing broccoli and you run your tongue over the stalk and can tell that it is still a stalk or over the floret and you can tell that it is still a floret, don't swallow. You need to keep on chewing until you can't tell the stalk from the floret.

The benefits of thoroughly chewing your food will extend beyond improved digestion. It will cause you to slow down when you are eating, making more space for the enjoyment of your meal. Food will begin to taste even better when there is more focus and concentration on the process and act of eating. By chewing your food well, you will be able to better enjoy the benefits of the World's Healthiest Foods—their abundance of nutrients and great, lively tastes.

# walnuts

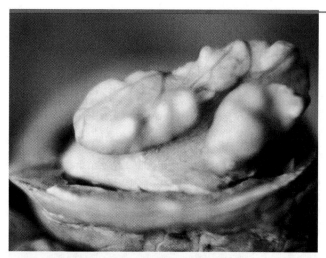

## nutrient-richness chart

Total Nutrient-Richness: **8**
One quarter cup (25 grams) of Walnuts contains 164 calories

| NUTRIENT | AMOUNT | %DV | DENSITY | QUALITY |
|---|---|---|---|---|
| Omega-3 Fatty Acids | 2.3 g | 90.8 | 10.0 | excellent |
| Manganese | 0.9 mg | 42.5 | 4.7 | very good |
| Copper | 0.4 mg | 20.0 | 2.2 | good |
| Tryptophan | 0.1 g | 15.6 | 1.7 | good |

| PHYTOSTEROLS: | | |
|---|---|---|
| Campesterol | 2 mg | Daily values for these nutrients have not yet been established. |
| Beta-Sitosterol | 32 mg | |

For more on "Total Nutrient-Richness," "%DV," "Density," and The World's Healthiest Foods "Quality" Rating System, see page 805.

O riginating in Persia, Walnuts are one of the oldest tree foods and were prized by the Romans who referred to them as the "Royal Nut of Jove." (Jove was the king of their mythological gods.) Today, they remain highly esteemed not only for their delicious flavor, but also for their nutritional value. Add them to a salad in place of croutons, toss them into a "Healthy Sauté," use them as a topping for both vegetables and desserts and enjoy their many health-promoting benefits as part of your "Healthiest Way of Eating."

## why walnuts should be part of your healthiest way of eating

Walnuts are a rich source of heart-healthy monounsaturated fats and an excellent source of those hard-to-find omega-3 fatty acids in the form of alpha-linolenic acid (ALA). Among numerous other benefits, diets rich in ALA have been found to be cardio-protective and provide anti-inflammatory benefits. (For more on the *Health Benefits of Walnuts* and a complete analysis of their content of over 60 nutrients, see page 532.)

### highlights

| | |
|---|---|
| AVAILABILITY: | Year-round |
| REFRIGERATE: | Yes |
| SHELF LIFE: | 6 months in refrigerator; 1 year in freezer |
| PREPARATION: | Minimum |

## varieties of walnuts

It is no surprise that the regal and delicious Walnut comes from an ornamental tree that is highly prized for its beauty. The Walnut kernel consists of two bumpy lobes that look like abstract butterflies. While there are numerous species of Walnut trees, three of the main types of Walnuts are:

### ENGLISH (PERSIAN)

The English Walnut *(Juglans regia)* originated in India and the regions surrounding the Caspian Sea; this is why it is also known as the Persian Walnut. It is the most popular type of Walnut in the United States, featuring a thinner shell than other varieties that is easily broken with a nutcracker. It is the variety featured in the photographs in this chapter.

### BLACK WALNUT

The Black Walnut *(Juglans nigra)* has a thicker shell, which is harder to crack, and a very pungent distinctive flavor.

### WHITE (BUTTERNUT)

The White Walnut *(Juglans cinerea)* features a sweeter and oilier taste than the other two varieties. However, they are not as widely available and may be more difficult to find in the marketplace.

## the peak season available year-round.

## 3 steps for the best tasting and most nutritious walnuts

Enjoying the best tasting Walnuts with the most nutrients is simple if you just follow my 3 easy steps:

1. The Best Way to Select
2. The Best Way to Store
3. The Best Way to Prepare

# 1. the best way to select walnuts

Walnuts are generally available in prepackaged containers as well as bulk bins. Walnuts stored in hermetically sealed containers will last longer than those sold in bulk since their exposure to heat, air and humidity is reduced. If I am going to buy Walnuts from bulk bins, I always check to make sure that the store where I buy Walnuts has a quick turnover of inventory and that the bulk containers are well sealed in order to ensure maximum freshness. The Walnuts should be uniform in color and not limp or shriveled. They should also smell sweet and nutty; be sure they do not smell rancid or musty.

When purchasing whole Walnuts that have not been shelled, I select ones that feel heavy for their size. Their shells should not be cracked, pierced or stained, as this is oftentimes a sign of mold developing on the nutmeat, which makes it unsafe for consumption. As with all nuts, I recommend selecting

organically grown Walnuts whenever possible. (For more on *Organic Foods*, see page 113.)

If you want Walnuts with a roasted flavor and texture, choose ones that have been "dry roasted" as they are not cooked in oil. The commercial roasting process of nuts is often a form of deep-frying, usually in saturated fat, such as coconut or palm kernel oil. Consumption of deep-fried foods has been linked to high levels of LDL (the "bad" form of cholesterol) and to thickening of larger artery walls.

Even "dry roasted" Walnuts may be cooked at high temperatures that damage their natural oils. It is important to read the label to be sure that no additional ingredients such as sugar, corn syrup or preservatives have been added. For the highest quality, least expensive "dry roasted" Walnuts, it's best to just roast them yourself using "The Healthiest Way to Dry Roast Walnuts" (See below.)

# 2. the best way to store walnuts

Due to their high polyunsaturated fat content, Walnuts are extremely perishable and care should be taken in their storage. Shelled Walnuts should be stored in an airtight container and placed in the refrigerator, where they will

keep for 6 months, or the freezer, where they will last for 1 year. Unshelled Walnuts should preferably be stored in a cool, dry, dark place where they will stay fresh for up to 6 months.

# 3. the best way to prepare walnuts

Whole shelled Walnuts can be chopped by hand or can be placed in a food processor. If using a food processor, it is best to pulse on and off a few times instead of running the

blade constantly, as this will help ensure that you end up with chopped Walnuts rather than Walnut butter.

---

### The Healthiest Way to Dry Roast Walnuts

**Dry Roasting Walnuts the healthiest way gives them a lightly roasted flavor and develops their sweetness. It is safe to dry roast Walnuts if done at a low temperature.**

2 cups Walnuts

1. Preheat oven to 160–170°F (70–75°C).
2. Place one layer of Walnuts on a cookie sheet.
3. Roast for 15–20 minutes.

To enhance the "roasted" flavor, try putting a little liquid aminos seasoning or tamari (soy sauce) into a spray bottle and misting the nuts before roasting.

Roasting Walnuts at a temperature higher than 170°F (75°C) will cause a breakdown of their fats and the production of free radicals. Commercially roasted Walnuts have been heated to high temperatures (over 350°F or

175°C) that damage the delicate oils in Walnuts resulting in the formation of free radicals and causing lipid peroxidation—the oxidizing of fats in your bloodstream that can trigger tiny injuries in artery walls—a first step in the buildup of plaque and cardiovascular disease.

Roasted Walnuts have a shorter shelf life and spoil more quickly than raw Walnuts because the unsaturated oils found in nuts oxidize more quickly after exposure to the heat of the roasting process.

Although some find raw nuts more difficult to digest than roasted nuts, this appears to vary greatly between individuals. For more information, see page 69.

# Coconut Walnut Balls

*These are like lemon candy!*
*These non-dairy treats require no baking.*

2 cups Walnuts
1 cup soft dates, pitted
3 TBS fresh lemon juice
1 TBS grated lemon rind
1/8 tsp sea salt
1/3 cup fine grated coconut for coating

1. Coarsely chop the nuts in the food processor.
2. Add dates, lemon juice, lemon rind and salt. Run until well combined, stopping when it starts to stick together but before it makes a ball.
3. Place coconut on a deep dessert plate or saucer.
4. Scoop out 1 TBS of the mixture. Form into a ball and roll in the coconut to coat the outside. Place the ball on a flat baking sheet or tray. Continue until all the dough has been rolled into balls. Let set in refrigerator for at least 1/2 hour to firm up. These will keep in the refrigerator in an airtight container for 1 month.

**Preparation Hints:** If you don't have a lemon zester, cut off thin slices of lemon peel and let the food processor mince it. Chopped nuts may also be used for the coating instead of grated coconut.

If you don't have a food processor, this recipe may be done by hand, which, of course, will take longer. Chop 1$\frac{1}{2}$ cups of Walnuts and 1$\frac{1}{2}$ cups of dates together in two or three batches until finely minced. Chopping them together keeps the dates from sticking together. Place the chopped mixture in a mixing bowl and add the salt, 2 TBS lemon rind and 3 TBS lemon juice, and mix thoroughly. Continue with the recipe as described in step 3.

**MAKES APPROXIMATELY 30 BALLS**

# Healthy Waldorf Chicken Salad

1 medium apple, diced
1 rib celery, diced
1 cup cooked chicken breast, diced
1/4 cup Walnuts, chopped
2 TBS fresh lemon juice
3 TBS extra virgin olive oil
Sea salt and pepper to taste

Combine all ingredients in a medium mixing bowl.

**VARIATIONS:**
• Substitute orange juice for lemon juice.
• Add diced jicama.
• Add 2 TBS dried cranberries.
• Add fresh minced dill.

---

**HEALTH-PROMOTING DISCOVERY**

**WALNUTS AND OMEGA-3 FATTY ACIDS**

Walnuts are an excellent source of alpha-linolenic acid (ALA), a form of omega-3 essential fatty acids that is noted as essential because the body cannot produce ALA on its own but must receive it through the diet. ALA has many important functions including being a readily used source of energy and playing a role in skin health; it also helps to combat inflammation and is a precursor to EDA and DMA. Walnuts' concentration of omega-3s (a quarter-cup provides more than 90% of the daily value for these essential fats) is one reason for their many health benefits, ranging from cardiovascular protection to anti-inflammatory effects. (For more on *Omega-Fatty-3 Acids*, see page 770.)

---

**Q** *I know that Walnuts are a source of omega-3s, but I also thought that they contained a lot of omega-6s as well. What is the ratio of Omega-6:3 in Walnuts and are they beneficial? I am trying to reduce the omega-6:3 ratio in my diet as I know it is better for my overall health.*

**A** Foods that contain omega-3 fatty acids (even salmon, one of the most renowned sources of these nutrients) will usually also contain omega-6 fatty acids as well. So, the fact that Walnuts contain them is no surprise. Yet, the ratio between omega-6 and omega-3 is about 4:1 in Walnuts, which is a much lower ratio than in many foods. Researchers estimate that many people who follow a Western diet have a omega-6:omega-3 ratio of about 20:1 and propose that closer to 2:1 would help reduce the incidence of inflammatory diseases. So, as you see, the ratio of these fatty acids in Walnuts falls within the overall target. This is why Walnuts are one of the recommended foods for individuals who are trying to increase their omega-3 intake, reduce their omega-6 intake, and shift the balance of essential fatty acids. It is important to remember that it is not just about adding the Walnuts, for example, to your diet, but trying to have them replace another food that may contain more omega-6s and less omega-3s.

There are other foods that are rich in omega-3s and have an even lower omega-6 to omega-3 ratio than Walnuts. These include flaxseeds (0.24:1) and cold-water fish such as salmon (0.18:1).

STEP-BY-STEP RECIPE
## The Healthiest Ways of Preparing Walnuts

# *Arugula Salad with Walnut Croutons*

*Top this quick and tasty salad with Walnut croutons.*

1/2 medium yellow onion, thinly sliced
1 cup hot water
2 TBS light vinegar
1 bunch arugula

Dressing:
2 medium cloves garlic, pressed
2 TBS chopped fresh parsley
1 TBS fresh lemon juice
2 TBS extra virgin olive oil
Sea salt and black pepper to taste

1/4 cup coarsely chopped Walnuts
Optional: 2 oz gorgonzola cheese

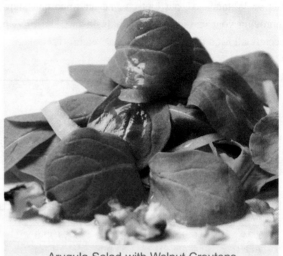

Arugula Salad with Walnut Croutons

1. Press garlic and let sit for 5 minutes (Why?, see page 261)

2. Slice onion thin and soak in hot water and vinegar while preparing rest of salad.

3. Whisk together the dressing ingredients, adding olive oil at the end, a little at a time.

4. Wash and dry arugula. Squeeze out excess liquid from onions. Combine onions and arugula and toss with dressing. Sprinkle salad with Walnuts just before serving. Top with cheese (optional).

**Preparation Hint:** Make sure your arugula is young and tender as older leaves can be quite bitter.

**SERVES 2**

Please write (address on back cover flap) or e-mail me at info@whfoods.org with your personal ideas for preparing Walnuts, and I will share them with others through our website at www.whfoods.org.

## 9 QUICK SERVING IDEAS for WALNUTS:

1. Add Walnuts, diced apple and cinnamon to cooked oatmeal.
2. Mix crushed Walnuts into plain yogurt and top with maple syrup.
3. Add Walnuts to green salads in place of croutons.
4. Garnish cooked grains with chopped Walnuts.
5. Sprinkle chopped Walnuts on your favorite vegetable dish.
6. **For an Energizing Snack:** Combine Walnuts, sunflower seeds, raisins and other favorite dried fruits such as dried cranberries or blueberries.
7. **Green Beans and Walnut Salad:** Combine 2 cups cold cooked green beans, slices of 1 orange, a thinly sliced medium-size red onion, 1 TBS fresh lemon juice, 3 TBS extra virgin olive oil, and sea salt and black pepper to taste. Top with 1 tsp minced tarragon and 3 TBS chopped Walnuts.
8. **Lentil Walnut Dip:** Purée 1 cup Walnuts, 1 cup cooked lentils and your favorite herbs and spices in a food processor. Add enough extra virgin olive oil to achieve a dip-like consistency. Season with sea salt and pepper to taste.
9. **Cranberry Walnut Chutney:** In a small mixing bowl, combine 1/3 cup dried cranberries and the juice of 1 orange. Combine 1/3 cup of chopped Walnuts and 1/2 finely diced apple and add to cranberry mixture. Add cinnamon and cayenne pepper to taste. Serve with cooked chicken breast or turkey.

# health benefits of walnuts

## Promote Heart Health

Adding Walnuts to your diet can be an important step in improving your cardiovascular health. In fact, the FDA has recently allowed the health claim that "eating 1.5 ounces per day of Walnuts as part of a diet low in saturated fat and cholesterol may reduce the risk of heart disease."

Walnuts are an excellent source of monounsaturated fats—approximately 15% of the fat found in Walnuts is healthful monounsaturated fat. A host of studies have shown that increasing the dietary intake of Walnuts has favorable effects on high cholesterol levels and other cardiovascular risk factors. Two recent studies compared individuals on a Mediterranean diet to those on a diet that contained the same calorie and fat content but where Walnuts were substituted for other monounsaturated fat-rich foods (such as olives and olive oil). It turns out that the individuals on the Walnut-rich diet showed lower levels of cardiovascular risk factors, including total cholesterol, LDL cholesterol, C-reactive protein and lipoprotein(a). In the study that measured arterial function, it was found to improve on the Walnut-rich diet.

The other cardio-protective nutrients for which Walnuts are a concentrated source include alpha-linolenic acid (ALA) and the amino acid l-arginine. Walnuts are an excellent source of omega-3 fatty acids in the form of ALA, which is a precursor to the EPA and DHA found in fish. Diets rich in ALA are associated with a reduced risk of heart disease as well as lower levels of cholesterol and triglycerides. Since Walnuts contain relatively high levels of the amino acid l-arginine, they may also be of special benefit when it comes to hypertension. In the body, l-arginine is converted into nitric oxide, a nutrient that helps keep the inner walls of blood vessels smooth and allows blood vessels to relax. (For more on plant-based *Omega-3 Fatty Acids*, see page 770.)

## Promote Optimal Health

Walnuts are a good source of copper and manganese, two minerals that are essential cofactors in a number of enzymes important in antioxidant defenses. For example, the key oxidative enzyme *superoxide dismutase* requires both copper and manganese. Walnuts are also a concentrated source of phytonutrients with researchers recently identifying 16 polyphenols in Walnuts with powerful antioxidant activity, including three new tannins. One of these compounds is ellagic acid, which seems to block the metabolic pathways that can lead to cancer. Ellagic acid not only helps protect healthy cells from free radical damage, but also helps detoxify potential cancer-causing substances and helps prevent cancer cells from replicating.

## Additional Health-Promoting Benefit of Walnuts

Walnuts are a concentrated source of sleep-promoting tryptophan.

### Nutritional Analysis of 1/4 cup of Walnuts:

| NUTRIENT | AMOUNT | % DAILY VALUE | NUTRIENT | AMOUNT | % DAILY VALUE |
|---|---|---|---|---|---|
| Calories | 163.50 | | Pantothenic Acid | 0.14 mg | 1.40 |
| Calories from Fat | 146.72 | | | | |
| Calories from Saturated Fat | 13.78 | | **Minerals** | | |
| Protein | 3.81 g | | Boron | — mcg | |
| Carbohydrates | 3.43 g | | Calcium | 26.00 mg | 2.60 |
| Dietary Fiber | 1.68 g | 6.72 | Chloride | 6.00 mg | |
| Soluble Fiber | 0.40 g | | Chromium | — mcg | — |
| Insoluble Fiber | 0.81 g | | Copper | 0.40 mg | 20.00 |
| Sugar – Total | 0.65 g | | Fluoride | — mg | — |
| Monosaccharides | 0.00 g | | Iodine | 2.25 mcg | 1.50 |
| Disaccharides | 0.53 g | | Iron | 0.73 mg | 4.06 |
| Other Carbs | 1.10 g | | Magnesium | 39.50 mg | 9.88 |
| Fat – Total | 16.30 g | | Manganese | 0.85 mg | 42.50 |
| Saturated Fat | 1.53 g | | Molybdenum | 7.38 mcg | 9.84 |
| Mono Fat | 2.23 g | | Phosphorus | 86.50 mg | 8.65 |
| Poly Fat | 11.79 g | | Potassium | 110.25 mg | |
| Omega-3 Fatty Acids | 2.27 g | 90.80 | Selenium | 1.15 mcg | 1.64 |
| Omega-6 Fatty Acids | 9.52 g | | Sodium | 0.50 mg | |
| Trans Fatty Acids | 0.00 g | | Zinc | 0.77 mg | 5.13 |
| Cholesterol | 0.00 mg | | | | |
| Water | 1.02 g | | **Amino Acids** | | |
| Ash | 0.45 g | | Alanine | 0.17 g | |
| | | | Arginine | 0.55 g | |
| **Vitamins** | | | Aspartate | 0.44 g | |
| Vitamin A IU | 10.25 IU | 0.20 | Cystine | 0.05 g | 12.20 |
| Vitamin A RE | 1.00 RE | | Glutamate | 0.68 g | |
| A - Carotenoid | 1.00 RE | 0.01 | Glycine | 0.20 g | |
| A - Retinol | 0.00 RE | | Histidine | 0.09 g | 6.98 |
| B1 Thiamin | 0.09 mg | 6.00 | Isoleucine | 0.15 g | 13.04 |
| B2 Riboflavin | 0.04 mg | 2.35 | Leucine | 0.28 g | 11.07 |
| B3 Niacin | 0.48 mg | 2.40 | Lysine | 0.10 g | 4.26 |
| Niacin Equiv | 1.23 mg | | Methionine | 0.06 g | 8.11 |
| Vitamin B6 | 0.13 mg | 6.50 | Phenylalanine | 0.17 g | 14.29 |
| Vitamin B12 | 0.00 mcg | 0.00 | Proline | 0.17 g | |
| Biotin | 4.75 mcg | 1.58 | Serine | 0.23 g | |
| Vitamin C | 0.33 mg | 0.55 | Threonine | 0.14 g | 11.29 |
| Vitamin D IU | 0.00 IU | 0.00 | Tryptophan | 0.05 g | 15.63 |
| Vitamin D mcg | 0.00 mcg | | Tyrosine | 0.10 g | 10.31 |
| Vitamin E Alpha Equiv | 0.74 mg | 3.70 | Valine | 0.18 g | 12.24 |
| Vitamin E IU | 1.10 IU | | | | |
| Vitamin E mg | 0.74 mg | | | | |
| Folate | 24.50 mcg | 6.13 | | | |
| Vitamin K | 0.68 mcg | 0.85 | | | |

(Note: "–" indicates data is unavailable. For more information, please see page 806.)

## Q&A

**Q** IS IT TRUE THAT WALNUTS AND FLAXSEEDS ARE NOT A GOOD SOURCE OF OMEGA-3s FOR SOME PEOPLE?

While walnuts and flaxseeds are rich in a type of omega-3 fats, they may not serve as a good source of omega-3s overall for some people. Understanding some of the basic issues involved with walnuts and flaxseeds—and in fact, any kind of plant food—and omega-3 nourishment can help you to optimize your nutritional intake and your overall health.

While walnuts and flaxseeds are an excellent source of omega-3 fat, they only contain one basic member of the omega-3 fat family. Virtually all of the omega-3 fat is found in the form of alpha-linolenic acid (ALA).

### The Omega-3 Assembly Line Starts With ALA

So that you can better understand how the fact that walnuts and flaxseeds feature a concentration of ALA impacts their potential ability to be an overall good source of omega-3s, let's start with a basic chemistry review of the omega-3 family of fats.

Omega-3s are a very diverse group of fats. Yet, all of the members fall into a basic pattern that can be imagined as a kind of metabolic assembly line.

Fats can be measured in length according to the number of carbon atoms that they contain. ALA, which is concentrated in walnuts and flaxseeds, has 18 carbons, making it the shortest of the omega-3 fats, and hence the simplest. It retains a position at the beginning of the assembly line with our omega-3 metabolism starting with this compound as a building block.

### ALA Gets Elongated Into Other Omega-3 Fatty Acids

If another pair of carbon atoms gets added on to ALA (a process called "elongation" in biochemistry, and a process that is carried out by enzymes called *elongases*), it gets ready to become EPA (eicosapentaenoic acid), another important member of the omega-3 family. If yet another pair of carbons are added to EPA, it gets ready to become DHA (docosahexaenoic acid), a third important member of the omega-3s.

### ALA Gets Desaturated Into Other Omega-3 Fatty Acids

The reason we say that these omega-3 fats "get ready" to turn into other forms is because getting longer is not the only requirement for conversion of one omega-3 into another. A second requirement is what's called "increased desaturation." During this process, the omega-3 fat gets altered chemically so that its carbon atoms are connected together in a new way that provides more flexibility to the fat. This new kind of connection is called double-bonding. For ALA to become EPA, two new double bonds must be added in addition to the two-carbon-atom increase in length.

### The Role of Other Nutrients in Omega-3 Metabolism

The process of lengthening and changing, of elongating and desaturating, the chemical bonds in omega-3 fat is complex, and many nutrients are required to bring it about. To get from ALA to EPA, for example, the required nutrients are vitamin B3, vitamin B6, vitamin C, zinc and magnesium.

### Nutrient Deficiencies Can Block Omega-3 Metabolism

What happens if an individual is deficient in one or more of the above nutrients? The answer is simple: that individual cannot convert ALA very efficiently (or at all) into the other omega-3 fats that are longer. In severe deficiency, the critical omega-3 fats, EPA and DHA, could simply not be made. People with known deficiencies in most of the above nutrients (vitamins B3, B6 and C, and the minerals zinc and magnesium) would not be able to get maximum benefit from walnuts and flaxseeds because they would not be able to convert the ALA into the other omega-3 fats.

In the above situation, many healthcare practitioners would ask for an increase in the omega-3 supportive nutrients (the B-complex vitamins, vitamin C, zinc and magnesium), and at the same time, they would ask for a different source of omega-3s, such as preformed EPA and DHA from salmon and other fish, until the nutrient deficiencies were resolved. Yet, in cases where the assembly line seems to be functioning properly, many healthcare practitioners opt for walnuts and flaxseeds since providing the body with the compound that is at the beginning of the assembly line allows the body to best decide the exact types and proportions of omega-3s it wants to create.

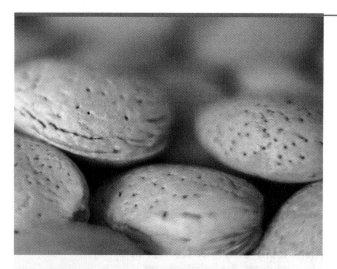

# almonds

## nutrient-richness chart

Total Nutrient-Richness: **7**
One-quarter cup (35 grams) of Almonds contains 213 calories

| NUTRIENT | AMOUNT | %DV | DENSITY | QUALITY |
|---|---|---|---|---|
| Manganese | 0.9 mg | 45.0 | 3.9 | very good |
| Vitamin E | 9.0 mg | 44.9 | 3.9 | very good |
| Magnesium | 98.7 mg | 24.7 | 2.2 | good |
| Tryptophan | 0.1 g | 21.9 | 1.9 | good |
| Copper | 0.4 mg | 20.0 | 1.7 | good |
| B2 Riboflavin | 0.3 mg | 17.6 | 1.5 | good |
| Phosphorus | 168.7 mg | 16.9 | 1.5 | good |

**PHYTOSTEROLS:**

| | | |
|---|---|---|
| Stigmasterol | 41 mg | Daily values for these nutrients have not yet been established. |
| Campesterol | 1 mg | |
| Beta-Sitosterol | 38 mg | |

For more on "Total Nutrient-Richness," "%DV," "Density," and
The World's Healthiest Foods "Quality" Rating System, see page 805.

Almonds have been revered by cultures throughout history. In Biblical times, Almonds were held in high regard as among "the best fruits of the land." The Romans considered them a sign of fertility, happiness and romance; they showered newlywed couples with Almonds for good health and fortune. In Israel, it is still common practice to plant an Almond tree as a memorial. Delicately flavored and versatile, Almonds can complement the flavors of almost any type of dish. They are satisfying, nutritious and easy to carry, making them the perfect snack and a great addition to your "Healthiest Way of Eating."

## why almonds should be part of your healthiest way of eating

Almonds are often referred to as "the King of Nuts" because of their high nutritional value. Nuts, such as Almonds, have actually received qualified health claim (QHC) status from the U.S. Food and Drug Administration, in recognition that eating 1.5 ounces (of most nuts) per day will provide special health benefits. Almonds are a very good source of vitamin E and, like other varieties of nuts, are a concentrated source of monounsaturated fats, which make them a very good food for a healthy heart. (For more on the *Health Benefits of Almonds* and a complete analysis of their content of over 60 nutrients, see page 538.)

## varieties of almonds

Almonds *(Prunus amygdalu)* were thought to have originated in regions of western Asia and North Africa. The Almond that we think of as a nut is technically the seed of the fruit of the Almond tree, a medium-size tree that bears fragrant pink and white flowers. Like its cousins, the peach, cherry and apricot trees, the Almond tree bears fruits with stone-like seeds (or pits) within. The seed of the Almond fruit is what we refer to as the Almond nut. Almonds are off-white in color, covered by a thin brownish skin, and encased in a hard shell. They are classified into two categories: sweet and bitter.

### SWEET ALMONDS

These are the edible variety of Almonds. They are oval in shape with a wonderfully buttery taste. They are available in markets in their shell or with their shell removed. Shelled Almonds are available whole, sliced or slivered in either their natural form with their skin or blanched with their skin removed. This is the variety featured in the photographs in this chapter.

#### Jordan Almonds

A Mediterranean variety imported from Spain. It has a semi-hard shell and a rich, sweet Almond flavor. It is the most popular variety of sweet Almonds.

**Nonpareil**

A variety cultivated in California that has a paper thin shell.

### BITTER ALMONDS

These are used to make Almond oil, a flavoring agent for foods and liqueurs such as Amaretto. They are otherwise inedible as they naturally contain toxic substances such as hydrocyanic acid. These compounds are removed in the manufacturing process.

### GREEN ALMONDS

The seed inside these furry green fruits is the actual Almond. When mature Almonds are harvested, the fruit portion is discarded, but when they are green, they can be eaten and have the crunch and taste of an unripe peach. At this stage, the seed or Almond has not yet hardened and is soft and jelly-like.

## the peak season

Almonds in the shell are the freshest and can be found most easily from fall to early winter. Packaged raw and roasted Almonds are available throughout the year.

## biochemical considerations

Almonds are a concentrated source of oxalates, which might be of concern to certain individuals. (For more on *Oxalates*, see page 725.)

## 3 steps for the best tasting and most nutritious almonds

Enjoying the best tasting Almonds with the most nutrients is simple if you just follow my 3 easy steps:

1. The Best Way to Select
2. The Best Way to Store
3. The Best Way to Prepare

# 1. the best way to select almonds

Almonds that are still in their shells have the longest shelf life. I look for shells that are not split, moldy or stained. Shelled Almonds that are stored in a hermetically sealed container will last longer than those that are sold in bulk bins since their exposure to heat, air and humidity is reduced. As with all nuts, I recommend selecting organically grown varieties whenever possible. (For more on *Organic Foods*, see page 113.)

If I am going to buy Almonds from bulk bins, I always check to make sure that the store where I buy Almonds has a quick turnover of inventory and that the bulk containers are well sealed in order to ensure maximum freshness. The Almonds should be uniform in color and not limp or shriveled. They should also smell sweet and nutty; if their odor is sharp or bitter, they are rancid.

If you want Almonds with a roasted flavor and texture, choose ones that have been "dry roasted" as they are not cooked in oil. The commercial roasting process of nuts is often a form of deep-frying, usually in saturated fat, such as coconut or palm kernel oil. Deep-fried foods have been linked to high levels of LDL (the "bad" form of cholesterol) and to thickening of larger artery walls.

Even "dry roasted" Almonds may be cooked at high temperatures that damage their natural oils. It is important to read the label to be sure that no additional ingredients such as sugar, corn syrup or preservatives have been added. For the highest quality, least expensive "dry roasted" Almonds, it's best to just roast them yourself using the "Healthiest Way to Dry Roast Almonds." (See page 536.)

# 2. the best way to store almonds

Since Almonds have a high fat content, it is important to store them properly in order to protect them from becoming rancid. Store shelled Almonds in a tightly sealed container in a cool dry place away from exposure to sunlight. Keeping them cold will further protect them from rancidity and prolong their freshness. Refrigerated Almonds will keep for 6 months, while Almonds stored in the freezer can be kept for up to 1 year. Shelled Almond pieces will become rancid more quickly than whole shelled Almonds. Almonds still in the shell have the longest shelf life.

# 3. the best way to prepare almonds

Whole shelled Almonds can be chopped by hand or can be placed in a food processor. If using a food processor, it is best to pulse on and off a few times instead of running the blade constantly, as this will help ensure that you end up with chopped Almonds rather than Almond butter. To peel Almonds, "blanch" them by bringing a small amount of water to a boil. Add Almonds and simmer for just about 2 minutes. Drain and slip off peels.

## The Healthiest Way to Dry Roast Almonds

**Dry Roasting Almonds the healthiest way brings out their flavor and develops their sweetness. It is safe to dry roast Almonds if done at a low temperature.**

2 cups Almonds

1. Preheat oven to 160–170°F (70–75°C).
2. Place one layer of Almonds on a cookie sheet.
3. Roast for 15–20 minutes.

To enhance the "roasted" flavor, try putting a little liquid aminos seasoning or tamari (soy sauce) into a spray bottle and misting the nuts before roasting.

Roasting Almonds at a temperature higher than 170°F (75°C) will cause a breakdown of their fats and the production of free-radicals. Commercially roasted Almonds have been heated to high temperatures (over 350°F or 175°C) that damage their delicate oils, resulting in the formation of free-radicals and causing lipid peroxidation—the oxidizing of fats in your bloodstream, which can trigger tiny injuries in artery walls—a first step in the buildup of plaque and cardiovascular disease.

Roasted Almonds have a shorter shelf life and spoil more quickly than raw Almonds because the unsaturated oils found in nuts oxidize more quickly after exposure to the heat of the roasting process.

Although some find raw nuts more difficult to digest than roasted nuts, this appears to vary greatly between individuals.

For more information, see page 69.

## 14 QUICK SERVING IDEAS for ALMONDS:

1. Top your morning cereal with chopped Almonds.
2. Add a crunch to plain yogurt by mixing in some chopped Almonds and dried fruit.
3. Add some Almond butter to a breakfast shake to boost its taste and protein content.
4. Spread Almond butter on apple slices or combine Almond butter with apple slices or whole grain crackers to make a wonderfully simple, on-the-go power snack.
5. Eat Almonds as a quick, substantial snack. Keep some in the car!
6. Sprinkle toasted or raw sliced Almonds onto your green salad.
7. Enhance the protein content of "Healthy Sautéed" vegetables with sliced Almonds.
8. Top your favorite fruit (apricots are great) with Lemon Sauce (see page 431) and sliced Almonds.
9. **Almond Energizer:** Stuff dried figs, dates or plums with whole Almonds.
10. **Rice Salad with Almonds:** Make a delightful cold rice salad with Almonds, fresh garden peas and currants.
11. **Almonds for Breakfast:** Serve blueberries or strawberries with almond milk (see next page) and chopped Almonds.
12. **Fish Amandine:** Combine sliced toasted Almonds with extra virgin olive oil and serve on white fish.
13. **Almond Butter:** Grind toasted Almonds in food processor until they achieve a pasty texture and the natural oils begin to appear from the Almonds. Spread on toast or fruit, such as apples and pears.
14. **Almond Butter and Banana Sandwich:** Make an open-faced sandwich of Almond butter and bananas drizzled with either maple syrup or honey and sprinkled with cinnamon.

**Q** *If you eat the blanched variety of Almonds, do you still enjoy the same health benefits as if you ate those with the skin?*

**A** While the blanched variety of Almonds will still provide you with many nutritional benefits, the skin does have additional properties. It is very rich in flavonoid phytonutrients that have powerful antioxidant properties. While there is some debate over the relationship between Almond skins, enzyme inhibitors and digestibility, I believe that Almond skins are worth eating as long as they don't bring along with them any evidence of poor digestion or allergic reaction.

**Q** *My friend told me that Almonds contain toxic compounds? Is that true?*

**A** Almonds are generally grouped into two classifications: sweet Almonds (*Prunus amygdaulus* var. *dulcis*) and bitter Almonds (*Prunus amygdalus* var. *amara*). The former is the type that we commonly eat and refer to as an "Almond." The latter is often used for its essential oil as the basis of almond essence for flavorings, including being used in the liqueur Amaretto. Yet, before extracting the oil from bitter Almonds, manufacturers have to remove the toxic substances that these Almonds contain. These substances include hydrocanic acid, which give these Almonds their bitter flavor. Potentially, it was these bitter Almonds to which your friend was referring.

STEP-BY-STEP RECIPES
## The Healthiest Ways of Preparing Almonds

# Almond Date Balls

*Special treat for any occasion.*

1 cup raw Almonds
1/2 cup pitted dates
1 TBS water
1½ tsp cinnamon
1/2 tsp almond extract
1/8 tsp sea salt
Optional: coconut flakes

1. Using a food processor with an S-blade, process the Almonds until they are in small pieces. Remove half of the Almonds and set aside.

2. Add dates to the remaining Almonds and process until the mixture is a fine meal.

3. Add remaining ingredients and process until the mixture begins to stick together. You may need to scrape down the bowl with a rubber spatula.

4. By hand, mix date mixture with the reserved Almond pieces.

5. Form 1-inch balls from the dough. Store in the refrigerator up to one week.

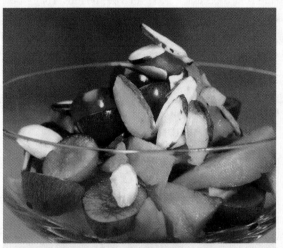

Top Your Favorite Fruit with Almonds

**Optional:** Roll the balls in coconut flakes.

**Preparation Hints:**
- You must use a food processor for this recipe.
- Rubbing a little oil on your hands will make rolling the balls easier.

MAKES **10–12** BALLS

# Almond Milk

*A great alternative to cow's milk or soy milk.*

1 cup Almonds, soaked overnight
3 pitted dates
Pinch of sea salt
3 cups water

1. Combine almonds, pitted dates, salt and water in a blender and blend on high for 2 minutes.

2. Strain through a cheesecloth-lined strainer into a large measuring cup or bowl. Store in a glass jar in the refrigerator for up to 3 days.

YIELDS ABOUT **4** CUPS

**Flavor Tips:** 1. Serve on cereal or berries.  2. Blend with a banana or apple.  3. Use in tea.

# Sweet and Hot Almond Dressing

*This is a hearty dressing for a vegetable salad.*

1/2 cup Almond butter
1 clove garlic, pressed
3 TBS maple syrup
2 TBS tamari (soy sauce)
1+ tsp hot chili sauce

In a small mixing bowl, whisk together all ingredients and add enough water to make the sauce the consistency of thick cream. Add more hot chili sauce for a spicier dressing.

HOW TO ENJOY SWEET AND HOT ALMOND DRESSING:
- Use as a dipping sauce for crudités.
- Spread on a vegetable wrap.
- Drizzle over broccoli or snow peas.
- Add 1 TBS of Dijon mustard to dressing and serve on top of cooked salmon or chicken breast.

SERVES **4–6**

Please write (address on back cover flap) or e-mail me at info@whfoods.org with your personal ideas for preparing Almonds, and I will share them with others through our website at www.whfoods.org.

# health benefits of almonds

## Promote Heart Health

A high-fat food that's good for your health? That's not an oxymoron, it's Almonds. In human feeding trials, substituting Almonds for more traditional fats has led to an 8–12% reduction of atherosclerosis-promoting LDL cholesterol. In addition, five large-scale human epidemiological studies all found that nut consumption is linked to a lower risk of heart disease.

One reason that Almonds may promote heart health is that they are high in monounsaturated fats, the same type of health-promoting fats as are found in olive oil; monounsaturated fats have been associated with lower levels of LDL cholesterol as well as reduced risk of heart disease. Almonds are also a very good source of vitamin E, which may also help to explain their cardiovascular-health-promoting properties since this nutrient can help to stop LDL oxidation, a process linked to atherosclerosis.

## Promote Healthy Weight

Preliminary research suggests that Almonds may benefit your waistline. Results from a recent study found that an Almond-enriched, low-calorie diet helped overweight individuals shed pounds more effectively than a low-calorie diet high in complex carbohydrates. Both test diets supplied the same number of calories and equivalent amounts of protein. Those eating Almonds experienced a 62% greater reduction in their weight/BMI (body mass index), 50% greater reduction in waist circumference and 56% greater reduction in body fat compared to those on the low-calorie, high-carbohydrate diet. Among those subjects who had type 1 diabetes, medication reductions were sustained or further reduced in 96% of those on the Almond-enriched diet versus in 50% of those on the complex carbohydrate diet.

## Promote Digestive System Health

In an animal study of the effect of Almonds on colon cancer, animals were exposed to a colon cancer-causing agent and fed Almond meal, Almond oil, whole Almonds or a control diet containing no Almonds. The animals given whole Almonds showed fewer signs of colon cancer, including fewer rapidly dividing cells. One reason may be the dietary fiber that is concentrated in Almonds.

Almonds' digestive health benefits may also extend to gallbladder health. Twenty years of dietary data found that women who eat at least one ounce of nuts, such as Almonds, or peanuts or peanut butter each week have a 25% lower risk of developing gallstones.

## Additional Health-Promoting Benefit of Almonds

Almonds are also a concentrated source of other nutrients providing additional health-promoting benefits. These include bone-building magnesium, manganese, copper and phosphorus; energy-producing vitamin B2 and sleep-promoting tryptophan.

### Nutritional Analysis of 1/4 cup of Almonds:

| NUTRIENT | AMOUNT | % DAILY VALUE |
|---|---|---|
| Calories | 205.96 | |
| Calories from Fat | 164.04 | |
| Calories from Saturated Fat | 12.57 | |
| Protein | 7.62 g | |
| Carbohydrates | 6.66 g | |
| Dietary Fiber | 4.07 g | 16.28 |
| Soluble Fiber | 0.45 g | |
| Insoluble Fiber | 3.62 g | |
| Sugar - Total | 1.69 g | |
| Monosaccharides | 0.01 g | |
| Disaccharides | 1.68 g | |
| Other Carbs | 0.89 g | |
| Fat–Total | 18.23 g | |
| Saturated Fat | 1.40 g | |
| Mono Fat | 11.61 g | |
| Poly Fat | 4.36 g | |
| Omega-3 Fatty Acids | 0.00 g | 0.00 |
| Omega-6 Fatty Acids | 4.36 g | |
| Trans fatty acids | 0.00 g | |
| Cholesterol | 0.00 mg | |
| Water | 0.90 g | |
| Ash | 1.10 g | |

| Vitamins | | |
|---|---|---|
| Vitamin A IU | 0.34 IU | 0.01 |
| Vitamin A RE | 0.03 RE | |
| A - Carotenoid | 0.03 RE | 0.00 |
| A - Retinol | 0.00 RE | |
| B1 Thiamin | 0.03 mg | 2.00 |
| B2 Riboflavin | 0.30 mg | 17.65 |
| B3 Niacin | 1.33 mg | 6.65 |
| Niacin Equiv | 2.44 mg | |
| Vitamin B6 | 0.04 mg | 2.00 |
| Vitamin B12 | 0.00 mcg | 0.00 |
| Biotin | 22.08 mcg | 7.36 |
| Vitamin C | 0.00 mg | 0.00 |
| Vitamin D IU | — IU | — |
| Vitamin D mcg | — mcg | |
| Vitamin E Alpha Equiv | 8.97 mg | 44.85 |
| Vitamin E IU | 13.37 IU | |
| Vitamin E mg | 8.97 mg | |
| Folate | 11.39 mcg | 2.85 |
| Vitamin K | 0.00 mcg | 0.00 |

| NUTRIENT | AMOUNT | % DAILY VALUE |
|---|---|---|
| Pantothenic Acid | 0.08 mg | 0.80 |

| Minerals | | |
|---|---|---|
| Boron | — mcg | |
| Calcium | 91.77 mg | 9.18 |
| Chloride | — mg | |
| Chromium | — mcg | — |
| Copper | 0.40 mg | 20.00 |
| Fluoride | — mg | — |
| Iodine | — mcg | — |
| Iron | 1.56 mg | 8.67 |
| Magnesium | 98.67 mg | 24.67 |
| Manganese | 0.90 mg | 45.00 |
| Molybdenum | 10.18 mcg | 13.57 |
| Phosphorus | 168.70 mg | 16.87 |
| Potassium | 257.37 mg | |
| Selenium | 0.97 mcg | 1.39 |
| Sodium | 0.34 mg | |
| Zinc | 1.22 mg | 8.13 |

| Amino Acids | | |
|---|---|---|
| Alanine | 0.35 g | |
| Arginine | 0.85 g | |
| Aspartate | 0.95 g | |
| Cystine | 0.10 g | 24.39 |
| Glutamate | 1.79 g | |
| Glycine | 0.51 g | |
| Histidine | 0.21 g | 16.28 |
| Isoleucine | 0.24 g | 20.87 |
| Leucine | 0.51 g | 20.16 |
| Lysine | 0.21 g | 8.94 |
| Methionine | 0.07 g | 9.46 |
| Phenylalanine | 0.40 g | 33.61 |
| Proline | 0.34 g | |
| Serine | 0.35 g | |
| Threonine | 0.23 g | 18.55 |
| Tryptophan | 0.07 g | 21.88 |
| Tyrosine | 0.18 g | 18.56 |
| Valine | 0.28 g | 19.05 |

(Note: "—" indicates data is unavailable. For more information, please see page 806.)

**Q** *Can you please confirm that the Almond is actually a fruit, the seed of which we eat, as opposed to a nut? What qualifies a nut as a real nut, and when is a nut really a fruit?*

**A** The Almond that we think of as a nut is technically the seed of the fruit of the Almond tree, a medium-size tree that bears fragrant pink and white flowers. Like its cousins, the peach, cherry and apricot tree, the Almond tree bears fruits with stone-like seeds (or pits) within. The seed of the Almond fruit is what we refer to as the Almond nut.

Yet, when are other "nuts" really nuts and when are they something other than a nut? I think it first depends upon how you use the term. For example, tomatoes and avocados are technically and botanically considered fruits, but in "culinary language" we call them vegetables.

In the botanical sense, a nut is a dry fruit with one (or sometimes two) seeds produced by plants in the botanical order *Fagales*. These include walnuts, chestnuts and pecans. But not all "nuts" are commonly edible, such as the nuts from the stone-oak tree, which is very bitter.

In terms of a more culinary and common definition, an oil-containing seed or kernel contained in a shell is often known as a nut. It is this category that is obviously more inclusive and contains such "non-nuts" as Almonds, peanuts and Brazil nuts.

**Q** *Do Almonds contain the "alpha tocopherol" type Vitamin E?*

**A** Almonds contain a range of naturally occurring forms of vitamin E, including the alpha-tocopherols, gamma-tocopherols and tocotrienols. That's one of the amazing benefits of eating a whole food—whole foods give us the widest variety of nutrients available.

## Q&A

**I LOVE ALMONDS. I USUALLY EAT 1 CUP PER DAY. IS IT HEALTHY TO EAT SO MANY IF I'M TRYING TO LOSE WEIGHT?**

Almonds are a very healthy food, providing good fats as well as important vitamins and minerals. Yet, a lot of a good thing is not necessarily a good thing. Eating that many almonds may stand in your way of losing a few pounds depending upon what the rest of your diet is like and what your overall caloric intake is.

Each cup of almonds contains 824 calories. Since reducing caloric intake by 3,500 calories would be associated with one pound of weight loss, reducing your intake of almonds but maintaining your current dietary intake would allow you to lose weight. For example, by cutting down to one-quarter cup of almonds each day you would reduce your caloric intake by 618 calories, which would allow you to lose one pound in about six days.

There is actually not a fixed amount of almonds that would be allowed or not allowed on a person's diet. The right amount depends upon the rest of the food consumed. Is there room in the diet for much fat? What vitamins and minerals are needed? Do almonds contain the nutrients that are needed? Unless you know the answers to these questions, you cannot make a helpful decision about the right amount of almonds to eat.

If these kinds of questions are unfamiliar to you, you may want to meet with a healthcare practitioner, such as a nutritionist, who can help you evaluate your nutritional needs. In general, it would be unusual to balance a diet that contained more than one-third cup of almonds. That amount would provide 275 calories and 24 grams of fat. The 275 calories would be about 14% of a 2,000-calorie diet—about as much as most people would want from a single food. But once again, these numbers are only a general description and cannot help you decide exactly what nutrients you need.

If you find that that you are eating that many almonds because you are a "boredom eater," you are definitely not alone. Many people eat to keep themselves occupied and to have a hand-to-mouth activity.

If you wanted to cut back on your almond snacking, I would suggest snacking on other foods that are lower in calories and that would provide other nutrients not provided by the almonds. For example, vegetables are a great snack. Some of my favorites are broccoli, carrots, cucumbers, bell peppers…the list goes on and on. The great thing about vegetables is that they take a while to chew and are very filling, while being nutrient-rich and low in calories.

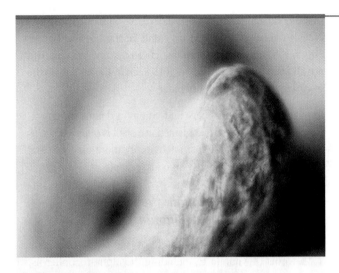

# peanuts

## highlights

| | |
|---|---|
| AVAILABILITY: | Year-round |
| REFRIGERATE: | Yes |
| SHELF LIFE: | 6 months in the refrigerator; 1 year in the freezer |
| PREPARATION: | Minimal |

## nutrient-richness chart

Total Nutrient-Richness: **6**

One-quarter cup (37 grams) of Peanuts contains 207 calories

| NUTRIENT | AMOUNT | %DV | DENSITY | QUALITY |
|---|---|---|---|---|
| Manganese | 0.7 mg | 35.5 | 3.1 | good |
| Tryptophan | 0.1 g | 28.1 | 2.4 | good |
| B3 Niacin | 4.4 mg | 22.0 | 1.9 | good |
| Folate | 87.5 mcg | 21.9 | 1.9 | good |
| Copper | 0.4 mg | 21.0 | 1.8 | good |
| Protein | 9.4 g | 18.8 | 1.6 | good |
| **PHYTOSTEROLS:** | | | Daily values for these nutrients have not yet been established. | |
| Phytosterols–Total | 80 mg | | | |

For more on "Total Nutrient-Richness," "%DV," "Density," and The World's Healthiest Foods "Quality" Rating System, see page 805.

Two individuals in the 19th century popularized Peanuts in the United States, and since that time, they have become ubiquitous in American culture. George Washington Carver not only invented more than 300 uses for Peanuts, he was instrumental in encouraging farmers to plant Peanuts when the boll weevil plague destroyed their cotton crops after the Civil War. During this same period, a St. Louis physician created a groundup paste made from Peanuts and prescribed this nutritious, high-protein, low-carbohydrate food to his patients—this was the precursor to the all-American favorite, Peanut butter!

## why peanuts should be part of your healthiest way of eating

Peanuts are another great way to add heart-healthy monounsaturated fats to your "Healthiest Way of Eating." They are also known for their resveratrol content, which contributes to Peanuts' antioxidant and anti-inflammatory properties.

Peanuts are also rich in niacin and folate, two B vitamins that are also important for a healthy heart. (For more on the *Health Benefits of Peanuts* and a complete analysis of their content of over 60 nutrients, see page 544.)

## varieties of peanuts

Peanuts originated in South America where they have existed for thousands of years. Technically, Peanuts are not nuts. They are, in botanical fact, legumes and are related to other foods in the legume family including peas, lentils, chickpeas and other beans. Their botanical name is *Arachis hypogeae*.

Peanuts grow in a very fascinating manner. They actually start out as an above ground flower that, due to its heavy weight, bends towards the ground. The flower eventually burrows underground, which is where the Peanut matures. The veined brown shell or pod of the Peanut contains two or three Peanut kernels. Each oval-shaped kernel or seed is comprised of two off-white lobes that are covered by brownish-red skin. Peanuts have a hardy, buttery and "nutty" taste.

Due to their high protein content and sweet, nutty taste, Peanuts are processed into a variety of different forms, including butter, oil, flour and flakes; some are oil roasted, dry roasted or blanched. While there are many varieties of Peanuts, the ones most commonly found in the marketplace include:

**VIRGINIA**

This variety is sold in the shell.

**SPANISH**

Small with reddish-brown skin.

**VALENCIA**

Sweeter, with the shell having three or four kernels inside. Popular in the South as it is mostly used for making boiled Peanuts.

## the peak season available year-round.

## biochemical considerations

Peanuts are a concentrated source of oxalates and goitrogens, which might be of concern to certain individuals. Peanuts are one of the foods most commonly associated with allergic reactions. (For more on *Oxalates*, see page 725; *Goitrogens*, see page 721; and *Food Allergies*, see page 719.)

## 3 steps for the best tasting and most nutritious peanuts

Enjoying the best tasting Peanuts with the most nutrients is simple if you just follow my 3 easy steps:

1. The Best Way to Select
2. The Best Way to Store
3. The Best Way to Prepare

# 1. the best way to select peanuts

Shelled Peanuts are generally available in prepackaged containers as well as bulk bins. Peanuts stored in a hermetically sealed container will last longer than those sold in bulk since their exposure to heat, air and humidity is reduced. If I am going to buy Peanuts from bulk bins, I always check to make sure that the store where I buy Peanuts has a quick turnover of inventory and that the bulk containers are well sealed in order to ensure maximum freshness. Whether purchasing Peanuts in bulk or in a packaged container, make sure that no evidence of moisture or insect damage is present. It is best to smell Peanuts, if possible, to ensure they do not have a rancid or musty odor.

Whole Peanuts still in their shell are usually available in bags or in bulk bins. If possible, I pick up a Peanut and shake it, looking for two signs of quality: (1) it should feel heavy for its size and (2) it should not rattle since a rattling sound suggests that the Peanut kernels have dried out. Additionally, the shells should be free from cracks, dark spots and insect damage. As with all nuts, I recommend selecting organically grown Peanuts whenever possible. (For more on *Organic Foods*, see page 113.)

If you want Peanuts with a roasted flavor and texture, choose ones that have been "dry roasted" as they are not cooked in oil. The commercial roasting process of nuts is often a form of deep-frying, usually in saturated fat, such as coconut or palm kernel oil. Deep-fried foods have been linked to high levels of LDL (the "bad" form of cholesterol) and to thickening of larger artery walls.

Even "dry roasted" Peanuts may be cooked at high temperatures that damage their natural oils. It is important to read the label to be sure that no additional ingredients such as sugar, corn syrup or preservatives have been added. For the highest quality, least expensive "dry roasted" Peanuts, it's best to just roast them yourself using "The Healthiest Way to Dry Roast Peanuts" (see page 542).

# 2. the best way to store peanuts

Shelled Peanuts should be stored in a tightly sealed container in the refrigerator or freezer since excess exposure to high temperatures, humidity or light will cause them to become rancid. Shelled Peanuts will keep in the refrigerator for about 6 months and in the freezer for up to 1 year. To prevent potential oxidation, it is best to chop Peanuts right before eating or using in a recipe rather than in advance. Chopping increases the amount of surface area that has contact with the air, which can increase the amount of oxidation.

Peanuts still in their shells can be kept in a cool, dry dark place, while keeping them in the refrigerator will extend their shelf life. Peanut butter should always be refrigerated once opened.

### How Proper Storage can Help Reduce the Growth of Aflatoxins

It is important to ensure that Peanuts are stored properly in a dry, cool environment to prevent the growth of aflatoxin, a toxic carcinogen produced by fungus that grows at temperatures of 86–96°F (30–36°C) and when the humidity is high. To help prevent aflatoxin ingestion, the FDA enforces a ruling that 20 parts per billion is the maximum aflatoxin permitted in all foods and animal foods, including Peanut butter and other Peanut products. Better storage and handling methods have virtually eliminated the risk of aflatoxin ingestion.

# 3. the best way to prepare peanuts

Shelled Peanuts can be chopped by hand using a knife and a cutting board or using a food processor. If using a food processor, it is best to pulse on and off a few times, instead of running the blade constantly, as this will help ensure that you end up with chopped Peanuts rather than chunky Peanut butter. If Peanut butter is what you want, grind Peanuts in a food processor until you have achieved the consistency you like.

---

### The Healthiest Way to Dry Roast Peanuts

**Dry Roasting Peanuts the healthiest way brings out their flavor and develops their sweetness. It is safe to dry roast Peanuts if done at a low temperature.**

2 cups shelled Peanuts

**1.** Preheat oven to 160–170°F (70–75°C).

**2.** Place one layer of Peanuts on a cookie sheet.

**3.** Roast for 15–20 minutes.

To enhance the "roasted" flavor, try putting a little liquid aminos seasoning or tamari (soy sauce) into a spray bottle and misting the nuts before roasting.

Roasting Peanuts at a temperature higher than 170°F (75°C) will cause a breakdown of their fats and the production of free radicals. Commercially dry roasted Peanuts have been heated to high temperatures (over 350°F or 175°C) that damage the delicate oils in Peanuts, resulting in the formation of free radicals and causing lipid peroxidation—the oxidizing of fats in your bloodstream that can trigger tiny injuries in artery walls—a first step in the buildup of atherosclerotic plaque and cardiovascular disease.

Roasted Peanuts have a shorter shelf life and spoil more quickly than raw Peanuts because the unsaturated oils found in nuts oxidize more quickly after exposure to the heat of the roasting process.

Although some find raw nuts more difficult to digest than roasted nuts, this appears to vary greatly between individuals.

For more information, see page 69.

---

### 8 QUICK SERVING IDEAS for PEANUTS:

1. Add chopped Peanuts to a green salad.
2. Instead of a Peanut butter and jelly sandwich, try Peanut butter and banana, Peanut butter and honey or Peanut butter, sliced apple or pear and/or raisins.
3. Sprinkle chopped Peanuts over curries.
4. **Trail Mix:** Combine roasted Peanuts, raisins, thickly grated coconut and dark organic chocolate bits.
5. **Peanut Butter and Apples:** Slice an apple, spread pieces with honey and Peanut butter, and dip in chopped Peanuts.
6. **Spicy Peanut Butter:** In a small bowl, mix 2 TBS Peanut butter with 1½ tsp of tamari (soy sauce) and hot sauce to taste.
7. **Asian Salad:** Combine sliced green cabbage, grated ginger, Serrano chilies and Peanuts. Toss with equal parts tamari (soy sauce) and rice vinegar and a sprinkle of sesame oil.
8. **Celery and Peanut Butter:** Fill a celery rib with Peanut Butter for a great lunch-bag addition or an afternoon snack.

---

**Q** *Does packaged nut milk provide the same health benefits as whole nuts?*

**A** Commercially purchased, prepackaged nut milk does not provide nearly the same benefits as whole nuts. It's not even close!

The first ingredient in most nuts milks is either water or "nut base." The latter generally refers to some form of blenderized and filtered nut water. Exactly how much nuts are contained in this "nut base" varies from manufacturer to manufacturer.

However, if you check the fiber content of your nut milk, that number will give you some clue about the likely amount of nuts involved. For example, there's about one gram of fiber in every seven almonds. Many almond milks contain zero grams of fiber per eight ounces! This is not to say that nut milks can't play a role in your "Healthiest Way of Eating" but rather to point out that they do not offer the same benefits that can be enjoyed by eating the nuts from which they were derived.

## The Healthiest Ways of Preparing Peanuts

# 10-Minute Peanut Bars

*This is a tasty, nutritious snack that takes only 10 minutes to prepare.*

> 1 cup raw or roasted Peanuts
> 1 TBS minced fresh ginger
> 2 TBS sesame seeds
> 1 cup raisins
> 2 TBS honey

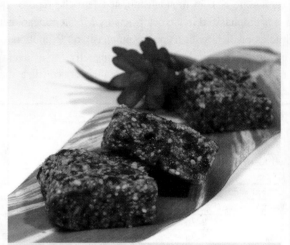

Peanut Bars

1. Grind all ingredients, except for the honey, in a food processor until fairly fine but still with some texture (you don't want it to have the consistency of Peanut butter).

2. Add honey and continue to process until mixed.

3. Press into a square about 3/4-inch thick on a plate or square pan and refrigerate for about an hour or more.

4. Cut into 2-inch squares.

**Preparation Tips:** You want to process ingredients until they press together and hold a shape without being completely smooth. Run your food processor on pulse, so you can stop and check often to avoid overprocessing.

### MAKES 8–12 BARS

# Indonesian Peanut Sauce

*A wonderfully tasty glaze for chicken, fish or tofu.*

> 1/4 cup Peanut butter
> 1 TBS tamari (soy sauce)
> 2 tsp honey
> 1 TBS lime juice
> 1 TBS water
> Hot sauce to taste

**Optional: Add chopped cilantro or chopped mint**

Whisk all ingredients together in a small mixing bowl.

### MAKES 1/3 CUP

## Flavor Tips: 5 ways to enjoy the Indonesian Peanut Sauce

1. Serve on "Healthy Sautéed" cabbage.
2. Stir into steamed carrots.
3. **Indonesian Chicken Wrap:** Spread Indonesian Peanut Sauce on a whole wheat tortilla and top with a romaine lettuce leaf, shredded chicken breast, grated carrot, avocado and chopped roasted Peanuts. Roll and enjoy!

4. **Indonesian Sauté:** Sauté vegetables and combine with Indonesian Peanut Sauce. Top with chicken or shrimp and chopped roasted Peanuts.
5. **Indonesian Marinade:** Use the Indonesian Peanut Sauce recipe as a marinade for tofu and tempeh.

Please write (address on back cover flap) or e-mail me at info@whfoods.org with your personal ideas for preparing Peanuts, and I will share them with others through our website at www.whfoods.org.

# health benefits of peanuts

## Promote Heart Health

Peanuts are rich in monounsaturated fats, the type of fat that is emphasized in the heart-healthy Mediterranean diet. Studies of diets with a special emphasis on Peanuts have shown that this little legume is a big ally for a healthy heart. In one study, a high-monounsaturated diet that emphasized Peanuts and Peanut butter decreased cardio-vascular disease risk by an estimated 21% compared to the average American diet.

In addition to their monounsaturated fat content, Peanuts feature an array of other nutrients that, in numerous studies, have been shown to promote heart health. Peanuts are good sources of niacin and folate. In addition, Peanuts provide resveratrol, the phenolic antioxidant also found in red grapes and red wine that is partially thought to be responsible for the French paradox: the fact that in France people consume a diet that is high in fat, but have a lower risk of cardiovascular disease compared to those in the United States. Peanuts are also packed with phytosterols, phytonutrients that help to reduce cholesterol levels. With all of the important nutrients provided by Peanuts, it is no wonder that numerous research studies have found that frequent Peanut consumption is related to reduced risk of cardiovascular disease.

## A Good Source of Protein

Peanuts are a good source of low-cost high-quality protein. We rely on dietary protein for our supply of amino acids. Our bodies use amino acids for a multitude of functions, including manufacturing muscles, tissues, enzymes and nutrient-carrying protein molecules.

## Promote Brain Health

Recent research suggests that regular consumption of niacin-rich foods, like Peanuts, provides protection against age-related cognitive decline. When researchers tested thousands of individuals aged 65 years and older, they found that those who got the most niacin from their food were 70% less likely to have developed Alzheimer's disease than those consuming the least; their rate of age-related cognitive decline was also significantly less.

## Promote Digestive Health

A landmark 20-year study has shown that women who eat at least one ounce of nuts, Peanuts or Peanut butter each week have a 25% lower risk of developing gallstones. Since one ounce is only about 30 nuts or about two table-spoons of nut butter, preventing gallbladder disease may be as easy as packing one Peanut butter and jelly sandwich (be sure to use whole wheat bread for its fiber, vitamins and minerals) for lunch each week.

## Additional Health-Promoting Benefits of Peanuts

Peanuts are also a concentrated source of other nutrients providing additional health-promoting benefits. These nutrients include free-radical-scavenging copper and manganese and sleep-promoting tryptophan.

### Nutritional Analysis of 1/4 cup of Peanuts:

| NUTRIENT | AMOUNT | % DAILY VALUE |
|---|---|---|
| Calories | 206.96 | |
| Calories from Fat | 161.75 | |
| Calories from Saturated Fat | 22.45 | |
| Protein | 9.42 g | |
| Carbohydrates | 5.89 g | |
| Dietary Fiber | 3.10 g | 12.40 |
| Soluble Fiber | 0.87 g | |
| Insoluble Fiber | 2.23 g | |
| Sugar – Total | 1.13 g | |
| Monosaccharides | — g | |
| Disaccharides | — g | |
| Other Carbs | 1.66 g | |
| Fat – Total | 17.97 g | |
| Saturated Fat | 2.49 g | |
| Mono Fat | 8.92 g | |
| Poly Fat | 5.68 g | |
| Omega-3 Fatty Acids | 0.00 g | 0.00 |
| Omega-6 Fatty Acids | 5.69 g | |
| Trans Fatty Acids | 0.00 g | |
| Cholesterol | 0.00 mg | |
| Water | 2.37 g | |
| Ash | 0.85 g | |
| **Vitamins** | | |
| Vitamin A IU | 0.00 IU | 0.00 |
| Vitamin A RE | 0.00 RE | |
| A - Carotenoid | 0.00 RE | 0.00 |
| A - Retinol | 0.00 RE | |
| B1 Thiamin | 0.23 mg | 15.33 |
| B2 Riboflavin | 0.05 mg | 2.94 |
| B3 Niacin | 4.40 mg | 22.00 |
| Niacin Equiv | 5.90 mg | |
| Vitamin B6 | 0.13 mg | 6.50 |
| Vitamin B12 | 0.00 mcg | 0.00 |
| Biotin | 26.28 mcg | 8.76 |
| Vitamin C | 0.00 mg | 0.00 |
| Vitamin D IU | 0.00 IU | 0.00 |
| Vitamin D mcg | 0.00 mcg | |
| Vitamin E Alpha Equiv | 3.33 mg | 16.65 |
| Vitamin E IU | 4.97 IU | |
| Vitamin E mg | 3.65 mg | |
| Folate | 87.53 mcg | 21.88 |
| Vitamin K | 0.00 mcg | 0.00 |

| NUTRIENT | AMOUNT | % DAILY VALUE |
|---|---|---|
| Pantothenic Acid | 0.64 mg | 6.40 |
| **Minerals** | | |
| Boron | — mcg | |
| Calcium | 33.58 mg | 3.36 |
| Chloride | 2.56 mg | |
| Chromium | — mcg | — |
| Copper | 0.42 mg | 21.00 |
| Fluoride | — mg | — |
| Iodine | 7.30 mcg | 4.87 |
| Iron | 1.67 mg | 9.28 |
| Magnesium | 61.32 mg | 15.33 |
| Manganese | 0.71 mg | 35.50 |
| Molybdenum | 10.77 mcg | 14.36 |
| Phosphorus | 137.24 mg | 13.72 |
| Potassium | 257.33 mg | |
| Selenium | 2.63 mcg | 3.76 |
| Sodium | 6.57 mg | |
| Zinc | 1.19 mg | 7.93 |
| **Amino Acids** | | |
| Alanine | 0.37 g | |
| Arginine | 1.12 g | |
| Aspartate | 1.14 g | |
| Cystine | 0.12 g | 29.27 |
| Glutamate | 1.95 g | |
| Glycine | 0.56 g | |
| Histidine | 0.24 g | 18.60 |
| Isoleucine | 0.33 g | 28.70 |
| Leucine | 0.61 g | 24.11 |
| Lysine | 0.34 g | 14.47 |
| Methionine | 0.11 g | 14.86 |
| Phenylalanine | 0.48 g | 40.34 |
| Proline | 0.41 g | |
| Serine | 0.46 g | |
| Threonine | 0.32 g | 25.81 |
| Tryptophan | 0.09 g | 28.13 |
| Tyrosine | 0.38 g | 39.18 |
| Valine | 0.39 g | 26.53 |

(Note: "–" indicates data is unavailable. For more information, please see page 806.)

## Q&A
### WHY THE WORLD'S HEALTHIEST FOODS CAN HELP YOU DETOXIFY AND CLEANSE

The World's Healthiest Foods have detoxifying and cleansing properties. By eating nutrient-rich foods, such as the World's Healthiest Foods, our body is able to cleanse and regenerate all the time. That's because these foods contains abundant amounts of the full range of health-supportive nutrients. Unlike processed foods that are nutrient depleted and may rob your body of nutrients in order to digest them, nutrient-rich whole foods provide additional nutrients so that your body can continually support itself. Plus, since they do not contain synthetic additives, and notably if they are organically grown and do not have pesticide residues, they won't have these toxins that your body needs to detoxify. Therefore, I think it's important to remember that eating nutrient-rich foods and following the "Healthiest Way of Eating" is probably the best thing you can do if you are interested in detoxifying and cleansing your body.

### World's Healthiest Foods Help with Cleansing and Detoxification

Salads and green leafy vegetables are some of the best foods included among the World's Healthiest Foods to help cleanse and detoxify the body.  They can help remove wastes, reduce acids in the body, alkalize the body and control obesity by reducing excess body fat. The chlorophyll found in salads and green leafy vegetables may help cleanse and purify the blood and boost the immune system.

Here's how some of the other World's Healthiest Foods can assist with cleansing and detoxification:

- Lemon juice detoxifies and cleanses the digestive tract and balances pH
- Cilantro can detoxify and reduce mercury levels
- Prunes help cleanse and detoxify the digestive system and help prevent constipation
- Grains, high in fiber, cleanse the digestive tract
- Fibers such as beta-glucan, found in oats and barley, help eliminate excess cholesterol

By placing special emphasis on enjoying the World's Healthiest fruits and vegetables to help cleanse and detoxify your body, you will start to feel cleaner and lighter, become more mentally clear and have more energy.

### Detoxification

Our body has a wide variety of processes for helping us eliminate potential toxins. Some of those processes take place in our digestive tract. Others take place in our skin, our lymphatic vessels and our liver. We're able to sweat out certain toxins, breathe out certain toxins, and, of course, excrete toxins in our urine or in a bowel movement. It's important not to overlook the role of any detox process if you are considering any kind of "cleanse," even if you plan to make dietary changes the center of your cleansing plan.

Most of the toxins found in food are fat soluble, and if they cannot be eliminated directly in a bowel movement, they are sent from our digestive tract to our liver for detox processing. When you want to cleanse your body of food toxins, it's therefore important to have optimal digestive and liver support. These two organ systems— your liver and your digestive tract—are especially important when it comes to cleansing and detoxification.

### How the Liver Detoxifies Potentially Harmful Chemicals

There are usually two steps required for the liver to detoxify a potentially harmful chemical. Since many potential toxins are fat soluble, the liver cells must typically turn these fat-soluble substances into water-soluble substances in order for them to be excreted from the body. This conversion process requires two steps. In the first step, the potential toxin is made more chemically reactive. In the second step, this more reactive form of the substance is chemically combined with another molecule, creating a new substance that is water soluble and can be excreted from the body. The first step often requires a good supply of antioxidant nutrients, including vitamins C and E, flavonoids and other molecules. The second step requires a good supply of amino acids (the building blocks of protein) together with other unique nutrients that are sometimes overlooked in the world of nutrition.

### Sulfur Is Especially Important In Detox and Cleansing

The mine\ral sulfur is critical for the detoxification of many potential toxins. Sulfur-rich foods can therefore be a mainstay in detox support. The Allium vegetables— onions, garlic and leeks—are all great sources of sulfur. So are the cruciferous vegetables including broccoli, cauliflower and Brussels sprouts. In fact, one of the most well-known crucifers, cabbage, has been found to be so health-promoting in its ability to support the liver that one study suggested that it was this common vegetable that was responsible for protecting women from developing breast cancer in a study that explored the reasons why women emigrating from Poland to the United States dramatically increased their risk of breast cancer. It turns out that eating cabbage was one of the dietary habits they left behind when they emigrated. Their intake of cabbage once they began living in the United States dropped to one-third of their typical amount while their risk of breast cancer rose 300%! (For more on this topic, see page 153.)

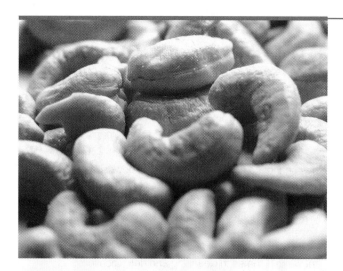

# cashews

### highlights

| | |
|---|---|
| AVAILABILITY: | Year-round |
| REFRIGERATE: | Yes |
| SHELF LIFE: | 6 months in the refrigerator; 1 year in the freezer |
| PREPARATION: | Minimal |

## nutrient-richness chart

Total Nutrient-Richness: **5**

One-quarter cup (34 grams) of Cashews contains 197 calories

| NUTRIENT | AMOUNT | %DV | DENSITY | QUALITY |
|---|---|---|---|---|
| Copper | 0.8 mg | 38.0 | 3.5 | very good |
| Magnesium | 89.1 mg | 22.3 | 2.0 | good |
| Tryptophan | 0.1 g | 21.9 | 2.0 | good |
| Phosphorus | 167.8 mg | 16.8 | 1.5 | good |
| **PHYTOSTEROLS:** | | | Daily values for these nutrients have not yet been established. | |
| Phytosterols–Total | 54 mg | | | |

For more on "Total Nutrient-Richness," "%DV," "Density," and The World's Healthiest Foods "Quality" Rating System, see page 805.

Cashews are indigenous to the Americas but are widely cultivated in India and Africa. Surprisingly, they belong to the same family as mangos as well as other nuts such as pistachios. Cashews are a great out-of-hand snack, making them an easy addition to your "Healthiest Way of Eating." They go well in salads, add rich, buttery flavor and extra nutrition to sautéed dishes and can be ground into healthy and delicious Cashew butter.

## why cashews should be part of your healthiest way of eating

Cashews are a tasty heart-healthy food. They have a lower fat content than most other nuts with approximately 58% of their total fat being oleic acid, the heart-healthy monounsaturated fat that has made olive oil famous. They are extremely rich in copper, important for supporting joint integrity, and magnesium, a mineral essential for both bone and heart health. (For more on the *Health Benefits of Cashews* and a complete analysis of their content of over 60 nutrients, see page 548.)

## varieties of cashews

The true fruit of the Cashew tree is the nut that encases the inner kidney-shaped kernel we enjoy as Cashews. From one end of the nut develops a plump, fleshy, pear-shaped "pseudofruit," or false fruit, because it is easily mistaken for the fruit of the tree; it is known as the Cashew apple. Juicy and fibrous with an acidic taste, Cashew apples, while not widely known in the United States, are regarded as delicacies in Brazil and the Caribbean. Cashews are known botanically as *Anacardium occidentale.*

## the peak season available year-round.

## biochemical considerations

Cashews are a concentrated source of oxalates, which might be of concern to certain individuals. (For more on *Oxalates,* see page 725.)

## 3 steps for the best tasting and most nutritious cashews

Enjoying the best tasting Cashews with the most nutrients is simple if you just follow my 3 easy steps:

1. The Best Way to Select
2. The Best Way to Store
3. The Best Way to Prepare

# 1. the best way to select cashews

Cashews are generally available in prepackaged containers as well as bulk bins. Cashews stored in a hermetically sealed container will last longer than those sold in bulk since their exposure to heat, air and humidity is reduced. If I am going to buy Cashews from bulk bins, I always check to make sure that the store where I buy Cashews has a quick turnover of inventory and that the bulk containers are well sealed in order to ensure maximum freshness. The Cashews should be uniform in color and not limp or shriveled. They should also smell sweet and nutty; if their odor is sharp or bitter, they are rancid. As with all nuts, I recommend selecting organically grown Cashews whenever possible. (For more on *Organic Foods*, see page 113.)

If you want Cashews with a roasted flavor and texture, choose ones that have been "dry roasted" as they are not cooked in oil. The commercial roasting process of nuts is often a form of deep-frying, usually in saturated fat, such as coconut or palm kernel oil. Deep-fried foods have been linked to high levels of LDL (the "bad" form of cholesterol) and to thickening of larger artery walls.

Even "dry roasted" Cashews may be cooked at high temperatures that damage their natural oils. It is important to read the label to be sure that no additional ingredients such as sugar, corn syrup or preservatives have been added. For the highest quality, least expensive "dry roasted" Cashews, it's best to just roast them yourself the using "The Healthiest Way to Dry Roast Cashews." (See below.)

# 2. the best way to store cashews

Due to their high content of oleic acid, the oils in Cashews are more stable than those in most other nuts; however, Cashews should still be stored in a tightly sealed container in the refrigerator, where they will keep for about

6 months, or in the freezer, where they will keep for about 1 year. Cashew butter should always be refrigerated once it is opened.

# 3. the best way to prepare cashews

Whole shelled Cashews can be chopped by hand or can be placed in a food processor. If using a food processor, it is best to pulse on and off a few times, instead of running the

blade constantly, as this will help ensure that you end up with chopped Cashews rather than Cashew butter.

---

### The Healthiest Way to Dry Roast Cashews

**Dry Roasting Cashews the healthiest way brings out their flavor and develops their sweetness. It is safe to dry roast nuts if done at a low temperature.**

2 cups Cashews

1. Preheat oven to 160–170°F (70–75°C).
2. Place one layer of Cashews on a cookie sheet.
3. Roast for 15–20 minutes.

To enhance the "roasted" flavor, try putting a little liquid aminos seasoning or tamari (soy sauce) into a spray bottle and misting the nuts before roasting.

Roasting Cashews at a temperature higher than 170°F (75°C) will cause a breakdown of their fats and the production of free radicals. Commercially dry roasted Cashews have been heated to high temperatures (over 350°F or 175°C) that dam-

age their delicate oils, resulting in the formation of free radicals and causing lipid peroxidation—the oxidizing of fats in your bloodstream, which can trigger tiny injuries in artery walls—a first step in the buildup of plaque and cardiovascular disease.

Roasted Cashews have a shorter shelf life and spoil more quickly than raw Cashews because the unsaturated oils found in nuts oxidize more quickly after exposure to the heat of the roasting process.

Although some find raw nuts more difficult to digest than roasted nuts, this appears to vary greatly between individuals. For more information, see page 69.

# health benefits of cashews

## Promote Heart Health

Not only do Cashews have a lower fat content than most other nuts, but approximately 76% of their total fat is unsaturated fatty acids, with 76% of their unsaturated fatty acid content being oleic acid, the same heart-healthy monounsaturated fat found in olive oil. Studies show that oleic acid promotes good cardiovascular health, even in individuals with diabetes. Studies of diabetic patients show that monounsaturated fat, when added to a low-fat diet, can help to reduce high triglyceride levels. Cashews are also a good source of magnesium, a mineral that helps regulate nerve and muscle tone. As such, insufficient magnesium has been found to contribute to high blood pressure and muscle spasms (including spasms of the heart muscle). Additionally, Cashews are rich in phytosterols, phytonutrients that help to block cholesterol absorption and lower cholesterol levels in the body.

## Promote Bone Health

Cashews are rich in nutrients that help to maintain bone density. As noted above, they are a good source of magnesium. This mineral helps to give bone its physical structure. It is part of the crystal lattice that serves as "scaffolding" that supports the integrity of bone. Also part of this crystal lattice is the mineral phosphorus of which Cashews are a good source. Phosphorus binds with calcium to form calcium phosphate, a component of hydroxyapatite, a mineral complex that gives bones strength and structure. Additionally, Cashews are a very good source of copper, which is a cofactor of enzymes necessary for proper bone metabolism.

## Promote Digestive Health

Twenty years of dietary data collected on tens of thousands of women shows that women who eat at least one ounce of nuts, peanuts or peanut butter each week have a 25% lower risk of developing gallstones. Since one ounce is only about 30 nuts, preventing gallbladder disease may be as easy as having a handful of Cashews as an afternoon pick-me-up at least once a week.

## Additional Health-Promoting Benefits of Cashews

Cashews are also a concentrated source of sleep-promoting tryptophan.

### Nutritional Analysis of 1/4 cup of Cashews:

| NUTRIENT | AMOUNT | % DAILY VALUE |
|---|---|---|
| Calories | 196.60 | |
| Calories from Fat | 142.87 | |
| Calories from Saturated Fat | 28.23 | |
| Protein | 5.24 g | |
| Carbohydrates | 11.20 g | |
| Dietary Fiber | 1.03 g | 4.12 |
| Soluble Fiber | 0.55 g | |
| Insoluble Fiber | 0.48 g | |
| Sugar - Total | 2.43 g | |
| Monosaccharides | 0.07 g | |
| Disaccharides | 2.06 g | |
| Other Carbs | 7.74 g | |
| Fat - Total | 15.87 g | |
| Saturated Fat | 3.14 g | |
| Mono Fat | 9.36 g | |
| Poly Fat | 2.68 g | |
| Omega-3 Fatty Acids | 0.06 g | 2.40 |
| Omega-6 Fatty Acids | 2.62 g | |
| Trans Fatty Acids | 0.00 g | |
| Cholesterol | 0.00 mg | |
| Water | 0.58 g | |
| Ash | 1.35 g | |
| **Vitamins** | | |
| Vitamin A IU | 0.00 IU | 0.00 |
| Vitamin A RE | 0.00 RE | |
| A - Carotenoid | 0.00 RE | 0.00 |
| A - Retinol | 0.00 RE | |
| B1 Thiamin | 0.07 mg | 4.67 |
| B2 Riboflavin | 0.07 mg | 4.12 |
| B3 Niacin | 0.48 mg | 2.40 |
| Niacin Equiv | 1.60 mg | |
| Vitamin B6 | 0.09 mg | 4.50 |
| Vitamin B12 | 0.00 mcg | 0.00 |
| Biotin | 4.45 mcg | 1.48 |
| Vitamin C | 0.00 mg | 0.00 |
| Vitamin D IU | 0.00 IU | 0.00 |
| Vitamin D mcg | 0.00 mcg | |
| Vitamin E Alpha Equiv | 0.20 mg | 1.00 |
| Vitamin E IU | 0.29 IU | |
| Vitamin E mg | 2.55 mg | |
| Folate | 23.70 mcg | 5.92 |
| Vitamin K | 11.88 mcg | 14.85 |

| NUTRIENT | AMOUNT | % DAILY VALUE |
|---|---|---|
| Pantothenic Acid | 0.42 mg | 4.20 |
| **Minerals** | | |
| Boron | — mcg | |
| Calcium | 15.41 mg | 1.54 |
| Chloride | 167.83 mg | |
| Chromium | — mcg | — |
| Copper | 0.76 mg | 38.00 |
| Fluoride | — mg | — |
| Iodine | 3.77 mcg | 2.51 |
| Iron | 2.06 mg | 11.44 |
| Magnesium | 89.05 mg | 22.26 |
| Manganese | 0.28 mg | 14.00 |
| Molybdenum | 10.10 mcg | 13.47 |
| Phosphorus | 167.83 mg | 16.78 |
| Potassium | 193.51 mg | |
| Selenium | 4.01 mcg | 5.73 |
| Sodium | 5.48 mg | |
| Zinc | 1.92 mg | 12.80 |
| **Amino Acids** | | |
| Alanine | 0.22 g | |
| Arginine | 0.54 g | |
| Aspartate | 0.47 g | |
| Cystine | 0.09 g | 21.95 |
| Glutamate | 1.13 g | |
| Glycine | 0.25 g | |
| Histidine | 0.12 g | 9.30 |
| Isoleucine | 0.23 g | 20.00 |
| Leucine | 0.40 g | 15.81 |
| Lysine | 0.25 g | 10.64 |
| Methionine | 0.09 g | 12.16 |
| Phenylalanine | 0.25 g | 21.01 |
| Proline | 0.22 g | |
| Serine | 0.26 g | |
| Threonine | 0.18 g | 14.52 |
| Tryptophan | 0.07 g | 21.88 |
| Tyrosine | 0.15 g | 15.46 |
| Valine | 0.32 g | 21.77 |

(Note: "—" indicates data is unavailable. For more information, please see page 806.)

### Carrot Cashew Paté

**Combine in a food processor:** 2 medium chopped carrots, 1 cup Cashews, 2 tsp fresh chopped ginger, 5 tsp fresh lemon juice, 2 tsp tamari (soy sauce), 4 tsp extra virgin olive oil and 1/2–1 tsp sea salt. Blend until a smooth paste forms, scraping down the sides of the food processor bowl periodically. Add 2 tsp chopped parsley or cilantro and pulse to mix it in. Use paté in wraps with shredded vegetables, put a scoop on salads or serve as a dip with celery and bell pepper pieces.

STEP-BY-STEP RECIPE
## The Healthiest Way of Preparing Cashews

# Sautéed Vegetables with Cashews

*Makes a great side dish with fish or poultry.*

1/2 cup chicken or vegetable broth
1 cup each red and yellow bell peppers,
    sliced 1/2 inch thick
1 cup onion, sliced 1/2 inch thick
1 cup snow peas
1/4 cup cashews

Dressing:
3 TBS extra virgin olive oil
2 tsp lemon juice
2 cloves garlic
Sea salt and pepper to taste

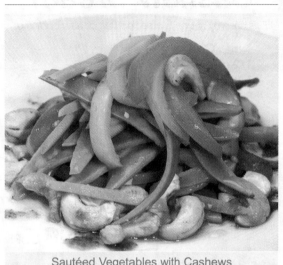

Sautéed Vegetables with Cashews

1. Chop or press garlic, slice onions and let sit for 5 minutes. (Why? See page 261.)

2. Heat broth in a stainless steel skillet over medium heat.

3. When broth is steaming, add bell peppers and onions, **cover** and sauté for 5 minutes.

4. Add snow peas and sauté **covered** for 2 minutes.

5. Transfer vegetable mixture to a serving bowl and toss with Cashews and dressing ingredients.

**SERVES 2**

Please write (address on back cover flap) or e-mail me at info@whfoods.org with your personal ideas for preparing Cashews, and I will share them with others through our website at www.whfoods.org.

## 11 QUICK SERVING IDEAS for CASHEWS:

1. Add Cashews to your morning cereal.

2. Cashews with a little bit of maple syrup make a great topping for waffles, pancakes or hot cereals.

3. Eat Cashews as a quick, substantial snack. Keep some in the car!

4. Add Cashews to vegetable salads.

5. Add a handful of Cashews to your favorite Asian-style stir-fried vegetables.

6. Add Cashews to make a special chicken salad.

7. Spread Cashew butter on toast or fruit, such as apples and pears.

8. **Cashew Shake:** Add Cashew butter to breakfast soy or rice milk shakes to increase their protein content and give them a creamy, nutty taste.

9. **Papaya Salad with Cashews:** Combine diced medium papaya and 1/2 cup of chopped Cashews. Mix with 1 TBS honey.

10. **Thai Shrimp with Cashews:** "Healthy Sauté" 2 cups green beans in 3 TBS broth for 3 minutes, **covered**. Add 1/2 cup red bell pepper and sauté **covered**, for 3 minutes. Add 1 tsp Thai curry paste, 1 tsp grated ginger, 1 tsp minced garlic and one 15 oz can coconut milk. Simmer for 3–5 minutes. Add 1 1/2 cups medium raw shrimp, 1/2 cup whole Cashews, 1/2 cup torn basil leaves, and tamari (soy sauce) and lime juice to taste. Sauté for 3 minutes **uncovered.** Serve over hot brown rice.

11. **Cashew Trail Mix:** Combine 1/2 cup of Cashews, 1/2 cup raisins, 1/4 cup sunflower seeds and 1/2 cup chopped dark chocolate. A great snack.

# Cashew Cream

*This creamy sauce is great on fruit or as a pudding.*

1 cup Cashews
1/2 cup water
1 TBS maple syrup or to taste
Pinch of sea salt

1. Blend all ingredients in blender on high speed until smooth (2–3 minutes).

2. Add additional water in small amounts to create desired consistency.

**Optional:** Soak the Cashews in water for 2 hours before blending for a creamier consistency.

### YIELDS ABOUT 1–1 1/2 CUPS

## Variations...
- Add 1 1/2 tsp almond or vanilla extract for a different flavor.
- Add cinnamon to recipe.

# Cashew Milk

*Enjoy over cereal, in a smoothie or in coffee or tea.*

1 cup Cashews
3 pitted dates
Pinch of sea salt
3 cups water

1. Combine all ingredients in a blender and blend on high for 3 minutes.

2. Strain through a cheesecloth-lined strainer into a large measuring cup or bowl. Store in a glass jar in the refrigerator for up to 3 days

**Optional:** Soak the Cashews in water for 2 hours before blending for a creamier consistency.

### YIELDS ABOUT 4 CUPS

*(Continued from Page 505)*

inflammatory response are called "pro-inflammatory." Eicosanoids that decrease the response are called "anti-inflammatory." In general, many eicosanoids that have potential anti-inflammatory effects (including thromboxane A3, prostaglandin I3 and leukotriene E5) are made from EPA. Similarly, many eicosanoids that have potential pro-inflammatory effects (including thromboxanes A2 and B2, as well as prostaglandin E2) are made not from any omega-3 fatty acid, but from an omega-6 fatty acid called arachidonic acid. It's therefore correct to think about omega-3 fat as the kind of fat that is potentially anti-inflammatory.

Since many anti-inflammatory molecules are made from EPA, it's reasonable to ask whether plant foods containing ALA are as helpful in preventing inflammation as animal foods containing preformed EPA. Some websites and supplement manufacturers have suggested that you cannot "fight" inflammation with ALA and plant food sources of omega-3 unless you consume 10 or 15 times as much ALA as EPA. Since a healthy body constantly decides on a second-by-second basis how much ALA to leave "as is," and how much to convert into EPA and DHA, there is no single amount of ALA that gets converted into EPA. Even more important, ALA itself is needed by the body and has established anti-inflammatory properties, and there are many other omega-3 fatty acids that may have anti-inflammatory properties as well. Just because EPA and DHA are currently the best studied and best represented fatty acids in the marketplace does not mean that they tell the whole story about the role of omega-3 fat and inflammation. And fortunately, we do not have to master all the biochemistry in order to make good food choices when it comes to omega-3s. Most of us would be well served to include more omega-3-rich foods of all kinds—both plant and animal—in our meal plan. And we would also be well served to focus on the overall quality of the food as well (for example, whether it was organically produced) and not get too sidetracked on one of the piece parts. It's the whole, natural context of our food that is going to keep us on target as we pursue a "Healthiest Way of Eating" geared towards vitality and health.

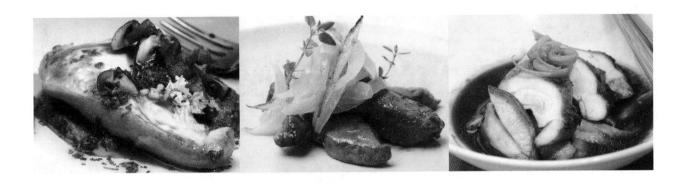

# poultry & lean meat

The numbers beside each food indicate their Total Nutrient-Richness. (For more details, see page 805.)

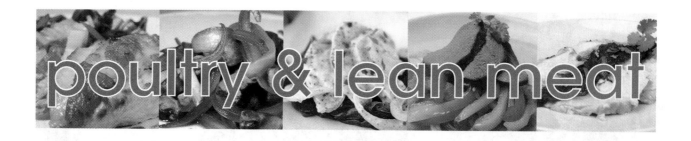

# poultry & lean meat

Poultry and lean meat can play an important role in the "Healthiest Way of Eating" for many people. A look at their nutritional profiles will quickly show you how these foods are incredibly concentrated sources of many nutrients, including zinc, iron and vitamin B12, which are more difficult to find in plant-based foods. Poultry and lean meat also provide complete protein, which means that they contain all of the amino acids required by the body.

There are two different forms of iron contained in the foods that we eat. Heme iron is found only in animal foods. About 40% of the iron in meat comes in the form of heme iron. Non-heme iron is found in both plant and animal foods. Studies on iron absorption have found that anywhere from 15–35% of heme iron can be absorbed by the body, whereas only 3–8% of non-heme iron is absorbed. This is another reason why poultry and lean meat in moderation may serve as an important dietary consideration for some people.

I believe that by including poultry and lean meat as a balanced part of a meal, as opposed to making them the main focus of the meal, you can enjoy their nutritional benefits while still subscribing to the "Healthiest Way of Eating."

### Poultry and Lean Meat: Definition

While the term poultry refers to any domesticated fowl, the two types of poultry that are included among the World's Healthiest Foods are chicken and turkey.

When I refer to lean meat, I mean the flesh and/or organ of a land animal that is consumed as food (not including poultry). Grass-fed beef, venison, lamb and calf's liver are the meats included among the World's Healthiest Foods.

### Importance of Organically Raised Poultry and Lean Meat

I recommend purchasing organically raised poultry and lean meat whenever possible. This is because commercially raised poultry and meat are usually infused with hormones, antibiotics and other drugs, and their diet is composed of conventionally grown grains that have been sprayed with pesticides. The concern is that residues from the use of antibiotics, hormones and feed pesticides can remain in the flesh and organs of commercially raised poultry and meat.

Organically raised poultry and lean meat, however, are not exposed to antibiotics and growth hormones and are fed a wholesome diet of organically raised foods. This leads to healthier muscles (the part of the "meat" that we eat) that also contain more moisture. They are also raised in a more humane manner in a less stressful environment, which may account for reduced levels of circulating hormones and may be the reason that many people feel they have a richer flavor than their conventionally raised counterparts. Organically raised poultry and meat are "certified organic" by the USDA. When you eat organically raised poultry and meat, you can feel confident that they are "safer" and "healthier."

### Fats, Saturated Fats and Cholesterol

Poultry and meat may be of concern because of their high levels of saturated fats and cholesterol; however, it is possible to enjoy these foods and still maintain a low-fat diet. One way to do this is to always use lean cuts of meat. The cuts surrounding the back leg bone are usually the leanest because the back legs of the animal have become more muscular, and muscular meat contains less fat. It is also easy to remove visible fat from some cuts of meat, as is the case with the fat found on lamb chops. The fat in chicken and turkey is found primarily in the skin; it can be easily removed, which reduces the fat content significantly. Venison is one of the leanest meats available and calf's liver has virtually no fat.

## Poultry: Chicken and Turkey

Chicken and turkey are both versatile and inexpensive. Chicken is the public's number one choice for animal food in the United States; we now eat more chicken than red meat. You can add chicken to salads, sandwiches, BBQs, stir-fries, sautés—the list goes on and on.

In 1970, 50% of all turkey was consumed during the holidays. Today, turkey is no longer reserved just for Thanksgiving and Christmas. With new cuts of turkey that are versatile and easy to prepare, you can enjoy turkey any time of the year. You can also find organic turkeys in many local markets. In addition to being delicious, turkey is also very versatile. There is a wide variety of turkey parts available (breasts, wings and thighs), so you can enjoy this food without having to roast an entire turkey.

### CHICKEN AND TURKEY SKIN

Removing the skin and visible fat from chicken and turkey can lower the fat content by about 50%! Since the skin of chicken and turkey is the major contributor of saturated fat and cholesterol, removing the skin is a good technique to reduce the fat content of chicken and turkey for people who are trying to eat lean.

The breast is the leanest portion of poultry, and removing the skin from a four-ounce serving of boneless chicken breast reduces the fat content from 8.8 grams to 4.0 grams. Four ounces of turkey breast without skin has less than 1 gram of fat. With the skin removed, both chicken and turkey have considerably less fat than beef, which has 1.5 grams for a four-ounce serving.

### WHEN TO REMOVE SKIN

I suggest cooking poultry with the skin on and removing it after cooking. This method does not significantly raise the fat content of the meat compared to cooking it with the skin removed. Skin will keep the meat insulated, allowing it to retain more of its natural moisture and flavors. This is particularly important when cooking the breast portion of poultry, which can easily become dry and tough. When you peel off the skin, the meat may look fatty; this is not actually fat, but moisture.

## Grass-Fed Beef

Grass-fed beef is beef that has been only fed grass and allowed to roam freely in green pastures. I have three suggestions when it comes to eating meat, including beef, all of which are principles that I discuss throughout the book. First, beef should be eaten in moderation, as a component of a meal and not its main focus. Second, always try to choose the leanest cut of beef, when possible. These cuts are generally from the back leg (round) bone and include top round, bottom round and eye of round. Third, I believe that beef should be grass-fed and/or organically raised whenever possible. To me, this is extremely important not only for humanitarian and environmental reasons, but for reasons of personal health.

Because beef can be high in fat and cholesterol, it may not be the best choice for individuals watching their fat intake and their cholesterol levels. Some individuals also report having difficulty digesting beef.

## Lamb

Many people still desire the rich taste of red meat, wanting an alternative to chicken and turkey, yet don't want to eat beef. Lamb is a delicious red meat that fits well in numerous recipes and provides intensity of flavor and texture. Lamb is one of the finest tasting meats available and can be even more tender and flavorful than beef when properly prepared.

One of lamb's nutritional signatures is that it is one of the best dietary sources of carnitine. This amino acid plays many important physiological functions including providing special benefits to the heart, transporting fatty acids into the mitochondria (the energy producing areas of the cell) and converting these fats into energy. Since much of this energy is used to fuel the muscles, athletes are usually especially interested in ensuring that their diet supplies them with adequate carnitine.

## Calf's Liver

Calf's liver has virtually no fat. It is a good source of protein and is very rich in vitamin B12, zinc, iron and powerful antioxidants such as vitamin A, vitamin C and selenium. Selecting organic calf's liver whenever possible provides the greatest assurance that the liver is free of pesticides, hormones and antibiotics. Calf's liver is also more tender and has better flavor than beef liver.

### Venison

Domesticated venison does not have the gamey flavor of wild venison and is becoming more readily available at the market. Domesticated venison is one of the leanest varieties of meats you can find.

### Enjoy Poultry and Lean Meat, But in Moderation

I recommend moderation and smaller portions of meat and poultry as the way to include these foods into your "Healthiest Way of Eating." Because a healthy diet is a diverse diet, I feel that meat and poultry can be enjoyed in moderate amounts and not relied upon as the main protein source of every meal. For example, instead of 8 ounces of chicken surrounded by a 1/2 cup each of vegetables and grains for dinner, I would suggest 4 ounces of chicken, 2 cups of vegetables and 1 cup of squash or brown rice. For most people, poultry and lean meat can be incorporated into their "Healthiest Way of Eating" by enjoying 3–4 servings per week. The serving size is 3–4 ounces, with skin removed from poultry and fat trimmed from meat.

### How to Use the Individual Poultry and Lean Meat Chapters

Each Poultry and Lean Meat chapter is dedicated to one of the World's Healthiest Poultry and Lean Meats and contains everything you need to know to enjoy and maximize its flavor and nutritional benefits. Each chapter is organized into two parts:

1. **POULTRY AND LEAN MEAT FACTS** describes each food and its different varieties and presents its unique nutritional profile. It also addresses biochemical considerations of each by describing unique compounds that may be potentially problematic for individuals with specific health problems. Detailed information of the health benefits of each of these foods can be found at the end of the chapter.

2. **THE 4 STEPS TO THE BEST TASTING AND MOST NUTRITIOUS POULTRY AND LEAN MEAT** include information on how to select, store, prepare and cook each one of the World's Healthiest Poultry and Lean Meats. While the 4 Steps provided in this Introduction can be used as an overview, more detail about the individual foods can be found in their dedicated chapters.

# 1. the best way to select poultry and lean meat

It is worth seeking out the best quality poultry and lean meat. I recommend selecting organically raised poultry and meat whenever possible because not only do they have the best flavor, but they are better for you (as well as the environment). By buying organic, you can reduce your exposure to the residues of hormones, antibiotics, pesticides and other chemicals that are found to be more concentrated in conventionally raised varieties. Additionally, in general, organically raised animals are raised in a more humane manner.

It is important to make sure that the poultry and lean meat you purchase are fresh, so try to find the packages with the latest use-by date or ask the staff at your market's meat department to give you the freshest piece possible.

By talking to the people that work in the meat departments of your local markets and asking them about where and how often they get their poultry and meat, you can determine which stores have the freshest selection.

It is important to remember that different cuts of meat are better suited to different cooking methods and recipes; in each of the recipes, I specify which type of cut to use. If you have questions regarding cuts to use for other recipes, you should ask the staff person in your market's meat department.

If you are having difficulties finding organically raised poultry and lean meats at your local supermarket or natural foods store, you may want to see if you can find a purveyor at your local farmer's market (if you have one).

# 2. the best way to store poultry and lean meat

How you store your poultry and lean meat is important to maintain their freshness, flavor and texture. In general, keep poultry and meat in the meat section of the refrigerator; the temperature should be 36–40°F (2–4°C). Defrost frozen poultry and meat only in the refrigerator; never defrost at room temperature because it will thaw more quickly, creating conditions that promote bacterial growth.

# 3. the best way to prepare poultry and lean meat

Poultry and lean meat require minimal preparation. Rinse with cold water and pat dry.

# 4. the healthiest way of cooking poultry and lean meat

Below are some general tips that can be applied to cooking poultry and lean meat.

## Healthy Cooking Times

Poultry and lean meat are easy to cook. Different cuts of poultry and meat require different cooking times for optimal flavor. Regardless of cooking method, if you overcook your poultry and meat, it will become dry and tough and lose its flavor. By not overcooking your poultry or meat, you will enjoy more flavor, moisture and nutrients. Each recipe in the chapters that follow has been created by considering the optimum cooking method and time for a particular cut of meat to give you the best results.

## Healthy Cooking Methods

I have created quick, easy and healthy cooking methods that will seal in the juices and flavor of poultry and lean meat. Since these creative cooking methods do not require the use of any fats or oils, they will help to reduce your fat intake without compromising your enjoyment of flavor. Below are general descriptions of these cooking methods; more details can be found in the recipes in which these methods are used.

### "QUICK BROIL"

The "Quick Broil" cooking method is a great technique that is very quick and easy. It is especially good for chicken breasts and lamb chops. It seals in moisture, creating meat that is juicy and flavorful. (For more on "*Quick Broil*," see page 60.)

### ROASTING

Roasting is used when you are cooking a larger piece of poultry or meat, such as a whole turkey or leg of lamb. It is very simple to do and produces meat that is infused with its own natural flavor and juices. (For more on "*Roasting*," see page 61.)

### "HEALTHY SAUTÉ"

If your recipe calls for poultry or meat cut into bite-size pieces sautéed with other ingredients (such as vegetables), you may want to use this cooking method. It cooks the poultry or meat quickly, requires no oil and makes a delicious simmering sauce. (For more on "*Healthy Sauté*," see page 57.)

## Cooking at High Temperature

High temperature cooking refers to cooking methods such as grilling and barbequing. When you use these methods, you will oftentimes notice that browning or charring occurs; this is a major source of carcinogenic compounds, known as heterocyclic amines (HCAs). These compounds are created from the interaction of the heat and the saturated fats contained in the meat. HCAs are found in cooked muscular meats and are very low or non-existent in liver and organ meats. It has been suggested that the consumption of meat cooked at high temperatures is linked to the development of certain types of chronic health conditions, including colon cancer.

Cooking methods that use lower temperatures such as "Healthy Sauté" form one-third less HCAs. Marinating meats in sauces that contain foods concentrated in antioxidant phytonutrients before broiling has also been shown to inhibit the production of HCAs; garlic-turmeric sauce and a mixture of olive oil, cider vinegar, garlic, mustard, lemon juice and salt are two examples of marinades that have been studied. Adding minced garlic to meat patties has also been found to reduce the development of HCAs. While vitamin C and citrus flavonoids act as antioxidants and have been shown to inhibit the activity of carcinogenic compounds, it has not been determined whether they will inhibit HCA formation; but at the very least, they will provide you with a delicious tasting meal with the potential of increased protection against HCAs.

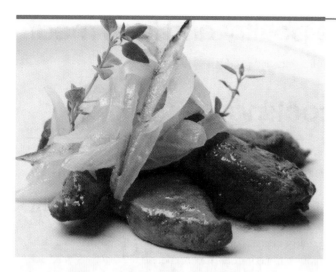

# calf's liver

| | |
|---|---|
| AVAILABILITY: | Year-round |
| REFRIGERATE: | Yes |
| SHELF LIFE: | 1–2 days refrigerated |
| PREPARATION: | Minimal |
| BEST WAY TO COOK: | "Healthy Sauté" |

## nutrient-richness chart

Total Nutrient-Richness: **41**

4 ounces (113 grams) of cooked Calf's Liver contains 187 calories

| NUTRIENT | AMOUNT | %DV | DENSITY | QUALITY |
|---|---|---|---|---|
| Vitamin B12 | 41.4 mcg | 689.8 | 66.4 | excellent |
| Vitamin A | 30485.3 IU | 609.7 | 58.7 | excellent |
| Copper | 9.0 mg | 450.5 | 43.3 | excellent |
| Folate | 860.7 mcg | 215.2 | 20.7 | excellent |
| B2 Riboflavin | 2.2 mg | 129.4 | 12.4 | excellent |
| Selenium | 57.8 mcg | 82.6 | 7.9 | excellent |
| Tryptophan | 0.3 g | 78.1 | 7.5 | excellent |
| Zinc | 10.8 mg | 72.0 | 6.9 | very good |
| Vitamin C | 35.2 mg | 58.6 | 5.6 | very good |
| Protein | 24.5 g | 49.1 | 4.7 | very good |
| B3 Niacin | 9.6 mg | 48.0 | 4.6 | very good |
| Phosphorus | 361.8 mg | 36.2 | 3.5 | very good |
| B6 Pyroxidine | 0.6 mg | 28.0 | 2.7 | good |
| B5 Pantothenic Acid | 2.6 mg | 25.9 | 2.5 | good |
| Iron | 3.0 mg | 16.5 | 1.6 | good |

For more on "Total Nutrient-Richness," "%DV," "Density," and The World's Healthiest Foods "Quality" Rating System, see page 805.

Although perhaps not a favorite of many people in the United States, liver is popular in cuisines in many other parts of the world. In European countries, including Italy, France, Austria and Germany, it is actually considered a delicacy. *Fegato alla Veneziana* (Venetian Liver) is one of the most famous dishes in the culinary history of the Italian city of Venice, while chopped liver is a mainstay of Jewish cooking. I would like to share with you how my quick and easy "Healthiest Way of Cooking" methods will help bring out the flavor and maximize the nutritional benefits of Calf's Liver, so you can make it an enjoyable addition to your "Healthiest Way of Eating."

## why calf's liver should be part of your healthiest way of eating

Lovers of Calf's Liver hold it in high regard not only for its delicious taste and texture, but because of its tremendous storehouse of nutrients. Its nutritional profile clearly shows why it is included among the list of the World's Healthiest Foods. Its wealth of B vitamins (especially vitamin B12) are important for a healthy heart, while its vitamin A and zinc help support the immune system; in addition, its vitamin C and selenium provide antioxidant protection against the oxidative damage to cells from free radicals. (For more on the *Health Benefits of Calf's Liver* and a complete analysis of its content of over 60 nutrients, see page 558.)

## varieties of calf's liver

The Liver from a calf is more tender and has a more delicate flavor than beef liver. Calf's Liver is from cows that are three to six months old, while beef liver is from animals six months and older. Calf's Liver has a paler color than beef liver, is more tender and has a more delicate flavor. Beef liver is darker in color and has a strong flavor.

## the peak season

Calf's Liver is available year-round.

## biochemical considerations

Calf's Liver contains purines and oxalates. It also is a concentrated source of cholesterol (4 ounces contain 636 mg of cholesterol), which may be of concern to certain individuals. (For more on *Purines*, see page 727; and *Oxalates*, see page 725).

## 4 steps for the best tasting and most nutritious calf's liver

Turning Calf's Liver into a flavorful dish with the most nutrients is simple if you just follow my 4 easy steps:

1. The Best Way to Select
2. The Best Way to Store
3. The Best Way to Prepare
4. The Healthiest Way of Cooking

# 1. the best way to select calf's liver

The best way to select Calf's Liver is to first check the sell-by date on the label and choose the one with the latest date. Calf's Liver should be shiny in appearance and have a pleasant smell. It is paler in color than beef liver and has a milder flavor.

It is particularly important to select Calf's Liver from organically raised animals, whenever possible. Calves that were raised organically will not have been exposed to pesticides, hormones and antibiotics like their conventionally raised counterparts; therefore, their livers will have less exposure to and accumulation of these toxins. Buying organic Calf's Liver will help assure you that you are feeding yourself and your family a delicious food from an animal that was raised in a more healthful and humane manner. (For more on *Organic Meats*, see page 565.)

Avoid Calf's Liver that has any unpleasant odor or a package that has passed its expiration date.

# 2. the best way to store calf's liver

Since Calf's Liver is very perishable, it should always be either refrigerated or frozen. Refrigerate the Calf's Liver in the original store packaging, if it is still intact and secure, as this will keep the amount of handling to a minimum. Calf's Liver will keep in the refrigerator for only one or two days.

If you will be unable to cook the Calf's Liver within one or two days of purchase, you can store it in the freezer, where it should keep for three to four months. Using a plastic freezer bag or freezer paper, wrap the Calf's Liver carefully so that it is packaged as tightly as possible.

# 3. the best way to prepare calf's liver

When handling raw Calf's Liver, be extremely careful that it does not come in contact with other foods, especially those that will be served uncooked because raw meats can contain bacteria. In fact, you should use a separate plastic cutting board for meats. If you don't use separate boards, make sure you wash your hands and cutting board very well with hot soapy water after handling Calf's Liver. It is a good idea to add two TBS of bleach to two cups of water in a spray bottle and use this mixture to clean your cutting board. Spray your cutting board with this mixture and let it sit for 20 minutes to let the bleach evaporate.

# 4. the healthiest way of cooking calf's liver

The "Healthiest Way of Cooking" Calf's Liver is by using methods that will keep it moist and tender. Since liver can be easily overcooked and become dry, be sure to watch your cooking times. "Healthy Sauté" is the method I have found to be the best to prepare Calf's Liver.

## Methods Not Recommended for Cooking Calf's Liver

### COOKING WITH OIL

I don't recommend cooking Calf's Liver in oil because high temperature heat can damage delicate oils and potentially create harmful free radicals. (For more on *Why it is Important to Cook Without Heated Oils*, see page 52).

# health benefits of calf's liver

## Promotes Heart Health

Calf's Liver is an excellent source of vitamin B12 and folic acid and a good source of vitamin B6, three nutrients needed to convert artery-damaging homocysteine into other, benign molecules. Vitamin B2, of which Calf's Liver is also an excellent source, is a cofactor in the reaction that regenerates glutathione, an antioxidant that protects lipids like cholesterol from free radical attack. Calf's Liver is also an excellent source of the mineral selenium and a very good source of vitamin C, two potent antioxidants found to be associated with reduced risk of cardiovascular disease.

## Promotes Optimal Immune Function

Calf's Liver is an excellent source of vitamin A and a very good source of zinc, two nutrients that support the functioning of the immune system. Vitamin A is critically important for the health of epithelial and mucosal tissues, the body's first line of defense against invading organisms and toxins. Zinc, the most critical mineral for immune function, acts synergistically with vitamin A, promotes the destruction of foreign particles and microorganisms, protects against free-radical damage and is required for proper white cell function. Zinc also inhibits replication of several viruses, including those associated with the common cold.

## Promotes Bone Health

Calf's Liver is an excellent source of copper. This trace mineral is an essential component of energy production and antioxidant defenses. It is also necessary for the activity of an enzyme that is involved in cross-linking collagen and elastin, both of which provide the ground substance for flexibility in blood vessels, bones and joints. Recent research findings have also suggested a correlation between low dietary intake of copper, low blood levels of zinc and osteoporosis at the hip and spine in men.

## Promotes Energy Production

Calf's Liver is also a very good source of niacin and a good source of pantothenic acid. Niacin helps promote blood sugar regulation via its actions as a component of a molecule called glucose tolerance factor, which optimizes insulin activity. Pantothenic acid plays an important role in the prevention of fatigue since it supports the function of the adrenal glands, particularly in times of stress. Calf's Liver is also a very good source of phosphorus, a component of the cellular fuel molecule, ATP.

## Additional Health-Promoting Benefits of Calf's Liver

Calf's Liver is also a concentrated source of other nutrients providing additional health-promoting benefits. These nutrients include muscle-building protein and sleep-promoting tryptophan.

### Nutritional Analysis of 4 ounces of cooked Calf's Liver:

| NUTRIENT | AMOUNT | % DAILY VALUE |
|---|---|---|
| Calories | 187.11 | |
| Calories from Fat | 70.43 | |
| Calories from Saturated Fat | 26.13 | |
| Protein | 24.53 g | |
| Carbohydrates | 3.08 g | |
| Dietary Fiber | 0.00 g | 0.00 |
| Soluble Fiber | 0.00 g | |
| Insoluble Fiber | 0.00 g | |
| Sugar – Total | 0.00 g | |
| Monosaccharides | 0.00 g | |
| Disaccharides | 0.00 g | |
| Other Carbs | 3.08 g | |
| Fat – Total | 7.83 g | |
| Saturated Fat | 2.91 g | |
| Mono Fat | 1.69 g | |
| Poly Fat | 1.24 g | |
| Omega-3 Fatty Acids | 0.09 g | 3.60 |
| Omega-6 Fatty Acids | 1.15 g | |
| Trans Fatty Acids | — g | |
| Cholesterol | 636.17 mg | |
| Water | 76.36 g | |
| Ash | 1.59 g | |
| **Vitamins** | | |
| Vitamin A IU | 30485.26 IU | 609.71 |
| Vitamin A RE | 9127.54 RE | |
| A - Carotenoid | 0.00 RE | 0.00 |
| A - Retinol | 9127.54 RE | |
| B1 Thiamin | 0.15 mg | 10.00 |
| B2 Riboflavin | 2.20 mg | 129.41 |
| B3 Niacin | 9.61 mg | 48.05 |
| Niacin Equiv | 13.91 mg | |
| Vitamin B6 | 0.56 mg | 28.00 |
| Vitamin B12 | 41.39 mcg | 689.83 |
| Biotin | — mcg | — |
| Vitamin C | 35.16 mg | 58.60 |
| Vitamin D IU | 13.61 IU | 3.40 |
| Vitamin D mcg | 0.35 mcg | |
| Vitamin E Alpha Equiv | 0.39 mg | 1.95 |
| Vitamin E IU | 0.57 IU | |
| Vitamin E mg | 0.41 mg | |
| Folate | 860.70 mcg | 215.18 |
| Vitamin K | — mcg | |

| NUTRIENT | AMOUNT | % DAILY VALUE |
|---|---|---|
| Pantothenic Acid | 2.59 mg | 25.90 |
| **Minerals** | | |
| Boron | — mcg | |
| Calcium | 7.93 mg | 0.79 |
| Chloride | — mg | |
| Chromium | — mcg | — |
| Copper | 9.01 mg | 450.50 |
| Fluoride | — mg | — |
| Iodine | — mcg | — |
| Iron | 2.97 mg | 16.50 |
| Magnesium | 21.55 mg | 5.39 |
| Manganese | 0.13 mg | 6.50 |
| Molybdenum | — mcg | — |
| Phosphorus | 361.75 mg | 36.17 |
| Potassium | 232.47 mg | |
| Selenium | 57.84 mcg | 82.63 |
| Sodium | 60.11 mg | |
| Zinc | 10.80 mg | 72.00 |
| **Amino Acids** | | |
| Alanine | 1.33 g | |
| Arginine | 1.17 g | |
| Aspartate | 2.27 g | |
| Cystine | 0.27 g | 65.85 |
| Glutamate | 2.93 g | |
| Glycine | 1.24 g | |
| Histidine | 0.53 g | 41.09 |
| Isoleucine | 1.08 g | 93.91 |
| Leucine | 2.00 g | 79.05 |
| Lysine | 1.11 g | 47.23 |
| Methionine | 0.39 g | 52.70 |
| Phenylalanine | 1.19 g | 100.00 |
| Proline | 1.07 g | |
| Serine | 1.04 g | |
| Threonine | 1.04 g | 83.87 |
| Tryptophan | 0.25 g | 78.13 |
| Tyrosine | 0.88 g | 90.72 |
| Valine | 1.37 g | 93.20 |

(Note: "–" indicates data is unavailable. For more information, please see page 806.)

STEP-BY-STEP RECIPE
## The Healthiest Ways of Cooking Calf's Liver

# *"Healthy Sautéed" Calf's Liver and Onions*

*Even if you think you don't like liver, you should try the "Healthy Sauté" method. Liver cooked this way has great flavor and you only need one skillet to cook both the Liver and onions. Liver should be sliced thin for the best taste.*

**For the onions:**
> 1 medium red onion
> 3 TBS low-sodium chicken broth

**For the Calf's Liver:**
> 3 TBS low-sodium chicken broth
> 3/4 lb Calf's Liver, sliced thin (1/4-inch)
> 2 tsp fresh lemon juice
> 2 tsp balsamic vinegar
> 1 clove garlic, chopped or pressed

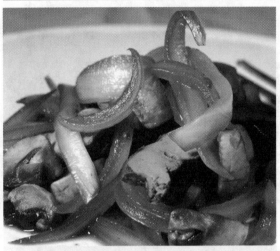

"Healthy Sautéed" Calf's Liver and Onions

1 TBS extra virgin olive oil
Sea salt and pepper to taste

1. Thinly slice the onion and let sit for 5 minutes. (Why? see page 276.)

2. Turn stove to medium. Heat 3 TBS low-sodium chicken broth in a stainless steel skillet.

3. When the broth begins to steam, add onions, **cover** and sauté for 4 minutes.

4. When the onions have lost most of their water content and have become dry, push them to the side of the skillet, leaving space in the center.

5. Heat the second 3 TBS broth in the center of the skillet, leaving the heat on medium.

6. When the broth begins to steam, add the sliced Calf's Liver and sauté **uncovered** for 3 minutes.

The pieces will be browned on one side, and the Liver will release liquid.

7. Turn the Liver pieces over and brown the other side for 3 minutes. When the liquid has evaporated, the Liver is done.

8. Remove the pan from the heat and drizzle the Liver and onions with balsamic vinegar, lemon juice, extra virgin olive oil, garlic and salt and pepper to taste.

9. Transfer to a serving plate and serve immediately.

**Cooking Hint:** Be sure not to overcook the Calf's Liver or it will get dry; it should still be a little pink in the middle for the best flavor and moistness.

**SERVES 2**

## Flavor Tips: Try these 8 great serving suggestions with the recipe above. ✳

1. Use white wine instead of broth for Berlin-style Calf's Liver.

2. Thyme and sage complement the flavor of Calf's Liver.

3. Add a few drops of tamari (soy sauce) to mellow the taste of Calf's Liver. If you add tamari, you will want to reduce the amount of sea salt you use.

4. Add dry mustard, 5 spice powder or curry powder while sautéing the onions.

5. Add tart sliced apples (such as Granny Smith) fresh thyme and cinnamon to taste when sautéing onions.

6. Top with "Healthy Sautéed" crimini mushrooms and fresh Italian herbs.

7. **Dijon Mustard Sauce:** Combine 1 TBS Dijon mustard with 3 TBS extra virgin olive oil for a tasty sauce.

8. **Liver Spread:** Mince leftover Calf's Liver recipe and boiled eggs for a delicious high protein spread.

Please write (address on back cover flap) or e-mail me at info@whfoods.org with your personal ideas for preparing Calf's Liver, and I will share them with others through our website at www.whfoods.org.

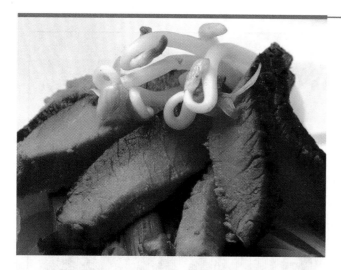

## nutrient-richness chart

Total Nutrient-Richness: **15**

4 ounces (113 grams) of cooked Beef tenderloin contains 240 calories

| NUTRIENT | AMOUNT | %DV | DENSITY | QUALITY |
|---|---|---|---|---|
| Tryptophan | 0.36 g | 112.5 | 8.4 | excellent |
| Protein | 32.04 g | 64.1 | 4.8 | very good |
| Vitamin B12 | 2.92 mcg | 48.7 | 3.6 | very good |
| Zinc | 6.33 mg | 42.2 | 3.2 | good |
| Selenium | 27.67 mcg | 39.5 | 3.0 | good |
| Phosphorus | 269.89 mg | 27.0 | 2.0 | good |
| B6 Pyridoxine | 0.49 mg | 24.5 | 1.8 | good |
| Iron | 4.05 mg | 22.5 | 1.7 | good |
| B3 Niacin | 4.44 mg | 22.2 | 1.7 | good |
| B2 Riboflavin | 0.35 mg | 20.6 | 1.5 | good |

For more on "Total Nutrient-Richness," "%DV," "Density," and
The World's Healthiest Foods "Quality" Rating System, see page 805.

For some people, Beef can play an important role in their "Healthiest Way of Eating" if eaten in moderation. That is why I have included it among the World's Healthiest Foods. But it is not just any Beef that is included; rather, I have chosen to include Grass-Fed Beef. That is because not only do many people feel that Grass-Fed Beef has superior flavor, but it offers some unique benefits over grain-fed Beef. One of the notable differences is its fatty acid profile as Grass-Fed Beef is suggested to have a higher omega-3 fatty acid content and lower total and saturated fat content than grain-fed Beef.

I also recommend Grass-Fed Beef that is organically raised, whenever possible, since this will give you greater assurance that the Beef you are eating is from an animal that was raised in a humane manner and without the use of unnecessary antibiotics and hormones. (For more on *Organic Meats*, see page 565.) I want to share with you how you can bring out the

# grass-fed beef

## highlights

| | |
|---|---|
| AVAILABILITY: | Year-round |
| REFRIGERATE: | Yes |
| SHELF LIFE: | 3–5 days refrigerated |
| PREPARATION: | Minimal |
| BEST WAY TO COOK: | Many ways |

maximum flavor and nutritional benefits of Grass-Fed Beef by using the "Healthiest Way of Cooking" Methods.

## why grass-fed beef should be part of your healthiest way of eating

Grass-Fed Beef is renowned as a very good source of protein and contains heme iron, a form of iron that is especially well absorbed by the body. It is a good source of zinc, an important mineral to support the immune system, and selenium, which provides antioxidant protection against the oxidative damage caused by free radicals. It is also a very good source of hard-to-find vitamin B12. (For more on the *Health Benefits of Grass-Fed Beef* and a complete profile of its content of over 60 nutrients, see page 564.)

## varieties of grass-fed beef

Grass-Fed Beef is available in a wide variety of cuts that can fulfill many different recipe needs. The different cuts range in texture and tenderness as well as in fat content, making Beef a very versatile food. The leanest cuts of Beef are taken from the back leg bone, called the round bone. These include eye of round, top round and bottom round. These cuts are the leanest (most muscular) because the cow uses its back legs as its primary means of movement. The underbelly—including rib, ribeye, spare rib and brisket—is the site of the fattiest cuts.

### VEAL

Veal is the meat of young calves. Many individuals have avoided veal because of the inhumane way that the calves have been raised. Now you can find veal from calves that have not been raised in confined pens but are raised humanely and allowed to roam the pasture with their mother. They drink their mother's milk and are not fed formula milk, which may contain antibiotics. "Calf's meat" rather than "veal" is the name now used by the USDA. The meat is from animals that are two to three months old and can be found in natural food stores.

There are organizations that are issuing labeling claims for humanely raised veal. Products from farms that meet their standards bear the label "Certified Humane Raised and Handled." You can find them at many natural food stores.

## the peak season

Grass-Fed Beef is available year-round.

## biochemical considerations

The saturated fat (4.28 g) and cholesterol (95.25 mg) content of Beef may be of concern to some individuals (amounts based on a 4-ounce serving). Grass-Fed Beef contains purines and is associated with food allergies, which may be problematic for some individuals. Scientists advise that red meat intake should be limited to less than three ounces per day. Grass-Fed Beef is not for everyone as some individuals have difficulty digesting Beef. (For more on *Purines*, see page 727; and *Food Allergies*, see page 719.)

## 4 steps for the best tasting and most nutritious grass-fed beef

Turning Grass-Fed Beef into a flavorful dish with the most nutrients is simple if you just follow my 4 easy steps:

1. The Best Way to Select
2. The Best Way to Store
3. The Best Way to Prepare
4. The Healthiest Way of Cooking

# 1. the best way to select grass-fed beef ———

There are a few clues you can look for that will help you choose fresher quality Grass-Fed Beef. Always examine the sell-by date on the label and choose the Beef with the latest date. The meat should be a red or purplish color. Purchase Beef that has the least amount of fat; any fat should be white in color.

Grades for Grass-Fed Beef include Prime, Choice and Select. Prime is the most tender and flavorful but also contains the highest fat content. While USDA inspection of Beef is mandatory, grading is voluntary; therefore not all Beef is graded.

Avoid Grass-Fed Beef that is brown (a sign that the meat has been excessively exposed to oxygen and is spoiled) or has yellow-colored fat (which indicates that it has come from an older animal and the meat is less tender). Choose organically raised Grass-Fed Beef whenever possible.

# 2. the best way to store grass-fed beef ———

Since Grass-Fed Beef is highly perishable, it should always be kept at cold temperatures, either refrigerated or frozen. Refrigerate Grass-Fed Beef in the original store packaging, if it is still intact and secure, as this will reduce the amount of handling involved. Length of storage varies with the cut of Grass-Fed Beef; larger pieces will have a longer shelf life than pieces with increased surface area, which increases the rate of oxidation that causes meat to spoil. Ground Grass-Fed Beef will keep for only one to two days (because of its larger surface area), steaks for two to three days and roasts for three to five days.

# 3. the best way to prepare grass-fed beef ———

When handling raw Grass-Fed Beef, be extremely careful that it does not come in contact with other foods, especially those that will be served uncooked, because raw meats can contain *E. coli* bacteria. In fact, you should use a separate plastic cutting board for meats. If you don't use a separate board, make sure you wash your hands and cutting board very well with hot soapy water after handling Grass-Fed Beef. It is a good idea to add two TBS of bleach to two cups of water in a spray bottle and use this mixture to clean your cutting board. Spray your cutting board with this mixture and let it sit for about 20 minutes to allow the bleach to evaporate.

If your recipe requires marinating, you should always do so in the refrigerator as Grass-Fed Beef is very sensitive to heat, which can increase the chances of spoilage. Discard the marinade after use because it contains raw juices, which may harbor bacteria.

Thaw uncooked frozen Grass-Fed Beef in the refrigerator. Thawing by refrigeration requires planning ahead and most likely allowing a 24-hour thawing period. After defrosting raw Grass-Fed Beef by this method, it will be safe in the refrigerator for up to four days before cooking, depending on cut.

To thaw Beef at room temperature be sure to place in cold water and leave the Grass-Fed Beef in its original wrapping or place it in a watertight plastic bag. Change the water every 30 minutes.

# 4. the healthiest way of cooking grass-fed beef

The "Healthiest Way of Cooking" Grass-Fed Beef is to use methods that will keep it moist and tender. Grass-Fed Beef can be easily overcooked and become dry, so be sure to watch your cooking times. Different cuts of Grass-Fed Beef can be prepared using almost any cooking method.

While grilled Grass-Fed Beef tastes great, make sure it does not burn. Cut away and discard any burnt areas. It is best to grill Grass-Fed Beef on an area without a direct flame as the temperatures directly above or below the flame can reach as high as 500°F to 1000°F (260°C to 538°C). Burning Grass-Fed Beef can damage nutrients and create free radicals that can be harmful to your health. (For more on *Grilling*, see page 61.)

Using a thermometer is the only reliable way to ensure safety and to determine the "doneness" of Grass-Fed Beef. When cooking whole cuts or parts of Grass-Fed Beef, the thermometer should be inserted into the thickest part of the meat, away from the bone, fat and gristle. The thermometer may be inserted sideways if necessary. The USDA recommends cooking to a minimum internal temperature of 160°F (71°C) for medium-cooked whole cuts of fresh Beef and 170°F (77°C) for well-done cuts.

**GROUND BEEF:** Ground Beef must be cooked thoroughly to kill harmful *E. coli* bacteria. Unlike whole muscle meat, whose interior meat is sterile, the grinding process exposes the interior meat in ground Grass-Fed Beef to bacteria, which may be on the surface, in the air, on the equipment or on people's hands. Food safety experts have one major rule of thumb to kill these bacteria—cook ground Beef to at least 160°F (71°C) or to well-done with no sign of pink coloration.

## Methods Not Recommended for Cooking Grass-Fed Beef

### PARTIAL COOKING OR COOKING WITH OIL

Never brown or partially cook Beef, then refrigerate and finish cooking later because any bacteria present will not have been destroyed. I don't recommend cooking Grass-Fed Beef in oil because high temperature heat can damage delicate oils and potentially create harmful free radicals. (For more on *Why it is Important to Cook Without Heated Oils*, see page 52.)

Here are questions I received from readers of the whfoods.org website about Grass-Fed Beef:

**Q** *I've read several claims on the Internet by producers of Grass-Fed Beef claiming that Grass-Fed Beef has an Omega-6:3 ratio comparable to fish. Is there any truth to this?*

**A** I have seen some research that Grass-Fed Beef has a higher omega-3 content than grain-fed Beef. Yet, I have not seen any research that shows that they provide the same Omega-6:3 ratio as fish.

**Q** *What is the healthiest cut of meat to eat?*

**A** The differences you find in Beef are related to differences in fat distribution and tenderness. The nutritional composition of the meat such as vitamins, minerals and protein do not vary. Because Beef can be high in saturated fat, one of the criteria for "healthy" would be to look for a lean cut. The leanest cuts of Beef are taken from the back leg bone, called the round bone. These include eye of round, top round and bottom round. These cuts are the leanest (most muscular) because the cow uses its back legs as its primary means of movement. The site of the fattiest cuts of meat include the rib, ribeye, spare rib and brisket.

STEP-BY-STEP RECIPE
## The Healthiest Ways of Cooking Grass-Fed Beef

# *"Healthy Sautéed"* Grass-Fed Beef and Vegetables

*Thinly sliced Grass-Fed Beef takes only minutes to prepare!*

- 1 medium onion, cut in half and sliced medium thick
- 1 bunch asparagus, cut into 1-inch lengths, discard bottom fourth (about 2 cups when cut)
- 1/2 cup red bell pepper, thinly sliced
- 1 small carrot, sliced on the diagonal
- 3 TBS low-sodium chicken broth
- 1 TBS minced fresh ginger
- 3 medium cloves garlic
- 3/4 lb Grass-Fed Beef sliced thin (1/4-inch)
- 2 TBS tamari (soy sauce)
- 1 TBS rice vinegar

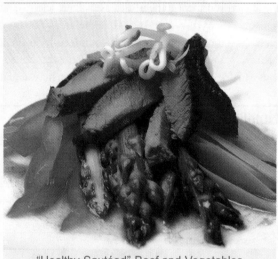

"Healthy Sautéed" Beef and Vegetables

Pinch red chili flakes
2–3 TBS extra virgin olive oil
Sea salt and pepper to taste

1. Slice onion and press garlic, and let sit for 5 minutes (Why?, see page 276.)

2. Heat 3 TBS broth in a 12-inch skillet until it begins to steam.

3. Add onion, carrot and bell pepper to the broth and sauté **covered** for about 3 minutes over medium heat.

4. Add ginger, garlic, asparagus and Beef, and continue to sauté for another 3–4 minutes, stirring constantly.

5. Add tamari (soy sauce), vinegar and red chili flakes. Stir together and **cover**. Cook for another 2–3 minutes. It may take a few extra minutes to make sure the vegetables are cooked. Season with salt and pepper to taste and sprinkle with the olive oil. **SERVES 2**

---

**Flavor Tips:** Try these 2 great serving suggestions with the recipe above. ✳

1. Add orange zest and juice from one medium orange to the "Healthy Sautéed" Grass-Fed Beef recipe and heat through.

2. Add toasted sesame oil and sesame seeds to "Healthy Sautéed" Grass-Fed Beef after cooking.

---

Please write (address on back cover flap) or e-mail me at info@whfoods.org with your personal ideas for preparing Grass-Fed Beef, and I will share them with others through our website at www.whfoods.org.

---

## QUICK SERVING IDEA for GRASS-FED BEEF:

**Marinated Grass-Fed Beef Salad:** In a large covered bowl, combine strips of cooked lean Grass-Fed Beef (2 inches x 1/4 inch), 6 whole small crimini mushrooms, 8 bell pepper strips, 1 small sliced sweet onion, 4 tomato wedges and 1 TBS of fresh oregano. Cover with Mediterranean dressing (see page 331). Let marinate 1–12 hours in the refrigerator. Stir occasionally. Serve over romaine leaves for a nutritious light meal. Add olive oil for more flavor.

# health benefits of grass-fed beef

Lately, red meat has been getting a lot of bad press. Studies have linked red meat to heart disease, atherosclerosis and even some types of cancer. But while the greasy, charcoal-burned bacon cheeseburger served with deep-fried French fries is a bad idea, a little bit of Grass-Fed Beef, added to stews, stir-fries or your favorite burrito recipe, may actually be healthy for you. Grass-Fed Beef is not only a very good source of protein but is also a concentrated source of numerous other health-promoting nutrients.

## Promotes Energy Production

Grass-Fed Beef is a good source of iron, a mineral of vital importance to health, especially to pregnant women and children. Severe iron depletion leads to anemia, but even before anemia develops, people may experience iron deficiency, with symptoms of lethargy, forgetfulness and depression among others. This is because one of the vital roles of iron is that it is a component of hemoglobin, a molecule that transports energy-producing oxygen to the cells of the body.

## Provides a Very Good Source of Protein

Grass-Fed Beef is a very good source of protein, a macronutrient vital to so many of our body's functions. From dietary protein, our body makes numerous other molecules that guide our body's processes. These include structural proteins such as those that make up muscles, connective tissue and skin, antibodies that help keep our immune system strong, and transport proteins that deliver oxygen and nutrients throughout the body.

## Promotes Bone Health

In addition to its numerous important physiological functions, dietary protein may be important in preventing bone loss in older people. In one study, the 70 to 90 year old men and women with the highest protein intakes lost significantly less bone over a four-year period than those who consumed less protein. Animal protein, as well as overall protein intake, was associated with preserving bone. Grass-Fed Beef contains high concentrations of the mineral zinc. In addition to playing a vital role in immune system health, recent research is focusing on zinc's role in promoting bone health. A recent study found a correlation between low dietary intake of zinc, low blood levels of zinc and osteoporosis in men.

## Additional Health-Promoting Benefits of Grass-Fed Beef

Grass-Fed Beef is also a concentrated source of many other nutrients providing additional health-promoting benefits. These nutrients include free-radical-scavenging selenium; heart-healthy vitamin B6, vitamin B12 and niacin; energy-producing vitamin B2 and phosphorus; and sleep-promoting tryptophan.

### Nutritional Analysis of 4 ounces of cooked lean Beef tenderloin:

| NUTRIENT | AMOUNT | % DAILY VALUE | NUTRIENT | AMOUNT | % DAILY VALUE |
|---|---|---|---|---|---|
| Calories | 240.41 | | Pantothenic Acid | 0.43 mg | 4.30 |
| Calories from Fat | 103.08 | | | | |
| Calories from Saturated Fat | 38.57 | | **Minerals** | | |
| Protein | 32.04 g | | Boron | — mcg | |
| Carbohydrates | 0.00 g | | Calcium | 7.93 mg | 0.79 |
| Dietary Fiber | 0.00 g | 0.00 | Chloride | — mg | |
| Soluble Fiber | 0.00 g | | Chromium | — mcg | — |
| Insoluble Fiber | 0.00 g | | Copper | 0.20 mg | 10.00 |
| Sugar – Total | 0.00 g | | Fluoride | — mg | |
| Monosaccharides | 0.00 g | | Iodine | — mcg | — |
| Disaccharides | 0.00 g | | Iron | 4.05 mg | 22.50 |
| Other Carbs | 0.00 g | | Magnesium | 34.03 mg | 8.51 |
| Fat – Total | 11.45 g | | Manganese | 0.01 mg | 0.50 |
| Saturated Fat | 4.28 g | | Molybdenum | 3.85 mcg | 5.13 |
| Mono Fat | 4.32 g | | Phosphorus | 269.89 mg | 26.99 |
| Poly Fat | 0.43 g | | Potassium | 475.15 mg | |
| Omega-3 Fatty Acids | 0.04 g | 1.60 | Selenium | 27.67 mcg | 39.53 |
| Omega-6 Fatty Acids | 0.39 g | | Sodium | 71.44 mg | |
| Trans Fatty Acids | — g | | Zinc | 6.33 mg | 42.20 |
| Cholesterol | 95.25 mg | | | | |
| Water | 67.81 g | | **Amino Acids** | | |
| Ash | 1.48 g | | Alanine | 1.93 g | |
| | | | Arginine | 2.03 g | |
| **Vitamins** | | | Aspartate | 2.93 g | |
| Vitamin A IU | 0.00 IU | 0.00 | Cystine | 0.36 g | 87.80 |
| Vitamin A RE | 0.00 RE | | Glutamate | 4.81 g | |
| A - Carotenoid | 0.00 RE | 0.00 | Glycine | 1.75 g | |
| A - Retinol | 0.00 RE | | Histidine | 1.09 g | 84.50 |
| B1 Thiamin | 0.15 mg | 10.00 | Isoleucine | 1.44 g | 125.22 |
| B2 Riboflavin | 0.35 mg | 20.59 | Leucine | 2.53 g | 100.00 |
| B3 Niacin | 4.44 mg | 22.20 | Lysine | 2.67 g | 113.62 |
| Niacin Equiv | 10.41 mg | | Methionine | 0.81 g | 109.46 |
| Vitamin B6 | 0.49 mg | 24.50 | Phenylalanine | 1.25 g | 105.04 |
| Vitamin B12 | 2.92 mcg | 48.67 | Proline | 1.41 g | |
| Biotin | — mcg | — | Serine | 1.23 g | |
| Vitamin C | 0.00 mg | 0.00 | Threonine | 1.40 g | 112.90 |
| Vitamin D IU | 13.61 IU | 3.40 | Tryptophan | 0.36 g | 112.50 |
| Vitamin D mcg | 0.35 mcg | | Tyrosine | 1.08 g | 111.34 |
| Vitamin E Alpha Equiv | 0.23 mg | 1.15 | Valine | 1.56 g | 106.12 |
| Vitamin E IU | 0.33 IU | | | | |
| Vitamin E mg | 0.23 mg | | (Note: "–" indicates data is unavailable. For more information, please see page 806.) | | |
| Folate | 7.93 mcg | 1.98 | | | |
| Vitamin K | — mcg | — | | | |

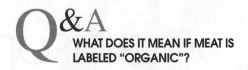

## Q&A
### WHAT DOES IT MEAN IF MEAT IS LABELED "ORGANIC"?

The term "organic" can be applied to a variety of different kinds of foods. The term can be used on agricultural products and on meat, poultry, eggs and dairy products. And it also applies to the methods used to process organically grown foods in preparing them for market or to retard spoilage.

## Organic Livestock Production

Standards for organic livestock production are meant to assure both an organic product to the consumer and living conditions for farm animals that limit stress and promote good health. They address substances used in health care and feeding, as well as herd or flock management and housing.

Livestock includes cattle, sheep, goats, swine, poultry, fish, wild or domesticated game and horses raised for slaughter or used as draft animals. There are even standards for organic bee-keeping.

Regardless of whether they're raised as breeding stock, as dairy animals or for slaughter, all livestock is covered by the Organic Foods Production Act.

## What are the Basic Organic Standards for Livestock (Animals)?

Quite simply, organic livestock must be fed organic feed.

The National Organic Standards Board (NOSB) recommends that conventional feed be allowed only if the organic feed supply has been compromised by a national, state or local weather emergency, or by fire or flood on an organic farm. Growth promoters and hormones, and plastic pellets for roughage in feed are prohibited. Synthetic vitamins and minerals are allowed.

The following are some of the standards that meat and poultry (as well as eggs and dairy products) need to meet for them to be labeled as "organic":

- Livestock must be fed rations composed of agricultural products, pasture and forage that are organically produced and, if applicable, handled.
- Prohibitions regarding animal feed include:
  - Administering of animal drugs in the absence of illness
  - Use of hormones to promote growth
  - Use of supplements in amounts above those for adequate nutrition
  - Use of mammal or poultry slaughter by-products for feed
  - Excessive use of feed additives
  - Routinely administering synthetic parasiticides

- Producers must provide conditions to maintain and promote the health and welfare of livestock including:
  - Sufficient nutritional feed rations
  - Appropriate housing, pasture and sanitation conditions
  - Conditions allowing for exercise, freedom of movement and minimizing stress of the animals
  - Administration of veterinary care
- Origin of livestock:
  - Organic livestock must be from livestock under continuous organic management from the last third of gestation or hatching
  - Organic poultry must be under continuous organic management beginning no later than the second day of life
  - Milk or milk products must be from animals that have been under continuous organic management beginning no later than one year prior to milk production.

Organic production is managed with the intent to integrate cultural, biological and mechanical practices to promote the cycling of resources and promote ecological balance and biodiversity. These practices help to protect the soil and groundwater, provide health-promoting conditions for animals and ultimately help promote the health of the consumer.

The following highlights address some of the questions most frequently asked about the NOSB Recommendations for Organic Livestock Standards.

**HOUSING AND HEALTH CARE FOR ORGANIC LIVESTOCK**
Healthy living conditions and attentive care are considered first steps in the prevention of illness. Therefore, animals must not be overcrowded and must be allowed periodic access to the outdoors and direct sunlight. Antibiotics, wormers and other medications may not be used routinely as preventive measures.

**WHY ARE ANTIBIOTICS ALLOWED IN ORGANIC LIVESTOCK PRODUCTION?**
Organic feed, good living conditions and attentive care are usually enough to support animals without medication. However, animals do get sick, and it would be contrary to the underlying values of organic production to let an animal suffer or die when treatment is available. The NOSB therefore recommends that antibiotics be allowed only for the treatment of a sick animal, not as a growth promoter or preventive measure, and never on a routine basis. If an animal intended for slaughter must be given antibiotics, it can no longer be considered organic. If a breeding animal, dairy cow or laying hen must be given antibiotics, the NOSB recommends it be taken out of the organic production system for an appropriate withdrawal period.

# venison

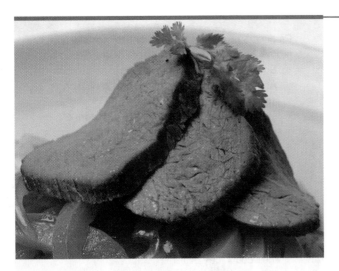

## nutrient-richness chart

Total Nutrient-Richness: **14**
4 ounces (113 grams) of cooked Venison contains 179 calories

| NUTRIENT | AMOUNT | %DV | DENSITY | QUALITY |
|---|---|---|---|---|
| Protein | 34.25 g | 68.5 | 6.9 | very good |
| Vitamin B12 | 3.60 mcg | 60.0 | 6.0 | very good |
| B2 Riboflavin | 0.68 mg | 40.0 | 4.0 | very good |
| B3 Niacin | 7.61 mg | 38.0 | 3.8 | very good |
| Iron | 5.07 mg | 28.2 | 2.8 | good |
| Phosphorus | 256.28 mg | 25.6 | 2.6 | good |
| B6 Pyridoxine | 0.43 mg | 21.5 | 2.2 | good |
| Selenium | 14.63 mcg | 20.9 | 2.1 | good |
| Zinc | 3.12 mg | 20.8 | 2.1 | good |
| Copper | 0.35 mg | 17.5 | 1.8 | good |

For more on "Total Nutrient-Richness," "%DV," "Density," and
The World's Healthiest Foods "Quality" Rating System, see page 805.

Venison is a highly prized, wonderfully delicious and nutritious meat that can come from either wild or farm-raised deer. Historians suggest that Venison has been consumed as a food longer than the other meats we enjoy today. The ancient Greeks seemed to be the first civilization that printed a guide to hunting with the ancient Romans lauding the pleasures of hunting and consuming wild game. Today, Venison is enjoyed by many cultures that enjoy hunting. While the flavor of the meat is directly related to the animal's diet, Venison is typically described as having a strong flavor that is somewhat akin to a deeply woody, yet berry-like, red wine and a texture that is supple and tender. If you are not a hunter, you can now find Venison in the frozen food or refrigerated section of the market.

## highlights

| | |
|---|---|
| AVAILABILITY: | Year-round |
| REFRIGERATE: | Yes |
| SHELF LIFE: | 3–5 days refrigerated |
| PREPARATION: | Minimal |
| BEST WAY TO COOK: | "Healthy Sauté" |

## why venison should be part of your healthiest way of eating

The concern over eating meat is often related to its high concentration of saturated fats. Unlike other meats, Venison is very low in saturated fat while providing a good source of protein. It is also a rich source of heme iron, the type of iron readily absorbed by the body, as well as the heart-healthy B-vitamins, B6 and B12. (For more on the *Health Benefits of Venison* and a complete profile of its content of over 60 nutrients, see page 568.)

## varieties of venison

Venison is more dense and less fatty than beef and will not have a gamey taste if it is properly prepared. Like beef, it comes in many different cuts, such as steaks, roasts, brisket, stew meat and ground Venison. The meat from the ribs and loin sections are more tender than cuts from the rump and shoulder. Chuck and shoulder are tasty and make good pot roast or can be tenderized and enjoyed as steak. Ribs and rib-eye steaks are tender and can be broiled or grilled. Shank and heel of round are bony leg cuts that are good for making soup stock.

## the peak season

Venison is available year-round.

## biochemical considerations

Venison contains purines, which may be of concern to certain individuals. (For more on *Purines*, see page 727.)

## 4 steps for the best tasting and most nutritious venison

Turning Venison into a flavorful dish with the most

nutrients is simple if you just follow my 4 easy steps:

1. The Best Way to Select
2. The Best Way to Store
3. The Best Way to Prepare
4. The Healthiest Way of Cooking

# 1. the best way to select venison

There are a few clues you can look for that will help you choose fresher quality Venison. Venison from younger animals will have darker, more finely grained flesh and whiter fat; it will offer the most flavorful taste. The rib and loin sections are the most tasty cuts of Venison. Always examine the sell-by date on the label, if there is one, and choose the package with the latest date. Venison is generally available fresh and frozen.

# 2. the best way to store venison

Since Venison is highly perishable, it should always be kept at cold temperatures, either refrigerated or frozen. Refrigerate the Venison in the original store packaging, if it is still intact and secure, as this will reduce the amount of handling involved.

Follow the use-by date as a gauge to how long Venison will remain fresh. If the package does not have a use-by date, follow these simple guidelines: stored in store packaging or repackaged in a similar fashion, Venison roasts and chops can stay fresh in the refrigerator for 3 to 5 days, while ground Venison will only stay fresh for up to 2 days.

To help Venison remain fresh and extend its storage life, put it in a plastic storage bag, place it in a bowl and cover it with ice to reduce its temperature.

# 3. the best way to prepare venison

As with other meats, be careful when handling raw Venison so that it does not come in contact with other foods, especially those that will be served uncooked. Wash the cutting board, utensils and even your hands very well with hot soapy water after handling the meat. It is a good idea to add two TBS of bleach to two cups of water in a spray bottle and use this mixture to clean your cutting board. Spray your cutting board with this mixture and let it sit for about 20 minutes to allow the bleach to evaporate.

If your recipe requires marinating, you should always do so in the refrigerator as the meat is very sensitive to heat, which increases the chances of spoilage. When defrosting frozen Venison, do so in the refrigerator and not at room temperature. Place it on a plate to capture any liquid drippings.

# 4. the healthiest way of cooking venison

The "Healthiest Way of Cooking" Venison is to use methods that will keep it moist and tender. Venison can be easily overcooked and become dry, so be sure to watch your cooking times. Different cuts of Venison are best prepared using different methods.

I have found that "Healthy Sauté" is the best way to cook Venison steaks. Tender cuts can be roasted or broiled, while tougher cuts like the leg and shoulder are best braised. (For more on *"Healthy Sauté,"* see page 57.)

## Methods Not Recommended for Cooking Venison

### COOKING WITH OIL

I don't recommend cooking Venison in oil because high temperature heat can damage delicate oils and potentially create harmful free radicals. (For more on *Why it is Important to Cook Without Heated Oils*, see page 52.)

# health benefits of venison

## Very Good Low-Fat Source of Protein

Venison is a very good source of protein. Unlike most meats, it tends to be fairly low in fat, especially saturated fat. In fact, only 7% of its calories come from saturated fat. (For comparison, lean beef provides 16% of its calories from saturated fat, and chicken breast 10%.)

### Nutritional Analysis of 4 ounces of cooked Venison:

| NUTRIENT | AMOUNT | % DAILY VALUE | NUTRIENT | AMOUNT | % DAILY VALUE |
|---|---|---|---|---|---|
| Calories | 179.17 | | Pantothenic Acid | 0.36 mg | 3.60 |
| Calories from Fat | 32.56 | | | | |
| Calories from Saturated Fat | 12.76 | | **Minerals** | | |
| Protein | 34.25 g | | Boron | — mcg | |
| Carbohydrates | 0.00 g | | Calcium | 7.93 mg | 0.79 |
| Dietary Fiber | 0.00 g | 0.00 | Chloride | — mg | |
| Soluble Fiber | 0.00 g | | Chromium | 0.00 mcg | 0.00 |
| Insoluble Fiber | 0.00 g | | Copper | 0.35 mg | 17.50 |
| Sugar – Total | 0.00 g | | Fluoride | — mg | — |
| Monosaccharides | 0.00 g | | Iodine | — mcg | — |
| Disaccharides | 0.00 g | | Iron | 5.07 mg | 28.17 |
| Other Carbs | 0.00 g | | Magnesium | 27.21 mg | 6.80 |
| Fat – Total | 3.61 g | | Manganese | 0.05 mg | 2.50 |
| Saturated Fat | 1.41 g | | Molybdenum | — mcg | — |
| Mono Fat | 1.00 g | | Phosphorus | 256.28 mg | 25.63 |
| Poly Fat | 0.71 g | | Potassium | 379.89 mg | |
| Omega-3 Fatty Acids | 0.11 g | 4.40 | Selenium | 14.63 mcg | 20.90 |
| Omega-6 Fatty Acids | 0.60 g | | Sodium | 61.24 mg | |
| Trans Fatty Acids | 0.00 g | | Zinc | 3.12 mg | 20.80 |
| Cholesterol | 127.01 mg | | | | |
| Water | 73.97 g | | **Amino Acids** | | |
| Ash | 1.72 g | | Alanine | 2.13 g | |
| | | | Arginine | 2.47 g | |
| **Vitamins** | | | Aspartate | 3.17 g | |
| Vitamin A IU | 0.00 IU | 0.00 | Cystine | 0.39 g | 95.12 |
| Vitamin A RE | 0.00 RE | | Glutamate | 4.97 g | |
| A - Carotenoid | 0.00 RE | 0.00 | Glycine | 1.75 g | |
| A - Retinol | 0.00 RE | | Histidine | 1.69 g | 131.01 |
| B1 Thiamin | 0.20 mg | 13.33 | Isoleucine | 1.36 g | 118.26 |
| B2 Riboflavin | 0.68 mg | 40.00 | Leucine | 2.91 g | 115.02 |
| B3 Niacin | 7.61 mg | 38.05 | Lysine | 2.99 g | 127.23 |
| Niacin Equiv | 7.61 mg | | Methionine | 0.84 g | 113.51 |
| Vitamin B6 | 0.43 mg | 21.50 | Phenylalanine | 1.40 g | 117.65 |
| Vitamin B12 | 3.60 mcg | 60.00 | Proline | 1.76 g | |
| Biotin | — mcg | — | Serine | 1.45 g | |
| Vitamin C | 0.00 mg | 0.00 | Threonine | 1.61 g | 129.84 |
| Vitamin D IU | 13.61 IU | 3.40 | Tryptophan | 0.00 g | 0.00 |
| Vitamin D mcg | 0.35 mcg | | Tyrosine | 1.21 g | 124.74 |
| Vitamin E Alpha Equiv | 0.28 mg | 1.40 | Valine | 1.60 g | 108.84 |
| Vitamin E IU | 0.43 IU | | | | |
| Vitamin E mg | 0.28 mg | | | | |
| Folate | 5.35 mcg | 1.34 | | | |
| Vitamin K | — mcg | — | | | |

(Note: "–" indicates data is unavailable. For more information, please see page 806.)

## Promotes Heart Health

Venison is rich in B vitamins. It is a very good source of vitamin B12, riboflavin and niacin and a good source of vitamin B6. Vitamin B12 and vitamin B6 are both needed to prevent a build up of a potentially dangerous molecule, called homocysteine, in the body. High levels of homocysteine can cause damage to blood vessels, contribute to the development and progression of atherosclerosis and diabetic heart disease and greatly increase the risk of heart attack or stroke. Homocysteine is also associated with osteoporosis, and a recent study found that osteoporosis occurred more frequently among women whose vitamin B12 status was deficient or marginal compared with those who had normal B12 status.

## Promotes Energy Production

In comparison to beef, a well-known source of iron, Venison provides well-absorbed iron for less calories and fat. Particularly for menstruating women, who are more at risk for iron deficiency, boosting iron stores is a good idea. Iron is an integral component of hemoglobin, which transports oxygen from the lungs to all body cells, and is also part of key enzyme systems for energy production and metabolism. Women who are pregnant or lactating as well as growing children and adolescents need to pay particular attention to their dietary iron intake.

Venison's B vitamins are also integrally important for maintaining optimal energy production. Two unique forms of niacin (known as NAD and NADP) are essential for conversion of the body's proteins, fats and carbohydrates into usable energy. Niacin is also used to synthesize starch that can be stored in the body's muscles and liver for eventual use as an energy source. Riboflavin protects oxygen-containing molecules from being damaged through its ability to recycle the antioxidant glutathione; therefore, like its fellow B-complex vitamins, it is important in energy production. Venison is also a good source of the mineral phosphorus, which is an active component of ATP, the molecule that fuels the activity of our cells.

## Promotes Optimal Antioxidant Status

Venison is a good source of three important antioxidant minerals—selenium, zinc and copper. These minerals help to promote overall health by helping to neutralize free radicals, which can cause damage to cells and tissues and compromise physiological function.

STEP-BY-STEP RECIPE
## The Healthiest Ways of Cooking Venison

# *"Healthy Sautéed" Venison with Peppers*

6 oz Venison steak
3 TBS + 3 TBS low-sodium chicken broth
3/4 cup red bell pepper, sliced thin
3/4 cup yellow bell pepper, sliced thin
1 small yellow onion, sliced thin
1/2 cup raisins
Extra virgin olive oil to taste
Sea salt and pepper to taste

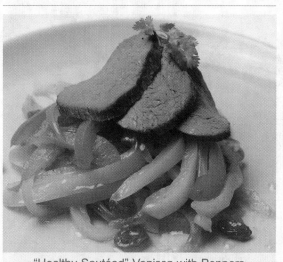

"Healthy Sautéed" Venison with Peppers

1. Slice onions and let sit for 5 minutes. (Why?, see page 276.)

2. Heat 3 TBS chicken broth on medium in a stainless steel skillet.

3. When the broth begins to steam, add Venison steak and sauté for 3 minutes on one side, then turn and sauté for 2 minutes on the other side. Remove from the pan, set aside and **cover**.

4. In the same skillet, heat remaining 3 TBS chicken broth and add onions, bell peppers and raisins. **Cover** and sauté for 7 minutes.

5. While the vegetables are cooking, slice Venison.

6. When the vegetables are done, toss them with extra virgin olive oil, and sea salt and pepper to taste. Top with sliced Venison.

**SERVES 2**

Please write (address on back cover flap) or e-mail me at info@whfoods.org with your personal ideas for preparing Venison, and I will share them with others through our website at www.whfoods.org.

---

Here is a question I received from a reader of the whfoods.org website about Venison:

**Q** *A friend recently told me that beef is better than Venison because Venison has less protein in it than beef. I had never heard that before. Can you tell me if it is true or not?*

**A** In the case of any animal, the meat we eat for food is mostly a mixture of proteins found in the muscle of the animal and fats in the surrounding tissue. The muscles of a deer (the animal from which Venison is derived) have the same basic protein structure as the muscles of a cow. An ounce of roasted Venison contains about 8.5 grams of protein. An ounce of broiled round steak contains this same amount of protein.

If you took an ounce of rib roast, however, and compared it to most any cut of Venison, you'd find more fat and less protein per ounce because the rib area of the cow is an especially fatty area. The deer does not have any area that reaches this high a fat percentage. That would be a situation opposite of the one described by your friend. In the example above with 8.5 grams of protein, I used the round bone cut of beef because the round bone (back leg bone) of the cow is one of the most muscular and least fatty regions of the cow's body.

In general, it would not make sense to talk about a food being better or worse than another food because it had more or less protein. Whether a food is good or bad for us would depend on how much protein we needed and what other wanted or unwanted nutrients/substances were present in the food.

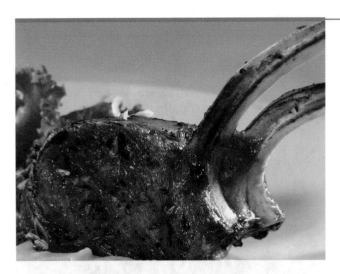

# lamb

| | |
|---|---|
| AVAILABILITY: | Year-round |
| REFRIGERATE: | Yes |
| SHELF LIFE: | 3–5 days refrigerated |
| PREPARATION: | Minimal |
| BEST WAY TO COOK: | "Quick Broiled" |

## nutrient-richness chart

Total Nutrient-Richness: **12**
4 ounces (113 grams) of roasted Lamb loin contains 229 calories

| NUTRIENT | AMOUNT | %DV | DENSITY | QUALITY |
|---|---|---|---|---|
| Tryptophan | 0.35 g | 109.4 | 8.6 | excellent |
| Protein | 30.15 g | 60.3 | 4.7 | very good |
| Selenium | 34.36 mcg | 49.1 | 3.9 | very good |
| Vitamin B12 | 2.45 mcg | 40.8 | 3.2 | good |
| B3 Niacin | 7.75 mg | 38.8 | 3.0 | good |
| Zinc | 4.60 mg | 30.7 | 2.4 | good |
| Phosphorus | 233.60 mg | 23.4 | 1.8 | good |

For more on "Total Nutrient-Richness," "%DV," "Density," and
The World's Healthiest Foods "Quality" Rating System, see page 805.

L amb is considered the most flavorful of all the meats. While Lamb is currently the most abundant form of livestock in the world and one of the most popular sources of meat, this delicious, tender meat has not yet been fully appreciated in the United States. In fact, the yearly consumption of Lamb per person is equivalent to the amount of beef found in four quarter-pound hamburgers! However, in many other countries and regions of the world, including Spain, Portugal, Italy, Southern France, Greece, the Middle East, India, Australia, New Zealand and North Africa, Lamb is a dietary staple with consumption upwards of 60 pounds per person per year. I want to share with you how to prepare Lamb easily and quickly and bring out its flavor by using the "Healthiest Way of Cooking" methods.

## why lamb should be part of your healthiest way of eating

Trim off the visible fat from a Lamb chop and you will have meat that is more tender and lean than beef and a great addition to your "Healthiest Way of Eating." Lamb may be more expensive than other meats, but its nutrition and taste make it well worth the extra cost. Lamb is rich in vitamin B12 and selenium zinc nutrients, important for immune function. (For more on the *Health Benefits of Lamb* and a complete profile of its content of over 60 nutrients, see page 574.)

## varieties of lamb

Sheep were originally domesticated in the Middle East and Asia more than 10,000 years ago. What we usually call Lamb is the pinkish meat from young sheep that are usually between five to six months old (but can be up to one year old. Varieties of Lamb can be categorized by age, season or how they have been fed:

**BABY LAMB**
Lamb that is milk fed.

**YEARLING**
This is the meat from an animal that is between one and two years of age.

**MUTTON**
The meat from an animal that is older than two years. Mutton has red meat and yellow-colored fat; it is less tender and has a stronger flavor than Lamb. It is difficult to find mutton in the United States.

**SPRING LAMB**
Spring Lamb means that it is brought to market during the spring and summer months, which was formerly the peak season for fresh Lamb. However, Lamb is now available throughout the year, and the label Spring Lamb does not necessarily connote additional quality.

**MILK-FED LAMB**

This is from very young Lamb and is found primarily during the spring. It is the most tender, free of hormones and antibiotics but also very expensive.

**GRASS-FED LAMB**

Generally, grass-fed Lamb is fed grass for three to six months after they are taken off of milk. The meat from Lamb that has been grass-fed until it is a year old and never fed any grain will not contain any hormones or antibiotics. Grass-fed Lamb is much more widely produced in New Zealand and Australia, and your chances of getting grass-fed, hormone-free Lamb increases when it comes from these countries. Ask your butcher for names of companies that produce grass-fed or organically raised Lamb.

**GRAIN-FED LAMB**

Most U.S. Lamb is fed grain before it is sold. Grain-fed Lamb can be labeled "Select," "Choice," or "Prime."

**ORGANIC**

Organically raised Lamb has been fed an organically grown diet and raised without the use of hormones or antibiotics.

The best Lamb is milk-fed, grass-fed and/or certified organic.

Range-fed Lamb does not necessarily mean it has only been grass-fed or that it is organic. There are six cuts of Lamb, as well as ground Lamb (for details, see Step 4 on next page).

## the peak season

Lamb is available year-round.

## biochemical considerations

Lamb contains purines, which may be problematic for certain individuals. The saturated fat (4.2 g) and cholesterol (99 mg) content of 4 ounces of Lamb may be of concern to some individuals. (For more on *Purines*, see page 727.)

## 4 steps for the best tasting and most nutritious lamb

Turning Lamb into a flavorful dish with the most nutrients is simple if you just follow my 4 easy steps:

1. The Best Way to Select
2. The Best Way to Store
3. The Best Way to Prepare
4. The Healthiest Way of Cooking

# 1. the best way to select lamb

The best tasting Lamb is the meat from animals that are five months to one year old. The best way to select Lamb is to look for meat that is firm, finely textured and pink in color. Its fatty portion should be white. I recommend selecting milk-fed, grass-fed and/or certified organic Lamb whenever possible. (For more on *Organic Meats*, see page 565.)

Grades for Lamb include Prime, Choice and Select. Prime is the most tender and flavorful but also contains the highest fat content. While USDA inspection of Lamb is

mandatory, grading is voluntary; therefore, not all Lamb is graded.

Avoid Lamb with any yellow (rather than white) fat surrounding or marbled throughout the meat.

Darker fat indicates that the meat is actually mutton from an older animal and therefore does not have the delicate flavor of Lamb. Check the use-by date to be sure that the Lamb is still fresh.

# 2. the best way to store lamb

Since Lamb is highly perishable, it should always be kept at cold temperatures, either refrigerated or frozen. Refrigerate the Lamb in the original store packaging, if it is still intact and secure, as this will reduce the amount of handling involved.

Follow the use-by date as a gauge of how long Lamb will remain fresh. If the package does not have a use-by date,

follow these simple guidelines: Lamb roasts and chops can stay fresh in the refrigerator for 3 to 5 days while ground Lamb will only stay fresh for up to 2 days.

To help Lamb remain fresh and extend its storage life, put it in a storage bag, place it in a bowl and cover it with ice to further reduce its temperature in the refrigerator.

# 3. the best way to prepare lamb

When handling raw Lamb, be extremely careful that it does not come in contact with other foods, especially those that will be served uncooked because raw meats can contain *E. coli* bacteria. In fact, you should use a separate plastic cutting board for meats. If you don't use a separate board, make sure you wash your hands and cutting board very well with hot soapy water after handling Lamb. It is a good idea to add two TBS of bleach to two cups of water in a spray bottle and use this mixture to clean your cutting board. Spray your cutting board with this mixture and let it sit 20 minutes to allow the bleach to evaporate.

If your recipe requires marinating, you should always do so in the refrigerator as Lamb is very sensitive to heat, which can increase the chances of spoilage. Discard the marinade after use because it contains raw juices, that may harbor bacteria.

Thaw uncooked frozen Lamb in the refrigerator. Thawing by refrigeration requires planning ahead and most likely allowing a 24-hour thawing period. After defrosting raw Lamb by this method, it will be safe in the refrigerator for up to four days before cooking, depending on cut.

To thaw Lamb at room temperature be sure to place in cold water and leave the Lamb in its original wrapping or place it in a watertight plastic bag. Change the water every 30 minutes.

I always trim the fat from my Lamb before cooking it. Not only is the fat unhealthy, but it can give Lamb an overly strong flavor.

# 4. the healthiest way of cooking lamb

The "Healthiest Way of Cooking" Lamb is to use methods that will keep it moist and tender. Lamb can be easily overcooked and become dry, so be sure to watch your cooking times. Different cuts of Lamb are best prepared using different methods:

**SHOULDER:** Best to make stew and cooked medium-well.

---

## *Moroccan Lamb Chops*

*If you like Moroccan spices, give this recipe a try.*

4 Lamb chops, medium size
1/2 tsp cinnamon
1 tsp curry powder
1 tsp fresh ginger, minced
1/4 cup apple juice
2 tsp cider vinegar
1 tsp tamari (soy sauce)
2 TBS extra virgin olive oil

1. In a large bowl, marinate Lamb chops for 1 hour in the spices, apple juice, vinegar and tamari.

2. Cook according to "Quick Broiled" Lamb recipe (see page 573).

3. Drizzle with extra virgin olive oil before serving.

**SERVES 2**

---

**SHANK / BREAST:** Best braised and cooked well-done.
**LEG:** Best roasted and cooked well-done.
**LOIN (LAMB CHOPS):** Best "Quick Broiled." (For more on *"Quick Broil,"* see page 60.)
**RACK OF LAMB:** Best roasted or "Quick Broiled" medium-rare.
**GROUND LAMB:** Best "Healthy Sautéed" and cooked well. It has a greater amount of surface area exposed to the air and is therefore more susceptible to spoilage. I therefore recommend cooking it on the same day it is purchased.

While grilled Lamb tastes great, make sure it does not burn. It is best to grill Lamb on an area without a direct flame as the temperatures directly above or below the flame can reach as high as 500°F to 1000°F (260°–538°C). Burning Lamb can damage nutrients and create free radicals that can be harmful to your health. (For more on *Grilling*, see page 61.)

## Roasting Lamb

Roasting works best for rolled and tied boneless leg and shoulder roasts or for bone-in leg of Lamb. (Boneless is easiest to carve.) Ideally, it should be marinated in fresh lemon juice, garlic, salt and pepper (rosemary is also a good addition) for 24 hours before roasting. Preheat oven to 350°F (175°C). Cook until internal temperature is 145°F (63°C) for medium-rare Lamb. A 4-pound leg of Lamb will take from 45 minutes to 1 hour to cook.

STEP-BY-STEP RECIPE
## The Healthiest Ways of Cooking Lamb

# Rosemary "Quick Broiled" Lamb

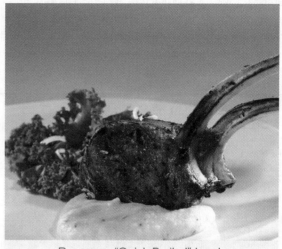

Rosemary "Quick Broiled" Lamb

*If you have extra time, marinating Lamb will give it great flavor. This easy preparation seals in the juices, and the skillet requires no oil.*

**4 Lamb chops, medium size**

**Marinade:**
**5 cloves garlic**
**3 TBS fresh lemon juice**
**2 TBS fresh rosemary, removed from stem and chopped**
**Sea salt and pepper to taste**

1. Press garlic and let sit for 5 minutes. (Why? See page 261.)

2. Combine the marinade ingredients and Lamb chops in a bowl or plastic bag with seal. Marinate in refrigerator 2 hours to overnight. If you don't have time to marinate, let the Lamb chops sit in marinade for at least 10 minutes.

3. Preheat the broiler on high and place an all stainless steel skillet (be sure the handle is also stainless steel) or cast iron pan under the heat for about 10 minutes to get it very hot. The pan should be about 5–7 inches from the heat source.

4. Remove Lamb chops from marinade. Using a hot pad, pull the pan out from the broiler, place the Lamb chops on the pan and return to the broiler. They cook very quickly as they are cooking on both sides simultaneously. Do not turn.

5. Broil for 7–10 minutes for medium-rare, depending on the thickness of the chops. They are done when the internal temperature is 135°F (57°C). For medium-well chops, cook 2–3 minutes longer.

**SERVES 2**

---

## Flavor Tips: Try these 4 great serving suggestions with the recipe above. ✳

1. Lamb is enhanced by mint, thyme, cinnamon and oregano.
2. Chopped mint leaves or mint jelly and finely sliced scallions (green onions) complement the flavor of Lamb.
3. Serve the "Quick Broiled" Lamb Recipe with Puréed Navy Beans (see page 627).
4. **Lamb with Dijon Mustard:** Combine Dijon mustard and fresh thyme with extra virgin olive oil and serve on "Quick Broiled" Lamb recipe.

---

Please write (address on back cover flap) or e-mail me at info@whfoods.org with your personal ideas for preparing Lamb, and I will share them with others through our website at www.whfoods.org.

---

## 2 QUICK SERVING IDEAS for LAMB:

1. **Middle Eastern Wrap:** On a flour tortilla, place a romaine leaf, fresh mint leaves, low-fat yogurt, a dash of ground cumin and strips of cooked Lamb loin.

2. **Lamb Burger with Yogurt:** Ground Lamb makes a delicious burger. Try it seasoned with dried spices such as cumin or rosemary and salt and pepper to taste. Top with low-fat yogurt and sliced scallions.

# health benefits of lamb

## Provides a Very Good Source of Protein

Lamb is a very good source of protein. The structure of the human body is built on protein. Animal and plant sources of protein provide amino acids that the body rearranges into patterns the body can use. The proteins synthesized by the body have a variety of very impor-tant functions including the production of: structural pro-teins that maintain the integrity of the muscles, connective tissues, hair, skin and nails; enzymes and hormones, nec-essary to spark chemical reactions in the body; transport proteins, which carry substances, such as oxygen and nutrients, to body tissues; and antibodies, which play an important role in the immune system.

## Promotes Healthy Immune Function

Lamb is a good source of zinc, a mineral that plays a criti-cal role in supporting immune function. It protects against free-radical damage, is required for proper white cell function, promotes the destruction of foreign particles and microorganisms and is necessary for the activation of serum thymic factor—a thymus hormone with profound immune-enhancing actions. It also inhibits replication of several viruses, including those that cause the common cold.

## Promotes Heart Health

Lamb is a very good source of selenium, a mineral that has powerful antioxidant activity. In many instances of heart disease, for example, where oxidative stress has been shown to be the source of blood vessel damage, low intake of selenium has been identified as a contributing factor to the disease. In addition, Lamb is a good source of vitamin B12, which is important for keeping homocysteine levels in check. Since homocysteine directly damages artery walls, the vitamin B12 provided by Lamb may help to reduce risk of cardiovascular disease.

## A Hypoallergenic Food

Lamb is considered to be a hypoallergenic food. Most people do not have adverse food sensitivity reactions to Lamb as they may to beef or poultry. As such, Lamb is usually included on elimination diets and other hypo-allergenic diets.

## Additional Health-Promoting Benefits of Lamb

Lamb is also a concentrated source of other nutrients pro-viding additional health-promoting benefits. These nutri-ents include energy-producing niacin and phosphorus, and sleep-promoting tryptophan.

### Nutritional Analysis of 4 ounces of roasted Lamb loin:

| NUTRIENT | AMOUNT | % DAILY VALUE |
| --- | --- | --- |
| Calories | 229.07 | |
| Calories from Fat | 99.61 | |
| Calories from Saturated Fat | 37.97 | |
| Protein | 30.15 g | |
| Carbohydrates | 0.00 g | |
| Dietary Fiber | 0.00 g | 0.00 |
| Soluble Fiber | 0.00 g | |
| Insoluble Fiber | 0.00 g | |
| Sugar – Total | 0.00 g | |
| Monosaccharides | 0.00 g | |
| Disaccharides | 0.00 g | |
| Other Carbs | 0.00 g | |
| Fat – Total | 11.07 g | |
| Saturated Fat | 4.22 g | |
| Mono Fat | 4.48 g | |
| Poly Fat | 0.98 g | |
| Omega-3 Fatty Acids | 0.16 g | 6.40 |
| Omega-6 Fatty Acids | 0.82 g | |
| Trans Fatty Acids | 0.00 g | |
| Cholesterol | 98.66 mg | |
| Water | 71.17 g | |
| Ash | 1.53 g | |
| **Vitamins** | | |
| Vitamin A IU | 0.00 IU | 0.00 |
| Vitamin A RE | 0.00 RE | |
| A - Carotenoid | 0.00 RE | 0.00 |
| A - Retinol | 0.00 RE | |
| B1 Thiamin | 0.11 mg | 7.33 |
| B2 Riboflavin | 0.31 mg | 18.24 |
| B3 Niacin | 7.75 mg | 38.75 |
| Niacin Equiv | 13.62 mg | |
| Vitamin B6 | 0.18 mg | 9.00 |
| Vitamin B12 | 2.45 mcg | 40.83 |
| Biotin | 2.27 mcg | 0.76 |
| Vitamin C | 0.00 mg | 0.00 |
| Vitamin D IU | 13.61 IU | 3.40 |
| Vitamin D mcg | 0.34 mcg | |
| Vitamin E Alpha Equiv | 0.18 mg | 0.90 |
| Vitamin E IU | 0.27 IU | |
| Vitamin E mg | 0.18 mg | |
| Folate | 28.35 mcg | 7.09 |
| Vitamin K | — mcg | — |

| NUTRIENT | AMOUNT | % DAILY VALUE |
| --- | --- | --- |
| Pantothenic Acid | 0.77 mg | 7.70 |
| **Minerals** | | |
| Boron | — mcg | |
| Calcium | 19.28 mg | 1.93 |
| Chloride | — mg | |
| Chromium | — mcg | — |
| Copper | 0.15 mg | 7.50 |
| Fluoride | — mg | — |
| Iodine | — mcg | — |
| Iron | 2.77 mg | 15.39 |
| Magnesium | 30.62 mg | 7.66 |
| Manganese | 0.03 mg | 1.50 |
| Molybdenum | 3.86 mcg | 5.15 |
| Phosphorus | 233.60 mg | 23.36 |
| Potassium | 302.78 mg | |
| Selenium | 34.36 mcg | 49.09 |
| Sodium | 74.84 mg | |
| Zinc | 4.60 mg | 30.67 |
| **Amino Acids** | | |
| Alanine | 1.81 g | |
| Arginine | 1.79 g | |
| Aspartate | 2.65 g | |
| Cystine | 0.36 g | 87.80 |
| Glutamate | 4.38 g | |
| Glycine | 1.47 g | |
| Histidine | 0.95 g | 73.64 |
| Isoleucine | 1.45 g | 126.09 |
| Leucine | 2.35 g | 92.89 |
| Lysine | 2.66 g | 113.19 |
| Methionine | 0.77 g | 104.05 |
| Phenylalanine | 1.23 g | 103.36 |
| Proline | 1.26 g | |
| Serine | 1.12 g | |
| Threonine | 1.29 g | 104.03 |
| Tryptophan | 0.35 g | 109.38 |
| Tyrosine | 1.01 g | 104.12 |
| Valine | 1.63 g | 110.88 |

(Note: "–" indicates data is unavailable. For more information, please see page 806.)

(Continued from Page 44)

dinner will help you feel satiated more quickly so you will eat fewer calories over the entire meal. For example, one study found that woman who ate a large low-calorie salad ate 12% less pasta even when they were offered as much as they wanted. Not only will your appetite be more satisfied by enjoying a daily salad but you'll also greatly benefit from all of the important nutrients it has to offer. Studies have shown that people who ate one salad a day with dressing also had high levels of vitamin C, E, folic acid, lycopene and other carotenoids than those who did not add salad as part of their daily menu. You can readily make your salads versatile and even have them be the centerpiece of a meal but topping them with some chicken, fish or beans; you'll have a substantial meal that will provide you with less calories than meals you may regularly consume.

Another example of a feature of the Plan that can help you lose weight is green tea. Studies show that three cups of green tea a day can reduce body weight and waist circumference by 5% in three months. Not only does it inhibit the breakdown of fats, it also increases your metabolism.

## Nutrient-Richness Means that Foods Don't Have Excessive Calories

While the science of weight management is discovering exciting new findings that will one day substantiate a more complex picture, there is an undeniable fact that we can't get away from: weight gain and loss is related to calories—calorie intake and calorie expenditure. If you expend more calories than you take in, you'll lose weight. If you take in more calories than you expend, you'll gain weight.

Since the World's Healthiest Foods are nutrient-rich foods that don't contain excess calories, they'll be a much better option for low-calorie foods than others. For example, eating two cups of green vegetables rather a baked potato with butter or margarine will save you over 300 calories while a fruit parfait made with low-fat yogurt and berries will save you 200 calories compared to eating one cup of ice cream. Since it takes about 3,500 calories to make a pound, you can see how these caloric savings can quickly add up to weight loss.

While nutrient-rich foods, like the World's Healthiest Foods, contain a concentration of nutrients for the calories they contain, some do contain more calories than others. Therefore, I'd suggest making these foods the foundation of your menu plans but looking through the detailed nutritional analysis profiles in each food chapter to not only see the nutrients that the foods offer but the calories they contain. This way you can make the best choices to support your personal needs. For example, while salmon is a wonderful fish that contains great amount of nutrients, if you chose to substitute cod for a salmon recipe one day, you'd save 150 calories per each 4-ounce serving.

## Feeling Great, Looking Great, Losing Weight

You will be amazed and delighted by your body's responsiveness when you begin to follow the "Healthiest Way of Eating" and eat more nutrient-rich World's Healthiest Foods. Within days you will probably begin to see improvements. You may feel more alert and have a surge in energy, sleep better and digest your food more easily. Within a week or so, you may even experience those excess pounds melting away. Consider each day a gift to your body and one more step along the path of a lifetime of vibrant health and energy.

## Letters From Readers of WHFoods.org About Losing Weight with the World's Healthiest Foods

*The World's Healthiest Foods have changed my life for the better. Your recipes deliver every time and the facts are there to back them up. I've lost over 50 pounds, and I doubt there's a recipe I haven't tried. The recipes are great but what's really important is I've learned to cook much healthier. The whole idea behind the "Healthiest Way of Eating" is to pay attention first to health but without compromising taste—nobody else does it! —Kerry*

*The World's Healthiest Foods is possibly the cure to the American problems of obesity. From my own experience, I decided to change my diet in the New Year. I was obese—at 5'8" I was about 240 lbs. Now six months later, I have lost 32 pounds and am still losing. I feel and look a lot better. I hope to lose another 28 lbs...and with exercise and your great recipes, I should be able to do it. THANKS A LOT! —Astrida*

*Since I have started eating the World's Healthiest Foods, my sugar has stabilized, and I have lost 50 lbs! I have truly turned my life around. Thank you so much. — Cindy*

*I used to eat pasta and ice cream for dinner until I stumbled upon the World's Healthiest Foods about six months ago. Since then, I've been working out and eating healthier than ever before in my life, resulting in a fit and 35-pound lighter self! —Amy*

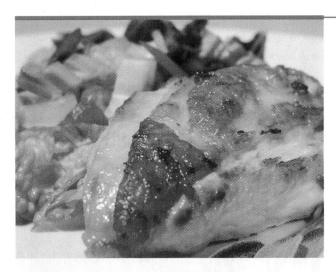

# chicken

## nutrient-richness chart

Total Nutrient-Richness: **11**
4 oz (113 grams) of roasted Chicken contains 223 calories

| NUTRIENT | AMOUNT | %DV | DENSITY | QUALITY |
|---|---|---|---|---|
| Tryptophan | 0.4 g | 121.9 | 9.8 | excellent |
| B3 Niacin | 14.4 mg | 72.0 | 5.8 | very good |
| Protein | 33.8 g | 67.6 | 5.4 | very good |
| Selenium | 28.0 mcg | 40.0 | 3.2 | good |
| B6 Pyridoxine | 0.6 mg | 32.0 | 2.6 | good |
| Phosphorus | 242.7 mg | 24.3 | 2.0 | good |

For more on "Total Nutrient-Richness," "%DV," "Density," and
The World's Healthiest Foods "Quality" Rating System, see page 805.

If there is one word that describes Chicken, it is versatility. Roasted, broiled or sautéed, Chicken can be combined with a wide range of herbs and spices to make a delicious, flavorful and nutritious meal. From southern fried Chicken to tandoori Chicken to homemade Chicken soup, Chicken is appreciated and valued by people of all ages and diverse ethnic backgrounds. The "Healthiest Way of Cooking" methods will help you prepare moist and flavorful Chicken with the greatest nutritional value.

## why chicken should be part of your healthiest way of eating

If you are looking for a way to reduce the fat content of your meals by almost half, try substituting lean, skinned Chicken breast for red meat as part of your "Healthiest Way of Eating." Chicken is a great source of protein and a very good source of niacin, an important B vitamin that may help protect against genetic (DNA) damage. (For more on the *Health Benefits of Chicken* and a complete analysis of its content of over 60 nutrients, see page 580.)

## varieties of chicken

The practice of raising Chickens for food is ancient, with the first domestication of poultry thought to have occurred in southern Asia over 4,000 years ago. Today, the most popular varieties of Chicken include:

### ORGANIC

Organically grown Chickens have been fed an organically grown diet without the use of hormones or antibiotics. They have been raised under humane conditions; they are not allowed to be overcrowded and must have periodic access to the outdoors and direct sunlight.

### FREE-RANGE CHICKENS

They have been allowed to run freely in the farmyard rather than being raised in coops. Some believe that this method of raising Chickens makes for more flavorful meat. Free-Range Chickens are not necessarily organic.

### BROILER/FRYERS

Not limited to just broiling or frying, these all-purpose Chickens can also be poached, steamed, grilled or roasted. They are, however, not a good choice for stewing. Broiler/Fryers average in weight from two and one-half to five pounds and are approximately eight weeks old when brought to market.

### ROASTERS

This variety can be roasted, grilled, braised or stewed. They average from three and one-half to five pounds and are brought to market when they are three to five months old.

### STEWING CHICKENS

Tough, but flavorful, they are best for stewing, braising and making stock. Stewing Chickens are mature Chickens that weigh from four to six pounds and are usually about one year old.

**CAPONS**

These are surgically castrated male Chickens. This procedure results in birds that can weigh about 10 pounds at a very young age. They have a large proportion of white meat but the thick layer of fat under the skin makes them fattier than most other varieties. They are best roasted.

**CORNISH GAME HENS**

This is a hybrid cross between a Cornish Game Cock and a White Plymouth Rock Chicken. They weigh from three quarters to two pounds, are very low in fat and can be roasted, broiled, braised or sautéed.

## the peak season

Chicken is available year-round.

## biochemical considerations

Chicken is a food associated with allergic reactions, which may be of concern to some individuals. (For more on *Food Allergies*, see page 719.)

## 4 steps for the best tasting and most nutritious chicken

Turning Chicken into a flavorful dish with the most nutrients is simple if you just follow my 4 easy steps:

1. The Best Way to Select
2. The Best Way to Store
3. The Best Way to Prepare
4. The Healthiest Way of Cooking

# 1. the best way to select chicken

You can select the best Chicken by choosing ones that have a solid and plump shape with a rounded breast and a fresh smell. Whether purchasing a whole Chicken or Chicken parts, the Chicken should feel pliable when gently pressed. The color of the Chicken's skin, white or yellow, does not have any bearing on its nutritional value. Regardless of color, the skin should be opaque and not spotted.

If possible, purchase Chicken that has been organically raised or that is "free-range" since these methods of poultry raising are both more humane and produce Chickens that are tastier and

healthier to eat. You will also not have concerns over the presence of hormone and antibiotics in organically raised Chicken.

Check the sell-by date on the package, and be sure that it has not expired.

If purchasing frozen Chicken, I make sure that it is frozen solid and does not have any ice deposits or freezer burn. Additionally, avoid frozen Chicken that has frozen liquid in the package as this is an indication that it has been defrosted and refrozen.

# 2. the best way to store chicken

Chicken should be stored in the coldest section of your refrigerator. Do not remove Chicken from its packaging until you are ready to prepare it. Check to see if the packaging leaks before storing. If it leaks, rewrap it securely before storing. This is very important to make sure that the

Chicken does not contaminate other foods in the refrigerator. Refrigerated raw Chicken can keep for 2 to 3 days.

Place fresh Chicken in a storage bag, place in a bowl and cover it with ice or an ice pack to reduce its temperature; this will help it remain fresh and extend its storage time.

# 3. the best way to prepare chicken

When handling raw Chicken, be extremely careful that it does not come in contact with other foods, especially those that will be served uncooked, because raw poultry can contain *Salmonella* bacteria. In fact, you should use a separate plastic cutting board for meats. If you don't use a separate board, make sure you wash your hands and cutting board very well with hot soapy water after handling Chicken. It is a good idea to add two TBS of bleach to two cups of water in a spray bottle and use this mixture to

clean your cutting board. Spray your cutting board with this mixture and let it sit for 20 minutes to allow the bleach to evaporate.

If your recipe requires marinating, you should always do so in the refrigerator as the meat is very sensitive to heat, which increases the chances of spoilage. When defrosting a frozen Chicken, do so in the refrigerator and not at room temperature. Place it on a plate to capture any liquid drippings.

# 4. the healthiest way of cooking chicken

The "Healthiest Way of Cooking" Chicken is to use methods that keep it moist and tender. While it is important not to overcook Chicken as it dries out and gets tough quickly, it is also important not to undercook Chicken because of the risk of *Salmonella* poisoning. Test for an interior temperature of 165°F (74°C) to ensure that Chicken is done.

I have found "Quick Broil" to be the best method when cooking whole pieces (e.g., breasts) of Chicken. The Chicken cooks quickly and leaving the skin on while cooking helps retain moisture and keeps the pieces tender. Remove the skin before serving. (For more on *"Quick Broil,"* see page 60.)

"Healthy Roasting" is the best method when cooking a whole Chicken. It is best to leave the skin on to retain moisture; remove the skin before serving. (For more on *Roasting,* see page 61.)

"Healthy Sautéing" is best when cooking small, cut-up pieces of Chicken. The pieces take just minutes to cook, and it is a great way to combine Chicken with a variety of vegetables for a complete meal. (For more on *"Healthy Sautéing,"* see page 57.)

While grilled Chicken tastes great, make sure it does not burn. It is best to grill Chicken on an area without a direct flame as the temperatures directly above or below the flame can reach as high as 500°F to 1000°F (260°–538°C). Extra care should be taken when grilling as burning Chicken can damage nutrients and create free radicals that can be harmful to your health. (For more on *Grilling,* see page 61.)

*(Continued on Page 581)*

---

## 7-Minute "Healthy Sautéed" Chicken with Asparagus

*This is a quick and easy way to prepare Chicken with a vegetable for a one-dish meal. Preheating the pan helps to seal the juices in the Chicken.*

- 3/4 lb Chicken breast
- 2 TBS + 1 TBS Chicken broth
- 1 lb asparagus, ends removed, stalks cut into 2-inch pieces
- 2 cloves garlic
- 3 TBS extra virgin olive oil
- 1 + 1 tsp fresh lemon juice
- Salt and pepper to taste

1. Press or chop garlic and let it sit for 5 minutes. (Why?, see page 261.)
2. Bring 2 TBS Chicken broth to a boil over medium heat in a stainless steel skillet.
3. While broth is heating, rub the Chicken breast with 1 tsp fresh lemon juice, salt and pepper, and cut into 1-inch cubes.
4. When broth begins to bubble, place the Chicken in skillet and stir frequently for 3 minutes until golden brown.
5. Add asparagus and remaining 1 TBS broth to the Chicken, **cover**, and cook for 4 minutes, stirring occasionally.
6. Dress with garlic, 1 tsp lemon juice, extra virgin olive oil, and salt and pepper to taste.

**SERVES 2**

*For an Asian flavor, add tamari (soy sauce), ginger, and rice vinegar, and replace black pepper with white pepper.*

---

## Homemade Low-Fat Chicken Broth

*Many recipes in this book call for Chicken broth as a replacement for oil. Now you can make your own broth and store it in the freezer in handy amounts.*

- 2–3 lb whole Chicken, cut into serving pieces
- 6 cups of water
- 1 medium onion, halved and pierced with 2 cloves garlic
- 1 carrot, halved
- 1 stalk celery including leaves, halved
- 2 bay leaves
- 3 sprigs parsley
- 1/2 tsp dried basil, sage or thyme

1. Place Chicken pieces and water in a large soup pot. Bring to a boil, reduce heat and skim off particles that rise to the surface.
2. Add remaining ingredients and simmer gently **uncovered** for 2 hours.
3. Strain broth through a fine sieve. Discard vegetables. Save Chicken for another use.
4. Let broth stand at room temperature until lukewarm, then refrigerate for several hours or overnight. Before using, skim off all the fat that has risen to the surface.

**MAKES 3 CUPS**

STEP-BY-STEP RECIPE
## The Healthiest Ways of Cooking Chicken

# 7-Minute "Quick Broiled" Chicken

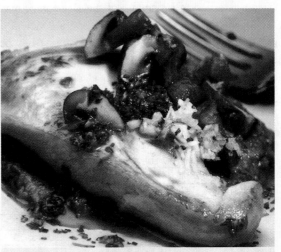
"Quick Broiled" Chicken

*For the best flavor and moistness, I recommend the "Quick Broil" method to cook boneless Chicken breasts. Be sure to leave the skin on while cooking.*

2 6-oz boneless Chicken breasts
2 tsp fresh lemon juice
Sea salt and pepper to taste

**Dressing:**
2 cloves garlic, chopped
3 TBS extra virgin olive oil
2 tsp fresh lemon juice
Sea salt and pepper to taste
**Optional: Add rosemary, sage or Dijon mustard to dressing**

1. Preheat the broiler on high and place an all stainless steel skillet (be sure the handle is also stainless steel) or cast iron pan about 6 inches from the heat source for about 10 minutes to get it very hot.

2. While the pan is heating, rinse Chicken, pat it dry and season it with lemon juice, salt and pepper.

3. Leaving the skin on, place the breast (skin side up) on the hot pan. It is not necessary to turn the breast because it is cooking on both sides at once. Depending on the size, it should be cooked in about 7 minutes. Remove the skin before serving; it is left on to keep it moist while broiling. The breast is done when it is moist, yet its liquid runs clear when pierced. The inside temperature needs to reach 165°F (74°C).

4. Dress with garlic, lemon juice, extra virgin olive oil, and salt and pepper to taste. Add rosemary, sage or Dijon mustard to the dressing for a tasty variation.

**COOKING HINT:**
This recipe is best if the Chicken breasts are small. Larger breasts will take longer to cook. If you use thighs for this recipe, be sure to use boneless thighs or they will take much longer to cook.

**SERVES 2**

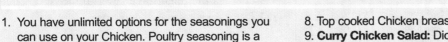

**Flavor Tips:** Try these 10 great serving suggestions with the recipe above. ✳

1. You have unlimited options for the seasonings you can use on your Chicken. Poultry seasoning is a traditional favorite. Add seasonings to the dressing.
2. Smother cooked Chicken with "Healthy Sautéed" onions, red peppers and thyme.
3. Coat skinned Chicken with Dijon or honey mustard before broiling.
4. Top cooked Chicken breasts with salsa and diced avocado.
5. Add capers to the dressing recipe.
6. "Quick Broiled" Chicken breast topped with an herbal vinaigrette (see page 143) over mixed salad greens makes a great lunch.
7. Add boneless, skinless Chicken pieces to your vegetable stir-fry for a healthy addition of protein.
8. Top cooked Chicken breasts with pesto.
9. **Curry Chicken Salad:** Dice the 7-Minute "Quick Broiled" Chicken. Combine with sliced dried apricots, dried cranberries, diced celery, chopped almonds, lemon juice, extra virgin olive oil, curry powder, and sea salt and cayenne pepper to taste.
10. **Chicken Salad:** Combine cooked Chicken chunks, corn kernels, cooked green beans, fresh basil strips and Mediterranean dressing (page 331). Toss together and serve over fresh greens.

**COOKING HINT:**
For boneless breasts, the internal temperature should read 165°F (74°C). For a whole Chicken, the internal breast temperature should read 180°F (82°C).

---

Please write (address on back cover flap) or e-mail me at info@whfoods.org with your personal ideas for preparing Chicken, and I will share them with others through our website at www.whfoods.org.

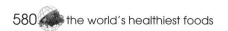

# health benefits of chicken

## Promotes Optimal Health

Chicken is a very good source of the B vitamin, niacin. Components of DNA require niacin, and a deficiency of niacin (as well as other B-complex vitamins) has been directly linked to genetic (DNA) damage. Chicken is also a good source of the trace mineral, selenium, an essential component of several major metabolic pathways, including thyroid hormone metabolism, antioxidant defense systems and immune function. Accumulated evidence from prospective studies, intervention trials and studies on animal models of cancer has suggested a strong inverse correlation between selenium intake and cancer incidence.

## Promotes Energy Production

Chicken is also a good source of vitamin B6. Its concentration of niacin and vitamin B6 makes Chicken helpful in supporting energy metabolism because these B vitamins are involved as cofactors that help enzymes throughout the body guide metabolic reactions. Niacin is essential for the conversion of the body's proteins, fats and carbohydrates into usable energy and helps optimize blood sugar regulation. Vitamin B6 is essential for the body's processing of carbohydrates, especially the breakdown of glycogen. Chicken is also a good source of phosphorus, a mineral that is an essential part of the ATP molecule that fuels the activities of our cells.

## Promotes Heart Health

In addition to its role in energy metabolism, vitamin B6 plays a pivotal role in the basic cellular process of methylation, through which methyl groups are transferred from one molecule to another. When levels of B6 are inadequate, the availability of methyl groups is also reduced. This has a variety of effects, including that potentially dangerous molecules that would normally be quickly changed into other benign molecules not only do not change, but accumulate. One such molecule, homocysteine, is so damaging to blood vessel walls that high levels are considered a significant risk factor for cardiovascular disease.

## Promotes Bone Health

Chicken is a very good source of protein. In addition to its numerous important physiological functions, dietary protein may be important in preventing bone loss in older people. In one study, the 70 to 90 year old men and women with the highest protein intakes lost significantly less bone over a four-year period than those who consumed less protein. Animal protein, as well as overall protein intake, was associated with preserving bone.

## Additional Health-Promoting Benefit of Chicken

Chicken is also a concentrated source of sleep-promoting tryptophan.

### Nutritional Analysis of 4 ounces of roasted Chicken breast:

| NUTRIENT | AMOUNT | % DAILY VALUE | NUTRIENT | AMOUNT | % DAILY VALUE |
|---|---|---|---|---|---|
| Calories | 223.40 | | Pantothenic Acid | 1.06 mg | 10.60 |
| Calories from Fat | 79.40 | | | | |
| Calories from Saturated Fat | 22.35 | | **Minerals** | | |
| Protein | 33.79 g | | Boron | — mcg | |
| Carbohydrates | 0.00 g | | Calcium | 15.88 mg | 1.59 |
| Dietary Fiber | 0.00 g | 0.00 | Chloride | — mg | |
| Soluble Fiber | 0.00 g | | Chromium | — mcg | — |
| Insoluble Fiber | 0.00 g | | Copper | 0.06 mg | 3.00 |
| Sugar – Total | 0.00 g | | Fluoride | — mg | — |
| Monosaccharides | 0.00 g | | Iodine | — mcg | — |
| Disaccharides | 0.00 g | | Iron | 1.21 mg | 6.72 |
| Other Carbs | 0.00 g | | Magnesium | 30.62 mg | 7.66 |
| Fat – Total | 8.82 g | | Manganese | 0.02 mg | 1.00 |
| Saturated Fat | 2.48 g | | Molybdenum | — mcg | — |
| Mono Fat | 3.44 g | | Phosphorus | 242.68 mg | 24.27 |
| Poly Fat | 1.88 g | | Potassium | 277.83 mg | |
| Omega-3 Fatty Acids | 0.11 g | 4.40 | Selenium | 28.01 mcg | 40.01 |
| Omega-6 Fatty Acids | 1.68 g | | Sodium | 80.51 mg | |
| Trans Fatty Acids | — g | | Zinc | 1.16 mg | 7.73 |
| Cholesterol | 95.26 mg | | | | |
| Water | 70.81 g | | **Amino Acids** | | |
| Ash | 1.12 g | | Alanine | 1.91 g | |
| | | | Arginine | 2.08 g | |
| **Vitamins** | | | Aspartate | 3.01 g | |
| Vitamin A IU | 105.46 IU | 2.11 | Cystine | 0.44 g | 107.32 |
| Vitamin A RE | 30.62 RE | | Glutamate | 4.99 g | |
| A - Carotenoid | 0.00 RE | 0.00 | Glycine | 1.95 g | |
| A - Retinol | 30.62 RE | | Histidine | 1.02 g | 79.07 |
| B1 Thiamin | 0.07 mg | 4.67 | Isoleucine | 1.73 g | 150.43 |
| B2 Riboflavin | 0.13 mg | 7.65 | Leucine | 2.49 g | 98.42 |
| B3 Niacin | 14.41 mg | 72.05 | Lysine | 2.80 g | 119.15 |
| Niacin Equiv | 20.84 mg | | Methionine | 0.92 g | 124.32 |
| Vitamin B6 | 0.64 mg | 32.00 | Phenylalanine | 1.33 g | 111.76 |
| Vitamin B12 | 0.36 mcg | 6.00 | Proline | 1.53 g | |
| Biotin | — mcg | — | Serine | 1.18 g | |
| Vitamin C | 0.00 mg | 0.00 | Threonine | 1.41 g | 113.71 |
| Vitamin D IU | 13.61 IU | 3.40 | Tryptophan | 0.39 g | 121.88 |
| Vitamin D mcg | 0.34 mcg | | Tyrosine | 1.11 g | 114.43 |
| Vitamin E Alpha Equiv | 0.30 mg | 1.50 | Valine | 1.66 g | 112.93 |
| Vitamin E IU | 0.45 IU | | | | |
| Vitamin E mg | 0.65 mg | | | | |
| Folate | 4.54 mcg | 1.14 | | | |
| Vitamin K | 0.17 mcg | 0.21 | | | |

(Note: "—" indicates data is unavailable. For more information, please see page 806.)

*(Continued from Page 578)*

## Methods Not Recommended for Cooking Chicken

### COOKING WITH OIL

I don't recommend cooking Chicken in oil because high temperature heat can damage delicate oils and potentially create harmful free radicals. (For more on *Why it is Important to Cook Without Heated Oils*, see page 52.)

Here are questions I received from readers of the whfoods.org website about Chicken:

**Q** *How much nutrition is destroyed in Chicken if I stew it in a Dutch oven on the stove and then freeze small servings to be used later?*

**A** Since eating raw Chicken is not an option, your question really focuses on two issues: using a Dutch oven versus other types of cooking method and the impact of freezing. I'll answer it from these perspectives.

In the context of an overall meal plan, Chicken is a noteworthy source of protein (and the amino acid tryptophan), several B vitamins (including B3 and B6) and the mineral selenium. I don't see any need to worry about your Dutch oven, or your freezing of servings, when it comes to the protein content. With respect to the B vitamins, there is definitely more nutrient loss with prolonged heating than with minimal heating of the Chicken, so if your Dutch oven recipes take less time than other methods, it may offer nutritional benefits. Freezing should not have that much of an effect on the B vitamin content.

**Q** *What is the best way to cook Chicken? I think it's boiling while my friend says it's grilling.*

**A** If "best" means nutritionally the best, boiling or grilling are probably fairly comparable. Boiling Chicken does not lose nutrients the same way as when you boil vegetables. If "best" also includes taste, grilling is probably more tasty.

Chicken is prepared in different ways for different types of dishes. Boiling Chicken is usually best when you are preparing a soup and you want the Chicken flavor to transfer to the liquid to make a tasty soup stock.

Grilling concentrates the flavor of the Chicken as the juices are locked inside the meat. However, grilled Chicken can be easily burnt and burnt meat contains compounds that have been found to be harmful to your health. If you want to grill your Chicken try to keep it away from direct flames and be careful not to burn it.

No matter how you prepare your Chicken, it is best to remove the skin before eating since the skin is rich in saturated fats. But cook your Chicken with the skin on and remove it after cooking, so it will remain moist. This is especially important when cooking breasts, which tend to be dry.

**Q** *Can you please tell me more about the relationship of protein intake to bone loss and osteoporosis? Some of what I've read indicates that any animal-source food (including dairy products) contributes to the loss of calcium via calcium drain through the kidneys.*

**A** It is true that excess protein intake increases a person's risk of osteoporosis. This is because bones work best in a slightly alkaline body, but high-protein diets require the body to release more acids as a means of helping to digest the protein. When these acids are released, and the body becomes more acidic, the body then responds and tries to buffer this acidity by withdrawing alkaline minerals like calcium from the bones. In clinical research studies, raising daily protein intake from 47 to 142 grams doubles the excretion of calcium in the urine. If you think about the intake of protein in the U.S., for example, it is pretty concentrated mainly because of the high consumption of animal meats.

I think that it may be OK for people who are not sensitive to dairy products, who like these foods and for whom they are not contraindicated to consume "some" cow's milk, yogurt and cheese since these foods are concentrated sources of calcium (which meats are not). The "some" reflects a balance in intake—not having it be a main feature of a diet but rather an accessory to the diet.

With a balanced approach to consuming dairy products, you will not consume nearly as much protein as you would from animal products. Eight ounces of low-fat yogurt has about 13 grams of protein while four ounces of lean meat has over 32 grams.

That is not to say that I promote the use of dairy products for everyone, and I respect that many people, for various reasons, do not want to consume them. I also believe that a person can help support their bone health through a balanced plant-based diet (without the addition of dairy products). That is because many vegetables and legumes are rich in not only calcium but also other nutrients that are intrinsically important to bone health—magnesium, copper, zinc and manganese, to name a few.

# turkey

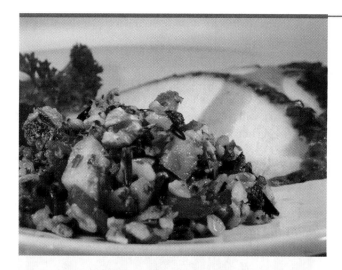

## highlights

| | |
|---|---|
| AVAILABILITY: | Year-round |
| REFRIGERATE: | Yes |
| SHELF LIFE: | 5–7 days refrigerated |
| PREPARATION: | Minimal |
| BEST WAY TO COOK: | Roasting |

## nutrient-richness chart

Total Nutrient-Richness: **11**
4 oz (113 grams) of roasted Turkey breast contains 214 calories

| NUTRIENT | AMOUNT | %DV | DENSITY | QUALITY |
|---|---|---|---|---|
| Tryptophan | 0.4 g | 109.4 | 9.2 | excellent |
| Protein | 32.6 g | 65.1 | 5.5 | very good |
| Selenium | 33.0 mcg | 47.1 | 4.0 | very good |
| B3 Niacin | 7.2 mg | 36.1 | 3.0 | good |
| B6 Pyridoxine | 0.5 mg | 27.0 | 2.3 | good |
| Phosphorus | 238.1 mg | 23.8 | 2.0 | good |

For more on "Total Nutrient-Richness," "%DV," "Density," and
The World's Healthiest Foods "Quality" Rating System, see page 805.

Turkeys have long played a role in the history of the United States. Benjamin Franklin so revered the Turkey that he wanted it to be the national bird and was disappointed when the eagle was chosen instead. For most Americans, Turkey evokes images of the Pilgrims, the first Thanksgiving dinner and the holiday season, although it is no longer reserved for just special occasions. From sandwiches to salads to the popular Turkey burger, we now enjoy this low-fat, high-quality protein food year-round. I want to share with you how the "Healthiest Way of Cooking" Turkey can help bring out its flavor, maximize its nutritional benefits and make it a quick, easy and nutritious addition to your "Healthiest Way of Eating."

## why turkey should be part of your healthiest way of eating

Turkey is a concentrated source of protein. One of the great advantages of Turkey is that the fat from Turkey can be easily removed, thereby making it one of the leanest sources of protein with about half the saturated fat found in red meat.

Turkey also contains vitamin B6 and niacin, which are important for energy production. (For more on the *Health Benefits of Turkey* and a complete analysis of its content of over 60 nutrients, see page 586.)

## varieties of turkey

Turkeys are native to the United States and Mexico and were a traditional food of the Native Americans. Christopher Columbus took Turkeys back with him to Europe from the New World, and by the 16th century, they were domestically raised in Italy, France and England. The rise in popularity of Turkey has spurred the availability of different varieties and cuts of Turkey:

### FRYER/ROASTER

Weighing from five to nine pounds, these are the youngest and most tender of the Turkey varieties. They are good roasted or broiled.

### HENS

This variety is thought to contain a greater proportion of white meat. Weighing from eight to eighteen pounds, they are good roasted or broiled.

### TOM TURKEYS

Tom Turkeys weigh up to twenty-four pounds, and some people believe that they are tastier than Hen Turkeys. They can be roasted or broiled.

### TURKEY PARTS

Today, Turkey parts such as breasts, breast steaks, cutlets, tenderloins, thighs, drumsticks and wings are readily available.

### GROUND TURKEY

If made from light meat, ground Turkey can be a leaner substitute for ground beef. Most ground Turkey, however, contains dark meat, and a large percentage of its calories are derived from fat. If purchasing frozen ground Turkey, read the label to ensure that there are no additives or preservatives included.

### ORGANIC

Organically raised Turkeys have been fed an organically grown diet, are not routinely treated with hormones or antibiotics and are raised under humane conditions. They are not allowed to be overcrowded and must have periodic access to the outdoors and direct sunlight.

### WILD TURKEY

Recently domesticated Wild Turkeys are smaller and have darker meat, a richer and more intense flavor, and firmer texture than Hen or Tom Turkeys.

## the peak season

Turkey is available year-round.

## biochemical considerations

Turkey can be a significant source of dietary cholesterol (84 mg in a 4-ounce serving). Almost all of the fat in Turkey is found in the skin, and dark meat is higher in fat than light meat. Check labels carefully if you use Turkey cold cuts because food processors may combine the dark meat of the animal along with organ meats like heart and gizzards, which increases the fat content.

## 4 steps for the best tasting and most nutritious turkey

Turning Turkey into a flavorful dish with the most nutrients is simple if you just follow my 4 easy steps:

1. The Best Way to Select
2. The Best Way to Store
3. The Best Way to Prepare
4. The Healthiest Way of Cooking

# 1. the best way to select turkey

You can select the most flavorful Turkey by looking for ones that have a solid and plump shape with a rounded breast. Whether purchasing a whole Turkey or Turkey parts, the Turkey should feel pliable when gently pressed. The color of the Turkey's skin, white or yellow, does not have any bearing on its nutritional value. Regardless of color, the skin should be opaque and not spotted.

If possible, purchase Turkey that has been organically raised or that is "free-range" since these methods of poultry raising are both more humane and produce Turkeys that are tastier and healthier to eat. Organically raised Turkeys are not administered hormones or antibiotics like most of their conventionally raised counterparts. (For more on *Organic Meats*, see, page 565.)

Avoid Turkey that has an "off" smell. Check the sell-by date on the package, and be sure that it has not expired.

If purchasing frozen Turkey, I make sure that it is frozen solid and does not have any ice deposits or freezer burn. Additionally, avoid frozen Turkey that has frozen liquid in the package as this is an indication that it has been defrosted and refrozen.

# 2. the best way to store turkey

Turkey should be stored in the coldest section of your refrigerator (usually at the bottom and towards the back). If the store packaging is intact and secure, store it this way since this will reduce the amount of handling. If the packaging is not secure, and it seems as if the Turkey liquid will leak, rewrap it securely before storing. This is very important to make sure that the Turkey does not contaminate other foods in the refrigerator. If you buy a whole Turkey with giblets, remove the giblets because they spoil quickly; store them in another container and rewrap the Turkey. Remember to always store the Turkey meat separately from any stuffing or gravy you have prepared. Raw Turkey will last about 5–7 days if refrigerated.

# 3. the best way to prepare turkey

Make sure you defrost your frozen Turkey in the refrigerator with a plate under it to catch the liquid as it defrosts.

When handling raw Turkey, be extremely careful that it does not come in contact with other foods, especially those that will be served uncooked, because raw poultry can contain *Salmonella* bacteria. In fact, you should use a separate plastic cutting board for meats. If you don't use separate boards, make sure you wash your hands and cutting board very well with hot soapy water after handling Turkey.

It is a good idea to add two TBS of bleach to two cups of water in a spray bottle and use this mixture to clean your cutting board. Spray your cutting board with this mixture and let sit for 20 minutes to allow the bleach to evaporate.

# 4. the healthiest way of cooking turkey

The "Healthiest Way of Cooking" Turkey is to use methods that keep it moist and tender. Turkey dries out and gets tough quickly, so it is important not to overcook it. It is also important to not undercook Turkey because of the risk of *Salmonella* poisoning. Turkey with no stuffing takes 15 minutes per pound at 350°F (175°C). Turkey with stuffing will take 20 minutes per pound at 350°F (175°C). For example, a 10 pound Turkey that is not stuffed will take about 2½ hours to roast. A stuffed 10 pound Turkey will take about 3 hours. Test to be sure the thickest part of the thigh reaches a temperature of 165°F to 170°F (74–77°C) to ensure that your Turkey is done.

I have found roasting to be the best way to prepare Turkey. Although roasting takes a long time, it is the most flavorful way of preparing Turkey.

## Methods Not Recommended for Cooking Turkey

### COOKING WITH OIL

I don't recommend cooking Turkey in oil because high temperature heat can damage delicate oils and potentially create harmful free radicals. (For more on *Why it is Important to Cook Without Heated Oils*, see page 52.)

Here is a question I received from a reader of the whfoods.org website about Turkey:

**Q** *I was wondering what the best way to eat Turkey was. More specifically, how does organic ground Turkey compare to a plain slice of white meat Turkey?*

**A** As your question addresses two separate issues, I will address them that way. One is the question of organic versus conventionally raised poultry and the other is how ground Turkey compares to a slice of white meat Turkey.

I always recommend organically raised varieties of meats and poultry over conventionally raised varieties. Organically raised poultry have not been given hormones to promote growth, excessive amounts of feed additives, drugs in the absence of illness or supplements above those required for adequate nutrition. Organic production is managed with the intent to integrate cultural, biological and mechanical practices to promote the cycling of resources and to promote ecological balance and biodiversity. These practices help to protect the soil and groundwater and provide health-promoting conditions for animals, all of which ultimately help promote the health of the consumer. These are some of the reasons that I strongly urge people to consume meats, such as Turkey that are organically raised .

The nutritional profile of white meat versus ground Turkey does vary. While there may still be a place in your "Healthiest Way of Eating" for ground Turkey, it has more calories, saturated fat and protein than white Turkey meat.

---

## 5-Minute Asian Turkey Sauté

*A tasty dish in minutes!*

2 TBS + 2 TBS low-sodium chicken broth
1/2 small red onion, diced fine
2 cups shiitake mushrooms, diced fine
6 snow peas, diced
6 ounces ground Turkey
2 tsp + 1 tsp fresh minced ginger
1 tsp + 1 tsp minced garlic
1 TBS + 1 TBS tamari (soy sauce)
2 TBS extra virgin olive oil
Optional: 1 avocado, diced

1. Mince garlic and let sit for 5 minutes. (Why?, see page 261.)

2. Heat 2 TBS broth in a 12-inch stainless steel skillet until it begins to steam.

3. Add onion, mushrooms and snow peas. Sauté in the broth for about 1 minute over medium-high heat, stirring constantly.

4. Add 2 TBS chicken broth, 1 TBS tamari, ground Turkey, 2 tsp ginger and 1 tsp garlic. Continue to sauté for 2 minutes, breaking up Turkey pieces and cooking until all the pink is gone from the meat.

5. Remove from the burner and season with 1 TBS tamari, 1 tsp garlic, 1 tsp ginger, ground pepper and extra virgin olive oil.

   This dish is best served cold with the diced avocado. Try it in a wrap!

STEP-BY-STEP RECIPE
## The Healthiest Ways of Cooking Turkey

# *Roasted Turkey*

*I recommend roasting Turkey to bring out its best flavor, although you will have to allot several hours for cooking. Add 15 minutes for each pound of Turkey to calculate cooking time for Turkey larger than 15 pounds.*

**1 hen Turkey, approximately 12–15 lbs**
**3 TBS fresh lemon juice**
**Sea salt and pepper to taste**

1. Rub lemon juice and salt and pepper on the outside of the Turkey, then lift up the skin where you can and rub these seasonings directly on the flesh.

2. Preheat the oven to 350°F (175°C). Place the Turkey, breast side down, in a shallow roasting pan. Roast 15 minutes for each pound.

3. Turn the Turkey over 30–60 minutes (depending on size) before it is done. The internal temperature should read 125°F (74°C) when you turn it. Turn the heat up to 400°F (200°C) for the remaining roasting time.

   When the Turkey is done, its internal temperature should read about 165°F to 170°F (74°C to 77°C) with thermometer inserted in the mid-thigh. Remove

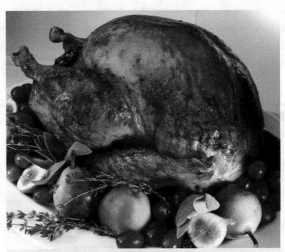

Roasted Turkey

the bird to a platter, and let sit for 15–20 minutes before carving to allow the juices to be redistributed and the meat to become moist throughout.

For roasted boneless breasts, the internal temperature should read 170°F (77°C).

## SERVES 10–12

---

## Flavor Tips: Try these 9 great serving suggestions with the recipe above. ✳

1. Serve with Cranberry Relish (see page 413).

2. Sage, thyme and curry powder complement Turkey.

3. Serve Turkey with cooked spinach and grated low-fat Parmesan cheese.

4. A mixture of low-fat plain yogurt and Dijon mustard makes a creamy topping for sliced Turkey or a tasty sauce for a Turkey burger.

5. Make a chutney to serve with cooked Turkey. Combine strips of 8 dried apricots, 1 tsp curry powder, 1 TBS fresh minced ginger, 1 TBS apple juice, 1 tsp of cider vinegar and 3 TBS extra virgin olive oil. Let marinate until apricots are hydrated.

6. **Romaine Turkey Wrap:** Combine 1 cup of Turkey breast strips, 1 TBS dried cranberries, 1 medium avocado cut into 1/2-inch cubes, 1/4 cup diced celery, 1 TBS lemon, 3 TBS juice and extra virgin olive oil. Wrap in romaine leaves.

7. **Tortilla-Free Wrap:** Drizzle 2 slices of cooked Turkey breast, sliced tomatoes, sprouts and thinly sliced sweet onion with Mediterranean dressing (see page 331). Roll up in a collard green leaf and enjoy!

8. **Turkey Hash:** "Healthy Sauté" 2 TBS diced red onion, 1/2 medium-size diced red pepper, 1 cup diced Roast Turkey, and salt and pepper to taste. Add hot chili sauce if desired. Serve with a poached egg on top.

9. **Turkey with Ravigote Sauce:** Top cold cooked Turkey with a sauce made by mixing 2 TBS fresh lemon juice, 3 TBS extra virgin olive oil, 3 TBS minced parsley, 1/4 minced sweet onion, 1 finely chopped sour pickle, 1 TBS rinsed capers, and sea salt and pepper to taste.

---

Please write (address on back cover flap) or e-mail me at info@whfoods.org with your personal ideas for preparing Turkey, and I will share them with others through our website at www.whfoods.org.

# health benefits of turkey

### A Very Good Source of Protein

Turkey is a very good source of protein. The structure of the human body is built on protein obtained from plant and animal sources. Once consumed, the amino acids found in proteins are rearranged into patterns that can be used by the body. The proteins synthesized by the body have a variety of very important functions including the production of structural proteins, enzymes, hormones, transport proteins and antibodies.

### Promotes Optimal Health

Turkey is a very good source of the trace mineral, selenium, which is an essential component of several major metabolic pathways, including thyroid hormone metabolism, antioxidant defense systems and immune function. Accumulated evidence from numerous human and animal studies on cancer has suggested a strong inverse correlation between selenium intake and the incidence of cancer. Turkey is also a good source of niacin, which helps to preserve cellular integrity. Components of DNA require niacin, and a deficiency of niacin (as well as other B-complex vitamins) has been directly linked to genetic (DNA) damage.

### Promotes Heart Health

While meats naturally contain fat, Turkey's total fat accounts for only 35% of its calories with 10% of its calories coming from saturated fat, amounts within the overall target range recommended by the 2005 U.S. Dietary Guidelines. Turkey is a good source of vitamin B6, necessary to metabolize homocysteine into other benign molecules. This has heart-health benefits since homocysteine can damage artery walls.

### Promotes Energy Production

Both niacin and vitamin B6 are important for energy production. In addition to helping prevent damage to DNA, niacin is essential for the conversion of the body's proteins, fats and carbohydrates into usable energy. As a component of a molecule called glucose tolerance factor, which optimizes insulin activity, niacin also plays an important role in blood sugar regulation. Vitamin B6 is essential for the body's processing of carbohydrates, especially the breakdown of glycogen, the form in which sugar is stored in muscle cells and to a lesser extent in our liver. Turkey is a good source of phosphorus, which is a component of ATP, the energy molecule that fuels our cellular activities.

### Additional Health-Promoting Benefit of Turkey

Turkey is also a concentrated source of sleep-promoting tryptophan.

## Nutritional Analysis of 4 ounces of roasted Turkey breast:

| NUTRIENT | AMOUNT | % DAILY VALUE | NUTRIENT | AMOUNT | % DAILY VALUE |
|---|---|---|---|---|---|
| Calories | 214.33 | | Pantothenic Acid | 0.72 mg | 7.20 |
| Calories from Fat | 75.63 | | | | |
| Calories from Saturated Fat | 21.43 | | **Minerals** | | |
| Protein | 32.56 g | | Boron | — mcg | |
| Carbohydrates | 0.00 g | | Calcium | 23.81 mg | 2.38 |
| Dietary Fiber | 0.00 g | 0.00 | Chloride | — mg | |
| Soluble Fiber | 0.00 g | | Chromium | — mcg | — |
| Insoluble Fiber | 0.00 g | | Copper | 0.05 mg | 2.50 |
| Sugar – Total | 0.00 g | | Fluoride | — mg | — |
| Monosaccharides | 0.00 g | | Iodine | — mcg | — |
| Disaccharides | 0.00 g | | Iron | 1.59 mg | 8.83 |
| Other Carbs | 0.00 g | | Magnesium | 30.62 mg | 7.66 |
| Fat – Total | 8.40 g | | Manganese | 0.02 mg | 1.00 |
| Saturated Fat | 2.38 g | | Molybdenum | 3.86 mcg | 5.15 |
| Mono Fat | 2.78 g | | Phosphorus | 238.14 mg | 23.81 |
| Poly Fat | 2.04 g | | Potassium | 326.59 mg | |
| Omega-3 Fatty Acids | 0.12 g | 4.80 | Selenium | 33.00 mcg | 47.14 |
| Omega-6 Fatty Acids | 1.83 g | | Sodium | 71.44 mg | |
| Trans Fatty Acids | — g | | Zinc | 2.30 mg | 15.33 |
| Cholesterol | 83.92 mg | | | | |
| Water | 71.69 g | | **Amino Acids** | | |
| Ash | 1.17 g | | Alanine | 2.04 g | |
| | | | Arginine | 2.26 g | |
| **Vitamins** | | | Aspartate | 3.10 g | |
| Vitamin A IU | 0.00 IU | 0.00 | Cystine | 0.35 g | 85.37 |
| Vitamin A RE | 0.00 RE | | Glutamate | 5.15 g | |
| A - Carotenoid | 0.00 RE | 0.00 | Glycine | 1.88 g | |
| A - Retinol | 0.00 RE | | Histidine | 0.97 g | 75.19 |
| B1 Thiamin | 0.06 mg | 4.00 | Isoleucine | 1.62 g | 140.87 |
| B2 Riboflavin | 0.15 mg | 8.82 | Leucine | 2.51 g | 99.21 |
| B3 Niacin | 7.22 mg | 36.10 | Lysine | 2.94 g | 125.11 |
| Niacin Equiv | 13.07 mg | | Methionine | 0.91 g | 122.97 |
| Vitamin B6 | 0.54 mg | 27.00 | Phenylalanine | 1.26 g | 105.88 |
| Vitamin B12 | 0.41 mcg | 6.83 | Proline | 1.47 g | |
| Biotin | — mcg | — | Serine | 1.42 g | |
| Vitamin C | 0.00 mg | 0.00 | Threonine | 1.41 g | 113.71 |
| Vitamin D IU | 13.61 IU | 3.40 | Tryptophan | 0.35 g | 109.38 |
| Vitamin D mcg | 0.34 mcg | | Tyrosine | 1.23 g | 126.80 |
| Vitamin E Alpha Equiv | 0.20 mg | 1.00 | Valine | 1.68 g | 114.29 |
| Vitamin E IU | 0.30 IU | | | | |
| Vitamin E mg | 0.20 mg | | | | |
| Folate | 6.80 mcg | 1.70 | | | |
| Vitamin K | — mcg | — | | | |

(Note: "–" indicates data is unavailable. For more information, please see page 806.)

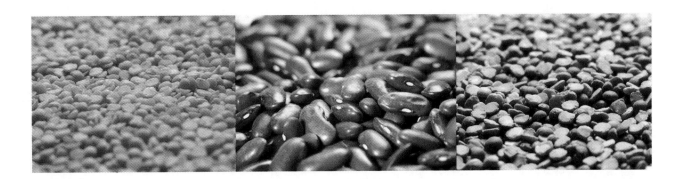

# beans & legumes

The numbers beside each food indicate their Total Nutrient-Richness. (For more details, see page 805.)

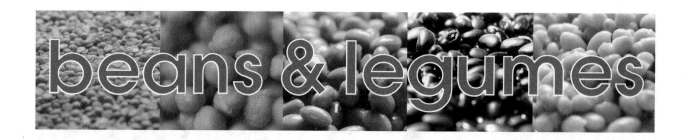

# beans & legumes

More people are eating ethnic cuisines, which feature a high regard for beans and legumes. The popularity of legumes—whether they appear as a bean burrito, chili, bean enchilada, dahl, edamame, sukiyaki or sweet and sour tofu—means they are now included on the menu in many restaurants, from fast food to gourmet. During a stroll through the supermarket, you are certain to see rows of canned beans and probably an ample selection of soy products.

It is no surprise that these ancient foods, among the first plants to ever be cultivated, are being embraced by our food culture. In addition to being low-fat, low-calorie, no-cholesterol, vegetarian sources of high-quality protein and fiber, they are also inexpensive, easy to store, versatile and delicious foods. Since more people are substituting beans and legumes for meat because of their high supply of low-fat protein, I want to share with you new ways of preparing them that will only take you a few minutes.

## Definition: Beans and Legumes

Common beans (*Phaseolus vulgaris*) such as kidney, black and navy beans fall into the plant category called legumes, whose other members also include broad beans, lentils, soybeans and peanuts (since most people think of peanuts more as a "nut," I present them in the Nuts and Seeds section.) Technically speaking, legumes are plants that have edible seeds contained in pods, with the term referring both to the plant itself as well as to the seeds. Oftentimes, they are referred to as "pulses." If you think about how black beans, for example, are actually the seed of the plant, with the nutrients and energy capable of creating a new plant, it is no wonder that legumes are so nutrient-rich—packed with protein, dietary fiber, phytonutrients (plant nutrients), vitamins and minerals.

## Why Beans and Legumes Help You Stay Slim, Energized and Healthy

Adding beans and legumes to your diet not only promotes optimal health, but also helps you maintain an optimal weight. That's because these foods are nutrient-rich, delivering protein, many vitamins, minerals and phytonutrients as well as a storehouse of dietary fiber.

Beans and legumes are a hearty food that satisfy even the hardiest of appetites, while their rich flavor satisfies the most demanding tastes. Since they are so rich in protein, they can be a great substitute for meat as a meal's main dish. You'll receive protein and beneficial nutrients while avoiding the concentrated saturated fat and cholesterol contained in many animal foods. Not only will your waistline benefit, but so will your pocketbook since beans and legumes are less expensive than meat. They contain more protein (amino acids) than any other type of plant-based food. To get the full benefit of this protein, however, you need to combine them with other plant foods, like grains, over the course of the day. Beans and rice is a good example of this combination.

Another important feature of beans and legumes that is inherently linked to maintaining a healthy weight is that they are a concentrated source of dietary fiber. Fiber contributes to healthy weight through a variety of means. As it helps to slow the rate at which food leaves the stomach, fiber promotes a sense of satiety, or fullness, after a meal; this helps to prevent overeating and weight gain. Dietary fiber also helps to promote bowel regularity. Legumes are low glycemic-index foods.

Legumes, such as black beans, are also recognized as a rich source of health-promoting phytonutrients called anthocyanins, which can act as powerful antioxidants. The darker the beans, the more anthocyanins they contain.

## It is Easy to Eat 5 Servings of Beans and Legumes Per Week

Leading health organizations recommend we eat 5 servings of beans and legumes per week. That's not difficult since they are an incredibly versatile food. Need a hearty side dish in winter when many fresh vegetables are scarce? Think beans and legumes. Want a great addition to a winter stew? Think beans and legumes. Interested in making a high-protein summer salad? Think beans and legumes. Looking for a zesty, crunchy sprout? Think beans and legumes. An ingredient in stuffing, dips, sauces, vegetable patés… the list goes on and on. While beans and legumes make the perfect accompaniment to many foods, they can also be featured as the main ingredient of a dish. A steaming plate of seasoned vegetables and beans or other type of legume is one of my favorite meals. As you can see, there are numerous opportunities to incorporate these beneficial foods into your diet.

While most people are used to cooking just the seeds of the beans and legumes, there are some varieties where both seeds and pods are cooked. Edamame, the whole soybean pod, is one example. Enjoying surging popularity, edamame is not only found as an appetizer in many Japanese restaurants, but it is becoming a typical offering in the freezer section of many grocery stores.

## Serving size of Beans and Legumes:

The recommended serving size for beans and legumes is 1/2 cup cooked.

## What You Will Find in Each Chapter

Each chapter is dedicated to one of the World's Healthiest Beans and Legumes and contains everything you need to know to enjoy and maximize their flavor and nutritional benefits. Each chapter is organized into two parts:

1. **BEAN AND LEGUME FACTS** describes each food and its different varieties and its peak season. It also addresses biochemical considerations of each bean and legume by describing any of its unique compounds that may be potentially problematic to individuals with specific health problems. Detailed information about the health benefits of each food can be found at the end of each chapter as can a complete nutritional profile.

2. **4 STEPS TO THE BEST TASTING AND MOST NUTRITIOUS BEANS AND LEGUMES** includes information about how to best select, store, prepare and cook each one of the World's Healthiest Beans and Legumes. Since many of the beans share similiar approaches to these steps, I put detailed information in one—black beans (page 610) because it is the most popular—to which I refer you in the chapters of the others. While specific information for individual beans and legumes is given in each of the specific chapters, here are the 4 Steps that can be applied to beans and legumes in general, including those not on the list of the World's Healthiest Foods.

# 1. the best way to select beans and legumes—

Adding delicious and nutritious beans and legumes to your diet begins with selecting those that are preferably organically grown and minimally processed since these will have retained the maximum amount of nutrients.

Even though the beans and legumes you buy may be dried, you can still tell the difference between those that are fresh and those that are stale. In order to ensure the freshest quality, it is best to purchase those in bulk from a store that has a high product turnover, such as a natural foods store. Dried beans and legumes should be similar in size and shape and somewhat glossy. Avoid faded, wrinkled, cracked and dry looking

ones, which are likely to be older and have lost some of their nutritional value. Additionally, make sure there is no evidence of moisture or insect damage.

Since beans and legumes are harvested in late summer, try buying a new batch each fall, so that you'll have the best chance of getting the year's freshest crop. (When the summertime comes, you can use up your dried beans and legumes by sprouting them or including them in cold salads.) This general practice will enable you to enjoy beans and legumes that contain the most flavor and nutrition and also take the least amount of time to cook.

# 2. the best way to store beans and legumes —

Store dried beans and legumes in an airtight container to best preserve their freshness.

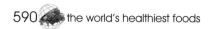

# 3. the best way to prepare beans and legumes

How beans and legumes are prepared will affect the length of time that is required to cook them as well as your enjoyment after they have been cooked.

## Soak in the Nutritional Benefits

Legumes should always be cooked because most contain a potentially toxic substance called phytohemaglutinin when they are raw. This is especially true of kidney beans. When they are cooked, the concentration of this compound is reduced. Other potentially toxic compounds found in raw beans are called cyanogenic glycosides — compounds that can produce cyanide. Raw beans that contain these compounds include lima beans, kidney beans and garbanzo beans (chickpeas).

Legumes should also always be sorted and rinsed before cooking. Before washing them, spread them out on a light-colored plate or cooking surface to check for and remove damaged legumes as well as small stones or debris that may have accompanied them from the farm to the market. After this process, place them in a strainer, rinsing them thoroughly under cool running water.

I highly recommend that you soak dried legumes overnight before you cook them. While it may only reduce the time that it takes for them to cook by about 30 minutes or less, the great benefit is that it will make the legumes much easier to digest, less gas forming and more nutritious.

Beans contain complex sugars that can cause flatulence because they are not easily broken down in the gastrointestinal tract. Soaking beans has been shown to reduce the content of these sugars, known as raffinose-type oligosaccharides, allowing you to consume more beans with less worry about intestinal discomfort. In addition, soaking beans has been shown to reduce the levels of phytates in beans, which can bind minerals such as iron and zinc, making them less bioavailable. Therefore, the process of soaking may increase the amount of minerals available for absorption.

## Sprout Your Way to Health

Sprouting is a great way to enjoy legumes. Not only do sprouts have a zesty taste and crunchy texture, but they are a concentrated source of nutrients. They are high in nutrient vitality because sprouts contain the nutrients that will eventually support the growth of the rest of the plant. Therefore, when you eat the sprouts, you get to enjoy the additional concentration of certain nutrients. Sprouting has been shown to increase protein availability and decrease phytates, thereby increasing the availability of some minerals. Some of my favorite legumes to sprout are garbanzos, lentils and peas. (For more on *Sprouts*, see page 141.)

# 4. the healthiest way of cooking beans and legumes

The way you cook your beans and legumes can affect their taste, texture and digestibility.

## The Effect of Using Salt and Acidic Substances When Cooking Legumes

As a general rule, do not add seasonings that are salty or acidic until after the legumes have cooked. Adding salt before they have cooked will prevent them from becoming tender and greatly increase the cooking time. Acidic substances, such as lemon juice or tomatoes, will also slow down the cooking time. Yet, one benefit of adding acidic substances to your legumes is that they help them to maintain their well defined shape and not turn soft and mushy. If your recipe calls for this type of texture and you want to have the legumes infused with the flavor that the acidic substance will impart (and you have some extra time), you can cook 4to helThur++them with these ingredients.

## Ready to Eat

One of the great things about legumes is their versatility and convenience. If you don't have time to cook up a pot of beans, you can always use ones that are ready to eat from a can. Since canned beans have been cooked for a long period of time, they are also easier to digest and less likely to cause flatulence. A wide variety of canned beans line shelves of markets throughout the country. And more and more stores are also now carrying brands that offer organically grown varieties. As always, look for canned foods that don't have extra salt or additives.

Beans from a can are easily heated and added to any hot soup or entrée. They can also be used right out of the can (after rinsing them well) for cold salads, bean dips and spreads. They even make great snacks that require little preparation. I know many people who love to eat cold beans, such as garbanzos, with just a touch of salt and pepper.

# beans and legumes cooking chart

| QUANTITY: 1 CUP | SOAK OR NOT | WATER TO BEAN RATIO | SIMMERING TIME | PRESSURE COOKING TIME | WATER TO BEAN RATIO |
|---|---|---|---|---|---|
| **Black Beans** | 8 hrs or overnight | 3:1 | 1–1$^1$/2 hrs | 30–40 min | 2:1 |
| **Garbanzo Beans** | 8 hrs or overnight | 3:1 | 1–1$^1$/2 hrs | 40–50 min | 2:1 |
| **Kidney Beans** | 8 hrs or overnight | 3:1 | 1–1$^1$/2 hrs | 30–35 min | 2:1 |
| **Lentils** | Not required | 3:1 | 20–30 min | 15–25 min  not recommended for red lentils | 3:1 |
| **Lima Beans** | Not required | 3:1 | 40–50 min | 20–30 min | 2:1 |
| **Navy Beans** | 8 hrs or overnight | 3:1 | 1–1$^1$/2 hrs | 30–35 min | 2:1 |
| **Pinto Beans** | 8 hrs or overnight | 3:1 | 1–1$^1$/2 hrs | 25–30 min | 2:1 |
| **Soybeans** | 8 hrs or overnight | 3:1 | 1–1$^1$/2 hrs | 35–40 min | 2:1 |
| **Split Peas**  (green) | Not required | 3:1 | 30 min | 10–15 min | 3:1 |
|   (yellow) | Not required | 3:1 | 30–35 min | 15 min | 3:1 |

*\* Please use this chart as a general guide. Cooking times may vary depending on the freshness of your legumes, differences in stovetop temperatures, etc. If using a pressure cooker, it is best to follow the cooking times recommended by the manufacturer.*

Q *Which nutrients are thrown out with the soaking water when beans are soaked?*

A There is limited research on the overall nutritional effects of presoaking dried beans. But the available research points in two clear directions.

First involves the digestibility of the beans. One type of carbohydrates—called oligosaccharides—definitely leaches into the soaking water in significant amounts. The loss of these oligosaccharides (like raffinose and stachyose) into the soaking water increases the digestibility of the beans because these compound sugar molecules are fairly resistant to digestion.

However, research on oligosaccharides also shows that these carbohydrates can provide us with important health benefits for exactly the same reason. By resisting digestion, oligosaccharides can make it all the way down through our digestive tract to our large intestine and serve as fuel for friendly bacteria (like Bifidobacteria and Lactobacilli).

If your were having trouble with digestion and were trying to minimize the impact of eating on your digestive tract, soaking beans and losing some oligosaccharides might make sense. It also might make sense if you were sensitive to beans from a gas-forming standpoint, since the oligosaccharides in beans have been associated with the problem of flatulence related to beans. If your digestive tract was working well, however, and you did not have bean-related gas problems, soaking might make less sense in order to leave the oligosaccharides more intact for the benefit of friendly bacteria in your large intestine.

The second area of research involves overall nutrient loss that takes place as a result of soaking. The degree of nutrient loss depends primarily on the length of soaking time. In general, the nutrient loss is moderate, but since dried beans cannot be eaten as is, it's not really relevant to compare the nutrient content of dry versus soaked beans. What matters more is the nutrient content of soaked-cooked beans versus cooked-only beans. Here the overall difference does not seem great. Although many of the lost nutrients could be found in the soaking water, I believe it is better to discard this water rather than reusing it when cooking the beans. Some dried beans (like red kidney beans) release potentially toxic substances into the water when soaking, and most beans release oligosaccharides, as just discussed.

One nutrient that shows greater loss from cooked-only versus soaked-cooked beans is protein. The reason here involves the prolonged heat exposure that is required for cooked-only beans. This prolonged heat exposure further denatures proteins found in the beans. The overnight cold water soaking method has the advantage of shortening the total time of heat exposure when cooking the beans and reducing nutrient loss in this way.

# lentils

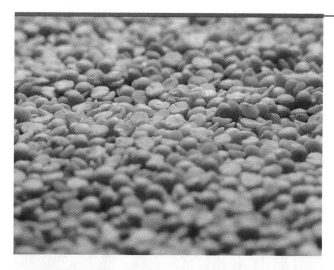

## nutrient-richness chart

Total Nutrient-Richness: **20**  GI: **42**

One cup (198 grams) of cooked Lentils contains 230 calories

| NUTRIENT | AMOUNT | %DV | DENSITY | QUALITY |
|---|---|---|---|---|
| Molybdenum | 148.5 mcg | 198.0 | 15.5 | excellent |
| Folate | 358.0 mcg | 89.5 | 7.0 | excellent |
| Dietary Fiber | 15.6 g | 62.6 | 4.9 | very good |
| Tryptophan | 0.2 g | 50.0 | 3.9 | very good |
| Manganese | 1.0 mg | 49.0 | 3.8 | very good |
| Iron | 6.6 mg | 36.6 | 2.9 | good |
| Protein | 17.9 g | 35.7 | 2.8 | good |
| Phosphorus | 356.4 mg | 35.6 | 2.8 | good |
| Copper | 0.5 mg | 25.0 | 2.0 | good |
| B1 Thiamin | 0.3 mg | 22.0 | 1.7 | good |
| Potassium | 730.6 mg | 20.9 | 1.6 | good |

For more on "Total Nutrient-Richness," "%DV," "Density," and
The World's Healthiest Foods "Quality" Rating System, see page 805.

For more on GI, see page 342.

The culinary enjoyment of Lentils dates back to prehistoric times, as far back as the Bronze Age. One of the first foods to be cultivated, Lentils were used by the ancient Greeks for both medicinal and culinary purposes. Today they are a dietary staple in India where they are prepared as dahl, a delicious spicy dish made from Lentils, onions, garlic, cumin and oil. Unlike other members of the legume family, Lentils do not need to be soaked before cooking, so they are a relatively quick and easy way to add nutrient-rich legumes to your "Healthiest Way of Eating."

## why lentils should be part of your healthiest way of eating

Like other varieties of legumes, Lentil's rich concentration of dietary fiber and folate makes them an excellent choice for a

**highlights**

| | |
|---|---|
| AVAILABILITY: | Year-round |
| REFRIGERATE: | No |
| SHELF LIFE: | Up to 12 months |
| PREPARATION: | Minimal |
| BEST WAY TO COOK: | Canned beans require no cooking |

healthy heart. Lentils also contain polyphenolic phytonutrients, including proanthocyanins and catechins, which provide powerful antioxidant protection to cellular structures from the oxidative damage caused by free radicals. (Lentils' health benefits and nutritional profile are similiar to black beans. For more information, see page 615.)

## varieties of lentils

Both dried and canned Lentils are available (same as black beans, see page 610). Lentils come in a variety of colors including green, brown, yellow and pink.

## the peak season available year-round.

## biochemical considerations

Same as black beans (see page 611).

## the best way to select lentils

Same as black beans (see page 611).

## the best way to store lentils

Same as black beans (see page 611).

## the best way to prepare lentils

Same as black beans (see page 612) except that Lentils require no soaking prior to cooking.

## the healthiest way of cooking lentils

For details about cooking, see black bean recipe (page 614). Red Lentils take 20 minutes to cook and green Lentils take 30 minutes.

STEP-BY-STEP RECIPE
## The Healthiest Ways to Prepare Lentils

# 5-Minute Lentils– No Cooking

*Many brands of organic canned Lentils are now available. You can use dried Lentils if you have time to cook them (see page 614 for directions).*

1 15-oz can Lentils, preferably organic
2 TBS extra virgin olive oil
2 cloves garlic
Sea salt and pepper to taste
Optional: Add 1/2 medium red onion, chopped

1. Press or mince garlic and let sit for 5 minutes. (Why?, see page 261.)

2. Drain liquid from Lentils and rinse under cold running water; this helps prevent intestinal gas.

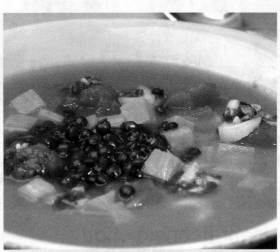
Vegetable Soup with Lentils

3. Combine all ingredients, mix and enjoy! For added flavor, you may want to add more olive oil.

**SERVES 2**

## Flavor Tips: Try these 8 great serving suggestions with the recipe above. ✱

1. Add cumin, oregano, basil and thyme to complement the flavor of Lentils.

2. Roasted peppers go well with Lentils.

3. Top Lentils with yogurt spiced with mint and red pepper flakes.

4. **Lentil Yogurt Salad:** Combine 5-Minute Lentils recipe, low-fat yogurt, brown rice, ground cumin and red pepper flakes to taste. Serve in a romaine leaf and garnish with chopped mint.

5. **Puréed Lentils:** "Healthy Sauté" 1 small minced onion in a large sauce pan. On low speed, blend together the sautéed onion, 5-Minute Lentils recipe and 2 TBS vegetable or chicken broth until smooth. Make sure you don't fill the blender more than half full. You will have to stop the blender a couple times and scrape the sides with a rubber spatula. Puréed Lentils are a great healthy alternative to mashed potatoes served with chicken or lamb.

6. **Lentil Salad:** Combine 5-Minute Lentils recipe (using green Lentils), chopped tomatoes, chopped bell pepper, minced sweet onion and minced mint. Toss with Mediterranean Dressing (page 331) and top with crumbled feta cheese and minced parsley.

7. **Lentil Soup with Curry:** Cook 5-Minute Lentils with onion, garlic, ginger and curry powder to taste, and 3–4 cups chicken or vegetable broth for an easy and flavorful soup. Garnish with chopped tomatoes and cilantro.

8. **Vegetable Soup with Lentils:** Add protein to a vegetable soup by adding the 5-Minute Lentils near the end of the cooking time (pictured above).

Please write (address on back cover flap) or e-mail me at info@whfoods.org with your personal ideas for preparing Lentils, and I will share them with others through our website at www.whfoods.org.

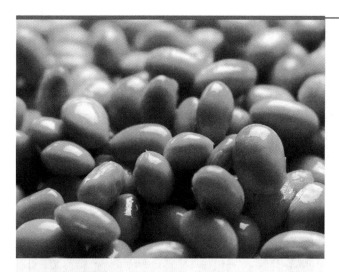

# soybeans

## highlights

| | |
|---|---|
| AVAILABILITY: | Year-round |
| REFRIGERATE: | No |
| SHELF LIFE: | Up to 12 months |
| PREPARATION: | Minimal |
| BEST WAY TO COOK: | Canned beans require no cooking |

## nutrient-richness chart

Total Nutrient-Richness: **20**     GI: **25**

One cup (172 grams) of cooked Soybeans contains 298 calories

| NUTRIENT | AMOUNT | %DV | DENSITY | QUALITY |
|---|---|---|---|---|
| Molybdenum | 129.0 mcg | 172.0 | 10.4 | excellent |
| Tryptophan | 0.4 g | 115.6 | 7.0 | excellent |
| Manganese | 1.4 mg | 71.0 | 4.3 | very good |
| Protein | 28.6 g | 57.2 | 3.5 | very good |
| Iron | 8.8 mg | 49.1 | 3.0 | good |
| Phosphorus | 421.4 mg | 42.1 | 2.5 | good |
| Dietary Fiber | 10.3 g | 41.3 | 2.5 | good |
| Vitamin K | 33.0 mcg | 41.3 | 2.5 | good |
| Omega-3 Fatty Acids | 1.0 g | 41.2 | 2.5 | good |
| Magnesium | 147.9 mg | 37.0 | 2.2 | good |
| Copper | 0.7 mg | 35.0 | 2.1 | good |
| B2 Riboflavin | 0.5 mg | 28.8 | 1.7 | good |
| Potassium | 885.8 mg | 25.3 | 1.5 | good |

For more on "Total Nutrient-Richness," "%DV," "Density," and
The World's Healthiest Foods "Quality" Rating System, see page 805.

The Soybean is native to China where it has been cultivated for over 3,000 years. The Chinese name for Soybean translates to "greater bean," a fitting name for a bean that offers such a wealth of nutritional benefits and culinary versatility. It wasn't until the early 1800s that Soybeans arrived in the United States as ballast aboard a ship! And it wasn't until the 1940s that the farming of Soybeans actually became popular. The texture of Soybeans is so adaptable that they can be processed in a host of different ways, making it easy for you to enjoy them in your daily diet. There are fresh Soybeans (also known as edamame), dried Soybean seeds, soymilk, soynuts, tofu, tempeh, soy flour… the list goes on and on. And with their delicious, slightly nutty flavor and wonderful nutritional profile, this legume known scientifically as *Glycine max* can offer you maximum enjoyment and health and be a great addition to your "Healthiest Way of Eating."

## why soybeans should be a part of your healthiest way of eating

Today, Soybeans are the most widely grown and utilized legumes in the world and one of the most well-researched health-promoting foods available! Rich in many vitamins and minerals, as well as protein and dietary fiber, Soybeans easily earn their place among the World's Healthiest Foods. Soybeans also contain powerful health-promoting isoflavone phytonutrients, including genistein and daidzen, which are especially important for women's health and a healthy heart. (For more on the *Health Benefits of Soybeans* and a complete analysis of their content of over 60 nutrients, see page 601.)

## variety of soybeans

Like other beans, Soybeans grow in pods, featuring edible seeds. While we are most familiar with green Soybeans, the seeds can also be yellow, brown or black. The texture of Soybeans is very adaptable, so they can be processed in a variety of different ways:

### EDAMAME

Fresh green Soybeans cooked in the pod.

### TOFU

Sometimes called the "cheese of Asia" because the methods used to produce tofu are similar to those used to make cheese. (For more information, see Tofu chapter, page 618.)

### TEMPEH

Originating in Indonesia, it is used as a meat substitute. To make tempeh, Soybeans are usually cooked with a grain and then aged with a special culture, resulting in a firm substance that can either be sliced or made into patties.

### SOYMILK

Made from grinding Soybeans with water, it is often used by individuals allergic to cow's milk and vegans who do not consume any animal products.

### MISO

Originating in Japan, it is a salty, fermented paste made from a combination of Soybeans and a grain (usually barley or rice).

### DRIED AND READY-TO-EAT SOYBEANS

Beans, such as Soybeans, are available dried, which require cooking, or in a can, which are fully prepared and ready to use. Unlike canned vegetables, which have lost much of their nutritional value, there is little difference in the nutritional value between canned Soybeans and those you cook yourself. Canning lowers vegetables' nutritional value since they are best lightly cooked for a short period of time, while their canning process requires a long cooking time at high temperatures. On the other hand, beans require a long time to cook whether they are from a can or you cook them yourself, so there is little difference in their nutritional value. You can now also find good quality canned Soybeans made from organically grown beans, which have better flavor and texture (not mushy and excellent for use in salads and cold dishes) and do not contain additives or extra salt. Canned Soybeans may cost slightly more than dried beans, but the time you save in preparation makes them well worth it.

# the peak season

Both dried and canned Soybeans are available throughout the year.

# biochemical considerations

Soybeans contain oxalates and goitrogens, which may be of concern to certain individuals and can be associated with allergic reactions. (For more on *Oxalates*, see page 725; *Goitrogens*, see page 721; and *Food Allergies*, see page 719.)

## Phytic Acid and Iron Absorption

Most beans contain phytic acid. This naturally occurring substance can work as an antioxidant in plants and has been shown to have some cancer-preventing and lipid-lowering effects in animal studies. A good bit of attention has been given to the relationship between phytic acid and iron absorption from food. This relationship is controversial. In some studies, phytates appear to lower iron absorption by as little as 3–4%. In other studies, this percentage is more like 45–50%. Since most people don't rely upon Soybeans as their primary source of dietary iron—rather it comes from other foods in the meal plan—any impact of the phytates found in Soybeans on iron absorption should not be of major concern for most people.

Soybeans are a good source of protein and at 29 grams per cup can provide a significant amount of our daily requirement. Phytic acid is sometimes regarded as interfering with protein digestibility, but the research I've seen suggests otherwise; it is partly because of their great protein benefits that I encourage incorporating Soybeans into the "Healthiest Way of Eating."

## Intestinal Gas

Legumes, like Soybeans, cause intestinal gas because humans cannot digest the oligosaccharides (sugars) found in beans. These sugars are consumed by bacteria in the large intestine and form gas. The gas-forming compounds can be reduced by draining off the water used to soak the dried beans and replacing it with fresh water before cooking. For canned Soybeans, drain off the liquid in the can and rinse with fresh water before using.

There is anecdotal evidence that cooking beans with kombu (a type of sea vegetable) and plenty of spices can improve the digestibility of beans. Adding kombu to your beans will also increase their nutritional value by adding trace minerals to your dish. Cumin, fennel and ginger are among the spices that are especially effective in preventing the formation of gas, but any of your favorite aromatic spices may help by inhibiting bacteria and stimulating digestion.

# 4 steps for the best tasting and most nutritious soybeans

Turning Soybeans into a flavorful dish with the most nutrients is simple if you just follow my 4 easy steps:

1. The Best Way to Select
2. The Best Way to Store
3. The Best Way to Prepare
4. The Healthiest Way of Cooking

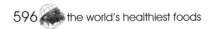

# 1. the best way to select soybeans

When purchasing canned Soybeans, it is preferable to select those that feature organically grown beans and do not contain extra salt or additives; dried beans should also be organically grown whenever possible.

As with other foods purchased in the bulk section at the local market, make sure that the bins containing dried Soybeans are covered and that the store has a good product turnover to ensure their maximal freshness. Whether purchasing Soybeans in bulk or in packaged containers, it is important that no evidence of moisture or insect damage is present and that they are whole and not cracked.

Fresh Soybeans, or edamame, should be deep green in color with firm pods that are not bruised. Edamame can be found in many supermarkets as well as in natural foods stores and Asian markets. They are usually available in the frozen food section, although some stores offer precooked edamame in their refrigerated display cases.

# 2. the best way to store soybeans

Store dried Soybeans in an airtight container in a cool, dry, dark place where they will keep for up to 12 months. If you purchase Soybeans at different times, store and cook them separately; legumes increase in dryness the longer they are stored, resulting in differences in required cooking time.

Cooked or unused portions of canned Soybeans will ferment and go sour if kept at room temperature. Store them in the refrigerator where they will keep for about 3 days.

Fresh edamame should be stored in the refrigerator and eaten within 2 days. Frozen edamame can be stored for a few months.

# 3. the best way to prepare soybeans

Properly preparing canned or dried Soybeans helps ensure that they will have the best flavor and retain the greatest number of nutrients.

### Rinsing Ready-to-Eat Soybeans

Rinse ready-to-eat canned Soybeans under cold running water. Most canned Soybeans have not been soaked before cooking, so they contain higher amounts of oliogosaccharides and thus may be more likely to cause indigestion. For information about how beans were prepared, you can call the manufacturer. Rinsing will help eliminate some of canned beans' oligosaccharides. If you still experience flatulence, experiment with different brands until you find one that agrees with you.

### Washing Dried Soybeans

Before washing Soybeans, spread them out on a light-colored plate or cooking surface to remove small stones, debris or damaged beans. Put beans in a large bowl of water and swish around. Discard any beans that float to the top. Place beans in a strainer and rinse thoroughly under cool running water.

### Washing Fresh Soybeans (Edamame)

Rinse under cold running water before cooking.

### Soaking Dried Soybeans

Add 4 cups water to 1 cup Soybeans, and soak for 8 hours or overnight. Drain and rinse again.

# 4. the healthiest way of cooking soybeans ———

The length of time required to cook dried Soybeans will vary depending on their freshness. Recently harvested beans cook much more quickly than those that have been stored for a long period of time.

## Cooking Tips for Soybeans

- Do not add salt to the cooking water or Soybeans will become tough. Add salt only after the beans are completely cooked.

- If your recipe calls for acidic ingredients, such as tomatoes, vinegar or wine, add them after the beans are cooked since adding them during cooking will cause the beans to become tough; acid reacts with the starch in the beans and prevents them from swelling.

- The flavor of Soybeans is complemented by cooking with 3 bay leaves or 10 peppercorns. Remove these spices before serving. It is best to add spices, such as garlic, onion, ginger, or chili powder 5 to 10 minutes before the end of cooking.

---

## The Healthiest Way of Cooking Soybeans

*If you have time to cook Soybeans at home, it's well worth the effort.*

**1 cup of dried Soybeans**
**4 cups water to soak**
**3 cups of water or salt-free broth**
**Sea salt and extra virgin olive oil to taste**

1. Place Soybeans in a large pot, **cover** the beans with 4 cups water and let soak overnight or for at least 8 hours.

2. Drain and rinse Soybeans, add 3 cups water or salt-free broth, **cover loosely** and bring to a boil.

3. Reduce heat to low and simmer for approximately 1 to 1½ hours or until soft. (Cooking time varies depending on the freshness of the Soybeans.) Stir occasionally and skim off foam as necessary.

4. Test Soybeans for doneness. If they are still hard and no more water remains in the pot, add ½–1 cup hot water and continue to cook until soft. Drain liquid if beans have cooked and excess water remains. If purchasing packaged dried Soybeans, it is best to follow the instructions on the package.

5. Add salt and extra virgin olive oil to taste after the beans are cooked.

**SERVES 2**

## Cooking Soybeans in a Pressure Cooker

*Presoaked Soybeans will cook much more quickly using a pressure cooker, which exposes the beans to a higher temperature but for a shorter period of time. Overcooking Soybeans will increase their glycemic index (GI).*

**1 cup dried Soybeans (4 cups water to soak)**
**2 cups water**
**Sea salt and extra virgin olive oil to taste**

1. Place Soybeans in a large pot, add 4 cups water and let soak overnight or for at least 8 hours.

2. Pressure cookers vary in the amount of pressure they produce and therefore in the amount of time needed to cook various beans. Before cooking Soybeans in your pressure cooker, read the manufacturer's instructions.

3. Drain and rinse beans and place them and 2 cups water in pressure cooker. **Do not fill it more than half full.**

4. Attach lid and bring up to pressure on medium heat. You should hear a soft hissing sound.

5. Lower heat and let Soybeans cook the amount of time recommended for them in your pressure cooker instruction book or approximately 35–40 minutes.

6. Add salt and extra virgin olive oil to taste after the beans are cooked.

For more ideas, see Flavor Tips on Page 599.

**SERVES 2**

**Q** *I've just started to eat Soybeans, and I am unsure as to what texture they should be after they are cooked. Should they be like other beans (such as navy beans) or should they be more firm?*

**A** Cooked Soybeans should be soft. They should be similar to navy beans or maybe just a tiny bit firmer.

**Q** *Are Soybeans a vegetable and therefore would help meet the "5-A-Day" requirement for health?*

**A** While Soybeans are technically plant foods, most nutrition recommendations categorize them as legumes, and they are usually viewed as a protein source. That is why they fall in the "meat and beans" category of the USDA's new Food Pyramid. Not only are they a concentrated source of protein but they also have phytonutrients such as isoflavones. Yet, unlike "vegetables" such as leafy greens, root vegetables and others, Soybeans are not rich sources of vitamin C, vitamin A and phytonutrients such as carotenoids and flavonoids and, as such, I wouldn't consider them as contributors to the "5-A-Day" requirement for fruits and vegetables.

**Q** *Do soynuts have the same nutritional benefits as Soybeans?*

**A** Soynuts do not have the same nutritional benefits as regular Soybeans. No processed food has the same benefits as the original whole food. In the case of soynuts, a large number of nutrients are lost. Included in this loss are the minerals copper, magnesium, manganese, phosphorus, potassium, selenium and zinc; the vitamins B1, B2, B3, B5, B6, folate and C; and the omega-3 fatty acid linolenic acid. That is not to say that you can't enjoy soynuts. They certainly are delicious and can play a part in the "Healthiest Way of Eating." It's just that they feature a different nutrient matrix.

**Q** *I have been making my own soy/nut butter, grinding Soybeans and mixed nuts. Is it harmful to use raw Soybeans?*

**A** I would recommend cooked Soybeans over raw Soybeans since cooking can reduce levels of certain components that can cause adverse effects in certain people if consumed in high levels. These include protease inhibitors, phytates and hemaglutinins.

**Q** *What exactly is soy sauce and is it nutritionally similar to Soybeans?*

**A** It is difficult to actually compare the nutritional value of soy sauce and Soybeans because they are consumed and used in such different ways. Soybeans can be a great addition to your "Healthiest Way of Eating," and there is a continual abundance of research providing evidence of their health-promoting properties.

Soy sauce, also known as tamari, is used in a totally different way than Soybeans. It is a popular condiment used in small quantities to enhance the flavor of food rather than as a primary source of nutrients in your "Healthiest Way of Eating." It was developed from the salty fermented paste derived from Soybeans, called miso. This development occurred during the Edo period (1603–1867) when extra water was added to the miso paste to create a thick, dark sauce. Later, changes in the process added wheat to the paste's ingredients, and today, tamari can be purchased as either wheat-containing or wheat-free. Tamari is dark brown in color and usually slightly thicker than regular soy sauce, but both provide the same nutritional value.

One tablespoon of soy sauce (tamari) contains 42% of your daily value for sodium, 5% DV for niacin, 3.4% DV for protein, 3% DV for phosphorus, 2.3% DV for iron, 2.3% DV for riboflavin and 2.3% DV for manganese. As you can see, it is very high in sodium and should be used in moderation for those who are on a low-sodium diet.

**Q** *How do you roast Soybeans?*

**A** The basic method for roasting Soybeans involves two steps. First, the beans should be soaked overnight. Begin by rinsing the beans well and then combining 4 cups of filtered water for every 1 cup of beans. In addition, use about 2 teaspoons of baking soda for every 4 cups of water. You should do your soaking in the refrigerator and let the beans soak overnight (for at least 8 hours). At this point, drain and rinse the beans thoroughly. Second, spread the soaked and rinsed beans on baking sheets. About 2 cups' worth of beans will fit on a baking sheet in a single layer. Preheat the oven to 350°F (175°C), and bake the beans for approximately 25–35 minutes, stirring the beans every 10–15 minutes and watching them closely to avoid burning them. Each cup of unroasted beans will produce about 1/2 cup of roasted ones.

STEP-BY-STEP RECIPE

## The Healthiest Ways to Prepare Soybeans

# 5-Minute Soybeans – No Cooking

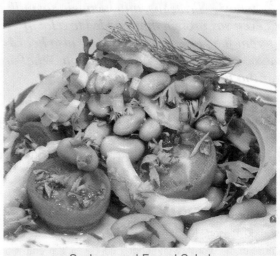

Soybean and Fennel Salad

*You can now enjoy organically grown ready-to-eat canned Soybeans that are healthier and tastier, and they only take minutes to prepare. If you have time to cook Soybeans, see page 597.*

1 15-oz can Soybeans, preferably organic
2 TBS extra virgin olive oil
2 cloves garlic
Sea salt and pepper to taste
Optional: Add tamari (soy sauce), ginger and
    sesame seeds for an Asian flavor

1. Press or mince garlic and let sit for 5 minutes (Why?, see page 261.)

2. Drain liquid from canned Soybeans and rinse under cold running water; this helps prevent intestinal gas.

3. Combine all ingredients, mix and enjoy!

For added flavor, you may want to add more olive oil.

**SERVES 2**

---

### Flavor Tips: Try these 4 great serving suggestions with the recipe above. ✳

1. Add miso, ginger, scallions, onions or wasabi.
2. Add a small, minced red onion and 1 TBS lemon juice or a few drops of balsamic vinegar for a Mediterranean flair.
3. Soybeans are best served with grains (such as rice), dairy, meat or vegetables for complete nutrition.
4. **Soybean Spread:** For wonderful flavor, blend the 5-Minute Soybeans recipe with mint and thyme.

**ADDITIONAL RECIPE:**

**Soybean and Fennel Salad:** Combine in a large bowl: 2 15-oz cans rinsed soybeans, 1 1/2 cups thinly sliced fennel bulb, 12 halved cherry tomatoes, 1/4 cup minced red onion, 2 cloves pressed garlic, 4 TBS lemon juice, 3 TBS chopped parsley, 1/2 cup extra virgin olive oil, 1/2–1 tsp sea salt and 1/4 tsp black pepper. This salad gets better as it marinates.

**EDAMAME (Whole Soybean Pods)**

To cook frozen edamame, just add the Soybean pods to lightly salted water and boil for about 15 minutes. Fresh edamame will take about 10 minutes longer. For both fresh and frozen edamame, it is best to follow the directions on the package.

- Add edamame to your favorite green salad.

- A small bowl full of edamame makes a wonderful appetizer or first course.

- Add cooked edamame to your favorite vegetable dish for added protein.

- **Edamame Salad:** Dress edamame with Mediterranean dressing (page 331) and minced mint leaves.

---

Please write (address on back cover flap) or e-mail me at info@whfoods.org with your personal ideas for preparing Soybeans, and I will share them with others through our website at www.whfoods.org.

**Q** *Soyfoods have been hailed as a healing food, and soy protein is everywhere today—Soybeans, tofu, tempeh, soymilk and even soy protein that's added to a lot of different food products. Yet, I have also heard that too much soy can be bad for you. What are your thoughts about soy?*

**A** You ask a very good question that is on the minds of many people. As soy is a healthy food, it is becoming more and more popular and therefore showing up in many different foods. All the while, there have been reports circulating on the Internet that soy foods are not healthy. Here are my thoughts on the subject:

I've included soy as one of the World's Healthiest Foods, and for good reason. It's the most widely grown and utilized legume in the world, with about 13,000 years of cultivation and over 5,000 research studies. There are studies that show soy to help regulate blood sugar, blood pressure, and estrogen balance. And there are studies showing soy intake to help prevent colon, breast, and prostate cancer, as well as atherosclerosis and post-menopausal hip fracture. It's seldom the case that a whole, natural food can be this widely used and studied for such a long period of time and have a predominantly negative impact on our health.

Yet, soy does have components that can compromise health in some circumstances. Soy contains goitrogens, for example, and in some individuals, goitrogens can decrease thyroid function and increase the possibility of depression. Soy also contains hemaglutinins that can sometimes increase the likelihood of our red blood cells clumping together. If that happened, our circulation could become compromised—including the blood flow to our brain. Soy also contains phytates that can sometimes decrease mineral absorption, including absorption of the minerals calcium, magnesium, iron and zinc. Each of these minerals has a role to play in our health. So yes, it's possible that soy can have a negative impact on our health in certain circumstances and for certain individuals. Yet, for the majority of people, soy is a good match healthwise.

Like all foods, soy is not a "magic bullet" and needs to be incorporated into a person's overall meal plan in a balanced and logical way. I believe that it needs to be eaten in moderation like all foods, as it is in Asia where it has been linked with promoting health. In Japan, for example, they don't usually consume large quantities of soy at one time, like many in the West have begun to do. I do not believe that more of a good thing is always a good thing, and this applies to eating soy. Like for everything, I believe in balance. What I observed in Japan was that while they enjoy soy almost daily, their portions are very small. They only use a few cubes of tofu in miso soup, enjoy small portions of edamame (fresh soy beans in pods) and when they drink soymilk, their servings are small.

At this point, no public health organization in the U.S. has recommended daily intake of soy products, including the National Cancer Institute, the American Heart Association or the American Dietetics Association. In 1995 in Japan, with all soy food products taken into account, the average intake was 50–70 total grams per day (not grams of soy protein, but of the entire food), which would translate into two ounces per day. This is potentially the highest daily average intake and seems to be less than the amount ordinarily used in the case of using soymilk and tofu in stir-fries. It is difficult to actually create a limit for individual daily consumption because the answer to that question can be best found by looking at a person's individual diet and health status.

**Q** *Do sprouted or soaked and boiled Soybeans provide more nutrients? Is there a difference in their ability to be digested?*

**A** All three practices you mentioned—sprouting, soaking and cooking—help make Soybeans more digestible. All three processes also impact the nutritional composition of the Soybeans. Some water-soluble nutrients are lost during the soaking process while some are lost during the cooking process; in addition, nutrient patterns are changed during sprouting. In general, although not always, cooked foods are easier to digest than raw foods, and I would expect cooked Soybeans to be more easily digested than raw sprouted Soybeans. At the same time, however, cooked foods are usually lower in nutrients than raw ones. In the case of Soybeans, I like the trade-off between digestibility and overall nutrient composition that occurs during cooking. However, for individuals accustomed to uncooked foods, raw sprouted Soybeans can also make important nutritional contributions to a meal. There is no absolute, single, correct way to prepare Soybeans. In all cases, however, I recommend organically grown Soybeans as the version that can provide you with optimal nourishment.

# health benefits of soybeans

## Promote Heart Health

In recent years, soy protein has been found to be excellent for a number of different conditions, one of the most important ones being its ability to help prevent heart disease. Soy protein has been shown in some studies to be able to lower total cholesterol levels by 30% and to lower levels of LDL, or "bad" cholesterol, by as much as 35–40%. Some studies have even shown that soy protein may be able to raise HDL ("good") cholesterol levels. It has also been found to increase the size of LDL cholesterol. This may have heart-health benefits since small, dense LDL is the most dangerous form of cholesterol, while large LDL, especially when accompanied by adequate supplies of HDL, is less risky.

Soy protein has also been shown to reduce the stickiness of platelets, possibly because Soybeans are a good source of omega-3 essential fatty acids. When platelets get overly sticky, they are more likely to clump together to form blood clots. Soybeans and other soy foods may also provide benefit for blood pressure as shown by a study that found men consuming soy in their diet had significant reductions in both diastolic and systolic blood pressure. In addition to their beneficial form of protein, Soybeans also contain very good amounts of fiber, which has been shown to reduce cholesterol levels.

Research suggests that diets rich in soy foods are cardioprotective, yet soy isoflavones alone (including its genistein and daidzein phytoestrogens) do not produce much effect. Therefore, incorporating soy foods like Soybeans into your diet (as compared to consuming soy supplements) may be the best way to approach optimizing heart health.

## Promote Women's Health

Soy foods seem to have a protective effect against breast cancer. In one study in Japan, women with the highest intakes of isoflavones—compounds in soy foods that can bind to estrogen receptors in the body and block out human estrogen, thus lessening its effects—had a 54% lower risk of developing breast cancer compared to those whose intake of isoflavones was lowest.

New research suggests that eating soy foods may also be one reason Asian women have the lowest incidence in the world of endometrial cancer, another hormone-dependent form of cancer. Soy's concentration of isoflavones and dietary fiber may be the reason that it has this protective effect: the isoflavones, genistein and daidzen, bind to estrogen receptors in the body and block out human estrogens, while dietary fiber has been found to lower estrogen levels.

Although these and other studies have supported a connection between soy food consumption and reduced risk of breast and endometrial cancer, some people have raised the question as to whether soy isoflavones, with their estrogenic activity, are safe. Even though the estrogenic potential of soy isoflavones is only 1/1,000th the potency of human estrogens, these

## Nutritional Analysis of 1 cup of cooked Soybeans:

| NUTRIENT | AMOUNT | % DAILY VALUE |
|---|---|---|
| Calories | 297.56 | |
| Calories from Fat | 138.86 | |
| Calories from Saturated Fat | 20.08 | |
| Protein | 28.62 g | |
| Carbohydrates | 17.06 g | |
| Dietary Fiber | 10.32 g | 41.28 |
| Soluble Fiber | 4.23 g | |
| Insoluble Fiber | 6.09 g | |
| Sugar – Total | 5.16 g | |
| Monosaccharides | 0.52 g | |
| Disaccharides | 0.86 g | |
| Other Carbs | 1.58 g | |
| Fat – Total | 15.43 g | |
| Saturated Fat | 2.23 g | |
| Mono Fat | 3.41 g | |
| Poly Fat | 8.71 g | |
| Omega-3 Fatty Acids | 1.03 g | 41.20 |
| Omega-6 Fatty Acids | 7.68 g | |
| Trans Fatty Acids | 0.00 g | |
| Cholesterol | 0.00 mg | |
| Water | 107.59 g | |
| Ash | 3.29 g | |

| Vitamins | | |
|---|---|---|
| Vitamin A IU | 15.48 IU | 0.31 |
| Vitamin A RE | 1.72 RE | |
| A - Carotenoid | 1.72 RE | 0.02 |
| A - Retinol | 0.00 RE | |
| B1 Thiamin | 0.27 mg | 18.00 |
| B2 Riboflavin | 0.49 mg | 28.82 |
| B3 Niacin | 0.69 mg | 3.45 |
| Niacin Equiv | 6.87 mg | |
| Vitamin B6 | 0.40 mg | 20.00 |
| Vitamin B12 | 0.00 mcg | 0.00 |
| Biotin | — mcg | — |
| Vitamin C | 2.92 mg | 4.87 |
| Vitamin D IU | 0.00 IU | 0.00 |
| Vitamin D mcg | 0.00 mcg | |
| Vitamin E Alpha Equiv | 3.35 mg | 16.75 |
| Vitamin E IU | 5.00 IU | |
| Vitamin E mg | 3.35 mg | |
| Folate | 92.54 mcg | 23.14 |
| Vitamin K | 33.02 mcg | 41.28 |

| NUTRIENT | AMOUNT | % DAILY VALUE |
|---|---|---|
| Pantothenic Acid | 0.31 mg | 3.10 |

| Minerals | | |
|---|---|---|
| Boron | — mcg | |
| Calcium | 175.44 mg | 17.54 |
| Chloride | — mg | |
| Chromium | — mcg | — |
| Copper | 0.70 mg | 35.00 |
| Fluoride | — mg | — |
| Iodine | — mcg | — |
| Iron | 8.84 mg | 49.11 |
| Magnesium | 147.92 mg | 36.98 |
| Manganese | 1.42 mg | 71.00 |
| Molybdenum | 129.00 mcg | 172.00 |
| Phosphorus | 421.40 mg | 42.14 |
| Potassium | 885.80 mg | |
| Selenium | 12.56 mcg | 17.94 |
| Sodium | 1.72 mg | |
| Zinc | 1.98 mg | 13.20 |

| Amino Acids | | |
|---|---|---|
| Alanine | 1.28 g | |
| Arginine | 2.10 g | |
| Aspartate | 3.41 g | |
| Cystine | 0.44 g | 107.32 |
| Glutamate | 5.24 g | |
| Glycine | 1.25 g | |
| Histidine | 0.73 g | 56.59 |
| Isoleucine | 1.31 g | 113.91 |
| Leucine | 2.21 g | 87.35 |
| Lysine | 1.80 g | 76.60 |
| Methionine | 0.36 g | 48.65 |
| Phenylalanine | 1.41 g | 118.49 |
| Proline | 1.58 g | |
| Serine | 1.57 g | |
| Threonine | 1.18 g | 95.16 |
| Tryptophan | 0.37 g | 115.63 |
| Tyrosine | 1.03 g | 106.19 |
| Valine | 1.35 g | 91.84 |

(Note: "—" indicates data is unavailable. For more information, please see page 806.)

individuals base their concern on the fact that hormone replacement therapy has been found to increase breast cancer risk. A recent animal study has found that consuming the amount of soy phytoestrogens that would be ingested when soy foods are included in the diet (in women, about 129 mg/day of isoflavones) does not increase risk of breast or uterine cancer and does appear to be protective. Yet, while it seems that soy foods themselves may be protective, concern may be justified when it comes to taking purified isoflavone supplements since isolated soy isoflavone products have been found to stimulate the growth of pre-existing estrogen-dependent breast tumors. This is yet another example (as is discussed in the Promote Heart Health section) of how a whole food, with its natural matrix of ingredients, can support health in ways that isolated food ingredient dietary supplements cannot. For more on this topic, please see the Q&A on page 603.

Soybeans may also help to alleviate many symptoms associated with menopause. Studies have shown that women who consume soy foods report a significant reduction in the amount of hot flashes and other symptoms that they experience. There is also some evidence that soy foods may even be able to help reduce the bone loss that typically occurs after menopause. And as women's risk for heart disease significantly increases at menopause, Soybeans' numerous beneficial cardiovascular effects make it a particularly excellent food to consume as menopause approaches.

## Promote Men's Health

In epidemiological studies, genistein has been consistently linked to lower incidence of prostate cancer. A recent study of human prostate cancer cells demonstrated some of the mechanisms behind genistein's anti-prostate cancer effects. Genistein not only induced chemicals that block cell cycling, thus preventing the proliferation of cancerous cells in the prostate, but at high concentrations, actually induced apoptosis, the self-destruct sequence the body uses to eliminate worn out or abnormal cells.

In addition to genistein, the soy isoflavone daidzein has also demonstrated protective action against prostate cancer. A study in China found that men consuming the most tofu had a 42% lower risk of developing prostate cancer compared to those consuming the least. When researchers checked the relationship between the soy isoflavones, genistein and daidzein, which are found not only in tofu, but in Soybeans and other foods made from them, those consuming the most genistein were found to have a 47% lower risk for prostate cancer, while those consuming the most daidzein had a 44% lower risk.

## Promote Digestive Health

In areas of the world where Soybeans are eaten regularly, rates of colon cancer tend to be low, which is not surprising considering that Soybeans contain a variety of compounds that may have benefit on digestive health. They are a good source of dietary fiber, which is able to bind to cancer-causing toxins and remove them from the body, so they can't damage colon cells. Soy also contains a lipid (fat) known as soy glucosylceramide, which has been found to protect animals from colon cancer proliferation. Additionally, a recent animal study suggests that colon cancer may be a hormone-responsive cancer and that soy protein can not only help prevent its occurrence but can have a very positive effect on the number and size of tumors that do occur. Soybean fiber may also be able to reduce the symptoms of diarrhea or constipation.

## Promote Healthy Weight Control

New research suggests that the active isoflavone compounds found in soy, specifically genistein, may help us stay lean by causing us to produce fewer and smaller fat cells. In this study, animals eating genistein-rich diets created less and smaller fat cells than animals eating regular food. In human terms, a comparable amount of genistein to that which the animals were given could easily be consumed by simply including traditional soy foods as part of a healthy, whole foods eating plan.

## Promote Balanced Blood Sugar

Another condition for which Soybeans can be very beneficial is diabetes, particularly type 2 diabetes mellitus. The protein in Soybeans, and also in other legumes, is excellent for diabetic individuals, who tend to have problems with animal sources of protein. The protein and fiber in Soybeans can also prevent high blood sugar levels and help in keeping blood sugar levels under control.

## Additional Health-Promoting Benefits of Soybeans

Soybeans are also a concentrated source of many other nutrients providing additional health-promoting benefits. These nutrients include bone-building calcium, magnesium, copper and manganese; energy-producing iron and phosphorus; free-radical-scavenging selenium; and sleep-promoting tryptophan.

## Q *Does soymilk have the same or at least similar nutritional value as Soybeans?*

A Although soymilk is produced from Soybeans, the first ingredient you will find listed on a container of soymilk will be water. The large quantities of water added to produce soymilk greatly diminishes its nutritional value when compared to eating Soybeans in their natural form. And while you may see soymilk advertised as being rich in certain nutrients, many of the nutrients are additives used to enrich the milk. In addition, soymilk usually contains some form of oil to give it its "milky" consistency as well as sweetener (regarding soymilk sweeteners, I much prefer evaporated cane sugar to corn syrup), making soymilk less nutrient-rich. All that being said, there may be a place in the diet for soymilk as a dairy-free beverage alternative. Yet, I don't see soymilk necessarily as a nutritional alternative to Soybeans.

## Q *Is it true that fermented Soybean foods are better for you?*

A In many Asian traditions, Soybeans have always undergone the processes of fermentation and aging before they have been consumed. Soy sauces, soy curds (made into tofu), soy pastes (made into miso) and other soy products like tempeh have all been traditionally produced through methods that take time and revolve around the ability of microorganisms (mostly friendly bacteria) to convert the cooked Soybeans into a more digestible, nutrient-rich and health-supportive food.

I've seen studies, for example, comparing soy foods fermented with the bacterium Bifidobacterium to non-fermented soy foods. In these studies (conducted on laboratory animals), the fermented foods were able to support health in a way that the non-fermented products were not. Two phytoestrogens, genistein and daidzen, were also found to be present in the fermented foods but not detectable in the non-fermented versions.

Research has clearly shown that soy proteins become more digestible with fermentation. A significant percentage of soy proteins get broken down into shorter protein strands (called polypeptides) or even into single amino acids during the process of fermentation. These protein forms require less chemical activity in our digestive tract and are much better prepared for digestion than whole intact proteins.

I've also seen studies that examined traditional fermentation process used to make soy sauce (shoyu), and these studies suggest that the antioxidant properties of soy sauce and its potentially cancer-preventive properties are both related to the process of fermentation. In addition, these studies show that the risk of allergy to soy is decreased through the process of fermentation. This conclusion makes sense to me, because many food allergies involve our immune system's response to food proteins, and the proteins in soy are clearly changed during the fermentation process.

## Q *I was told to avoid Soybeans because they are genetically engineered. Is that true?*

A Fifteen years ago, no genetically engineered food crops had been planted in the United States. Today, one of the top genetically engineered food crops is Soybeans.

There is no solid research evidence that genetic engineering of Soybeans is harmful to our health, but the reason for this lack of evidence is lack of studies. Genetically engineered foods are allowed into the marketplace without studies testing their safety. There's every reason to think that our digestive tracts and our immune systems would react differently to genetically modified foods due to the abrupt presence of new proteins in these foods that would be difficult for our organ systems to evaluate. I am concerned about this type of uncontrolled experiment with a widely consumed food crop, and it's one of the reasons I support consumption of certified organic soy products. Genetic engineering is prohibited in the production of any certified organic food.

## Q *Is there a concern about the phytoestrogens in soy and their effect on breast cancer?*

A I have some specific concerns based on the most recent research with soy. First is the mixed results I've see with respect to the phytoestrogens found in soy, particularly genistein and daidzein. Most of the earlier research in this area showed consumption of these phytoestrogens to be preventive of breast cancer in women who had not yet reached the age of menopause. However, more recent research has shown that in women who are postmenopausal, these same phytoestrogens can be potentially detrimental. In addition, they can increase the rate of tumor growth in women who have already been diagnosed with estrogen-dependent breast cancer. These mixed results with respect to soy phytoestrogens and breast cancer mean that a blanket statement about the cancer-preventive effects of soy foods is no longer accurate and that menopausal status is important when evaluating the benefits of these foods. Because the clinical issues here can be different from individual to individual, I'd recommend the advice of a healthcare practitioner for women of menopausal age considering the role of soy foods in their diet.

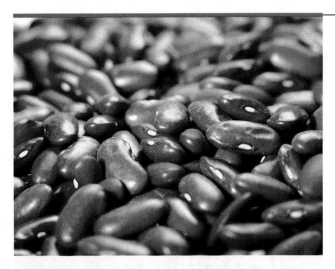

# kidney beans

| | |
|---|---|
| AVAILABILITY: | Year-round |
| REFRIGERATE: | Yes |
| SHELF LIFE: | Up to 12 months |
| PREPARATION: | Minimal |
| BEST WAY TO COOK: | Canned beans require no cooking |

## nutrient-richness chart

Total Nutrient-Richness: **19**      GI: **39**

One cup (177 grams) of cooked Kidney Beans contains 225 calories

| NUTRIENT | AMOUNT | %DV | DENSITY | QUALITY |
|---|---|---|---|---|
| Molybdenum | 132.8 mcg | 177.0 | 14.2 | excellent |
| Folate | 229.4 mcg | 57.3 | 4.6 | very good |
| Tryptophan | 0.2g | 56.3 | 4.5 | very good |
| Dietary Fiber | 11.3 g | 45.3 | 3.6 | very good |
| Manganese | 0.8 mg | 42.0 | 3.4 | very good |
| Protein | 15.4 g | 30.7 | 2.5 | good |
| Iron | 5.2 mg | 28.9 | 2.3 | good |
| Phosphorus | 251.3 mg | 25.1 | 2.0 | good |
| Copper | 0.4 mg | 21.5 | 1.7 | good |
| Potassium | 713.3 mg | 20.4 | 1.6 | good |
| Magnesium | 79.7 mg | 19.9 | 1.6 | good |
| B1 Thiamin | 0.3 mg | 18.7 | 1.5 | good |

For more on "Total Nutrient-Richness," "%DV," "Density," and
The World's Healthiest Foods "Quality" Rating System, see page 805.

For more on GI, see page 342.

Kidney Beans derived their name from their kidney-like shape. Native to Central and South America, the variety popular in the United States and Europe is a deep glossy red, while those popular in the Caribbean, Portugal and Spain are light pink in color. It's hard to imagine a good chili without the rich full-bodied flavor of Kidney Beans. For a meatless chili that is a great addition to your "Healthiest Way of Eating," combine Kidney Beans with a whole grain, such as rice, to transform this southwestern favorite into virtually fat-free, high quality protein.

## why kidney beans should be part of your healthiest way of eating

Like most varieties of legumes, Kidney Beans' rich supply of dietary fiber makes them valuable for both heart and digestive health. Their soluble fiber also makes them an excellent food to help maintain healthy blood sugar levels, while their manganese and copper help provide antioxidant protection from free radicals that can damage cellular structures. (Kidney Beans' health benefits and nutritional profile are similiar to black beans. For more information, see page 615.)

## varieties of kidney beans

Dried and canned Kidney Beans are available (same as black beans, see page 610).

## the peak season available year-round.

## biochemical considerations

Same as black beans (see page 611).

## the best way to select kidney beans

Same as black beans (see page 611).

## the best way to store kidney beans

Same as black beans (see page 611).

## the best way to prepare kidney beans

Same as black beans (see page 612).

## the healthiest way of cooking kidney beans

For details about cooking, see black bean recipe (page 614). Kidney Beans take 1 to $1^{1}/2$ hours to cook.

STEP-BY-STEP RECIPE
## The Healthiest Ways to Prepare Kidney Beans

# 5-Minute Kidney Beans – No Cooking

*Since dried Kidney Beans need soaking and substantial cooking time, I suggest using organic canned Kidney Beans. This recipe takes just minutes to prepare. If you have time to cook Kidney Beans, see page 614 for directions.*

1 15-oz can Kidney Beans, preferably organic
2 TBS extra virgin olive oil
2 cloves garlic
Sea salt and pepper to taste
Optional: Top with cilantro and grated cheese

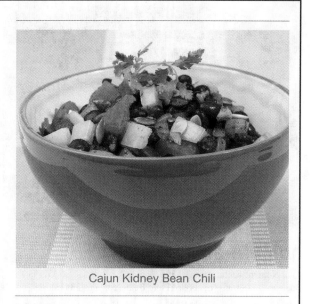
Cajun Kidney Bean Chili

1. Press or mince garlic and let sit for 5 minutes. (Why?, see page 261.)

2. Drain liquid from Kidney Beans and rinse under cold running water, which helps prevent intestinal gas.

3. Combine all ingredients, mix and enjoy!
For added flavor, you may want to add more olive oil.

SERVES **2**

## Flavor Tips: Try these 9 great serving suggestions with the recipe above. ✱

1. Add chili peppers, chili powder, cumin or oregano to complement the flavor of Kidney Beans.
2. Combine with chopped boiled egg, diced avocado, chopped tomato, chopped sweet onion and lime juice. Roll up in a flour tortilla and serve with salsa.
3. **Kidney Bean Romaine Wrap:** Wrap 5-Minute Kidney Beans recipe, avocado slices, shredded lettuce, chopped tomatoes and cilantro leaves in a large romaine lettuce leaf and add your favorite salsa.
4. **Kidney Bean Pasta:** "Healthy Sauté" a medium-size diced onion and medium-size diced green pepper. Add a large diced tomato, 1/2 tsp dried oregano, the 5-Minute Kidney Beans recipe, cooked whole wheat pasta shells, and salt and pepper to taste. Heat through. Top with 1/2 cup grated low-fat mozzarella cheese.
5. **Kidney Bean Salad:** Combine the 5-Minute Kidney Bean recipe with a medium-size diced sweet onion, medium-size diced green pepper, 1 cup of fresh minced cilantro and juice of 1/2–1 lime.
6. **Three Bean Salad:** Combine the 5-Minute Kidney Beans recipe with equal amounts of canned black beans and white beans to make a colorful three bean salad. Mix with tomatoes and scallions, and dress with olive oil, lemon juice and black pepper.
7. **Cajun Kidney Bean Chili:** "Healthy Sauté" 1 medium diced onion and 1 diced yellow or red bell pepper for 5 minutes. Add 3 cloves pressed garlic, 1 tsp paprika, 1 TBS chili powder, 1/2 tsp each dried thyme, oregano and fennel seeds, 1 tsp cumin and 1/8 tsp cayenne. Then add a 15-oz can diced tomatoes and a 15-oz can Kidney Beans. Cover and simmer 15–20 minutes. Season to taste with salt, pepper and olive oil (pictured above). Optional: add cooked ground turkey.
8. **Kidney Bean Dip:** In a food processor or blender, combine the 5-Minute Kidney Beans recipe with 1 tsp cumin and 1/2 tsp chili flakes (dried red chili peppers) for a delicious spread that can be used as a crudité dip or sandwich filling.
9. **Kidney Bean Taco:** Make tacos with a vegetarian twist by using the 5-Minute Kidney Beans recipe in place of ground meat.

Please write (address on back cover flap) or e-mail me at info@whfoods.org with your personal ideas for preparing Kidney Beans, and I will share them with others through our website at www.whfoods.org.

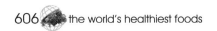

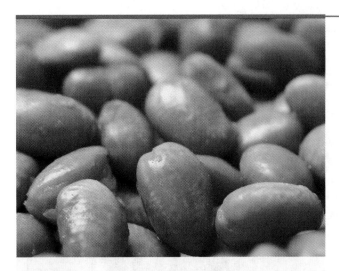

# pinto beans

## nutrient-richness chart

Total Nutrient-Richness: **19**    GI: **55**
One cup (171 grams) of cooked Pinto Beans contains 234 calories

| NUTRIENT | AMOUNT | %DV | DENSITY | QUALITY |
|---|---|---|---|---|
| Molybdenum | 128.3 mcg | 171.0 | 13.1 | excellent |
| Folate | 294.1 mcg | 73.5 | 5.6 | very good |
| Dietary Fiber | 14.7 g | 58.8 | 4.5 | very good |
| Tryptophan | 0.2 g | 53.1 | 4.1 | very good |
| Manganese | 1.0 mg | 47.5 | 3.6 | very good |
| Protein | 14.0 g | 28.1 | 2.2 | good |
| Phosphorus | 273.6 mg | 27.4 | 2.1 | good |
| Iron | 4.5 mg | 24.8 | 1.9 | good |
| Magnesium | 94.1 mg | 23.5 | 1.8 | good |
| Potassium | 800.3 mg | 22.9 | 1.8 | good |
| Copper | 0.4 mg | 22.0 | 1.7 | good |
| B1 Thiamin | 0.3 mg | 21.3 | 1.6 | good |

For more on "Total Nutrient-Richness," "%DV," "Density," and
The World's Healthiest Foods "Quality" Rating System, see page 805.

For more on GI, see page 342.

Pinto Beans are the most popular variety of beans in the United States. When cooked, the characteristic "painted" appearance of Pinto Beans disappears, and they become a beautiful reddish-tan color with a delightfully creamy texture. Like other beans, you can combine Pinto Beans with whole grains, such as rice, and add virtually fat-free, high quality protein to your "Healthiest Way of Eating."

## why pinto beans should be part of your healthiest way of eating

Pinto Beans provide great value—both in terms of price and nutrition. They are usually the least expensive of the different types of legumes, yet still contain similar health-promoting benefits to other varieties of beans. They are a concentrated

## highlights

| AVAILABILITY: | Year-round |
|---|---|
| REFRIGERATE: | No |
| SHELF LIFE: | Up to 12 months |
| PREPARATION: | Minimal |
| BEST WAY TO COOK: | Canned beans require no cooking |

source of dietary fiber, folate, magnesium and potassium, all of which make them a great choice for promoting heart health. (Pinto Beans' health benefits and nutritional profile are similiar to black beans. For more information see page 615.)

## varieties of pinto beans

Dried and canned Pinto Beans are available (same as black beans, see page 610).

## the peak season available year-round.

## biochemical considerations

Same as black beans (see page 611).

## the best way to select pinto beans

Same as black beans (see page 611).

## the best way to store pinto beans

Same as black beans (see page 611).

## the best way to prepare pinto beans

Same as black beans (see page 612).

## the healthiest way of cooking pinto beans

For details about cooking, see black bean recipe (page 614). Pinto Beans take 1 to 1 1/2 hours to cook.

STEP-BY-STEP RECIPE
## The Healthiest Ways to Prepare Pinto Beans

# 5-Minute Pinto Beans – No Cooking

*Since dried Pinto Beans need soaking and substantial cooking time, I suggest using organic canned Pinto Beans. This recipe takes just minutes to prepare. If you have time to cook Pinto Beans, see page 614 for directions.*

**1 15-oz can Pinto Beans, preferably organic**
**2 TBS extra virgin olive oil**
**2 cloves garlic**
**Sea salt and pepper to taste**
**Optional: Top with diced avocado and salsa**

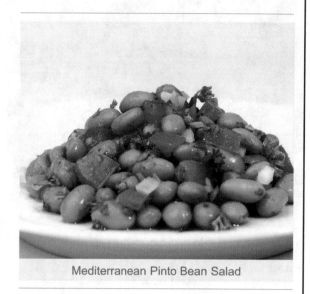

Mediterranean Pinto Bean Salad

1. Press or mince garlic and let sit for 5 minutes (Why?, see page 261.)

2. Drain liquid from Pinto Beans and rinse under cold running water; this helps prevent intestinal gas.

3. Combine all ingredients, mix and enjoy!

For added flavor, you may want to add more olive oil.

**SERVES 2**

---

## Flavor Tips: Try these 10 great serving suggestions with the recipe above. ✱

1. For spicy Pinto Beans, combine with minced jalapeños or red chili flakes, minced garlic and lime juice.

2. Serve heated 5-Minute Pinto Beans with grated cheese, corn tortillas and rice.

3. Combine with cilantro pesto (see Pesto Recipe, page 525, and substitute cilantro for basil).

4. Add to your favorite salad for more protein and fiber.

5. **Mediterranean Pinto Bean Salad:** Add diced tomatoes and red onions, chopped herbs (such as rosemary, flat-leaf parsley, oregano and basil), fresh lemon juice and more olive oil to the 5-Minute Pinto Beans recipe (pictured above).

6. **Puréed Pinto Beans with Poached Egg:** "Healthy Sauté" a small minced onion. Blend sautéed onions, the 5-Minute Pinto Beans recipe and 2 TBS chicken or vegetable broth until smooth. Make sure you don't fill the blender more than half full. Start on low speed. You will have to stop the blender a couple times and scrape the sides with a rubber spatula. Serve with a poached egg and top with your favorite salsa or hot sauce.

7. **Pinto Bean Taco:** Mash 5-Minute Pinto Beans recipe and combine with 6 chopped black olives. Finely shred 2 cups of cabbage and 1/2 cup cheese. Chop a medium tomato and cube a small avocado. Serve desired amounts of each ingredient in a corn tortilla and top with salsa.

8. **Chili Pasta:** "Healthy Sauté" diced onions and diced green peppers for 2 minutes. Add chopped tomatoes, minced fresh oregano, minced jalapeño pepper, minced garlic and sea salt. Cook 1 minute on high heat. Add equal amounts of cooked whole wheat macaroni and 5-Minute Pinto Beans recipe. Cook for 3 minutes on medium heat or until warm.

9. **Pinto Bean Corn Salad:** Combine 5-Minute Pinto Beans recipe, corn kernels and pre-made salsa. For more flavor, add Mediterranean Dressing and red pepper flakes. Serve on a bed of romaine lettuce.

10. **Pinto Bean Chili:** Pinto Beans are great for making chili. "Healthy Sauté" a medium diced onion. Add a 15-oz can of diced canned tomatoes (do not drain), 2 TBS chili powder and the 5-Minute Pinto Beans recipe. **Cover** and simmer for about 20 minutes. Add chopped cilantro and ground cumin at the end of the cooking time.

---

Please write (address on back cover flap) or e-mail me at info@whfoods.org with your personal ideas for preparing Pinto Beans, and I will share them with others through our website at www.whfoods.org.

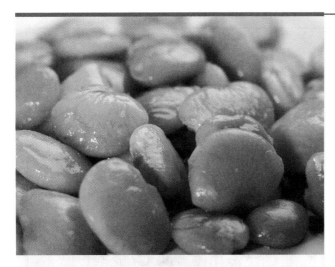

# lima beans

| | |
|---|---|
| AVAILABILITY: | Year-round |
| REFRIGERATE: | No |
| SHELF LIFE: | Up to 12 months |
| PREPARATION: | Minimal |
| BEST WAY TO COOK: | Canned beans require no cooking |

## nutrient-richness chart

Total Nutrient-Richness: **18**    GI: **n/a**

One cup (188 grams) of cooked Lima Beans contains 216 calories

| NUTRIENT | AMOUNT | %DV | DENSITY | QUALITY |
|---|---|---|---|---|
| Molybdenum | 141.0 mcg | 188.0 | 15.7 | excellent |
| Tryptophan | 0.2 g | 53.1 | 4.4 | very good |
| Dietary Fiber | 13.2 g | 52.6 | 4.4 | very good |
| Manganese | 1.0 mg | 48.5 | 4.0 | very good |
| Folate | 156.2 mcg | 39.1 | 3.3 | good |
| Protein | 14.7 g | 29.3 | 2.4 | good |
| Potassium | 955.0 mg | 27.3 | 2.3 | good |
| Iron | 4.5 mg | 24.9 | 2.1 | good |
| Copper | 0.4 mg | 22.0 | 1.8 | good |
| Phosphorus | 208.7 mg | 20.9 | 1.7 | good |
| Magnesium | 80.8 mg | 20.2 | 1.7 | good |
| B1 Thiamin | 0.3 mg | 20.0 | 1.7 | good |

For more on "Total Nutrient-Richness," "%DV," "Density," and
The World's Healthiest Foods "Quality" Rating System, see page 805.

For more on GI, see page 342.

Named after the capital of Peru where they have been cultivated for over 7,000 years, Lima Beans are a delicately flavored bean with a somewhat starchy texture. Sometimes called "butter beans," they have a mild flavor that makes them a suitable addition to a wide variety of recipes. Combined with whole grains, Lima Beans, like most other beans, provide a virtually fat-free, full-spectrum protein, making them a great addition to your "Healthiest Way of Eating."

## why lima beans should be part of your healthiest way of eating

Like other legumes, Lima Beans are a rich source of protein and cholesterol-lowering fiber. Dietary fiber, along with the folate, potassium and magnesium found in Lima Beans, also makes them a very heart-healthy food. (Lima Beans' health benefits and nutritional profile are similiar to black beans. For more information, see page 615.)

## varieties of lima beans

Dried and canned Lima Beans are available (same as black beans, see page 610). Photo on this page is of frozen Lima Bean.

## the peak season available year-round.

## biochemical considerations

Same as black beans (see page 611).

## the best way to select lima beans

Same as black beans (see page 611).

## the best way to store lima beans

Same as black beans (see page 611).

## the best way to prepare lima beans

Same as black beans (see page 612).

## the healthiest way of cooking lima beans

For details about cooking, see black bean recipe (page 614). Lima Beans take 40 to 50 minutes to cook.

STEP-BY-STEP RECIPE
## The Healthiest Ways to Prepare Lima Beans

# 5-Minute Lima Beans – No Cooking

*Lima Beans often don't get the credit they deserve. Try this quick, tasty recipe using organic, canned Lima Beans. If you have time to cook Lima Beans, see page 614 for directions.*

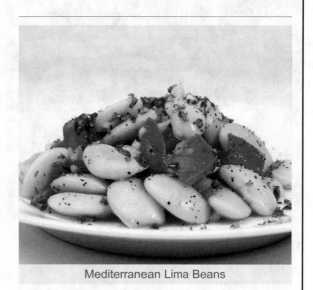

Mediterranean Lima Beans

**1 15-oz can Lima Beans, preferably organic**
**2 TBS extra virgin olive oil**
**2 cloves garlic**
**Sea salt and pepper to taste**
**Optional: Top with low-fat Parmesan cheese**

**1.** Press or mince garlic and let sit for 5 minutes (Why?, see page 261.)

**2.** Drain liquid from Lima Beans and rinse under cold running water; this helps prevent intestinal gas.

**3.** Combine all ingredients, mix and enjoy!

For added flavor, you may want to add more olive oil.

**SERVES 2**

## Flavor Tips: Try these 8 great serving suggestions with the recipe above. ✱

1. **Mediterranean Lima Beans:** Mix 5-Minute Lima Beans recipe with 1 diced tomato, 1 TBS lemon juice and minced fresh or dried thyme, rosemary and parsley.

2. **Lima Bean Salsa:** Combine 1 cup of the 5-Minute Lima Beans recipe with 1 diced tomato, 2 TBS minced sweet onion, 1/2 cup corn, 1/4 cup minced cilantro, 2 tsp lime juice, 1 tsp cumin and sea salt and cayenne pepper to taste.

3. **Mexican Succotash:** Combine 1 cup of the 5-Minute Lima Beans recipe with 1 cup of corn, 1 TBS minced jalapeño pepper (seeds removed), 1/4 cup chopped red bell peppers, 2 TBS fresh oregano, and sea salt and pepper to taste.

4. **Quick Lima Bean Soup:** Blend 2 cups of hot chicken broth, 1 cup of the 5-Minute Lima Beans recipe, 1 TBS tahini, and tamari (soy sauce) and pepper to taste until smooth. Garnish with fresh thyme.

5. **Asian Lima Beans:** Combine 5-Minute Lima Beans recipe with 2 sliced scallions, 1 TBS sesame seeds, 1 TBS brown rice vinegar, 2 additional TBS extra virgin olive oil and 1 TBS tamari (soy sauce). Serve with fish or seafood (such as shrimp or scallops).

6. **Lima Bean Hummus:** Blend the 5-Minute Lima Beans recipe with 1/4 cup tahini and 2 TBS lemon juice. Add water as needed to make a smooth paste. Add sea salt to taste. Serve in a bowl, sprinkle with paprika and drizzle with olive oil. Serve with crudités.

7. **Puréed Lima Beans:** Purée the 5-Minute Lima Beans recipe with your favorite fresh herbs and use as a sandwich spread or a dip for crudités.

8. **Lima Bean Burritos:** Fill corn tortillas with 5-Minute Lima Beans and corn kernels, then top with chopped tomatoes, avocado and scallions.

Please write (address on back cover flap) or e-mail me at info@whfoods.org with your personal ideas for preparing Lima Beans, and I will share them with others through our website at www.whfoods.org.

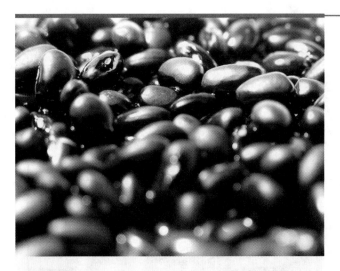

# black beans

| | |
|---|---|
| AVAILABILITY: | Year-round |
| REFRIGERATE: | No |
| SHELF LIFE: | Up to 12 months |
| PREPARATION: | Minimal |
| BEST WAY TO COOK: | Canned beans require no cooking |

## nutrient-richness chart

Total Nutrient-Richness: **16**      GI: **n/a**

One cup (172 grams) of cooked Black Beans contains 277 calories

| NUTRIENT | AMOUNT | %DV | DENSITY | QUALITY |
|---|---|---|---|---|
| Molybdenum | 129.0 mcg | 172.0 | 13.6 | excellent |
| Folate | 255.9 mcg | 64.0 | 5.1 | very good |
| Dietary Fiber | 15.0 g | 59.8 | 4.7 | very good |
| Tryptophan | 0.2 g | 56.3 | 4.5 | very good |
| Manganese | 0.8 mg | 38.0 | 3.0 | good |
| Protein | 15.2 g | 30.5 | 2.4 | good |
| Magnesium | 120.4 mg | 30.1 | 2.4 | good |
| B1 Thiamin | 0.4 mg | 28.0 | 2.2 | good |
| Phosphorus | 240.8 mg | 24.1 | 1.9 | good |
| Iron | 3.6 mg | 20.1 | 1.6 | good |

For more on "Total Nutrient-Richness," "%DV," "Density," and
The World's Healthiest Foods "Quality" Rating System, see page 805.

For more on GI, see page 342.

Known as *frijoles negro* in Spanish, Black Beans remain an inexpensive source of protein for many cultures throughout the world and are synonymous with the rich flavors of Hispanic cuisine. Favorites in Mexico, South America and the Caribbean, Black Beans' popularity has been increasing in the United States as we grow to enjoy the influence of these regions' cuisines on our taste buds. I want to share with you how you can easily transform Black Beans into a great dish for a "South of the Border" influence on your "Healthiest Way of Eating."

## why black beans should be part of your healthiest way of eating

While all beans are exceptionally healthy foods when it comes to their protein and fiber content, it's the color coat on Black Beans that makes them particularly nutritionally interesting in contrast to other beans. Researchers have found at least eight different flavonoids, including anthocyanins, in the Black Bean's color coat, which bestow this little bean with the potent antioxidant power that provides cells protection from the damage caused by free radicals. (For more on the *Health Benefits of Black Beans* and a complete analysis of their content of over 60 nutrients, see page 615.)

## varieties of black beans

Beans, such as Black Beans, are available dried, which require cooking, or canned, which are fully prepared and ready to use. Unlike canned vegetables, which have lost much of their nutritional value, there is little difference in the nutritional value between canned Black Beans and those you cook yourself. Canning lowers vegetables' nutritional value since they are best lightly cooked for a short period of time, while their canning process requires a long cooking time at high temperatures. On the other hand, beans require a long time to cook whether they are canned or you cook them yourself, so there is little difference in their nutritional value. You can now also find good quality organically grown canned Black Beans, which have better flavor and texture (not mushy and excellent for use in salads and cold dishes) and do not contain additives or extra salt. Canned Black Beans may cost slightly more than dried beans, but the time you save in preparation makes them well worth it.

## the peak season

Both dried and canned Black Beans are available throughout the year.

## biochemical considerations

Black Beans contain purines, which may be of concern to certain individuals. (For more on *Purines*, see page 727.)

### Phytic Acid and Iron Absorption

Most beans contain phytic acid. This naturally occurring substance can work as an antioxidant in plants and has been shown to have some cancer-preventing and lipid-lowering effects in animal studies. A good bit of attention has been given to the relationship between phytic acid and iron absorption from food. This relationship is controversial. In some studies, phytates appear to lower iron absorption by as little as 3–4%. In other studies, this percentage is more like 45–50%. Since most people don't rely upon Black Beans as their primary source of dietary iron—rather it comes from other foods in the meal plan—any impact of the phytates found in Black Beans on iron absorption should not be of major concern for most people.

Black Beans are a good source of protein and at 15 grams per cup can provide a significant amount of our daily requirement. Phytic acid is sometimes regarded as interfering with protein digestibility, but the research I've seen suggests otherwise; it is partly because of their great protein benefits that I continue to encourage incorporating Black Beans into your "Healthiest Way of Eating."

### Intestinal Gas

Legumes, like Black Beans, cause intestinal gas because humans cannot digest the oligosaccharides (sugars) found in beans. These sugars are consumed by bacteria in the large intestine and form gas. The gas-forming compounds can be reduced by draining off the water used to soak the dried beans and replacing it with fresh water before cooking. For canned Black Beans, drain off the liquid in the can and rinse with fresh water before using.

There is anecdotal evidence that cooking beans with kombu (a type of sea vegetable) and plenty of spices can improve the digestibility of beans. Adding kombu to your beans will also increase their nutritional value by adding trace minerals to your dish. Cumin, fennel and ginger are among the spices that are especially effective in preventing the formation of gas, but any of your favorite aromatic spices may help by inhibiting bacteria and stimulating digestion.

## 4 steps for the best tasting and most nutritious black beans

Turning Black Beans into a flavorful dish with the most nutrients is simple if you just follow my 4 easy steps:

1. The Best Way to Select
2. The Best Way to Store
3. The Best Way to Prepare
4. The Healthiest Way of Cooking

# 1. the best way to select black beans

When purchasing canned Black Beans, it is preferable to choose those that feature organically grown beans and do not contain extra salt or additives; dried beans should also be organically grown whenever possible.

As with other foods purchased in the bulk section of the market, make sure that the bins containing dried Black Beans are covered and that the store has a good product turnover to ensure their maximal freshness. Whether purchasing Black Beans in bulk or in packaged containers, it is important that no evidence of moisture or insect damage is present and that they are whole and not cracked.

# 2. the best way to store black beans

Store dried Black Beans in an airtight container in a cool, dry, dark place where they will keep up to 12 months. If you purchase Black Beans at different times, store and cook them separately as legumes increase in dryness the longer they are stored, resulting in differences in required cooking time.

Unused portions of cooked or canned Black Beans will keep fresh in the refrigerator for about 3 days if placed in a covered container.

# 3. the best way to prepare black beans

Properly preparing canned Black Beans or dried Black Beans helps ensure that they will have the best flavor and retain the greatest number of nutrients.

### Rinsing Ready-to-Eat Black Beans

Rinse canned Black Beans under cold running water. Most canned Black Beans have not been soaked before cooking, so they contain higher amounts of oligosaccharides and thus may be more likely to cause indigestion. For information about how beans were prepared, you can call the manufacturer. Rinsing will help eliminate some of canned beans' oligosaccharides. If you still experience flatulence, experiment with different brands until you find one that agrees with you.

### Washing Dried Black Beans

Before washing Black Beans, spread them out on a light-colored plate or cooking surface to remove small stones, debris or damaged beans. Put beans in a large bowl of water and swish around. Discard any beans that float to the top. Place beans in a strainer and rinse thoroughly under cool running water.

### Soaking Dried Black Beans

Add 4 cups water to 1 cup Black Beans, and soak for 8 hours or overnight. Drain and rinse again before cooking.

# 4. the healthiest way of cooking black beans

The length of time required to cook Black Beans will vary depending on their freshness. Recently harvested beans cook much more quickly than those that have been stored for a long period of time.

### Cooking Tips for Black Beans

*   Do not add salt to the cooking water or Black Beans will become tough. Add salt only after the beans are completely cooked.
*   If your recipe calls for acidic ingredients, such as tomatoes, vinegar or wine, add them after the beans are cooked since adding them during cooking will cause the beans to become tough; acid reacts with the starch in the beans and prevents them from swelling.
*   The flavor of Black Beans is complemented by cooking with 3 bay leaves, 2 dried chipotle peppers or 10 peppercorns. Remove these spices before serving. It is best to add spices, such as cumin, coriander, paprika or chili pepper 5–10 minutes before the end of cooking.
*   Black Beans are best served with grains (for example, rice) to make a complete protein.

---

## *10-Minute Huevos Rancheros*

2 omega-3-rich eggs
1/2 can black beans, drained and mashed
2 TBS extra virgin olive oil
1 tsp lemon juice
Sea salt and pepper to taste
1/4 avocado, sliced
Salsa from a jar
3 TBS grated low-fat cheddar cheese
Chopped cilantro
Optional: cayenne pepper

1.  Poach eggs.
2.  Heat beans in a skillet while eggs are cooking.
3.  Remove beans from heat and mix in olive oil, lemon juice, salt and pepper. Add a pinch of cayenne for spicy beans.
4.  Place beans on plate, top with poached eggs, avocado, salsa, cheese and cilantro.

SERVES 1

STEP-BY-STEP RECIPE
## The Healthiest Ways to Prepare Black Beans

# 5-Minute Black Beans – No Cooking

*You can now find many brands of organic, ready-to-eat canned Black Beans that are healthier and tastier than conventionally produced Black Beans. This recipe takes just minutes to prepare. If you have time to cook Black Beans, see page 614 for directions.*

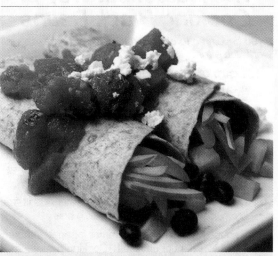
Spicy Black Bean Burrito

> 1 15-oz can Black Beans,
>     preferably organic
> 2 TBS extra virgin olive oil
> 2 cloves garlic
> **Sea salt and pepper to taste**
> **Optional: Top with salsa**

1. Press or mince garlic and let sit for 5 minutes (Why?, see page 261.)
2. Drain liquid from canned Black Beans and rinse under cold running water; this helps prevent intestinal gas.
3. Combine all ingredients, mix and enjoy!

   For added flavor, you may want to add more olive oil.

**SERVES 2**

## Flavor Tips: Try these 13 great serving suggestions with the recipe above. ✳

1. Add herbs like rosemary, ginger, thyme and oregano to complement the flavor of Black Beans.
2. Add chopped chili peppers.
3. Black Beans taste great with garlic and pepper.
4. Add 1/2 small chopped red onion, 1 TBS lemon juice or a few drops of balsamic vinegar.
5. A squeeze of lime juice will add a refreshing taste.
6. **Black Bean Breakfast Wrap:** On a whole wheat tortilla, place a scrambled egg, a spoonful of the 5-Minute Black Beans recipe, chopped tomato, 2 avocado slices and minced cilantro. Add hot sauce if you like. Roll it up and enjoy!
7. **Black Bean and Romaine Salad:** Combine the 5-Minute Black Beans recipe, 1 TBS salsa, 3 TBS extra virgin olive oil, cider vinegar, ground cumin and red pepper flakes to taste. Serve in romaine leaves.
8. **Quick Black Bean Soup:** Blend the 5-Minute Black Beans recipe with 2 cups of hot chicken broth and chili powder, sea salt and cayenne pepper to taste. Put a dollop of yogurt on top.
9. **Black Bean Dip:** In a blender, purée the 5-Minute Black Beans recipe, using 1/4 cup extra virgin olive oil, 1 tsp chili powder, and salt and pepper to taste.
10. **Black Bean Salad:** Combine a 15-oz can Black Beans with 1 small chopped bell pepper, 1/2 cup sweet corn, 1 medium chopped tomato, 1/2 cup minced cilantro, 1 TBS lime juice, 1/2 cup of extra virgin olive oil, and salt and pepper to taste.
11. **Black Bean Chili:** Black Beans are great for making chili. "Healthy Sauté" 1 medium diced onion. Add a 15-oz can of diced canned tomatoes (do not drain), 2 TBS chili powder and the 5-Minute Black Beans recipe. **Cover** and simmer for about 20 minutes. Add fresh chopped cilantro and cumin at the end of the cooking time.
12. **Black Beans and Butternut Squash:** For a quick vegetarian meal, "Healthy Steam" 1 medium cubed butternut squash. Mix with 5-Minute Black Beans, 1 tsp cumin, 1/4 tsp cinnamon, a pinch cayenne and sea salt to taste. Sprinkle with sliced green onion.
13. **Spicy Black Bean Burrito:** "Healthy Sauté" 1/2 diced red onion and 1 diced yellow or red bell pepper. Add 5-Minute Black Beans recipe, 2 tsp chili powder and 1/8 tsp cayenne pepper. Wrap mixture in a large whole wheat tortilla with low-fat cheese. Top with your favorite salsa (pictured above).

Please write (address on back cover flap) or e-mail me at info@whfoods.org with your personal ideas for preparing Black Beans, and I will share them with others through our website at www.whfoods.org.

## The Healthiest Way of Cooking Black Beans

*If you have time to cook Black Beans at home, it's well worth the effort.*

**1 cup of dried Black Beans**
**4 cups of water to soak**
**3 cups of water or salt-free broth**
**3 TBS extra virgin olive oil**
**Sea salt and pepper to taste**

1. Place Black Beans in a large pot, cover the beans with 4 cups water and let soak overnight or for at least 8 hours.

2. Drain off water, add 3 cups fresh water or salt-free broth, **cover** loosely and bring to a boil.

3. Reduce heat to low and simmer for approximately 1 to 1$^1$/2 hours or until soft. (Cooking time varies depending on the freshness of the Black Beans.) Stir occasionally and skim off foam as necessary.

4. Test Black Beans for doneness. If they are still hard and no more water remains in the pot, add 1/2–1 cup hot water and continue to cook until soft. Drain liquid if beans have cooked and excess water remains. If purchasing packaged dried Black Beans, it is best to follow the instructions on the package.

5. Add olive oil, salt and pepper to taste after the Black Beans are cooked.

**SERVES 2**

## Cooking Black Beans in a Pressure Cooker

*Presoaked Black Beans will cook much more quickly using a pressure cooker, which exposes the beans to a higher temperature but for a shorter period of time. Overcooking Black Beans will increase their glycemic index (GI).*

**1 cup presoaked Black Beans (soak**
 **8 hours to overnight, rinse well)**
**2 cups water**
**3 TBS extra virgin olive oil**
**Sea salt and pepper to taste**

1. Pressure cookers vary in the amount of pressure they produce and therefore in the amount of time needed to cook various types of beans. Before cooking Black Beans in your pressure cooker, read the manufacturer's instructions.

2. Place beans and water in pressure cooker. **Do not fill it more than half full.**

3. Attach lid and bring up to pressure on medium heat. You should hear a soft hissing sound.

4. Lower heat and let Black Beans cook the amount of time recommended for them in your pressure cooker instruction book or 30–40 minutes.

5. Add olive oil, salt and pepper to taste after cooking.

**Q** *How do you keep Black Beans as black as possible? Mine are a purple color, but sometimes at restaurants their color is of a deep black.*

**A** The jet black glossy color on Black Beans is actually not black, but very dark purple. This dark purple color reflects the beans' concentration of antioxidant phytonutrients, such as anthocyanins.

I am not sure how the restaurants' beans became so dark in color. Potentially they used canned beans that had a preservative that helped retain the deep color, as there are a good number of additives that can promote color retention in canned foods. I've seen EDTA, for example, used to preserve the color in black-eyed peas and ferrous gluconate used to preserve the color of canned black olives.

Another explanation for the darker color beans is that they used a different variety of Black Bean as I've seen research indicating that different varieties of Black Beans are better at retaining their color during the cooking process; I've seen at least one experimental Black Bean, called the Phantom, being reported as better-than-average when it comes to color retention. Therefore, you may want to experiment with the variety of Black Beans you buy. Natural foods groceries should have a couple of alternatives for you to try; sampling Black Beans from a couple of different groceries may even turn up the desired result.

When cooking beans from scratch, I have seen recommendations for soaking Black Beans from 4 hours to overnight and then cooking them in this same soaking liquid to retain color. I dislike this preparation method as a way of retaining color and always recommended discarding the water in which the beans were soaked, rinsing them and cooking them in a fresh pot of water. The reason is to remove potential toxins that can naturally be present in dried beans that may have leeched into the water.

**Q** *Are Black Beans and black-eye beans the same bean?*

**A** Even though Black Beans and black-eyed beans both belong to the same botanical family (Leguminosae), they are not the same plant. Black Beans are black (or dark purple) in color and are known botanically as Phaseolus vulgaris. Black-eyed beans are more often called black-eyed peas, reflecting the dark-colored eye that they have on their tan-colored skin; they are also known as field peas, lobiya and chawli. Their botanical name is Vigna unguiculata, indicating that they belong to a different genus of plant than Black Beans.

# health benefits of black beans

## Promote Heart Health

Black Beans are a great food for promoting heart health. They are a concentrated source of both dietary fiber, which helps to reduce cholesterol, and folic acid, which lowers blood concentrations of homocysteine, a compound that damages artery walls. The magnesium they contain improves the flow of blood, oxygen and nutrients throughout the body. In addition, their polyphenolic antioxidant phytonutrients protect cholesterol from becoming oxidized, inhibiting atherosclerosis development.

## Promote Energy Production

Black Beans are a protein-rich source of soluble dietary fiber; they provide sustainable energy while promoting stabilized blood sugar levels. They contain vitamin B1, which is instrumental in converting sugar into usable energy, as well as phosphorus, which is a component of ATP, the fuel molecule that powers the body's cells. Additionally, Black Beans' manganese, through its role as a cofactor of the *superoxide dismutase* antioxidant, protects the energy-producing mitochondria from free-radical damage. Finally, the iron found in Black Beans is an integral component of hemoglobin, a molecule that transports oxygen throughout the body.

## Promote Optimal Health

A recent study suggests that Black Beans may help protect against cancer. When researchers fed laboratory animals a 20% Black Bean diet, a clear reduction in the number of precancerous cells was seen, even in animals that were simultaneously given a chemical known to promote cancer. In addition, preliminary observational studies have found that individuals who eat legumes, such as Black Beans, may be at a reduced risk for developing cancer of the breast, prostate and pancreas.

## Provide Powerful Antioxidant Protection

A recent study has found that Black Beans are as rich in polyphenolic antioxidant phytonutrient compounds called anthocyanins as grapes and cranberries, fruits long considered antioxidant superstars. When researchers analyzed different types of beans, they found that the darker the bean's seed coat, the higher its level of antioxidant activity. Gram for gram, Black Beans were found to have the most antioxidant activity, followed in descending order by red, brown, yellow and white beans. Overall, the level of antioxidants found in Black Beans in this study was approximately 10 times that found in an equivalent amount of oranges and comparable to that found in an equivalent amount of grapes or cranberries.

## Additional Health-Promoting Benefits of Black Beans

Black Beans are also a concentrated source of other nutrients providing additional health-promoting benefits. These nutrients include sulfite-detoxifying molybdenum and sleep-promoting tryptophan.

### Nutritional Analysis of 1 cup of cooked Black Beans:

| NUTRIENT | AMOUNT | % DAILY VALUE | NUTRIENT | AMOUNT | % DAILY VALUE |
|---|---|---|---|---|---|
| Calories | 227.04 | | Pantothenic Acid | 0.42 mg | 4.20 |
| Calories from Fat | 8.36 | | | | |
| Calories from Saturated Fat | 2.15 | | **Minerals** | | |
| Protein | 15.24 g | | Boron | — mcg | |
| Carbohydrates | 40.78 g | | Calcium | 46.44 mg | 4.64 |
| Dietary Fiber | 14.96 g | 59.84 | Chloride | — mg | |
| Soluble Fiber | 4.13 g | | Chromium | — mcg | — |
| Insoluble Fiber | 10.84 g | | Copper | 0.36 mg | 18.00 |
| Sugar – Total | 3.78 g | | Fluoride | — mg | — |
| Monosaccharides | — g | | Iodine | — mcg | — |
| Disaccharides | — g | | Iron | 3.61 mg | 20.06 |
| Other Carbs | 22.03 g | | Magnesium | 120.40 mg | 30.10 |
| Fat – Total | 0.93 g | | Manganese | 0.76 mg | 38.00 |
| Saturated Fat | 0.24 g | | Molybdenum | 129.00 mcg | 172.00 |
| Mono Fat | 0.08 g | | Phosphorus | 240.80 mg | 24.08 |
| Poly Fat | 0.40 g | | Potassium | 610.60 mg | |
| Omega-3 Fatty Acids | 0.18 g | 7.20 | Selenium | 2.06 mcg | 2.94 |
| Omega-6 Fatty Acids | 0.22 g | | Sodium | 1.72 mg | |
| Trans Fatty Acids | 0.00 g | | Zinc | 1.93 mg | 12.87 |
| Cholesterol | 0.00 mg | | | | |
| Water | 113.07 g | | **Amino Acids** | | |
| Ash | 1.98 g | | Alanine | 0.64 g | |
| | | | Arginine | 0.94 g | |
| **Vitamins** | | | Aspartate | 1.84 g | |
| Vitamin A IU | 10.32 IU | 0.21 | Cystine | 0.17 g | 41.46 |
| Vitamin A RE | 1.72 RE | | Glutamate | 2.32 g | |
| A - Carotenoid | 1.72 RE | 0.02 | Glycine | 0.60 g | |
| A - Retinol | 0.00 RE | | Histidine | 0.42 g | 32.56 |
| B1 Thiamin | 0.42 mg | 28.00 | Isoleucine | 0.67 g | 58.26 |
| B2 Riboflavin | 0.10 mg | 5.88 | Leucine | 1.22 g | 48.22 |
| B3 Niacin | 0.87 mg | 4.35 | Lysine | 1.05 g | 44.68 |
| Niacin Equiv | 3.88 mg | | Methionine | 0.23 g | 31.08 |
| Vitamin B6 | 0.12 mg | 6.00 | Phenylalanine | 0.82 g | 68.91 |
| Vitamin B12 | 0.00 mcg | 0.00 | Proline | 0.65 g | |
| Biotin | — mcg | — | Serine | 0.83 g | |
| Vitamin C | 0.00 mg | 0.00 | Threonine | 0.64 g | 51.61 |
| Vitamin D IU | 0.00 IU | 0.00 | Tryptophan | 0.18 g | 56.25 |
| Vitamin D mcg | 0.00 mcg | | Tyrosine | 0.43 g | 44.33 |
| Vitamin E Alpha Equiv | 0.14 mg | 0.70 | Valine | 0.80 g | 54.42 |
| Vitamin E IU | 0.20 IU | | | | |
| Vitamin E mg | 1.03 mg | | | | |
| Folate | 255.94 mcg | 63.98 | | | |
| Vitamin K | — mcg | | | | |

(Note: "—" indicates data is unavailable. For more information, please see page 806.)

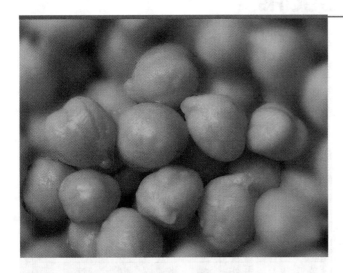

# garbanzo beans
## (chickpeas)

| | |
|---|---|
| AVAILABILITY: | Year-round |
| REFRIGERATE: | No |
| SHELF LIFE: | 12 months |
| PREPARATION: | Minimal |
| BEST WAY TO COOK: | Canned beans require no cooking |

## nutrient-richness chart

Total Nutrient-Richness: **16**      GI: **39**

One cup (164 grams) of cooked Garbanzo Beans contains 269 calories

| NUTRIENT | AMOUNT | %DV | DENSITY | QUALITY |
|---|---|---|---|---|
| Molybdenum | 123.0 mcg | 164.0 | 11.0 | excellent |
| Manganese | 1.7 mg | 84.5 | 5.7 | excellent |
| Folate | 282.1 mcg | 70.5 | 4.7 | very good |
| Dietary Fiber | 12.5 g | 49.8 | 3.3 | good |
| Tryptophan | 0.1 g | 43.8 | 2.9 | good |
| Protein | 14.5 g | 29.1 | 1.9 | good |
| Copper | 0.6 mg | 29.0 | 1.9 | good |
| Phosphorus | 275.5 mg | 27.6 | 1.8 | good |
| Iron | 4.7 mg | 26.3 | 1.8 | good |

For more on "Total Nutrient-Richness," "%DV," "Density," and
The World's Healthiest Foods "Quality" Rating System, see page 805.

For more on GI, see page 342.

Enjoyed as far back as in ancient Greece and Rome, Garbanzo Beans, also known as chickpeas, originated in the Middle East, the region of the world where they are still enjoyed and relied upon as a valuable dietary staple. Although not as popular in the United States, Garbanzo Beans are the most widely consumed legume in the world. Their delicious nutlike taste and buttery, yet somewhat starchy, texture is a wonderful addition to your "Healthiest Way of Eating." Top your favorite salad with Garbanzo Beans for extra taste and nutrition.

## why garbanzo beans should be part of your healthiest way of eating

Garbanzo Beans' rich supply of dietary fiber makes them valuable for both heart and digestive health. Their soluble fiber content also makes them an excellent food to help maintain healthy blood sugar levels. (Garbanzo Beans' health benefits and nutritional profile are similiar to black beans. For more information, see page 615.)

## varieties of garbanzo beans

Dried and canned Garbanzo Beans are available (same as black beans, see page 610).

## the peak season available year-round.

## biochemical considerations

Same as black beans (see page 611).

## the best way to select garbanzo beans

Same as black beans (see page 611).

## the best way to store garbanzo beans

Same as black beans (see page 611).

## the best way to prepare garbanzo beans

Same as black beans (see page 612).

## the healthiest way of cooking garbanzo beans

For details about cooking, see black bean recipe (page 614). Garbanzo Beans take 1 to 1$^1$/2 hours to cook.

**STEP-BY-STEP RECIPES**

## The Healthiest Ways to Prepare Garbanzo Beans

# 5-Minute Garbanzo Beans – No Cooking

*Since dried Garbanzo Beans need soaking and substantial cooking time, I suggest using organic canned Garbanzo Beans. This recipe takes just minutes to prepare. If you have time to cook Garbanzo Beans, see page 614 for directions.*

1 15-oz can Garbanzo Beans,
    preferably organic
2 TBS extra virgin olive oil
2 cloves garlic
Sea salt and pepper to taste
Optional: Add 1 TBS lemon juice and
    1/2 medium chopped red onion

1. Press or mince garlic and let sit for 5 minutes (Why?, see page 261.)
2. Drain liquid from Garbanzo Beans and rinse under

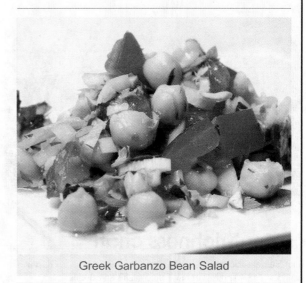

Greek Garbanzo Bean Salad

cold running water; this helps prevent intestinal gas.
3. Combine all ingredients, mix and enjoy!

For added flavor, you may want to add more olive oil.

**SERVES 2**

---

### Flavor Tips: Try these 8 great serving suggestions with the recipe above. ✱

1. Add sage, oregano, thyme or paprika to complement the flavor of Garbanzo Beans.
2. Extra virgin olive oil, garlic, curry powder and cumin also complement the flavor of Garbanzo Beans.
3. Garbanzo Beans are a great source of protein when added to your salads.
4. **Mediterranean Garbanzo Beans:** Add the 5-Minute Garbanzo Beans recipe, ground cumin and a pinch of cloves to chopped tomatoes and onions.
5. **Hummus or Middle Eastern Spread:** Purée the 5-Minute Garbanzo Beans recipe with 1 TBS sesame tahini and 1 TBS fresh lemon juice in a blender. Add 3 TBS of extra virgin olive oil, a little at a time, through the feed hole as the mixture is blending. Season to taste with sea salt.
6. **Hummus Wrap:** Spread Hummus recipe on a whole wheat tortilla, lettuce or cabbage leaf and garnish with raw vegetables, like red bell pepper or cucumber. Drizzle with Mediterranean dressing (see page 331) and roll up.
7. **Greek Garbanzo Bean Salad:** In a bowl, combine 5-Minute Garbanzo Beans recipe, 2/3 cup minced green onion, 1 diced tomato, 2 TBS fresh lemon juice and 3 TBS minced fresh parsley. Optional: top with 1/4 cup feta cheese and serve over chopped romaine lettuce (pictured above).
8. **Quick Chana Masala:** "Healthy Sauté" one medium onion. Add one cup tomato sauce, the 5-Minute Garbanzo Beans recipe, and curry powder and cayenne to taste. Sprinkle with minced parsley.

---

## 8-Minute Creamy Garbanzo Bean Soup

1 recipe of 5-Minute Garbanzo Beans
2 tsp lemon juice
1 TBS tahini
1 1/2 cups water

1. Boil water.
2. Add Garbanzo Beans, lemon juice and tahini to the blender. Then add hot water.
3. Blend until smooth, starting on low speed so the blender will not overflow.
4. Add sea salt, pepper and olive oil to taste, if desired. Pour into soup bowls.
5. Optional: Add 1/2 cup of your favorite cooked grain to the soup bowl.

**SERVES 2**

---

Please write (address on back cover flap) or e-mail me at info@whfoods.org with your personal ideas for preparing Garbanzo Beans, and I will share them with others through our website at www.whfoods.org.

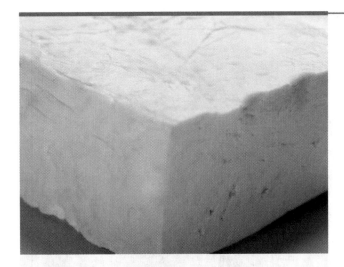

# tofu

| | |
|---|---|
| AVAILABILITY: | Year-round |
| REFRIGERATE: | Yes |
| SHELF LIFE: | Up to one week |
| PREPARATION: | Minimal |
| BEST WAY TO COOK: | "Healthy Sauté" |

## nutrient-richness chart

| Total Nutrient-Richness: | **16** | | | GI: **n/a** |
|---|---|---|---|---|

4 ounces (113.40 grams) of raw Tofu contains 86 calories

| NUTRIENT | AMOUNT | %DV | DENSITY | QUALITY |
|---|---|---|---|---|
| Tryptophan | 0.1 g | 43.8 | 9.1 | excellent |
| Manganese | 0.7 mg | 34.5 | 7.2 | very good |
| Iron | 6.1 mg | 33.8 | 7.1 | very good |
| Protein | 9.2 g | 18.3 | 3.8 | very good |
| Selenium | 10.1 mcg | 14.4 | 3.0 | good |
| Omega-3 Fatty Acids | 0.4 g | 14.4 | 3.0 | good |
| Copper | 0.2 mg | 11.0 | 2.3 | good |
| Phosphorus | 110.0 mg | 11.0 | 2.3 | good |
| Calcium | 100.0 mg | 10.0 | 2.1 | good |
| Magnesium | 34.0 mg | 8.5 | 1.8 | good |

For more on "Total Nutritional Density," "%DV," "Density" and
The World's Healthiest Foods "Quality" Rating System, see page 805.

For more on GI, see page 342.

Discovered over 2,000 years ago by the Chinese, Tofu is sometimes called "the cheese of Asia" because of its physical resemblance to a block of farmer's cheese. While the details of its discovery are uncertain, legend has it that it was discovered by accident when a Chinese cook added a type of sea vegetable to a pot of soybean milk, which caused it to curdle and produce what we now know as Tofu. Unlike cheese, Tofu has very little flavor; yet, because it readily absorbs the flavors of the other ingredients in a dish, its neutral flavor actually increases its versatility. A traditional mainstay of Chinese, Japanese and Korean cuisines, Tofu can now be found in a host of foods—frozen meals, sandwiches and salads—available in food markets as well as on the menus of many different types of restaurants. I want to share with you how to add some of your favorite seasonings to Tofu so you will want to make it a regular part of your "Healthiest Way of Eating."

## why tofu should be part of your healthiest way of eating

Tofu began receiving widespread attention in the 1960s and has skyrocketed in popularity since then as increasing evidence supports its many health benefits. It is rich in many nutrients including selenium, calcium, magnesium and omega-3 fatty acids, nutrients essential for a healthy heart. Tofu also contains phytoestrogens, specifically the isoflavones genistein and daidzein, which also have cardiovascular health benefits. (For more on the *Health Benefits of Tofu* and a complete analysis of its content of over 60 nutrients, see page 622.)

## varieties of tofu

Tofu is a highly nutritious, protein-rich food that is made from soybeans. Soybeans are first mixed with water and ground to produce soymilk. A mineral compound is then added to the soymilk that coagulates the protein in the soymilk to produce curds, which are then pressed into blocks. Tofu is labeled soft, firm or silken depending on its texture. Tofu is a staple in the cuisines of many Asian countries. Tofu is its Japanese name, while in China it is known as *doufa*.

### SILKEN TOFU

Similar to custard, it usually comes in aseptic packages and is available as soft, firm or extra firm. There are also low-fat and lite versions of silken Tofu. Easily puréed, it is a good substitute for milk, sour cream or yogurt depending on the texture.

### REGULAR TOFU

Also available in soft, firm and extra firm, but its texture is more granular than silken Tofu. Sold either in bulk or in water-packed plastic containers, it can be used in sautés, stir-fries, soups and salads. Calciuim sulfate is the coagulant usually used to make regular Tofu, which is why it is a concentrated source of calcium.

## the peak season available year-round.

## biochemical considerations

Tofu is a concentrated source of oxalates and goitrogens, which might be of concern to certain individuals. Tofu is also a food to which some people have allergic reactions.

(For more on *Oxalates*, see page 725; *Goitrogens*, see page 721; and *Food Allergies*, see page 719.)

## 4 steps for the best tasting and most nutritious tofu

Turning Tofu into a flavorful dish with the most nutrients is simple if you just follow my 4 easy steps:

1. The Best Way to Select
2. The Best Way to Store
3. The Best Way to Prepare
4. The Healthiest Way of Cooking

# 1. the best way to select tofu

Tofu is available refrigerated in individual packages or in bulk. Non-refrigerated varieties of silken Tofu can be found in aseptically sealed containers. Look for Tofu that is not made from genetically modified soybeans; since organic soybeans cannot be genetically modified, organic Tofu is a

great choice. Check to make sure the expiration date on the package has not passed. If your recipe calls for sliced or cubed Tofu, purchase the firm or extra firm variety. If you are making a sauce or dip, silken Tofu or soft Tofu would be better.

# 2. the best way to store tofu

While aseptically packaged Tofu need not be refrigerated until it is opened, all other forms of Tofu should be refrigerated in their container. Once the packages are open, all varieties of Tofu should be rinsed well, kept in a container covered with water and placed in the refrigerator. Changing the water daily will help keep the Tofu fresh for up to one week.

Tofu can also be frozen in its original packaging and will keep this way for up to five months. This process will actually

alter its texture and color, making it more spongy, absorbent and yellow in color. These changes in its physical properties are actually very suitable for certain types of recipes. Be sure to squeeze the water from thawed Tofu before using.

Firm Tofu usually contains the highest fat content. Soft Tofu contains the lowest amount of fat. If you are looking for Tofu with high calcium content, look for products that specifically say "calcium-precipitated" on the label, which indicates that calcium was used to help coagulate the Tofu.

# 3. the best way to prepare tofu

Rinse Tofu under cool running water before using.

# 4. the healthiest way of cooking tofu

Tofu can be eaten raw, so cooking is primarily to heat it and enhance its ability to absorb the seasonings in the recipe. If you want to heat Tofu and combine it with a

variety of vegetables, the best way to prepare it is by using the "Healthy Sauté" method of cooking (see page 57).

# Q Why is Tofu white?

A Actually, not all Tofu is white. The color of Tofu depends on several key factors. First is the type of soybean (white-eyed or black-eyed) used as the Tofu's starting point. The white-eyed soybeans used for production of most Tofus in the U.S. are off-white, beige and slightly grayish in color. During the production of Tofu, however, following cooking, the outer husk is removed from the creamy inner part and along with the husk goes some of the non-white color. What's left is a lighter, whiter-colored product.

# Q Are there any dairy products used in the making of Tofu? I ask because I am sensitive to dairy.

A Tofu cheese and soy cheese very often contain casein, a milk protein found in cow's milk, as it is used to help create the foods' consistency. Yet, blocks of Tofu themselves generally don't contain casein. The coagulated texture of Tofu is a result of the proteins in the soy itself as well as the addition of other ingredients such as magnesium or calcium sulfate.

# Q There is research linking Tofu consumption with dementia. I get most of my protein from soybean foods and am now wondering whether I should keep eating Tofu. What's your opinion about the research?

A I am currently only aware of two studies on the relationship between Tofu intake and cognitive function. Both are epidemiological studies that looked at large groups of individuals over long periods of time. In one of the studies, intake of Tofu more than twice a week during midlife (ages 40–55) was associated with increased prevalence of cognitive impairment and brain atrophy later in life (ages 70–90). It's impossible to come to any hard and fast conclusions about Tofu and dementia from this kind of study. We simply don't know enough about the study participants and what they did and didn't have in common (besides their higher Tofu intake). In addition to the non-clinical nature of these studies, many health experts have reason to believe that Tofu intake can make individuals healthier in later life. Evidence from countries where soy products are eaten regularly throughout life suggests that late-life dementia is less problematic than it is in the United States. So I would say that the jury is definitely out here.

# Q Is it true that "lite" Tofu has virtually no omega-3 fatty acids?

A Unfortunately, the listing for "lite" Tofu in the USDA National Nutrient Database for Standard Reference does not contain measurements of omega-3 fatty acids. Yet, it seems that "lite" Tofu has about one-third the amount of total polyunsaturated fats (PUFAs) as regular Tofu. Assuming the reduction in total PUFAs is consistent across types of PUFAs, and based upon the Tofu profile featured on the World's Healthiest Foods website, a "lite" version might have about 0.12 mg omega-3 fatty acids (in the form of linolenic acid). While this is a small amount, it still provides about 5% of the Daily Value for omega-3 fatty acids.

# Q I see that you use silken Tofu in some of your recipes. What is it exactly?

A "Silken" refers to the texture and consistency of the Tofu. It is a form of Tofu that is velvety-smooth, which is what makes it so good for use in dips, puddings and sauces. If you are making a recipe that calls for silken Tofu and you can't find it in your local supermarket or natural foods store, I would recommend that you purchase the least firm type of Tofu available. You may just need to adjust the recipe by adding more liquid—either water or oil—to achieve the smooth consistency that you would like the sauce to have.

# Q Does eating Tofu burgers and hotdogs harm one's health? I find that eating these foods is easier for me as they are very convenient, but if I knew they could be harmful, I would change my eating habits.

A While ideally I prefer food in more of its unprocessed state, in reality, given such circumstances as convenience, time, resources, variety and even taste, there are times when a food that is more processed is still a very good choice for a person's diet. The foods that you mention are based upon whole foods, such as Tofu, vegetables and grains. If by eating these foods, you enjoy your food and find it easier to eat healthy, then I think that they can therefore be supportive of your health. I would just suggest two things: 1) purchase brands of these foods that feature organic ingredients and contain no/minimal additives, if possible and 2) eat them as part of a balanced diet.

STEP-BY-STEP RECIPE
## The Healthiest Ways to Prepare Tofu

# 3-Minute Gingered Tofu – No Cooking

*Tofu needs no cooking, so it can be prepared in minutes!*

2 cups of firm Tofu, cubed
3 TBS tamari (soy sauce)
3 TBS extra virgin olive oil
1 TBS fresh ginger, grated
1/4 cup scallions
Optional: Sprinkle with toasted
          sesame seeds

1. Cut Tofu into cubes.
2. Mix with rest of ingredients. Serve with brown rice and vegetables.

**SERVES 2**

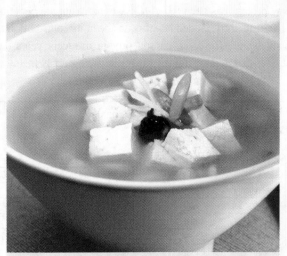
Miso Tofu Soup

**PREPARATION TIP FOR TOFU:**

Make sure you use firm Tofu when recipes call for cubed tofu, so that it will not crumble or fall apart.

Please write (address on back cover flap) or e-mail me at info@whfoods.org with your personal ideas for preparing Tofu, and I will share them with others through our website at www.whfoods.org.

## 8 QUICK SERVING IDEAS for TOFU:

1. **Mediterranean Tofu:** Mix 1 1/2 cups cubed firm Tofu, 1 tsp capers, 1 medium chopped tomato, 6 chopped olives, extra virgin olive oil, and sea salt and pepper to taste.
2. **Sweet Firecracker Tofu:** Marinate Tofu slices in hot chili sauce, honey, extra virgin olive oil and sea salt to taste for 6 hours. Serve as a side dish or in a salad or wrap. Use any leftover marinade as a sauce.
3. **Classic Tofu Scramble:** "Healthy Sauté" 1 medium diced onion and 1 cup sliced mushrooms. Add 1 1/2 cups mashed soft Tofu, 1 tsp turmeric and sauté 2 minutes covered. Add 2 TBS extra virgin olive oil and tamari (soy sauce) to taste. Garnish with chopped parsley or scallions.
4. **Italian Tofu Spread:** Blend 1 cup soft or silken tofu with 1/2 cup pre-made pesto, 1/2 cup chopped sundried tomatoes (packed in olive oil), and salt and pepper to taste. Spread on crackers or in a lettuce wrap.
5. **Sweet and Sour Tofu:** Make a sauce combining 2 TBS tamari, 1 TBS vinegar, 2 TBS honey, 3 TBS extra virgin olive oil, a pinch of red pepper flakes and 1/4 cup pineapple juice. "Healthy Sauté" sliced onion and 2 cups red and green peppers for 2 minutes and then add 2 cups firm Tofu cubes, 1 cup pineapple chunks and the sauce. Simmer for 3 minutes. Add more tamari as needed. Tofu will pick up the flavor of the sauce.
6. **Tofu Ginger Dressing:** Blend 1 package silken Tofu, 1 TBS plus 1 tsp tamari, 1 TBS extra virgin olive oil, 2 tsp fresh ginger, 1 clove garlic, 1 TBS white or red miso, 1 TBS rice or apple cider vinegar, 1 tsp honey and cayenne to taste. Use on romaine lettuce and hearty vegetables like jicama, carrots and radishes.
7. **Creamy Tofu Dressing** (non-dairy): Blend together 1 package silken Tofu, 1 TBS olive oil, 1 TBS lemon juice, 1 1/2 TBS Dijon mustard, 2 TBS fresh herbs (such as basil, dill or parsley), 1/2 tsp sea salt and pepper to taste. Use as a dip for vegetables or a salad dressing.
8. **Miso Tofu Soup:** Add Tofu to a miso broth with scallions and ginger for a quick and easy soup (pictured above).

# health benefits of tofu

## Promotes Heart Health

Soy protein has been found to have many unique benefits. One of its most lauded benefits has been its contribution to heart health. Research on soy protein in recent years has shown that regular intake of soy protein can help lower total cholesterol levels by as much as 30%, lower LDL ("bad" cholesterol) levels by as much as 35–40%, lower triglyceride levels, reduce the tendency of platelets to form blood clots and possibly even raise levels of HDL ("good" cholesterol).

Tofu's benefits on heart health are also related to it being a good source of omega-3 fatty acids, specifically alpha-linolenic acid (ALA). ALA is considered an "essential fatty acid" since the body cannot make it, so we must get it from our diet. ALA's heart-health benefit comes not only from it being a precursor of EPA and DHA, the fatty acids found in cold-water fish that have trigclyeride- and blood pressure-lowering properties, but ALA itself has been found to be cardioprotective. It has been found to reduce levels of C-reactive protein, a risk factor for cardiovascular disease. In addition, it seems to have anti-arrhythmic properties, helping to stabilize the rhythmic beating of the heart.

Tofu is also a good source of other nutrients, such as selenium, calcium and magnesium, found to be important for heart health. For more details on the role of soy foods, such as Tofu, in cardiovascular health, please see Health Benefits of Soybeans on page 601.

## Promotes Women's Health

Most types of Tofu are enriched with calcium, which can help build bone density and prevent the accelerated bone loss for which women are at risk during menopause. Plus, it is a very good source of manganese and a good source of magnesium, copper and phosphorus, four other minerals important for promoting bone health.

Soy has also been shown to be helpful in alleviating symptoms associated with menopause. Soy foods, like Tofu, contain phytoestrogens, specifically the isoflavones genistein and daidzein. In a woman's body, these compounds can dock at estrogen receptors and act like very weak estrogens. During perimenopause, when a woman's estrogen fluctuates, rising to very high levels and then dropping below normal, soy's phytoestrogens can help her maintain balance, blocking out estrogen when levels rise excessively high and filling in for estrogen when levels are low. When women's production of natural estrogen drops at menopause, soy's isoflavones may provide just enough estrogenic activity to prevent or reduce uncomfortable symptoms, like hot flashes. While the exact mechanisms through which they work their effects remain under investigation, the results of intervention trials suggest that soy isoflavones may also inhibit the resorption of bone and therefore help prevent post-menopausal osteoporosis.

### Nutritional Analysis of 4 ounces of raw Tofu:

| NUTRIENT | AMOUNT | % DAILY VALUE |
|---|---|---|
| Calories | 86.18 | |
| Calories from Fat | 48.78 | |
| Calories from Saturated Fat | 7.05 | |
| Protein | 9.16 g | |
| Carbohydrates | 2.13 g | |
| Dietary Fiber | 0.34 g | 1.36 |
| Soluble Fiber | 0.20 g | |
| Insoluble Fiber | 0.14 g | |
| Sugar – Total | 0.45 g | |
| Monosaccharides | 0.00 g | |
| Disaccharides | 0.00 g | |
| Other Carbs | 1.34 g | |
| Fat – Total | 5.42 g | |
| Saturated Fat | 0.78 g | |
| Mono Fat | 1.20 g | |
| Poly Fat | 3.06 g | |
| Omega-3 Fatty Acids | 0.36 g | 14.40 |
| Omega-6 Fatty Acids | 2.70 g | |
| Trans Fatty Acids | — g | |
| Cholesterol | 0.00 mg | |
| Water | 95.88 g | |
| Ash | 0.82 g | |
| **Vitamins** | | |
| Vitamin A IU | 96.39 IU | 1.93 |
| Vitamin A RE | 10.21 RE | |
| A - Carotenoid | — RE | — |
| A - Retinol | — RE | |
| B1 Thiamin | 0.09 mg | 6.00 |
| B2 Riboflavin | 0.06 mg | 3.53 |
| B3 Niacin | 0.22 mg | 1.10 |
| Niacin Equiv | 2.60 mg | |
| Vitamin B6 | 0.05 mg | 2.50 |
| Vitamin B12 | 0.00 mcg | 0.00 |
| Biotin | — mcg | — |
| Vitamin C | 0.11 mg | 0.18 |
| Vitamin D IU | — IU | — |
| Vitamin D mcg | — mcg | |
| Vitamin E Alpha Equiv | 0.01 mg | 0.05 |
| Vitamin E IU | 0.02 IU | |
| Vitamin E mg | 0.01 mg | |
| Folate | 17.01 mcg | 4.25 |
| Vitamin K | — mcg | |

| NUTRIENT | AMOUNT | % DAILY VALUE |
|---|---|---|
| Pantothenic Acid | 0.08 mg | 0.80 |
| **Minerals** | | |
| Boron | — mcg | |
| Calcium | 100.00 mg | 10.00 |
| Chloride | — mg | |
| Chromium | — mcg | — |
| Copper | 0.22 mg | 11.00 |
| Fluoride | — mg | — |
| Iodine | — mcg | — |
| Iron | 6.08 mg | 33.78 |
| Magnesium | 34.02 mg | 8.51 |
| Manganese | 0.69 mg | 34.50 |
| Molybdenum | — mcg | — |
| Phosphorus | 110.00 mg | 11.00 |
| Potassium | 137.21 mg | |
| Selenium | 10.09 mcg | 14.41 |
| Sodium | 7.94 mg | |
| Zinc | 0.91 mg | 6.07 |
| **Amino Acids** | | |
| Alanine | 0.38 g | |
| Arginine | 0.61 g | |
| Aspartate | 1.01 g | |
| Cystine | 0.13 g | 31.71 |
| Glutamate | 1.58 g | |
| Glycine | 0.36 g | |
| Histidine | 0.27 g | 20.93 |
| Isoleucine | 0.45 g | 39.13 |
| Leucine | 0.70 g | 27.67 |
| Lysine | 0.60 g | 25.53 |
| Methionine | 0.12 g | 16.22 |
| Phenylalanine | 0.45 g | 37.82 |
| Proline | 0.49 g | |
| Serine | 0.43 g | |
| Threonine | 0.37 g | 29.84 |
| Tryptophan | 0.14 g | 43.75 |
| Tyrosine | 0.31 g | 31.96 |
| Valine | 0.46 g | 31.29 |

(Note: "—" indicates data is unavailable. For more information, please see page 806.)

## Promotes Men's Health

A study in China found that men consuming the most Tofu had a 42% lower risk of developing prostate cancer compared to those consuming the least. In other epidemiological studies, intake of soy isoflavones, like those found in Tofu, has also been linked to lower incidence of prostate cancer. For more details on the role of soy foods, such as Tofu, in men's health, please see Health Benefits of Soybeans on page 601.

## Promotes Energy Production

Tofu is not only a concentrated source of high quality protein, but is also a very good source of iron. While this important mineral plays many roles in the body, its most well-known one is being at the core of hemoglobin, a molecule essential to energy production since it is responsible for transporting and releasing oxygen throughout the body. Hemoglobin synthesis also relies on copper, so without this trace mineral, iron cannot be properly utilized in red blood cells. As is often the case in whole foods, Nature supplies complementary nutrients; Tofu is a good source of copper as well.

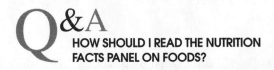

## Q&A HOW SHOULD I READ THE NUTRITION FACTS PANEL ON FOODS?

The Nutrition Facts panel, required on most packaged foods in the United States, is one of the most informative and detailed of such labels worldwide. Taking a little time to become familiar with it can be a very empowering way to evaluate and compare foods' nutritional values. However, it is important to be aware that it is not comprehensive and that each person must interpret it individually.

The intent of the Nutrition Facts panel is to provide nutrition information, per serving of food, deemed pertinent to individuals with particular health conditions or nutritional needs, as well as to provide consumers with the means to make wise food choices. A few examples of the types of information provided include:

- cholesterol and saturated fat content of foods, meaningful to people concerned with cardiovascular health (which means virtually every American!)

- sodium content of foods, for individuals with sodium-sensitive high blood pressure

- dietary fiber content of foods, for those trying to increase their fiber intake (again, this should include virtually every American!)

- "Percentage Recommended Daily Intake" (or "%RDI") for all recognized essential nutrients, based on a diet of a particular calorie count (usually 2000), which must be interpreted according to each individual's average daily calorie intake

The Nutrition Facts panel provides a bounty of detail that pertains to "an average serving" of the food, the amount of which is defined at the top of the label. This means that the information provided must be quantitatively compared to how much you actually eat of that food. For example, if "an average serving" of a cracker product is FOUR crackers but you actually eat TEN crackers, you must remember that you are receiving 2.5 times as much of every nutrient on the label as is listed—sodium, cholesterol, fat, calories, vitamins, fiber, and so on.

The following nutrients are required on the Nutrition Facts panel if the nutrient is present above a certain defined minimum level per defined serving of the food:

- total calories

- total fat, calories from fat, calories from saturated fat, saturated fat, trans fats, polyunsaturated fat, monounsaturated fat

- cholesterol

- sodium and potassium

- total carbohydrates, dietary fiber, soluble fiber, insoluble fiber, sugar, sugar alcohols (such as xylitol and sorbitol), and other carbohydrates (the difference between total carbohydrates and the sum of dietary fiber, sugars, and sugar alcohols)

- protein

- vitamin A and percent as beta-carotene

- vitamin C, calcium, iron, and all other recognized essential vitamins and minerals

Despite the considerable detail provided by the Nutrition Facts panel, other useful information has not yet been included, such as:

- subtotals of essential omega-3 and omega-6 polyunsaturated fats

- the glycemic indices of carbohydrate-containing foods (to provide a comparative gauge of how quickly the food releases its energy)

All in all, however, the Nutrition Facts panel is an excellent tool that can help you make deliberate and informed decisions about the foods you choose to eat.

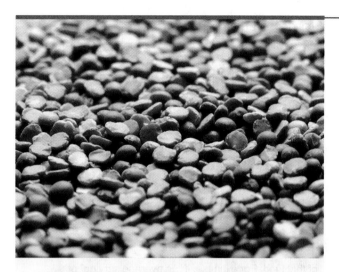

# split peas

| | |
|---|---|
| AVAILABILITY: | Year-round |
| REFRIGERATE: | No |
| SHELF LIFE: | Up to 12 months |
| PREPARATION: | Minimal |
| BEST WAY TO COOK: | Simmer |

## nutrient-richness chart

Total Nutrient-Richness: **14**  GI: **45**
One cup (196 grams) of cooked Split Peas contains 231 calories

| NUTRIENT | AMOUNT | %DV | DENSITY | QUALITY |
|---|---|---|---|---|
| Molybdenum | 147.0 mcg | 196.0 | 15.3 | excellent |
| Dietary Fiber | 16.3 g | 65.1 | 5.1 | very good |
| Tryptophan | 0.2 g | 56.3 | 4.4 | very good |
| Manganese | 0.8 mg | 39.0 | 3.0 | good |
| Protein | 16.4 g | 32.7 | 2.5 | good |
| Folate | 127.2 mcg | 31.8 | 2.5 | good |
| B1 Thiamin | 0.4 mg | 24.7 | 1.9 | good |
| Potassium | 709.5 mg | 20.3 | 1.6 | good |
| Phosphorus | 194.0 mg | 19.4 | 1.5 | good |

For more on "Total Nutrient-Richness," "%DV," "Density," and
The World's Healthiest Foods "Quality" Rating System, see page 805.

For more on GI, see page 342.

Split Peas are produced by drying the peapods of the fully mature garden pea. Peas are known scientifically as *Pisum sativum* and are believed to have been cultivated for more than 20,000 years! For thousands of years, it was dried Split Peas that were consumed rather than the fresh varieties of peas that we enjoy today. Although they belong to the same family as beans and lentils, they are usually distinguished as a separate group because of their usage and spherical shape. Their hardy flavor makes Split Pea soup a winter favorite and a nutritious and delicious addition to your "Healthiest Way of Eating."

## why split peas should be part of your healthiest way of eating

Split Peas are a great source of important heart-healthy nutrients including dietary fiber, potassium and folate. They also contain the isoflavone phytonutrient, daidzein, which acts as a phytoestrogen and promotes heart health. (Split Peas' health benefits and nutritional profile are similiar to black beans. For more information, see page 615.)

## varieties of split peas

Split Peas are available in green and yellow, with the former more popular in North America. Black-eyed peas are cream-colored with a black spot and are not related to Split Peas.

## the peak season available year-round.

## biochemical considerations
Same as black beans (see page 611).

## the best way to select split peas
Same as black beans (see page 611).

## the best way to store split peas
Same as black beans (see page 611).

## the best way to prepare split peas

Same as black beans (see page 612) except that Split Peas require no soaking prior to cooking. Whole peas will require 8 hours of soaking.

## the healthiest way of cooking split peas

For details about cooking, see black bean recipe (page 614). Split peas take about 30 minutes to cook.

STEP-BY-STEP RECIPE
## The Healthiest Ways of Cooking Split Peas

# Healthy Cooked Split Peas

*Split Peas do not take long to cook.*

**1 cup dried Split Peas (green or yellow)
3 cups water or salt-free broth
Sea salt and pepper to taste
Optional: 1 tsp dried thyme,
  at end of cooking**

1. Combine Split Peas in a large pot with 3 cups water or salt-free broth and bring to boil.

2. Simmer for 30 minutes. (Yellow Split Peas may take a little longer than green ones.) You will need to skim off the white foam periodically. The peas will be soft but still have their shape when they are done add salt and pepper to taste.

### PREPARATION TIPS FOR SPLIT PEAS

To prevent Peas from being tough, do not add any salt or salted ingredients (meat or fish) until Peas have already softened. Salt will prevent Peas from becoming tender.

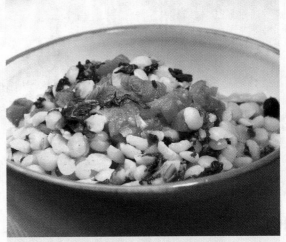

Indian Style Yellow Split Peas

**SERVES 4**

---

## Flavor Tips: Try these 7 great serving suggestions with the recipe above. ✳

1. Add extra virgin olive oil and chopped garlic to the Split Peas recipe.
2. Carrots, celery and onion complement the flavor of Split Peas.
3. Add curry or turmeric for great flavor.
4. **Asian Flavored Peas:** Combine Split Peas recipe with 1 tsp tamari (soy sauce), 1 TBS minced ginger and 2 cloves pressed garlic.
5. **Quick Indian-Style Yellow Split Peas:** "Healthy Sauté" 1 cup diced onion for 3 minutes. Add 2 cloves minced garlic, 1 tsp grated ginger, 1/2 tsp turmeric, 1/2 tsp salt, 1 cup canned diced tomatoes and 2 cups cooked yellow Split Peas (or canned lentils). Simmer **covered** for 5–7 minutes. Add 4 cups "Quick Boiled" fresh spinach or 1 cup frozen spinach. Serve over brown rice for a hearty vegetarian meal (pictured above).

6. **Split Pea Salad:** Combine the Split Peas recipe (or use canned black-eyed peas) with 1 medium-size finely chopped onion, 1 medium-size chopped green pepper, 1 boiled chopped egg and 1 medium-size chopped tomato. Toss with your favorite vinaigrette (see page 143).
7. **Split Peas with Kale or Spinach:** Combine the Split Peas recipe (or use canned black-eyed peas) with 2 cups "Healthy Steamed" kale or spinach, marinated onions,* and salt and pepper to taste. Serve with brown rice.

* To marinate onions, place 1 medium sliced onion in a bowl with 1 cup water and 2 TBS apple cider vinegar. Let sit for 20–30 minutes and then drain, squeezing out excess moisture.

---

Please write (address on back cover flap) or e-mail me at info@whfoods.org with your personal ideas for preparing Split Peas, and I will share them with others through our website at www.whfoods.org.

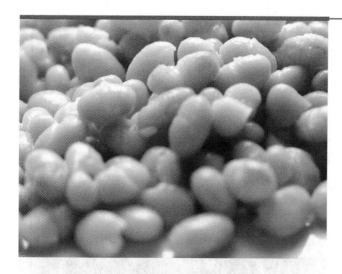

# navy beans

## highlights

| | |
|---|---|
| AVAILABILITY: | Year-round |
| REFRIGERATE: | No |
| SHELF LIFE: | 12 months |
| PREPARATION: | Minimal |
| BEST WAY TO COOK: | Canned beans require no cooking |

## nutrient-richness chart

Total Nutrient-Richness: **13**    GI: **53**

One cup (182 grams) of cooked Navy Beans contains 258 calories

| NUTRIENT | AMOUNT | %DV | DENSITY | QUALITY |
|---|---|---|---|---|
| Folate | 254.6 mcg | 63.7 | 4.4 | very good |
| Tryptophan | 0.2 g | 59.4 | 4.1 | very good |
| Manganese | 1.0 mg | 50.5 | 3.5 | very good |
| Dietary Fiber | 11.7 g | 46.6 | 3.2 | good |
| Protein | 15.8 g | 31.7 | 2.2 | good |
| Phosphorus | 285.7 mg | 28.6 | 2.0 | good |
| Copper | 0.5 mg | 27.0 | 1.9 | good |
| Magnesium | 107.4 mg | 26.8 | 1.9 | good |
| Iron | 4.51 mg | 25.1 | 1.7 | good |
| B1 Thiamin | 0.4 mg | 24.7 | 1.7 | good |

For more on "Total Nutrient-Richness," "%DV," "Density," and
The World's Healthiest Foods "Quality" Rating System, see page 805.

For more on GI, see page 342.

These small white beans were once a staple on U.S. Naval ships; hence came the name, Navy Bean. Also known as Boston beans or Yankee beans, they are the beans of choice to make baked beans because they do not break up when they are cooked. Navy Beans are the official vegetable of Massachusetts, known as the baked bean state. The smooth texture and delicate flavor of Navy Beans is a great addition to your "Healthiest Way of Eating."

## why navy beans should be part of your healthiest way of eating

As with other varieties of legumes, combining Navy Beans with a whole grain, such as brown rice, provides a virtually fat-free, high-quality protein. Their good supply of dietary fiber promotes a healthy heart and helps maintain healthy blood sugar levels. (Navy Beans' health benefits and nutritional profile are similiar to black beans. For more information, see page 615.)

## varieties of navy beans

Dried and canned Navy Beans are available (same as black beans, see page 610).

## the peak season available year-round.

## biochemical considerations

Same as black beans (see page 611).

## the best way to select navy beans

Same as black beans (see page 611).

## the best way to store navy beans

Same as black beans (see page 611).

## the best way to prepare navy beans

Same as black beans (see page 612).

## the healthiest way of cooking navy beans

For details about cooking, see black bean recipe (page 614). Navy Beans take 1 to 1$^1$/2 hours to cook.

STEP-BY-STEP RECIPE
## The Healthiest Way to Prepare Navy Beans

# 5-Minute Navy Beans – No Cooking

*Dried Navy Beans require soaking and substantial cooking time, but this recipe makes use of canned organic Navy Beans and takes just minutes to prepare. If you have time to cook Navy Beans, see page 614 for directions.*

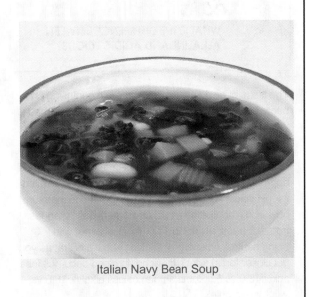

Italian Navy Bean Soup

1 15-oz can Navy Beans, preferably organic
2 TBS extra virgin olive oil
2 cloves garlic
Sea salt and pepper to taste
Optional: Add 1/2 medium red onion, chopped

1. Press or mince garlic and let sit for 5 minutes (Why?, see page 261.)

2. Drain liquid from Navy Beans and rinse under cold running water; this helps prevent intestinal gas.

3. Combine all ingredients, mix and enjoy!

For added flavor, you may want to add more olive oil.

**SERVES 2**

## Flavor Tips: Try these 7 great serving suggestions with the recipe above. ✻

1. Add lemon juice or zest to give Navy Beans an extra zip.

2. Oregano, rosemary, thyme, basil and sage complement the flavor of Navy Beans.

3. Combine 5-Minute Navy Beans and Olive Tapenade (see page 325) or pesto (see page 508).

4. **Puréed Navy Beans:** Puréed Navy Beans are a great substitute for potatoes or rice. "Healthy Sauté" 1 small minced onion in a large saucepan. Blend sautéed onions, the 5-Minute Navy Beans recipe and 2 TBS vegetable or chicken broth until smooth. Make sure you don't fill the blender more than half full. Start on low speed. You will have to stop the blender a couple times and scrape the sides with a rubber spatula.

5. **Navy Bean Pesto Dip:** Blend the 5-Minute Navy Beans recipe with 1/4 cup pesto.

6. **Mediterranean Navy Bean Salad:** Combine the 5-Minute Navy Beans recipe, 1/4 chopped medium onion, 6 chopped olives, 1 TBS chopped fresh thyme leaves, 3 TBS extra virgin olive oil, 1 TBS fresh lemon juice, and sea salt and pepper to taste.

7. **Italian Navy Bean Soup:** "Healthy Sauté" 1 diced onion, 1 diced carrot and 2 stalks diced celery in a large soup pot for 5 minutes. Add 5 cloves pressed garlic and sauté 1 minute. Add 4 cups chicken or vegetable broth, 4 cups minced kale, a 15-oz can diced tomatoes, 1 tsp fresh rosemary and 2 TBS fresh oregano. Cover and simmer 30 minutes. Add two 15-oz cans drained Navy Beans and sea salt and pepper to taste (pictured above).

Please write (address on back cover flap) or e-mail me at info@whfoods.org with your personal ideas for preparing Navy Beans, and I will share them with others through our website at www.whfoods.org.

# Q&A

## WHAT IS THE DIFFERENCE BETWEEN ALKALINE AND ACIDIC FOODS?

The issue of acid and alkaline foods is a confusing one, because there are several different ways of using these words with respect to food.

### Acidic and alkaline foods

In food chemistry textbooks that take a Western science approach to foods, every food has a value that is called its "pH value." pH is a special scale created to measure how acidic or alkaline a fluid or substance is. It ranges from 0.0 (most acidic) to 14.0 (most alkaline) with 7.0 being neutral. One way of thinking about it is that as you get closer to 7.0 from either end, the food becomes less acidic (6.0 vs 5.0, for example) or less alkaline (8.0 vs 9.0, for example).

Limes, for example, have a very low pH of 2.0 and are highly acidic according to the pH scale. Lemons are slightly less acidic at a pH of 2.2. Egg whites are not acidic at all and have a pH of 8.0. Meats are also non-acidic, with a pH of about 7.0.

Many vegetables lie somewhere in the middle of the pH range. For example: asparagus, 5.6; sweet potatoes, 5.4; cucumbers, 5.1; carrots, 5.0; green peas, 6.2; and corn, 6.3. Tomatoes have a lower pH than most other vegetables with their pH ranging from 4.0 to 4.6. Tomatoes also have a higher pH (are less acidic) than some fruits such as pears (3.9), peaches (3.5), strawberries (3.4) and plums (2.9).

### Acid-forming and acid-ash, alkaline-ash foods

Another way to talk about food acidity is not to measure the acidity of the food itself but the body's acidity once the food has been eaten. In other words, from this second perspective, a food is not labeled as "acidic," but instead as "acid-forming."

Similar to this "acid-forming" concept is the "acid-ash, alkaline-ash" concept, in which a food is not chemically broken down in the body, but instead burned, leaving an ash residue, which is then measured for its mineral content. Acid-ash foods are foods that leave high concentrations of chloride, phosphorus or sulfur in their ash. These foods are called "acid-ash" because chloride, phosphorus and sulfur are minerals that are used to make acids in the body (namely, hydrochloric acid, phosphoric acid and sulfuric acid). Alkaline-ash foods are foods that leave high concentrations of magnesium calcium and potassium in their ash. These foods are called "alkaline-ash" because these minerals are used to form alkaline compounds (called bases) in the body (including magnesium hydroxide, calcium hydroxide and potassium hydroxide).

The acid-ash model of measuring food acidity is not, of course, what happens inside a living person. We don't burn our food, and ash is not all that's left after we eat. In fact, the whole concept of acid-forming foods is a much more complicated idea than the pH idea, since "acid-forming" is a process that happens inside a living body.

How well a food is digested, for example, can influence the degree to which it is acid-forming or not. Many foods have preformed acids in their composition that would normally be altered during digestion. However, in a person with problematic digestion, these acids might not get transformed, and their acid-forming properties would be increased.

### Research on the Acid-Forming and Acid-Ash, Alkaline-Ash Foods Principles

Although there are many popular diets that revolve around the principle of acid-forming foods, there are virtually no research studies that have focused on this issue. A survey about dietary patterns and lifestyles carried out in China in the early 1990s has shown that higher intake of animal foods and animal-derived proteins results in increased loss of calcium and acids in the urine, while increased intake of plant foods and plant proteins results in lower calcium and acid loss. Presumably, the loss of acids in the urine reflected increased formation of acids in the body that needed to be excreted, and decreased urine acids reflected less formation of acids in the body. Vegetables were one of the major groups of plant foods focused on in the study; vegetables have been described in many alternative dietary approaches as being non-acid-forming.

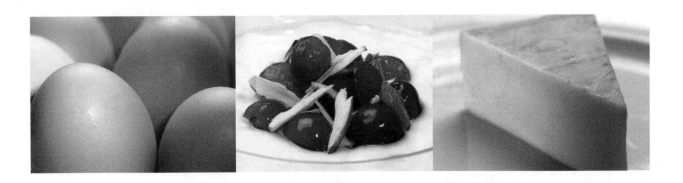

# dairy & eggs

The numbers beside each food indicate their Total Nutrient-Richness. (For more details, see page 805.)

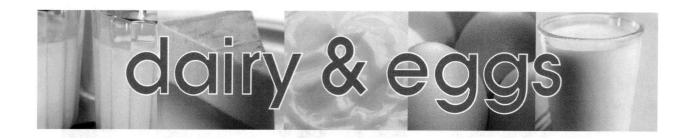

# dairy & eggs

**D**airy products are among the most widely consumed foods in the United States—and for good reason. Just consider the array of delicious dairy foods that we enjoy—a cold glass of milk, a rich piece of cheese, creamy yogurt, cottage cheese or ice cream topped with fresh fruit— and it's easy to see why they are an integral part of our food culture. Not only do these foods taste great and add a flavorful flair to many meals and snacks, but they are also a concentrated source of many important nutrients.

Think about the all-American breakfast, and eggs will probably come to mind. Scrambled, poached, boiled, baked or made into an omelet… the ways to prepare and enjoy eggs are many and varied. And because eggs provide a source of complete, inexpensive protein and also supply many other important nutrients, they provide your body with energy and vitality.

While I feel that most people can enjoy dairy products and eggs as an important component of the "Healthiest Way of Eating," I believe that these foods should be consumed in moderation. The reason for this is that many people have sensitivities to dairy and eggs and in addition to concentrating many nutrients, these foods can also be high in saturated fat and cholesterol.

### Definition: Dairy and Eggs

Dairy products come from the milk of cows and other animals. While the dairy products used in the United States are primarily made from cow's milk, products from goat's and sheep's milk are growing in popularity in the United States and are widely consumed in other parts of the world.

Although many different types of birds lay eggs, that can be consumed as food, in this book I am referring to chicken eggs.

### Dairy and Eggs are Rich in Health-Promoting Nutrients

Dairy products and eggs contain a wealth of vital nutrients that can help support health. Not only are they protein-rich foods, but they also deliver concentrated amounts of vitamins such as D, B2, B12, K and biotin as well as minerals like calcium, selenium, iodine and phosphorus.

Because one of the concerns surrounding dairy products is their high fat content, I recommend using low-fat milk, cheese and yogurt; enjoyed in moderation they will help you stay energized and healthy. While dairy products are often high in fat, egg whites contain no fat and are a rich source of protein. The yolk is the fat-containing portion of the egg with about 5–6 grams of total fat; approximately one-third of this fat is saturated fat. But when eating eggs in moderation, don't avoid the yolk—egg yolk is a very rich source of choline, a key component of healthy cell membranes, nerves and brain cells. Egg yolks also provide lutein, a carotenoid that protects against macular degeneration and cataracts.

### Why Dairy and Eggs Should be Heated to Be Safe to Eat

Eggs have a fairly high concentration of biotin, but before they are heated, the biotin is bound to a protein called avidin that reduces its absorption by the body. Heating breaks the bond and actually increases the bioavailability of biotin.

Heating or cooking eggs for a sufficient length of time and at a sufficiently high temperature also kills bacteria such as *Salmonella*. Therefore, soft-cooked, sunny-side up or raw eggs carry greater risk of contracting salmonellosis than poached, scrambled or hard-boiled eggs. It's been estimated that *Salmonella* bacteria may be present in 1 out of every 30,000 eggs produced in the United States, and since almost 100 billion eggs are produced in the United States each year, that means there are over 3,000 potentially contaminated eggs. So remember to cook your eggs well.

Unheated, raw milk may also be contaminated with bacteria such as *Salmonella, E. coli, Campylobacter, Listeria* or *Yersinia*. Although some people prefer to drink raw milk because they believe it is more natural or nutrient-rich in terms of enzymes and other nutrients, pasteurization kills the potentially harmful microbes making it safer to drink. If you wish to consume raw dairy foods, you may want to consider raw milk cheese as it falls into a somewhat different category than raw milk, since cheese has a naturally longer shelf life. Some producers of raw milk cheese still expose their products to a short period of heat treatment, which comes very close to, but falls short of, the pasteurization threshold. I would choose raw milk cheese that has been aged for at least 60 days, because this destroys the bacteria.

## Calcium—Are Dairy Products the Best Source of Calcium?

Since dairy products are a concentrated source of calcium, people concerned about bone health and preventing osteoporosis tend to include lots of milk and milk products in their diets with the hope of meeting their calcium requirements. While dairy products have been widely emphasized as the primary source of calcium, it is important to remember that they are by no means the only foods that provide significant amounts of this important mineral. Virtually all dark green leafy vegetables, including spinach, Swiss chard, mustard greens and collard greens contain calcium. Practically all nuts and seeds—especially sesame seeds—contain calcium as do most beans, including navy, pinto, kidney and black beans. And tofu that has been prepared with calcium chloride is also an excellent source of this nutrient. Therefore, a diet that preserves bone health need not be solely dependent on dairy products for calcium but should also emphasize calcium-rich plant foods.

## Dairy and Eggs May Not Be for Everyone

While dairy products are an important component of a health-promoting diet for most people, many individuals have difficulty tolerating dairy products. For example, people who are lactose intolerant do not have sufficient amounts of the enzyme *lactase*, which is necessary to break down the milk sugar, lactose, found in dairy products, and therefore have problems digesting these foods. Yet even if a person produces sufficient *lactase*, dairy products may still be a challenge since dairy products, as well as eggs, are amongst the foods most associated with allergic and delayed hypersensitivity reactions. (For more on *Food Allergies*, see page 719.)

Many people who are sensitive to cow's milk can tolerate goat's milk, a food that I have included among the World's Healthiest Foods. That is because while goat's milk contains casein, researchers have found that it generally only has trace amounts of a specific casein, alpha-s1-casein, which is thought to be one of the main proteins in cow's milk responsible for eliciting sensitivity reactions.

## The Importance of Organically Produced Dairy and Eggs

As with all of the World's Healthiest Foods, I recommend purchasing organic varieties of the World's Healthiest Dairy Products and Eggs whenever possible. This is because organic dairy products and eggs are not only better for our health, but they are also produced in a way that provides a less stressful and more humane environment for the animals from which they come. Here is some background information on what constitutes "organic" dairy products and eggs:

The term organic is related to both the way in which the food was handled in production and the way in which the animals that produced the milk or eggs were raised. According to the organic regulations, organic cows, goats and chickens can only be fed organically produced foods and never receive mammal or poultry slaughter by-products for feed (an important consideration when we think of potential problems such as mad cow disease and hoof-and-mouth disease). They cannot be given growth-promoting hormones, administered drugs in the absence of illness or be given supplements in amounts above those for adequate nutrition. Plus, they must be treated in a humane manner. Their health and welfare must be maintained and promoted; they must be given sufficient nutritional feed rations, appropriate housing, pasture and sanitation conditions, and freedom of movement. Additionally, the stress placed on them must be minimized.

## How to Use the Individual Dairy and Eggs Chapters

Each chapter is dedicated to one of the World's Healthiest Dairy Products or Eggs and contains everything you need to know to enjoy and maximize their flavor and nutritional benefits. Each chapter is organized into two parts:

1. **DAIRY AND EGGS FACTS** describes eggs or each dairy product and its different varieties and peak season. It also addresses biochemical considerations of each food by describing unique compounds each contains that may be potentially problematic to individuals with specific health problems. Detailed information about the health benefits of the dairy product and eggs can be found at the end of the chapter devoted to each individual food, as can a complete nutritional profile.

2. **THE 3 STEPS TO THE BEST TASTING AND MOST NUTRITIOUS DAIRY PRODUCTS AND THE 4 STEPS TO THE BEST TASTING AND MOST NUTRITIOUS EGGS** includes information about how to best select, store and prepare each one of these World's Healthiest Foods.

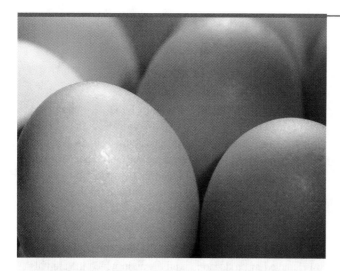

# eggs

## highlights

| | |
|---|---|
| AVAILABILITY: | Year-round |
| REFRIGERATE: | Yes, in carton |
| SHELF LIFE: | Up to 1 month |
| PREPARATION: | Minimal |
| BEST WAY TO COOK: | Boil, poach or frittata |

## nutrient-richness chart

Total Nutrient-Richness:  **18**
One whole (44 grams) boiled hen Egg contains 68 calories

| NUTRIENT | AMOUNT | %DV | DENSITY | QUALITY |
|---|---|---|---|---|
| Tryptophan | 0.07 g | 21.9 | 5.8 | very good |
| Selenium | 13.55 mcg | 19.4 | 5.1 | very good |
| Iodine | 23.76 mcg | 15.8 | 4.2 | very good |
| B2 Riboflavin | 0.23 mg | 13.5 | 3.6 | very good |
| Protein | 5.54 g | 11.1 | 2.9 | good |
| Molybdenum | 7.48 mcg | 10.0 | 2.6 | good |
| Vitamin B12 | 0.49 mcg | 8.2 | 2.2 | good |
| Phosphorus | 75.68 mg | 7.6 | 2.0 | good |
| B5 Pantothenic Acid | 0.62 mg | 6.2 | 1.6 | good |
| Vitamin D | 22.88 IU | 5.7 | 1.5 | good |
| **CAROTENOIDS**: | | Daily values for these nutrients have not yet been established. | | |
| Lutein + Zeaxanthin | 146 mcg | | | |

For more on "Total Nutrient-Richness," "%DV," "Density," and
The World's Healthiest Foods "Quality" Rating System, see page 805.

Although Eggs have long been referred to as the "perfect food," cholesterol-conscious Americans have recently been shying away from them. An increasing number of studies, however, are now supporting high saturated-fat intake as more closely related to elevated cholesterol levels than the dietary intake of cholesterol-rich foods such as Eggs. Nutritious, versatile and easy to prepare, they are a great addition to your "Healthiest Way of Eating."

## why eggs should be part of your healthiest way of eating

Eggs are one of the highest quality sources of protein. Egg whites contain adequate amounts of all essential amino acids and are used as the standard against which all protein is measured. Eggs are not only a good source of inexpensive protein, they are also a very good source of iodine, important for healthy thyroid function. Egg yolks contain the carotenoid phytonutrient lutein, which has been found to be important for eye health. They are also one of the few excellent sources of the B vitamin, choline, a key nutrient for brain function and health. Eggs are an ideal food to add to your "Healthiest Way of Eating" not only because they are high in nutrients, but also because they are low in calories: one Egg contains only 68 calories. (For more on the *Health Benefits of Eggs* and a complete analysis of their content of over 60 nutrients, see page 636.)

## varieties of eggs

Some of the types of hen Eggs available in the market include:

### ORGANIC

Produced following the organic food guidelines. From chickens not treated with any antibiotics or hormones.

### OMEGA-3 ENRICHED EGGS

Eggs produced by chickens that have been fed a diet containing higher levels of omega-3 fatty acids. Although the Eggs have enhanced levels of omega-3s, they are not intended to be the sole source of this essential fatty acid.

### BROWN EGGS

Produced by a special breed of chickens. The color of these Eggs does not necessarily confer a significant nutritional benefit.

Some markets also carry duck, goose and quail Eggs, all of which have yet to gain mainstream popularity.

## the peak season

Eggs are available throughout the year.

## biochemical considerations

Eggs are one of the foods most often associated with allergic reactions. (For more on *Food Allergies*, see page 719.)

### Handling of Eggs

Health safety concerns about Eggs center on salmonellosis (*Salmonella*-caused food poisoning). *Salmonella* bacteria from the chicken's intestines may be found even in clean uncracked Eggs. Formerly, these bacteria were found only in Eggs with cracked shells. Safe food handling techniques, like washing the Eggs before cracking them, may not protect you from infection. To kill the *Salmonella*, eggs must reach an internal temperature of 160°F (71°C), effectively pasteurizing them. Soft-cooked or sunny-side-up Eggs should be cooked until the yolk is firm. There is no risk of salmonellosis when Eggs are hard-boiled, scrambled or poached (make sure to refrigerate hard-boiled Eggs at most 2 hours after cooking). Raw Eggs, however, do carry risk of *Salmonella*-caused food poisoning.

Dishes and utensils used when preparing Eggs (as well as meat and poultry) should be washed in warm water separately from other kitchenware, and washing your hands with warm, soapy water is essential after handling Eggs. Any surfaces that might have potentially come into contact with raw Eggs should be washed and can be sanitized with a solution of one teaspoon chlorine bleach mixed with one quart water.

### Cholesterol in Eggs

Eggs yolks are high in cholesterol, which may be of concern to some individuals. (Egg whites are cholesterol-free.) One Egg contains 187 mg of cholesterol.

## 4 steps for the best tasting and most nutritious eggs

Turning Eggs into a flavorful dish with the most nutrients is simple if you just follow my 4 easy steps:

1. The Best Way to Select
2. The Best Way to Store
3. The Best Way to Prepare
4. The Healthiest Way of Cooking

## 1. the best way to select eggs

Eggs are often classified according to the USDA grading system and bear a label of AA, A or B; however, not all Eggs are labeled or graded because it is not legally mandatory. The grading system is an indicator of quality parameters including freshness. I always try to purchase the freshest and best quality Eggs, which means selecting AA Eggs. Farm fresh Eggs from a local purveyor are often not labeled. If this is the case, familiarize yourself with the reputation of the person selling the Eggs and make sure the Eggs have been kept refrigerated. Eggs are also labeled according to their size—extra large, large, medium and small.

Inspect Eggs for breaks or cracks before purchasing them and remain aware of their fragility while packing them into a shopping bag for the trip home. As with all foods, I recommend selecting organically produced Eggs whenever possi-

## 2. the best way to store eggs

Do not wash Eggs before storing as this can remove the protective coating on the shells, making them more susceptible to bacterial contamination. Be sure that they are stored with their pointed end facing downward as this will help to prevent the air chamber and the yolk from being displaced. Although many refrigerators feature an Egg container on the door, this is not the best place to store Eggs since this exposes them to too much warm air each time the refrigerator door is opened and closed. Store your Eggs in the back of the refrigerator where they will keep for up to one month. You can check the container for the date they were packed.

It is best to leave Eggs in their original carton or place them in a covered container so that they will not absorb odors or lose any moisture.

## 3. the best way to prepare eggs

Make sure your Eggs are fresh. Yolks of fresh Eggs will float on top of the Egg white. Cracking each Egg individually into a bowl before adding it to your recipe will allow you to determine whether it is old or spoiled. It helps if you bring refrigerated Eggs to room temperature for certain cooking methods. For instance, when you boil Eggs, the shells are not as likely to crack if they start at room temperature. Also, Egg whites will not peak well if they are cold. Be sure to throw away cracked Eggs as they may be contaminated.

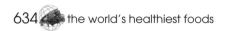

# 4. the healthiest way of cooking eggs

When cooking Eggs, it is important to watch that they are cooked long enough that the Egg whites are no longer translucent. The best ways to cook Eggs is by boiling, poaching or making a frittata with broth instead of oil. These methods ensure your Eggs will be well cooked.

**METHODS NOT RECOMMENDED FOR COOKING EGGS**

I don't recommend cooking Eggs in oil because high temperature heat can damage delicate oils and potentially create harmful free radicals. (For more on *Why it is Important to Cook Without Heated Oils*, see page 52.)

Here are questions I received from readers of the whfoods.org website about Eggs:

**Q** *Can Eggs be eaten raw? Will they still be nutritious?*

**A** As far as I see it, the main concern about raw versus cooked Eggs is not so much issues of nutrients but of safety. Eating raw Eggs brings with it the risk of poisoning from *Salmonella*, a bacteria that is destroyed by thoroughly cooking Eggs. To kill the *Salmonella*, Eggs must reach an internal temperature of 160°F (71°C) or be cooked at 140°F (60°C) for at least three minutes, effectively pasteurizing them. This translates to a 7-minute boiled Egg, a 5-minute poached Egg or a 3-minute per side fried Egg. Now, this is not to say that eating raw Eggs is a definite way to ingest *Salmonella*, but it does carry this risk. Restaurants that serve raw Eggs in certain recipes (such as Caesar salads) normally use Eggs that have been pasteurized, a process that helps to kill bacteria.

The main nutritional concern regarding consuming raw Egg whites is that Egg whites contain a compound called avidin that binds the B-vitamin biotin which can lead to a deficiency of this nutrient in certain people. Cooking the Egg white deactivates the avidin.

**Q** *Does the cholesterol in Egg come from the yolk only or is it present in the Egg whites as well?*

**A** All of the cholesterol in the Egg comes from the yolk, so eating only the whites will not contribute any cholesterol to your diet.

**Q** *Do the whites of Eggs absorb the chemicals fed to chickens?*

**A** Both the whites and yolks of Eggs absorb chemicals consumed by chickens. Since the whites are mostly composed of protein, they tend to absorb more of the heavy metals (like mercury) and less of the pesticides (which are mostly fat soluble). The yolks tend to absorb more of the pesticides and other fat-soluble contaminants since they are composed primarily of fat. However, there has been research showing various types of contaminants in both whites and yolks. All of these potential problems are avoided, of course, by choosing certified organic Eggs produced by organically raised chickens.

---

## *Poached Eggs*

*Poached Eggs are a quick, easy and nutritious way to prepare Eggs in a matter of minutes. It is best to use organic omega-3-rich Eggs.*

1. Bring 1 quart of water to a medium boil in a sauce pan. Add a few drops of light vinegar, such as wine or apple cider vinegar (use about one-quarter teaspoon per quart of water). Vinegar helps to hold Egg whites together. Don't add salt to the water as it dissolves Egg whites.

2. Crack Eggs into a small bowl one at a time and slip them into the simmering water.

3. Cook 5 minutes, until the white is set and the yolk has filmed over. Remove with a slotted spoon.

## *Boiled Eggs*

*Boiled Eggs can be either hard or soft boiled and enjoyed for breakfast or packed for lunch. It is best to use organic omega-3-rich Eggs.*

1. Fill a pan with enough water to completely cover the Eggs.

2. Add a little vinegar, and bring the water to a boil.

3. Once the water has come to a boil, add Eggs. Cook for 5 minutes for soft boiled Eggs and 10 minutes for hard boiled Eggs. Egg whites should no longer be translucent.

**PREPARATION HINTS FOR EGGS:**

To bring Eggs to room temperature quickly, crack them into a stainless steel bowl and place that bowl inside another slightly larger bowl of warm water.

Research is now showing that a very small percentage of people experience an increase in cholesterol levels if they eat foods high in cholesterol.

STEP-BY-STEP RECIPE
## The Healthiest Ways of Cooking Eggs

# Healthy Breakfast Frittata

*This great tasting frittata is full of health benefits and will keep your energy level high for hours.*

> 1/2 medium onion
> 4 medium cloves garlic
> 1/4 lb ground lamb or turkey
> 1 TBS + 2 TBS chicken broth
> 3 cups rinsed and finely chopped kale
>     (stems removed)
> 5 omega-3 enriched Eggs
> Sea salt and black pepper to taste

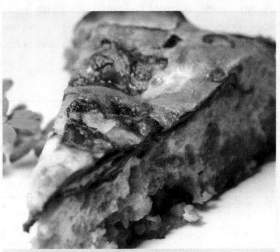

Healthy Breakfast Frittata

1. Chop garlic, mince onions and let sit for 5 minutes. (Why?, see pages 261 and 276.)

2. Preheat broiler on low.

3. Heat 1 TBS broth in a 9–10 inch stainless steel skillet. You will need a pan with a steel handle. "Healthy Sauté" onion over medium-low heat for about 3 minutes, stirring often. (For how to "Healthy Sauté," see page 57.)

4. Add garlic and ground lamb or turkey and cook for another 3 minutes, breaking up clumps.

5. Add kale and 2 TBS broth. Reduce heat to low and continue to cook **covered** for about 5 more minutes. Season with salt and pepper.

6. Beat Eggs, season with a pinch of salt and pepper, and pour on top of mixture evenly. Cook on low for another 2 minutes without stirring.

7. Place skillet under the broiler on a rack in the middle of the oven, about 7 inches from the heat source so it has time to cook without the top burning. As soon as the Eggs are firm, it is done; this should take about 2–3 minutes.

**SERVES 2**

Please write (address on back cover flap) or e-mail me at info@whfoods.org with your personal ideas for preparing Eggs and I will share them with others through our website at www.whfoods.org.

## 7 QUICK SERVING IDEAS for EGGS:

1. Boiled Eggs make a quick, high-protein snack for morning or afternoon.

2. Add sliced or quartered boiled Eggs to green salads.

3. Egg salad is a great filling for sandwiches. Plain yogurt and mustard are a good substitute for the mayonnaise typically used.

4. **Poached Eggs over Greens:** Place poached Eggs on top of steamed kale, Swiss chard or collard greens for an energizing meal any time of day.

5. **Marinated Beet Salad and Eggs:** Add chopped boiled eggs to the Marinated Beet Salad recipe on page 248.

6. **Spicy Vegetable Fried Rice:** In a large stainless steel sauté pan, "Healthy Sauté" diced carrots, diced celery and diced onion for 2 minutes. Drain and put in a mixing bowl. Add cooked brown rice, peas, beaten Eggs, tamari (soy sauce) and red pepper flakes. Put back in the pan and cook over medium heat stirring constantly until the Eggs are cooked.

7. **Egg Crepe Filled with Veggies:** Make a thin crepe batter by whisking 2 TBS of water with an Egg and sea salt and pepper to taste. Add 2 TBS of chicken broth to a stainless steel sauté pan. Pour batter mix into pan. Quickly turn the pan until the bottom is coated. Cook over medium heat until top is firm. Remove to a serving plate, fill with your favorite combination of cooked vegetables and roll to cover the vegetables.

# health benefits of eggs

## A Good Source of Protein

Eggs are a good source of low-cost, high-quality protein. Dietary protein provides us with amino acids that we use to make our muscles, tissues, skin, immune system antibodies, nutrient-carrying transport proteins and a host of other compounds vital to physiologic function.

## Nutritional Analysis of 1 whole boiled hen Egg:

| NUTRIENT | AMOUNT | % DAILY VALUE | NUTRIENT | AMOUNT | % DAILY VALUE |
|---|---|---|---|---|---|
| Calories | 68.20 | | Pantothenic Acid | 0.62 mg | 6.20 |
| Calories from Fat | 42.02 | | | | |
| Calories from Saturated Fat | 12.94 | | **Minerals** | | |
| Protein | 5.54 g | | Boron | 0.66 mcg | |
| Carbohydrates | 0.49 g | | Calcium | 22.00 mg | 2.20 |
| Dietary Fiber | 0.00 g | 0.00 | Chloride | 70.40 mg | |
| Soluble Fiber | 0.00 g | | Chromium | — mcg | — |
| Insoluble Fiber | 0.00 g | | Copper | 0.01 mg | 0.50 |
| Sugar – Total | 0.49 g | | Fluoride | — mg | — |
| Monosaccharides | 0.49 g | | Iodine | 23.76 mcg | 15.84 |
| Disaccharides | 0.00 g | | Iron | 0.52 mg | 2.89 |
| Other Carbs | 0.00 g | | Magnesium | 4.40 mg | 1.10 |
| Fat – Total | 4.67 g | | Manganese | 0.01 mg | 0.50 |
| Saturated Fat | 1.44 g | | Molybdenum | 7.48 mcg | 9.97 |
| Mono Fat | 1.79 g | | Phosphorus | 75.68 mg | 7.57 |
| Poly Fat | 0.62 g | | Potassium | 55.44 mg | |
| Omega-3 Fatty Acids | 0.03 g | 1.20 | Selenium | 13.55 mcg | 19.36 |
| Omega-6 Fatty Acids | 0.59 g | | Sodium | 54.56 mg | |
| Trans Fatty Acids | 0.00 g | | Zinc | 0.46 mg | 3.07 |
| Cholesterol | 186.56 mg | | | | |
| Water | 32.83 g | | **Amino Acids** | | |
| Ash | 0.48 g | | Alanine | 0.31 g | |
| | | | Arginine | 0.33 g | |
| **Vitamins** | | | Aspartate | 0.56 g | |
| Vitamin A IU | 246.40 IU | 4.93 | Cystine | 0.13 g | 31.71 |
| Vitamin A RE | 73.92 RE | | Glutamate | 0.72 g | |
| A - Carotenoid | 0.00 RE | 0.00 | Glycine | 0.19 g | |
| A - Retinol | 73.92 RE | | Histidine | 0.13 g | 10.08 |
| B1 Thiamin | 0.03 mg | 2.00 | Isoleucine | 0.30 g | 26.09 |
| B2 Riboflavin | 0.23 mg | 13.53 | Leucine | 0.47 g | 18.58 |
| B3 Niacin | 0.03 mg | 0.15 | Lysine | 0.40 g | 17.02 |
| Niacin Equiv | 1.15 mg | | Methionine | 0.17 g | 22.97 |
| Vitamin B6 | 0.05 mg | 2.50 | Phenylalanine | 0.29 g | 24.37 |
| Vitamin B12 | 0.49 mcg | 8.17 | Proline | 0.22 g | |
| Biotin | 7.04 mcg | 2.35 | Serine | 0.41 g | |
| Vitamin C | 0.00 mg | 0.00 | Threonine | 0.27 g | 21.77 |
| Vitamin D IU | 22.88 IU | 5.72 | Tryptophan | 0.07 g | 21.88 |
| Vitamin D mcg | 0.57 mcg | | Tyrosine | 0.23 g | 23.71 |
| Vitamin E Alpha Equiv | 0.46 mg | 2.30 | Valine | 0.34 g | 23.13 |
| Vitamin E IU | 0.69 IU | | | | |
| Vitamin E mg | 0.46 mg | | (Note: "–" indicates data is unavailable. For more information, please see page 806.) | | |
| Folate | 19.36 mcg | 4.84 | | | |
| Vitamin K | 0.10 mcg | 0.13 | | | |

## Promote Healthy Thyroid Function

Eggs are a very good source of iodine, which is a component of the thyroid hormones, thyroxine (T4) and tri-iodothyronine (T3). Without sufficient supplies of iodine, the body cannot synthesize these hormones. Eggs are also a very good source of selenium, which is also necessary for thyroid hormone metabolism.

## Promote Brain Health

Another health benefit of Eggs is their contribution to the diet as a source of choline. Although our bodies can produce some choline, we cannot synthesize enough to make up for an inadequate supply in our diets. Choline deficiency can cause a deficiency of folic acid, another B vitamin critically important for health. Since choline is a component of not only phosphatidylcholine and sphingomyelin, two fat-like molecules in the brain that account for an unusually high percentage of the brain's total mass, but also of the neurotransmitter acetylcholine, choline is particularly important for brain function and health.

## Promote Heart Health

Although Egg yolks are high in cholesterol, and health experts in the past had counseled patients with cholesterol problems to avoid this food, nutrition experts now suggest that some people on a low-fat diet can eat one or two Eggs a day without measurable changes in their blood cholesterol levels. This information is supported by a statistical analysis of 224 dietary studies carried out over the past 25 years that investigated the relationship between diet and blood cholesterol levels in thousands of subjects. (For more on this subject, see page 637.)

## Promote Eye Health

Eggs contain concentrated amounts of the carotenoid lutein, for which leafy green vegetables like spinach and kale are well-known. Lutein is an antioxidant found concentrated in the eyes, where it helps to prevent free-radical-scavenging. Consumption of lutein-rich diets is associated with a reduced risk of age-related macular degeneration and cataracts.

## Additional Health-Promoting Benefits of Eggs

Eggs are also a concentrated source of many other nutrients providing additional health-promoting benefits. These nutrients include bone-building vitamin D, vitamin K and phosphorus; energy-producing vitamin B2 and vitamin B5; sulfite-detoxifying molybdenum; and sleep-promoting tryptophan.

# Q *What is the latest research on Eggs and cholesterol?*

A Several dozen high-quality studies confirm the lack of negative effects on blood lipids from mild to moderate consumption of whole Eggs. One of the key issues seems to be that about 70% of U.S. adults can be classified as "hyporesponders," meaning that they experience very mild or no increase at all in their serum cholesterol when consuming significant amounts of cholesterol in their diet.

The research on Eggs and cholesterol, however, is not all one-sided. Dietary cholesterol (as found in Egg yolks) raises the ratio of total-to-HDL cholesterol. This shift is not something we want because it increases our risk of heart disease. In addition, for individuals who have high intakes of dietary cholesterol—in the 200–400 mg per day range—a drop in dietary cholesterol of about 100 mg per day can lower the level of blood cholesterol by about 10 mg per deciliter of blood. This drop may be protective for individuals with high blood cholesterol levels.

Yet, the nutrition research is finding that while there are some people who are sensitive to dietary cholesterol, for many others, dietary cholesterol—as found in Eggs—may not be a key element in raising risk of coronary heart disease (CHD). As the author of a recent review study (Kratz M. Dietary cholesterol, atherosclerosis and coronary heart disease. Handb Exp Pharmacol. 2005;(170):195-213.) notes: "These studies suggest that the association between dietary cholesterol and CHD is small, as most subjects can effectively adapt to higher levels of cholesterol intake." Yet, the author also refers to "a subgroup of individuals who are highly responsive to changes in cholesterol intake." Follow-up research has further suggested that the responsiveness of this subgroup may involve their genetics: it seems that some people carry genes that make them sensitive to dietary cholesterol while others don't. This is the state of the present research understanding as far as I understand it.

# Q *How can I tell whether an Egg is bad?*

A I don't recommend using appearance alone as your Egg safety test as it is not the best way to measure safety. Particularly with respect to an Egg that has been cracked open, there can be a good number of discolorations in the white or yolk that do not represent food safety concerns. However, with that context in mind, there are certain types of Egg inspection that also make sense when trying to determine whether an Egg has gone bad or not.

First, I would look to ensure that there are no cracks in the shell. If there are cracks, then I would dispose of the Egg. Once you have cracked the shell, smell the Egg and see if it smells fine. If it doesn't, I would throw it away. If the raw white of the Egg has turned pinkish, green or black, you should also definitely toss out the Egg.

In terms of determining quality from an uncracked Egg, in his classic book "On Food and Cooking," Harold McGee discusses how better quality Eggs have smaller air cells; he notes that in a fresh Egg, the space is about 1/8-inch deep and has the diameter of a dime. To test the size without cracking it, he writes that you should put the whole Egg in a bowl of water; if the air cell is much larger than the size noted above, the wide end of the Egg will rise above the narrow end. If your Egg does this, it would then be a reflection that it is not that fresh.

McGee's freshness test is also related to a long-time folklore belief about the degree to which an Egg will float in water. According to this belief, a spoiled Egg will float all the way to the surface, but a safe Egg will not. While this belief is not completely accurate, it does harbor one important element of truth. If the pores in an Eggshell have become sufficiently large, or if the shell has been cracked, it is possible not only for air but also for additional bacteria to enter into the Egg, become metabolically active and create gas inside the Eggshell. This additional gas could cause the Egg to do more floating. (However, other factors could also cause the Egg to float, including simple transfer of air through larger pores, even if no bacteria had migrated into the Egg.)

The bottom line: While you may want to try the float test for fun or the "wide end up" float test for freshness, I would judge whether an Egg is safe to eat by the smell and discoloration of the opened Egg as described above, or by noticing if there are cracks in the shell of the unopened Egg.

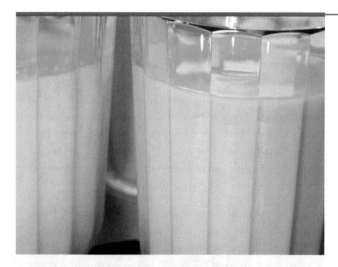

# low-fat milk

## highlights

| | |
|---|---|
| AVAILABILITY: | Year-round |
| REFRIGERATE: | Yes |
| SHELF LIFE: | Check use-by date |
| PREPARATION: | Minimal |

## nutrient-richness chart

Total Nutrient-Richness: **17**
One cup (244 grams) of Low-Fat Milk contains 121 calories

| NUTRIENT | AMOUNT | %DV | DENSITY | QUALITY |
|---|---|---|---|---|
| Iodine | 58.6 mcg | 39.0 | 5.8 | very good |
| Tryptophan | 0.1 g | 31.3 | 4.6 | very good |
| Calcium | 296.7 mg | 29.7 | 4.4 | very good |
| Vitamin D | 97.6 IU | 24.4 | 3.6 | very good |
| B2 Riboflavin | 0.4 mg | 23.5 | 3.5 | very good |
| Phosphorus | 232.0 mg | 23.2 | 3.4 | very good |
| Protein | 8.1 g | 16.3 | 2.4 | good |
| Vitamin B12 | 0.9 mcg | 14.8 | 2.2 | good |
| Vitamin K | 9.8 mcg | 12.2 | 1.8 | good |
| Potassium | 376.7 mg | 10.8 | 1.6 | good |
| Vitamin A | 500.2 IU | 10.0 | 1.5 | good |

For more on "Total Nutrient-Richness," "%DV," "Density," and
The World's Healthiest Foods "Quality" Rating System, see page 805.

Although the practice of drinking Cow's Milk is thought to date back as early as 6,000-8,000 BC, it wasn't until the 14th century that the demand for Cow's Milk became greater than the demand for goat's or sheep's Milk. In the United States, Cow's Milk is so ubiquitous that it needs no description and is most likely already included in the "Healthiest Way of Eating" of most Americans. Few of us have grown up without the promise of strong teeth and bones from drinking Milk. Served with breakfast cereals or enjoyed as a cold beverage, Milk is a staple in the American diet.

## why low-fat milk should be part of your healthiest way of eating

There is little doubt that Milk is a highly nutritious food; however, increasing awareness of its high concentration of saturated fats, a major contributor to heart disease, has led to debate over how much we should consume. Low-fat varieties help resolve this dilemma by providing a satisfying alternative to whole Milk without giving up any nutritional benefits. Its rich supply of calcium and vitamin D (most Milk is fortified with vitamin D) is the reason it is renowned as an excellent choice for healthy bones. (For more on the *Health Benefits of Low-Fat Milk* and a complete analysis of its content of over 60 nutrients, see page 640.)

## varieties of milk

Milk is available in a variety of forms that are often differentiated by their fat content. It is the basis for a variety of different dairy products including cheese, yogurt, kefir and ice Milk.

### ORGANIC MILK

Organic Milk is from cows raised without the use of steroids, antibiotics, pesticides or synthetic growth hormones. It is processed using techniques that minimize harmful effects on the environment. It is often of higher quality than non-organic varieties.

### 2% MILK

The 2% designation refers to the percent of fat by weight that the Milk contains. It is often referred to as reduced-fat Milk, since it contains less fat than the 3.5% found in whole Milk.

### 1% AND NON-FAT MILK:

Containing about 3 grams of fat per cup, 1% Milk has 99% of its fat removed. Non-Fat Milk contains less than 1% Milk fat and less than 1/2 gram of fat per cup. The FDA requires that reduced fat Milk be fortified with vitamin A, a fat-soluble vitamin that is lost with the removal of the Milk fat.

### RAW MILK

Since Raw Milk is not pasteurized, it is not heated before being taken to market. Dairies selling Raw Milk must be certified, must follow rigid standards and the cows must be inspected on a regular basis.

### LACTASE-TREATED OR REDUCED-LACTOSE MILK

Many adults experience bloating, diarrhea and cramps after drinking Milk. Individuals with these symptoms may suffer from lactose intolerance, a condition caused by a deficiency of an enzyme called *lactase* that is necessary to digest lactose or Milk sugars. *Lactase*-treated Milk has the enzyme *lactase* added to help lactose-intolerant individuals digest Milk sugars.

### Pasteurization

Milk is pasteurized to ensure it is free from bacterial contamination. The type of pasteurization affects the taste of the Milk product:

### VAT PASTEURIZED MILK

Heated to low boiling and held for 30 minutes, Milk treated with this method retains the most flavor and nutrients.

### HIGH TEMPERATURE SHORT TIME PASTEURIZATION (HTST)

The most common method of pasteurization. Milk is heated to up to 161°F (71°C) and then cooled rapidly.

### ULTRA HEAT TREATMENT (UHT)

Milk is heated to a very high temperature (up to 307°F or 153°C) and held for only two to six seconds before it is packaged into sterilized containers. Packages can be kept unrefrigerated until they are opened. The nutrient content is comparable to HTST-treated Milk; however, the high temperature creates a product with a slightly bitter and scalded taste.

## the peak season

Low-Fat Milk is available throughout the year.

## biochemical considerations

The Milk sugar, lactose, found in Low-Fat Milk is associated with lactose intolerance, which may be of concern for some individuals. Individuals may also be allergic to Milk. There has been some concern over cows treated with a compound called recombinant bovine growth hormone, rBGH. The best way to ensure that the Milk you buy is not from cows treated with rBGH is to buy organic dairy products. (For more on *Lactose Intolerance*, see page 722; *Food Allergies*, see page 719; and *rBGH*, see page 728.)

## 3 steps for the best tasting and most nutritious low-fat milk

Enjoying the best tasting Low-Fat Milk with the most nutrients is simple if you just follow my 3 easy steps:
1. The Best Way to Select
2. The Best Way to Store
3. The Best Way to Prepare

# 1. the best way to select low-fat milk —————

When purchasing Milk, use the "sell-by" date as a guide to its shelf life. Smell the top of the container to make sure that the Milk does not smell spoiled. This could have been caused by being stored for a period of time outside of the refrigerator. Select Milk from the coldest part (the lowest sections) of the refrigerator case.

I have found Milk in translucent plastic jugs to have an off-taste. In addition, these plastic jugs and clear glass bottles expose the Milk to light, which can destroy up to 90% of its vitamin A and 14% of its riboflavin content. Buying Milk in opaque cardboard cartons avoids these problems. I highly recommend buying organic milk, or at least rBGH-Free milk, whenever possible.

# 2. the best way to store low-fat milk —————

Milk should always be refrigerated (34–40°F or 1–4°C) since warm temperatures can cause it to turn sour quickly. Always seal or close the Milk container when storing it to prevent the Milk from absorbing the aromas of other foods

in the refrigerator. Avoid storing Milk in the refrigerator door since this exposes it to too much warm air each time the refrigerator is opened and closed.

# 3. the best way to prepare low-fat milk —————

Milk requires no preparation and can be used as an ingredient in a variety of different types of recipes. Follow the

instructions on individual recipes for the best results.

# health benefits of low-fat milk

## Promotes Bone Health

Low-Fat Milk promotes strong bones by being a very good source of calcium, phosphorus and vitamin D and a good source of vitamin K—four nutrients essential to bone health. In a process known as bone mineralization, calcium joins with phosphorus to form calcium phosphate, which is a major component of the mineral complex hydroxyapatite, which gives structure and strength to bones. Calcitriol, the most metabolically active form of vitamin D, works with parathyroid hormone (PTH) to maintain proper levels of calcium in the blood. Vitamin K1 activates osteocalcin, the major non-collagen protein in bone, which anchors calcium molecules inside of the bone. Therefore, without enough vitamin K1, osteocalcin levels are inadequate and bone mineralization is impaired.

## A Good Source of Protein

Low-Fat Milk is a good source of low-cost, high-quality protein. The structure of humans and animals is built on protein. We rely on animal and vegetable protein for our supply of amino acids, and then our bodies rearrange them to create the pattern of amino acids we require. These amino acids are used in a vast number of ways, doing everything from comprising our muscles and tissues to serving as the basis for enzymes and nutrient-carrying protein molecules.

## Promotes Optimal Health

Low-Fat Milk produced by grass-fed cows also contains a beneficial fatty acid called conjugated linoleic acid (CLA). Research suggests that CLA may help lower cholesterol and prevent atherosclerosis. Animal research has found that this fatty acid inhibits several types of cancer in laboratory animals. In test tubes, this compound has been found to kill human skin cancer, colorectal cancer and breast cancer cells.

## Promotes Healthy Thyroid Function

Low-Fat Milk is a very good source of iodine, which is a component of the thyroid hormones thyroxine (T4) and triiodothyronine (T3); without sufficient iodine, your body cannot synthesize these hormones. Because these thyroid hormones regulate metabolism in every cell of the body and play a role in virtually all physiological functions, consuming adequate amounts of dietary iodine is vitally important to maintaining health.

## Additional Health-Promoting Benefits of Low-Fat Milk

Low-Fat Milk is a concentrated source of other nutrients providing additional health-promoting benefits. These nutrients include immune system-supporting vitamin A; heart-healthy vitamin B12 and potassium; energy-producing vitamin B2; muscle-building protein; and sleep-promoting tryptophan.

### Nutritional Analysis of 1 cup of Low-Fat Milk:

| NUTRIENT | AMOUNT | % DAILY VALUE |
|---|---|---|
| Calories | 121.20 | |
| Calories from Fat | 42.16 | |
| Calories from Saturated Fat | 26.24 | |
| Protein | 8.13 g | |
| Carbohydrates | 11.71 g | |
| Dietary Fiber | 0.00 g | 0.00 |
| Soluble Fiber | 0.00 g | |
| Insoluble Fiber | 0.00 g | |
| Sugar – Total | 11.71 g | |
| Monosaccharides | 0.00 g | |
| Disaccharides | 11.71 g | |
| Other Carbs | 0.00 g | |
| Fat – Total | 6.68 g | |
| Saturated Fat | 2.92 g | |
| Mono Fat | 1.35 g | |
| Poly Fat | 0.17 g | |
| Omega-3 Fatty Acids | 0.07 g | 2.80 |
| Omega-6 Fatty Acids | 0.10 g | |
| Trans Fatty Acids | 0.13 g | |
| Cholesterol | 18.30 mg | |
| Water | 217.67 g | |
| Ash | 1.81 g | |
| **Vitamins** | | |
| Vitamin A IU | 500.20 IU | 10.00 |
| Vitamin A RE | 139.08 RE | |
| A - Carotenoid | 9.76 RE | 0.13 |
| A - Retinol | 129.32 RE | |
| B1 Thiamin | 0.10 mg | 6.67 |
| B2 Riboflavin | 0.40 mg | 23.53 |
| B3 Niacin | 0.21 mg | 1.05 |
| Niacin Equiv | 1.94 mg | |
| Vitamin B6 | 0.10 mg | 5.00 |
| Vitamin B12 | 0.89 mcg | 14.83 |
| Biotin | 4.88 mcg | 1.63 |
| Vitamin C | 2.32 mg | 3.87 |
| Vitamin D IU | 97.60 IU | 24.40 |
| Vitamin D mcg | 2.44 mcg | |
| Vitamin E Alpha Equiv | 0.17 mg | 0.85 |
| Vitamin E IU | 0.25 IU | |
| Vitamin E mg | 0.17 mg | |
| Folate | 12.44 mcg | 3.11 |
| Vitamin K | 9.76 mcg | 12.20 |
| Pantothenic Acid | 0.78 mg | 7.80 |
| **Minerals** | | |
| Boron | 3.66 mcg | |
| Calcium | 296.70 mg | 29.67 |
| Chloride | 244.00 mg | |
| Chromium | — mcg | — |
| Copper | 0.02 mg | 1.00 |
| Fluoride | — mg | — |
| Iodine | 58.56 mcg | 39.04 |
| Iron | 0.12 mg | 0.67 |
| Magnesium | 33.35 mg | 8.34 |
| Manganese | 0.00 mg | 0.00 |
| Molybdenum | 4.88 mcg | 6.51 |
| Phosphorus | 232.04 mg | 23.20 |
| Potassium | 376.74 mg | |
| Selenium | 5.37 mcg | 7.67 |
| Sodium | 121.76 mg | |
| Zinc | 0.95 mg | 6.33 |
| **Amino Acids** | | |
| Alanine | 0.27 g | |
| Arginine | 0.28 g | |
| Aspartate | 0.59 g | |
| Cystine | 0.07 g | 17.07 |
| Glutamate | 1.62 g | |
| Glycine | 0.16 g | |
| Histidine | 0.21 g | 16.28 |
| Isoleucine | 0.47 g | 40.87 |
| Leucine | 0.76 g | 30.04 |
| Lysine | 0.61 g | 25.96 |
| Methionine | 0.20 g | 27.03 |
| Phenylalanine | 0.37 g | 31.09 |
| Proline | 0.75 g | |
| Serine | 0.42 g | |
| Threonine | 0.35 g | 28.23 |
| Tryptophan | 0.10 g | 31.25 |
| Tyrosine | 0.37 g | 38.14 |
| Valine | 0.52 g | 35.37 |

(Note: "—" indicates data is unavailable. For more information, please see page 806.)

STEP-BY-STEP RECIPE
## The Healthiest Ways to Use Low-Fat Milk

# *Healthy Creamed Corn*

*An easy way to make creamed corn in just minutes!*

**1 cup Low-Fat Milk**
**1 + 1 cups corn kernels (fresh or frozen)**
**1 TBS honey**
**Sea salt and pepper to taste**

1. Combine 1 cup of Milk, 1 cup of corn and 1 TBS honey in blender. Add sea salt and pepper to taste. Blend on medium speed for 1 minute.

2. In a mixing bowl, combine remaining cup of corn kernels with the corn purée.

3. On stove, heat on medium for 5 minutes.

4. Garnish with minced parsley or toasted sunflower seeds. Serve with chicken or any type of seafood (such as shrimp, scallops or fish).

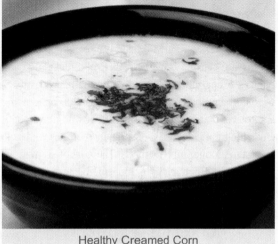
Healthy Creamed Corn

**SERVES 2**

Please write (address on back cover flap) or e-mail me at info@whfoods.org with your personal ideas for preparing Low-Fat Milk, and I will share them with others through our website at www.whfoods.org.

## 10 QUICK SERVING IDEAS for LOW-FAT MILK:

1. Pour Low-Fat Milk over your favorite whole grain cereal. Don't forget to also add 1 TBS of ground flaxseed for added omega-3s.

2. Add Low-Fat Milk to coffee, tea, cream sauces and soups instead of cream.

3. **Chocolate Shake:** Mix together chocolate syrup, malt powder and Low-Fat Milk.

4. **Fruit Shake:** Blend together 1 cup of Low-Fat Milk, medium banana and a mixture of any of your favorite fruits for a delicious shake.

5. **Yummy Pink Milk:** Blend 4 strawberries, 2 tsp honey and 1 cup of Low-Fat Milk in a blender on medium speed for 1 minute. Children will love this recipe!

6. **Rice Pudding:** Add Low-Fat Milk, raisins, cinnamon and nutmeg to a pot of cooked brown rice and heat gently to make rice pudding.

7. **Peanut Butter Banana Shake:** Blend 1 cup Low-Fat Milk, 1 TBS peanut butter, 1 small banana, 2–3 ice cubes and 2 tsp honey until smooth.

8. **Hot Chocolate:** Heat 1 cup Low-Fat Milk over low heat. In a cup, combine 2 TBS unsweetened dark chocolate cocoa and 1 TBS honey to make a paste. Stir mixture into the hot milk.

9. **Cinnamon Milk:** Heat 1 cup Low-Fat Milk with 1 tsp cinnamon, 1/2 tsp cardamon, 3 fresh ginger slices, 3 whole peppercorns and 2 TBS honey over low heat for 15–20 minutes. (The more ginger and peppercorns, the spicier it will be.) Strain into a mug for a warming brew.

10. **Cream of Vegetable Soup:** In a blender, combine 1 cup each of steamed peas and broccoli with 2 cups warm Low-Fat Milk, and salt and pepper to taste. Blend for 2 minutes until creamy. Serve as a delicious soup.

## Q What can you tell me about Milk pasteurization and raw Milk?

A In the U.S, 46 out of 50 states have adopted the Pasteurized Milk Ordinance that was first proposed in 1924 by the U.S. Public Health Service. This ordinance calls for the pasteurization of Milk as a way of killing any potentially disease-causing bacteria in the Milk, including campylobacter, escherichia, listeria, salmonella, yersinia and brucella. Today there are more pasteurization options in the marketplace than there were in 1924, and these options include high-temperature, short time methods, as well as low-temperature, longer time methods. The goal of all methods is the same: to kill potentially pathogenic bacteria that may be present in the Milk or Milk product (like cheese or yogurt).

There's no debate about the effectiveness of pasteurization for killing unwanted bacteria. There's also no doubt that pasteurization gives dairy products a longer shelf life by lowering the presence of bacteria that cause spoilage. But pasteurization also kills desirable bacteria found in fresh Milk, and it denatures Milk enzymes that may be active in the human digestive tract when fresh Milk is consumed. There is little research, however, to determine what nutritional benefits are lost when Milk is pasteurized. I've seen speculation about changes in protein structure, calcium, amino acid and vitamin C bioavailability all being triggered by pasteurization, but I have not seen research that confirms or rejects these occurrences.

In the majority of states, dairy farms are free to produce raw (unpasteurized) Milk as long as they adhere to the conditions and restrictions set out in state law. The safety of unpasteurized Milk depends on the quality of the cow's life, including the immediate environment and feeding. It also depends on the quality of handling facilities once the cow has been milked. For these reasons, I recommend a very careful look at any dairy farm's procedures, track record and publicly available information before considering becoming a consumer of its unpasteurized Milk. Because freshness is at a premium, and the product shelf life is greatly shortened (not necessarily bad factors), the dairy is most likely to be in driving distance of your residence and could be visited in person.

## Q Does eating more lower fat products really help you lose weight?

A If you currently consume whole Milk dairy products on a daily basis, switching to lower fat dairy products might help you lose weight. The reason is fairly simple. If the rest of your meal plan stayed exactly the same, the switch to non-fat milk, for example, would lower your calorie intake. One glass of whole Milk contains about 150 calories, while one glass of non-fat contains about 90 calories. If you consume 3 cups per day, you will save about 180 calories per day, or 1,260 calories per week. Over the course of a year, this savings in calories consumed would translate into a loss of about 17 pounds. However, it is not usually helpful to approach weight loss by focusing on one single type of food. It's your overall meal plan that really counts.

## Q Are there any health risks associated with the homogenization of Milk?

A Beginning in the 1960's and continuing through the 1980's, an MD named Kurt Oster published a series of articles questioning the health safety of homogenized Milk and hypothesized a connection between homogenization and the development of heart disease. According to Oster's hypothesis, an enzyme called xanthine oxidase (XO) was naturally associated with the fat globules in Milk. Homogenization was theorized to trap XO in the new micro-droplets and prevent this enzyme from being metabolized in the digestive tract. Oster was convinced that because of homogenization, unmetabolized XO was being absorbed from the digestive tract to the bloodstream where it could trigger immune reactions and cause damage to blood vessel walls. The result was described as plaque formation—the very same plaque formation that gives rise to atherosclerosis in many U.S. adults.

Research studies have yet to conclusively prove, or disprove, Oster's hypothesis. While there continues to be strong interest in XO, however, and its relationship to heart problems, the contribution of homogenization to these problems is still a research hypothesis and not a research conclusion.

Non-homogenized Milks are becoming increasingly available in the U.S. I support their consumption, even though I have not seen research that confirms the connection between homogenization and risk of heart disease, or the mechanism of XO damage.

Milk is put under high pressure to force homogenization—the splitting of the fat globules into very small molecules that will be dispersed in the Milk. But it's possible to produce Milk, including low-fat and non-fat Milk varieties, without this homogenization process by letting whole Milk naturally separate into non-fat Milk and cream. Homogenization is carried out for convenience and texture, not for nourishment or safety. Even though homogenization moves us away from the whole, natural food and could be objected to on these grounds—and I definitely support the availability and consumption of non-homogenized Milk—in the absence of better research, it's impossible for me to take a stand against the consumption of homogenized Milk for health reasons.

# Q&A

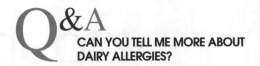

### CAN YOU TELL ME MORE ABOUT DAIRY ALLERGIES?

Many people find that they are sensitive to dairy products, experiencing a host of symptoms including flatulence (gas), diarrhea, skin rash and fatigue when they consume milk and other dairy products. Yet, because adverse reactions to foods don't necessarily occur right after the consumption of these foods, sometimes occurring hours or even days after the food has been eaten, many people are uncertain which specific food may have triggered the unforeseen and unwanted symptoms. Additionally, there are so many "hidden" sources of dairy-derived ingredients that it takes a concerted effort to figure out whether you may be sensitive to dairy.

## Lactose and Casein Found in Many Processed Foods

The problem is that lactose, one of the primary sugars in cow's milk, and casein, one of the primary proteins in cow's milk, are both added to a wide variety of foods; lactose is added for flavor while casein is often added for emulsification, texture and protein supplementation. For example, foods that may contain casein include: bakery glazes, breath mints, coffee whiteners, fortified cereals, high-protein beverage powders, ice cream, infant formulas, nutrition bars, processed meats, salad dressings and whipped toppings. Therefore, the only way to tell for sure whether it is added to a food product is to read the food label.

## Food Allergy Versus Food Intolerance

It is important to realize that sensitivity to certain foods may not always be caused by a food allergy but may be the result of food intolerance. This differentiation is important since these two types of sensitivities occur as a result of two distinct physiological events.

## Dairy Allergy

Food allergies are reactions that involve the immune system. Typically, reactions to the casein in dairy products will involve a full-fledged immune response, manifesting in a manner as specific as a skin rash or as general as fatigue. What happens during an allergic reaction is that your immune system cells will bind to the offending molecule, such as casein, triggering a cascade of physiological events that will activate other components of the immune system. Inflammation and the creation of immune complexes that disrupt normal physiological functioning may ensue as a result.

## Dairy Intolerance

Unlike allergies, some adverse reactions to food do not involve the immune system. These types of responses are called food intolerances with lactose intolerance being the most common food intolerance in the United States, affecting as many as 30% of adult Americans. Individuals who have lactose intolerance are sensitive to the milk sugar lactose that is found in dairy products. This intolerance may occur because they do not produce enough of the digestive, enzyme, *lactase*, which functions to break down lactose in the small intestines. If the lactose does not get digested, it makes its way into the large intestine, causing a host of symptoms, including flatulence and/or diarrhea.

## Hidden Culprits: Dairy in Soy and Meat Products

### DAIRY-BASED REACTIONS TO SOY FOODS

As many consumers have chosen to replace some of their beef, chicken and pork meals with soy-based products, manufacturers of soy-based products often try to place products in the marketplace that match up closely with meat-containing foods (soy hot dogs and sausages are two examples). To boost up the protein content of their soy products, manufacturers often add dairy-based proteins, with the most common of these proteins being casein. Casein, caseinates and sodium caseinate are all words that you might see on a soy food label, and they always indicate the presence of a dairy-based component.

### DAIRY-BASED REACTIONS TO MEAT

A second common overlap between processed non-dairy foods and dairy components involves the processing of meat itself. Lactose—one of the key sugars that is found in cow's milk—is often included in processed meats for flavor; and just as with soy products, sodium caseinate is often added as an emulsifier. Frankfurters, Vienna sausages, luncheon meats, chicken sausages and patés all fall victim to such practices. Caseinate is added to ham brine for improved slicing ability.

## Contaminants in Cow's Milk

If you haven't already switched to organic dairy products in your meal plan, you'll definitely need to do so in order to determine if you have an adverse reaction to cow's milk. The reason is quite simple: about a dozen pesticide residues are commonly found in non-organic cow's milk. (The source of these pesticides, of course, is the food that the cows were given to eat.) Also commonly found are antibiotics, as well as hormonal residues from hormones that were given to the cows prior to milking. Residues of plastic packaging from cow's milk products like cheese, cream or butter can be found in the dairy products. These residues are called packaging migrants, and they include the substances DEHP and DEHA (diethylhexyl phthalate and diethylhexyl adipate). Unless you switch over to organic dairy products when trying to determine a dairy reaction, you won't know whether your reaction is occurring due to components of the cow's milk itself or to these contaminant residues.

# yogurt

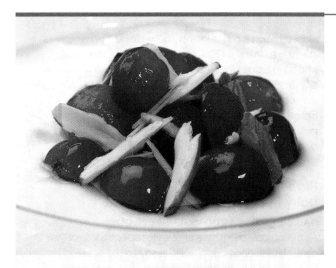

## highlights

| | |
|---|---|
| AVAILABILITY: | Year-round |
| REFRIGERATE: | Yes |
| SHELF LIFE: | Check use-by date |
| PREPARATION: | Minimal |

## nutrient-richness chart

Total Nutrient-Richness: **15**
One cup (245 grams) of low-fat Yogurt contains 209 calories

| NUTRIENT | AMOUNT | %DV | DENSITY | QUALITY |
|---|---|---|---|---|
| Iodine | 87.2 mcg | 58.1 | 6.8 | very good |
| Calcium | 447.4 mg | 44.7 | 5.2 | very good |
| Phosphorus | 351.6 mg | 35.2 | 4.1 | very good |
| B2 Riboflavin | 0.5 mg | 30.6 | 3.6 | very good |
| Protein | 12.9 g | 25.7 | 3.0 | good |
| Vitamin B12 | 1.4 mcg | 23.0 | 2.7 | good |
| Tryptophan | 0.1 g | 18.8 | 2.2 | good |
| Potassium | 572.8 mg | 16.4 | 1.9 | good |
| Molybdenum | 11.3 mcg | 15.0 | 1.7 | good |
| Zinc | 2.2 mg | 14.5 | 1.7 | good |
| B5 Pantothenic Acid | 1.5 mg | 14.5 | 1.7 | good |

For more on "Total Nutrient-Richness," "%DV," "Density," and
The World's Healthiest Foods "Quality" Rating System, see page 805.

Middle Eastern civilizations used the fermenting process to produce Yogurt as far back as 2,000 BC. Yogurt and other fermented dairy products have also long been dietary staples in Asia, Russia and Eastern European countries, such as Bulgaria. In the United States, Yogurt was once relegated to a "health food," but today is enjoyed by people of all walks of life. Because Yogurt makes a quick, easy and nutritious breakfast, lunch or between-meal snack, it is a great addition to your "Healthiest Way of Eating."

## why yogurt should be part of your healthiest way of eating

The recognition of Yogurt's special health benefits did not become apparent until the 20th century, when research was conducted on the health-promoting benefits of the lactic-acid-producing bacteria found in Yogurt. This was followed by research reports that Bulgarian peasants, whose diets included a high consumption of Yogurt, have extraordinary lifespans. While it may still be questionable whether Yogurt is the secret to long life, it is certain that its many health-promoting nutrients make it a great addition to your "Healthiest Way of Eating." (For more on the *Health Benefits of Yogurt* and a complete analysis of its content of over 60 nutrients, see page 646.)

## varieties of yogurt

Yogurt is a fermented dairy product made by adding bacterial cultures to milk, which causes the transformation of the milk's sugar, lactose, into lactic acid. This process gives Yogurt its refreshingly tart flavor and unique pudding-like texture, a quality that is reflected in its original Turkish name, *Yoghurmak*, which means "to thicken." The lactic acid bacteria that are traditionally used to make Yogurt — *Lactobacillus bulgaricus* and *Streptococcus thermophilus* —also confer Yogurt with many of its health benefits. Yogurt and low-fat Yogurt are available in a variety of different flavors and styles:

**PLAIN**
This is the original, unflavored variety and the most nutritious and versatile of the Yogurts. It also contains the least number of calories.

**SUNDAE-STYLE YOGURT**
This version has fruit at the bottom, which must be stirred into the Yogurt before eating. It is higher in sugar content than plain Yogurt.

**SWISS OR FRENCH STYLE YOGURT**
Fruit and flavors are blended into the Yogurt.

**YOGURT DRINKS**

A drink made of Yogurt mixed with fruit flavoring.

**FROZEN YOGURT**

Yogurt in a frozen form, similar to ice cream (for more, see page 654).

## the peak season

Yogurt is available throughout the year.

## biochemical considerations

Some people do not have enough *lactase*, an enzyme that breaks down the lactose sugar found in milk, and therefore may have adverse reactions to eating dairy foods such as Yogurt. Some individuals are also allergic to the casein found in dairy products. There has been some concern over cows that may be treated with a compound called recombinant bovine growth hormone, rBGH. The best way to ensure that the Yogurt you buy is not made from milk from cows treated with rBGH is to buy organic dairy products. (For more on *Food Allergies*, see page 719: and *rBGH*, see page 728.)

## 3 steps for the best tasting and most nutritious yogurt

Enjoying the best tasting yogurt is simple if you just follow my 3 easy steps:

1. The Best Way to Select
2. The Best Way to Store
3. The Best Way to Prepare

## 1. the best way to select yogurt

Some Yogurt manufacturers pasteurize their Yogurt products, while others do not. Although the aim of pasteurization is to kill any harmful bacteria, it also kills the beneficial lactic acid bacteria in the Yogurt, substantially reducing its health benefits. Therefore, I look for Yogurt that features "live active cultures" or "living Yogurt cultures" (indicated on the label) and preferably varieties made from organic milk.

It is best to check the expiration date on the side of the Yogurt container to make sure that it is still fresh. Avoid Yogurt that has artificial colors, flavorings or sweeteners. While fruit-filled Yogurt and frozen Yogurt can be a delicious treat, be aware that these products can often contain excessive amounts of sugar.

## 2. the best way to store yogurt

It is best to keep Yogurt in its original container stored in the refrigerator. Most Yogurt labels include a use-by date, which will provide you with information on how long it can be stored.

## 3. the best way to prepare yogurt

Yogurt requires no preparation. You can enjoy it right out of the container!

---

Here are questions I received from readers of the whfoods.org website about Yogurt:

**Q** *How much lactose is there in Yogurt compared to the amount found in milk?*

**A** The amount of lactose present in Yogurt depends upon the Yogurt preparation method. An 8-ounce glass of 2% cow's milk contains about 10–12 grams of lactose. An 8-ounce serving of many commercial low-fat Yogurts will contain about the same, or even slightly more lactose, because there is less water content in the 8-ounce serving of Yogurt than fluid milk.

Some companies cite much lower levels of lactose per cup of live culture Yogurt due to the *lactase* enzymes produced by the living microorganisms added to the Yogurt, although I have not seen published research to verify this (that doesn't mean it isn't true, though). Therefore, I think it is safe to say that Yogurts vary in their lactose content, with some being higher than milk on an ounce-for-ounce basis, and that live culture Yogurts may contain a lower level of lactose, which would make them much easier to digest than milk in terms of their lactose content.

**Q** *Why does Yogurt provide such little vitamin D when its source, milk, is quite a good source?*

**A** While milk is usually fortified with vitamin D (this nutrient is added to the milk during the packaging process), most dairy products, including Yogurt, are not fortified with vitamin D. That is why you will find that milk has a higher amount of vitamin D than Yogurt.

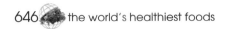

# health benefits of yogurt

## Promotes Optimal Health with Beneficial Bacteria

The highest quality Yogurt in your grocery store contains live bacteria that provide a host of health benefits. Make sure that the label of the Yogurt you purchase indicates that it contains *Lactobacillus bulgaricus* and *Streptococcus thermopholis*, the lactic acid bacteria used in the U.S.

These bacterial cultures may help you to live longer and may fortify your immune system. Research studies have shown that increased Yogurt consumption, particularly in immuno-compromised populations such as the elderly, may enhance the immune response, which would in turn increase resistance to immune-related diseases. This may be why one study found that eating Yogurt and milk more than three times per week imparted a 38% increase in survival rate compared to the survival rate of those who ate those foods less than once a week.

Additionally, recent research also suggests that Yogurt's probiotic (friendly) bacteria may offer other health benefits. One study found that animals that received *Lactobacillus*-containing Yogurt had less arthritic inflammation than those receiving milk or even Yogurt without *Lactobacillus*. Another study found that in individuals receiving Yogurt-containing probiotics, the activity of *H. pylori*, the bacterium responsible for most ulcers, was suppressed.

## Promotes Healthy Weight Control

A recent study found consumption of calcium-rich foods, such as Yogurt, to be inversely correlated with body fat. Earlier studies have also reported an inverse association between calcium intake and body fat accumulation during childhood and between calcium intake and body weight at midlife.

These benefits may extend to overweight adults as well. In a study of obese subjects, all of whom consumed an equal number of calories, those who ate the diet with the most calcium lost the most amount of weight as well as the most amount of fat from their midsection.

## Promotes Women's Health

Eating Yogurt may help to prevent vaginal yeast infections. In one study, when women who had frequent yeast infections ate one cup of Yogurt daily for six months, they experienced a threefold decrease in infections. The benefits probably come from the beneficial bacteria contained in the Yogurt.

## Additional Health-Promoting Benefits of Yogurt

Yogurt is a concentrated source of many other nutrients providing additional health benefits. These nutrients include free-radical-scavenging zinc; thyroid-health-supporting iodine; heart-healthy vitamin B12 and potassium; energy-producing vitamin B2, vitamin B5 and phosphorus; muscle-building protein; sulfite-detoxifying molybdenum; and sleep-promoting tryptophan.

## Nutritional Analysis of 1 cup of low-fat Yogurt:

| NUTRIENT | AMOUNT | % DAILY VALUE | NUTRIENT | AMOUNT | % DAILY VALUE |
|---|---|---|---|---|---|
| Calories | 155.05 | | Pantothenic Acid | 1.45 mg | 14.50 |
| Calories from Fat | 34.18 | | | | |
| Calories from Saturated Fat | 22.05 | | **Minerals** | | |
| Protein | 12.86 g | | Boron | — mcg | |
| Carbohydrates | 17.25 g | | Calcium | 447.37 mg | 44.74 |
| Dietary Fiber | 0.00 g | 0.00 | Chloride | 367.50 mg | |
| Soluble Fiber | 0.00 g | | Chromium | — mcg | — |
| Insoluble Fiber | 0.00 g | | Copper | 0.03 mg | 1.50 |
| Sugar – Total | 17.25 g | | Fluoride | — mg | — |
| Monosaccharides | 4.21 g | | Iodine | 87.22 mcg | 58.15 |
| Disaccharides | 11.17 g | | Iron | 0.20 mg | 1.11 |
| Other Carbs | 0.00 g | | Magnesium | 42.75 mg | 10.69 |
| Fat – Total | 43.80 g | | Manganese | 0.01 mg | 0.50 |
| Saturated Fat | 2.45 g | | Molybdenum | 11.27 mcg | 15.03 |
| Mono Fat | 1.04 g | | Phosphorus | 351.58 mg | 35.16 |
| Poly Fat | 0.11 g | | Potassium | 572.81 mg | |
| Omega-3 Fatty Acids | 0.03 g | 1.20 | Selenium | 8.09 mcg | 11.56 |
| Omega-6 Fatty Acids | 0.08 g | | Sodium | 171.99 mg | |
| Trans Fatty Acids | 0.08 g | | Zinc | 2.18 mg | 14.53 |
| Cholesterol | 14.95 mg | | | | |
| Water | 208.42 g | | **Amino Acids** | | |
| Ash | 2.67 g | | Alanine | 0.50 g | |
| | | | Arginine | 0.35 g | |
| | | | Aspartate | 0.93 g | |
| **Vitamins** | | | Cystine | 0.11 g | 26.83 |
| Vitamin A IU | 161.70 IU | 3.23 | Glutamate | 2.30 g | |
| Vitamin A RE | 39.20 RE | | Glycine | 0.28 g | |
| A - Carotenoid | 2.45 RE | 0.03 | Histidine | 0.29 g | 22.48 |
| A - Retinol | 36.75 RE | | Isoleucine | 0.64 g | 55.65 |
| B1 Thiamin | 0.11 mg | 7.33 | Leucine | 1.18 g | 46.64 |
| B2 Riboflavin | 0.52 mg | 30.59 | Lysine | 1.05 g | 44.68 |
| B3 Niacin | 0.28 mg | 1.40 | Methionine | 0.35 g | 47.30 |
| Niacin Equiv | 1.30 mg | | Phenylalanine | 0.64 g | 53.78 |
| Vitamin B6 | 0.12 mg | 6.00 | Proline | 1.39 g | |
| Vitamin B12 | 1.38 mcg | 23.00 | Serine | 0.73 g | |
| Biotin | 7.35 mcg | 2.45 | Threonine | 0.48 g | 38.71 |
| Vitamin C | 1.96 mg | 3.27 | Tryptophan | 0.06 g | 18.75 |
| Vitamin D IU | 3.90 IU | 0.98 | Tyrosine | 0.59 g | 60.82 |
| Vitamin D mcg | 0.10 mcg | | Valine | 0.97 g | 65.99 |
| Vitamin E Alpha Equiv | 0.10 mg | 0.50 | | | |
| Vitamin E IU | 0.15 IU | | | | |
| Vitamin E mg | 0.10 mg | | | | |
| Folate | 27.44 mcg | 6.86 | | | |
| Vitamin K | 0.49 mcg | 0.61 | | | |

(Note: "–" indicates data is unavailable. For more information, please see page 806.)

STEP-BY-STEP RECIPE
## The Healthiest Ways of Preparing Yogurt

# *Ginger Yogurt with Fruit*

*The ginger adds a delicious twist to the blend of banana and Yogurt.*

1 large papaya, diced
1 banana, sliced
1 cup seedless grapes
1/4 cup sliced almonds

Sauce:
3/4 cup low-fat plain Yogurt
2 large ripe bananas
2 tsp fresh ginger, grated

1. Blend together Yogurt, 2 bananas and ginger in blender.
2. Divide papaya, banana and grapes between two bowls.
3. Pour blended Yogurt over fruit and top with sliced almonds.

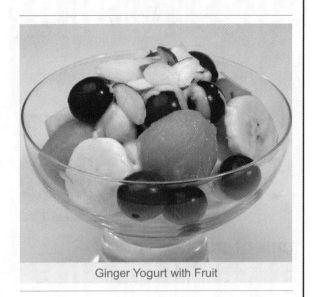
Ginger Yogurt with Fruit

**Preparation Hint:** For best flavor, make sure you use ripe bananas. Using two large ones makes this blend thicker and richer.

**SERVES 2**

Please write (address on back cover flap) or e-mail me at info@whfoods.org with your personal ideas for preparing Yogurt, and I will share them with others through our website at www.whfoods.org.

## 11 QUICK SERVING IDEAS for YOGURT:

1. Mix cold cereal or granola with Yogurt for a twist on the traditional cereal and milk breakfast.
2. Top waffles or pancakes with a dollop (or two) of plain Yogurt and then sprinkle on your favorite nuts and fruits.
3. **Fruit Smoothie:** Blend sliced banana, strawberries and ice cubes with Yogurt.
4. **Spicy Smoothie:** In a blender, combine 1 cup Yogurt, 1 tsp chopped fresh ginger, 1 medium banana, 1 tsp ground cardamom, 1 TBS honey, 1 TBS cocoa powder and 3 TBS water to cover. Blend on medium speed for 1 minute.
5. **Yogurt Chocolate Sauce:** Combine 1 cup Yogurt, 3 TBS cocoa powder and 1 TBS honey for a quick chocolate sauce—delicious served with strawberries or as a pudding!
6. **Yogurt Parfait:** Yogurt parfaits are a visual as well as delicious treats. In a large wine glass, alternate layers of Yogurt and your favorite fruit.
7. **Yogurt Salad Dressing:** Yogurt is a great base for salad dressings. Simply place plain Yogurt in the blender with a little water. With the blender running, slowly pour in extra virgin olive oil to achieve desired consistency. Add your favorite herbs and spices, and sea salt and pepper to taste.
8. **Creamy Mediterranean Salad Dressing:** Stir 2 TBS of low-fat plain Yogurt into the Healthy Vinaigrette Dressing (see page 143) to make it creamy.
9. **Tangy Yogurt Sauce:** Add 1 tsp fennel seeds, 1 tsp cumin seeds and a pinch of red pepper flakes to 1 cup plain Yogurt and let set in the refrigerator for at least 1/2 hour. It makes a tasty sauce for poultry and vegetables.
10. **Indian Cucumber and Yogurt Salad (Raita):** Add 1 large finely chopped cucumber and 1/2 tsp dill weed to 2 cups plain Yogurt. Season with sea salt and pepper. Eat this delicious and cooling salad as is or use as an accompaniment to grilled chicken or lamb.
11. **Creamy Virgin Mary:** Blend 2 fresh ripe tomatoes, 2 stalks celery, flesh of a small jalapeño pepper, juice of 1/2 lemon or lime, 1/2 cup water, 1/2 cup low-fat plain Yogurt, tamari (soy sauce) and cayenne pepper to taste. Blend on high for 2 minutes for a refreshing cocktail.

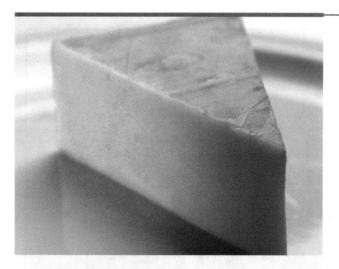

# low-fat cheese

| | |
|---|---|
| AVAILABILITY: | Year-round |
| REFRIGERATE: | Yes |
| SHELF LIFE: | Check use-by date |
| PREPARATION: | Minimal |

## nutrient-richness chart

Total Nutrient-Richness: **9**
One oz-wt (28.35 grams) of Low-Fat Mozzarella Cheese contains
72 calories

| NUTRIENT | AMOUNT | %DV | DENSITY | QUALITY |
|---|---|---|---|---|
| Tryptophan | 0.08 g | 25.0 | 6.2 | very good |
| Calcium | 183.06 mg | 18.3 | 4.6 | very good |
| Protein | 6.88 g | 13.8 | 3.4 | very good |
| Phosphorus | 131.26 mg | 13.1 | 3.3 | good |
| Iodine | 10.09 mcg | 6.7 | 1.7 | good |
| Selenium | 4.08 mcg | 5.8 | 1.5 | good |

"%DV" based on daily intake of 1,800 calories
For more on "Total Nutrient-Richness," "%DV," "Density," and
The World's Healthiest Foods "Quality" Rating System, see page 805

The discovery of creating Cheese from milk is believed to date back more than 10,000 years. The legend tells of an Arabian traveler who placed milk in a canteen made from sheep's stomach that he was carrying during a journey across the desert. To his surprise, after several hours he found that the sun's heat and the coagulating enzymes in the milk had changed the milk into Cheese curds. Today, Cheese is one of the most prized and enjoyed foods in the world and a quick and easy addition to your "Healthiest Way of Eating." With over 1,000 different varieties of Cheese available, varying in flavor, aroma and nutritional value, a Cheese can be found to suit almost any taste. I want to share with you how to select and store your Cheese to maintain its freshness and flavor and to maximize your enjoyment of this wonderful food.

## why low-fat cheese should be part of your healthiest way of eating

While Cheese is a rich source of protein, vitamins and minerals, its one drawback can be its high fat content. That is why it is specifically Low-Fat Cheese that has been included as one of the World's Healthiest Foods. Low-Fat Cheese provides the nutritional benefits of whole-fat Cheese with less concern over excessive amounts of fat, especially saturated fat. Like other milk products, Low-Fat Cheese is a very good source of the calcium that is important for bone health. (For more on the *Health Benefits of Low-Fat Cheese* and a complete analysis of its content of over 60 nutrients, see page 650.)

## varieties of low-fat cheese

The process of making Cheese is considered an art, akin to winemaking. While all Cheese is made from the same raw ingredient—the milk of an animal, such as a cow, sheep or goat—there are many different varieties of Cheese throughout the world, all of which feature unique tastes, textures and processing methods. New varieties of Low-Fat and Fat-Free Cheese can often be found at the market. Some of the most popular and familiar varieties include:

**LOW-FAT MOZZARELLA CHEESE**
You can also find this in a fat-free version.

**LOW-FAT CREAM CHEESE**
You can also find this in a fat-free version.

**LOW-FAT COTTAGE CHEESE**
You can also find this in a fat-free version.

**LOW-FAT RICOTTA CHEESE**
You can also find this in a fat-free version.

**LOW-FAT SWISS AND CHEDDAR CHEESE AND OTHERS**
The low-fat versions of these familiar cheeses are becoming tastier and more readily available.

1. The Best Way to Select
2. The Best Way to Store
3. The Best Way to Prepare

## the peak season
Low-Fat Cheese is available throughout the year.

## biochemical considerations
The milk sugar, lactose, found in cow's milk from which Cheese is made is associated with hypersensitivity reactions for some individuals. Some individuals are also allergic to the casein found in dairy products. There has been some concern over cows that may be treated with a compound called recombinant bovine growth hormone, rBGH. The best way to ensure that the Low-Fat Cheese you buy is not made from milk from cows treated with rBGH is to buy organic dairy products. (For more on *Food Allergies*, see page 719; and *rBGH*, see page 728.)

## 3 steps for the best tasting and most nutritious low-fat cheese
Enjoying the best tasting Low-Fat Cheese is simple if you just follow my 3 easy steps:

---

**THE AMOUNT OF LACTOSE IN DIFFERENT TYPES OF CHEESE**

Cow's milk contains a special sugar called lactose. An enzyme called *lactase* is needed to digest this special sugar. Many individuals throughout the world do not produce large enough supplies of this enzyme to keep up with their intake of dairy products containing lactose.

While a cup of cow's milk contains about 10–12 grams of lactose, the bacteria used to produce cheese and the time required for cheese to ferment both work to lower lactose levels. Soft cheeses typically have only half as much lactose as the milk from which they are made, and sometimes even less. Aged cheeses, including most hard cheeses, have less lactose still. For example, an ounce of Swiss cheese or cheddar cheese typically has less than one gram of lactose (Parmesan cheese has even less)—a safe level of lactose intake for most individuals, even those who are lactose intolerant.

---

# 1. the best way to select low-fat cheese

If your market has a Cheese department, speak with the person who specializes in Cheese. She or he can help you select the best quality Low-Fat Cheese as well as introduce you to different varieties of Low-Fat Cheese, which will help expand your repertoire and increase your appreciation for this wonderful food. Low-Fat Cheese from organic milk is becoming more widely available.

# 2. the best way to store low-fat cheese

All Cheese, regardless of variety, should be well wrapped and kept in the warmest section of the refrigerator. (The refrigerator door is often one of the warmest spots). Shelf life is related to the moisture content of the Cheese; therefore, soft Cheese will not keep as long as firm or semi-firm Cheese. In general, firm and semi-firm Cheese will keep for two weeks while soft, bleu and grated Cheese will keep for about one week. It is best to follow the use-by date on the package.

# 3. the best way to prepare low-fat cheese

If your recipe calls for grated Low-Fat Cheese, use Cheese that has a firm texture since it is the only kind suitable for grating. It will be easier to grate if it is has been kept cold in the refrigerator.

For all other purposes, it is best to remove Cheese from the refrigerator at least thirty minutes before using as Cheese has better flavor when it is a bit warmer.

If you are using Mozzarella, add lemon juice or white wine when cooking to prevent it from getting stringy.

To help cut Mozzarella, use an egg slicer. Place the Mozzarella ball in the cradle and slice it. Turn the sliced Cheese around 90 degrees (at a right angle) to get julienned pieces.

# health benefits of low-fat cheese

## Promotes Bone Health

Low-Fat Cheese is a very good source of calcium, a mineral vital to promoting optimal bone health. When dietary intake of calcium is too low to maintain adequate blood levels of calcium, calcium stores are drawn out of the bones to maintain normal blood concentrations. If a person's diet does not supply adequate calcium for many years, this situation can result in osteoporosis. Since calcium also plays a role in many other vital physiological activities, including blood clotting, nerve conduction, muscle contraction, regulation of enzyme activity and cell membrane function, eating calcium-rich foods like Low-Fat Cheese also has many other beneficial health-promoting effects.

## Important Protein Source

Low-Fat Cheese is a very good source of low-cost, high-quality protein. Our body needs protein to build its structure —including muscles and tissues—as well as compounds such as enzymes and molecules that transport nutrients throughout the body. Plus, protein provides us with a source of slow-burning energy to power our cells.

## Promotes Healthy Thyroid Function

Low-Fat Cheese is a good source of iodine, which is a component of the thyroid hormones thyroxine (T4) and tri-iodothyronine (T3). Without sufficient supplies of iodine, the body cannot synthesize these hormones. Because thyroid hormones regulate metabolic activity in every cell of the body and play a role in virtually all physiological functions, an iodine deficiency can have a devastating impact on health and well-being. Low-Fat Cheese is also a good source of selenium, which is necessary for thyroid hormone metabolism.

## Promotes Optimal Health

In addition to its role in thyroid hormone metabolism, the selenium provided by Low-Fat Cheese is also an essential component of other major metabolic pathways, including antioxidant defense systems and immune function. Accumulated evidence from prospective studies, intervention trials and studies on animal models of cancer has suggested a strong inverse correlation between selenium intake and cancer incidence.

## Promotes Energy Production

Low-Fat Cheese is also a good source of the mineral phosphorus. One of the key roles that phosphorus plays is promoting efficient energy production by being an integral component of the molecule ATP (adenosine triphosphate). ATP is the molecule that fuels the chemical reactions in our body's cells.

## Additional Health-Promoting Benefit of Low-Fat Cheese

Low-Fat Cheese contains sleep-promoting tryptophan.

### Nutritional Analysis of 1 oz-wt of low-fat Mozzarella Cheese:

| NUTRIENT | AMOUNT | % DAILY VALUE | NUTRIENT | AMOUNT | % DAILY VALUE |
|---|---|---|---|---|---|
| Calories | 72.08 | | Pantothenic Acid | 0.02 mg | 0.20 |
| Calories from Fat | 40.62 | | | | |
| Calories from Saturated Fat | 25.81 | | **Minerals** | | |
| Protein | 6.88 g | | Boron | — mcg | |
| Carbohydrates | 0.79 g | | Calcium | 183.06 mg | 18.31 |
| Dietary Fiber | 0.00 g | 0.00 | Chloride | 238.14 mg | |
| Soluble Fiber | 0.00 g | | Chromium | — mcg | — |
| Insoluble Fiber | 0.00 g | | Copper | 0.01 mg | 0.50 |
| Sugar – Total | 0.79 g | | Fluoride | — mg | — |
| Monosaccharides | 0.00 g | | Iodine | 10.09 mcg | 6.73 |
| Disaccharides | 0.00 g | | Iron | 0.06 mg | 0.33 |
| Other Carbs | 0.00 g | | Magnesium | 6.58 mg | 1.65 |
| Fat – Total | 4.51 g | | Manganese | 0.00 mg | 0.00 |
| Saturated Fat | 2.87 g | | Molybdenum | 1.30 mcg | 1.73 |
| Mono Fat | 1.28 g | | Phosphorus | 131.26 mg | 13.13 |
| Poly Fat | 0.13 g | | Potassium | 23.73 mg | |
| Omega-3 Fatty Acids | 0.04 g | 1.60 | Selenium | 4.08 mcg | 5.83 |
| Omega-6 Fatty Acids | 0.09 g | | Sodium | 132.11 mg | |
| Trans Fatty Acids | — g | | Zinc | 0.78 mg | 5.20 |
| Cholesterol | 16.39 mg | | | | |
| Water | 15.25 g | | **Amino Acids** | | |
| Ash | 0.93 g | | Alanine | 0.19 g | |
| | | | Arginine | 0.27 g | |
| **Vitamins** | | | Aspartate | 0.45 g | |
| Vitamin A IU | 165.56 IU | 3.31 | Cystine | 0.04 g | 9.76 |
| Vitamin A RE | 50.18 RE | | Glutamate | 1.46 g | |
| A - Carotenoid | 11.34 RE | 0.15 | Glycine | 0.12 g | |
| A - Retinol | 38.84 RE | | Histidine | 0.23 g | 17.83 |
| B1 Thiamin | 0.01 mg | 0.67 | Isoleucine | 0.30 g | 26.09 |
| B2 Riboflavin | 0.09 mg | 5.29 | Leucine | 0.61 g | 24.11 |
| B3 Niacin | 0.03 mg | 0.15 | Lysine | 0.63 g | 26.81 |
| Niacin Equiv | 1.35 mg | | Methionine | 0.17 g | 22.97 |
| Vitamin B6 | 0.02 mg | 1.00 | Phenylalanine | 0.33 g | 27.73 |
| Vitamin B12 | 0.23 mcg | 3.83 | Proline | 0.64 g | |
| Biotin | 1.11 mcg | 0.37 | Serine | 0.36 g | |
| Vitamin C | 0.00 mg | 0.00 | Threonine | 0.24 g | 19.35 |
| Vitamin D IU | 1.40 IU | 0.35 | Tryptophan | 0.08 g | 25.00 |
| Vitamin D mcg | 0.03 mcg | | Tyrosine | 0.36 g | 37.11 |
| Vitamin E Alpha Equiv | 0.12 mg | 0.60 | Valine | 0.39 g | 26.53 |
| Vitamin E IU | 0.18 IU | | | | |
| Vitamin E mg | 0.18 mg | | | | |
| Folate | 2.49 mcg | 0.62 | | | |
| Vitamin K | — mcg | — | | | |

(Note: "–" indicates data is unavailable. For more information, please see page 806.)

STEP-BY-STEP RECIPE
## The Healthiest Ways to Use Low-Fat Cheese

### Mexican Cheese Salad

*Add extra nutrition to your salad by adding grated Low-Fat Cheese.*

1 head romaine lettuce
1 15-oz can black or pinto beans,
    rinsed and drained
1 medium avocado, cubed
1 medium tomato, diced
2 oz Low-Fat Cheddar Cheese, grated
Salsa
Lime wedges

1. Chop lettuce and place on salad plate. Sprinkle beans, avocado and tomato over lettuce.

2. Top with Cheddar Cheese, your favorite salsa and the juice of lime wedges.    **SERVES 2**

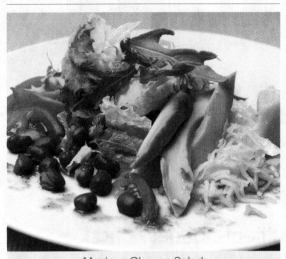
Mexican Cheese Salad

Please write (address on back cover flap) or e-mail me at info@whfoods.org with your personal ideas for preparing Low-Fat Cheese, and I will share them with others through our website at www.whfoods.org.

### 12 QUICK SERVING IDEAS for LOW-FAT CHEESE:

*It is best to serve cheese at room temperature.*

1. **Most Popular: Classic Italian Salad.** Arrange slices of Low-Fat Mozzarella Cheese, thinly sliced red or sweet onion and tomato on a platter. Top with thinly sliced fresh basil leaves, olive oil and balsamic vinegar, and sprinkle with sea salt and black pepper.

2. For breakfast, add Low-Fat Cheese to a frittata or use as a topping on poached eggs.

3. Grated Low-Fat Cheese is delicious on cooked greens.

4. Marinate Low-Fat Cheese (such as feta or goat cheese), oregano and basil in extra virgin olive oil. Serve with olives as an appetizer or accompaniment to salad.

5. Combine Low-Fat Cottage Cheese with chili powder, ground cumin and cayenne pepper to taste. Serve with celery and cucumber sticks.

6. Add your favorite Low-Fat Cheese to a green salad for a nutritious, quick meal.

7. **Orange and Fennel Salad:** Combine 1 thinly sliced fennel bulb and pieces of 1 orange and top with grated Low-Fat Parmesan Cheese.

8. **Healthy Pizza:** Sprinkle Low-Fat Mozzarella Cheese on a whole wheat pita, top with tomato sauce and your favorite vegetables and cook in toaster oven until the Cheese melts.

9. **Stuffed Tomato and Low-Fat Cottage Cheese:** Combine Low-Fat Cottage Cheese with plenty of fresh herbs or pesto. Spoon into a hollowed out tomato.

10. **Lentil Salad:** Combine 2 oz grated Low-Fat Cheese with 2 cups chilled cooked lentils, 1/2 minced medium red onion, 1 diced small green bell pepper and Healthy Vinaigrette (see page 143) for a delicious cold salad.

11. **Cheese and Fruit:** Low-Fat Cheese makes a delightful pairing with fruits such as apples, pears and melons. Serve as an appetizer or dessert.

12. **Summer Fruit Sundae:** Make a fruit salad using ripe summer fruits, and top with a scoop of Low-Fat Cottage Cheese, fresh mint leaves and walnuts.

Q *What would you recommend as the healthiest type of Cheese to eat, both plain and on sandwiches and salads?*

A Since most of the concern with Cheese is its high fat content, I recommend selecting a Low-Fat Cheese, such as Low-Fat Mozzarella, to include in your diet. Low-Fat Mozzarella can be eaten plain and on sandwiches and salad.

Hard Cheeses (such as fresh Parmesan) are usually lower in fat than soft Cheeses, but they are best used for grating. They can be used for salads, but they are not practical for sandwiches. If you are not overly concerned with your saturated fat intake and cholesterol levels, you can probably enjoy a variety of different types of Cheeses if consumed in moderation. When possible, I like to buy organic Cheese.

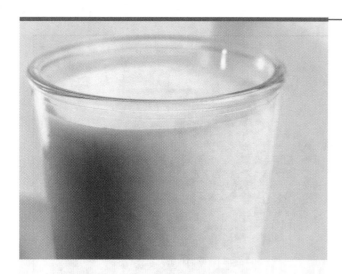

## nutrient-richness chart

Total Nutrient-Richness: **8**
One cup (244 grams) of Goat's Milk contains 168 calories

| NUTRIENT | AMOUNT | %DV | DENSITY | QUALITY |
|---|---|---|---|---|
| Tryptophan | 0.1 g | 34.4 | 3.7 | very good |
| Calcium | 325.7 mg | 32.6 | 3.5 | very good |
| Phosphorus | 270.1 mg | 27.0 | 2.9 | good |
| B2 Riboflavin | 0.3 mg | 20.0 | 2.1 | good |
| Protein | 8.7 g | 17.4 | 1.9 | good |
| Potassium | 498.7 mg | 14.2 | 1.5 | good |

For more on "Total Nutrient-Richness," "%DV," "Density," and
The World's Healthiest Foods "Quality" Rating System, see page 805.

Goat's Milk and cheese were so highly revered in ancient Egypt that they were among the many treasures placed in the burial chambers of the pharaohs. Although Americans are traditionally brought up on cow's milk, Goat's Milk is actually more widely consumed in most other parts of the world. The fat globules in cow's milk tend to separate to the surface, but the globules in Goat's Milk are much smaller and will remain suspended in solution, so unlike cow's milk, Goat's Milk does not need to be homogenized. Goat's Milk has a delicious slightly sweet, slightly salty taste and can be used as a substitute for cow's milk in your "Healthiest Way of Eating."

## why goat's milk should be part of your healthiest way of eating

Goat's Milk can serve as an alternative to cow's milk, and some individuals who cannot tolerate cow's milk can sometimes drink Goat's Milk. It also contains more calcium and protein than cow's milk. (For more on the *Health Benefits of Goat's Milk* and a complete analysis of its content of over 60 nutrients, see page 653.)

# goat's milk

## highlights

| | |
|---|---|
| AVAILABILITY: | Year-round |
| REFRIGERATE: | Yes |
| SHELF LIFE: | Check use-by date |
| PREPARATION: | Minimal |

## varieties of goat's milk

### GOAT'S MILK
Goat's Milk comes with different amounts of butterfat and is available fresh, powdered, as canned evaporated milk or as ultra heat treated (UHT) milk in aseptic containers.

### GOAT CHEESE
Goat Cheese has fewer calories than cheese made from cow's milk and has a stronger flavor. Young Goat Cheese has a pleasant tartness with a slightly gummy texture. Goat Cheese increases in gumminess as it is aged.

### GOAT YOGURT
Goat Yogurt has a fuller flavor than yogurt made from cow's milk.

## the peak season

Goat's Milk is available throughout the year.

## biochemical considerations

The milk sugar, lactose, and the small amount of casein found in Goat's Milk may be associated with allergic reactions for some individuals. Goat's Milk is slightly lower in lactose than cow's milk, with 4.1% milk solids as lactose versus 4.7% in cow's milk. (For more on *Lactose Intolerance*, see page 722.)

## 3 steps for the best tasting and most nutritious goat's milk

Enjoying the best tasting Goat's Milk is simple if you just follow my 3 easy steps:

1. The Best Way to Select
2. The Best Way to Store
3. The Best Way to Prepare

# 1. the best way to select goat's milk

When purchasing Goat's Milk, use the "sell-by" date as a guide to the shelf life of the milk. Smell the top of the container to make sure that the milk does not smell spoiled as it may have been stored for a period of time outside of the refrigerator. Select Goat's Milk from the lowest part of the refrigerator case as this is usually the coldest section.

Although Goat's Milk comes in a variety of forms, fresh is best for drinking and for making delicate desserts. Dried, canned and those in aseptic packages pick up an unpleasant caramelized flavor when they're heated for packaging.

# 2. the best way to store goat's milk

Goat's Milk should always be refrigerated (34–40°F or 1–4°C) because warm temperatures can cause it to turn sour quickly. Always seal or close the milk container when storing it to prevent it from absorbing the aromas of other foods in the refrigerator. Avoid storing Goat's Milk in the refrigerator door since this exposes it to too much warm air each time the refrigerator is opened and closed.

# 3. the best way to prepare goat's milk

Fresh Goat's Milk requires no preparation; just pour it from the container.

# health benefits of goat's milk

## Allergy-Free Alternative to Cow's Milk

In addition to being a concentrated source of many nutrients, one of the great benefits of Goat's Milk is that many people who cannot tolerate cow's milk can often drink Goat's Milk without any problems. Allergy to cow's milk has been related to conditions such as recurrent ear infections, asthma, eczema and even rheumatoid arthritis. Replacing cow's milk with Goat's Milk may help reduce some of the symptoms associated with these conditions. Additionally, Goat's Milk provides more protein per cup than cow's milk.

Goat's Milk can sometimes be used as a replacement for cow's milk in formulas designed for infants that have difficulties with dairy products, although it is lacking in several nutrients that are necessary for growing infants. Therefore, parents interested in substituting Goat's Milk for cow's milk-based formula for their infants should ask their pediatrician or other qualified healthcare practitioner for recipes and ways to provide the missing nutrients.

## Promotes Bone Health

Goat's Milk is a very good source of calcium, a mineral that is extremely important for maintaining the strength and structure of our bones. When our diets do not contain enough calcium, it leaches from our bones into our bloodstream to support physiological functions in other parts of our body. Since this can lead to a weakening of the bones, maintaining an adequate dietary supply of calcium is very important to health.

## Important Protein Source

Goat's Milk is a good source of high-quality protein. Our bodies use dietary protein to build our muscles and tissues as well as chemicals such as enzymes and transport proteins that are integral to optimal health. Protein also gives us slow burning energy that helps us to feel our best.

## Promotes Heart Health

Goat's Milk is a good source of potassium, a mineral essential for maintaining normal blood pressure and heart function. The effectiveness of potassium-rich foods in lowering blood pressure has been demonstrated by a number of studies.

## Promotes Energy Production

Goat's Milk is a good source of two nutrients important in the production of cellular energy—phosphorus and vitamin B2 (riboflavin). Phosphorus is needed to make ATP (adenosine triphosphate), the molecule that serves as the fuel for cellular activity. Riboflavin is a component of the flavoprotein enzymes that allow oxygen-based energy production to occur. In addition, riboflavin-based enzymes also have antioxidant activity.

## Additional Health-Promoting Benefits from Goat's Milk

Goat's Milk is also a concentrated source of sleep-promoting tryptophan.

*(Nutritional Analysis Chart follows on the next page.)*

# Q Is Goat's Milk better for us than cow's milk?

A Goat's Milk is a nutrient-rich food, which is why I included it as one of the World's Healthiest Foods. According to the Food Rating System, Goat's Milk is a very good source of calcium and tryptophan, and a good source of protein, vitamin B2, potassium and phosphorus.

## Nutritional Analysis of 1 cup of Goat's Milk:

| NUTRIENT | AMOUNT | % DAILY VALUE | NUTRIENT | AMOUNT | % DAILY VALUE |
|---|---|---|---|---|---|
| Calories | 167.90 | | Pantothenic Acid | 0.76 mg | 7.60 |
| Calories from Fat | 90.91 | | | | |
| Calories from Saturated Fat | 58.57 | | **Minerals** | | |
| Protein | 8.69 g | | Boron | — mcg | |
| Carbohydrates | 10.86 g | | Calcium | 325.74 mg | 32.57 |
| Dietary Fiber | 0.00 g | 0.00 | Chloride | 427.00 mg | |
| Soluble Fiber | 0.00 g | | Chromium | — mcg | |
| Insoluble Fiber | 0.00 g | | Copper | 0.11 mg | 5.50 |
| Sugar – Total | 10.86 g | | Fluoride | — mg | — |
| Monosaccharides | — g | | Iodine | — mcg | — |
| Disaccharides | — g | | Iron | 0.12 mg | 0.67 |
| Other Carbs | 0.00 g | | Magnesium | 34.09 mg | 8.52 |
| Fat – Total | 10.10 g | | Manganese | 0.04 mg | 2.00 |
| Saturated Fat | 6.51 g | | Molybdenum | — mcg | — |
| Mono Fat | 2.71 g | | Phosphorus | 270.11 mg | 27.01 |
| Poly Fat | 0.36 g | | Potassium | 498.74 mg | |
| Omega-3 Fatty Acids | 0.10 g | 4.00 | Selenium | 3.42 mcg | 4.89 |
| Omega-6 Fatty Acids | 0.27 g | | Sodium | 121.51 mg | |
| Trans Fatty Acids | 0.29 g | | Zinc | 0.73 mg | 4.87 |
| Cholesterol | 27.82 mg | | | | |
| Water | 212.35 g | | **Amino Acids** | | |
| Ash | 2.00 g | | Alanine | 0.29 g | |
| | | | Arginine | 0.29 g | |
| **Vitamins** | | | Aspartate | 0.51 g | |
| Vitamin A IU | 451.40 IU | 9.03 | Cystine | 0.11 g | 26.83 |
| Vitamin A RE | 136.64 RE | | Glutamate | 1.53 g | |
| A - Carotenoid | 0.00 RE | 0.00 | Glycine | 0.12 g | |
| A - Retinol | 136.64 RE | | Histidine | 0.22 g | 17.05 |
| B1 Thiamin | 0.12 mg | 8.00 | Isoleucine | 0.51 g | 44.35 |
| B2 Riboflavin | 0.34 mg | 20.00 | Leucine | 0.77 g | 30.43 |
| B3 Niacin | 0.68 mg | 3.40 | Lysine | 0.71 g | 30.21 |
| Niacin Equiv | 2.46 mg | | Methionine | 0.20 g | 27.03 |
| Vitamin B6 | 0.11 mg | 5.50 | Phenylalanine | 0.38 g | 31.93 |
| Vitamin B12 | 0.16 mcg | 2.67 | Proline | 0.90 g | |
| Biotin | 8.54 mcg | 2.85 | Serine | 0.44 g | |
| Vitamin C | 3.15 mg | 5.25 | Threonine | 0.40 g | 32.26 |
| Vitamin D IU | 29.28 IU | 7.32 | Tryptophan | 0.11 g | 34.38 |
| Vitamin D mcg | 0.73 mcg | | Tyrosine | 0.44 g | 45.36 |
| Vitamin E Alpha Equiv | 0.22 mg | 1.10 | Valine | 0.59 g | 40.14 |
| Vitamin E IU | 0.33 IU | | | | |
| Vitamin E mg | 0.22 mg | | | | |
| Folate | 1.46 mcg | 0.36 | | | |
| Vitamin K | 0.73 mcg | 0.91 | | | |

(Note: "–" indicates data is unavailable. For more information, please see page 806.)

Generally speaking, it is not necessarily better than cow's milk nor is cow's milk necessarily better. That is because "which one is better" depends upon the individual consuming it and their nutrient needs. For example, for individuals who are allergic to cow's milk, Goat's Milk can serve as a great dairy alternative. Other people, including those for whom cow's milk is not a problem, may enjoy this food and the many nutrients that it includes, some of which are at a higher level than found in cow's milk.

Yet, please remember that Goat's Milk is lacking in several nutrients that are necessary for growing infants, so parents interested in trying Goat's Milk instead of cow's milk-based formula for their infants should ask their pediatricians or other qualified healthcare practitioners for recipes and ways to add these important and vital nutrients to their child's diet.

# Q Does Goat's Milk contain the protein casein?

A Goat's Milk does contain casein. Yet, researchers have found that it generally has only trace amounts of a specific casein, alpha-s1-casein, which is thought to be one of the main proteins in cow's milk responsible for eliciting sensitivity reactions. This may be one of the reasons responsible for the finding that many people who are sensitive to cow's milk can tolerate Goat's Milk.

# Q How long can regular Milk be left unrefrigerated and still be OK to drink?

A While variables like temperature affect exactly how long Milk can be kept outside of the refrigerator, a few hours would be the maximum. Smelling the Milk may be your best test to see whether it has gone bad. If it smells sour or acidic, it would be best to discard it.

# Q Does frozen yogurt contain the same levels of live bacteria and other healthy characteristics as yogurt?

A The important thing when it comes to frozen yogurt (and all foods, actually) is to read the ingredients label. For example, many frozen yogurt products are really not all that different than frozen ice cream desserts. They are loaded with sugars, calories and fats—I would not consider healthy treats.

Yet, you can find some frozen yogurts that are of good
(Continued on bottom of Page 655)

STEP-BY-STEP RECIPE

## The Healthiest Ways to Use Goat's Milk, Goat Cheese, and Goat Yogurt

# Goat Cheese and Pear Salad

*Goat Cheese is a great addition to almost any salad.*

1 medium pear, sliced
1 Granny Smith apple, sliced
1 head romaine lettuce
2 oz Goat Cheese
2 TBS pumpkin seeds, chopped
2 TBS walnuts, chopped
Healthy Vinaigrette dressing (see page 143)

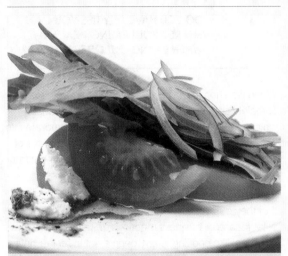

Tomato and Dandelion Greens with Goat Cheese

1. Slice pear and apple and chop lettuce.

2. Combine pear, apple and lettuce.

3. Top with crumbled Goat Cheese, pumpkin seeds and walnuts.

4. Toss with your favorite Healthy Vinaigrette (page 143).

SERVES **2**

Please write (address on backcover flap) or e-mail me at info@whfoods.org with your personal ideas for preparing Goat's Milk, and I will share them with others through our website at www.whfoods.org.

## 8 QUICK SERVING IDEAS for GOAT'S MILK, GOAT CHEESE and GOAT YOGURT:

1. **Most Popular: Goat Cheese Sauce for Vegetables:** Combine Goat Cheese thinned with low-fat milk, minced garlic, finely shredded basil and plenty of ground black pepper. Toss with cooked green beans or broccoli until well coated and serve with chicken or seafood (such as shrimp, scallops or fish).

2. Top your morning cereal with Goat's Milk or Goat's Milk Yogurt and your favorite fresh or dried fruit.

3. Add extra taste and protein to a vegetable sandwich by including some Goat Cheese.

4. Spread Goat Cheese on celery sticks, slices of fruit or whole grain crackers/bread.

5. Create an omelet filled with Goat Cheese, tomatoes and fresh thyme.

6. Fill a pita bread with shredded lettuce, chopped vegetables and crumbled Goat Cheese.

7. **Tomato and Dandelion Greens with Goat Cheese:** Make a pungent salad with tomatoes, avocado, dandelion greens, Goat Cheese and red onions. Toss with your favorite Vinaigrette (see page 143). (Pictured above.)

8. **Goat Cheese Appetizer:** Mix 1 cup Goat Cheese with 1/2 cup minced sundried tomatoes (oil-packed) and 2 TBS parsley or basil. Add salt and pepper to taste. Serve on toasted whole grain bread or crackers.

*(Continued from Page 654)*

quality. I would look for ones made from organic milk and those that state that they include active cultures. These active cultures — beneficial bacteria — do survive in cold temperatures, such as that of frozen yogurt. They remain in the dormant state and become active when they are exposed to suitable conditions, such as the higher temperature of our intestines, where they will grow and multiply.

# Q&A

**DO YOU HAVE ANY TIPS YOU CAN SHARE ABOUT EATING HEALTHY WHEN EATING OUT OR TRAVELING?**

When we shop for and cook our own food, we have complete control over what we eat. We can choose which of the World's Healthiest Foods to incorporate into our meals and decide which of the "Healthiest Ways of Cooking" methods we want to use to create a meal that will be brimming with taste and nutrient-richness.

Yet, for most people, home is not the only place that they eat. Whether it be for social gatherings, celebrations or business meetings or just because they don't feel like cooking, many people eat in restaurants where they can enjoy the experience of being served delicious meals. While eating out can be a delightful experience, it can also seem like a surefire way to not eat healthy since we don't have as much control over the ingredients and cooking preparation techniques as we do in our own kitchens.

Here are some tips on how you can continue to enjoy your "Healthiest Way of Eating" while eating out:

- If you have diet restrictions (i.e., vegetarian, salt-sensitive), communicate these to the waitstaff before ordering or call the restaurant ahead of time and ask the host if the chef will be able to accommodate your needs. Many restaurants will gladly accommodate a patron's specific needs, if they are reasonable and within the abilities of the kitchen, so you should not feel ashamed asking.

- If possible, avoid refined grain products such as bread, rolls and crackers. Oftentimes, a bread-basket will offer whole grain alternatives. If you usually butter your bread, ask for some olive oil instead into which you can dip your bread.

- Look for foods that are prepared with healthier cooking techniques. These include baked, broiled, poached, steamed, grilled or dry-sautéed. Yet, many times chefs will still use butter when preparing foods with these techniques. Ask the wait-person if butter is used and whether it can be limited or eliminated or a healthier type of oil can be substituted.

- Restaurants can be a great place to eat your vegetables. Ordering a vegetable side dish and a salad or vegetable-focused appetizer is sure to provide you with several servings of these nutrient-rich foods. If you feel that you have eaten adequate amounts of protein throughout the day or if your appetizer contains a good amount of protein, consider ordering an entrée that is vegetable-centric.

- The serving sizes of most restaurants are bigger than most people can, and should, eat. And while we may feel that we are getting our money's worth by ordering and eating large portions, we are also, unfortunately, getting our waistline's worth since we are consuming an overabundance of calories, and oftentimes fat. Remembering that the recommended size of a serving of meat, for example, is about the size of a deck of cards will help you to realize that the average restaurant's meal can provide you with meals for days to come.

- While salads made with organic baby greens have long been a favorite of many chefs who appreciate their superior quality of taste and appearance, more and more restaurants are featuring other organically grown ingredients on their menus. Ask the waitperson if any items on the menu are made with organically grown ingredients. Even if they are not, asking will communicate interest and may spur the restaurant to begin to incorporate organic ingredients into its menu.

- Many restaurants offer a starch side dish with their entrées. Inquire whether the restaurant offers whole grains, like brown rice, as an alternative. Your next best starch bet in terms of nutrition would be a baked potato with skin (holding the sour cream, of course) over other options such as French fries or white rice. Or skip the grain/starch side dish altogether.

- It is oftentimes hard to desert dessert. Yet, since the lively taste of fresh fruit is oftentimes just what our palate craves after a meal, what a delightful way to not only cap off a good meal but to provide our bodies with bursting amounts of nutrients than to enjoy a dessert of fresh fruit.

- Remember that each meal you eat, whether it be at a restaurant, friend's house or at your own home, is an opportunity not only for your senses to enjoy the gustatory experience of food but for your body to enjoy the benefits of foods that are nutrient-rich. Yet, it is also important to remember that each meal is just that—one meal. If you go to a restaurant and don't eat as many of the World's Healthiest Foods as you would have liked, remember that this meal does not stand alone. Each meal should be viewed not in isolation but as a part of a well-balanced diet, remembering that tomorrow brings yet another opportunity to enjoy the delicious taste of the nutrient-rich World's Healthiest Foods.

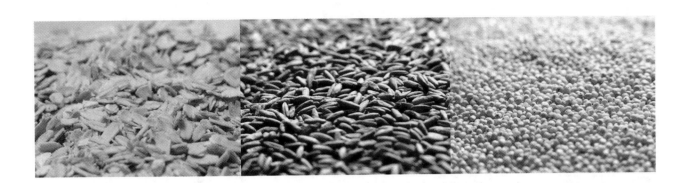

# whole grains

| NUTRIENT-RICHNESS | NAME | PAGE |
|---|---|---|
| 12 | Oats | 664 |
| 10 | Rye | 668 |
| 7 | Quinoa | 672 |
| 7 | Brown Rice | 676 |
| 7 | Whole Wheat | 682 |
| 5 | Buckwheat | 686 |

The numbers beside each food indicate their Total Nutrient-Richness. (For more details, see page 805.)

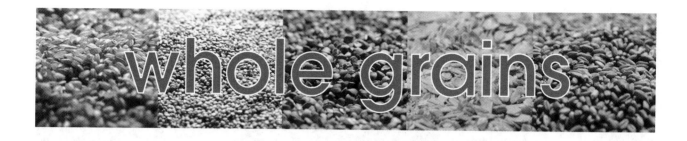

# whole grains

Creamy oatmeal, crunchy popcorn, crusty breads, snappy crackers, plates of pasta and steamy bowls of rice are just some of the grain-based foods that make frequent appearances in our daily meals.

Because high-carbohydrate diets have recently come under a lot of criticism in the popular press, and because grains are often viewed as key sources of carbohydrates, they have been called into question as contributors to obesity and diabetes. I feel that the problem isn't so much grains themselves (although I suspect that we've been routinely overconsuming them) but the fact that most of the grains eaten in the U.S. are overprocessed.

It is important to remember that all grain products are not created equal. For example, while whole wheat is one of the World's Healthiest Foods, refined wheat (referred to as "wheat" on food labels and used to make "white bread" and "wheat pasta") is not. Refined grains have been stripped of their germ and bran (the parts of the grain where their vitamins, minerals, healthy fats and fiber are concentrated) until virtually all that remains is starch; yet whole grains retain their full range of health-promoting nutrients. So, when choosing grains, it is important to remember one of the primary criteria that distinguish the World's Healthiest Foods—they are whole, unprocessed foods that provide the maximum nutritional value as well as the best flavor.

## Definition: Grains

Botanically speaking, grains such as wheat, rice and rye are the edible seeds of plants that belong to the grass family. However, when I refer to grains, I use a broader definition, which includes other "grain-like" foods, such as buckwheat and quinoa, that do not belong to the grass family.

## How Whole Grains Keep You Energized and Healthy

Whole grains provide an array of important nutrients including dietary fiber, vitamin E and minerals such as magnesium, iron and zinc. You can also count on most grains to be a rich source of the B complex vitamins, which is important because these vitamins work together synergistically to promote health. Additionally, whole grains are a low-fat source of many essential amino acids (although most do not contain much lysine); for example, a quarter cup of uncooked quinoa contains over 5 grams of protein and less than 160 calories.

Incorporating a variety of whole grains as a regular part of your menu is essential for providing energy and vitality. While it is well-known that athletes consume large quantities of complex carbohydrates like pasta and breads to provide them with extra energy resources, what is not well-known is that it's not only the carbohydrates that help their performance. Unless athletes are eating *whole* grain pastas and *whole* grain breads, however, they will not get the benefits of the essential energy-releasing nutrients found in the grain! Starchy complex carbohydrates, by themselves, aren't enough. It takes the vitamins and minerals that are locked in the germ and bran of grains to catalyze their transformation into usable energy. (For more on *Energy Production*, see page 76.)

## Potent Antioxidant Activity in Grains from Phytonutrients

The whole story of whole grains can't be told without appreciating the important health contribution of the newly discovered phytonutrients (plant nutrients) that they contain. These important nutrients are contained in the germ and bran of whole grains. Included among these phytonutrient compounds are ferulic and caffeic acids, saponins and lignans. Each of these phytonutrients has unique and varied health-promoting properties, including potent antioxidant activity. This is yet another reason why whole grains are so much better for you than refined, processed grains.

## It is Important to Read the Label

When it comes to bread, label reading is especially important. Bread can be sold as "whole wheat" even if 99% of its wheat flour is not made from whole wheat. As long as some of the bread is made from the whole grain, the bread can be sold as "whole wheat." Don't let this labeling loophole fool you! Be sure to choose bread that is labeled "100% whole wheat" instead of one that simply says "whole wheat." Always check the ingredient list. If "whole wheat flour" is not the only, or at least the first, flour ingredient listed, then the bread is made primarily of refined flour. "Wheat flour," the standard flour used in the U.S., is refined and bleached. "Unbleached flour" is simply refined flour that has not also been bleached; it is not a whole grain flour. (For more on this subject, see page 690.)

## Grains and Legumes— A Great Complete Protein Combination

Proteins are made up of building blocks called amino acids, all but nine of which our bodies can manufacture on its own. Called essential amino acids, these nine must be obtained from the food we eat. Most animal products, such as fish, eggs and dairy products, contain all the essential amino acids in sufficient amounts to form any needed protein and are therefore said to provide complete proteins. Most proteins from vegetables also contain all essential amino acids, yet they are usually very low in one or two, which is why they are called incomplete proteins.

For grains to be used to form a complete protein, they must be combined with other foods that can supply the amino acids in which they are low. For example, legumes will complement the amino acid profile of grains by supplying the amino acid lysine in which the grains are lacking. At the same time, most grains complement the amino acid profile of legumes by supplying the amino acid methionine in which legumes are usually low. Interestingly, the traditional meals of cultures around the world naturally combine foods that supply complete proteins. Beans and rice are enjoyed in Mexico, rice and soybeans in Asian countries and dried peas and rice in Mediterranean countries. So, not only do "beans and grains" make great nutritional sense, they make a tasty combination as well. It's not surprising when you think about the number of cultures throughout the world that rely upon this inexpensive combination of foods as their traditional protein source.

## Easy Ways to Eat 3–4 Servings of Whole Grains Per Day

The Food Guide Pyramid, developed by the United States Department of Agriculture (USDA) recommends a total of 6 to 11 servings of grains each day. However, people in Mediterranean countries, who are some of the healthiest in the world, eat 3 to 4 servings of grains per day.

## Serving Size of Whole Grains

1/2 cup cooked grains
slice of whole grain bread
1 cup of cooked whole grain pasta

## Glycemic Index

The glycemic index of a food is a measure of how fast insulin rises after 100 grams of the food have been eaten. As you might expect, whole grains have very different glycemic index values when compared to processed grains. Whole grains—and products made from them, like 100% whole grain breads—are slower to digest than processed grains, partly because of the fiber contained in the germ and the bran and partly because of their greater overall nutrient density. Because they are slower to leave the stomach and be digested, whole grains have a much lower glycemic index than processed grains. In addition, there is a "double whammy" effect on the glycemic index of products when they are made from processed grains and are also extensively cooked, as is the case with a plain bagel. A plain bagel made from highly processed (65% extraction) flour, which is both baked and boiled (as is the case with most bagels), will show up on the glycemic index in the 70–75 point range, whereas a slice of 100% whole wheat bread can show up as low as 50–55. (For more on the *Glycemic Index*, see page 342.)

## Every Grain May Not Be Good for Everybody

Wheat, one of the most popular grains, is one of the most widely consumed foods in the Western diet. It is also one of the foods most commonly associated with food allergies and food sensitivities. This can be very problematic because wheat is not only found in breads, baked goods and pastas, but it is also a common "hidden" ingredient in many processed foods. Wheat's ubiquitous nature may be one of the reasons that many people find they are increasingly sensitive to this food. (For more on *Food Allergies*, see page 719.)

One reason for including so many different grains among the World's Healthiest Foods is so you will have a wide selection of delicious whole grains to incorporate into your diet. It is important to not be overly reliant on any one grain. Not only will this make your diet more versatile and interesting, but it will reduce the chances that you will too frequently consume any one grain, which increases your likelihood of becoming sensitive to it.

## Familiar Grains Not Included as One of the World's Healthiest Foods

I have included six of the most commonly enjoyed grains on the list of the World's Healthiest Foods and described them in detail in their individual chapters. The two grains I describe below—barley and millet—are familiar to many people, but they are not as commonly used as the grains included on the list. Because they are both delicious and health-promoting grains, I did not want to totally neglect them in this book.

### BARLEY

Barley is one of the oldest domesticated grains and was held in such high esteem for its ability to increase strength that the Roman gladiators were known as *hordearii*, or "eaters of Barley." Barley is an especially good source of soluble fiber, including beta-glucan, which helps reduce cholesterol levels and support digestive health. Its concentration of dietary fiber and selenium also protect against various degenerative diseases.

Barley can be cooked with minimal effort. Combine 1 cup Barley, 3 cups water, add sea salt to taste, cover and bring to boil. Simmer for about 1 1/2 hours. If you are using prepackaged Barley, it is best to follow the directions on the package.

Here are some tips on how to enhance the flavor of Barley:

- Combine with your favorite nuts and seeds and fresh or dried fruit. Serve with soy or almond milk for an energizing breakfast.

- **BARLEY PILAF:** Prepare Barley with chicken or vegetable broth. After it's cooked, add extra virgin olive oil and "Healthy Sautéed" mushrooms to enhance its flavor. Top with toasted sesame seeds or almonds.

- **BARLEY STUFFED CABBAGE:** Season cooked Barley with chopped tomatoes, sliced scallions, chili powder, sea salt and pepper. Roll mixture in a steamed cabbage leaf.

### MILLET

While not widely consumed in the United States, Millet has been cultivated for 8,000 years and is an extremely important food staple in Africa, where finely ground Millet is used to make a traditional flatbread known as *injera*. Millet is a good source of both manganese and phosphorus, important minerals for bone health. It is also considered a gluten-free grain, so it can be enjoyed by those who cannot tolerate gluten-containing grains, such as wheat and rye.

Millet can be fluffy like rice or creamy like mashed potatoes. It makes a great side dish. Combine 1 cup Millet, 2 1/2 cups water or broth and sea salt to taste in a saucepan and bring to a boil. Turn heat to low, cover and simmer for about 20 minutes. If you are using prepackaged Millet, it is best to follow the directions on the package.

Here are some tips on how to enhance the flavor of Millet:

- Combine with your favorite nuts and seeds, fresh or dried fruit and serve with soy or almond milk for an energizing breakfast.

- **MILLET SALAD:** Combine cooked Millet with minced scallion, diced tomato, cucumbers sliced into 1/8-inch pieces, feta cheese, chopped mint and your favorite vinaigrette.

- **CREAMY INDIAN-STYLE MILLET:** If you want the Millet to have a more creamy consistency, stir it frequently, adding a little water every now and then. Combine with curry powder, tamari (soy sauce) and extra virgin olive oil. Toss in cooked peas and carrots.

## What's Old is New: The Growing Popularity of Ancient Grains

In the past few years, there has been an emergence of new varieties of whole grains into the marketplace. The increasing array of ancient grains into our modern-day market shelves is a welcome addition for those who are interested in healthy eating and are looking for an alternative to traditional wheat products. While I have not addressed these grains in their own individual chapters, owing to the fact that they are not yet as widely available, one of the criteria for a food to be included as a World's Healthiest Food, I wanted to make mention of them here in the Whole Grains Introduction. If you have a chance to try them, I suggest you do. They will add versatility, excitement and great nutritional value to your "Healthiest Way of Eating."

# whole grain cooking chart

| GRAINS (1 CUP DRY) | | WATER (CUPS) | TIME TO COOK (STOVETOP) |
|---|---|---|---|
| **Barley:** | | | |
| | **Pearled** | 3 C | 30–40 min |
| | **Hulled** | 3 C | 1$^1$/2 hrs |
| **Buckwheat Groats:** | | | |
| | **Toasted or raw** | 2 C | 30 min |
| **Millet** | | 2–3 C | 25 min |
| **Oats:** | | | |
| | **Instant** (no cooking) | 1–1$^1$/2 C | Steep in hot water for 5 min |
| | **Steel cut** | 2–3 C | 30 min |
| | **Old fashioned** (rolled) **oats** | 2–3 C | 10–15 min |
| | **Groats** | 3 C | 50 min |
| **Quinoa** (rinse first) | | 2 C | 15–25 min |
| **Brown Rice:** | | | |
| | **Long grain** | 2–2$^1$/2 C | 45 min |
| | **Short/medium grain** | 2 C | 45 min |
| **Rye:** | | | |
| | **Berries** | 2$^1$/2 C | 1–1$^1$/2 hrs |
| | **Flakes** | 3 C | 30 min |
| **Wheat:** | | | |
| | **Berries** | 3 C | 1–1$^1$/2 hrs |
| | **Bulgur** (no cooking) | 2–2$^1$/2 C | Steep in hot water for 15–20 min |
| **Couscous** (no cooking) | | 1$^1$/4 C | Steep in hot water for 10–15 min |

- *Please use this chart as a general guide. Actual cooking times may vary depending on freshness, stovetop temperatures, etc. For best results, follow the cooking instructions on the package.*
- *Soaking whole grains overnight will make them easier to digest and decrease cooking time.*
- *If you are using a pressure cooker to cook whole grains, it is best to follow the manufacturer's directions.*

### AMARANTH: AN ANCIENT GRAIN FOR A MODERN WORLD

I traveled the world searching for amaranth, the super grain which had once been a staple in the diets of pre-Columbian Aztecs. With the arrival of Cortez and the Spanish conquistadors, all crops of amaranth were burned; its use was forbidden, and possession of amaranth was cause for severe punishment. Amaranth became a "lost" grain. After 300 years of it being in obscurity, I rediscovered amaranth in Mexico where I was honored to share it on ceremonial days with the descendents of the Aztecs, who believed it provided them with supernatural power. Therefore, it is not surprising to me when people say they are not familiar with amaranth as it was only in the 1970s that I reintroduced this ancient grain to the United States.

Amaranth is assuming its rightful position as a highly lauded "grain" (it is actually a seed) and beginning to be discovered by more and more people—and for good reason since Amaranth is incredibly nutrient-rich. While it can be served like a grain, it features something that many other grains don't—a good supply of the essential amino acid lysine (approximately twice as much as wheat), making it more like a whole protein source. In addition, amaranth is a concentrated source of numerous other nutrients: for example, one quarter cup of uncooked amaranth contains 75 mg calcium, 3.7 mg iron, 130 mg magnesium, 1.1 mg manganese, 1.5 mg zinc and 4.5 grams fiber, all for only 182 calories.

Amaranth can be simmered like other grains and has a porridge-like texture. It can be combined with other grains if you desire a more "rice-like" dish. It can also be popped in a skillet like popcorn, which gives it a nutty flavor and crunchy texture.

The reason that I don't include amaranth as one of the 100 World's Healthiest Foods is because it is not as widely available as the other grains that I do include.

### EMMER/FARRO

A variety of wheat with a long and impressive heritage (it played an important role in ancient Roman culture), emmer/faro is now making a comeback. It is similar to spelt, but has a hearty, firm and chewy texture when cooked.

### KAMUT

An ancient strain of wheat whose popularity is being revived thanks to concentrated efforts of farmers focused on its cultivation. Although kamut does contain gluten, many with wheat allergies have reported that they are able to tolerate it. It has a higher protein content than common wheat; research suggests that it may also have a lower glycemic index value than common wheat.

### SPELT

A wonderfully nutritious ancient grain with a deep nutlike flavor, spelt is a cousin to wheat that has recently been receiving renewed recognition. Some individuals who are sensitive to wheat can tolerate spelt.

### TEFF

A tiny grain that plays a large role in Ethiopian cuisine, Teff is a type of millet that has a sweet flavor. It can be used to make baked goods or cooked like oatmeal. It is especially rich in minerals, such as iron and calcium.

### TRITICALE

A cross between durum wheat and rye, triticale is one of the newest grains available, dating back to the beginning of the 20th century. The protein content of triticale is more bioavailable than wheat.

## How to Use the Individual Grain Chapters

Each chapter is dedicated to one of the World's Healthiest Whole Grains and contains everything you need to know to enjoy and maximize its flavor and nutritional benefits. Each chapter is organized into two parts:

1. **WHOLE GRAIN FACTS** describes each grain and its different varieties and presents its unique nutritional profile. This section also addresses the biochemical considerations of each grain by describing unique compounds that may be potentially problematic for individuals with specific health problems. Detailed information of the health benefits of each grain can be found at the end of the chapter.

2. **THE 4 STEPS TO THE BEST TASTING AND MOST NUTRITIOUS WHOLE GRAINS** includes information on how to best select, store, prepare and cook each one of the World's Healthiest Grains. By following these 4 steps, you can be assured that you will enjoy grains with the best taste and greatest number of nutrients. Each step is simple, and you will enjoy your food so much more if you follow them.

Here are some questions I received from readers of the whfoods.org website about Whole Grains:

### Q *Are the various types of oatmeal—instant, quick, old fashioned, steel cut—the same as far as nutrition is concerned?*

A Different types of oatmeal are actually not at all the same in terms of nutrition. The very outermost portion of the oat—called the hull—is always removed before the oat is eaten. Once the hull has been removed, there are several additional processing steps that can be taken. The least processed forms for oats are oat groats and steel cut oats. Oat groats consist of the hulled, but unflattened and unchopped oat kernels. Steel cut oats are the same as oat groats, except for being chopped with steel blades. Because they are the least processed, these two forms of oats are also the most nutritious. Old fashioned oats are both chopped, steamed, and rolled to give them their flatter shape. Because they are more processed, they are less nourishing than oat groats or steel cut oats. However, they are still better sources of nourishment than most quick-cooking oats or instant oatmeals. Quick and instant oatmeals usually have their oat bran—the layer of the grain that's just beneath the hull—removed. Many vitamins and much of the oat's fiber are contained within the bran, and so its removal is particularly problematic when it comes to nutritional value. Oat groats, steel cut oats and, to a slightly lesser extent, old fashioned or rolled oats would be your best choices; quick and instant oatmeals are usually less nourishing because they are more processed and have their bran layer removed.

### Q *Is cereal considered a whole grain?*

A It would depend upon what is in the cereal. A quick look at the ingredients list can provide you with the answer. If the ingredients include whole wheat and other grains (for example, barley) then it would be considered a whole grain. But if the cereal ingredients are primarily "refined wheat" or even just "wheat," even though the cereal may be enriched with nutrients, I would not consider it to be a whole grain.

Whole grain cereals can be found in most supermarkets; again it is best to do a little label reading. While you are reading the label, though, do take into account the amount of sugar that may be present. I always prefer to buy unsweetened (or naturally sweetened) cereals so that I can avoid the empty calories offered by sugar. If you buy unsweetened cereal, you can always sweeten it at home with a more natural sweetener such as honey or evaporated cane juice.

natural sweetener such as honey or evaporated can juice. Additionally, more and more cereals are being made with organically grown whole grains, which I think is great.

## Q Is it essential to cook oats before eating to benefit from all the nutrients? I ask because I usually add raw rolled oats to my yogurt instead of a granola and was wondering whether I was receiving its full benefit.

A Oats are highly nutritious and filled with cholesterol-fighting soluble fiber and also have a pleasant nutty flavor. Since rolled oats are made from oat groats that are steamed and rolled, you do not have to cook them before eating. That being said, it is a good idea to chew well when eating uncooked oats. This will help to make them easier to digest and maximize the benefits you derive from them.

## Q Everyone says eat more "whole" grains, but how do you do it?

A Whole grains are grains that have not been processed and refined. For example, white flour is not a whole grain, but whole wheat flour is. Brown rice is considered to be a whole grain while white rice is not. Processing into refined grain products removes many nutrients: fiber (which is in the bran portion) and many B vitamins, for example.

Whole grains would include such grains as brown rice, barley, buckwheat, quinoa, rye and whole wheat (and products made from them). To increase the amount of whole grains you eat, you could prepare one of these grains for a side dish with your dinner entrée. For example, a bowl of steaming brown rice or quinoa seasoned with your favorite herbs and spices makes a nice accompaniment to fish, meat and vegetarian entrées. A popular food that is considered to be a whole grain is oats, and so a bowl of oatmeal is an easy way to eat whole grains (I prefer whole oats to instant oats if possible). You could also make hot cereal with any of the whole grains listed above, adding milk, fruit, nuts, seeds, cinnamon or any other ingredient that you would normally add to a bowl of oatmeal.

## Q Is using oatmeal in the package bad if you don't have time to make regular oatmeal?

A No, using prepackaged oatmeal isn't bad if you are running short of time. However, it would still be important for you to select high quality oatmeal even if purchasing it in prepackaged form. I'll give you a quick example. There are some high-quality manufacturers who make whole grain, organic, prepackaged oatmeals, whose products often offer about 4–5 grams of fiber and 5–6

grams of protein per packet. While not quite as good as the "from scratch" version, these prepackaged oatmeals are definitely high-quality and worth including in a meal plan from a convenience standpoint. On the other hand, you can also purchase prepackaged oatmeals that are non-organic and more processed. These oatmeals will usually contain pesticide and other unwanted chemical residues and will also contain less fiber, protein and vitamins, usually in the range of 25%–33% less. While instant oatmeal may be ready in an "instant," don't forget that it only takes 10 minutes to cook a bowl of oatmeal using old fashioned oats.

## Q Should I soak oats overnight to reduce the level of phytic acid that they contain?

A Oats are actually a little lower in phytic acid content than some of their fellow grains. For example, whole wheat flours have shown as much as 20 mg of phytic acid per gram while oat flours have 4 to 7 mg of phytic acid per gram. Since I don't consider oats to be particularly high in phytic acid, I would not consider the soaking of oats necessary in creating an optimally nourishing meal that contained this health-promoting grain.

## Q How do the different parts of the wheat grain compare in terms of their contribution of nutrients?

A There are three parts to the grain: the endosperm, germ and bran. The germ and bran are a concentrated source of fiber and many vitamins while the endosperm mainly contains starch (carbohydrates). When grains such as wheat are processed, the bran and germ are removed. That is why whole grains, such as whole wheat, offer so many more nutrients. Below is a chart that shows the percentage of nutrients found in the wheat grain's three components; this chart will help to further elucidate why whole grains are nutritionally far superior to refined grains.

| | BRAN | GERM | ENDOSPERM |
|---|---|---|---|
| Fiber | 85% | 15% | 0% |
| Fats | 15% | 65% | 20% |
| Vitamin B1 (thiamin) | 33% | 64% | 3% |
| Vitamin B2 (riboflavin) | 42% | 26% | 32% |
| Vitamin B3 (niacin) | 86% | 2% | 12% |
| Vitamin B5 (pantothenic acid) | 50% | 7% | 43% |
| Vitamin B6 (pyridoxine) | 73% | 21% | 6% |

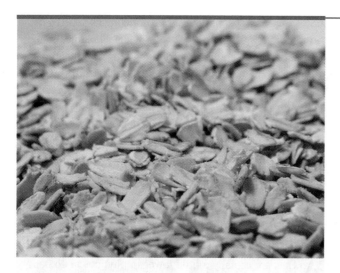

# oats

| | |
|---|---|
| AVAILABILITY: | Year-round |
| REFRIGERATE: | Yes |
| SHELF LIFE: | 2 months |
| PREPARATION: | Minimal |
| BEST WAY TO COOK: | Simmer |

## nutrient-richness chart

Total Nutrient-Richness: **12**      GI: **81**

One cup (234 grams) of whole grain Oats contains 145 calories

| NUTRIENT | AMOUNT | %DV | DENSITY | QUALITY |
|---|---|---|---|---|
| Manganese | 1.4 mg | 68.5 | 8.5 | excellent |
| Selenium | 19.0 mcg | 27.1 | 3.4 | very good |
| Tryptophan | 0.1 g | 25.0 | 3.1 | good |
| Phosphorus | 177.8 mg | 17.8 | 2.2 | good |
| B1 Thiamin | 0.3 mg | 17.3 | 2.2 | good |
| Dietary Fiber | 4.0 g | 15.9 | 2.0 | good |
| Magnesium | 56.2 mg | 14.0 | 1.7 | good |
| Protein | 6.1 g | 12.2 | 1.5 | good |
| **CAROTENOIDS:** | | | Daily values for these nutrients have not yet been established. | |
| Lutein + Zeaxanthin | 421.0 mcg | | | |

For more on "Total Nutrient-Richness," "%DV," "Density," and The World's Healthiest Foods "Quality" Rating System, see page 805.

For more on GI, see page 342.

Oats are a hardy cereal grain able to withstand poor soil conditions in which other crops are unable to thrive. Their natural fortitude seems to transfer to those who consume this nutrient-rich grain. Today, Oats are enjoyed and recognized as a delicious food that also has many health-promoting qualities. A steaming bowl of freshly cooked Oatmeal is a great way to start your day. Not only is it hearty and satisfying, but it is sure to provide the strength and energy you need to carry you through a hectic morning schedule.

## why oats should be part of your healthiest way of eating

Although Oats are hulled like many other types of grains, this process does not strip away their bran and their germ, so they remain a rich source of dietary fiber and other nutrients. Oats have been found to be a heart-healthy food. They not only contain a form of dietary fiber known as beta-glucan, which has been found to help lower cholesterol levels, but also unique phenolic phytonutrients called avenanthramides, which act as powerful antioxidants. (For more on the *Health Benefits of Oats* and a complete analysis of their content of over 60 nutrients, see page 666.)

## varieties of oats

The Oats we enjoy today originated from the wild red oat native to Asia. Part of their distinctive flavor can be attributed to the roasting process they undergo after they have been harvested and cleaned. Different processing methods are used to produce Oat products such as breakfast cereals, baked goods and stuffing. Oats are known botanically as *Avena sativa*.

### OAT GROATS (SCOTTISH OATS OR IRISH OATMEAL)

Unflattened kernels that can be used as a breakfast cereal or for stuffing.

### STEEL CUT OATS

Produced by running the grain through steel blades, which thinly slices them. Steel Cut Oats have a dense and chewy texture.

### OLD FASHIONED OATS

Oat Groats that are steamed, rolled and flattened.

### QUICK-COOKING OATS

Processed in the same way as Old Fashioned Oats, but they are cut very fine before rolling.

### INSTANT OATMEAL

Oats that are partially cooked and then rolled very thin; most of the bran is removed in the processing. Instant Oatmeal has a higher GI value than Old Fashioned Oats and therefore may be more likely to cause elevations in blood sugar levels.

### OAT BRAN

The outer layer of the kernel that resides under the hull, Oat Bran is also available as a separate product and is added to recipes or cooked to make a hot cereal. Oat Groats and Steel Cut Oats have retained most of the bran portion of the grain.

### OAT FLOUR

Used in baking, it is oftentimes combined with wheat or other gluten-containing flours when making leavened bread.

## the peak season available year-round.

## biochemical considerations

Oats are a concentrated source of purines, which might be of concern to certain individuals. Oats have traditionally been included among the "gluten grains"—grains that may be problematic for individuals allergic to the gluten found in wheat. More recently, though, the idea of grouping grains under one umbrella has come into question with some healthcare practitioners having reservations about drawing a conclusion that other "gluten grains" elicit the same physiological response as wheat. (For more information on *Purines*, see page 727; and *Gluten Intolerance*, see page 720.)

## 4 steps to the best tasting and most nutritious oats

Turning Oats into a flavorful dish with the most nutrients is simple if you just follow my 4 easy steps:

1. The Best Way to Select
2. The Best Way to Store
3. The Best Way to Prepare
4. The Healthiest Way of Cooking

## 1. the best way to select oats

It is best to purchase small quantities of Oats at one time since this grain has a slightly higher fat content than other grains and will go rancid more quickly. Oats are generally available in prepackaged containers as well as in bulk bins. As with other foods you may purchase in the bulk section, make sure that the bins containing the Oats are covered and that the store has a good product turnover to ensure their maximal freshness. Whether purchasing Oats in bulk or in a packaged container, it is important that no evidence of moisture is present. As with all grains, I recommend selecting organically grown Oats whenever possible. (For more on *Organic Foods*, see page 113.)

If you purchase prepared Oat products such as Oatmeal, look at the ingredients to ensure that the product does not contain any salt, sugar or other additives.

## 2. the best way to store oats

Oats should be kept in an airtight container. It is best to keep them in the refrigerator, where they will keep fresh for 2 months.

## 3. the best way to prepare oats

Oats require a minimal amount of preparation.

## 4. the healthiest way of cooking oats

Different types of Oats require slightly different cooking methods for making hot cereal or porridge. However, it is best to add all varieties of Oats to cold water and then to simmer them.

Note: See page 662 and 663 for interesting questions from Readers on Oats.

# health benefits of oats

## Promote Heart Health

Oats, Oat Bran and Oatmeal contain a specific type of fiber known as beta-glucan. Since 1963, study after study has proven its beneficial effects on cholesterol levels. Studies show that in individuals with high cholesterol (above 220 mg/dl), consuming just three grams of soluble Oat fiber per day (an amount found in one bowl of Oatmeal) typically lowers total cholesterol by 8–23%.

Oats' cardioprotective effect may not be limited to their fiber but may also be due to the unique phenolic phytonutrients, avenanthramides, that Oats contain. Avenanthramides are unique antioxidants that can protect LDL cholesterol from oxidation, therefore curbing a mechanism involved in atherosclerosis. A recent study also showed that Oat avenanthramides could significantly suppress the production of several types of molecules involved in the attachment of immune cells to the arterial wall—the first step in the development of atherosclerosis. In addition, Oats are a good source of magnesium, a mineral that promotes heart health by keeping blood vessels relaxed.

## Promote Blood Sugar Balance

Studies show that beta-glucan also has beneficial effects on diabetes. Type 2 diabetic patients given foods high in this type of Oat fiber, Oatmeal or Oat Bran-rich foods, experienced much lower rises in blood sugar compared to those who were given white rice or bread. Starting out your day with a blood-sugar-stabilizing food, such as Oats, may help to keep blood sugar levels under control the rest of the day, especially if the rest of the day is also supported with nourishing fiber-rich foods.

## Celiac Disease Substitute

Although treatment of celiac disease has been thought to require lifelong avoidance of the protein gluten, recent studies of adults have suggested that Oats, despite the small amount of gluten they contain, are well-tolerated. A recent double-blind, multi-center study suggests that Oats are a good grain choice for children with celiac disease as well. The children were randomly assigned to receive either the standard gluten-free diet or a gluten-free diet with some wheat-free Oat products. At the end of the year-long study, all the children were doing well. In both groups, the mucosal lining of the small intestine (which is damaged by wheat gluten in celiac disease) had healed, and the immune system (which is excessively reactive in celiac patients) had returned to normal.

## Additional Health-Promoting Benefits of Oats

Oats are also a concentrated source of other nutrients providing additional health-promoting benefits. These nutrients include muscle-building protein, free-radical-scavenging selenium and manganese, energy-producing vitamin B1 and phosphorus, and sleep-promoting tryptophan.

## Nutritional Analysis of 1 cup of whole grain Oats:

| NUTRIENT | AMOUNT | % DAILY VALUE | NUTRIENT | AMOUNT | % DAILY VALUE |
|---|---|---|---|---|---|
| Calories | 145.08 | | Pantothenic Acid | 0.47 mg | 4.70 |
| Calories from Fat | 21.06 | | | | |
| Calories from Saturated Fat | 3.79 | | **Minerals** | | |
| Protein | 6.08 g | | Boron | — mcg | |
| Carbohydrates | 25.27 g | | Calcium | 18.72 mg | 1.87 |
| Dietary Fiber | 3.98 g | 15.92 | Chloride | — mg | |
| Soluble Fiber | 2.34 g | | Chromium | — mcg | — |
| Insoluble Fiber | 1.64 g | | Copper | 0.13 mg | 6.50 |
| Sugar – Total | 0.94 g | | Fluoride | — mg | — |
| Monosaccharides | — g | | Iodine | — mcg | — |
| Disaccharides | — g | | Iron | 1.59 mg | 8.83 |
| Other Carbs | 20.36 g | | Magnesium | 56.16 mg | 14.04 |
| Fat – Total | 2.34 g | | Manganese | 1.37 mg | 68.50 |
| Saturated Fat | 0.42 g | | Molybdenum | — mcg | — |
| Mono Fat | 0.75 g | | Phosphorus | 177.84 mg | 17.78 |
| Poly Fat | 0.87 g | | Potassium | 131.04 mg | |
| Omega-3 Fatty Acids | 0.05 g | 2.00 | Selenium | 18.95 mcg | 27.07 |
| Omega-6 Fatty Acids | 0.82 g | | Sodium | 374.40 mg | |
| Trans Fatty Acids | — g | | Zinc | 1.15 mg | 7.67 |
| Cholesterol | 0.00 mg | | | | |
| Water | 199.60 g | | **Amino Acids** | | |
| Ash | 0.70 g | | Alanine | 0.32 g | |
| | | | Arginine | 0.43 g | |
| **Vitamins** | | | Aspartate | 0.52 g | |
| Vitamin A IU | 37.44 IU | 0.75 | Cystine | 0.15 g | 36.59 |
| Vitamin A RE | 4.68 RE | | Glutamate | 1.33 g | |
| A - Carotenoid | 4.68 RE | 0.06 | Glycine | 0.30 g | |
| A - Retinol | 0.00 RE | | Histidine | 0.15 g | 11.63 |
| B1 Thiamin | 0.26 mg | 17.33 | Isoleucine | 0.25 g | 21.74 |
| B2 Riboflavin | 0.05 mg | 2.94 | Leucine | 0.46 g | 18.18 |
| B3 Niacin | 0.30 mg | 1.50 | Lysine | 0.25 g | 10.64 |
| Niacin Equiv | 1.71 mg | | Methionine | 0.11 g | 14.86 |
| Vitamin B6 | 0.05 mg | 2.50 | Phenylalanine | 0.32 g | 26.89 |
| Vitamin B12 | 0.00 mcg | 0.00 | Proline | 0.33 g | |
| Biotin | — mcg | — | Serine | 0.27 g | |
| Vitamin C | 0.00 mg | 0.00 | Threonine | 0.21 g | 16.94 |
| Vitamin D IU | 0.00 IU | 0.00 | Tryptophan | 0.08 g | 25.00 |
| Vitamin D mcg | 0.00 mcg | | Tyrosine | 0.21 g | 21.65 |
| Vitamin E Alpha Equiv | 0.23 mg | 1.15 | Valine | 0.33 g | 22.45 |
| Vitamin E IU | 0.35 IU | | | | |
| Vitamin E mg | 0.23 mg | | | | |
| Folate | 9.36 mcg | 2.34 | | | |
| Vitamin K | — mcg | — | | | |

(Note: "–" indicates data is unavailable. For more information, please see page 806.)

STEP-BY-STEP
## Recipes for Enjoying Oatmeal

# 10-Minute Energizing Oatmeal

*This is a delicious, complete breakfast and a perfect way to start your day.*

1 cup Old Fashioned Rolled Oats
2 cups water
Sea salt to taste
1/2 tsp cinnamon
1/2 cup raisins
1/4 cup chopped walnuts
Soymilk or skim milk
Sweetener such as molasses or honey

1. Bring the water and salt to a boil in a saucepan, then turn the heat to low and add the Oats.

2. Cook for about 5 minutes, stirring regularly so that the Oatmeal will not clump together. Add cinnamon, raisins, and walnuts, stir, **cover** the pan and turn off heat. Let sit for 5 minutes. Serve with milk and sweetener.

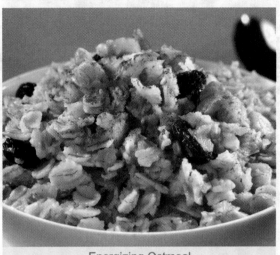

Energizing Oatmeal

**Preparation Hint:** If you are using prepackaged Oats, it is best to follow the directions on the package.

**SERVES 2**

## Flavor Tips: Try these 3 great serving suggestions with the recipe above. ✳

1. Use dried cranberries, dried figs or other dried fruits instead of raisins to add unique flavor and nutrition to this wonderful morning meal.
2. Ground flaxseeds make a great addition to Energizing Oatmeal.

3. You can also make Energizing Oatmeal with Oat Groats. To make Oat Groats Oatmeal, you need to use 3 parts water to 1 part Oats, bring them to a boil, turn heat to low and then simmer for approximately 50 minutes.

# Swiss Oatmeal – No Cooking

*This traditional Swiss breakfast, also known as muesli, is a hearty breakfast.*

1 cup Old Fashioned Rolled Oats
1 cup boiling water
1/4 cup dried apricots
1 TBS honey
1/4 cup unsweetened coconut
1/2 cup raisins
Cinnamon and vanilla to taste

1. Pour 1 cup of boiling water over Oats. Let stand overnight. In the morning, divide Oats into two bowls.

2. Top with remaining ingredients (one-half of the amount for each bowl). Add cinnamon and vanilla to taste. Swiss Oatmeal also tastes great served with yogurt or soymilk and your favorite nuts.

**SERVES 2**

# Granola with Fruit and Nuts

4 cups Old Fashioned Rolled Oats
1 cup mixture of nuts, seeds and dried fruit (use your favorite)
Soymilk or almond milk
Honey

1. Preheat oven to 350°F (175°C).
2. In baking pan, toast Oats for 15 minutes.
3. Mix with nut, seed and fruit mixture.
4. Serve with soymilk or almond milk and honey.

Please write (address on back cover flap) or e-mail me at info@whfoods.org with your personal ideas for preparing Oats, and I will share them with others through our website at www.whfoods.org.

# rye

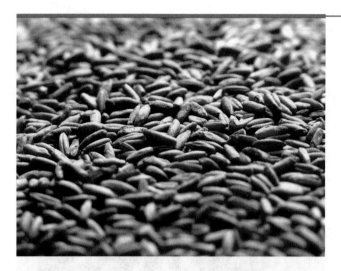

## nutrient-richness chart

Total Nutrient-Richness: **10**    GI: **48**
One-third cup (56.33 grams) of Whole Grain Rye (1 cup cooked)

| NUTRIENT | AMOUNT | %DV | DENSITY | QUALITY |
|---|---|---|---|---|
| Manganese | 1.5 mg | 75.5 | 7.2 | excellent |
| Dietary Fiber | 8.2 g | 32.9 | 3.1 | good |
| Selenium | 19.9 mcg | 28.4 | 2.7 | good |
| Tryptophan | 0.1 g | 28.1 | 2.7 | good |
| Phosphorus | 210.7 mg | 21.1 | 2.0 | good |
| Magnesium | 68.2 mg | 17.0 | 1.6 | good |
| Protein | 8.3 g | 16.6 | 1.6 | good |

For more on "Total Nutrient-Richness," "%DV," "Density," and
The World's Healthiest Foods "Quality" Rating System, see page 805.

For more on GI, see page 342.

I n the United States where wheat products are so prevalent, baked goods made from Rye are rarely given prominent shelf space at the market. But hopefully, out of sight does not mean out of mind because foods made from whole Rye are worth looking for, not only for their hardy, deep flavor, but also for their numerous health benefits. Rye is most well-known as the main ingredient in traditional Rye and pumpernickel breads. It is one of the premier grains enjoyed in the food cultures of Scandinavia and Eastern Europe, where it plays a very important culinary role.

## why rye should be part of your healthiest way of eating

Unlike wheat, it is very difficult to separate the germ and bran from the endosperm of Rye; therefore, the flour used to prepare Rye breads retains a large quantity of nutrients, making these baked goods an excellent substitute for wheat-based breads in your "Healthiest Way of Eating." Like other grains, Rye is a good source of dietary fiber. In addition, Rye

## highlights

| | |
|---|---|
| AVAILABILITY: | Year-round |
| REFRIGERATE: | No |
| SHELF LIFE: | 6 months |
| PREPARATION: | Minimal |
| BEST WAY TO COOK: | Simmer |

also contains lignan phytonutrients with phytoestrogenic and antioxidant properties. (For more on the *Health Benefits of Rye* and a complete analysis of its content of over 60 nutrients, see page 670.)

## varieties of rye

Rye is a cereal grain, known botanically as *Secale cereale*. Similar to wheat in appearance, the Rye grain is longer and more slender. Rye's color varies from yellowish-brown to grayish-green. It is generally available in its whole or cracked grain form, as flour or as flakes, which look like old-fashioned oats. Because Rye contains less gluten than wheat, it holds less gas during the leavening process, so breads made with Rye flour are more compact and dense.

### RYE GROATS OR WHOLE RYE BERRIES

Similar to wheat berries, they can be added to soups, prepared as a side dish or as a main dish casserole.

### CRACKED RYE

This form of Rye cooks more quickly than whole Rye Groats. It makes a good addition to soups and can be prepared as a side dish or as a hot cereal.

### RYE FLAKES

These are similar to rolled oats and produced by the same process. Rye Flakes are steamed and pressed. They can be prepared as cooked hot cereal or mixed into bread or muffin recipes.

### RYE FLOUR

Rye Flour is made by milling Rye Berries. While it looks like wheat flour, it contains less gluten. It comes in dark and light color. The bran and germ have been sifted out of light Rye Flour, depleting it of most of its nutrients.

**the peak season** available year-round.

## biochemical considerations

Rye has traditionally been included among the "gluten grains"—grains that may be problematic for individuals allergic to the gluten found in wheat. More recently, though, the idea of grouping grains under one umbrella has come into question with some healthcare practitioners having reservations about drawing a conclusion that other "gluten grains" elicit the same physiological response as wheat. (For more on *Gluten Intolerance*, see page 720.)

## 4 steps to the best tasting and most nutritious rye

Turning Rye into a flavorful dish with the most nutrients is simple if you just follow my 4 easy steps:

1. The Best Way to Select
2. The Best Way to Store
3. The Best Way to Prepare
4. The Healthiest Way of Cooking

# 1. the best way to select rye

Rye is generally available in prepackaged containers as well as bulk bins. Just as with any other food that you may purchase in the bulk section, make sure that the bins containing the Rye are covered and that the store has a good product turnover to ensure its maximal freshness. Whether purchasing Rye in bulk or in a packaged container, it is important that no evidence of moisture is present. As with all grains, I recommend selecting organically grown Rye whenever possible. (For more on *Organic Foods*, see page 113.)

When shopping for Rye bread, make sure to read the labels because "Rye bread" can often be wheat bread colored with caramel coloring and contain very little Rye.

# 2. the best way to store rye

Store Rye Groats, Cracked Rye and Rye Flakes in an airtight container in a cool, dry and dark place where they will keep for several months. Because it is perishable, store Rye Flour in an airtight container in the freezer, where it can keep for 1 month. You can use it right from the freezer.

# 3. the best way to prepare rye

As with other grains, thoroughly rinse Rye before cooking. Remember that Rye contains less gluten than wheat, so when using Rye Flour, the texture of your baked goods will be more dense. Rye flour is often combined with wheat flour in baked goods.

# 4. the healthiest way of cooking rye

Rye Flakes can be cooked similar to oats. Rye Berries and Cracked Rye can be cooked similar to rice (Cracked Rye takes less time to prepare). It is best to add the Rye to cold water and then cook at a simmer. (For cooking instructions for oats, see page 667; for rice, see page 679.)

**Q** *I want to increase my consumption of Rye. Besides Rye bread, what other products should I look for?*

**A** Rye is available in a variety of products. You can find whole Rye Berries, Cracked Rye and Rye Flakes, all of which can be cooked like cereal. If you are a baker, you may want to try Rye Flour in your next recipe. Many stores often carry several varieties of Rye crackers as well. While supermarkets may carry some Rye products, natural food stores may be your best bet as they usually carry a wide array. Many Rye products are oftentimes found in the bulk bin section.

# health benefits of rye

### Promotes Women's Health

Similar to flaxseeds, Rye contains lignan phytonutrients that have phytoestrogenic activity. In the body, phytoestrogens act a little like natural estrogens, and although their effect is much weaker, they can help normalize estrogenic activity. For some women, the phytoestrogens in Rye are just strong enough to help prevent or reduce uncomfortable symptoms that may accompany menopause, like hot flashes, which are thought to be due to plummeting estrogen levels. On the other hand, when too much estrogen is around, Rye's lignans can occupy estrogen receptors and block out the much more powerful human estrogens, causing a lowering in estrogenic activity and providing protection against breast cancer.

### Promotes Blood Sugar Balance

A recent study found that bread made from Rye triggers a lower insulin response than wheat bread does. Since a few different types of Rye bread were tested, and they all had a similar response, the researchers suggested that the lower after-meal insulin response could, therefore, not be attributed only to the fiber content of the Rye breads but was also due to the uniqueness of Rye's starch granules. For a grain, Rye is incredibly rich in protein. Its matrix of protein and carbohydrates may also contribute to its potential benefits on blood sugar balance.

### Promotes Heart Health

The soluble fiber found in Rye also helps to lower cholesterol by binding to bile acids and removing them from the body. When they are excreted along with the fiber, the liver must manufacture new bile acids and uses up more cholesterol, therefore lowering the amount of cholesterol in circulation. Soluble fiber may also reduce the amount of cholesterol manufactured by the liver. Rye's lignan phytonutrients are also thought to be protective of heart health.

### Promotes Healthy Weight Control

Rye is a good source of dietary fiber. Rye fiber is richly endowed with non-cellulose polysaccharides, which have exceptionally high water-binding capacity and quickly give a feeling of fullness and satiety, making Rye bread a real help for anyone trying to lose weight.

### Promotes Digestive Health

Studies have found that diets rich in high-fiber foods, such as Rye, may help to prevent colon cancer. In fact, a recent study showed that subjects who replaced white wheat bread with whole meal Rye bread had greatly improved digestive functions, improvements that have been linked to lower risk of colon cancer. In addition, eating the Rye bread resulted in favorable changes in colonic enzymes and short chain fatty acids, again reflecting cancer protection.

### Additional Health-Promoting Benefits of Rye

Rye is also a concentrated source of other nutrients providing additional health-promoting benefits. These nutrients include bone-building magnesium and phosphorus, free-radical-scavenging manganese and selenium, and sleep-promoting tryptophan.

## Nutritional Analysis of 1/3 cup of Whole Grain Rye (1 cup cooked):

| NUTRIENT | AMOUNT | % DAILY VALUE | NUTRIENT | AMOUNT | % DAILY VALUE |
|---|---|---|---|---|---|
| Calories | 188.72 | | Pantothenic Acid | 0.82 mg | 8.20 |
| Calories from Fat | 12.68 | | | | |
| Calories from Saturated Fat | 1.46 | | **Minerals** | | |
| Protein | 8.31 g | | Boron | — mcg | |
| Carbohydrates | 39.30 g | | Calcium | 18.59 mg | 1.86 |
| Dietary Fiber | 8.22 g | 32.88 | Chloride | — mg | |
| Soluble Fiber | 0.96 g | | Chromium | — mcg | — |
| Insoluble Fiber | 7.27 g | | Copper | 0.25 mg | 12.50 |
| Sugar – Total | 2.31 g | | Fluoride | — mg | — |
| Monosaccharides | — g | | Iodine | — mcg | — |
| Disaccharides | — g | | Iron | 1.50 mg | 8.33 |
| Other Carbs | 28.76 g | | Magnesium | 68.16 mg | 17.04 |
| Fat – Total | 1.41 g | | Manganese | 1.51 mg | 75.50 |
| Saturated Fat | 0.16 g | | Molybdenum | — mcg | — |
| Mono Fat | 0.17 g | | Phosphorus | 210.69 mg | 21.07 |
| Poly Fat | 0.63 g | | Potassium | 148.72 mg | |
| Omega-3 Fatty Acids | 0.09 g | 3.60 | Selenium | 19.89 mcg | 28.41 |
| Omega-6 Fatty Acids | 0.54 g | | Sodium | 3.38 mg | |
| Trans Fatty Acids | — g | | Zinc | 2.10 mg | 14.00 |
| Cholesterol | 0.00 mg | | | | |
| Water | 6.17 g | | **Amino Acids** | | |
| Ash | 1.14 g | | Alanine | 0.40 g | |
| | | | Arginine | 0.46 g | |
| **Vitamins** | | | Aspartate | 0.66 g | |
| Vitamin A IU | 0.00 IU | 0.00 | Cystine | 0.19 g | 46.34 |
| Vitamin A RE | 0.00 RE | | Glutamate | 2.06 g | |
| A - Carotenoid | 0.00 RE | 0.00 | Glycine | 0.39 g | |
| A - Retinol | 0.00 RE | | Histidine | 0.21 g | 16.28 |
| B1 Thiamin | 0.18 mg | 12.00 | Isoleucine | 0.31 g | 26.96 |
| B2 Riboflavin | 0.14 mg | 8.24 | Leucine | 0.55 g | 21.74 |
| B3 Niacin | 2.41 mg | 12.05 | Lysine | 0.34 g | 14.47 |
| Niacin Equiv | 3.85 mg | | Methionine | 0.14 g | 18.92 |
| Vitamin B6 | 0.17 mg | 8.50 | Phenylalanine | 0.38 g | 31.93 |
| Vitamin B12 | 0.00 mcg | 0.00 | Proline | 0.84 g | |
| Biotin | — mcg | — | Serine | 0.38 g | |
| Vitamin C | 0.00 mg | 0.00 | Threonine | 0.30 g | 24.19 |
| Vitamin D IU | 0.00 IU | 0.00 | Tryptophan | 0.09 g | 28.13 |
| Vitamin D mcg | 0.00 mcg | | Tyrosine | 0.19 g | 19.59 |
| Vitamin E Alpha Equiv | 1.05 mg | 5.25 | Valine | 0.42 g | 28.57 |
| Vitamin E IU | 1.57 IU | | | | |
| Vitamin E mg | 1.05 mg | | | | |
| Folate | 33.80 mcg | 8.45 | | | |
| Vitamin K | — mcg | — | | | |

(Note: "–" indicates data is unavailable. For more information, please see page 806.)

STEP-BY-STEP
## Recipes for Enjoying Rye

# *The Healthiest Way of Cooking Rye*

*Cooked Rye Berries make a great pilaf and complement almost any meal.*

**1 cup Rye Berries, rinsed**
**2 1/2 cups water**
**Sea salt to taste**

1. Add water and a pinch of salt to a sauce pan. **Cover** and bring to boil. Add Rye Berries to boiling water. After it has returned to a boil, turn down the heat, **cover** and then simmer for 1–1 1/2 hours. When the Rye Berries are done cooking, drain off any excess liquid.

   Rye Berries will cook more quickly if they are soaked overnight. Discard soaking water.

2. Test Rye for doneness. Rye should be not too soft or too chewy. If it is not done and no water is left in the pan, add a couple of TBS of water, cover and cook a few more minutes. If water still remains in the pan,

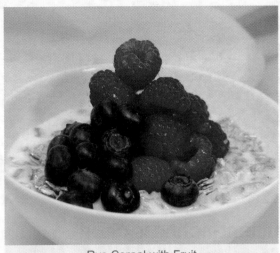
Rye Cereal with Fruit

turn off the heat and let Rye sit until the excess water is absorbed.

**Preparation Hint:** If you are using prepackaged Rye Berries, it is best to follow the directions on the package.

**SERVES 3**

## Flavor Tips: Try these 8 great serving suggestions with the recipe above. ✱

1. When serving Rye for lunch or dinner as a pilaf, try cooking it with chicken or vegetable broth instead of water and serve with extra virgin olive oil to enhance its flavor.
2. Sprinkle cooked Rye with lots of freshly minced parsley, sage, cilantro, chives and/or garlic, and lemon juice, cider or balsamic vinegar and extra virgin olive oil.
3. Rye goes well with "Healthy Sautéed" leeks and celery and seasoned with caraway seeds.
4. Top Rye with toasted sesame seeds or chopped toasted almonds.
5. **Rye Cereal with Fruit:** Top cooked rye berries with soy or almond milk, blueberries, raspberries and honey. For more flavor and nutrition, add raisins or dried cranberries, almonds, walnuts, pumpkin seeds, flaxseeds or cinnamon to your cereal (pictured above).
6. **Rye Spinach Salad:** Combine cooked Rye, feta cheese, minced onion and fresh or dried oregano, chopped tomato and low-fat yogurt. Serve on a bed of baby spinach.
7. **Rye Wrap:** Put cooked Rye Berries, romaine lettuce dressed with vinaigrette, and pinto beans in a whole wheat tortilla and enjoy this twist on a traditional burrito.
8. **Rye Stuffed Cabbage:** Season cooked Rye Berries with chopped tomatoes, sliced scallions, caraway seeds, and sea salt and pepper to taste in a mixing bowl. Roll up the mixture in a lightly steamed cabbage leaf.

Please write (address on back cover flap) or e-mail me at info@whfoods.org with your personal ideas for preparing Rye, and I will share them with others through our website at www.whfoods.org.

# quinoa

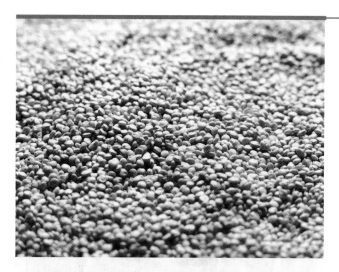

## nutrient-richness chart

Total Nutrient-Richness: **7**  GI: **n/a**

One-quarter cup (42.50 grams) of uncooked Quinoa contains 159 calories (1 cup cooked)

| NUTRIENT | AMOUNT | %DV | DENSITY | QUALITY |
|---|---|---|---|---|
| Manganese | 0.96 mg | 48.0 | 5.4 | very good |
| Magnesium | 89.25 mg | 22.3 | 2.5 | good |
| Iron | 3.93 g | 21.8 | 2.5 | good |
| Tryptophan | 0.06 mg | 18.8 | 2.1 | good |
| Copper | 0.35 mg | 17.5 | 2.0 | good |
| Phosphorus | 174.25 mg | 17.4 | 2.0 | good |

For more on "Total Nutrient-Richness," "%DV," "Density," and The World's Healthiest Foods "Quality" Rating System, see page 805.

For more on GI, see page 342.

Quinoa has been a staple food in the diet of South American Indians for thousands of years. The Incas and Aztecs considered Quinoa a sacred food, with the Incas referring to it as the "mother seed" and the Aztecs recognizing its value in increasing the stamina of their warriors. With the advent of the Spanish conquerors, who burned the Quinoa fields and made its harvest illegal, came the decline of Quinoa. Yet, the cultivation of this superfood and cultural icon could not be extinguished forever. In the 1980s, two Americans, discovering the concentrated nutritional potential of Quinoa, began importing it to the United States and cultivating it in Colorado. Since then, Quinoa has become more and more popular as people realize that it is both delicious and exceptionally beneficial for their health. While commonly referred to as a grain, it is not technically a grain; rather, Quinoa is the seed of a plant that is related to leafy green vegetables like spinach and Swiss chard. The health benefits and delicious, fluffy, creamy texture and somewhat nutty flavor of this quick-cooking grain make it a great choice as a mainstay of your "Healthiest Way of Eating."

## highlights

| | |
|---|---|
| AVAILABILITY: | Year-round |
| REFRIGERATE: | Yes |
| SHELF LIFE: | 6 months |
| PREPARATION: | Minimal |
| BEST WAY TO COOK: | Simmer |

## why quinoa should be part of your healthiest way of eating

Not only does Quinoa supply significant protein, a rare occurrence for a food that can be prepared like a grain, but the protein it supplies is complete protein, meaning that it includes all nine essential amino acids. Its amino acid profile is well balanced making it a good choice for vegans concerned about adequate protein intake, and it is also especially well-endowed with the amino acid lysine, which is essential for tissue growth and repair. In addition, Quinoa is a concentrated source of many important minerals. (For more on the *Health Benefits of Quinoa* and a complete analysis of its content of over 60 nutrients, see page 674.)

## varieties of quinoa

While relatively new to the United States, Quinoa (*Chenopodium quinoa*) has been cultivated in the Andean mountain regions of Peru, Chile and Bolivia for more than 5,000 years and has long been a staple food in the diets of the native Indians. While these are the lands where much of the world's supply of Quinoa grows, it is also now cultivated in other places, including areas in the West Coast of the United States.

Quinoa is not technically a cereal grain, but rather is the seed of an herbaceous plant. While the most popular type of Quinoa is a transparent yellow color, other varieties feature a rainbow palette of colors including orange, pink, red, purple and black. Quinoa is typically classified as bitter, medium or sweet, although in other places besides South America, only one general type is usually available.

Quinoa can be found in the market in various forms:

**WHOLE SEEDS**

The grain that we call Quinoa is actually a seed. It can be prepared like grains, similar to rice, or as porridge.

**QUINOA FLOUR**

Usually available in natural foods supermarkets, Quinoa flour is gluten-free and has a pumpkin-seed-like flavor that imparts a wonderful taste to baked goods.

**QUINOA PASTA**

Pasta made from Quinoa flour, it is a delicious alternative for those who are gluten-intolerant.

**QUINOA LEAVES**

Although often difficult to find in the marketplace, the leaves of the Quinoa plant are edible, with a taste similar to its green-leafed relatives—spinach, Swiss chard and beets.

**the peak season** available year-round.

## 4 steps to the best tasting and most nutritious quinoa

Turning Quinoa into a flavorful dish with the most nutrients is simple if you just follow my 4 easy steps:

1. The Best Way to Select
2. The Best Way to Store
3. The Best Way to Prepare
4. The Healthiest Way of Cooking

# 1. the best way to select quinoa

Quinoa is generally available in prepackaged containers as well as bulk bins. Just as with any other food that you may purchase in the bulk section, make sure that the bins containing the Quinoa are covered and that the store has a good product turnover to ensure its maximal freshness. Whether purchasing Quinoa in bulk or in a packaged container, make sure that no evidence of moisture is present. When deciding upon the amount to purchase, remember that Quinoa expands during the cooking process to three to five times its original size. If you cannot find Quinoa or products made from it (such as flour and pasta) in your local supermarket, look for it at natural foods stores. As with all grains, I recommend selecting organically grown Quinoa whenever possible. (For more on *Organic Foods*, see page 113.)

# 2. the best way to store quinoa

Store Quinoa in an airtight container in the refrigerator where it will keep for up to 6 months.

# 3. the best way to prepare quinoa

Quinoa is coated with saponin compounds, a natural insect repellent that can impart a rather soapy taste to this otherwise delicious food. While the processing methods used in commercial cultivation remove most of the saponins, it is still necessary to thoroughly wash the seeds to remove any remaining saponin residue. Place Quinoa in a large bowl and cover with water and swish around. The soapy residue will float to the top. Then place in a fine-meshed strainer and run cold water over it, gently rubbing the seeds together with your hands. Usually, this process must be repeated several times for the rinse water to become completely clear. To ensure that the saponins have been completely removed, taste a few seeds. If they still have a bitter taste, continue the rinsing process.

# 4. the healthiest way of cooking quinoa

Prepare Quinoa like you would prepare other grains or cook it with more water to make porridge. It can also be added to soups and stews. Quinoa flour can be used in baked goods, but must be combined with a gluten-containing flour, such as that from wheat, to make leavened baked goods.

Here is a question I received from a reader of the whfoods.org website about Quinoa:

**Q** *I just made Quinoa for the first time (it was delicious, by the way). I rinsed it before I cooked it, and the water got all soapy looking. Why is that?*

**A** Quinoa seeds are coated with compounds called saponins. When saponins come in contact with water, they form a soapy resin that lathers. While I think it is important to rinse all grains before cooking, it is especially important to do so with Quinoa since not only do saponins have a soapy texture, but they will impart a soapy flavor to your delicious Quinoa if not first washed away.

# health benefits of quinoa

## A Plant Food That Offers Complete Protein

Not only is Quinoa very high in protein, but the protein it supplies is complete protein, which means that it includes all nine essential amino acids. Its amino acid profile is well balanced, making it a good choice for vegans (or anyone else who is restricting their intake of animal foods) concerned about adequate protein intake. Additionally, Quinoa is especially well-endowed with the amino acid lysine, which is essential for tissue growth and repair.

## Promotes Energy Production

Not only is Quinoa a unique plant-based food since it is a complete protein, but it is also a concentrated source of dietary iron. This mineral is integral to energy production. It is a component of hemoglobin, which transports oxygen from the lungs to all body cells. Additionally, iron is an essential part of several enzymes necessary for energy production and metabolism. Quinoa is also a good source of phosphorus, a mineral that is an integral component of adenosine triphosphate (ATP), the energy currency of the body, which powers the operations of our body's cells. In addition, phosphorus promotes bone health by joining with calcium to form calcium phosphate, which enhances bone density.

## Promotes Heart Health

Dietary fiber, as found in Quinoa, helps reduce total cholesterol, especially LDL ("bad" cholesterol) levels. Additionally, Quinoa is a good source of magnesium, the mineral that relaxes blood vessels. Since low dietary levels of magnesium are associated with increased rates of hypertension, ischemic heart disease and heart arrhythmias, this ancient grain can offer yet another way to promote cardiovascular health.

## Promotes Optimal Health

Quinoa is a very good source of manganese and a good source of copper, two minerals that are necessary for the functioning of the enzyme *superoxide dismutase*. This enzyme plays a key role in protecting the body from free-radical-scavenging. Both of these nutrients also have many other important roles. For example, they play an important role in supporting bone density.

## Additional Health-Promoting Benefit of Quinoa

Quinoa also contains sleep-promoting tryptophan.

### Nutritional Analysis of 1/4 cup of uncooked Quinoa (1 cup cooked):

| NUTRIENT | AMOUNT | % DAILY VALUE | NUTRIENT | AMOUNT | % DAILY VALUE |
|---|---|---|---|---|---|
| Calories | 158.95 | | Pantothenic Acid | 0.44 mg | 4.40 |
| Calories from Fat | 22.19 | | | | |
| Calories from Saturated Fat | 2.26 | | **Minerals** | | |
| Protein | 5.57 g | | Boron | 0.00 mcg | |
| Carbohydrates | 29.28 g | | Calcium | 25.50 mg | 2.55 |
| Dietary Fiber | 2.51 g | 10.04 | Chloride | 0.59 mg | |
| Soluble Fiber | — g | | Chromium | — mcg | — |
| Insoluble Fiber | — g | | Copper | 0.35 mg | 17.50 |
| Sugar – Total | — g | | Fluoride | — mg | — |
| Monosaccharides | — g | | Iodine | — mcg | — |
| Disaccharides | — g | | Iron | 3.93 mg | 21.83 |
| Other Carbs | — g | | Magnesium | 89.25 mg | 22.31 |
| Fat – Total | 2.47 g | | Manganese | 0.96 mg | 48.00 |
| Saturated Fat | 0.25 g | | Molybdenum | — mcg | — |
| Mono Fat | 0.65 g | | Phosphorus | 174.25 mg | 17.43 |
| Poly Fat | 1.00 g | | Potassium | 314.50 mg | |
| Omega-3 Fatty Acids | 0.06 g | 2.40 | Selenium | — mcg | — |
| Omega-6 Fatty Acids | 0.94 g | | Sodium | 8.93 mg | |
| Trans Fatty Acids | — g | | Zinc | 1.40 mg | 9.33 |
| Cholesterol | 0.00 mg | | | | |
| Water | 3.95 g | | **Amino Acids** | | |
| Ash | 1.23 g | | Alanine | 0.26 g | |
| | | | Arginine | 0.39 g | |
| **Vitamins** | | | Aspartate | 0.41 g | |
| Vitamin A IU | 0.00 IU | 0.00 | Cystine | 0.16 g | 39.02 |
| Vitamin A RE | 0.00 RE | | Glutamate | 0.66 g | |
| A - Carotenoid | 0.00 RE | 0.00 | Glycine | 0.29 g | |
| A - Retinol | 0.00 RE | | Histidine | 0.13 g | 10.08 |
| B1 Thiamin | 0.08 mg | 5.33 | Isoleucine | 0.20 g | 17.39 |
| B2 Riboflavin | 0.17 mg | 10.00 | Leucine | 0.33 g | 13.04 |
| B3 Niacin | 1.25 mg | 6.25 | Lysine | 0.31 g | 13.19 |
| Niacin Equiv | 2.27 mg | | Methionine | 0.11 g | 14.86 |
| Vitamin B6 | 0.09 mg | 4.50 | Phenylalanine | 0.23 g | 19.33 |
| Vitamin B12 | 0.00 mcg | 0.00 | Proline | 0.17 g | |
| Biotin | — mcg | — | Serine | 0.21 g | |
| Vitamin C | 0.00 mg | 0.00 | Threonine | 0.20 g | 16.13 |
| Vitamin D IU | 0.00 IU | 0.00 | Tryptophan | 0.06 g | 18.75 |
| Vitamin D mcg | 0.00 mcg | | Tyrosine | 0.16 g | 16.49 |
| Vitamin E Alpha Equiv | 2.07 mg | 10.35 | Valine | 0.25 g | 17.01 |
| Vitamin E IU | 3.08 IU | | | | |
| Vitamin E mg | 2.07 mg | | | | |
| Folate | 20.83 mcg | 5.21 | | | |
| Vitamin K | — mcg | — | | | |

(Note: "—" indicates data is unavailable. For more information, please see page 806.)

STEP-BY-STEP

## Recipes for Enjoying Quinoa

# *The Healthiest Way of Cooking Quinoa*

*Quinoa's fluffy texture and creamy, yet slightly nutty, flavor can serve as a basis for many delightful meals.*

**1 cup Quinoa**
**2 cups water or broth**
**Sea salt to taste**

1. Place well-rinsed Quinoa with water and salt in a saucepan, **cover** and bring to a boil.

2. Turn the heat to low, keep covered, and simmer for 15 minutes.

   When cooking is complete, the grains become translucent, and the white germ will partially detach itself, appearing like a spiraled tail.

   If you want the Quinoa to have a nuttier flavor, you can dry roast it for five minutes in a skillet, stirring constantly, before cooking.

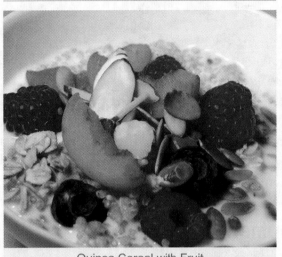
Quinoa Cereal with Fruit

**Preparation Hint:** If you are using prepackaged Quinoa, it is best to follow the directions on the package.

**SERVES 4**

## Flavor Tips: Try these 10 great serving suggestions with the recipe above. ✱

1. When serving Quinoa for lunch or dinner, it is best to prepare it with chicken or vegetable broth and serve with extra virgin olive oil to enhance its flavor.
2. Top cooked vegetables with Quinoa.
3. Sprinkle with lots of freshly minced parsley, sage, chives and/or garlic.
4. Combine with "Healthy Sautéed" onions.
5. Quinoa goes well with "Healthy Sautéed" leeks and celery.
6. Top with tahini (sesame seed butter).
7. **Quinoa Cereal with Fruit:** For a high-protein breakfast, combine cooked Quinoa with rolled oats (uncooked), your favorite fruits, pumpkin seeds and slivered almonds. Top with soy or almond milk and honey (pictured above).
8. **Quinoa Wrap:** Combine the Quinoa recipe with black beans, cilantro and salsa. Wrap in a whole wheat tortilla for an alternative to traditional burritos.
9. **Quinoa Salad:** Combine 1 cup cooked Quinoa with 1 small minced sweet onion, 1 small diced red pepper, 1/4 cup corn kernels and 1/4 chopped cashews or walnuts. Toss with your favorite vinaigrette.
10. **Alternate Quinoa Salad:** Combine 1 cup warm (not hot or cold) Quinoa recipe with 4 thinly sliced scallions, 1/2 cup finely chopped flat leaf parsley, 1/4 cup finely chopped fresh mint, 1 small diced red pepper and 1/4 cup lightly toasted pine nuts. Whisk together extra virgin olive oil and lemon juice to taste. Toss ingredients with dressing and sea salt and pepper to taste. Cooked beans, crumbled feta cheese and diced cucumber (seeds removed) are also great additions to this salad.

Please write (address on back cover flap) or e-mail me at info@whfoods.org with your personal ideas for preparing Quinoa, and I will share them with others through our website at www.whfoods.org.

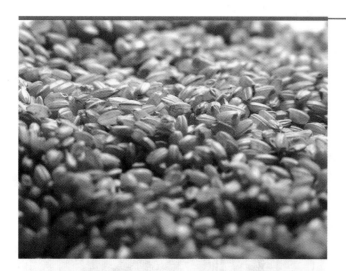

## nutrient-richness chart

Total Nutrient-Richness: **7**  GI: **77**

One cup (195 grams) of cooked Brown Rice contains 216 calories

| NUTRIENT | AMOUNT | %DV | DENSITY | QUALITY |
|---|---|---|---|---|
| Manganese | 1.8 mg | 88.0 | 7.3 | excellent |
| Selenium | 19.1 mcg | 27.3 | 2.3 | good |
| Magnesium | 83.9 mg | 21.0 | 1.7 | good |
| Tryptophan | 0.1 g | 18.8 | 1.6 | good |

For more on "Total Nutrient-Richness," "%DV," "Density," and
The World's Healthiest Foods "Quality" Rating System, see page 805.

For more on GI, see page 342.

Although we have known that the people of Asia have been eating Brown Rice since antiquity, it has only been through recent archeological findings that we are discovering how long they have actually been dependent on rice as a source of food. Rice was first believed to have been cultivated in China 6,000 years ago, but primitive rice seeds and ancient farm tools have been found that date back as far as 9,000 years! It is no wonder that in Asian countries like Thailand rice is so highly valued that the translation of the word "to eat" literally means "to eat rice." Today, rice is one of the most important food staples in the world, supplying as much as half of the daily calories for half of the world's population. Asked to name the types of rice they are familiar with, people may be able to recall one or two. Yet, in actuality, there is an abundance of different types of rice—over 8,000 varieties.

## why brown rice should be part of your healthiest way of eating

All rice is not created equal. That is why only Brown Rice has been included among the World's Healthiest Foods. White rice goes through a complete milling and polishing process that results in a loss of 70–90% of its B vitamins, not

# brown rice

## highlights

| | |
|---|---|
| AVAILABILITY: | Year-round |
| REFRIGERATE: | Yes |
| SHELF LIFE: | 6 months in the refrigerator |
| PREPARATION: | Minimal |
| BEST WAY TO COOK: | Simmer |

to mention large amounts of phosphorus, iron and manganese. Although the United States requires that white rice be enriched with some B vitamins and iron, there are at least eleven other nutrients that are lost and never replaced! That's why it is important to be sure that it is Brown Rice (or unrefined rice) you are enjoying as part of your "Healthiest Way of Eating." (For more on the *Health Benefits of Brown Rice* and a complete analysis of its content of over 60 nutrients, see page 678.)

## varieties of rice

Rice *(Oryza sativa)* is often categorized by the size of the grain: short, medium or long. Short grain rice, which has the highest starch content, makes the stickiest rice, while long grain rice is lighter with grains that tend to remain separate when cooked. The qualities of medium grain fall between the other two.

### SOME VARIETIES OF SPECIALTY RICE INCLUDE:

**BASMATI**

An aromatic rice that has a nutlike fragrance, delicate flavor and light texture. It is available as unrefined brown Basmati rice and refined white Basmati rice.

**JASMINE**

A soft-textured, long grain, aromatic rice that is available in both brown (unrefined) and white (refined) varieties.

**BHUTANESE RED RICE**

Grown in the Himalayas, this red-colored rice has a nutty, earthy taste.

**FORBIDDEN RICE**

A black-colored rice that turns purple upon cooking and has a sweet taste and sticky texture.

**POPULAR VARIETIES OF REFINED (POLISHED) RICE INCLUDE:**

**ARBORIO**

A round, starchy white rice, it is traditionally used to make the Italian dish *risotto*.

**SWEET RICE**

Almost translucent when it is cooked, this very sticky rice is traditionally used to make the Japanese dish mochi.

**WILD RICE**

Not a true rice, but the seed of a grass from a completely different botanical family. It has a nut-like flavor and is chewy when cooked. It is good to mix with Brown Rice.

## the peak season

Brown Rice is harvested in the fall but is available throughout the year.

## 4 steps to the best tasting and most nutritious brown rice

Turning Brown Rice into a flavorful dish with the most nutrients is simple if you just follow my 4 easy steps:

1. The Best Way to Select
2. The Best Way to Store
3. The Best Way to Prepare
4. The Healthiest Way of Cooking

# 1. the best way to select brown rice

Brown Rice is available prepackaged as well as in bulk containers. The best way to select prepackaged Brown Rice is by the checking the use-by date on the package. It is important to not use Brown Rice past its expiration date since it contains natural oils, which have the potential to become rancid if kept too long. As with all grains, I recommend selecting organically grown Brown Rice whenever possible. (For more on *Organic Foods*, see page 113.)

When purchasing Brown Rice in bulk, make sure that the bins containing the Brown Rice are covered and that the store has a good product turnover to ensure its maximal freshness. Whether purchasing Brown Rice in bulk or in a packaged container, it is important that there is no evidence of moisture.

# 2. the best way to store brown rice

Since Brown Rice still features an oil-rich germ, it is more susceptible to becoming rancid than white rice and therefore should be stored in the refrigerator. Stored in an airtight container, Brown Rice will keep fresh for about 6 months.

# 3. the best way to prepare brown rice

Before cooking rice, especially if it is sold in bulk, rinse it thoroughly under running water and then remove any dirt or debris that you may find.

# 4. the healthiest way of cooking brown rice

Brown Rice is a favorite side dish that complements almost any meal and also makes a great breakfast cereal. When cooking my Brown Rice, I prefer a water to rice ratio of 2 to 1 (2$^{1}$/2 to 1 for long grain rice). But if you want your Brown Rice to take on more of a porridge-like texture, like the Chinese dish *congee*, you can use more water (up to 6 parts to 1 part Brown Rice) and cook it until the grain becomes very soft.

**Q** *Can you tell me more about wild rice?*

**A** Like many grains, wild rice is a rich source of fiber, minerals and B vitamins. Interestingly, wild rice belongs to a completely different family than regular rice (i.e., Brown Rice, white rice). Its scientific name is *Zizania aquatica* while rice's is *Oryza sativa*.

**Q** *Is it OK to eat instant Brown Rice or has it lost some of the nourishment of regular Brown Rice?*

**A** It is fine to eat instant Brown Rice, which is Brown Rice that has been precooked and dried. While it loses some of its nutritional value in the process, the loss is minimal, and it is a convenient substitute for rice when there is little time to cook.

# health benefits of brown rice

## Promotes Optimal Weight Control

Eating Brown Rice may help in maintaining optimal weight. A recent large-scale study found that weight gain was inversely associated with the intake of high-fiber whole-grain foods but positively related to the intake of refined-grain foods. Not only did women who consumed more whole grains consistently weigh less than those who ate less of these fiber-rich foods, but those consuming the most dietary fiber from whole grains were 49% less likely to gain weight compared to those eating foods made from refined grains.

## Promotes Optimal Health

Brown Rice is rich in phytonutrients that have shown promising health benefits. Among them is ferulic acid, an antioxidant that has been found to scavenge free radicals and protect against radiation-induced cellular oxidative damage. Ferulic acid and other phytonutrients in Brown Rice have been researched for their potential to control high blood pressure, protect against kidney stones and prevent cancer in experimental animals. Since they are found in the bran and germ of rice, you get their maximal benefits by eating Brown, but not white, rice.

Brown Rice also contains minerals with strong antioxidant activity. It is an excellent source of manganese, a component of an antioxidant enzyme called *superoxide dismutase,* which protects the mitochondria against damage from the free radicals produced during energy production. Brown Rice also features concentrated amounts of selenium, which acts as an antioxidant, protecting cells from compounds that may promote cancer. Selenium is also important for maintaining thyroid hormone metabolism.

## Promotes Heart Health

Another reason to incorporate Brown Rice into your diet is that it may protect your cardiovascular health. In many instances of heart disease, where oxidative stress has been shown to be the source of blood vessel damage, low intake of selenium, of which Brown Rice is a good source, has been identified as a contributing factor to the disease. Brown Rice is also a good source of magnesium, a mineral that relaxes nerves and muscles, promoting the optimal functioning of blood vessels. As noted above, Brown Rice's ferulic acid has been shown to have promising cardiovascular benefits. Research in animals suggests that it may reduce blood pressure and protect against the oxidation of lipids, one of the first steps in the development of atherosclerosis.

## Promotes Digestive Health

Like other whole grains, Brown Rice provides ample amounts of dietary fiber, a nutrient critical for promoting normalized bowel function and keeping the gastrointestinal system healthy. Dietary fiber also helps to keep blood sugar levels under control.

## Additional Health-Promoting Benefit of Brown Rice

Brown Rice is a concentrated source of sleep-promoting tryptophan.

### Nutritional Analysis of 1 cup of cooked Brown Rice:

| NUTRIENT | AMOUNT | % DAILY VALUE | NUTRIENT | AMOUNT | % DAILY VALUE |
|---|---|---|---|---|---|
| Calories | 216.45 | | Pantothenic Acid | 0.56 mg | 5.60 |
| Calories from Fat | 15.80 | | | | |
| Calories from Saturated Fat | 3.16 | | **Minerals** | | |
| Protein | 5.03 g | | Boron | — mcg | |
| Carbohydrates | 44.77 g | | Calcium | 19.50 mg | 1.95 |
| Dietary Fiber | 3.51 g | 14.04 | Chloride | 448.50 mg | |
| Soluble Fiber | 0.39 g | | Chromium | — mcg | — |
| Insoluble Fiber | 3.12 g | | Copper | 0.20 mg | 10.00 |
| Sugar — Total | 0.39 g | | Fluoride | — mg | — |
| Monosaccharides | 0.00 g | | Iodine | — mcg | — |
| Disaccharides | 0.39 g | | Iron | 0.82 mg | 4.56 |
| Other Carbs | 40.87 g | | Magnesium | 83.85 mg | 20.96 |
| Fat – Total | 1.76 g | | Manganese | 1.76 mg | 88.00 |
| Saturated Fat | 0.35 g | | Molybdenum | — mcg | — |
| Mono Fat | 0.64 g | | Phosphorus | 161.85 mg | 16.18 |
| Poly Fat | 0.63 g | | Potassium | 83.85 mg | |
| Omega-3 Fatty Acids | 0.03 g | 1.20 | Selenium | 19.11 mcg | 27.30 |
| Omega-6 Fatty Acids | 0.60 g | | Sodium | 9.75 mg | |
| Trans Fatty Acids | — g | | Zinc | 1.23 mg | 8.20 |
| Cholesterol | 0.00 mg | | | | |
| Water | 142.53 g | | **Amino Acids** | | |
| Ash | 0.90 g | | Alanine | 0.29 g | |
| | | | Arginine | 0.38 g | |
| **Vitamins** | | | Aspartate | 0.47 g | |
| Vitamin A IU | 0.00 IU | 0.00 | Cystine | 0.06 g | 14.63 |
| Vitamin A RE | 0.00 RE | | Glutamate | 1.02 g | |
| A - Carotenoid | 0.00 RE | 0.00 | Glycine | 0.25 g | |
| A - Retinol | 0.00 RE | | Histidine | 0.13 g | 10.08 |
| B1 Thiamin | 0.19 mg | 12.67 | Isoleucine | 0.21 g | 18.26 |
| B2 Riboflavin | 0.05 mg | 2.94 | Leucine | 0.42 g | 16.60 |
| B3 Niacin | 2.98 mg | 14.90 | Lysine | 0.19 g | 8.09 |
| Niacin Equiv | 4.05 mg | | Methionine | 0.11 g | 14.86 |
| Vitamin B6 | 0.28 mg | 14.00 | Phenylalanine | 0.26 g | 21.85 |
| Vitamin B12 | 0.00 mcg | 0.00 | Proline | 0.24 g | |
| Biotin | 1.54 mcg | 0.51 | Serine | 0.26 g | |
| Vitamin C | 0.00 mg | 0.00 | Threonine | 0.19 g | 15.32 |
| Vitamin D IU | 0.00 IU | 0.00 | Tryptophan | 0.06 g | 18.75 |
| Vitamin D mcg | 0.00 mcg | | Tyrosine | 0.19 g | 19.59 |
| Vitamin E Alpha Equiv | 1.40 mg | 7.00 | Valine | 0.29 g | 19.73 |
| Vitamin E IU | 2.09 IU | | | | |
| Vitamin E mg | 1.40 mg | | | | |
| Folate | 7.80 mcg | 1.95 | | | |
| Vitamin K | 1.17 mcg | 1.46 | | | |

(Note: "—" indicates data is unavailable. For more information, please see page 806.)

STEP-BY-STEP
## Recipes for Enjoying Brown Rice

# *The Healthiest Way of Cooking Brown Rice*

*This traditional way of cooking Brown Rice provides the foundation for a wide variety of rice dishes—or just enjoy as is!*

**1 cup short or medium grain Brown Rice**
**2 cups water or broth**
**(for long grain Brown Rice**
**add 1/2 cup more water)**
**Sea salt to taste**

1. Bring water and salt to a boil. While water is heating, wash rice under cool running water, which not only cleans it but prevents it from sticking together.

2. Add rice to boiling water and return water to a boil. Turn down the heat to low and **cover**.

3. Simmer for about 45 minutes.

**Preparation Hints:**
You can also follow this recipe to prepare Brown

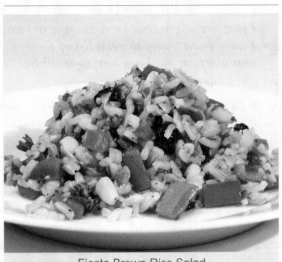
Fiesta Brown Rice Salad

Basmati Rice, which has a lighter, fluffier texture (and a wonderfully sweet aroma). Before putting any type of Brown Rice in the pot, soak it in a bowl of cool water, stirring frequently and replace the water four or five times until the water no longer has a milky appearance.

If you are using prepackaged Brown Rice, it is best to follow the directions on the package.

**SERVES 3**

---

## Flavor Tips: Try these 7 great serving suggestions with the recipe above. ✱

1. Top Brown Rice with nuts, sesame seeds, "Healthy Sautéed" mushrooms, scallions or raisins.
2. For optimal nutrition, it is best to serve Brown Rice with beans, dairy or nuts and seeds to make a complete protein.
3. **Fiesta Brown Rice Salad:** Combine 4 cups cooked brown rice, 1 diced red and 1 diced green bell pepper, 1 cup of corn and 1 cup of black beans. Toss with Healthy Vinaigrette (see page 143). Mix 1 tsp turmeric to dressing. Sprinkle rice salad with chopped cilantro (pictured above).
4. **Sesame Rice:** Combine cooked Brown Rice recipe

with 1 TBS toasted sesame oil, 1½ TBS sesame seeds, 1 cup thinly sliced scallions (green onions) and 1–2 TBS of tamari (soy sauce). Toss all together. Serve with fish or chicken.
5. **Rice Pudding:** Heat up cooked Brown Rice and cover with milk or soymilk. Add cinnamon, nutmeg, raisins and honey for a delicious rice pudding.
6. **Vegetable Sushi Rolls:** Wrap Brown Rice and your favorite vegetables in nori sheets. Dip in tamari (soy sauce) and wasabi.
7. **Sea Vegetable Rice:** Combine Brown Rice with soaked sea vegetables, such as dulse, hijiki or arame.

---

Please write (address on back cover flap) or e-mail me at info@whfoods.org with your personal ideas for preparing Brown Rice, and I will share them with others through our website at www.whfoods.org.

Here are questions I received from readers of the <u>whfoods.org</u> website about Brown Rice:

**Q** *I just found out that I am allergic to rice. I have been trying to get a list of foods that contain rice, but I am having trouble. Can you help me?*

**A** Regarding rice-containing products, what is going to be very important to do is to read labels. Fortunately, rice is easier to identify than wheat- or dairy-containing foods where a host of ingredients that don't bear the name wheat or dairy do, in fact, appear in these foods. So, read the labels of packaged food, and if you buy food at a deli counter, ask the clerk whether there is rice in it. Do the same thing when in a restaurant. Depending upon the seriousness of your allergy, you may want to make sure that the food that you order is not cooked in the same cookware as rice-containing recipes.

In terms of foods and ingredients, here are some that come to mind—rice, rice cakes, rice milk, mochi, rice starch, rice protein and sake, the Japanese alcoholic drink. This list may not be comprehensive but it is a great start.

Depending upon the seriousness of your allergy, you may also want to ensure that the other grains that you purchase were not packaged in a factory that also packaged rice. You can ask your grocer for help in this arena, or if you buy packaged grains, call the company and ask them. Chances are this may not be an issue, but you may want to check just to be safe.

**Q** *I was recently told that chemicals are now being added to Brown Rice to give it the brown color. I have difficulty believing this is true but wanted to check.*

**A** I am not aware of any manufacturers adding coloring agents to Brown Rice in order to alter its color. The brown color is a natural part of most unpolished rice and is, in fact, a sign that the rice has not been heavily processed. At the same time, however, I'm aware of no regulation that would prevent a rice manufacturer from adding a coloring agent to Brown Rice. Rice-containing mixes that include spices and seasonings along with the rice (and are designed to be used as part of a stir-fry, for example) often contain artificial coloring agents, such as caramel color, that will help produce a golden brown color. Since artificial coloring agents are not allowed in the production of organically grown foods, including organically grown Brown Rice, the purchase of organic Brown Rice would be one way to make sure that no artificial coloring agents were involved.

**Q** *How long does cooked Brown Rice stay fresh in the refrigerator?*

**A** In general, I like the idea of preparing a very limited amount of Brown Rice—only the amount that you will be consuming on that same day, or at most, by the end of the following day. One night of refrigeration is really all I recommend. My thinking is very conservative here, and I realize that many organizations support refrigeration of rice for as many as four to seven days.

However, I believe that there are some unnecessary risks worth avoiding in the case of cooked rice. These risks all involve the presence of moisture, time, temperature, bacteria, fungi or spores. The growth of toxin-producing fungi is probably the greatest of these risks. It appears that some fungi can turn one of the amino acids (tryptophan) in rice into alpha-picolinic acid; this substance, when excessive, can cause hypersensitivity reactions to rice in some persons. Another mycotoxin (fungus-triggered toxin) called T-2 can also be produced in rice by the fungus Fusarium. While these fungus-related problems are fairly unlikely to occur, their risk of occurrence will increase along with increased storage time for the cooked rice. I believe the added inconvenience of preparing rice more frequently is worth the effort. For increased safety, I would also recommend letting your cooked rice cool to room temperature before placing it in the refrigerator. I'd also recommend storing it in a tightly sealed container.

**Q** *Can I substitute rice flour one for one in a cookie recipe that calls for wheat flour?*

**A** That is a very good question you ask since replacing one type of flour for another is not always on a one-to-one ratio. However, in this case, you can use one cup of rice flour in place of each one cup of regular wheat flour called for in the cookie recipe and it should be fine. Yet, if you find that the mixture looks a bit too soft, you may want to add just a little bit more rice flour.

**Q** *What is cargo rice?*

**A** "Cargo" is a term used to classify rice according to the degree of milling that it undergoes. Cargo rice only has its outer hull removed and is therefore much more nutrient-rich than heavily milled rice such as white rice; Brown Rice is a cargo rice. There is also a red cargo rice, a Bhutanese rice grown in the Himalayas, which has recently become popular; it is a red-colored rice with a nutty, earthy taste.

Q *Can you tell me if Asian rice noodles are typically made from the whole rice grain?*

A There are so many different types of Asian rice noodles that it is difficult to say for certain. Most of the rice noodles I have seen seem to be white in color, which makes me think that they are from refined rice. The best thing to do would be to check the Nutrition Facts on the package to see what the fiber content is. This will give you a clue as to whether it is made from fiber-rich Brown Rice or fiber-depleted white rice. Additionally, if manufacturers use Brown Rice, they may note this in their ingredients listing, so you may want to check there as well.

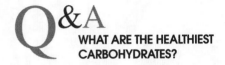

### Q&A
### WHAT ARE THE HEALTHIEST CARBOHYDRATES?

It would be difficult to find a hotter topic in the world of nutrition than carbohydrates (carbs). Or to be more specific: low-carb, no-carb and carb-smart foods.

Thanks to the Zone diet, the Atkins diet, the South Beach diet and the Paleolithic Prescription, many people have become aware of carbohydrates as a controversial part of the diet. Here are some basic facts you should know about carbs before you make up your mind about your own carb intake.

First and foremost, humans have always relied on carbs for part of their nourishment. Carbs include sugars, starches and most fibers, and carbs are found in virtually all plant foods. A cup of shredded iceberg lettuce has carbs (only 1 gram, however). A cup of green peas has 24 grams of carbs (6 grams of sugar, 10 grams of starch and 8 grams of fiber). Nuts and seeds are similar to lettuce insofar as they contain very few carbs, along the lines of 5 grams per ounce (3 grams of fiber, 1/2 gram of sugar, and 1½ grams of starch). Fruits, grains, beans, nuts, seeds—they all contain carbs.

Animal foods are another matter. Animals store some starch in their muscles and liver and have some circulating sugars, but not very much in comparison to plants. There are basically no carbs in an 8-ounce steak or in a chicken breast. For an egg, the carb level creeps up to 1/2 gram—but that's it. Not until we come to milk do we see the carb level increase. This time it's due to the milk sugar (lactose), which is found in cow's milk at approximately 10–12 grams per cup.

From my perspective, the biggest problem with the U.S. diet is not so much the total amount of carbs, but the quality of the carbs. We are averaging somewhere around 19% of our total calories from highly processed starch (wheat flour) products, which contain about 100 grams of very low-nutrient carbs. (The sugar adds about 80 more grams of carbs.) The total is 180 grams of carbs that brings very little to the plate in terms of nourishment. I recommend upgrading the quality of your carbs regardless of how many carbs you eat.

The question of how many carbs to eat does not have one clear-cut answer. Clearly, our understanding of "macronutrient balance" (the ratio of protein to carbohydrate to fat in our diet) has been changing over the past 20 years, and the very high-carb diets of the 1970s and 1980s with 75% of calories coming from carbohydrate are now being looked at much differently. There is a trend way from "white" grain consumption (refined flour prooducts) with vegetables gaining more emphasis as a carb source. High-carb diets may definitely be the wrong way for many people to lose weight. They may also be inappropriate for many people who have difficulty controlling their blood sugar. However, in the case of blood sugar, it's not the carbohydrate designation *per se,* but where the carbohydrate falls on the glycemic index, that seems most important. (The glycemic index is a rating given to foods based on their blood sugar impact.) Persons with certain hormonal patterns may also be better off staying away from high-carb intake.

Still, when it comes to carbs, "one size doesn't fit all." To a certain extent, our bodies are meant to run on sugars and starches, and extremely low-carb diets can be dangerous over long periods of time. Somewhere around 75 to 100 grams of carbs or less, our bodies tend to undergo a metabolic shift called ketosis, and while this shift is sometimes used therapeutically (to help control seizures, for example), it is not a natural state of affairs for our body over the long run.

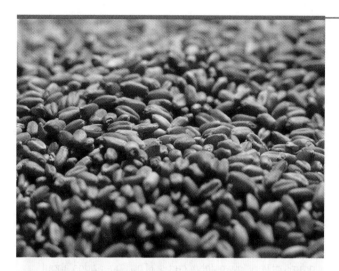

## nutrient-richness chart

Total Nutrient-Richness: **7**　　　　　　GI: **67**
One cup (182 grams) of cooked Wheat Bulgur contains 151 calories

| NUTRIENT | AMOUNT | %DV | DENSITY | QUALITY |
|---|---|---|---|---|
| Manganese | 1.1 mg | 55.5 | 6.6 | very good |
| Dietary Fiber | 8.2 g | 32.8 | 3.9 | very good |
| Tryptophan | 0.1 g | 28.1 | 3.4 | very good |
| Magnesium | 58.2 mg | 14.6 | 1.7 | good |
| **CAROTENOIDS:** | | | Daily values for these nutrients have not yet been established. | |
| Lutein + Zeaxanthin | 99.0 mcg | | | |

For more on "Total Nutrient-Richness," "%DV," "Density," and
The World's Healthiest Foods "Quality" Rating System, see page 805.

For more on GI, see page 342.

Considered the "Staff of Life" in the Bible, Wheat is believed to have been consumed for more than 12,000 years. Today, approximately one-third of the world's population depends on Wheat for nourishment. Kansas is known as the Wheat Capital of the World. In 1997, they harvested more than 490 million bushels of Wheat or enough to bake 36 billion loaves of bread! Wheat is ubiquitous in the United States with bread, pasta, pizza dough, bagels, crackers, cakes, cookies and muffins just part of a long list of popular Wheat products.

## why whole wheat should be part of your healthiest way of eating

Wheat, in its natural unrefined state, features a host of important nutrients. Unfortunately, most of the Wheat products in the United States have been processed into 60% extraction, which means that 40% of the original Wheat grain was removed, leaving only 60%. The problem with this is that the 40% that gets removed includes the bran and the germ of the

# whole wheat

## highlights

| | |
|---|---|
| AVAILABILITY: | Year-round |
| REFRIGERATE: | No |
| SHELF LIFE: | Several months |
| PREPARATION: | Minimal |
| BEST WAY TO COOK: | Simmer |

Wheat grain—its most nutrient-rich parts. The bran and germ include more than half of the vitamins B1, B2, B3 and E, as well as folic acid, calcium, phosphorus, zinc, copper, iron and fiber, all of which are subsequently lost in refined Wheat. While the law requires that processed Wheat is "enriched," not nearly as much of the nutrients are replaced as have been extracted. That is why it is very important to select 100% Whole Wheat products as part of your "Healthiest Way of Eating." (For more on the *Health Benefits of Whole Wheat* and a complete analysis of its content of over 60 nutrients, see page 684.)

## varieties of wheat

Wheat *(Triticum spp.)* is an ancient grain that is believed to have originated in southwestern Asia. Classes of Wheat are defined by their planting season and the hardness and color of the kernel (red or white):

### HARD RED WINTER/HARD RED SPRING

These are the most commonly used forms for milling all-purpose flour, especially for baking bread. The hardest variety of Wheat is Durham, which is processed into semolina to make pasta and couscous.

### SOFT RED WINTER/SOFT WHITE SPRING

Milled into flour for making cakes, cookies, pastries and crackers.

100% Whole Wheat contains the germ, bran and endosperm of the Wheat grain, while refined Wheat contains only the endosperm, or starchy portion of the grain. Varieties of 100% Whole Wheat include:

**WHOLE WHEAT BERRIES OR GROATS**

Whole Wheat berries that have not been processed. They can be used in a main dish featuring grains, as a side dish or as an addition to soups or yeast breads.

**BULGUR**

Whole Wheat berries that have been steamed, cooked, dried and cracked. They come in fine, medium and coarse grain. Coarse grain is usually used to make pilaf, the medium grain is generally used for cereal and the fine grain is used to make tabouli.

**CRACKED WHEAT BERRIES**

Whole Wheat berries that have been cracked into coarse, medium and fine granulations. Cracked Wheat can substitute for other grains or rice in recipes.

**ROLLED WHEAT BERRIES**

Similar to rolled oats but thicker and firmer. They can be used as a hot cereal or added to baked goods.

The chart on page 663 shows the percentage of the nutrients found in the three components of the Wheat grain and illustrates the small proportion of the nutrients you receive when selecting refined Wheat products that only contain the endosperm.

Other forms of Wheat that are not 100% Whole Wheat include:

**WHEAT GERM**

The sprouting portion of the Wheat grain. It is rich in nutrients, especially vitamin E, and should be kept refrigerated.

**WHEAT BRAN**

The protective outer layer of the Wheat grain, it is rich in minerals and high in insoluble fiber. Since it is high in the WGA lectin, people with very mild Wheat allergies may have more problems with isolated Wheat germ than they would with consumption of the whole grain.

**COUSCOUS**

Made from semolina flour, the same type of flour used to make pasta (semolina flour is not whole wheat). Couscous is steamed and dried. Quick-cooking Couscous requires only steaming for a fluffy texture or just add boiling water for a denser texture.

## the peak season available year-round.

## biochemical considerations

The germ of Wheat is a concentrated source of oxalates, which might be of concern to certain individuals. Wheat is also one of the foods most commonly associated with allergic reactions. Wheat contains gluten proteins to which some people have intolerance. (For more on *Oxalates*, see page 725; *Food Allergies*, see page 719; and *Gluten Intolerance*, see page 720.)

# 1. the best way to select whole wheat —————

Whole Wheat flour, berries and bulgur are generally sold in bulk. Just as with any other food that you may purchase in the bulk section, make sure that the bins containing the Wheat are covered and that the store has a good product turnover to ensure its maximal freshness. Whether purchasing Wheat in bulk or in a packaged container, it is important that no evidence of moisture is present.

Wheat germ is highly perishable. When purchasing Wheat germ, always look for packages in sealed containers (especially those that are vacuum packaged) as they will be more protected from potential oxidation and rancidity. Wheat germ in sealed containers that are not vacuum packed should be kept in the store's refrigerator section. Wheat germ should have a slightly sweet, nutty taste; a bitter undertaste is a sign it has become rancid and should be thrown away.

# 2. the best way to store whole wheat —————

Wheat berries should be stored in an airtight container in a cool, dry and dark place. The optimal way to store Wheat products such as flour, bulgur, bran and germ is in an air-tight container in the refrigerator as a cooler temperature will help to prevent them from becoming rancid.

# 3. the best way to prepare whole wheat —————

Whole Wheat products bought in bulk, except for flour, should be washed before cooking. Packaged products do not require rinsing.

# 4. the healthiest way of cooking whole wheat —

For making hot cereal or porridge, it is best to add the Wheat berries or rolled Whole Wheat kernels to boiling water and then simmer. Bulgur requires no cooking. Wheat berries can be sprouted by soaking berries overnight.

# health benefits of whole wheat

## Promotes Digestive Health

Wheat bran is a popular bulk laxative. For most people, a third of a cup per day is all that is necessary to promote healthy, regular bowel movements. A study examining the effects of fiber on bowel regularity found that 89% of the participants eating a fiber-rich diet primarily composed of Whole Wheat breads, cereals high in bran and supplemental "miller's bran" alleviated the symptoms of diverticular disease (i.e., pain, nausea, flatulence, distension and constipation).

## Promotes Healthy Weight Control

A recent large-scale study found that weight gain was inversely associated with the intake of high-fiber whole-grain foods, such as Whole Wheat, but positively related to the intake of refined-grain foods, such as products made from refined wheat. Not only did the female study subjects who consumed more whole grains consistently weigh less than those who ate less of these fiber-rich foods, but those consuming the most dietary fiber from whole grains were 49% less likely to gain weight compared to those eating foods made from refined grains.

## Promotes Balanced Blood Sugar

In addition to helping maintain balanced weight, eating more whole grain foods, like Whole Wheat, has been also linked to protecting against insulin resistance (the precursor of Type 2 diabetes) and the metabolic syndrome (a strong predictor of both diabetes and cardiovascular disease); eating refined grains and the foods made from them has been linked to an increased risk of both conditions as well as weight gain. In a recent study, the prevalence of both insulin resistance and the metabolic syndrome was significantly lower among those eating the most cereal fiber from whole grains compared to those eating the least.

## Promotes Optimal Health

A recent study suggests that eating foods high in insoluble fiber, such as cereals and breads made from Whole Wheat, may help women avoid gallstones. Researchers found that female study participants who consumed the most fiber overall (both soluble and insoluble) had a 13% lower risk of developing gallstones compared to women consuming the fewest fiber-rich foods. Those eating the most foods rich in insoluble fiber, such as that found in Whole Wheat, gained even more protection against gallstones: a 17% lower risk compared to women eating the least. And the protection was dose-related: a 5-gram increase in insoluble fiber intake dropped risk by 10%.

## Additional Health-Promoting Benefits of Whole Wheat

Whole Wheat is also a concentrated source of other nutrients providing additional health-promoting benefits. These nutrients include free-radical-scavenging manganese, muscle-relaxing magnesium and sleep-promoting tryptophan.

### Nutritional Analysis of 1 cup of cooked Wheat Bulgur:

| NUTRIENT | AMOUNT | % DAILY VALUE | NUTRIENT | AMOUNT | % DAILY VALUE |
|---|---|---|---|---|---|
| Calories | 151.06 | | Pantothenic Acid | 0.63 mg | 6.30 |
| Calories from Fat | 3.93 | | | | |
| Calories from Saturated Fat | 0.69 | | **Minerals** | | |
| Protein | 5.61 g | | Boron | — mcg | |
| Carbohydrates | 33.82 g | | Calcium | 18.20 mg | 1.82 |
| Dietary Fiber | 8.19 g | 32.76 | Chloride | — mg | |
| Soluble Fiber | 1.38 g | | Chromium | — mcg | — |
| Insoluble Fiber | 6.81 g | | Copper | 0.14 mg | 7.00 |
| Sugar – Total | 0.36 g | | Fluoride | — mg | — |
| Monosaccharides | — g | | Iodine | — mcg | — |
| Disaccharides | 0.83 g | | Iron | 1.75 mg | 9.72 |
| Other Carbs | 25.26 g | | Magnesium | 58.24 mg | 14.56 |
| Fat – Total | 0.44 g | | Manganese | 1.11 mg | 55.50 |
| Saturated Fat | 0.08 g | | Molybdenum | — mcg | — |
| Mono Fat | 0.06 g | | Phosphorus | 72.80 mg | 7.28 |
| Poly Fat | 0.18 g | | Potassium | 123.76 mg | |
| Omega-3 Fatty Acids | 0.01 g | 0.40 | Selenium | 1.09 mcg | 1.56 |
| Omega-6 Fatty Acids | 0.17 g | | Sodium | 9.10 mg | |
| Trans Fatty Acids | — g | | Zinc | 1.04 mg | 6.93 |
| Cholesterol | 0.00 mg | | | | |
| Water | 141.52 g | | **Amino Acids** | | |
| Ash | 0.62 g | | Alanine | 0.20 g | |
| | | | Arginine | 0.26 g | |
| **Vitamins** | | | Aspartate | 0.29 g | |
| Vitamin A IU | 0.00 IU | 0.00 | Cystine | 0.13 g | 31.71 |
| Vitamin A RE | 0.00 RE | | Glutamate | 1.77 g | |
| A - Carotenoid | 0.00 RE | 0.00 | Glycine | 0.23 g | |
| A - Retinol | 0.00 RE | | Histidine | 0.13 g | 10.08 |
| B1 Thiamin | 0.10 mg | 6.67 | Isoleucine | 0.21 g | 18.26 |
| B2 Riboflavin | 0.05 mg | 2.94 | Leucine | 0.38 g | 15.02 |
| B3 Niacin | 1.82 mg | 9.10 | Lysine | 0.15 g | 6.38 |
| Niacin Equiv | 3.28 mg | | Methionine | 0.09 g | 12.16 |
| Vitamin B6 | 0.15 mg | 7.50 | Phenylalanine | 0.26 g | 21.85 |
| Vitamin B12 | 0.00 mcg | 0.00 | Proline | 0.58 g | |
| Biotin | — mcg | — | Serine | 0.26 g | |
| Vitamin C | 0.00 mg | 0.00 | Threonine | 0.16 g | 12.90 |
| Vitamin D IU | 0.00 IU | 0.00 | Tryptophan | 0.09 g | 28.13 |
| Vitamin D mcg | 0.00 mcg | | Tyrosine | 0.16 g | 16.49 |
| Vitamin E Alpha Equiv | 0.05 mg | 0.25 | Valine | 0.25 g | 17.01 |
| Vitamin E IU | 0.08 IU | | | | |
| Vitamin E mg | 0.55 mg | | | | |
| Folate | 32.76 mcg | 8.19 | | | |
| Vitamin K | 0.91 mcg | 1.14 | | | |

(Note: "—" indicates data is unavailable. For more information, please see page 806.)

## Recipes for Enjoying Whole Wheat

# Mediterranean Tabouli Salad

*Bulgur does not need to be cooked, just softened, because it has already been steamed, dried and cracked. It is a traditional ingredient in Tabouli Salad.*

2 cups Wheat Bulgur
3 cups parsley, minced
1/2 medium onion, minced
1 medium tomato, chopped
3 TBS extra virgin olive oil
1 TBS fresh lemon juice or wine vinegar
2 cloves garlic, pressed or chopped
Sea salt and pepper to taste

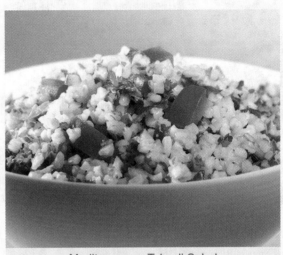

Mediterranean Tabouli Salad

**To prepare Bulgur:** Place 1 cup Wheat Bulgur and salt to taste in a bowl. Pour 2 cups boiling water or broth over the Bulgur, stir once and let sit for 15–20 minutes until liquid is absorbed.

Combine all ingredients and mix well.

For added flavor you may want to add more olive oil and lemon juice.

**SERVES 4**

## Flavor Tips: 2 Ways to Enjoy Wheat Bulgur

1. Bulgur goes well with "Healthy Sautéed" leeks and celery.

2. For breakfast, add sliced almonds, chopped walnuts, dried apricots, currants or dried cranberries, and soymilk and honey to bulgur.

# The Healthiest Way of Cooking Whole Wheat Berries

*For an energizing breakfast, cooked Whole Wheat Berries are a great way to start the day because they are hearty and have a nut-like flavor. Combine with raisins or dried cranberries, your favorite fresh fruit and nuts and seeds, such as almonds, walnuts, sunflower seeds or pumpkin seeds. Serve with soy or almond milk and add honey and cinnamon to taste.*

1 cup Whole Wheat Berries, rinsed
3 cups water
Pinch of sea salt

Add water and a pinch of salt to a sauce pan, cover and bring to boil. Add Wheat Berries to boiling water. After water has returned to a boil, reduce heat, **cover**, simmer for 1–1$^{1}$/2 hours and drain.

**SERVES 3**

**Preparation Hints:**
Wheat Berries will cook more quickly if they are soaked overnight; discard soaking water. If you are using prepackaged Whole Wheat Berries, it is best to follow the directions on the package.

Whole Wheat is best known as the main ingredient in baking bread, pizza dough, pie crust, sour dough bread, muffins and desserts. There are hundreds of great books written on how to prepare these foods, and therefore I have not included recipes for them here.

Please write (address on back cover flap) or e-mail me at <u>info@whfoods.org</u> with your personal ideas for preparing Whole Wheat, and I will share them with others through our website at <u>www.whfoods.org</u>.

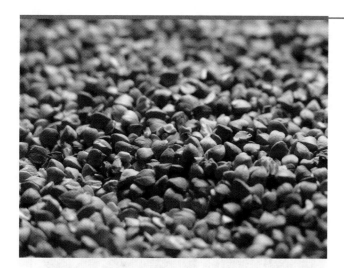

## nutrient-richness chart

| Total Nutrient-Richness: | 5 | | | GI: 76 |
|---|---|---|---|---|

One cup (168 grams) of cooked Buckwheat Groats contains 154 calories

| NUTRIENT | AMOUNT | %DV | DENSITY | QUALITY |
|---|---|---|---|---|
| Manganese | 0.7 mg | 34.0 | 4.0 | very good |
| Tryptophan | 0.1 g | 25.0 | 2.9 | good |
| Magnesium | 85.67 mg | 21.4 | 2.5 | good |
| Dietary Fiber | 4.5 g | 18.2 | 2.1 | good |

| **CAROTENOIDS:** | | Daily values for these nutrients have not yet been established. |
|---|---|---|
| Lutein + Zeaxanthin | 101.0 mcg | |

For more on "Total Nutrient-Richness," "%DV," "Density," and The World's Healthiest Foods "Quality" Rating System, see page 805.

For more on GI, see page 342.

**B**uckwheat is actually not a true grain but a fruit seed that is related to rhubarb. Energizing and nutritious, it is gluten-free and therefore can serve as a grain substitute for individuals sensitive to wheat and other grains that contain the protein gluten. The name Buckwheat is believed to have been derived from the Dutch word *bockweit*, which means "beech wheat," reflecting its beechnut-like shape and its wheat-like characteristics. The French are famous for their buckwheat crepes, and the Russians for *blinis*, their version of a buckwheat crepe that is usually filled with caviar. Buckwheat has a unique flavor that is stronger than any other grain.

## why buckwheat should be part of your healthiest way of eating

The flavonoid phytonutrients found in Buckwheat, such as quercetin and kaempferol, provide powerful antioxidant protection against damage from free radicals. Buckwheat is

# buckwheat

## highlights

| | |
|---|---|
| AVAILABILITY: | Year-round |
| REFRIGERATE: | No |
| SHELF LIFE: | 6 months |
| PREPARATION: | Minimal |
| BEST WAY TO COOK: | Simmer |

also a very good source of manganese, a trace mineral necessary to help protect the mitochondria—the energy-production factories in our cells—from free-radical-scavenging. (For more on the *Health Benefits of Buckwheat* and a complete analysis of its content of over 60 nutrients, see page 688.)

## varieties of buckwheat

Buckwheat is known botanically as *Polygonum fagopyrum* and is native to both Northern Europe as well as Asia. Since Buckwheat does not contain gluten, it is necessary to mix Buckwheat flour with some type of gluten-containing flour (such as wheat) for baking bread or other leavened foods.

Buckwheat is sold either unroasted or roasted. Unroasted Buckwheat has a soft, subtle flavor, while roasted Buckwheat has more of an earthy, nutty taste. Its color ranges from tannish-pink to brown after roasting.

### BUCKWHEAT GROATS

These are raw Buckwheat kernels with their shells removed. They are unroasted and often referred to as whole white Buckwheat Groats. White Groats can be substituted in recipes calling for rice.

### KASHA

Since the Russian porridge dish known as kasha is often-times made with roasted Buckwheat Groats, this form of Buckwheat is usually called by this name. Kasha can come in coarse, medium or fine granules and is an excellent accompaniment to meat dishes or can be combined with vegetables for a main dish. It has a sweeter, nuttier flavor than unroasted Buckwheat Groats.

**BUCKWHEAT GRITS**

These are finely ground unroasted Buckwheat Groats. They cook quickly and are sold as Buckwheat cereal or cream of Buckwheat.

**BUCKWHEAT FLOUR AND SOBA NOODLES**

Buckwheat is also ground into flour and available in either light or dark forms; the darker variety is more nutritious. Buckwheat flour is used in pancakes, muffins, cakes, cookies, Italian pasta and Japanese soba noodles. True soba noodles are made from 100% Buckwheat flour, but check label ingredients as many noodles labeled "Buckwheat" also contain wheat flour.

**the peak season** available year-round.

## 4 steps to the best tasting and most nutritious buckwheat

Turning Buckwheat into a flavorful dish with the most nutrients is simple if you just follow my 4 easy steps:

1. The Best Way to Select
2. The Best Way to Store
3. The Best Way to Prepare
4. The Healthiest Way of Cooking

# 1. the best way to select buckwheat ———

Just as with any other food that you may purchase in the bulk section, make sure that the bins containing the Buckwheat are covered and that the store has a good product turnover to ensure its maximal freshness. Whether purchasing Buckwheat in bulk or in a packaged container, it is important that no evidence of moisture is present.

Buckwheat products like soba noodles often contain wheat, so be sure to read the labels carefully if you are trying eliminate wheat from your diet.

# 2. the best way to store buckwheat ———

Place Buckwheat in an airtight container and store in a cool, dry place. Buckwheat flour should always be stored in the refrigerator, while other Buckwheat products should be kept refrigerated if you live in a warm climate or during periods of warmer weather.

Stored properly, whole Buckwheat can last for 6 months, while the flour will keep fresh for 3 months.

# 3. the best way to prepare buckwheat ———

Before cooking Buckwheat, rinse it thoroughly under running water, then remove any dirt or debris you may find.

# 4. the healthiest way of cooking buckwheat ——

Cooked Buckwheat is a delicious substitute for brown rice and can be cooked in a similiar manner (see page 679).

Q *Is Buckwheat actually a grain?*

A Buckwheat is technically not a grain, although many people (including myself) colloquially refer to it as such since it is prepared the same way as grains. All cereal grains are found in the plant family of grasses called *Gramineae*. This family includes wheat, rye, barley, oat, rice and corn. Buckwheat does not belong to the *Gramineae* family but rather to an entirely different botanical family, called *Polygonacea*. The plants in this Buckwheat family are shrubs rather than grasses.

# health benefits of buckwheat

## Promotes Blood Sugar Balance

New evidence suggests that Buckwheat may be helpful in the management of diabetes. A single dose of Buckwheat seed extract lowered blood glucose levels by 12–19% when fed to laboratory animals with chemically-induced diabetes, while no reduction was seen in animals given a placebo. The component in Buckwheat responsible for these effects appears to be chiro-inositol, which has been shown in other animal and human studies to play a significant role in glucose metabolism and cell signaling.

Whole grains seem to have great benefits for maintaining blood sugar. One study found that women who consumed an average of three servings of whole grains daily had a 21% lower risk of diabetes compared to those who ate one serving per week.

## Promotes Heart Health

Diets that contain Buckwheat have been linked to a lowered risk of developing high cholesterol and high blood pressure. One study evaluated individuals in China who consumed a diet high in Buckwheat. Researchers found that Buckwheat intake was associated with lower total serum cholesterol, lower LDL levels and a higher ratio of HDL to total cholesterol in these individuals. Buckwheat's concentration of dietary fiber and magnesium—it's a good source of both of these nutrients—may help to partially explain Buckwheat's heart-health-protecting qualities. Fiber has been found to reduce cholesterol levels, while magnesium helps to promote blood vessel relaxation and blood circulation.

## Promotes Optimal Health

Buckwheat is a unique grain in that it is a concentrated source of phytonutrients called flavonoids, including rutin, quercetin and kaempferol. These flavonoids are strong antioxidants, protecting cells from the harmful effects of free radicals. Flavonoids also protect against disease by prolonging the activity of vitamin C. Buckwheat's ability to promote cardiovascular health may be due, in part, to its flavonoid compounds. These compounds appear to keep platelets from clumping and protect LDL from oxidizing into damaging cholesterol oxides.

Buckwheat is also a very good source of manganese. This trace mineral is a cofactor in *superoxide dismutase* (SOD), a very powerful antioxidant. SOD protects our cells' mitochondria from free-radical-scavenging that can occur during the process of energy production.

## Celiac Disease Substitute

Buckwheat can be eaten by people who have celiac disease. This intestinal disease is associated with sensitivity to grains or other foods that contain the protein gluten. In unleavened products, Buckwheat can be substituted for gluten-containing grains, such as wheat or rye.

## Additional Health-Promoting Benefit of Buckwheat

Buckwheat also contains sleep-promoting tryptophan.

### Nutritional Analysis of 1 cup of cooked Buckwheat Groats:

| NUTRIENT | AMOUNT | % DAILY VALUE |
| --- | --- | --- |
| Calories | 154.56 | |
| Calories from Fat | 9.38 | |
| Calories from Saturated Fat | 2.02 | |
| Protein | 5.68 g | |
| Carbohydrates | 33.50 g | |
| Dietary Fiber | 4.54 g | 18.16 |
| Soluble Fiber | — g | |
| Insoluble Fiber | — g | |
| Sugar – Total | 1.52 g | |
| Monosaccharides | — g | |
| Disaccharides | — g | |
| Other Carbs | 27.46 g | |
| Fat – Total | 1.04 g | |
| Saturated Fat | 0.22 g | |
| Mono Fat | 0.32 g | |
| Poly Fat | 0.32 g | |
| Omega-3 Fatty Acids | 0.02 g | 0.80 |
| Omega-6 Fatty Acids | 0.30 g | |
| Trans Fatty Acids | — g | |
| Cholesterol | 0.00 mg | |
| Water | 127.06 g | |
| Ash | 0.72 g | |

| Vitamins | | |
| --- | --- | --- |
| Vitamin A IU | 0.00 IU | 0.00 |
| Vitamin A RE | 0.00 RE | |
| A - Carotenoid | 0.00 RE | 0.00 |
| A - Retinol | 0.00 RE | |
| B1 Thiamin | 0.06 mg | 4.00 |
| B2 Riboflavin | 0.06 mg | 3.53 |
| B3 Niacin | 1.58 mg | 7.90 |
| Niacin Equiv | 2.96 mg | |
| Vitamin B6 | 0.12 mg | 6.00 |
| Vitamin B12 | 0.00 mcg | 0.00 |
| Biotin | — mcg | — |
| Vitamin C | 0.00 mg | 0.00 |
| Vitamin D IU | 0.00 IU | 0.00 |
| Vitamin D mcg | 0.00 mcg | |
| Vitamin E Alpha Equiv | 0.40 mg | 2.00 |
| Vitamin E IU | 0.60 IU | |
| Vitamin E mg | 0.40 mg | |
| Folate | 23.52 mcg | 5.88 |
| Vitamin K | 3.19 mcg | 3.99 |

| NUTRIENT | AMOUNT | % DAILY VALUE |
| --- | --- | --- |
| Pantothenic Acid | 0.60 mg | 6.00 |

| Minerals | | |
| --- | --- | --- |
| Boron | — mcg | |
| Calcium | 11.76 mg | 1.18 |
| Chloride | — mg | |
| Chromium | — mcg | — |
| Copper | 0.24 mg | 12.00 |
| Fluoride | — mg | — |
| Iodine | — mcg | — |
| Iron | 1.34 mg | 7.44 |
| Magnesium | 85.68 mg | 21.42 |
| Manganese | 0.68 mg | 34.00 |
| Molybdenum | — mcg | — |
| Phosphorus | 117.60 mg | 11.76 |
| Potassium | 147.84 mg | |
| Selenium | 3.70 mcg | 5.29 |
| Sodium | 6.72 mg | |
| Zinc | 1.02 mg | 6.80 |

| Amino Acids | | |
| --- | --- | --- |
| Alanine | 0.32 g | |
| Arginine | 0.42 g | |
| Aspartate | 0.48 g | |
| Cystine | 0.10 g | 24.39 |
| Glutamate | 0.88 g | |
| Glycine | 0.44 g | |
| Histidine | 0.14 g | 10.85 |
| Isoleucine | 0.22 g | 19.13 |
| Leucine | 0.36 g | 14.23 |
| Lysine | 0.28 g | 11.91 |
| Methionine | 0.08 g | 10.81 |
| Phenylalanine | 0.22 g | 18.49 |
| Proline | 0.22 g | |
| Serine | 0.30 g | |
| Threonine | 0.22 g | 17.74 |
| Tryptophan | 0.08 g | 25.00 |
| Tyrosine | 0.10 g | 10.31 |
| Valine | 0.30 g | 20.41 |

(Note: "—" indicates data is unavailable. For more information, please see page 806.)

STEP-BY-STEP
## Recipes for Enjoying Buckwheat

# The Healthiest Way of Cooking Buckwheat

*Buckwheat makes a great cereal or side dish, known as kasha. It has a toasty flavor and will go well with your favorite entrée.*

**1 cup Buckwheat, roasted or raw**
**2 cups water or broth**
**Sea salt to taste**

1. Combine all ingredients in a saucepan, **cover** and bring to a boil.

2. Turn the heat to low and simmer for about 30 minutes. Whole Groats will take longer to cook.

**SERVES 3**

**Preparation Hint:**
Test Buckwheat for doneness. Buckwheat should not be not too soft or too chewy. If it is not done and no water remains in the pan, add a couple of TBS of hot water, **cover** and cook a few more minutes. If water

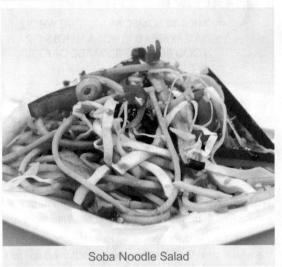

Soba Noodle Salad

is still left in the pan, turn off the heat, **cover** and let Buckwheat sit until the excess water is absorbed.

If you are using prepackaged Buckwheat, it is best to follow the directions on the package.

## Flavor Tips: 7 Ways to Enjoy Buckwheat

1. Buckwheat Kasha makes an energizing breakfast and is a great way to start the day. Combine with raisins or dried cranberries, your favorite fresh fruit, and nuts and seeds, such as almonds, walnuts, sunflower seeds or pumpkin seeds. Top with soy or almond milk. Add honey and cinnamon to taste.

2. Use chicken or vegetable broth instead of water when preparing Buckwheat Kasha for lunch or dinner. Add extra virgin olive oil to enhance its flavor.

3. Garnish with finely sliced scallions or onions.

4. Combine with minced cilantro or basil.

5. **Buckwheat Salad:** Combine the cooked Buckwheat recipe with minced onion, diced red

pepper, snow peas sliced into 1-inch pieces, fresh corn kernels and your favorite vinaigrette.

6. **Buckwheat Tabouli:** Substitute cooked Buckwheat for bulgur wheat in the tabouli recipe (page 685) for a tasty Mediterranean salad. Add diced avocados for an extra treat.

7. **Soba Noodle Salad:** Combine cooked Buckwheat soba noodles, shredded cabbage, sliced red bell pepper, sliced cucumber, green onions and chopped cilantro. Make a dressing from 1/4 cup tamari (soy sauce), 1/4 cup rice vinegar, 1/2 cup olive oil, 2 tsp toasted sesame oil and 1/4 tsp red chili flakes. Drizzle desired amount of dressing on noodle mixture (pictured above).

Please write (address on back cover flap) or e-mail me at info@whfoods.org with your personal ideas for preparing Buckwheat, and I will share them with others through our website at www.whfoods.org.

**Q** *I want to reduce the amount of wheat in my diet. I just learned about soba noodles. Is it true that they are made from Buckwheat?*

**A** Soba noodles are oftentimes just made from Buckwheat flour, but it is important to read the package label because some are made with Buckwheat flour and wheat flour. You can find varieties of soba noodles that contain other ingredients as well, including tea leaves, wild yam flour and mugwort.

## Q&A

**I HEARD SOMEONE SAY THAT WHOLE-WHEAT BREAD IS NOT A WHOLE-GRAIN FOOD BECAUSE IT'S MADE OF FLOUR. IS THAT TRUE?**

No, what you heard is not true. The fact that bread is made from flour does not automatically mean that it's not whole grain.

There are many different ways of making flour from grain. Most of these ways can be classified according to a measurement system called "percent extraction." When a grain is harvested, it's essentially whole in nature. The flour must then be extracted from the grain.

When flour is classified as 100% extraction, 100% of the whole grain that went into the extraction equipment is recovered in the flour itself. This type of extraction flour is therefore completely whole grain and is considered 100% whole grain wheat.

Unfortunately, the vast majority of breads in the supermarket aren't anything close to 100% extraction. Most of them are much closer to 60% extraction, which means that only 60% of the whole grain ends up in the flour. The other 40% of the whole grain (mostly the germ and bran portion) never makes it into the final flour at all.

Unfortunately, no breads on the grocery store shelf will tell you their percent extraction. The labeling of bread in the United States has long been a source of confusion for consumers, and even though the U.S. Food and Drug Administration (FDA) issued some new voluntary policy guidelines for bread in February 2006, the non-binding nature of these guidelines is unlikely to make bread labeling much clearer.

With respect to wheat, many breads simply carry the label "wheat bread" in very large letters. That label tells you absolutely nothing about the whole grain content of the bread. (Most of the time, in fact, there is no whole grain content in breads that are simply labeled as "wheat bread.") The label "whole wheat bread" may help a little bit, but please note that companies are allowed to use the label "whole wheat bread" even when a very, very small amount of 100% extraction wheat flour has been used to make the bread. In strictly legal terms, a "whole wheat bread" could contain very, very little whole wheat.

The label "100% whole wheat bread" is another story. In this case, all of the wheat flour in the bread would be 100% extraction. Therefore, "100% whole wheat bread" would indeed be the most nutritious wheat bread available—provided, of course, that it was also made from organically grown wheat.

In its 2006 guidance statement on the labeling of grain products, the FDA recommended that the principle components of a grain (including the bran, germ and starchy main portion, called the endosperm) be present in a whole grain flour "in the same relative proportions as they exist in the intact grain" in order for the flour to be considered "whole grain." While this recommendation did help to clarify the intended use of the term "whole grain," it also left some room for manufacturers to use something less than 100% extraction wheat flour in a bread and still refer to that bread as whole grain. More important, this guidance statement carried with it no mandatory action. Companies were not required to limit their labeling claims, just asked to voluntarily adopt a general labeling approach.

You best bet is to look for wheat breads that advertise themselves as being "100% whole wheat" and that also carry the USDA's symbol of being certified organic. That same principle would apply to all other whole grain breads as well (not just those made from wheat).

For more information on the FDA's definition of whole grains, please see their website at: http://www.cfsan.fda.gov/~dms/flgragui.html

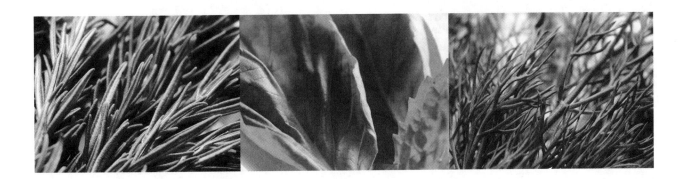

# herbs & spices

The numbers beside each food indicate their Total Nutrient-Richness. (For more details, see page 805.)

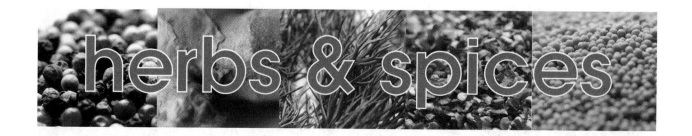

herbs & spices

When I think of the value of herbs and spices in the "Healthiest Way of Eating," the phrase "big things come in small packages" always comes to mind. That's because you only need to add a small amount of herbs and spices to transform an ordinary meal into an extraordinary one from both a flavor and nutritional perspective.

Herbs and spices have been a revered component of culinary traditions for thousands of years, not only for the flavor that they contribute, but also for their healing properties. While more and more people are turning to herbs and spices as healing compounds in the form of dietary supplements, I believe that by regularly incorporating them into the food we prepare, we can do great things for our health.

Cultures throughout time have known this. For example, while research into turmeric's health benefits has been making headlines recently, it has been used in India as a vital part of curry spice mixes and Ayurvedic medicine for thousands of years. Additionally, dating back to the times of ancient Greece and Rome, you can find numerous examples of both physicians and laypersons extolling the many virtues of culinary plants, including rosemary, dill and oregano.

So, add some spice to your meals and spice up your health by regularly using herbs and spices as a part of your "Healthiest Way of Eating."

### Definition: Herbs and Spices

Herbs and spices are plants that are used as seasonings. Herbs are seasonings from green, leafy plants, such as rosemary, peppermint and parsley. Spices are aromatic plants, with the part used generally not the leaf, but rather the seed, fruit, root or other part. Examples include ginger, black pepper and cinnamon.

### Why Herbs and Spices Can Help You Stay Slim, Energized and Healthy

Think about the satisfaction that you would receive from a plate of plain brown rice and steamed vegetables, and then think about the satisfaction you would receive from that same dish if it were prepared with your favorite seasonings. Your enjoyment of their taste is directly related to the fulfillment you'll feel, increasing the satiety you'll experience. If you enjoy meals with robust flavors, you'll also be less likely to crave the intense flavors offered by empty-calorie processed snack foods. In addition, spices such as cayenne pepper are actually being researched for their ability to promote weight loss.

Investigating the health benefits of herbs and spices is currently one of the most exciting research arenas, with scientific studies supporting the efficacy of their traditional uses. For example, in study after study, turmeric has been shown to have potent anti-inflammatory properties, while ginger has been found to help alleviate nausea.

Many of the benefits of herbs and spices seem to be related to their incredibly rich concentration of antioxidant phytonutrients. These include unique flavonoids such as quercetin, apigenin, luteolin, kaempferol and orientin.

What I find so interesting about this is that some of their antioxidant power comes from their volatile oil phytonutrients that also give them their fragrant aromas. For example, the volatile oils thymol and carvacol in basil have been found to have antimicrobial activity. So, once again, the nose knows…the potent fragrance of herbs and spices is actually related to the benefits that they will provide to your health.

### A World of Herbs and Spices

While I have included 11 herbs and spices in this book, please don't think that these are the only ones that I appreciate. There are many others that I use and consider as valuable additions to the "Healthiest Way of Eating." Examples of these include, but are definitely not limited to:

| | |
|---|---|
| ANISE | NUTMEG |
| CARDAMOM | OREGANO |
| CLOVES | SAFFRON |
| CUMIN | SAGE |
| HORSERADISH | TARRAGON |
| MARJORAM | THYME |

When considering which of the herbs and spices to include in the book, I reflected not only on their health benefits, but their versatility, popularity and availability. You can find more information on other herbs and spices not included in the book at the World's Healthiest Foods website, www.whfoods.org.

## what you will find in each herb and spice chapter

In each of the individual Herb and Spice chapters, you will find a nutritional profile as well as information on the health benefits of that culinary plant. In order for you to best enjoy them and readily incorporate them into your "Healthiest Way of Eating," I have created, and included in each chapter, the 4 Steps for the Best Tasting and Most Nutritious Herbs and Spices. These are tips on selecting, storing, preparing and cooking with each specific herb or spice as well as some ways to enjoy them.

In order for you to enjoy a fuller repertoire of herbs and spices, I wanted to include the 4 Steps that can be generally applied to them, so that you can feel confident in purchasing and using other health-promoting seasonings in your "Healthiest Way of Eating."

## 1. the best way to select herbs and spices

When purchasing fresh green herbs, look for ones that are deep in color and avoid those that are yellowing, have dark spots or excessive holes.

It is best to buy dried herbs and spices from the bulk section of your grocery or natural food store in small amounts, purchasing only what you will need over the next month. Use your sense of smell to evaluate their condition before purchasing. Look for ones that have an aromatic fragrance.

I recommend purchasing organically grown fresh or dried herbs and spices, whenever possible. (For more on *Organic Foods*, see page 113.)

## 2. the best way to store herbs and spices

To preserve freshness and the greatest number of nutrients, fresh herbs should be stored in the refrigerator either in their original packaging or loosely wrapped in a damp paper towel. You can also freeze many fresh whole or chopped herbs; just be sure to place them in an airtight container. If you are going to be using them for flavoring soups, you can also chop up fresh herbs and place them with some water in ice cube trays, which can be stored in the freezer.

Store dried herbs and spices in an airtight container in a cool, dark place. Do not store your dried seasonings above the stove or near a source of heat or moisture. Even though they have been dried, spices and seasonings are heat sensitive. Exposure to steam from a teapot or simmering pot of water can increase the risk of bacterial or fungal contamination.

## 3. the best way to prepare herbs and spices

It is best to gently wash fresh herbs and pat dry with a towel before you use them rather than before storing. The stems of some herbs are woody. For these it is best to separate the leaves and discard the stems.

Dried herbs generally require no preparation unless your recipe requires them to be ground. Sometimes dried spices that are in seed form are used in their whole form, but usually they are crushed before adding to a recipe. A mortar and pestle, available in kitchenware stores, is the best for this and one of my favorite and most used kitchen tools.

## 4. the healthiest way of cooking with herbs and spices

Most fresh herbs are delicate and lose their flavor if exposed to too much heat. Therefore, many are added towards the end of cooking, although there are some exceptions. Some recipes call for sprinkling fresh, uncooked, chopped or whole herbs on top after cooking.

Dried herbs and spices are usually added towards the beginning of cooking time since it takes a while for their flavor to bloom and infuse throughout the recipe. Some people like to crush the dried herbs between their fingers before adding to a recipe in order to release more of the fragrant oils.

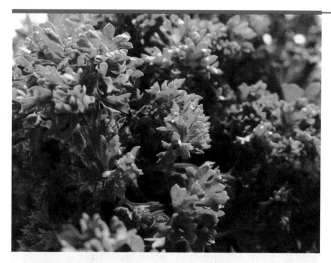

# parsley

## highlights

| | |
|---|---|
| AVAILABILITY: | Year-round |
| REFRIGERATE: | Yes |
| SHELF LIFE: | 14 days refrigerated |
| PREPARATION: | None |

## nutrient-richness chart

Total Nutrient-Richness: **21**
2 tablespoons (8 grams) of fresh Parsley contains 3 calories

| NUTRIENT | AMOUNT | %DV | DENSITY | QUALITY |
|---|---|---|---|---|
| Vitamin K | 123.0 mcg | 153.8 | 1025.0 | excellent |
| Vitamin C | 10.0 mg | 16.6 | 110.8 | excellent |
| Vitamin A | 631.8 IU | 12.6 | 84.2 | excellent |
| Folate | 11.4 mcg | 2.9 | 19.0 | good |
| Iron | 0.5 mg | 2.6 | 17.0 | good |
| **CAROTENOIDS:** | | | | |
| Beta-Carotene: | 379.1 mcg | | | |
| Lutein + Zeaxanthin: | 417.1 mcg | | | |
| **FLAVONOIDS:** | | | | |
| Apigenin: | 22.9 mg | | | |
| Myricetin: | 0.6 mg | | | |

Daily values for these nutrients have not yet been established.

For more on "Total Nutrient-Richness," "%DV," "Density," and The World's Healthiest Foods "Quality" Rating System, see page 805.

Parsley was held sacred by the ancient Greeks, who used it to adorn athletic victors. The Romans were the first to enjoy it as a food and used it as a salad vegetable. Today, it is one of the world's most popular seasonings, adding its flavor to many recipes. It is also enjoyed as a main ingredient as in the popular Middle Eastern salad known as Tabouli (see page 685).

## why parsley should be part of your healthiest way of eating

Parsley is an ideal food to add to your "Healthiest Way of Eating" not only because it is rich in nutrients, but also because it is low in calories: two tablespoons of fresh Parsley contain only 3 calories!

## varieties of parsley

Parsley is native to the Mediterranean region of Southern Europe. It derives its name from the Greek word, *petroselinum*, meaning "rock celery" (Parsley is a relative of celery), and is a biennial plant that will return to the garden year after year once it is established. The most familiar varieties of Parsley include Curly Parsley and Italian Parsley. Curly Parsley is a common variety with bright green leaves and long stems. This is the variety featured in the photographs. Italian Parsley is characterized by it fragrant flat leaves; it is less bitter than Curly Parsley.

## the peak season available year-round.

## biochemical considerations

Parsley is a concentrated source of oxalates, which might be of concern to certain individuals. (For more on *Oxalates*, see page 725.)

## 1. the best way to select parsley

You can select the best tasting Parsley by looking for dark-green-colored leaves that look fresh and crisp.

## 2. the best way to store parsley

Parsley will remain fresh for up to 14 days when properly stored:

- Place Parsley in a plastic storage bag before refrigerating.
- Do not wash Parsley before refrigeration.

## 3. the best way to prepare parsley

Just rinse under cold running water.

Blend Pesto into sauce for fish, poultry and soup.

## 4. the healthiest way of cooking with parsley

### TIPS: 3 Ways to Enjoy Parsley

1. Make Tabouli (see page 685).

2. Chop and sprinkle on fish, poultry and soup.

3. **PARSLEY PESTO:** In a food processor, process 3 cloves garlic, 1/2 cup fresh basil leaves, 1 cup Parsley leaves, 1/4 cup walnuts, 1/2 tsp sea salt, and 1/2 tsp grated lemon rind. When well mixed, add 3 TBS extra virgin olive oil slowly through the feed hole. Serve over steamed vegetables or whisk 2 TBS of pesto into an oil and vinegar dressing.

# health benefits of parsley

### Long History of Benefits

Parsley has been honored for its health benefits since the days of the ancient Greeks and Romans, who used Parsley for many different applications. They would chew on a sprig to refresh their breath, eat the leaves when they wanted to relieve digestive upset or make Parsley tea to enjoy its diuretic properties. These traditional uses are still recommended by many natural-medicine-oriented healthcare practitioners.

### Promotes Optimal Health

While Parsley is a concentrated source of traditional vitamins and minerals, its unique phytonutrients may also contribute to its longstanding reputation of being a health-promoting food. Parsley contains two types of distinctive phytonutrient components that provide unique health benefits.

The first is its volatile oil components—including myristicin, limonene, eugenol and alpha-thujene—that have been shown to inhibit tumor formation in animal studies. The activity of Parsley's volatile oils qualify it as a "chemoprotective" food, a food that can help neutralize particular types of carcinogens, such as the benzopyrenes that are found in cigarette smoke and charcoal grill smoke. The second is Parsley's flavonoids—including apiin, apigenin, crisoeriol, and luteolin. These flavonoids—especially luteolin—function as antioxidants that prevent oxygen-based damage to cells. In addition, animal studies have shown that extracts from Parsley help increase the antioxidant capacity of the blood.

### Additional Health-Promoting Benefits of Parsley

Parsley is also a concentrated source of many other nutrients providing additional health-promoting benefits. These nutri-ents include energy-producing iron; bone-building calcium and magnesium; heart-healthy potassium and dietary fiber; free-radical-scavenging vitamin E and manganese; and sleep-promoting tryptophan. Since fresh Parsley contains only 3 calories per 2 TBS serving, it is an ideal food for healthy weight control.

## Nutritional Analysis of 2 Tablespoons of fresh Parsley:

| NUTRIENT | AMOUNT | % DAILY VALUE |
|---|---|---|
| Calories | 2.70 | |
| Calories from Fat | 0.53 | |
| Calories from Saturated Fat | 0.09 | |
| Protein | 0.22 g | |
| Carbohydrates | 0.47 g | |
| Dietary Fiber | 0.25 g | 1.00 |
| Soluble Fiber | — g | |
| Insoluble Fiber | — g | |
| Sugar – Total | 0.06 g | |
| Monosaccharides | — g | |
| Disaccharides | — g | |
| Other Carbs | 0.16 g | |
| Fat – Total | 0.06 g | |
| Saturated Fat | 0.01 g | |
| Mono Fat | 0.02 g | |
| Poly Fat | 0.01 g | |
| Omega-3 Fatty Acids | 0.00 g | 0.00 |
| Omega-6 Fatty Acids | 0.01 g | |
| Trans Fatty Acids | 0.00 g | |
| Cholesterol | 0.00 mg | |
| Water | 6.58 g | |
| Ash | 0.17 g | |
| **Vitamins** | | |
| Vitamin A IU | 631.80 IU | 12.64 |
| Vitamin A RE | 63.15 RE | |
| A - Carotenoid | 63.15 RE | 0.84 |
| A - Retinol | 0.00 RE | |
| B1 Thiamin | 0.01 mg | 0.67 |
| B2 Riboflavin | 0.01 mg | 0.59 |
| B3 Niacin | 0.10 mg | 0.50 |
| Niacin Equiv | 0.15 mg | |
| Vitamin B6 | 0.01 mg | 0.50 |
| Vitamin B12 | 0.00 mcg | 0.00 |
| Biotin | — mcg | — |
| Vitamin C | 9.97 mg | 16.62 |
| Vitamin D IU | — IU | — |
| Vitamin D mcg | — mcg | |
| Vitamin E Alpha Equiv | 0.06 mg | 0.30 |
| Vitamin E IU | 0.08 IU | |
| Vitamin E mg | 0.06 mg | |
| Folate | 11.40 mcg | 2.85 |
| Vitamin K | 123.00 mcg | 153.75 |

| NUTRIENT | AMOUNT | % DAILY VALUE |
|---|---|---|
| Pantothenic Acid | 0.03 mg | 0.30 |
| **Minerals** | | |
| Boron | — mcg | |
| Calcium | 10.35 mg | 1.03 |
| Chloride | — mg | |
| Chromium | — mcg | — |
| Copper | 0.01 mg | 0.50 |
| Fluoride | — mg | — |
| Iodine | — mcg | — |
| Iron | 0.46 mg | 2.56 |
| Magnesium | 3.75 mg | 0.94 |
| Manganese | 0.01 mg | 0.50 |
| Molybdenum | — mcg | — |
| Phosphorus | 4.35 mg | 0.43 |
| Potassium | 41.55 mg | |
| Selenium | 0.01 mcg | 0.01 |
| Sodium | 4.20 mg | |
| Zinc | 0.08 mg | 0.53 |
| **Amino Acids** | | |
| Alanine | 0.01 g | |
| Arginine | 0.01 g | |
| Aspartate | 0.02 g | |
| Cystine | 0.00 g | 0.00 |
| Glutamate | 0.02 g | |
| Glycine | 0.01 g | |
| Histidine | 0.00 g | 0.00 |
| Isoleucine | 0.01 g | 0.87 |
| Leucine | 0.02 g | 0.79 |
| Lysine | 0.01 g | 0.43 |
| Methionine | 0.00 g | 0.00 |
| Phenylalanine | 0.01 g | 0.84 |
| Proline | 0.02 g | |
| Serine | 0.01 g | |
| Threonine | 0.01 g | 0.81 |
| Tryptophan | 0.00 g | 0.00 |
| Tyrosine | 0.01 g | 1.03 |
| Valine | 0.01 g | 0.68 |

(Note: "—" indicates data is unavailable. For more information, please see page 806.)

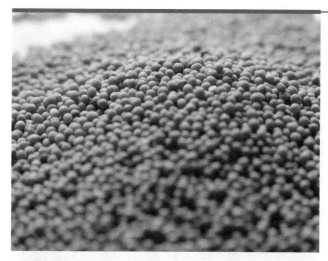

## nutrient-richness chart

Total Nutrient-Richness:    **15**
Two teaspoons (7 grams) of Mustard Seeds contain 35 calories

| NUTRIENT | AMOUNT | %DV | DENSITY | QUALITY |
|---|---|---|---|---|
| Selenium | 10.0 mcg | 14.2 | 7.3 | very good |
| Tryptophan | 0.04 g | 12.5 | 6.4 | very good |
| Omega-3 Fatty Acids | 0.2 g | 8.0 | 4.1 | very good |
| Phosphorus | 62.8 mg | 6.3 | 3.2 | good |
| Manganese | 0.1 mg | 6.0 | 3.1 | good |
| Magnesium | 22.3 mg | 5.6 | 2.9 | good |
| Dietary Fiber | 1.1 g | 4.3 | 2.2 | good |
| Iron | 0.8 mg | 4.2 | 2.2 | good |
| Calcium | 38.9 mg | 3.9 | 2.0 | good |
| Protein | 1.9 g | 3.8 | 1.9 | good |
| B3 Niacin | 0.6 mg | 3.0 | 1.5 | good |
| Zinc | 0.4 mg | 2.9 | 1.5 | good |
| **CAROTENOIDS:** | | | Daily values for these nutrients have not yet been established. | |
| Lutein+Zeaxanthin | 33.5 mcg | | | |

For more on "Total Nutrient-Richness," "%DV," "Density," and
The World's Healthiest Foods "Quality" Rating System, see page 805.

While Mustard Seeds were used for their culinary properties in ancient Greece, it is believed to have been the ancient Romans who invented a paste from the ground seeds, which was probably the ancestor of our modern day mustard condiment. Mustard Seeds are the seeds from which we get another of the World's Healthiest Foods—mustard greens, a cruciferous vegetable related to broccoli, Brussels sprouts and cabbage. Three varieties of Mustard Seeds include: white, from the Mediterranean; black, from Asia Minor; and brown, from India. If you are like most people, the word "mustard" probably conjures up images of ballparks and barbeques. Yet, once you add Mustard Seeds to your spice cabinet, the word will take on a whole new meaning as you will also relish the spicy, aromatic, rustic taste and fragrance that Mustard Seeds can add to your meals.

# mustard seeds

## highlights

| | |
|---|---|
| AVAILABILITY: | Year-round |
| REFRIGERATE: | No |
| SHELF LIFE: | 1 year |
| PREPARATION: | None |

## why mustard seeds should be part of your healthiest way of eating

Like other members of the *Brassica* family, Mustard Seeds contain glucosinolate phytonutrients that have been found to have anticarcinogenic properties. They are also rich in antioxidant nutrients including the mineral selenium as well as flavonoid antioxidants. Mustard Seeds are an ideal addition to your "Healthiest Way of Eating" not only because they are nutritious, but also because they are low in calories: 2 teaspoons of Mustard Seeds contain only 35 calories.

## biochemical considerations

Mustard Seeds contain goitrogens, which might be of concern to certain individuals. (For more on *Goitrogens*, see page 721.)

## 1. the best way to select mustard seeds

There are three types of Mustard Seeds: white, brown and black. Mustard Seeds are also available as ground powder.

Mustard Seeds are used to make different types of mustard condiments. Dijon mustard is a popular variety of mustard, which you can find in different flavors, including honey Dijon mustard.

I recommend purchasing organically grown varieties of Mustard Seeds and prepared mustards (such as Dijon mustard) whenever possible. (For more on *Organic Foods*, see page 113.)

## 2. the best way to store mustard seeds

To preserve the greatest number of nutrients and freshness, Mustard Seeds and ground Mustard should be kept in a tightly sealed container in a cool, dark and dry place. Prepared Mustard and Mustard oil should be refrigerated.

## 3. the best way to prepare mustard seeds

Mustard Seeds require no preparation.

It is impossible to make Dijon Mustard in the kitchen, since it requires special equipment.

## 4. the healthiest way of cooking with mustard seeds

It is best to add Mustard Seeds at the beginning of the cooking time, so they will have a chance to warm up and cook long enough to bring out their flavor.

### TIPS: 4 Ways to Enjoy Mustard Seeds

1. As an ingredient in many Mexican, Asian, South American and Thai Foods.
2. Add them to cilantro pesto.
3. Dry roast them and sprinkle on grains and vegetables.
4. Use them in curries and soups.

---

# health benefits of mustard seeds

## Promote Optimal Health

As a member of the *Brassica* family, Mustard Seeds contain plentiful amounts of phytonutrients called glucosinolates. They also contain *myrosinase* enzymes that can break apart the glucosinolates into isothiocyanates, phytonutrients that have been repeatedly studied for their anticancer effects. In animal studies—and particularly in studies involving the gastrointestinal tract—intake of isothiocyanates has been shown to inhibit growth of existing cancer cells and to be protective against the formation of such cells.

## Provide Powerful Antioxidant Protection

Mustard Seeds have been found to have high antioxidant capacity and a concentration of free-radical-scavenging flavonoids including quercetin, kaempferol, luteolin and pelargonidin. Mustard Seeds may promote detoxification as suggested by a study that found that Mustard Seeds enhanced the antioxidant potential in the livers of experimental animals.

## Additional Health-Promoting Benefits of Mustard Seeds

Mustard Seeds are also a concentrated source of heart-healthy omega-3 fatty acids, magnesium and dietary fiber; free-radical-scavenging selenium, zinc and manganese; energy-producing protein, iron, niacin and phosphorus; bone-building calcium; and sleep-promoting tryptophan.

### Nutritional Analysis of 2 teaspoons of Mustard Seeds:

| NUTRIENT | AMOUNT | % DAILY VALUE | NUTRIENT | AMOUNT | % DAILY VALUE |
|---|---|---|---|---|---|
| Calories | 35.04 | | Pantothenic Acid | — mg | — |
| Calories from Fat | 19.32 | | | | |
| Calories from Saturated Fat | 1.00 | | **Minerals** | | |
| Protein | 1.88 g | | Boron | — mcg | |
| Carbohydrates | 2.60 g | | Calcium | 38.92 mg | 3.89 |
| Dietary Fiber | 1.08 g | 4.32 | Chloride | — mg | |
| Soluble Fiber | — g | | Chromium | — mcg | — |
| Insoluble Fiber | — g | | Copper | 0.04 mg | 2.00 |
| Sugar – Total | — g | | Fluoride | — mg | — |
| Monosaccharides | — g | | Iodine | — mcg | — |
| Disaccharides | — g | | Iron | 0.76 mg | 4.22 |
| Other Carbs | — g | | Magnesium | 22.28 mg | 5.57 |
| Fat – Total | 2.16 g | | Manganese | 0.12 mg | 6.00 |
| Saturated Fat | 0.12 g | | Molybdenum | — mcg | — |
| Mono Fat | 1.48 g | | Phosphorus | 62.76 mg | 6.28 |
| Poly Fat | 0.40 g | | Potassium | 50.96 mg | |
| Omega-3 Fatty Acids | 0.20 g | 8.00 | Selenium | 9.96 mcg | 14.23 |
| Omega-6 Fatty Acids | 0.20 g | | Sodium | 0.32 mg | |
| Trans Fatty Acids | 0.00 g | | Zinc | 0.44 mg | 2.93 |
| Cholesterol | 0.00 mg | | | | |
| Water | 0.52 g | | **Amino Acids** | | |
| Ash | 0.32 g | | Alanine | 0.08 g | |
| | | | Arginine | 0.12 g | |
| **Vitamins** | | | Aspartate | 0.16 g | |
| Vitamin A IU | 4.64 IU | 0.09 | Cystine | 0.04 g | 9.76 |
| Vitamin A RE | 0.48 RE | | Glutamate | 0.36 g | |
| A - Carotenoid | 0.48 RE | 0.01 | Glycine | 0.08 g | |
| A - Retinol | 0.00 RE | | Histidine | 0.04 g | 3.10 |
| B1 Thiamin | 0.04 mg | 2.67 | Isoleucine | 0.08 g | 6.96 |
| B2 Riboflavin | 0.04 mg | 2.35 | Leucine | 0.12 g | 4.74 |
| B3 Niacin | 0.60 mg | 3.00 | Lysine | 0.12 g | 5.11 |
| Niacin Equiv | 1.24 mg | | Methionine | 0.04 g | 5.41 |
| Vitamin B6 | 0.04 mg | 2.00 | Phenylalanine | 0.08 g | 6.72 |
| Vitamin B12 | 0.00 mcg | 0.00 | Proline | 0.16 g | |
| Biotin | — mcg | — | Serine | 0.08 g | |
| Vitamin C | 0.24 mg | 0.40 | Threonine | 0.08 g | 6.45 |
| Vitamin D IU | — IU | — | Tryptophan | 0.04 g | 12.50 |
| Vitamin D mcg | — mcg | | Tyrosine | 0.04 g | 4.12 |
| Vitamin E Alpha Equiv | 0.20 mg | 1.00 | Valine | 0.08 g | 5.44 |
| Vitamin E IU | 0.28 IU | | | | |
| Vitamin E mg | 0.20 mg | | | | |
| Folate | 5.68 mcg | 1.42 | | | |
| Vitamin K | 0.36 mcg | 0.45 | | | |

(Note: "–" indicates data is unavailable. For more information, please see page 806.)

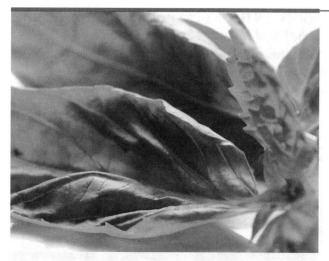

## nutrient-richness chart

Total Nutrient-Richness: **11**
Two teaspoons (3 grams) of ground Basil contain 8 calories

| NUTRIENT | AMOUNT | %DV | DENSITY | QUALITY |
|---|---|---|---|---|
| Vitamin K | 48.0 mcg | 60.0 | 143.6 | excellent |
| Iron | 1.3 mg | 7.1 | 17.0 | very good |
| Calcium | 63.4 mg | 6.3 | 15.2 | very good |
| Vitamin A | 281.2 IU | 5.6 | 13.5 | very good |
| Dietary Fiber | 1.2 g | 4.8 | 11.5 | good |
| Manganese | 0.1 mg | 4.0 | 9.6 | good |
| Magnesium | 12.7 mg | 3.2 | 7.6 | good |
| Vitamin C | 1.8 mg | 3.1 | 7.3 | good |
| Potassium | 103.0 mg | | | |
| **CAROTENOIDS:** | | | Daily values for these nutrients have not yet been established. | |
| Beta-Carotene | 156.4 mcg | | | |
| Lutein+Zeaxanthin | 32.2 mcg | | | |
| Lycopene | 11.0 mcg | | | |

For more on "Total Nutrient-Richness," "%DV," "Density," and
The World's Healthiest Foods "Quality" Rating System, see page 805.

B asil has a history as a token of love, an icon of hospitality and a passport to help the deceased enter Paradise. Like other members of the mint family to which it belongs, Basil has also been appreciated for its medicinal qualities as a digestive aid and antibacterial agent. Basil is a highly fragrant plant whose leaves are a familiar seasoning herb for a variety of different foods and is a favorite in the Mediterranean region. I want to share with you how Basil can add extra flavor and nutrition to your "Healthiest Way of Eating."

## why basil should be part of your healthiest way of eating

Basil contains powerful antioxidant flavonoids. It is also a concentrated source of volatile oil phytonutrients, which have been found to not only have antibiotic properties, but anti-inflammatory ones as well. Basil is an ideal addition

# basil

| | |
|---|---|
| AVAILABILITY: | Year-round |
| REFRIGERATE: | Yes |
| SHELF LIFE: | 5 days |
| PREPARATION: | Minimal |

to your "Healthiest Way of Eating" not only because it is nutritious, but also because it is low in calories: 2 teaspoons of dried Basil contain only 8 calories.

## varieties of basil

There are several varieties of Basil including: Sweet Basil, the Italian classic for making pesto and popularly served on top of tomatoes and mozzarella cheese; Sweet Thai Basil, which has an intensely rich aroma and is great with curries, fish and salad; Holy Basil, with its hint of mint is oftentimes served on top of noodles; Cinnamon Basil, used for making tea and potpourris; and Lime Basil, which has a tangy citrus taste and is a favorite in South Asian cooking.

## 1. the best way to select basil

**FRESH BASIL:** For the most nutritious and best tasting Basil, select fresh Basil with vibrantly colored leaves. Avoid leaves with darks spots or yellowing.

I recommend purchasing organically grown fresh or dried Basil whenever possible. (For more on *Organic Foods*, see page 113.)

## 2. the best way to store basil

**FRESH BASIL:** To preserve the greatest number of nutrients and freshness, wrap fresh Basil in a damp paper towel and place it in the warmest part of your refrigerator (the top shelf). It will keep for up to 5 days. The lower portion of your refrigerator is too cool and will cause the formation of brown spots on the leaves. Alternatively, you can freeze chopped Basil in ice cube trays covered with water or stock; these can then be easily added when preparing soups or stews.

**DRIED BASIL:** Should be kept in a tightly sealed glass container in a cool, dark, dry place where it will keep fresh for about 6 months. Keep track of freshness by writing the expiration date on your container.

## 3. the best way to prepare basil

To retain nutrients, it is best to wash fresh Basil under cold running water and pat dry with a paper towel. Do not soak Basil or the water-soluble nutrients will leach into the water. It is best to pull the leaves off of the stem as the stems have a bitter flavor.

## 4. the healthiest way of cooking with basil

**FRESH BASIL:** To retain the maximum number of nutrients and flavor, it is best to add fresh Basil to your dish at the end of the cooking time. Basil is a very delicate herb, which can be sprinkled on your dish after it has been cooked.

**DRIED BASIL:** I recommend using fresh Basil whenever possible since dried Basil has lost much of its flavor. Heating dried Basil will help release some of its flavor. It is best to add dried Basil after half of the cooking time has elapsed to allow it to warm up and add more flavor to your dish. Before using, rub dried Basil between your fingers to release its essential oils.

To substitute dried Basil leaves for fresh ones, use about one-third the amount of dried Basil as you would fresh. For example, substitute 1 tsp of dried Basil leaves for 1 TBS of fresh Basil. (To substitute ground basil for fresh use one-sixth of the amount.)

### TIPS: 3 Ways to Enjoy Basil

1. Pesto (see page 508).
2. Serve with tomatoes, fish and poultry.
3. Add to salads and serve as garnish for soups.

# health benefits of basil

### Provides Powerful Antioxidant Protection

Basil contains flavonoids, such as orientin and vicenin, which have been found to protect cell structures and chromosomes from radiation and oxygen-based damage.

### Provides Antimicrobial Protection

Lab studies have shown the effectiveness of Basil in restricting growth of numerous bacteria including *Staphylococcus aureus* and *Escherichia coli* as well as some bacterial strains found to be resistant to commonly used antibiotic drugs. This antimicrobial activity is thought to be due to its volatile oils such as eugenol, myrcene, limonene and others.

### Promotes Anti-Inflammatory Activity

Basil is considered an anti-inflammatory food since its volatile oil, eugenol, has been found to be able to block the activity of the *cyclooxygenase* (COX) enzyme. Many nonsteriodal over-the-counter anti-inflammatory medications (NSAIDS), including aspirin and ibuprofen, as well as the commonly used medicine acetaminophen, work by inhibiting this same enzyme.

### Additional Health-Promoting Benefits of Basil

Basil is also a concentrated source of energy-producing iron; bone-building calcium; heart-healthy potassium, magnesium and fiber; and free-radical-scavenging vitamin A, vitamin C and manganese.

### Nutritional Analysis of 2 teaspoons of ground Basil:

| NUTRIENT | AMOUNT | % DAILY VALUE | NUTRIENT | AMOUNT | % DAILY VALUE |
|---|---|---|---|---|---|
| Calories | 7.52 | | Pantothenic Acid | — mg | — |
| Calories from Fat | 1.08 | | | | |
| Calories from Saturated Fat | 0.08 | | **Minerals** | | |
| Protein | 0.44 g | | Boron | — mcg | |
| Carbohydrates | 1.84 g | | Calcium | 63.40 mg | 6.34 |
| Dietary Fiber | 1.20 g | 4.80 | Chloride | — mg | |
| Soluble Fiber | — g | | Chromium | — mcg | — |
| Insoluble Fiber | — g | | Copper | 0.04 mg | 2.00 |
| Sugar – Total | — g | | Fluoride | — mg | |
| Monosaccharides | — g | | Iodine | — mcg | — |
| Disaccharides | — g | | Iron | 1.28 mg | 7.11 |
| Other Carbs | — g | | Magnesium | 12.68 mg | 3.17 |
| Fat – Total | 0.12 g | | Manganese | 0.08 mg | 4.00 |
| Saturated Fat | 0.00 g | | Molybdenum | — mcg | — |
| Mono Fat | 0.00 g | | Phosphorus | 14.72 mg | 1.47 |
| Poly Fat | 0.08 g | | Potassium | 103.00 mg | |
| Omega-3 Fatty Acids | 0.04 g | 1.60 | Selenium | 0.08 mcg | 0.11 |
| Omega-6 Fatty Acids | 0.00 g | | Sodium | 1.04 mg | |
| Trans Fatty Acids | 0.00 g | | Zinc | 0.16 mg | 1.07 |
| Cholesterol | 0.00 mg | | | | |
| Water | 0.20 g | | **Amino Acids** | | |
| Ash | 0.44 g | | Alanine | 0.04 g | |
| | | | Arginine | 0.00 g | |
| **Vitamins** | | | Aspartate | 0.04 g | |
| Vitamin A IU | 281.24 IU | 5.62 | Cystine | 0.00 g | 0.00 |
| Vitamin A RE | 28.12 RE | | Glutamate | 0.04 g | |
| A - Carotenoid | 28.16 RE | 0.38 | Glycine | 0.04 g | |
| A - Retinol | 0.00 RE | | Histidine | 0.00 g | 0.00 |
| B1 Thiamin | 0.00 mg | 0.00 | Isoleucine | 0.00 g | 0.00 |
| B2 Riboflavin | 0.00 mg | 0.00 | Leucine | 0.04 g | 1.58 |
| B3 Niacin | 0.20 mg | 1.00 | Lysine | 0.00 g | 0.00 |
| Niacin Equiv | 0.32 mg | | Methionine | 0.00 g | 0.00 |
| Vitamin B6 | 0.04 mg | 2.00 | Phenylalanine | 0.04 g | 3.36 |
| Vitamin B12 | 0.00 mcg | 0.00 | Proline | 0.00 g | |
| Biotin | — mcg | — | Serine | 0.00 g | |
| Vitamin C | 1.84 mg | 3.07 | Threonine | 0.00 g | 0.00 |
| Vitamin D IU | 0.00 IU | 0.00 | Tryptophan | 0.00 g | 0.00 |
| Vitamin D mcg | 0.00 mcg | | Tyrosine | 0.00 g | 0.00 |
| Vitamin E Alpha Equiv | 0.04 mg | 0.20 | Valine | 0.04 g | 2.72 |
| Vitamin E IU | 0.08 IU | | | | |
| Vitamin E mg | 0.04 mg | | | | |
| Folate | 8.24 mcg | 2.06 | | | |
| Vitamin K | 48.01 mcg | 60.01 | | | |

(Note: "—" indicates data is unavailable. For more information, please see page 806.)

# turmeric

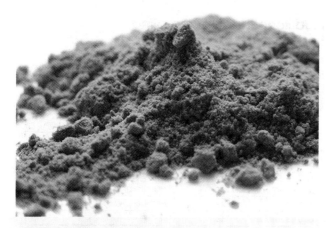

## nutrient-richness chart

Total Nutrient-Richness: **11**
Two teaspoons (5 grams) of ground Turmeric contain 16 calories

| NUTRIENT | AMOUNT | %DV | DENSITY | QUALITY |
|---|---|---|---|---|
| Manganese | 0.4 mg | 18.0 | 20.2 | excellent |
| Iron | 1.9 mg | 10.4 | 11.7 | excellent |
| B6 Pyridoxine | 0.1 mg | 4.0 | 4.5 | good |
| Dietary Fiber | 1.0 g | 3.8 | 4.3 | good |
| Potassium | 114.5 mg | 3.3 | 3.7 | good |

For more on "Total Nutrient-Richness," "%DV," "Density," and
The World's Healthiest Foods "Quality" Rating System, see page 805.

## highlights

| | |
|---|---|
| AVAILABILITY: | Year-round |
| REFRIGERATE: | No |
| SHELF LIFE: | 6 months |
| PREPARATION: | None |

Turmeric is native to Indonesia and southern India, where it has been harvested for more than 5,000 years. It was traditionally known as "Indian saffron" because of its similarity in color to this prized spice. Turmeric has been used throughout history as a condiment, healing remedy and textile dye. Peppery, warm and bittersweet, with a mild fragrance reminiscent of ginger to which it is related, Turmeric is well-known as one of the ingredients used to make curry powder.

## why turmeric should be part of your healthiest way of eating

Turmeric is a concentrated source of the unique phytonutrient curcumin, which has incredibly powerful anti-inflammatory properties and has been found to promote optimal liver function. Turmeric is also rich in minerals such as iron and manganese. Turmeric is an ideal addition to your "Healthiest Way of Eating" not only because it is nutritious, but also because it is low in calories: 2 teaspoons of Turmeric contain only 16 calories.

## 1. the best way to select turmeric

You can occasionally find fresh Turmeric rhizome in the refrigerated section of your local market. Turmeric powder is available prepackaged or in bulk; I prefer to purchase in bulk so that I can buy the exact amount I need.

**CURRY POWDER:** A blend of 20 different herbs, spices and seeds. Turmeric is one of the main ingredients and is responsible for the yellow color of curry powder.

I recommend purchasing organically grown Turmeric whenever possible. (For more on *Organic Foods*, see page 113.)

## 2. the best way to store turmeric

Turmeric powder should be kept in a tightly sealed glass container in a cool, dark, dry place where it will keep fresh for about 6 months. Fresh Turmeric rhizome should be kept in the refrigerator.

## 3. the best way to prepare turmeric

Turmeric powder requires no preparation. Be careful when using Turmeric or curry powder as they can easily stain things, including clothes and counter surfaces.

## 4. the healthiest way to cook with turmeric

It is best to add Turmeric powder at the end of cooking.

### TIPS: 5 Ways to Enjoy Turmeric

1. Give salad dressings extra nutritional value and an orange-yellow hue by adding some Turmeric powder to them.

2. Add Turmeric to egg salad to give it an even bolder yellow color and extra nutrition.

3. Mix brown rice with raisins and cashews and season with Turmeric or curry powder.

4. Although Turmeric is generally a staple ingredient in curry powder, some people like to add a little extra of this spice when preparing curries.

5. Turmeric or curry powder are great spices to complement the taste of lentils and of cauliflower.

# health benefits of turmeric

## Provides Powerful Anti-Inflammatory Protection

Turmeric is a powerful spice that has long been used in the Chinese and Indian systems of medicine as an anti-inflammatory agent. In numerous studies, the anti-inflammatory effects of its phytonutrient curcumin have been shown to be comparable to potent prescription and over-the-counter anti-inflammatory medicines.

## Promotes Joint Health

Turmeric's powerful antioxidant and anti-inflammatory capacities helps explain why many people with joint disease find relief when they use this spice regularly. In a recent study of patients with rheumatoid arthritis, curcumin produced a reduced duration of morning stiffness, lengthened walking time and reduced joint swelling.

## Promotes Optimal Health

Turmeric contributes to overall health in other ways including enhancing the liver's detoxification of nutritive substances, the inhibition of radiation-induced damage to chromosomes, and the inhibition of the formation of some cancer-causing chemicals in the body. The results of research with laboratory animals suggest that a combination of Turmeric and Brassica vegetables (like cauliflower, broccoli or kale) may help to prevent prostate cancer. Recent research also suggests that Turmeric's curcuminoid phytonutrients stimulate the macrophages of Alzheimer's patients' to clear out beta-amyloid plaques, which would otherwise contribute to the plaques characteristic of this disease.

## Promotes Heart Health

In a recent research study, 10 healthy volunteers who consumed 500 mg of curcumin per day for 7 days experienced a 12% reduction in total cholesterol, a 33% reduction of oxidized cholesterol and a 29% increase in HDL "good" cholesterol. For the most curcumin, be sure to use Turmeric rather than curry powder—a study analyzing curcumin content in 28 spice products described as Turmeric or curry powders found that pure Turmeric powder had the highest concentration of curcumin, averaging 3.14% by weight. The curry powder samples, with one exception, contained very small amounts of curcumin.

## Additional Health-Promoting Benefits of Turmeric

Turmeric is also a concentrated source of heart-healthy dietary fiber, vitamin B6 and potassium; energy-producing iron; and free-radical-scavenging manganese.

### Nutritional Analysis of 2 teaspoons of ground Turmeric:

| NUTRIENT | AMOUNT | % DAILY VALUE | NUTRIENT | AMOUNT | % DAILY VALUE |
|---|---|---|---|---|---|
| Calories | 16.04 | | Pantothenic Acid | — mg | — |
| Calories from Fat | 4.04 | | | | |
| Calories from Saturated Fat | 1.28 | | **Minerals** | | |
| Protein | 0.36 g | | Boron | — mcg | |
| Carbohydrates | 2.96 g | | Calcium | 8.28 mg | 0.83 |
| Dietary Fiber | 0.96 g | 3.84 | Chloride | — mg | |
| Soluble Fiber | — g | | Chromium | — mcg | — |
| Insoluble Fiber | — g | | Copper | 0.04 mg | 2.00 |
| Sugar – Total | — g | | Fluoride | — mg | — |
| Monosaccharides | — g | | Iodine | — mcg | — |
| Disaccharides | — g | | Iron | 1.88 mg | 10.44 |
| Other Carbs | — g | | Magnesium | 8.76 mg | 2.19 |
| Fat – Total | 0.44 g | | Manganese | 0.36 mg | 18.00 |
| Saturated Fat | 0.16 g | | Molybdenum | — mcg | — |
| Mono Fat | 0.08 g | | Phosphorus | 12.12 mg | 1.21 |
| Poly Fat | 0.08 g | | Potassium | 114.48 mg | |
| Omega-3 Fatty Acids | 0.04 g | 1.60 | Selenium | 0.20 mcg | 0.29 |
| Omega-6 Fatty Acids | 0.08 g | | Sodium | 1.72 mg | |
| Trans Fatty Acids | 0.00 g | | Zinc | 0.20 mg | 1.33 |
| Cholesterol | 0.00 mg | | | | |
| Water | 0.52 g | | **Amino Acids** | | |
| Ash | 0.28 g | | Alanine | — g | |
| | | | Arginine | — g | |
| **Vitamins** | | | Aspartate | — g | |
| Vitamin A IU | 0.00 IU | 0.00 | Cystine | — g | — |
| Vitamin A RE | 0.00 RE | | Glutamate | — g | |
| A - Carotenoid | 0.00 RE | 0.00 | Glycine | — g | |
| A - Retinol | 0.00 RE | | Histidine | — g | — |
| B1 Thiamin | 0.00 mg | 0.00 | Isoleucine | — g | — |
| B2 Riboflavin | 0.00 mg | 0.00 | Leucine | — g | — |
| B3 Niacin | 0.24 mg | 1.20 | Lysine | — g | — |
| Niacin Equiv | 0.24 mg | | Methionine | — g | — |
| Vitamin B6 | 0.08 mg | 4.00 | Phenylalanine | — g | — |
| Vitamin B12 | 0.00 mcg | 0.00 | Proline | — g | |
| Biotin | — mcg | — | Serine | — g | |
| Vitamin C | 1.16 mg | 1.93 | Threonine | — g | — |
| Vitamin D IU | 0.00 IU | 0.00 | Tryptophan | — g | — |
| Vitamin D mcg | 0.00 mcg | | Tyrosine | — g | — |
| Vitamin E Alpha Equiv | 0.00 mg | 0.00 | Valine | — g | — |
| Vitamin E IU | 0.00 IU | | | | |
| Vitamin E mg | 0.00 mg | | | | |
| Folate | 1.76 mcg | 0.44 | | | |
| Vitamin K | 0.59 mcg | 0.74 | | | |

(Note: "—" indicates data is unavailable. For more information, please see page 806.)

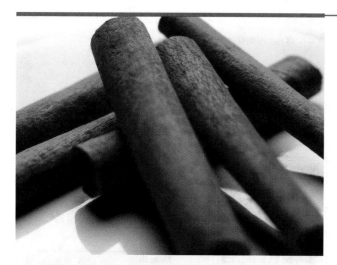

# cinnamon

| | |
|---|---|
| AVAILABILITY: | Year-round |
| REFRIGERATE: | No |
| SHELF LIFE: | 6 months to 1 year |
| PREPARATION: | None |

## nutrient-richness chart

Total Nutrient-Richness: **10**

Two teaspoons (5 grams) of ground Cinnamon contain 12 calories

| NUTRIENT | AMOUNT | %DV | DENSITY | QUALITY |
|---|---|---|---|---|
| Manganese | 0.8 mg | 38.0 | 57.8 | excellent |
| Dietary Fiber | 2.5 g | 9.9 | 15.1 | very good |
| Iron | 1.7 mg | 9.6 | 14.5 | very good |
| Calcium | 55.7 mg | 5.6 | 8.5 | very good |
| **CAROTENOIDS:** | | | | |
| Beta-Cryptoxanthin | 11.7 mcg | | | Daily values for these nutrients have not yet been established. |
| Lutein+Zeaxanthin | 19.0 mcg | | | |

For more on "Total Nutrient-Richness," "%DV," "Density," and The World's Healthiest Foods "Quality" Rating System, see page 805

Cinnamon is one of the oldest spices known to man and has been used as a botanical medicine since 2,700 BC with many of its healing properties attributed to its special essential oils. Long appreciated for its warming qualities, a quill (or stick) of Cinnamon added to a warm cup of hot apple cider is a welcome treat on a cold winter's day. And who can resist the smell of Cinnamon-rich apple pie? There are hundreds of varieties of Cinnamon, but Ceylon and Chinese Cinnamon are the most popular. Ceylon Cinnamon is also referred to as "true Cinnamon," while the Chinese variety is known as "cassia." While both feature a fragrant, sweet, warm taste, the flavor of the Ceylon variety is more refined and subtle.

## why cinnamon should be part of your healthiest way of eating

Cinnamon's phytonutrients provide it with many of its health-promoting properties, including blocking inflammation and bacterial growth as well as helping to regulate blood sugar. Cinnamon is ideal to add to your "Healthiest Way of Eating" not only because it is nutritious, but also because it is low in calories: 2 teaspoons of ground Cinnamon contain only 12 calories.

## 1. the best way to select cinnamon

For the most nutritious and best tasting Cinnamon, I like to smell it to make sure it has a sweet smell that ensures its freshness.

**CINNAMON POWDER:** Has a stronger flavor than sticks.

**CINNAMON STICKS:** Can be stored longer than the powder.

I recommend purchasing organically grown Cinnamon whenever possible. (For more on *Organic Foods*, see page 113.)

## 2. the best way to store cinnamon

To preserve freshness and its greatest number of nutrients, Cinnamon should be kept in a tightly sealed glass container in a cool, dark, dry place. Ground Cinnamon will keep for about six months, while Cinnamon sticks will stay fresh for about one year stored this way. Alternatively, you can extend their shelf life by storing them in the refrigerator.

## 3. the best way to prepare cinnamon

Cinnamon requires no preparation.

## 4. the healthiest way of cooking with cinnamon

To retain the maximum number of nutrients and flavor, add Cinnamon at the end of the cooking process since it loses its flavor and aroma if cooked too long. Cinnamon is commonly used in dessert and fruit dishes and complements the flavor of oatmeal, sweet potatoes, carrots and winter squash very nicely.

## TIPS: 5 Ways to Enjoy Cinnamon

1. Cinnamon toast with a healthy twist: Toast whole wheat bread and then sprinkle with Cinnamon and honey.

2. Simmer Cinnamon sticks with soymilk and honey for a deliciously warming beverage.

3. When poaching chicken or fish, add Cinnamon sticks to the poaching liquid.

4. Add ground Cinnamon to the black beans that you use for burritos or nachos.

5. "Healthy Sauté" lamb with eggplant, raisins and Cinnamon sticks to create a meal inspired by Middle Eastern flavors.

# health benefits of cinnamon

## Promotes Balanced Blood Sugar

Cinnamon may help people with type 2 diabetes. Both test tube and animal studies have shown that compounds in Cinnamon stimulate insulin receptors, increasing cells' ability to use glucose. Studies to confirm Cinnamon's beneficial actions in humans are currently underway with preliminary research showing that 1 gram per day (approximately 1/4 to 1/2 teaspoon) produced an approximately 20% drop in blood sugar levels in study participants.

## Provides Powerful Anti-Inflammatory Protection

Cinnamon contains cinnamaldehyde, a powerful anti-inflammatory phytonutrient. Cinnamaldehyde has been researched for its ability to prevent unwanted clumping of blood platelets, which has benefits on cardiovascular health.

## Provides Powerful Antimicrobial Protection

Cinnamon's essential oils—including cinnamaldehyde, cinnamyl acetate and cinnamyl alcohol—qualify it as an "antimicrobial" food. Cinnamon has been studied for its ability to help stop the growth of bacteria as well as fungi, including the commonly problematic yeast *Candida* as well as *H. pylori*, the bacteria that causes ulcers.

## Additional Health-Promoting Benefits of Cinnamon

Cinnamon is also a concentrated source of bone-building calcium and manganese; heart-healthy dietary fiber; and energy-producing iron.

### Nutritional Analysis of 2 teaspoons of ground Cinnamon:

| NUTRIENT | AMOUNT | % DAILY VALUE |
|---|---|---|
| Calories | 11.84 | |
| Calories from Fat | 1.28 | |
| Calories from Saturated Fat | 0.28 | |
| Protein | 0.16 g | |
| Carbohydrates | 3.60 g | |
| Dietary Fiber | 2.48 g | 9.92 |
| Soluble Fiber | — g | |
| Insoluble Fiber | — g | |
| Sugar – Total | — g | |
| Monosaccharides | — g | |
| Disaccharides | — g | |
| Other Carbs | — g | |
| Fat – Total | 0.16 g | |
| Saturated Fat | 0.04 g | |
| Mono Fat | 0.04 g | |
| Poly Fat | 0.04 g | |
| Omega-3 Fatty Acids | 0.00 g | 0.00 |
| Omega-6 Fatty Acids | 0.04 g | |
| Trans Fatty Acids | 0.00 g | |
| Cholesterol | 0.00 mg | |
| Water | 0.44 g | |
| Ash | 0.16 g | |

| Vitamins | AMOUNT | % DAILY VALUE |
|---|---|---|
| Vitamin A IU | 11.80 IU | 0.24 |
| Vitamin A RE | 1.16 RE | |
| A - Carotenoid | 1.16 RE | 0.02 |
| A - Retinol | 0.00 RE | |
| B1 Thiamin | 0.00 mg | 0.00 |
| B2 Riboflavin | 0.00 mg | 0.00 |
| B3 Niacin | 0.04 mg | 0.20 |
| Niacin Equiv | 0.04 mg | |
| Vitamin B6 | 0.00 mg | 0.00 |
| Vitamin B12 | 0.00 mcg | 0.00 |
| Biotin | — mcg | — |
| Vitamin C | 1.28 mg | 2.13 |
| Vitamin D IU | 0.00 IU | 0.00 |
| Vitamin D mcg | 0.00 mcg | |
| Vitamin E Alpha Equiv | 0.00 mg | 0.00 |
| Vitamin E IU | 0.00 IU | |
| Vitamin E mg | 0.00 mg | |
| Folate | 1.32 mcg | 0.33 |
| Vitamin K | 1.44 mcg | 1.80 |

| NUTRIENT | AMOUNT | % DAILY VALUE |
|---|---|---|
| Pantothenic Acid | — mg | — |
| **Minerals** | | |
| Boron | — mcg | |
| Calcium | 55.68 mg | 5.57 |
| Chloride | — mg | |
| Chromium | — mcg | — |
| Copper | 0.00 mg | 0.00 |
| Fluoride | — mg | — |
| Iodine | — mcg | |
| Iron | 1.72 mg | 9.56 |
| Magnesium | 2.52 mg | 0.63 |
| Manganese | 0.76 mg | 38.00 |
| Molybdenum | — mcg | — |
| Phosphorus | 2.80 mg | 0.28 |
| Potassium | 22.68 mg | |
| Selenium | 0.04 mcg | 0.06 |
| Sodium | 1.20 mg | |
| Zinc | 0.08 mg | 0.53 |
| **Amino Acids** | | |
| Alanine | — g | |
| Arginine | — g | |
| Aspartate | — g | |
| Cystine | — g | — |
| Glutamate | — g | |
| Glycine | — g | |
| Histidine | — g | |
| Isoleucine | — g | |
| Leucine | — g | — |
| Lysine | — g | — |
| Methionine | — g | |
| Phenylalanine | — g | — |
| Proline | — g | |
| Serine | — g | |
| Threonine | — g | — |
| Tryptophan | — g | — |
| Tyrosine | — g | — |
| Valine | — g | — |

(Note: "—" indicates data is unavailable. For more information, please see page 806.)

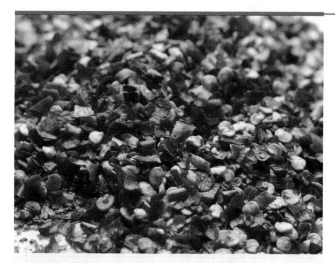

## nutrient-richness chart

Total Nutrient-Richness: **8**

Two teaspoons (4 grams) of Cayenne Pepper contain 11 calories

| NUTRIENT | AMOUNT | %DV | DENSITY | QUALITY |
|---|---|---|---|---|
| Vitamin A | 1470.2 IU | 29.4 | 47.3 | excellent |
| Vitamin C | 2.7 mg | 4.5 | 7.3 | good |
| Manganese | 0.1 mg | 4.0 | 6.4 | good |
| Vitamin B6 | 0.1 mg | 4.0 | 6.4 | good |
| Dietary Fiber | 1.0 g | 3.8 | 6.2 | good |
| **CAROTENOIDS:** | | | | |
| Beta-Carotene | 768.8 mcg | | | |
| Beta-Cryptoxanthin | 220.1 mcg | | | |
| Lutein+Zeaxanthin | 463.1 mcg | | | |

Daily values for these nutrients have not yet been established.

For more on "Total Nutrient-Richness," "%DV," "Density," and The World's Healthiest Foods "Quality" Rating System, see page 805.

It is not surprising that Cayenne and other Red Chili Peppers can trace their long history to Central and South America, regions whose cuisines are renowned for their hot and spicy flavors. They have been cultivated in these regions for more than 7,000 years, first as a decorative item and later as a foodstuff and medicine. Christopher Columbus brought the Cayenne Pepper, a type of Red Chili Pepper, back to Europe where it was used as a substitute for black pepper, which was very expensive at that time. Dried Red Chili Peppers add zest to flavorful dishes around the world and health benefits to those who enjoy their fiery heat.

## why cayenne and red chili peppers should be part of your healthiest way of eating

Cayenne and Red Chili Peppers are rich in antioxidant carotenoids such as beta-carotene as well as capsaicin, a unique phytonutrient that has anti-inflammatory and pain relief properties and provides the heat that may help you to burn excess fat. The latest studies are now finding capsaicin to actually induce the reduction of tumors. Cayenne and Red

# cayenne and red chili peppers

## highlights

| | |
|---|---|
| AVAILABILITY: | Year-round |
| REFRIGERATE: | No |
| SHELF LIFE: | 1 year |
| PREPARATION: | None |

Chili Peppers are ideal additions to your "Healthiest Way of Eating" not only because they are nutritious, but also because they are low in calories: 2 teaspoons of Cayenne Pepper contain only 11 calories.

## 1. the best way to select cayenne and red chili peppers

Cayenne Red Chili Peppers can be found either prepackaged or the bulk herbs and spice section of your local market.

**CAYENNE PEPPER:** Cayenne Pepper is made from the fresh pepper of the same name.

**DRIED RED CHILI PEPPERS:** Come in either flakes or power. The flakes are most often made from Anaheim chilies. True chili powder can be made from a variety of different types of chilies.

**COMMERCIAL CHILI POWDER:** A combination of dried chilies, garlic, oregano, cumin, coriander and cloves used to flavor chili.

Cayenne and dried Red Chili Peppers come in varying degrees of heat. Oftentimes, when they are sold in bulk, they are labeled with their heat intensity, measured in Scoville Units (SU). Comparing the heat rating of the different offerings of Cayenne and Red Chili Peppers can help you find the one that will best meet your taste preference and recipe needs.

I recommend purchasing organically grown Cayenne and dried Red Chili Peppers whenever possible. (For more on *Organic Foods*, see page 113.)

## 2. the best way to store cayenne and red chili peppers

To preserve the greatest number of nutrients and freshness,

Cayenne and Red Chili Peppers should be kept in a tightly sealed glass jar, away from direct sunlight.

## 3. the best way to prepare cayenne and red chili peppers

Cayenne and dried Red Chili Peppers require no preparation.

## 4. the healthiest way of cooking with cayenne and red chili peppers

To retain the maximum number of nutrients and flavor, add Cayenne and dried Red Chili Peppers at the end of the cooking process since they lose their flavor and aroma if cooked for too long. Both Cayenne and dried Red Chili Peppers are commonly used in Mexican, Indian and Chinese cooking. Only a pinch is necessary; they are very hot.

### TIPS: 4 Ways to Enjoy Chili Peppers

1. Add to soups, stews, curries and dressings.
2. Use in place of black pepper.
3. Mix with olive oil for a spicy oil that can be used on vegetables, meats, fish and beans.
4. Add a few pinches of Cayenne Pepper to Mediterranean dressing (page 331).

# health benefits of cayenne and red chili peppers

## Promote Natural Defenses Against Infections

Capsaicin is the phytonutrient in Cayenne and other dried Red Chili Peppers that not only gives them their heat but also delivers many of their health benefits. One of its functions is to break up mucus congestion in the nose and lungs. Their concentration of beta-carotene also contributes to their ability to support your immune system during cold and flu season.

## Promote Digestive Health

Capsaicin has anti-inflammatory and pain relief properties that may benefit digestive health. Additionally, the use of dried Red Chili Peppers, such as Cayenne, is associated with a reduced risk of stomach ulcers.

## Promote Heart Health

Cayenne Pepper has been shown to reduce blood cholesterol, triglyceride levels and platelet aggregation, while increasing the body's ability to dissolve fibrin, a substance integral to the formation of blood clots. Cultures where hot peppers like Cayenne are used liberally have a much lower rate of heart attack, stroke and pulmonary embolism.

## Promote Healthy Weight Control

Adding Cayenne and dried Red Chili Pepper to your food may help you to lose weight or maintain optimal weight.

Results from clinical and animal research studies suggest that hot peppers may not only speed up metabolic rate and thermogenesis (burning of fat) but may also act as mild appetite suppressants.

### Additional Health-Promoting Benefits of Cayenne and Red Chili Peppers

Cayenne Pepper is also a concentrated source of free-radical-scavenging vitamin A, vitamin C and manganese; and heart-healthy vitamin B6 and dietary fiber.

## Nutritional Analysis of 2 teaspoons of Cayenne Pepper:

| NUTRIENT | AMOUNT | % DAILY VALUE | NUTRIENT | AMOUNT | % DAILY VALUE |
|---|---|---|---|---|---|
| Calories | 11.20 | | Pantothenic Acid | — mg | — |
| Calories from Fat | 5.52 | | | | |
| Calories from Saturated Fat | 1.04 | | **Minerals** | | |
| Protein | 0.40 g | | Boron | — mcg | |
| Carbohydrates | 2.00 g | | Calcium | 5.28 mg | 0.53 |
| Dietary Fiber | 0.96 g | 3.84 | Chloride | — mg | |
| Soluble Fiber | — g | | Chromium | — mcg | — |
| Insoluble Fiber | — g | | Copper | 0.00 mg | 0.00 |
| Sugar – Total | — g | | Fluoride | — mg | — |
| Monosaccharides | — g | | Iodine | — mcg | — |
| Disaccharides | — g | | Iron | 0.24 mg | 1.33 |
| Other Carbs | — g | | Magnesium | 5.36 mg | 1.34 |
| Fat – Total | 0.64 g | | Manganese | 0.08 mg | 4.00 |
| Saturated Fat | 0.08 g | | Molybdenum | — mcg | — |
| Mono Fat | 0.08 g | | Phosphorus | 10.40 mg | 1.04 |
| Poly Fat | 0.32 g | | Potassium | 71.20 mg | |
| Omega-3 Fatty Acids | 0.00 g | 0.00 | Selenium | 0.32 mcg | 0.46 |
| Omega-6 Fatty Acids | 0.24 g | | Sodium | 1.04 mg | |
| Trans Fatty Acids | 0.00 g | | Zinc | 0.08 mg | 0.53 |
| Cholesterol | 0.00 mg | | | | |
| Water | 0.32 g | | **Amino Acids** | | |
| Ash | 0.24 g | | Alanine | — g | |
| | | | Arginine | — g | |
| **Vitamins** | | | Aspartate | — g | |
| Vitamin A IU | 1470.24 IU | 29.40 | Cystine | — g | — |
| Vitamin A RE | 147.04 RE | | Glutamate | — g | |
| A - Carotenoid | 147.04 RE | 1.96 | Glycine | — g | |
| A - Retinol | 0.00 RE | | Histidine | — g | — |
| B1 Thiamin | 0.00 mg | 0.00 | Isoleucine | — g | — |
| B2 Riboflavin | 0.00 mg | 0.00 | Leucine | — g | — |
| B3 Niacin | 0.32 mg | 1.60 | Lysine | — g | — |
| Niacin Equiv | 0.32 mg | | Methionine | — g | — |
| Vitamin B6 | 0.08 mg | 4.00 | Phenylalanine | — g | — |
| Vitamin B12 | 0.00 mcg | 0.00 | Proline | — g | |
| Biotin | — mcg | — | Serine | — g | |
| Vitamin C | 2.72 mg | 4.53 | Threonine | — g | — |
| Vitamin D IU | 0.00 IU | 0.00 | Tryptophan | — g | — |
| Vitamin D mcg | 0.00 mcg | | Tyrosine | — g | — |
| Vitamin E Alpha Equiv | 0.16 mg | 0.80 | Valine | — g | — |
| Vitamin E IU | 0.24 IU | | | | |
| Vitamin E mg | 0.16 mg | | | | |
| Folate | 3.76 mcg | 0.94 | | | |
| Vitamin K | — mcg | — | | | |

(Note: "–" indicates data is unavailable. For more information, please see page 806.)

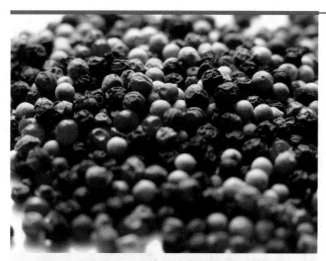

# black peppercorns

## highlights

| | |
|---|---|
| AVAILABILITY: | Year-round |
| REFRIGERATE: | No |
| SHELF LIFE: | 1 year |
| PREPARATION: | None |

## nutrient-richness chart

Total Nutrient-Richness: **7**
Two teaspoons (4 grams) of Black Pepper contains 11 calories

| NUTRIENT | AMOUNT | %DV | DENSITY | QUALITY |
|---|---|---|---|---|
| Manganese | 0.2 mg | 12.0 | 19.9 | excellent |
| Vitamin K | 6.9 mcg | 8.6 | 14.2 | very good |
| Iron | 1.2 mg | 6.9 | 11.4 | very good |
| Dietary Fiber | 1.1 g | 4.5 | 7.4 | good |

For more on "Total Nutrient-Richness," "%DV," "Density," and
The World's Healthiest Foods "Quality" Rating System, see page 805.

Pepper was historically used to honor the gods, pay taxes and ransoms, and as a measure of a man's wealth. Not only could its pungency spice up otherwise bland foods, but it could disguise a food's lack of freshness, the latter being an especially important quality in the times before efficient means of preservation. Pepper was in such demand that the quest for pepper is thought to have catalyzed much of the spice trade. Today, adding Pepper "to taste" is ubiquitous in almost any recipe, not only adding zest to your meal but also providing an array of nutritional benefits.

## why black pepper should be part of your healthiest way of eating

Black pepper contains piperine, a unique phytonutrient that has potent antioxidant activity as well as antibiotic properties. The nutrients in Black Pepper also have digestion-enhancing and diuretic properties. Black Pepper is an ideal addition to your "Healthiest Way of Eating" not only because it is nutritious, but also because it is low in calories: 2 teaspoons of Black Pepper contain only 11 calories.

## varieties of black pepper

Black, green and white peppercorns are actually the same fruit that is in different stages of development. Green is the least ripe, black is riper than green and white peppercorns are fully mature and ripe. White peppercorns are the hottest and are commonly used in Asian dishes. Pink peppercorns, with their sweet and aromatic taste, are actually a completely different plant species.

## 1. the best way to select black pepper

For the most nutritious and best flavor, I recommend purchasing whole peppercorns and grinding them yourself in a mill just before adding them to a recipe. In addition to superior flavor, buying whole peppercorns will help to ensure that you are purchasing unadulterated pepper since ground pepper is oftentimes mixed with other spices. Whole peppercorns should be heavy, compact and free of any blemishes. Black Pepper is also available crushed or ground into powder.

I recommend purchasing organically grown Black Pepper whenever possible. (For more on *Organic Foods*, see page 113.)

## 2. the best way to store black pepper

To preserve the greatest number of nutrients and freshness, Black Pepper should be kept in a tightly sealed glass container in a cool, dark and dry place. Whole peppercorns will keep for almost one year, while ground pepper will stay fresh for about three months.

# 3. the best way to prepare black pepper

Black Pepper requires no preparation.

# 4. the healthiest way of cooking with black pepper

To retain the maximum number of nutrients and flavor, add Pepper that you have freshly ground in a mill at the end of the cooking process or after the dish has completed cooking since it loses its flavor and aroma if cooked for too long. Add whole peppercorns to soup and stews and remove them before serving.

## TIPS: 4 Ways to Enjoy Black Pepper

1. Coat chicken or fish with fresh ground Pepper before cooking.
2. Add to soup as a great flavor enhancer.
3. Add to spreads, marinades and salad dressings.
4. Add whole peppercorns when making chicken or vegetable broth for added flavor.

# health benefits of black pepper

## Promotes Digestive Health

Black Pepper has long been recognized as a carminitive (a substance that helps prevent the formation of intestinal gas), a property likely due to its beneficial effect of stimulating hydrochloric acid production.

## Provides Powerful Antioxidant and Antimicrobial Protection

Black Pepper has demonstrated impressive antioxidant effects. Supplementation with Black Pepper and its phytonutrient, piperine, has been found to protect LDL from oxidation and enhance the liver's concentrations of glutathione, a powerful internal antioxidant. Research has found it to have effective antibiotic activity against an array of bacteria, supporting the traditional Ayurvedic use of Black Pepper as an antimicrobial agent.

## Promotes Healthy Weight Control

Preliminary research suggests that Black Pepper may stimulate the breakdown of fat cells. It has been traditionally known for its diaphoretic (promotes sweating) and diuretic (promotes urination) properties.

## Additional Health-Promoting Benefits of Black Pepper

Black pepper is also a concentrated source of energy-producing iron, heart-healthy dietary fiber, and free-radical-scavenging manganese.

### Nutritional Analysis of 2 teaspoons of ground Black Pepper:

| NUTRIENT | AMOUNT | % DAILY VALUE | NUTRIENT | AMOUNT | % DAILY VALUE |
|---|---|---|---|---|---|
| Calories | 10.88 | | Pantothenic Acid | —mg | — |
| Calories from Fat | 1.24 | | | | |
| Calories from Saturated Fat | 0.36 | | **Minerals** | | |
| Protein | 0.48 g | | Boron | —mcg | |
| Carbohydrates | 2.76 g | | Calcium | 18.64 mg | 1.86 |
| Dietary Fiber | 1.12 g | 4.48 | Chloride | —mg | |
| Soluble Fiber | —g | | Chromium | —mcg | — |
| Insoluble Fiber | —g | | Copper | 0.04 mg | 2.00 |
| Sugar –Total | —g | | Fluoride | —mg | — |
| Monosaccharides | —g | | Iodine | —mcg | — |
| Disaccharides | —g | | Iron | 1.24 mg | 6.89 |
| Other Carbs | —g | | Magnesium | 8.24 mg | 2.06 |
| Fat – Total | 0.12 g | | Manganese | 0.24 mg | 12.00 |
| Saturated Fat | 0.04 g | | Molybdenum | —mcg | — |
| Mono Fat | 0.04 g | | Phosphorus | 7.40 mg | 0.74 |
| Poly Fat | 0.04 g | | Potassium | 53.72 mg | |
| Omega-3 Fatty Acids | 0.00 g | 0.00 | Selenium | 0.12 mcg | 0.17 |
| Omega-6 Fatty Acids | 0.04 g | | Sodium | 1.88 mg | |
| Trans Fatty Acids | 0.00 g | | Zinc | 0.08 mg | 0.53 |
| Cholesterol | 0.00 mg | | | | |
| Water | 0.44 g | | **Amino Acids** | | |
| Ash | 0.20 g | | Alanine | —g | |
| | | | Arginine | —g | |
| **Vitamins** | | | Aspartate | —g | |
| Vitamin A IU | 8.12 IU | 0.16 | Cystine | —g | — |
| Vitamin A RE | 0.80 RE | | Glutamate | —g | |
| A - Carotenoid | 0.80 RE | 0.01 | Glycine | —g | |
| A - Retinol | 0.00 RE | | Histidine | —g | — |
| B1 Thiamin | 0.00 mg | 0.00 | Isoleucine | —g | — |
| B2 Riboflavin | 0.00 mg | 0.00 | Leucine | —g | — |
| B3 Niacin | 0.04 mg | 0.20 | Lysine | —g | — |
| Niacin Equiv | 0.04 mg | | Methionine | —g | — |
| Vitamin B6 | 0.00 mg | 0.00 | Phenylalanine | —g | — |
| Vitamin B12 | 0.00 mcg | 0.00 | Proline | —g | |
| Biotin | —mcg | — | Serine | —g | |
| Vitamin C | 0.88 mg | 1.47 | Threonine | —g | — |
| Vitamin D IU | 0.00 IU | 0.00 | Tryptophan | —g | — |
| Vitamin D mcg | 0.00 mcg | | Tyrosine | —g | — |
| Vitamin E Alpha Equiv | 0.04 mg | 0.20 | Valine | —g | — |
| Vitamin E IU | 0.08 IU | | | | |
| Vitamin E mg | 0.04 mg | | | | |
| Folate | 0.44 mcg | 0.11 | | | |
| Vitamin K | 6.88 mcg | 8.60 | | | |

(Note: "–" indicates data is unavailable. For more information, please see page 806.)

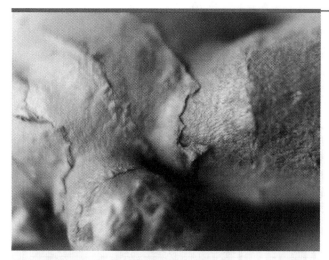

# ginger

| | |
|---|---|
| AVAILABILITY: | Year-round |
| REFRIGERATE: | Yes |
| SHELF LIFE: | 3 weeks |
| PREPARATION: | Peel, chop or grate |

## nutrient-richness chart

Total Nutrient-Richness: **5**

One oz wt (28 grams) of Ginger root contains 20 calories

| NUTRIENT | AMOUNT | %DV | DENSITY | QUALITY |
|---|---|---|---|---|
| Potassium | 117.7 mg | 3.4 | 3.1 | good |
| Magnesium | 12.2 mg | 3.0 | 2.8 | good |
| Copper | 0.1 mg | 3.0 | 2.8 | good |
| Manganese | 0.1 mg | 3.0 | 2.8 | good |
| B6 Pyridoxine | 0.1 mg | 2.5 | 2.3 | good |

For more on "Total Nutrient-Richness," "%DV," "Density," and
The World's Healthiest Foods "Quality" Rating System, see page 805.

Ginger was mentioned in ancient Chinese, Indian and Middle Eastern writings and has long been prized for its culinary and medicinal properties. The aromatic, pungent and hot taste of Ginger adds zest to a wide range of dishes from Asian stir-fries to tangy fruit desserts. The plant's botanical name is thought to be derived from its Sanskrit name *"singabera,"* which well describes its distinctive and characteristic "horn shape."

## why ginger should be part of your healthiest way of eating

Ginger contains special phytonutrients known as gingerols that have numerous health-promoting benefits, including potent anti-inflammatory properties. Ginger is also well-known for its ability to soothe the stomach and relieve nausea. Ginger is an ideal addition to your "Healthiest Way of Eating" not only because it is nutritious, but also because it is low in calories: 1 ounce of Ginger contains only 20 calories.

## 1. the best way to select ginger

**FRESH GINGER:** For the most nutritious and best tasting Ginger, I select fresh Ginger whenever possible. Fresh Ginger root should be firm, shiny and smooth. Avoid Ginger that is wrinkled, soft or cracked; it has lost much of its flavor and pungency. It is generally available in two forms: mature or young. Mature Ginger, the more widely available type, has a tough skin that requires peeling while young Ginger, usually only available in Asian markets, does not need to be peeled.

**DRIED GINGER:** Does not have the flavor of fresh Ginger.

**CRYSTALLIZED GINGER:** Candied Ginger is now very popular and readily available.

I recommend selecting organically grown varieties of fresh, dried and crystallized Ginger whenever possible. (For more on *Organic Foods*, see page 113.)

## 2. the best way to store ginger

**FRESH GINGER:** To preserve the greatest number of nutrients and freshness, fresh Ginger can be stored in the refrigerator, where it will keep for up to three weeks if it is left unpeeled. Stored unpeeled in the freezer, fresh Ginger will keep for up to six months.

**DRIED GINGER:** Ginger powder should be kept in a tightly sealed glass container in a cool, dark, dry place. Alternatively, you can store it in the refrigerator where it will enjoy an extended shelf life of about one year.

## 3. the best way to prepare ginger

Peel mature Ginger and chop or grate according to the recipe. You can peel Ginger with a knife or spoon. Young Ginger requires no peeling as the skin is very thin.

# 4. the healthiest way of cooking with ginger

**FRESH GINGER:** To retain the greatest number of nutrients and flavor, it is best to add fresh Ginger to your dish at the end of the cooking time. Ginger can also be sprinkled on your dish after it has been cooked.

**DRIED GINGER:** Has lost much of its original flavor. However, if you are using dried Ginger, it is best to add it at the beginning of the cooking time, so it will have a chance to warm up and cook long enough to bring out its flavor.

To substitute dried Ginger for fresh, use about one-third the amount of dried Ginger as you would fresh.

## TIPS: 5 Ways to Enjoy Ginger

1. Ginger can be used to flavor vegetables, chicken and fish dishes.
2. To make Ginger lemonade, combine freshly grated Ginger, lemon juice, cane juice or honey, and water.
3. Add extra inspiration to your rice side dishes by sprinkling grated Ginger, sesame seeds and strips of the sea vegetable, nori, on top.
4. Combine Ginger, tamari (soy sauce), sesame oil and garlic to make a wonderful salad dressing.
5. Spice up your "Healthy Sautéed" vegetables by adding freshly grated Ginger.

---

# health benefits of ginger

## Promotes Digestive Health

Historically, Ginger has a long tradition of use for alleviating symptoms of gastrointestinal distress and is known for its ability to relax the intestinal tract and reduce intestinal gas. Research studies have found it to be effective in preventing the symptoms of motion sickness, especially seasickness, as well as reducing the nausea and vomiting of pregnancy.

## Provides Powerful Anti-Inflammatory Protection

Ginger contains very potent anti-inflammatory compounds called gingerols. The presence of these substances may explain why so many people with arthritis experience reductions in their pain levels and improvements in their mobility when they consume Ginger regularly. In two clinical studies involving patients who responded to conventional drugs and those who didn't, physicians found that 75% of arthritis patients and 100% of patients with muscular discomfort experienced relief of pain and/or swelling after eating Ginger.

## Additional Health-Promoting Benefits of Ginger

Ginger is also a concentrated source of heart-healthy magnesium, vitamin B6 and potassium, and free-radical-scavenging manganese and copper.

## Nutritional Analysis of 1 oz-wt of fresh Ginger:

| NUTRIENT | AMOUNT | % DAILY VALUE | NUTRIENT | AMOUNT | % DAILY VALUE |
|---|---|---|---|---|---|
| Calories | 19.56 | | Pantothenic Acid | 0.06 mg | 0.60 |
| Calories from Fat | 1.86 | | | | |
| Calories from Saturated Fat | 0.52 | | **Minerals** | | |
| Protein | 0.49 g | | Boron | — mcg | |
| Carbohydrates | 4.28 g | | Calcium | 5.10 mg | 0.51 |
| Dietary Fiber | 0.57 g | 2.28 | Chloride | — mg | |
| Soluble Fiber | — g | | Chromium | — mcg | — |
| Insoluble Fiber | — g | | Copper | 0.06 mg | 3.00 |
| Sugar – Total | — g | | Fluoride | — mg | |
| Monosaccharides | — g | | Iodine | — mcg | — |
| Disaccharides | — g | | Iron | 0.14 mg | 0.78 |
| Other Carbs | — g | | Magnesium | 12.19 mg | 3.05 |
| Fat – Total | 0.21 g | | Manganese | 0.06 mg | 3.00 |
| Saturated Fat | 0.06 g | | Molybdenum | — mcg | — |
| Mono Fat | 0.04 g | | Phosphorus | 7.65 mg | 0.77 |
| Poly Fat | 0.04 g | | Potassium | 117.65 mg | |
| Omega-3 Fatty Acids | 0.01 g | 0.40 | Selenium | 0.20 mcg | 0.29 |
| Omega-6 Fatty Acids | 0.03 g | | Sodium | 3.69 mg | |
| Trans Fatty Acids | 0.00 g | | Zinc | 0.10 mg | 0.67 |
| Cholesterol | 0.00 mg | | | | |
| Water | 23.15 g | | **Amino Acids** | | |
| Ash | 0.22 g | | Alanine | 0.01 g | |
| | | | Arginine | 0.01 g | |
| **Vitamins** | | | Aspartate | 0.06 g | |
| Vitamin A IU | 0.00 IU | 0.00 | Cystine | 0.00 g | 0.00 |
| Vitamin A RE | 0.00 RE | | Glutamate | 0.05 g | |
| A - Carotenoid | 0.00 RE | 0.00 | Glycine | 0.01 g | |
| A - Retinol | 0.00 RE | | Histidine | 0.01 g | 0.78 |
| B1 Thiamin | 0.01 mg | 0.67 | Isoleucine | 0.01 g | 0.87 |
| B2 Riboflavin | 0.01 mg | 0.59 | Leucine | 0.02 g | 0.79 |
| B3 Niacin | 0.20 mg | 1.00 | Lysine | 0.02 g | 0.85 |
| Niacin Equiv | 0.26 mg | | Methionine | 0.00 g | 0.00 |
| Vitamin B6 | 0.05 mg | 2.50 | Phenylalanine | 0.01 g | 0.84 |
| Vitamin B12 | 0.00 mcg | 0.00 | Proline | 0.01 g | |
| Biotin | — mcg | — | Serine | 0.01 g | |
| Vitamin C | 1.42 mg | 2.37 | Threonine | 0.01 g | 0.81 |
| Vitamin D IU | 0.00 IU | 0.00 | Tryptophan | 0.00 g | 0.00 |
| Vitamin D mcg | 0.00 mcg | | Tyrosine | 0.01 g | 1.03 |
| Vitamin E alpha equiv | 0.07 mg | 0.35 | Valine | 0.02 g | 1.36 |
| Vitamin E IU | 0.11 IU | | | | |
| Vitamin E mg | 0.07 mg | | | | |
| Folate | 3.18 mcg | 0.80 | | | |
| Vitamin K | 0.03 mcg | 0.04 | | | |

(Note: "–" indicates data is unavailable. For more information, please see page 806.)

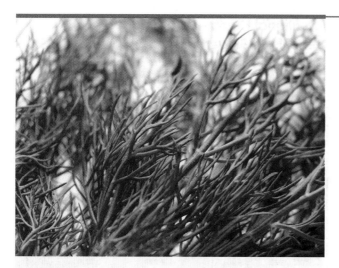

## nutrient-richness chart

Total Nutrient-Richness: **4**
2 teaspoons (2 grams) of dried Dill weed contain 5 calories

| NUTRIENT | AMOUNT | %DV | DENSITY | QUALITY |
|---|---|---|---|---|
| Iron | 0.98 mg | 5.4 | 19.4 | very good |
| Manganese | 0.08 mg | 4.0 | 14.2 | good |
| Calcium | 35.7 mg | 3.6 | 12.7 | good |

For more on "Total Nutrient-Richness," "%DV," "Density," and
The World's Healthiest Foods "Quality" Rating System, see page 805.

Dill has been recognized for both its culinary and medicinal benefits since antiquity. The Greeks and Romans regarded Dill as a sign of wealth and held it in high regard for its many healing properties. Dill's name comes from the old Norse word "*Dilla*" which means "to lull." This name reflects Dill's traditional uses as both a carminative stomach soother and an insomnia reliever. Dill is a unique herb in that both its leaves and seeds can be used as a seasoning. Dill's green leaves are wispy and fern-like and have a soft, sweet taste. The seeds are similar in taste to caraway; they can be used interchangeably. Dill seeds feature a flavor that is aromatic, sweet and citrus-like but also slightly bitter. Add Dill to your favorite vegetable and fish dishes for extra flavor and nutrition.

## why dill should be part of your healthiest way of eating

Dill is rich in antioxidant phytonutrients and volatile oils, which have antibacterial activity. Dill is an ideal addition to your "Healthiest Way of Eating" not only because it is nutritious, but also because it is low in calories: 2 teaspoons of dried Dill weed contains only 5 calories.

# dill

## highlights

| | |
|---|---|
| AVAILABILITY: | Year-round |
| REFRIGERATE: | Yes |
| SHELF LIFE: | 7 days |
| PREPARATION: | Minimal |

## 1. the best way to select dill

**FRESH DILL:** For the most nutritious Dill, select fresh Dill leaves that are feathery and green in color and that have a pungent odor. Dill leaves that are a little wilted are still acceptable since they usually droop very quickly after being picked. Avoid Dill leaves that have turned dark.

I recommend selecting organically grown fresh or dried Dill whenever possible. (For more on *Organic Foods*, see page 113.)

## 2. the best way to store dill

**FRESH DILL:** To preserve the greatest number of nutrients and freshness, fresh Dill should always be stored in the refrigerator either wrapped in a damp paper towel or with its stems placed in a container of water. Since it is very fragile, even if stored properly, Dill will only keep fresh for about seven days. Dill can be frozen, either whole or chopped, in airtight containers. Alternatively, you can freeze the Dill leaves in ice cube trays covered with water or stock; these can be easily added when preparing soups or stews.

**DRIED DILL AND DRIED DILL SEEDS:** Should be stored in a tightly sealed glass container in a cool, dry and dark place where they will keep fresh for about six months.

## 3. the best way to prepare dill

To retain nutrients, it is best to wash fresh Dill under cold running water and pat dry with a paper towel. Do not soak Dill or the water-soluble nutrients will leach into the water.

## 4. the healthiest way of cooking with dill

**FRESH DILL:** Because fresh Dill loses its flavor if it is cooked for a long period of time, it is best to add fresh Dill to your dish at the end of the cooking time. Dill is a very delicate herb, that can be sprinkled on your dish after it has been cooked.

**DRIED DILL:** Has lost some of its flavor which is why it is best to use fresh Dill whenever possible. Since heating dried Dill will help release its flavor, it is best to add it at the middle of the cooking time to allow the Dill to warm up and add more flavor to your dish. Both dried Dill leaves and seeds are aromatic. Dill is good in fish, beans, potato and cabbage dishes. The seeds are especially good for pickling. To substitute dried Dill for fresh, use about one-third the amount of dried Dill as you would fresh. Be careful not to overpower the flavor of food by adding too much Dill.

## TIPS: 5 Ways to Enjoy Dill

1. Combine Dill weed with plain yogurt and chopped cucumber for a delicious dip.

2. Use Dill when cooking fish, especially salmon and trout, as their flavors complement each other very well.

3. Use Dill weed as a garnish for sandwiches.

4. Since Dill seeds were traditionally used to soothe the stomach after meals, put some seeds in a small dish and place it on the dinner table for all to enjoy.

5. Add Dill to your favorite egg salad recipe.

# health benefits of dill

## Provides Powerful Antioxidant Protection

Dill is rich in flavonoid antioxidants such as kaempferol and vicenin. It also contains monoterpene phytonutrients such as carvone, limonene and anethofuran, which have been shown to activate one of the body's most powerful antioxidant compounds, glutathione, helping to prevent free-radical-scavenging. The activity of Dill's volatile oils helps neutralize particular types of carcinogens, such as the benzopyrenes that are part of cigarette smoke and charcoal grill smoke.

## Provides Powerful Antimicrobial Protection

Dill's volatile oil phytonutrients have also been studied for their ability to prevent bacterial overgrowth. In this respect, Dill shares the stage with garlic, which has also been shown to have "bacteriostatic" or bacteria-regulating effects.

## Additional Health-Promoting Benefits of Dill

Dill is also a concentrated source of bone-building calcium, magnesium and manganese; heart-healthy dietary fiber; and energy-producing iron.

### Nutritional Analysis of 2 teaspoons of dried Dill weed:

| NUTRIENT | AMOUNT | % DAILY VALUE | NUTRIENT | AMOUNT | % DAILY VALUE |
|---|---|---|---|---|---|
| Calories | 5.06 | | Pantothenic Acid | — mg | — |
| Calories from Fat | 0.78 | | | | |
| Calories from Saturated Fat | 0.04 | | **Minerals** | | |
| Protein | 0.40 g | | Boron | — mcg | |
| Carbohydrates | 1.12 g | | Calcium | 35.68 mg | 3.57 |
| Dietary Fiber | 0.27 g | 1.08 | Chloride | — mg | |
| Soluble Fiber | — g | | Chromium | — mcg | — |
| Insoluble Fiber | — g | | Copper | 0.01 mg | 0.50 |
| Sugar - Total | — g | | Fluoride | — mg | — |
| Monosaccharides | — g | | Iodine | — mcg | — |
| Disaccharides | — g | | Iron | 0.98 mg | 5.44 |
| Other Carbs | — g | | Magnesium | 9.02 mg | 2.25 |
| Fat - Total | 0.09 g | | Manganese | 0.08 mg | 4.00 |
| Saturated Fat | 0.00 g | | Molybdenum | — mcg | — |
| Mono Fat | 0.06 g | | Phosphorus | 10.86 mg | 1.09 |
| Poly Fat | 0.01 g | | Potassium | 66.16 mg | |
| Omega-3 Fatty Acids | 0.00 g | 0.00 | Selenium | 0.03 mcg | 0.04 |
| Omega-6 Fatty Acids | 0.01 g | | Sodium | 4.16 mg | |
| Trans Fatty Acids | 0.00 g | | Zinc | 0.07 mg | 0.47 |
| Cholesterol | 0.00 mg | | | | |
| Water | 0.15 g | | **Amino Acids** | | |
| Ash | 0.25 g | | Alanine | 0.02 g | |
| | | | Arginine | 0.14 g | |
| **Vitamins** | | | Aspartate | 0.03 g | |
| Vitamin A IU | 117.00 IU | 2.34 | Cystine | 0.00 g | 0.00 |
| Vitamin A RE | 11.72 RE | | Glutamate | 0.03 g | |
| A - Carotenoid | 11.72 RE | 0.16 | Glycine | 0.02 g | |
| A - Retinol | 0.00 RE | | Histidine | 0.01 g | 0.78 |
| B1 Thiamin | 0.01 mg | 0.67 | Isoleucine | 0.02 g | 1.74 |
| B2 Riboflavin | 0.01 mg | 0.59 | Leucine | 0.02 g | 0.79 |
| B3 Niacin | 0.06 mg | 0.30 | Lysine | 0.02 g | 0.85 |
| Niacin Equiv | 0.08 mg | | Methionine | 0.00 g | 0.00 |
| Vitamin B6 | 0.03 mg | 1.50 | Phenylalanine | 0.01 g | 0.84 |
| Vitamin B12 | 0.00 mcg | 0.00 | Proline | 0.03 g | |
| Biotin | — mcg | — | Serine | 0.02 g | |
| Vitamin C | 1.00 mg | 1.67 | Threonine | 0.01 g | 0.81 |
| Vitamin D IU | 0.00 IU | 0.00 | Tryptophan | 0.00 g | 0.00 |
| Vitamin D mcg | 0.00 mcg | | Tyrosine | 0.01 g | 1.03 |
| Vitamin E Alpha Equiv | — mg | — | Valine | 0.02 g | 1.36 |
| Vitamin E IU | — IU | | | | |
| Vitamin E mg | — mg | — | | | |
| Folate | — mcg | — | | | |
| Vitamin K | — mcg | — | | | |

(Note: "—" indicates data is unavailable. For more information, please see page 806.)

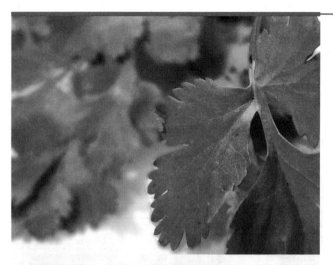

## nutrient-richness chart

Total Nutrient-Richness: **3**

Two tablespoons (2 grams) of fresh Cilantro contain less than 1 calorie

| NUTRIENT | AMOUNT | %DV | DENSITY | QUALITY |
|---|---|---|---|---|
| Vitamin K | 6.20 mcg | 7.8 | 303.3 | very good |
| Vitamin A | 135.0 IU | 2.7 | 105.6 | good |
| **CAROTENOIDS:** | | | | |
| Beta-Carotene | 78.6 mcg | | Daily values for these nutrients have not yet been established. | |
| Beta-Cryptoxanthin | 4.0 mcg | | | |
| Lutein + Zeaxanthin | 17.3 mcg | | | |

For more on "Total Nutrient-Richness," "%DV," "Density," and
The World's Healthiest Foods "Quality" Rating System, see page 805.

# cilantro

| | |
|---|---|
| AVAILABILITY: | Year-round |
| REFRIGERATE: | Yes |
| SHELF LIFE: | 1 week |
| PREPARATION: | Minimal |

Cilantro bears a strong resemblance to Italian flat leaf parsley and is sometimes called Chinese parsley. Native to the Mediterranean and Middle Eastern regions, its culinary use dates back to 5,000 BC. It was cultivated in ancient Egypt and even mentioned in the Old Testament. Today, Cilantro plays an important role not only in Indian and Chinese cuisines but also in the culinary traditions of Latin America, with Cilantro being one of the primary ingredients used in many salsas. Cilantro is also known as coriander; its seeds are used as a spice.

## why cilantro should be part of your healthiest way of eating

Cilantro contains numerous phytonutrients with antioxidant power including flavonoids such as quercetin, kaempferol, rhamnetin and apigenin and the phenolic acid compounds, caffeic and chlorogenic acid. It also features a compound called dodecenal, which has antimicrobial properties. Cilantro is an ideal addition to your "Healthiest Way of Eating" not only because it is nutritious, but also because it is low in calories: 2 tablespoons of fresh Cilantro contain less than 1 calorie.

## 1. the best way to select cilantro

For the most nutritious and best tasting Cilantro, look for leaves that are firm, vibrantly fresh smelling and green in color. Avoid leaves with yellow or brown spots. I recommend purchasing organically grown Cilantro whenever possible. (For more on *Organic Foods*, see page 113.)

## 2. the best way to store cilantro

To preserve the greatest number of nutrients and freshness, it is best to store fresh Cilantro in the refrigerator. If possible, it should be stored with its roots still attached; place the roots in a glass of water and cover the leaves with a loosely fitting plastic bag. If the roots have been removed, wrap the Cilantro leaves in a damp cloth or paper towel and place them in a perforated plastic bag. Cilantro with roots will last up to 1 week, while without roots it will last about 3 to 5 days.

Cilantro may also be frozen, either whole or chopped, in airtight containers; it should not be thawed before use since it will lose much of its crisp texture. Alternatively, you can place chopped Cilantro in ice cube trays covered with either water or stock and freeze. These Cilantro ice cubes can then be added when preparing soups or stews.

## 3. the best way to prepare cilantro

To retain nutrients, it is best to wash fresh Cilantro under cold running water and pat dry with a paper towel. Do not soak Cilantro leaves or the water-soluble nutrients will leach into the water.

# 4. the healthiest way of cooking with cilantro

Because fresh Cilantro loses its flavor if it is cooked for a long period of time, it is best to add it to your dish at the end of cooking or sprinkle it on top of your dish after it has been cooked. To substitute dried Cilantro for fresh, use about one-third the amount of dried Cilantro as you would fresh.

## TIPS: 6 Ways to Enjoy Cilantro

1. As an ingredient in many Mexican, Asian, South American and Thai Foods.
2. Substitute Cilantro for basil in a pesto recipe (see page 508).
3. Sprinkle on many foods as a garnish.
4. Add to salsa or guacamole.
5. Add to dressings.
6. Cilantro goes well with seafood, chicken and beans.

---

# health benefits of cilantro

## Provides Powerful Antioxidant Protection

Many of the above healing properties of Cilantro can be attributed to its exceptional phytonutrient content. Cilantro's volatile oil is rich in beneficial phytonutrients, including carvone, geraniol, limonene, borneol, camphor, elemol and linalool. Its flavonoids include quercitin, kaempferol, rhamnetin and epigenin. Plus, it contains active phenolic acid compounds, including caffeic and chlorogenic acid.

## Provides Powerful Antimicrobial Protection

Cilantro contains an antibacterial compound (called dodecenal), which the results of laboratory tests suggest is twice as effective as the commonly used antibiotic drug gentamicin at killing *Salmonella*. In addition to dodecenal, eight other antibiotic compounds were isolated from fresh Cilantro, inspiring the food scientists to suggest that Cilantro-based compounds might be developed as a tasteless food additive to prevent foodborne illness.

## Promote Heart Health

When Cilantro (Coriander) seeds were added to the diet of diabetic laboratory animals, it helped stimulate their secretion of insulin and lowered their blood sugar. In other research, Coriander seeds were found to reduce the amount of damaged fats (lipid peroxides) in animals' cell membranes and to lower levels of total cholesterol and LDL ("bad") cholesterol, while actually increasing levels of HDL ("good") cholesterol.

## Nutritional Analysis of 2 tablespoons of fresh Cilantro:

| NUTRIENT | AMOUNT | % DAILY VALUE | NUTRIENT | AMOUNT | % DAILY VALUE |
|---|---|---|---|---|---|
| Calories | 0.46 | | Pantothenic Acid | 0.01 mg | 0.10 |
| Calories from Fat | 0.09 | | | | |
| Calories from Saturated Fat | 0.00 | | **Minerals** | | |
| Protein | 0.04 g | | Boron | — mcg | |
| Carbohydrates | 0.07 g | | Calcium | 1.34 mg | 0.13 |
| Dietary Fiber | 0.06 g | 0.24 | Chloride | — mg | |
| Soluble Fiber | — g | | Chromium | — mcg | — |
| Insoluble Fiber | — g | | Copper | 0.00 mg | 0.00 |
| Sugar – Total | 0.02 g | | Fluoride | — mg | |
| Monosaccharides | — g | | Iodine | — mcg | — |
| Disaccharides | — g | | Iron | 0.04 mg | 0.22 |
| Other Carbs | 0.00 g | | Magnesium | 0.52 mg | 0.13 |
| Fat – Total | 0.01 g | | Manganese | 0.01 mg | 0.50 |
| Saturated Fat | 0.00 g | | Molybdenum | — mcg | — |
| Mono Fat | 0.01 g | | Phosphorus | 0.96 mg | 0.10 |
| Poly Fat | 0.00 g | | Potassium | 10.42 mg | |
| Omega-3 Fatty Acids | 0.00 g | 0.00 | Selenium | 0.02 mcg | 0.03 |
| Omega-6 Fatty Acids | 0.00 g | | Sodium | 0.92 mg | |
| Trans Fatty Acids | 0.00 g | | Zinc | 0.01 mg | 0.07 |
| Cholesterol | 0.00 mg | | | | |
| Water | 1.84 g | | **Amino Acids** | | |
| Ash | 0.03 g | | Alanine | — g | |
| | | | Arginine | — g | |
| **Vitamins** | | | Aspartate | — g | |
| Vitamin A IU | 134.96 IU | 2.70 | Cystine | — g | — |
| Vitamin A RE | 13.48 RE | | Glutamate | — g | |
| A - Carotenoid | 13.48 RE | 0.18 | Glycine | — g | |
| A - Retinol | 0.00 RE | | Histidine | — g | — |
| B1 Thiamin | 0.00 mg | 0.00 | Isoleucine | — g | — |
| B2 Riboflavin | 0.00 mg | 0.00 | Leucine | — g | — |
| B3 Niacin | 0.02 mg | 0.10 | Lysine | — g | — |
| Niacin Equiv | 0.02 mg | | Methionine | — g | — |
| Vitamin B6 | 0.00 mg | 0.00 | Phenylalanine | — g | — |
| Vitamin B12 | 0.00 mcg | 0.00 | Proline | — g | |
| Biotin | — mcg | — | Serine | — g | |
| Vitamin C | 0.54 mg | 0.90 | Threonine | — g | — |
| Vitamin D IU | — IU | — | Tryptophan | — g | — |
| Vitamin D mcg | — mcg | | Tyrosine | — g | — |
| Vitamin E Alpha Equiv | 0.05 mg | 0.25 | Valine | — g | — |
| Vitamin E IU | 0.07 IU | | | | |
| Vitamin E mg | 0.05 mg | | | | |
| Folate | 1.24 mcg | 0.31 | | | |
| Vitamin K | 6.20 mcg | 7.75 | | | |

(Note: "—" indicates data is unavailable. For more information, please see page 806.)

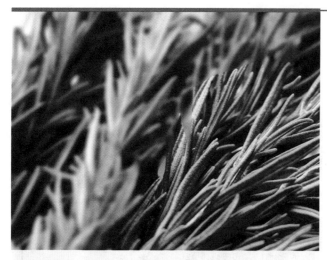

# rosemary

AVAILABILITY: Year-round
REFRIGERATE: Yes
SHELF LIFE: 5 days
PREPARATION: Minimal

## nutrient-richness chart

Total Nutrient-Richness:     3
Two teaspoons (2 grams) of dried Rosemary contain 7 calories

| NUTRIENT | AMOUNT | %DV | DENSITY | QUALITY |
|---|---|---|---|---|
| Dietary Fiber | 0.9 g | 3.7 | 9.1 | good |
| Iron | 0.6 mg | 3.6 | 8.8 | good |
| Calcium | 28.2 mg | 2.8 | 7.0 | good |

For more on "Total Nutrient-Richness," "%DV," "Density," and
The World's Healthiest Foods "Quality" Rating System, see page 805.

Part of Rosemary's popularity has come from the widespread belief that Rosemary stimulates and strengthens the memory, a quality for which it is still used today. In ancient Greece, students would place Rosemary sprigs in their hair when studying for exams. In England, Rosemary's ability to fortify the memory transformed it into a symbol of fidelity, and it played an important role in the costumes, decorations and gifts used at weddings. Rosemary's unique pine-like fragrant flavor balanced by a rich pungency is truly unforgettable. It grows on a small evergreen shrub and is related to mint. Its leaves look like flat pine-tree needles, deep green in color on top and silver-white on their underside. Rosemary is an especially great addition to chicken and lamb dishes.

## why rosemary should be part of your healthiest way of eating

Rosemary is a concentrated source of phytonutrients such as the flavonoids carnosol, rosmanol and rosmarinic acid that are powerful free radical scavengers. Rosemary has also been historically used for stimulating memory and increasing alertness. Rosemary is an ideal addition to your "Healthiest Way of Eating" not only because it is nutritious, but also because it is low in calories: 2 teaspoons of dried Rosemary contain only 7 calories.

## 1. the best way to select rosemary

Fresh Rosemary is a hearty herb. For the most nutritious and best tasting Rosemary, select sprigs of fresh Rosemary that look vibrantly fresh and deep sage green in color. Avoid Rosemary with dark spots or yellow coloration.

I recommend purchasing organically grown fresh or dried Rosemary whenever possible. (For more on *Organic Foods*, see page 113.)

## 2. the best way to store rosemary

**FRESH ROSEMARY:** To preserve freshness and the greatest number of nutrients, fresh Rosemary should be stored in the refrigerator either in its original packaging or wrapped in a slightly damp paper towel. It will keep for 5 days.

You can freeze either whole or chopped Rosemary by placing it in an airtight container. Alternatively, you can place chopped Rosemary in ice cube trays covered with water or stock and freeze; use the entire frozen cube in soups or stews.

**DRIED ROSEMARY:** Should be kept in a tightly sealed glass container in a cool, dark, dry place where it will keep fresh for about six months.

## 3. the best way to prepare rosemary

To retain nutrients, it is best to wash fresh Rosemary under cold running water and pat dry with a paper towel. Do not soak Rosemary or the water-soluble nutrients will leach into the water.

It is best to pull the leaves off of the stem as the stems are very woody. Chop Rosemary before adding it to recipes.

# 4. the healthiest way of cooking with rosemary

Both fresh and dried Rosemary have an aromatic scent.

**FRESH ROSEMARY:** To retain the maximum number of nutrients and flavor, it is best to add fresh Rosemary to your dish halfway through the cooking time.

**DRIED ROSEMARY:** If you are using dried Rosemary, it is best to add it at the beginning of the cooking time, so it will have a chance to warm up and cook long enough to bring out its flavor. Before using, rub dried Rosemary between your fingers to release its essential oils.

To substitute dried Rosemary for fresh, use about one-third the amount of dried Rosemary as you would fresh. For example, substitute 1 TBS of fresh Rosemary with 1 tsp of dried.

## TIPS: 3 Ways to Enjoy Rosemary

1. Add fresh Rosemary to omelets and frittatas.
2. Rosemary is a wonderful herb for seasoning chicken and lamb dishes.
3. Add Rosemary to tomato sauces and soups.

# health benefits of rosemary

## Provides Powerful Antioxidant and Anti-Inflammatory Protection

Rosemary contains a wealth of antioxidant phytonutrients, including flavonoids and the phenolic compounds carnosol, rosmanol and rosmarinic acid. Rosemary extract has shown the capacity to scavenge the peroxynitrite radical, one of the molecules responsible for causing lipid peroxidation, cell death and aging. Rosmarinic acid has been found to modulate the production of inflammatory molecules, promoting a reduced inflammatory state.

## Promotes Enhanced Memory

Rosemary's traditional use of stimulating and strengthening the memory is now being supported by research studies that have found that inhalation of its volatile oils, those that give it its memorable fragrance, help to enhance recall and increase alertness.

## Promotes Enhanced Detoxification

Rosemary and its phytonutrients have been found to enhance the action of liver enzymes responsible for metabolizing and detoxifying chemicals.

## Additional Health-Promoting Benefits of Rosemary

Rosemary is also a concentrated source of traditional nutrients such as bone-building calcium, heart-healthy dietary fiber and energy-producing iron.

### Nutritional Analysis of 2 teaspoons of dried Rosemary:

| NUTRIENT | AMOUNT | % DAILY VALUE | NUTRIENT | AMOUNT | % DAILY VALUE |
|---|---|---|---|---|---|
| Calories | 7.28 | | Pantothenic Acid | — mg | — |
| Calories from Fat | 3.00 | | | | |
| Calories from Saturated Fat | 1.44 | | **Minerals** | | |
| Protein | 0.12 g | | Boron | — mcg | |
| Carbohydrates | 1.40 g | | Calcium | 28.16 mg | 2.82 |
| Dietary Fiber | 0.92 g | 3.68 | Chloride | — mg | |
| Soluble Fiber | — g | | Chromium | — mcg | — |
| Insoluble Fiber | — g | | Copper | 0.00 mg | 0.00 |
| Sugar – Total | — g | | Fluoride | — mg | — |
| Monosaccharides | — g | | Iodine | — mcg | — |
| Disaccharides | — g | | Iron | 0.64 mg | 3.56 |
| Other Carbs | — g | | Magnesium | 4.84 mg | 1.21 |
| Fat – Total | 0.32 g | | Manganese | 0.04 mg | 2.00 |
| Saturated Fat | 0.16 g | | Molybdenum | — mcg | — |
| Mono Fat | 0.08 g | | Phosphorus | 1.56 mg | 0.16 |
| Poly Fat | 0.04 g | | Potassium | 21.00 mg | |
| Omega-3 Fatty Acids | 0.04 g | 1.60 | Selenium | 0.12 mcg | 0.17 |
| Omega-6 Fatty Acids | 0.04 g | | Sodium | 1.08 mg | |
| Trans Fatty Acids | 0.00 g | | Zinc | 0.08 mg | 0.53 |
| Cholesterol | 0.00 mg | | | | |
| Water | 0.20 g | | **Amino Acids** | | |
| Ash | 0.16 g | | Alanine | — g | |
| | | | Arginine | — g | |
| **Vitamins** | | | Aspartate | — g | |
| Vitamin A IU | 68.80 IU | 1.38 | Cystine | — g | — |
| Vitamin A RE | 6.88 RE | | Glutamate | — g | |
| A - Carotenoid | 6.88 RE | 0.09 | Glycine | — g | |
| A - Retinol | 0.00 RE | | Histidine | — g | — |
| B1 Thiamin | 0.00 mg | 0.00 | Isoleucine | — g | — |
| B2 Riboflavin | 0.00 mg | 0.00 | Leucine | — g | — |
| B3 Niacin | 0.04 mg | 0.20 | Lysine | — g | — |
| Niacin Equiv | 0.04 mg | | Methionine | — g | — |
| Vitamin B6 | 0.04 mg | 2.00 | Phenylalanine | — g | — |
| Vitamin B12 | 0.00 mcg | 0.00 | Proline | — g | |
| Biotin | — mcg | — | Serine | — g | |
| Vitamin C | 1.36 mg | 2.27 | Threonine | — g | — |
| Vitamin D IU | 0.00 IU | 0.00 | Tryptophan | — g | — |
| Vitamin D mcg | 0.00 mcg | | Tyrosine | — g | — |
| Vitamin E Alpha Equiv | 0.04 mg | 0.20 | Valine | — g | — |
| Vitamin E IU | 0.08 IU | | | | |
| Vitamin E mg | 0.04 mg | | | | |
| Folate | 6.76 mcg | 1.69 | | | |
| Vitamin K | — mcg | — | | | |

(Note: "—" indicates data is unavailable. For more information, please see page 806.)

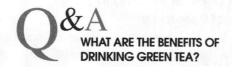

# Q&A

**WHAT ARE THE BENEFITS OF DRINKING GREEN TEA?**

Green tea has always been, and remains today, the most popular type of tea from China, where most historians and botanists believe the tea plant originated. Why is it so popular? Perhaps because green tea not only captures the taste, aroma and color of spring, but delivers this delightful bouquet along with a high concentration of beneficial phytonutrients.

Green tea is particularly rich in health-promoting flavonoids (which account for 30% of the dry weight of a leaf), including catechins and their derivatives. The most abundant catechin in green tea is epigallocatechin-3-gallate (EGCG), which is thought to play a pivotal role in green tea's anticancer and antioxidant effects. Catechins have been found to be more potent free radical scavengers than the well-known antioxidants vitamins E and C.

Most of the research showing the health benefits of green tea is based on the amount of green tea typically consumed in Asian countries—about three cups per day (which would provide 240–320 mg of polyphenols). Just one cup of green tea supplies 20–35 mg of EGCG, which has the highest antioxidant activity of all the green tea catechins.

## Health Benefits

The health benefits of green tea have been extensively researched. Green tea drinkers appear to have lower risk for a wide range of diseases, from simple bacterial or viral infections to chronic degenerative conditions including cardiovascular disease, cancer, stroke, osteoporosis and periodontal disease. The latest studies provide a deeper understanding of the ways in which green tea promotes some areas of health, including:

### PROTECTS AGAINST CORONARY ARTERY DISEASE

In Japanese studies, green tea consumption has been found to be an independent predictor for risk of coronary artery disease. In one study, those drinking five or more cups of green tea each day were found to be 16% less likely to suffer from coronary artery disease.

An elevation in the amount of free radicals in the arteries is a key event in many forms of cardiovascular disease. The latest research shows that green tea catechins inhibit the enzymes involved in the production of free radicals in the endothelial lining of the arteries. The arterial endothelium is a one-cell thick lining that serves as the interface between the bloodstream and the wall of the artery where plaques can form. By protecting the endothelium from free-radical-scavenging, green tea catechins help prevent the development of cardiovascular disease.

### PROTECTS AGAINST CANCER

In the last 10 years, green tea's cancer-preventive effects have been widely supported by epidemiological, cell culture, animal and clinical studies. For cancer prevention, the evidence is so promising that the Chemoprevention Branch of the National Cancer Institute has initiated a plan for developing tea compounds as cancer-chemopreventive agents in human trials.

### IMPROVES INSULIN SENSITIVITY IN TYPE 2 DIABETES

Population studies suggest that green tea consumption may help prevent type 2 diabetes. A number of animal studies are beginning to explain why. New studies suggest that green tea may improve glucose tolerance and insulin sensitivity in individuals with diabetes. In one study, after receiving green tea for 12 weeks, diabetic laboratory animals had lower fasting blood levels of glucose, insulin, triglycerides and free fatty acids compared to controls, and the ability of their adipocytes (fat cells) to respond to insulin and absorb blood sugar greatly increased.

### PREVENTS OSTEOPOROSIS AND PERIODONTAL DISEASES

Excessive bone loss is a characteristic feature not only of osteoporosis but also of periodontal disease. Green tea supports healthy bones and teeth both by protecting osteoblasts (the cells responsible for building bone) from destruction by free radicals and by inhibiting the formation of osteoclasts (the cells that break down bone).

## How to Select and Store Green Tea

Whenever possible, ask for a sample of tea before buying. Most high-quality teas will produce a pale green to yellow-green cup. To test loose tea for freshness, tightly squeeze a small amount and smell the aroma. The freshest, most flavorful tea will smell sweet and grassy. To test tea bags for freshness, remove the tea from one bag, place the empty bag in a cup, pour hot water over it and let it steep for two to three minutes. If the result tastes like plain hot water, the tea itself is likely fresh. If the tea bag water tastes like tea, the tea is old, and the paper has absorbed its flavor.

Since a single ounce of tea should produce 15 to 30 cups, the best way to ensure your tea is fresh is to purchase it in small amounts—two to four ounces at most. To retain freshness and flavor in both loose and bagged tea, store it in a tightly constructed opaque container to protect it from light, moisture and food odors.

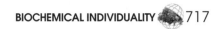

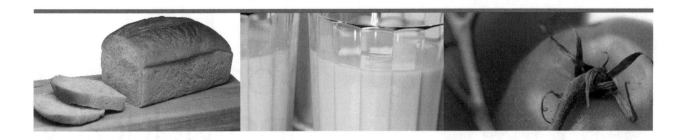

# PART 6

# biochemical individuality

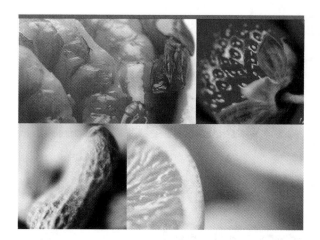

# biochemical individuality

## Everybody is Different

Have you ever noticed that there are some people who can eat just about anything and still feel great, while others may feel that their energy and vitality have just been zapped, even after eating foods that are generally considered "healthy"? For example, while I include low-fat dairy products in the list of the World's Healthiest Foods, certain people who are lactose-intolerant need to avoid consuming these foods, while others feel great after eating them and greatly benefit from these calcium-rich foods. The reason that individuals react differently to foods and their components is because of their biochemical individuality.

While two siblings with the same parents can eat the same meals together, one may stay slim, while the other may gain weight. Even though they are eating the same foods prepared at the same time, they may have different metabolisms; while they may consume the same number of calories, their bodies don't burn them at the same rate. The one whose body uses all the calories consumed stays slim, while the one whose body doesn't use them all stores the extra calories as fat. Sometimes it seems that when it comes to food, one person's "treasure" may be another's "poison" since a food may be health promoting for one person yet depleting for another. This is because genetic and biochemical differences among individuals result in different reactions to specific foods.

One of the central tenets of the George Mateljan Foundation is to eat nutrient-rich whole foods. I also recognize that the particular foods that may be of greatest benefit to different people may vary because every person is unique in his or her genetics and biochemical individuality. So, while I have created a list of 100 foods that I have deemed the World's Healthiest, I realize that each of these foods may not be equally beneficial for each individual.

Genetic individuality also determines the extent of the benefit that some foods can provide. For example, the extent of the benefits people derive by including flaxseeds in their "Healthiest Way of Eating" depends upon their genetic individuality. For some people, flaxseeds are a great source of a wide array of anti-inflammatory fatty acids. Yet, other people don't have the optimal enzyme activity to properly convert the seeds' alpha-linolenic acid (ALA) into eicosapentaenoic acid (EPA) and docosahexaenoic acid (DHA), the anti-inflammatory omega-3 fatty acids found in cold-water fish. While these people can still benefit from the many nutrients that flaxseeds have to offer, the amount of anti-inflammatory protection that they receive may be more limited. (For more on *Omega-3 Fatty Acids*, see page 770.)

The World's Healthiest Foods are a compendium of 100 nutrient-rich, health-promoting whole foods; yet those that may be of highest value to you may be different than those that best support another person. It is important to recognize your own biochemical individuality and honor your uniqueness when looking for the World's Healthiest Foods that are best for you. I have included information in the book that will help you determine which foods, if any, are not supportive of your health and help you design a healthy way of eating to better suit your individual needs.

## How to Use the Section on Biochemical Considerations

Each food chapter addresses the "Biochemical Considerations" of that particular food and includes information about whether the food is a significant source of oxalates, goitrogens, purines or other compounds that can cause challenges for individuals who have certain health concerns. Additionally, there are certain foods that are more likely to contain higher amounts of pesticide residues than others, while some foods more frequently cause allergic reactions than do others. If any of these potential concerns apply to a particular food, it is noted in that food's chapter.

This chapter explains the different "Biochemical Considerations" referenced in the food chapters. This information can be helpful in a few different ways. For example, if you know that you need to reduce your intake of goitrogenic foods owing to a thyroid condition, you will be able to see which foods have a significant amount of goitrogenic compounds. Or if you find that celery and strawberries make you feel fatigued after you eat them, and you do not regularly purchase the organically grown varieties of these foods, the information under "Pesticide Residues" will alert you to the fact that these foods are among those with the highest pesticide residues. You may then want to consider whether your body is reacting to the pesticide residues that remain on conventionally grown foods.

## Food Sensitivity

Biochemical Individuality helps us to understand why some individuals are sensitive to some foods, while others are not. It is possible to be sensitive to any food, and it is estimated that 60–70% of people are sensitive to one or more foods cited in the next column. People often believe that if they are not diagnosed as having a food allergy for a particular food then it is safe for them to eat that food; however, unlike food allergies, food sensitivities are not mediated by the immune system and cannot be detected through clinical analysis. Sensitivities to foods can involve many different physiological mechanisms, which is why the prevalence is higher than that cited for food allergies as discussed in the next section. For example, it is possible to have a sensitivity to milk and not be allergic to milk. As it turns out, even some of the World's Healthiest Foods can be problematic for some individuals. These include:

| BEEF | CHICKEN | CORN |
|---|---|---|
| COW'S MILK | EGGS | KIWIFRUIT |
| ORANGES | PEANUTS | SHELLFISH |
| SOYBEANS | SPINACH | STRAWBERRIES |
| TOMATOES | TREE NUTS | WHEAT |

Other foods not included among the World's Healthiest Foods most likely to cause adverse reactions include:

| ALCOHOL | CAFFEINE-CONTAINING BEVERAGES |
|---|---|
| CHOCOLATE | FERMENTED (HARD) CHEESE |
| PORK | SMOKED MEATS |
| SULFITES | VINEGAR |

Food sensitivities to food additives or preservatives have also been widely published; some of these potentially aggravating compounds include tartrazine (yellow dye #5), sulfites and the preservative BHT (butylated hydroxytoluene).

Any food has the potential of causing adverse reactions in specific individuals. The types of foods to which a person may have an adverse reaction can be as unique as each individual. Your unique biochemistry may be improved by eliminating some foods from your menu.

Clinical research is accumulating evidence that a food sensitivity can also increase the severity of the symptoms of several health conditions. These include rheumatoid arthritis, asthma and other diseases not normally considered food related.

One important tip: You need to avoid the food not only in its most obvious state (e.g., wheat in bread or pasta) but also when it is used as a component in prepared foods (e.g., wheat in soy sauce, soups, cereals and baked goods labeled as made from wheat). So, be sure to read labels and to order carefully when eating at restaurants.

One way to help determine the foods to which you may be sensitive to is to follow the Elimination Plan (page 821) with the guidance of a healthcare practitioner.

# food allergies ——————

Food allergies can elicit symptoms that range from mild (sneezing) to life-threatening (anaphylactic reaction) depending upon the individual. Researchers have estimated that over 3% of adults worldwide experience food allergies, with the prevalence even higher in children. As food allergies have compromising effects on health, it is important for individuals with known or suspected allergies to avoid foods to which they are sensitive.

## Food Allergies and Health

Food allergies are defined as toxic clinical reactions involving the immune system upon exposure to an "offending" substance found in a food. An allergic reaction to a food occurs when your body identifies molecules in that food as potentially harmful and toxic; these molecules are called antigens. Immune system cells bind to the antigens causing chemicals, such as histamine, to be released. These chemicals signal scavenger immune cells to come to the site of activity and destroy the antigens. An inflammatory process can result, which is the cause of many of the symptoms of food allergy reactions.

The most common symptoms for food allergies include eczema, hives, skin rash, headache, runny nose, itchy eyes, wheezing, diarrhea, vomiting and blood in stools. Symptoms can vary depending upon a number of variables including age, the type of allergen (antigen) and the amount of food consumed.

It may be difficult to associate the symptoms of an allergic reaction to a particular food because the response time can be highly variable. For example, an allergic response to eating seafood will usually occur within minutes after consumption in the form of a rash, hives or asthma, or a combination of these symptoms. However, the symptoms of an allergic reaction to cow's milk may be delayed for 24 to 48 hours after consuming the milk or milk-containing food; these symptoms may also be low-grade (feeling tired or a slight headache) and last for several days.

If this does not make diagnosis difficult enough, reactions to foods made from cow's milk may also vary depending on how it was produced and the portion of the milk to which you are allergic. (Casein is the protein portion of milk, which is responsible for most allergies to cow's milk.) Delayed allergic reactions to foods are difficult to identify without eliminating the food from your diet for at least several weeks, then slowly reintroducing it while taking note of any physical, emotional or mental changes that may occur.

It's also worth pointing out that some people have cravings for the foods to which they are most allergic. This also adds to the confusing aspect of identifying food allergies because the immune response to these foods produces histamines and cortisol, which may make you feel better while they are actually being detrimental to your health.

Although allergic reactions can occur to almost any food, research studies on food allergies have found that some foods are more closely associated with food allergies than others. The commonness of a food allergy appears to be country specific and is often related to foods most frequently eaten (for example, rice allergy in Japan).

## Foods That Can Cause Allergic Reactions

Although allergic reactions can occur to virtually any food, research studies on food allergy consistently report more problems with some foods than with others.

Foods most commonly associated with allergic reactions:

| MILK | WHEAT | SOY |
| SHELLFISH | EGGS | PEANUTS |
| FISH | TREE NUTS | |

Foods less commonly associated with allergic reactions:

| BEEF | CHICKEN | CORN |
| ORANGES | PORK | SPINACH |
| STRAWBERRIES | TOMATOES | |

## What To Do If You Suspect a Food Allergy

If you suspect food allergy to be an underlying factor in your health problems, you may want to avoid commonly allergenic foods. To do so, you may want to consider consulting a nutritionist or other healthcare practitioner well versed in nutrition who can assist you both in identifying the foods to which you may be allergic and in designing nutritious meal plans that avoid these foods. The Elimination Plan, on page 821, a wonderful tool for identifying foods that trigger adverse reactions, may be recommended.

# gluten intolerance —————

## Foods: Applies to Barley, Oats, Rye, Wheat

Certain grains, such as barley, oats, rye and wheat are often classified as members of a non-scientifically established grain group traditionally called the "gluten grains." The idea of grouping certain grains together under the label "gluten grains" has come into question in recent years as technology has given food scientists a way to look more

closely at the composition of grains. Some healthcare practitioners continue to group these grains together under the heading of "gluten grains" and to ask for elimination of the entire group on a wheat-free diet. Other practitioners now treat wheat separately from these other grains, based on recent research that does not support that these other grains elicit the same response as wheat, which is unquestionably a more common source of food allergies than any of the other "gluten grains." Although you may initially want to eliminate the non-wheat "gluten grains" from your meal planning if you are implementing a wheat-free diet, you may want to experiment at some point with reintroduction of these foods. You may be able to take advantage of their diverse nutritional benefits without experiencing an adverse reaction. Individuals with wheat-related conditions like celiac sprue or gluten-sensitive enteropathies should consult with their healthcare practitioner before experimenting with any of the "gluten grains."

# goitrogens

Some foods contain goitrogens, naturally occurring substances that can interfere with the function of the thyroid gland. Goitrogens get their name from the term "goiter," which means an enlargement of the thyroid gland. If the thyroid gland is having difficulty making thyroid hormones, it may enlarge as a way of trying to compensate for this inadequate hormone production. "Goitrogens" are compounds in foods that make it more difficult for the thyroid gland to create its hormones.

## Goitrogens and Health

In the absence of thyroid problems, no research evidence suggests that goitrogenic foods will negatively impact your health. In fact, the opposite is true: soy foods and cruciferous vegetables, two groups of foods that are known to contain goitrogens, have unique nutritional value and eating these foods has been associated with decreased risk of disease in many research studies.

Because carefully controlled research studies have yet to be done on the relationship between goitrogenic foods and thyroid hormone deficiency, healthcare practitioners differ greatly on their perspectives as to whether people who have thyroid problems, and notably a thyroid hormone deficiency, should limit their intake of goitrogenic foods. Most practitioners use words like "overconsumption" or "excessive" to describe the kind of goitrogen intake that would be a problem for individuals with thyroid hormone deficiency. Here the goal is not to eliminate goitrogenic foods from the meal plan, but to limit intake so that it falls within a reasonable range. A standard one cup serving of cruciferous vegetables two to three times per week and a standard four-ounce serving of tofu twice a week is likely to be tolerated by many individuals with thyroid hormone deficiency (although please get your doctor's perspective before undertaking this modification in an already suggested dietary plan).

## Food that Contain Goitrogens

Two general categories of foods have been associated with

disrupted thyroid hormone production in humans: soybean-related foods and cruciferous vegetables. In addition, a few other foods not included in these categories—such as peaches, strawberries and millet—also contain goitrogens. The following are some of the most well-known goitrogen-containing foods.

### SOYBEAN-RELATED FOODS

Included in the category of soybean-related foods are soybeans themselves, soy extracts and foods made from soy, including tofu and tempeh. While soy foods share many common ingredients, it is the isoflavones in soy that have been associated with decreased thyroid hormone output. Isoflavones are naturally occurring substances that belong to the flavonoid family of nutrients. Flavonoids, found in virtually all plants, are pigments that give plants their amazing array of colors. Most research studies in the health sciences have focused on the beneficial properties of flavonoids, and these naturally occurring phytonutrients have repeatedly been shown to be highly health supportive.

The link between isoflavones and decreased thyroid function is, in fact, one of the few areas in which flavonoid intake has been called into question as being problematic. Isoflavones like genistein appear to reduce thyroid hormone output by blocking activity of an enzyme called *thyroid peroxidase*, which is responsible for adding iodine to the thyroid hormones. (Thyroid hormones must have three or four iodine atoms added on to their structure in order to function properly.)

For individuals who need to limit their intake of goitrogenic foods, limiting the intake from soy foods is often much more problematic than with other foods since soy appears in so many combinations, and it is often a hidden ingredient in packaged food products. Ingredients like textured vegetable protein (TVP) and isolated soy concentrate may appear in foods that would rarely be expected to contain soy.

### CRUCIFEROUS VEGETABLES

A second category of foods associated with disrupted

thyroid hormone production is the cruciferous family of foods. Foods belonging to this family are called "crucifers" or *Brassica* vegetables and include broccoli, cauliflower, Brussels sprouts, cabbage, mustard, rutabagas, kohlrabi and turnips. Isothiocyanates are the category of substances in crucifers that have been associated with decreased thyroid function. Like the isoflavones, isothiocyanates appear to reduce thyroid function by blocking *thyroid peroxidase* and also by disrupting messages that are sent across the membranes of thyroid cells.

Goitrogen-containing foods include:

| | |
|---|---|
| BROCCOLI | KOHLRABI |
| BRUSSELS SPROUTS | MUSTARD |
| CABBAGE | RUTABAGA |
| CAULIFLOWER | TURNIPS |
| KALE | MILLET |
| PEACHES | PEANUTS |
| RADISHES | SPINACH |
| STRAWBERRIES | SOY PRODUCTS |

### The Effect of Cooking on Goitrogens

Although research studies are limited in this area, cooking may help inactivate the goitrogenic compounds found in food. Both isoflavones (found in soy foods) and isothiocyanates (found in cruciferous vegetables) seem to be heat sensitive, and cooking appears to lower the availability of these substances. In the case of isothiocyanates in cruciferous vegetables like broccoli, as much as one-third of this goitrogenic substance may be deactivated when broccoli is boiled in water. Unfortunately, boiling also depletes broccoli of such a high percentage of its other health-promoting nutrients that I cannot recommend this cooking method. Those with thyroid problems who have been advised by their healthcare practitioner to limit excessive consumption of goitrogen-containing foods should simply take care to consume no more than a one cup serving of crucifers two to three times per week. (Please check that your healthcare practitioner does not want you to limit it any further.)

# lactose intolerance

## Foods: APPLIES TO COW'S MILK, GOAT'S MILK, CHEESE, YOGURT

Lactose, or milk sugar, forms about 4.7% of the solids in cow's milk and 4.1% in goat's milk. Many individuals lack the enzyme, *lactase*, which is needed to digest lactose. For this reason, food intolerances to milk and dairy products are among the most common food intolerances seen by healthcare practitioners. Some individuals with lactose intolerance can better tolerate hard cheese and yogurt than other forms of dairy products.

The bacteria used to produce cheese and the time required for the cheese to ferment both work to lower lactose levels. Therefore, hard cheese may have much reduced lactose levels compared to milk (0–3 grams per ounce compared to 10–12 grams per cup of cow's milk). Because time is a factor in the reduction of lactose, as a hard cheese is aged, the lactose content will decrease towards the zero end of its range. Therefore, many individuals with lactose intolerance may be able to eat moderate amounts of hard, aged cheese without a problem. This does not apply to soft cheese, which may be identical to cow's milk in terms of lactose content, containing from 6–12 grams per ounce.

Some individuals with lactose intolerance may be able to also enjoy yogurt, as long as it is good quality yogurt made with active cultures. That is because these active cultures of beneficial bacteria predigest some of the lactose during the yogurt making process, and can also help digest it once inside your body. As noted above, this benefit only applies to yogurt with live active cultures as cultures that have been killed during the production process will not deliver the same benefit.

# latex food allergies

Between 30–50% of individuals who have allergies to latex may also have allergic reactions to certain plant foods. These allergic reactions may be either immediate or delayed hypersensitivity reactions, with symptoms ranging from hives to asthma to anaphylaxis.

Currently, the most conclusive evidence suggests that foods that cross-react with latex are those that contain enzymes called *chitinases*, which have similar protein structures to those found in latex. These include such foods as avocados, bananas and chestnuts. Researchers are also currently investigating other classes of compounds that may cross-react with latex, including patatin found in potatoes; however, this research is not yet as conclusive as that involving the *chitinase*-containing foods.

Latex food allergies have been found to be more prevalent in healthcare workers and those who have undergone medical procedures as these individuals have a greater exposure to medical supplies made of latex, including latex gloves.

### The Effect of Cooking

Usually, it is best for individuals with latex allergy to avoid eating potentially problematic foods; however, some evidence suggests that cooked forms of the foods may be acceptable. Preliminary research has shown that cooking can deactivate the enzymes that may be responsible for the cross-reaction with latex. Consult your healthcare practitioner for more guidance on this topic.

| DEGREE OF ASSOCIATION OR PREVALENCE | | | |
|---|---|---|---|
| HIGH | MEDIUM | LOW OR UNDETERMINED | |
| Avocado | Apple | Apricot | Peanut |
| Banana | Carrot | Cherry | Pear |
| Chestnut | Celery | Fig | Pineapple |
| | Kiwifruit | Grape | Plum |
| | Melons | Grasses | Ragweed |
| | Papaya | Hazelnut | Rye |
| | Potato | Mango | Soybean |
| | Tomato | Mugwort | Strawberry |
| | | Nectarine | Walnuts |
| | | Passion fruit | Wheat |
| | | Peach | |

### Foods Associated with Latex Food Allergies

According to the American Latex Allergy Association, the foods in the chart above have been found to have an association with latex food allergies.

# nightshades

Nightshades are a diverse group of foods, herbs, shrubs and trees belonging to the scientific order called *Polemoniales* and to the scientific family called *Solanaceae*. While this botanical family is very diverse, containing such plants as tobacco, mandrake and belladonna, it also contains commonly consumed vegetables such as the potato, pepper, tomato and eggplant.

### Nightshades and Health

Most of the health research on nightshades has focused on a special group of substances found in all nightshades called alkaloids. There are four basic types of alkaloids found in nightshade plants, but steroid alkaloids are those most commonly found in the nightshade plants that are consumed as food.

While nightshades may be of more concern to individuals with nerve-related or inflammatory health conditions, some healthcare practitioners recommend that individuals who don't have existing problems related to nightshade intake may want to still take precautions to avoid excessive intake of alkaloids from these foods.

### Effect of Steroid Alkaloids on the Nervous System

The steroid alkaloids in nightshade foods—primarily solanine and chaonine—have been studied for their ability to block activity of an enzyme in nerve cells called *cholinesterase*. If the activity of *cholinesterase* is too strongly blocked, the nervous system control of muscle movement becomes disrupted, and muscle twitching, trembling, paralyzed breathing or convulsions can result. The steroid alkaloids found in potato have clearly been shown to block *cholinesterase* activity, but this block does not usually appear strong enough to produce nerve-muscle disruptions like twitching or trembling.

### Effect of Steroid Alkaloids on Joint Health

It has also been suggested that nightshade alkaloids may alter mineral status and cause inflammation that can damage joints, but whether alkaloids can contribute to joint damage of this kind is not clear from current levels of research. Some researchers have speculated that nightshade alkaloids can contribute to excessive loss of calcium from bone and excessive deposition of calcium in soft tissue. For this reason, these researchers have recommended elimination of nightshade foods from the meal plans of all individuals with osteoarthritis, rheumatoid arthritis or other joint problems like gout. Other practitioners recommend that individuals with these inflammatory conditions eliminate nightshade foods from their meal plan for two to three weeks to determine whether these foods are contributing to joint problems (the same applies to individuals with existing nerve-muscle related problems).

## Effect of Nicotine Alkaloid on Health

Nicotine is another alkaloid compound found in nightshade plants. Although they contain dramatically less nicotine than tobacco, nightshade plants that we consume as foods do contain some nicotine; however, the levels of nicotine in all nightshade foods are so low that most healthcare practitioners have simply ignored its presence in these foods as a potential compromising factor in our health. I both agree and disagree with this conclusion. While the amount of nicotine in nightshade foods is very small, it still seems possible that some individuals might be particularly sensitive to the nicotine found in nightshades, and that even very small amounts might compromise function in the bodies of these individuals.

## Foods that Contain Nightshade Alkaloids

The most famous food members of the nightshade family include potatoes (*Solanum tuberosum*), tomatoes (*Lycopersicon lycopersicum*), many species of sweet and hot peppers (all species of *Capsicum*, including *Capsicum annum*) and eggplant (*Solanum melongena*). Less well-known, but equally genuine nightshade foods include ground cherries (all species of *Physalis*), tomatillos (*Physallis ixocapra*), garden huckleberry (*Solanum melanocerasum*), tamarillos (*Cyphomandra betacea*), pepinos (*Solanum muricatum*) and naranjillas (*Solanum quitoense*). Pimentos (also called pimientos) belong to the nightshade family and usually come from the pepper plant, *Capsicum annum*. Pimento cheese and pimento-stuffed olives are therefore examples of foods that should be classified as containing nightshade components. Although the sweet potato, whose scientific name is *Ipomoea batatas*, belongs to the same plant order as the nightshades (*Polemoniales*), it does not belong to the *Solanaceae* family found in this order; it belongs to a different plant family called *Convolvulaceae* and thus does not carry the same concerns.

The seasoning paprika is also derived from *Capsicum annum*, the common red pepper, and the seasoning cayenne comes from another nightshade, *Capsicum frutenscens*. Tabasco sauce, which contains large amounts of *Capsicum annum*, should also be considered as a nightshade food. It may be helpful to note here that black pepper, which belongs to the *Piperaceae* family, is not a member of the nightshade foods.

The following chart reflects the solanine alkaloid content of three of the most commonly consumed nightshade foods: peppers, eggplants and potatoes.

| VEGETABLE | SOLANINE CONTENT |
|---|---|
| | MILLIGRAMS PER 100 GRAM SERVING |
| Common peppers | 7.7–9.2 |
| Eggplant | 6.1–11.33 |
| Potatoes | 2–13 |
| Tomatoes | nv* |
| * NO QUANTIFIED DATA IS CURRENTLY AVAILABLE | |

## The Effect of Cooking and Preparation on Nightshade Alkaloids

Steaming, boiling and baking all help reduce the alkaloid content of nightshades. Alkaloids are only reduced, however, by about 40–50% from cooking. For non-sensitive individuals, the cooking of nightshade foods will often be sufficient to make the alkaloid risk from nightshade intake insignificant. However, for sensitive individuals, the remaining alkaloid concentration may still be enough to cause problems.

## Increased Alkaloid Content of Green and Sprouting Potatoes

Green spots on potatoes or sprouting on potatoes usually corresponds to increased alkaloid content; this increased alkaloid content is one of the main reasons for avoiding consumption of green or sprouted potatoes. Thoroughly cut out all green areas, especially green areas on the peel, before cooking potatoes. If you know you are sensitive to nightshades, it's best to discard the whole potato. A bitter taste in potatoes after they have been cooked is usually a good indication that excessive amounts of alkaloids are present.

# oxalates

Oxalates (oxalic acid) are naturally occurring substances found in plants, animals and humans. In nutritional terms, oxalates belong to a group of molecules called organic acids and are routinely made by plants, animals and humans. Our bodies always contain oxalates, and our cells routinely convert other substances into oxalates. For example, vitamin C is one of the substances that our cells routinely convert into oxalates. In addition to the oxalates our bodies make, oxalates can come into the body from the outside, from certain foods that contain them.

## Oxalates and Health

### CONDITIONS THAT REQUIRE STRICT OXALATE RESTRICTION

A few, relatively rare health conditions require strict oxalate restriction. These conditions include absorptive hypercalciuria type II, enteric hyperoxaluria and primary hyperoxaluria. Dietary oxalates are usually restricted to 50 milligrams per day in individuals with these conditions. These relatively rare health conditions are different than a more common condition called nephrolithiasis in which susceptibility to kidney stone formation is increased.

### OXALATES AND KIDNEY STONES (NEPHROLITHIASIS)

The formation of kidney stones containing oxalate is an area of controversy in clinical nutrition with respect to dietary restriction of oxalate. About 80% of kidney stones formed by adults in the U.S. are calcium oxalate stones. It is not clear from the research, however, that restriction of dietary oxalate helps prevent formation of calcium oxalate stones in individuals who have previously formed such stones. Since intake of dietary oxalate accounts for only 10–15% of the oxalate found in the urine of individuals who form calcium oxalate stones, many researchers believe that dietary restriction cannot significantly reduce risk of stone formation.

In addition to the above observation, recent research studies have shown that intake of protein, calcium and water influence calcium oxalate stone formation as much as, or more than, intake of oxalate. Finally, some foods that have traditionally been assumed to increase stone formation because of their oxalate content (like black tea) actually appear in more recent research to have a preventive effect. For all of the above reasons, when healthcare providers recommend restriction of dietary oxalates to prevent calcium oxalate stone formation in individuals who have previously formed stones, they often suggest "limiting" or "reducing" oxalate intake rather than setting a specific milligram amount that

should not be exceeded. "Reduce as much as can be tolerated" is another way that recommendations are often stated.

### OXALATES AND CALCIUM ABSORPTION

While the ability of oxalates to lower calcium absorption exists, it is actually relatively small and definitely does not outweigh the ability of oxalate-containing foods to contribute calcium to the meal plan. If your digestive tract is healthy, and you do a good job chewing and relaxing while you enjoy your meals, you will still get significant benefits—including absorption of calcium—from calcium-rich plant foods like soybeans and dark green leafy vegetables that also contain oxalic acid. Ordinarily, a healthcare practitioner would not discourage a person from eating these nutrient-rich foods because of their oxalate content.

### FOODS THAT CONTAIN OXALATES

For a detailed list of foods that contain concentrated levels

## World's Healthiest Foods Oxalate Values

| | MG OXALATE/ 100 GRAMS | | MG OXALATE/ 100 GRAMS |
|---|---|---|---|
| Spinach, boiled | 750.0** | Asparagus | 5.2* |
| Beet root, boiled | 675.0** | Currants, black | 4.3 |
| Chard, Swiss | 645.0** | Lima beans | 4.3 |
| Pepper | 419.0** | Carrots, canned | 4.0 |
| Wheat germ | 269.0** | Orange, raw | 4.0 |
| Peanuts, roasted | 187.0** | Apples, raw | 3.0 |
| Lime peel | 110.0** | Lettuce | 3.0 |
| Parsley | 100.0** | Onion, boiled | 3.0 |
| Leek | 89.0** | Pears | 3.0 |
| Lemon peel | 83.0** | Apricots | 2.8 |
| Collards | 74.0** | Mushrooms | 2.0 |
| Sweet potato | 56.0** | Tomato | 2.0 |
| Grapes, concord | 25.0* | Pears, Bartlett | 1.7 |
| Squash, summer | 22.0* | Plums, Golden Gage | 1.1 |
| Celery | 20.0* | Cauliflower, boiled | 1.0 |
| Currants, red | 19.0* | Cucumbers | 1.0 |
| Eggplant | 18.0* | Lemon juice | 1.0 |
| Pepper, green | 16.0* | Oatmeal | 1.0 |
| Berries, blueberries | 15.0* | Peas, canned | 1.0 |
| Berries, raspberries | 15.0* | Pineapple, canned | 1.0 |
| Green/snap beans | 15.0* | Milk | 0.15 |
| Kale | 13.0* | Banana, raw | trace |
| Berries, strawberries | 10.0* | Broccoli, boiled | trace |
| Plums, Damson | 10.0* | Lamb, roast | trace |
| Mustard greens | 7.7* | | |
| Liver | 7.1* | *Notably high level of oxalate | |
| Cranberry juice | 5.8* | **Very high level of oxalate | |
| Prunes, Italian | 5.8* | Source: LithoLink Corporation | |
| Corn, yellow | 5.2* | (www.litholink.com) | |

of oxalates, please see "Worlds Healthiest Foods Oxalate Values" chart on the previous page.

### THE EFFECT OF COOKING ON OXALATES

Cooking has a relatively small impact on the oxalate content of foods. Cooking has been shown to have negligible effects on oxalates when they are contained in the root or stalk of the plant. When oxalates are contained in the leaves, cooking has been shown to reduce their concentration, but not dramatically. A lowering of oxalate content by about 5–15% is the most you should expect when cooking a high-oxalate food. It does not make sense to me to overcook oxalate-containing foods in order to reduce their oxalate content. Because many vitamins and minerals are lost from overcooking more quickly than are oxalates, the overcooking of foods (particularly vegetables) will simply result in a far less nutritious diet that is minimally lower in oxalates.

# pesticide residues

For certain foods, it's important to buy organic whenever possible. These foods are those fruits and vegetables whose conventionally grown "alternatives" have been found to contain high levels of pesticide residues.

In the mid-1990s, the Environmental Working Group developed the "Dirty Dozen," a list of high-risk, pesticide-containing foods. In 2006, they updated this list. I suggest that if you must prioritize your purchasing of organic produce, you focus on avoiding those that are included in the "Dirty Dozen."

## The Dirty Dozen

The reason we want to reduce our exposure to pesticides is because many of these agricultural chemicals are known toxins. In fact, the U.S. Environmental Protection Agency has classified 73 pesticides authorized for agricultural use as potential carcinogens (cancer-causing agents). And while other pesticides that have not received classification as "toxin" are deemed "safe," the true nature of their impact may not really be known.

### THE "DIRTY DOZEN"

| VEGETABLES | FRUITS |
|---|---|
| Bell Peppers | Peaches |
| Celery | Apples |
| Spinach | Nectarines |
| Lettuce | Strawberries |
| Potatoes | Cherries |
| | Pears |
| | Grapes (imported) |

That is because many of the safety tests done focus on the effect of high doses of single pesticides rather than looking at more chronic low-dose impact, notably during times of development when an individual is more sensitive. Additionally, the effect of exposure to multiple chemical sources and the subsequent contamination that people experience (many of these chemicals are fat-soluble and therefore are stored in fatty deposits in the body) has not been studied as it is nearly impossible to assign specific health effects to one rather than another rather than the complex interplay of the chemicals.

Yet, independent research has been conducted focusing on exposure during fetal development and childhood, which has shown that pesticides can have life-long detrimental effects upon physical functioning. For more information about why organic foods, which are grown without pesticides and other agricultural chemicals, are better for health, please see page 171.

In their report (www.foodnews.org), the Environmental Working Group also identified the 12 fruits and vegetables least likely to have concentrated pesticide residues. If you are unable to purchase all organically grown produce, these are the conventionally grown varieties you can purchase with the least amount of concern.

### LEAST LIKELY TO CONTAIN PESTICIDE RESIDUES

| VEGETABLES | FRUITS |
|---|---|
| Onions | Pineapple |
| Avocados | Mangoes |
| Corn (sweet) | Kiwifruit |
| Asparagus | Bananas |
| Peas (sweet) | Papaya |
| Cabbage | |
| Broccoli | |

# phytic acid

Phytic acid, also referred to as phytate, is a naturally-occurring substance found in grains and beans. While this compound has been found to have some unique health-promoting properties, it has also garnered attention because of its ability to reduce absorption of certain minerals.

## Phytic Acid and Mineral Absorption

Concerns around phytic acid come from its ability to bind to minerals and lower their absorption. Researchers have suggested that in areas of the world where the diet is highly focused on grains to the exclusion of other foods, phytic acid may be responsible for the prevalence of mineral deficiencies. Therefore, there may be some concern as to the extent which ingesting phytic acid in whole grains and soybeans can impact the absorption of important dietary minerals, such as calcium, magnesium, iron, zinc and chromium.

While phytic acid may reduce mineral absorption, the amount to which it can really have a negative impact, given a well balanced diet that does not exclusively focus on grains and beans, is questionable. For most people, healthcare practitioners would not advise that individuals reduce their intake of whole grains or beans because of their phytic acid content. In addition, phytic acid has numerous health benefits.

## Health-Promoting Functions of Phytic Acid

Phytic acid has some very beneficial properties. It is a well-known antioxidant, able to scavenge free radicals that may cause oxidative damage to the body's cells. Researchers are also investigating its ability to promote genetic health and enhance immunity, two other functions which, in addition to its antioxidant activity, may help to explain why laboratory studies have found phytic acid to inhibit the formation of tumors in the colon and other locations. Other proposed benefits for phytic acid include helping balance blood sugar levels, decreasing plasma cholesterol and triglycerides, and chelating heavy metals.

## Effect of Cooking on Phytic Acid

The processing and cooking of grains and soybeans lowers their phytic acid content, often by more than 50%. The sprouting of raw grains also lowers their phytic acid content.

Since acidic conditions can reduce the amount of phytate, sourdough whole grain breads have been found to have lower phytate content and less impact on mineral absorption than other types of bread.

# purines

Purines are natural substances found in all of the body's cells and in virtually all foods. The reason for their widespread occurrence is simple: purines provide part of the structure of our genes and the genes of plants and other animals. A relatively small number of foods, however, contain concentrated amounts of purines. For the most part, these high-purine foods are also high-protein foods.

## Purines and Health

When purines get broken down completely, they form uric acid. In our blood, uric acid serves as an antioxidant and helps prevent damage to our blood vessel linings, so a continual supply of uric acid is important for protecting our blood vessels.

However, uric acid levels in the blood and other parts of the body can become too high under a variety of circumstances. Since our kidneys are responsible for helping keep blood levels of uric acid balanced, kidney problems can lead to excessive accumulation of uric acid in various parts of the body. Excessive breakdown of cells can also cause uric acid build-up. When uric acid accumulates, uric acid crystals can become deposited in our tendons, joints, kidneys and other organs. This accumulation of uric acid crystals is called gouty arthritis, or simply "gout."

Low-purine diets are often used to help treat conditions like gout in which excessive uric acid is deposited in the tissues of the body. The average daily diet for an adult in the U.S. contains approximately 600–1,000 milligrams of purines. In a case of severe or advanced gout, dietitians will often ask individuals to decrease their total daily purine intake to 100–150 milligrams.

Although, for most individuals, purines in the diet are of little concern and may actually be beneficial because of the antioxidant activity of uric acid, in several other conditions, in addition to gout, purines may present a problem. These are rare conditions in which purine metabolism is disrupted, leading to problems such as anemia, failure to thrive, autism, cerebral palsy, deafness, epilepsy, susceptibility to recurrent infection and the inability to walk or talk.

## Foods that Contain Purines

### FOODS WITH VERY HIGH PURINE LEVELS:

A 3.5-ounce serving of some foods can contain up to 1,000 milligrams (mg) of purines. These foods include:

- Anchovies
- Herring
- Liver
- Mackerel
- Meat extracts
- Mussels
- Sardines
- Yeast

### FOODS WITH HIGH AND MODERATELY HIGH PURINE LEVELS:

A 3.5-ounce serving of the following foods can contain 50–100 milligrams (mg) of purines:

- Beef
- Cod
- Lamb
- Lentils
- Scallops
- Bouillon (made from meat or poultry)
- Shrimp
- Turkey
- Venison

### FOODS WITH MODERATELY HIGH PURINE LEVELS:

A 3.5-ounce serving of the following foods can contain 5–50 milligrams (mg) of purines:

- Asparagus
- Cauliflower
- Chicken
- Kidney beans
- Lima beans
- Mushrooms
- Navy beans
- Oatmeal
- Peas
- Salmon
- Spinach
- Tuna

Recent research has shown that the impact of plant purines on gout risk is very different from the impact of animal purines. This research has demonstrated that purines from meat and fish clearly increase our risk of gout, while purines from vegetables fail to change our risk. In summary, this epidemiological research (on tens of thousands of men and women) makes it clear that all purine-containing foods are not the same and that plant purines are far safer than meat and fish purines in terms of gout risk.

If you are not at risk for gout or other health problems related to purine metabolism, you would be unlikely to consume greater than the U.S. average for purine intake even if you ate more than ten servings of the foods in the last group. If you have been placed on a low purine diet that calls for no more than 150 milligrams of dietary purines, you may still be able to consume a 3.5 ounce serving of these foods per day without exceeding the 150 milligram limit for your overall diet.

## The Effect of Cooking on Purines

Research on cooking and purine content is very limited. Animal studies in this area have shown definite changes in purine content following the boiling and broiling of purine-containing foods such as beef, beef liver, haddock and mushrooms. However, even though these cooking processes affect purine content, the nature of the changes is not clear.

On the one hand, boiling high-purine foods in water can cause breakdown of the purine-containing components (called nucleic acids) and eventual freeing up of the purines for absorption. For example, in some studies, when animals were fed cooked versus non-cooked foods, the animals eating the cooked version experienced greater absorption and excretion of purine-related compounds.

From this evidence, it might be tempting to conclude that cooking high-purine foods actually increases the amount of available purines. On the other hand, when foods were boiled, some of the purines were freed up into the cooking water and thus lost from the food (because the water in which the food was boiled was discarded after cooking). From this evidence, the exact opposite conclusion would make sense: cooking of high-purine-containing foods reduces the amount of purines they provide.

# rBGH and cow's milk——

Conventionally raised cows may be treated with a compound called recombinant bovine growth hormone (rBGH). Canada has banned the use of this hormone in cows, based on research from Canadian scientists. Their report on rBGH noted that cows injected with the growth hormone reportedly have an 18% increase in the risk of infertility, a 50% increase in the risk of lameness and a 25% increase in the risk of mastitis (one concern is that cows with mastitis are treated with antibiotics). Another independent Canadian scientific committee found there was no direct risk to human health.

rBGH increases the content of insulin-like growth factor (IGF-1) in cow's milk. IGF-1 in cow's milk is similar enough to the IGF-1 in humans to trigger biological activity. Our risk of breast and prostate cancer may be increased from routine consumption of cow's milk partly in relationship to this IGF-1 mechanism. However, the same mechanism may also reduce our risk of colon and lung cancer. All of the risks described above are still a matter of debate, however, in the research literature.

Several U.S. groups have opposed the use of the hormone. The best way to ensure that you buy milk that has not been treated with rBGH is to buy organic dairy products.

# sulfites

Sulfur-containing compounds (sulfites) are among the most frequently used preservatives in the U.S. food supply. Sulfites are used to extend the shelf life of dried fruits, wines, shellfish and many processed foods by preventing oxidation, reducing discoloration and inhibiting bacterial growth.

Unfortunately, many people cannot "tolerate" sulfites. It has been estimated that one out of every 100 people may have adverse reactions to sulfites. These reactions can be particularly acute for those who suffer from asthma; the U.S. Food and Drug Administration estimates that 5% of asthmatics may experience a reaction when exposed to sulfites.

## Sulfite-Containing Foods

The following is a list of foods that may contain sulfites. Only specific forms of some foods (such as bottled lemon juice) contain sulfites.

- Dried apricots, dried apples and other dried versions of fruits
- Grapes—as well as wine made from grapes
- Lemons—bottled lemon juice
- Potatoes—dehydrated and peeled raw potatoes
- Shrimp
- Scallops
- Cod (dried)
- Wheat—processed baked goods (may be used in the dough conditioner)

Foods that are classified as "organic" do not contain sulfites since federal regulations prohibit the use of these preservatives in organically grown or originally produced foods. Therefore, concern about sulfite exposure is yet another reason to purchase organic foods.

## How to Avoid Sulfites

As noted above, sulfites are not allowed to be used in organic foods. Therefore, if you want to avoid sulfites, it is best to purchase organic foods whenever possible, especially when it comes to foods listed above as well as processed foods.

There are some foods for which the sulfite-free version appears different than ones containing sulfites, For example, sulfite-free apricots are almost dark brown in color compared to the bright orange of apricots preserved with sulfites.

If you purchase foods that are not organically grown or organically produced, you will want to be diligent about reading packaged food labels to identify whether they contain sulfites. The following are the names of sulfite-containing preservatives as they may appear on the label:

- Sulfur dioxide
- Sodium sulfite
- Sodium bisulfute
- Potassium bisulfite
- Sodium metabisulfite
- Potassium metabisulfate

While preservatives need to be declared on the label, some foods are exempt from labeling laws. If you have questions about specific products, contact the manufacturer.

When eating in restaurants or purchasing foods from delis and other take-out locations, don't hesitate to ask whether the foods you are considering eating contain sulfites.

## Sulfites and Wine

Wines often contain sulfites. Migraine headaches and nasal and gastric discomfort are some of the symptoms associated with reactions to the sulfites contained in the wine. Conventional wines may also contain additional chemical additives to help protect against oxidation and bacterial spoilage to increase their shelf life. Selecting organic wines help some individuals avoid the headaches caused by conventionally produced wines.

### SELECTING RED WINES

Selecting organic red wines will help you avoid sulfites as well as help protect the environment because the grapes are grown without the use of chemical fertilizers, herbicides or insecticides. According to the USDA's National Organic Program, "organic" or "100% organic" wines cannot contain any sulfites to display the USDA organic seal. However, be careful not to confuse "organic" wines with those that indicate they are made from organically grown grapes. Wines produced from organically grown grapes may not have met the USDA guidelines for "organic" and therefore may still contain sulfites.

# biochemical considerations chart

## Vegetables

| | FOOD ALLERGIES | GLUTEN INTOLERANCE | GOITROGENS | LACTOSE INTOLERANCE | LATEX ALLERGIES | NIGHTSHADES | OXALATES | PESTICIDE RESIDUES | PURINES | SULFITES | WAX COATINGS |
|---|---|---|---|---|---|---|---|---|---|---|---|
| Asparagus | | | | | | | | | • | | |
| Avocados | | | | | • | | | | | | |
| Beets | | | | | | | • | | | | |
| Bell peppers | | | | | • | • | • | | | | |
| Broccoli | | | • | | | | | | | | |
| Cabbage | | | • | | | | | | | | |
| Carrots | | | | | • | | | | | | |
| Cauliflower | | | • | | | | | • | | | |
| Celery | | | | | • | | | • | | | |
| Collard greens | | | • | | | | • | | | | |
| Corn | • | | | | | | • | | | | |
| Crimini mushrooms | | | | | | | | • | | | |
| Cucumbers | | | | | | | | | | | • |
| Eggplant | | | | | | • | | | | | • |
| Fennel | | | | | | | | | | | |
| Garlic | | | | | | | | | | | |
| Green beans | | | | | | | • | | | | |
| Green peas | | | | | | | | • | | | |
| Kale | | | • | | | | | | | | |
| Leeks | | | | | | | • | | | | |
| Mustard greens | | | • | | | | • | | | | |
| Onions | | | | | | | | | | | |
| Potatoes | | | | | • | • | | • | | •[1] | |
| Olives | | | | | | | | | | | |
| Olive oil | | | | | | | | | | | |
| Romaine lettuce | | | | | | | | | | | |
| Sea vegetables | | | | | | | | | | | |
| Shiitake mushrooms | | | | | | | | | • | | |
| Spinach | • | | • | | | | • | • | • | | |
| Squash, summer | | | | | | | • | | | | |
| Squash, winter | | | | | | | | | | | |
| Sweet potato | | | | | | | • | | | | |
| Swiss chard | | | | | | | • | | | | |
| Tomatoes | • | | | | | • | • | | | | |

## Fruit

| | FOOD ALLERGIES | GLUTEN INTOLERANCE | GOITROGENS | LACTOSE INTOLERANCE | LATEX ALLERGIES | NIGHTSHADES | OXALATES | PESTICIDE RESIDUES | PURINES | SULFITES | WAX COATINGS |
|---|---|---|---|---|---|---|---|---|---|---|---|
| Apples | | | | | • | | | • | | •[2] | • |
| Apricots | | | | | | | | | | •[2] | |
| Bananas | | | | | • | | | | | •[2] | |
| Blueberries | | | | | | | | • | | •[2] | |
| Cantaloupe | | | | | • | | | | | | |
| Cranberries | | | | | | | • | | | •[2] | |
| Figs | | | | | | | | | | •[2] | |
| Grapefruit | | | | | | | | | | | • |
| Grapes | | | | | | | • | •[3] | | •[4] | |
| Kiwifruit | | | | | • | | | | | | |
| Lemons/limes | | | | | | | | • | | •[5] | • |
| Oranges | • | | | | | | | | | | • |
| Papaya | | | | | • | | | | | •[2] | |
| Pears | | | | | | | | | • | •[2] | |
| Plums | | | | | | | • | | | | |
| Prunes | | | | | | | • | | | •[2] | |
| Raisins | | | | | | | • | | | •[2] | |
| Raspberries | | | | | | | • | • | | •[2] | |
| Strawberries | | | | | | | • | • | | •[2] | |
| Watermelon | | | | | | | | | | | |

## Nuts/Seeds

| | FOOD ALLERGIES | GLUTEN INTOLERANCE | GOITROGENS | LACTOSE INTOLERANCE | LATEX ALLERGIES | NIGHTSHADES | OXALATES | PESTICIDE RESIDUES | PURINES | SULFITES | WAX COATINGS |
|---|---|---|---|---|---|---|---|---|---|---|---|
| Almonds | | | | | | | • | | | | |
| Cashews | | | | | | | • | | | | |
| Flaxseeds | | | •[8] | | | | | | | | |
| Peanuts | • | | • | | • | | | | | | |
| Pumpkin seeds | | | | | | | | | | | |
| Sesame seeds | | | | | | | | | | | |
| Sunflower seeds | | | | | | | | | | | |
| Walnuts | | | | | | | | | | | |

## Legumes

| | FOOD ALLERGIES | GLUTEN INTOLERANCE | GOITROGENS | LACTOSE INTOLERANCE | LATEX ALLERGIES | NIGHTSHADES | OXALATES | PESTICIDE RESIDUES | PURINES | SULFITES | WAX COATINGS |
|---|---|---|---|---|---|---|---|---|---|---|---|
| Black beans | | | | | | | | | • | | |
| Split peas | | | | | | | | | • | | |
| Garbanzo beans | | | | | | | | | • | | |

# biochemical considerations chart

| | FOOD ALLERGIES | GLUTEN INTOLERANCE | GOITROGENS | LACTOSE INTOLERANCE | LATEX ALLERGIES | NIGHTSHADES | OXALATES | PESTICIDE RESIDUES | PURINES | SULFITES | WAX COATINGS |
|---|---|---|---|---|---|---|---|---|---|---|---|
| Kidney beans | | | | | | | | • | | | |
| Lentils | | | | | | | | | • | | |
| Lima beans | | | | | | | | | • | | |
| Navy beans | | | | | | | | | • | | |
| Pinto beans | | | | | | | | | • | | |
| Soybeans | • | | • | | | | • | | • | | |
| Tofu | • | | • | | | | • | | • | | |
| | | | | | | | | | | | |
| **Grains** | | | | | | | | | | | |
| Brown Rice | | | | | | | | | | | |
| Buckwheat | | | | | | | | | | | |
| Oats | | • | | | | | | | • | | |
| Quinoa | | | | | | | | | | | |
| Rye | | • | | | | | | | | | |
| Wheat | • | • | | | | | •[6] | | | •[7] | |
| | | | | | | | | | | | |
| **Dairy** | | | | | | | | | | | |
| Cheese | • | | | • | | | | | | | |
| Eggs | • | | | | | | | | | | |
| Milk, cow | • | | | • | | | | | | | |
| Milk, goat | | | | • | | | | | | | |
| Yogurt | • | | | • | | | | | | | |
| | | | | | | | | | | | |
| **Fish/Shellfish** | | | | | | | | | | | |
| Cod | | | | | | | | | • | •[9] | |
| Salmon | | | | | | | | | • | | |
| Sardines | | | | | | | | | • | | |
| Scallops | • | | | | | | | | • | | |
| Shrimp | | | | | | | | | • | | |
| Tuna | | | | | | | | | • | | |

| Meat | FOOD ALLERGIES | GLUTEN INTOLERANCE | GOITROGENS | LACTOSE INTOLERANCE | LATEX ALLERGIES | NIGHTSHADES | OXALATES | PESTICIDE RESIDUES | PURINES | SULFITES | WAX COATINGS |
|---|---|---|---|---|---|---|---|---|---|---|---|
| Beef, grass-fed | • | | | | | | | | • | | |
| Calf's liver | | | | | | | | • | • | | |
| Chicken | • | | | | | | | | • | | |
| Lamb | | | | | | | | | • | | |
| Turkey | | | | | | | | | • | | |
| Venison | | | | | | | | | • | | |
| | | | | | | | | | | | |
| **Herbs and Spices** | | | | | | | | | | | |
| Basil | | | | | | | | | | | |
| Cayenne Pepper | | | | | | • | | | | | |
| Cilantro | | | | | | | | | | | |
| Cinnamon | | | | | | | | | | | |
| Dill | | | | | | | | | | | |
| Ginger | | | | | | | | | | | |
| Mustard Seeds | | | • | | | | | | | | |
| Parsley | | | | | | | • | | | | |
| Black Pepper | | | | | | | • | | | | |
| Rosemary | | | | | | | | | | | |
| Turmeric | | | | | | | | | | | |

1 dehydrated and peeled raw potatoes
2 may be found in commercially prepared, non-organic dried fruit
3 imported
4 wine
5 commercially prepared lemon/lime juice
6 wheat germ
7 processed baked goods (may be used in dough conditioner)
8 flaxseeds contain cyanogenic compounds that break down into isothiocyanates, which are goitrogenic compounds
9 dried cod

# wax coatings

Conventionally grown fruits and vegetables are often waxed to prevent moisture loss, protect them from bruising during shipping and increase their shelf life. Waxes are also said to help reduce greening in potatoes, but contrary to popular belief, waxes not only do not help reduce greening, but can actually increase potato decay by cutting down on gas exchange in and out of the potato.

When purchasing conventionally grown fruits and vegetables, you should ask your grocer about the kind of wax used even if you are going to peel the produce; carnauba wax (from carnauba palm tree), beeswax and shellac (from the lac beetle) are preferable to petroleum-based waxes, which contain solvent residues of wood rosins. Yet, it is not just the wax itself that may be of concern, but the other compounds often added to it: ethyl alcohol or ethanol for consistency, milk casein (a protein linked to milk allergy) as "film formers" and soaps as flowing agents.

Unfortunately, at this point in time, the only way I know of to remove the wax from conventionally grown produce is to remove the skin, as washing will not remove the wax or any bacteria trapped beneath it. If you choose to do this, use a peeler that takes off only a thin layer of skin, as many healthy vitamins and minerals lie below the skin.

Organically grown produce does not contain wax coatings, allowing you to enjoy all of the nutritional benefits offered by the skin.

**Q** *Is it true that some waxes used on vegetables may contain casein (milk protein) to which many people are allergic?*

**A** Many foods that have not been produced organically get subjected to treatments that make them easier to transport and have longer shelf lifes. In addition, conventionally grown foods can be packaged in materials that have been injected with additives designed to permeate the food. In many cases, coatings and packaging additives can be placed in a category of accidental additives that do not have to be disclosed. You'll find some fascinating discussion of the wax-and-casein issues in the websites below. The third website will give you an actual example of a produce wax available in the marketplace that contains casein.

(1) http://www.star-k.org/kashrus/kk-vegetables-wax.htm

(2) http://www.foodproductdesign.com/archive/1997/0497CS.html

(3) http://72.14.203.104/search?q=cache:hgyxEQw1wzMJ:www.cerexagri.com/pdfs/CitrusLustr402_MSDS.pdf+casein+food-grade+waxes&hl=en&gl=us&ct=clnk&cd=24

---

*(Continued from Page 42)*

to be an expensive way to get your full complement of nutrients and calories each day, a team of French and U.S. researchers found that they actually provided the greatest number of nutrients for the least amount of money. When 637 foods were analyzed using a nutrient-to-price ratio, fresh produce came in first as a nutritional bargain (based on daily values for 16 nutrients). The Dietary Guidelines for Americans 2005 recommends that consumers select nutrient-rich foods; foods that give you the greatest number of nutrients for the least number of calories. This study showed that not only were fruits and vegetables nutrient-rich in comparison to most high calorie foods, but in fact as the nutrient-to-price scores of nutrient-rich foods went up, the scores of high calorie foods went down. So enjoying more fruits and vegetables are not only good for your health but also good for your pocketbook. The list below will help you get the most for your money:

| Cost | Food |
| --- | --- |
| Highest: | desserts and other sweets |
| Above average: | grains, meats in general, composite dishes such as pizza or spaghetti and meatballs |
| Below average: | lean meats and dairy products |
| Bargain: | fruits and vegetables, especially oranges, bananas, carrots, cabbage, tomatoes, zucchini, celery and onions |

*Damon, N, Damon, M, Drewnowski, A. The nutrient density standard for vegetables and fruits: nutrients per calories and nutrients per unit cost. J Am Diabetic Assoc. 2005; 105(12):1881-1887.*

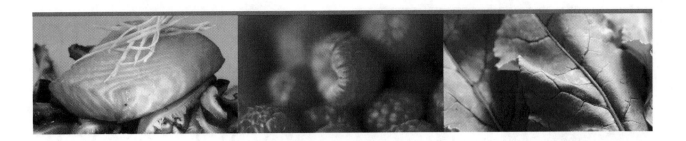

# PART 7

# health-promoting nutrients from the world's healthiest foods

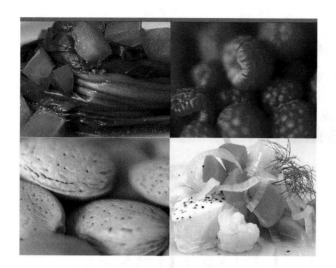

# how to select the best foods for you

What makes the World's Healthiest Foods so full of health-promoting potential is that they are nutrient-rich. What is so essential about these nutrients is that they are needed to sustain our body. An inadequate intake of these nutrients can cause a reduction in our physiological function, leading to poor health since the body doesn't have what it needs to work properly.

We must therefore rely upon our food to provide us with these important nutrients. The more our foods concentrate these nutrients, the better they are because they can give our body an abundance of what it needs to achieve optimal health. This is why nutrient-rich foods—the World's Healthiest Foods—form the foundation of our health.

The World's Healthiest Foods provides an abundance of the wide variety of nutrients you need for optimal function. It is important to remember that these nutrients do not work alone but in concert (synergistically) with other nutrients. Some set the stage for the activity of others or work in unison with them, while some neutralize or balance the effects of others. This is why study after study has shown that diets containing nutrient-rich foods, like the World's Healthiest Foods, are associated with better health.

## What You Will Find in Each Nutrient Chapter

The section on Health-Promoting Nutrients will give you detailed information about the function of an array of important nutrients and a list of the World's Healthiest Foods that provides the best sources of these nutrients. It will provide you with a variety of information on over 30 nutrients and why we need to include foods rich in each nutrient in our "Healthiest Way of Eating." It features the following information for each nutrient: the richest food sources of the nutrient; the nutrient's function; the impact that cooking, storage and processing has on it; public health recommendations; how it promotes health; the causes and symptoms of deficiency; and, whether you need to be concerned about consuming too much of it.

Each chapter includes a Health-Promoting Nutrient chart for that particular nutrient. These charts can serve as valuable tools for helping you to make decisions as to which foods can help you to meet your personal health and nutrition needs. Whether you want to increase your calcium intake to help reduce your risk of osteoporosis or increase your folic acid intake to reduce your risk of cardiovascular disease, these charts will be helpful to you. If you're looking to jump start your protective defenses during the winter season by consuming more vitamin C-rich foods or find easy ways to increase your content of dietary fiber, you can use the Health-Promoting Nutrient charts to see which foods are excellent, very good and good sources of the nutrient of interest.

*Note: If you want help determining your nutritional status and information regarding health-promoting nutrients, which ones may be deficient in your diet, and which foods will help fulfill your nutritional needs, I suggest you go to the home page of the www.whfoods.org website and click on the Food Advisor. The Food Advisor is an interactive program that cannot be replicated in this book. Many thousands of people have been helped by this short, unique questionnaire. It only takes a few minutes to be on your way to vibrant health.*

# antioxidants

**ANTIOXIDANTS ARE DIETARY COMPOUNDS**—such as vitamins, minerals, amino acids and phytonutrients—that directly bind to and destroy damaging free radicals. As metabolites of oxidation reactions, free radicals can negatively impact the structure and function of the body in various ways, including: damaging our DNA (see page 75) and causing mutations, which may lead to cancer; oxidizing LDL cholesterol, which is the initiating step in the progression of atherosclerosis; and causing joint damage that can lead to arthritis. As research continues to support the role that free radicals play in the progression of both chronic diseases and other signs of aging, such as the loss of skin elasticity and cognitive function, antioxidants are gaining an ever more important place in health-promoting diets.

## ANTIOXIDANT NUTRIENTS

Many people are familiar with the vitamins and minerals that are renowned for their antioxidant activity. The ACE vitamins—vitamins A, C and E—as well as the minerals selenium, zinc, copper and manganese are just some of the traditional nutrients that are important when it comes to fighting the damage caused by free radicals. These nutrient antioxidants do not work alone but rather in synergy, each depending upon others to help support its optimal function. Their synergistic relationship is one of the reasons that it is so important to not focus on single nutrient intake, but on intake of an array of nutrients, as offered in the World's Healthiest Foods.

## ANTIOXIDANT PHYTONUTRIENTS

In the past few years, there have been great contributions made to the arena of antioxidant nutrients, with researchers discovering special compounds in plants—known as phytonutrients—that have potent antioxidant potential. Their discovery of the wide array of phytonutrients, and the fact that so many of them have impressive abilities to prevent oxidative damage, has led researchers to suggest that the presence of these antioxidant phytonutrients may be one of the important reasons why diets rich in vegetables, fruits and other plant-based foods are consistently linked to promoting health and reducing risk of disease.

The wide spectrum of phytonutrients offered by plant-based foods such as fruits, vegetables, whole grains and legumes further supports the fact that these foods can make important contributions to our health. Some researchers estimate up to 40,000 phytonutrients will someday be fully catalogued and understood.

Plants are so rich in antioxidant phytonutrients for a reason: they provide plants with protection from the environmental challenges they face, such as damage from ultraviolet light, toxins, and pollution; when we consume plants rich in phytonutrients, they appear to provide humans with protection as well. Investigating the ways in which phytonutrients provide this protection is one of the most exciting areas in nutrition research today, and recent findings are providing science-based explanations as to how plant foods support our health and wellness.

Some of the major classes of phytonutrients that have antioxidant function include:

- Terpenoids: These include the basic terpenoids like limonene found in citrus foods and menthol, as well as the carotenoids (for more on *Carotenoids*, see page 740).
- Flavonoids: Flavonoids are the plant pigments that give plants their color. Flavonoids include the anthocyanins in blueberries and quercetin found in onions (for more on *Flavonoids*, see page 754).
- Isoflavonoids and lignans: Examples include genistein and daidzein found in soy foods, and the lignans in flaxseed and rye.
- Organic acids: Examples include ferulic acid, which is found in whole grains, and the coumarins, which are found in parsley and citrus fruits.

## HOW TO SELECT ANTIOXIDANT-RICH FOODS

Since many phytonutrients are also responsible for the deep pigments that color our food, one way to look for foods rich in antioxidants is to choose foods that feature a palette of colors. For example, red signals lycopene; yellow/orange, beta-carotene and beta-cryptoxanthin; blue/purple, anthocyanins; and green, chlorophyll. Enjoying a spectrum of different colored foods will allow you to enjoy the benefits of a spectrum of antioxidants.

To find foods rich in antioxidants, you can also use the nutrient chapters featured in this section. Look at the chapters for antioxidants such as vitamins A, C, and E, the antioxidant minerals, and carotenoids and flavonoids, and you will find charts that detail the World's Healthiest Foods that are the richest in those nutrients. In addition, I have also created a chart, located on page 804, which compiles the values of several antioxidant nutrients for some of World's Healthiest Foods. While this is not an all-inclusive chart, it can give you an idea of the measurement of some antioxidant nutrients in some of your favorite foods.

With the growing interest in antioxidants, researchers are developing ways to measure the overall antioxidant capacity of foods. Instead of measuring specific nutrients, they measure just how powerful different foods (and their compendium of nutrients) are at exerting antioxidant activity. One of the most well known is ORAC, which stands for Oxygen Radical Absorbance Capacity. While ORAC values have oftentimes been cited as a measurement of a food's inherent antioxidant potential, there are still very few studies published in Medline that review its use. Since I strongly believe that a food's antioxidant value is not linked to just one nutrient, but a compendium of its entire matrix, I look forward to more research on ORAC and other measurements of total antioxidant potential of food.

*(Continued on Page 804)*

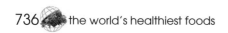

# biotin

Best Sources of Biotin from the *World's Healthiest Foods*

| FOOD | SERVING SIZE | CALS | AMOUNT (MG) |
|------|------|------|------|
| Peanuts | 0.25 cup | 207 | 26.3 |
| Almonds | 0.25 cup | 213 | 24.2 |
| Swiss chard | 1 cup | 35 | 10.5 |
| Goat's milk | 1 cup | 168 | 8.5 |
| Yogurt | 1 cup | 155 | 7.3 |
| Tomatoes | 1 cup | 38 | 7.2 |
| Eggs | 1 each | 68 | 7.0 |
| Carrots | 1 cup | 53 | 6.1 |
| Onions | 1 cup | 61 | 5.6 |
| Avocados | 1 cup | 235 | 5.3 |
| Milk, low-fat | 1 cup | 121 | 4.9 |
| Walnuts | 0.25 cup | 164 | 4.8 |
| Salmon | 4 oz-wt | 262 | 4.5 |
| Cashews | 0.25 cup | 197 | 4.5 |
| Sesame seeds | 0.25 cup | 206 | 4.0 |
| Bananas | 1 each | 109 | 3.1 |

## FUNCTIONS

What can biotin-rich foods do for you?
- Support healthy skin through proper fat production
- Help your body make efficient use of sugar
- Maintain an energy supply in your nerve cells

What events can indicate a need for more biotin-rich foods?
- Depression
- Nervousness
- Memory problems
- Red or sore tongue
- Tingling or numbness in feet
- Heart palpitations

## IMPACT OF COOKING, STORAGE & PROCESSING

Biotin is relatively stable when exposed to heat, light, and oxygen. Strongly acidic conditions, however, can denature this vitamin. In raw eggs, biotin is typically bound to a sugar-protein molecule (the glycoprotein called avidin), and cannot be absorbed into the body unless the egg is cooked, allowing the biotin to separate from the avidin protein.

## PUBLIC HEALTH RECOMMENDATIONS

In 1998, the Institute of Medicine at the National Academy of Sciences issued new Adequate Intake (AI) levels for biotin. The recommendations are as follows:
- 0–6 months: 5 mcg
- 6–12 months: 6 mcg
- 1–3 years: 8 mcg
- 4–8 years: 12 mcg
- 9–13 years: 20 mcg
- 14–18 years: 25 mcg
- 19 years and older: 30 mcg
- Pregnant females of any age: 30 mcg
- Lactating females of any age: 35 mcg

The FDA has set the Reference Value for Nutrition Labeling for biotin at 300 mcg. This is the recommended intake value used by the FDA to calculate the %Daily Value for biotin that may appear on food labels.

The Institute of Medicine did not establish a Tolerable Upper Intake Level (UL) for biotin.

## WHY WE NEED BIOTIN-RICH FOODS

Biotin plays an integral role in the metabolism of fats, sugars and amino acids. While bacteria in our digestive tract appear capable of making biotin, the extent and dependability of this process is still a matter of debate. For this reason, it's very important for us to get biotin from our food.

Biotin was discovered in the late 1930s and early 1940s and was originally referred to as "vitamin H." Egg yolks are one of the richest sources of biotin in the diet, but it is important to not eat whole eggs raw if you want to maximize your biotin consumption. That's because raw egg whites contain avidin, a sugar and protein-containing molecule that binds together with biotin and prevents its absorption.

Many foods that concentrate biotin also feature vitamin B5 (pantothenic acid), a nutrient that participates in many of the same chemical reactions as biotin.

## HOW DOES BIOTIN PROMOTE HEALTH?
### Energy Production
Biotin is involved in the metabolism of both sugar and fat. In sugar metabolism, biotin helps move sugar from its initial stages of processing to its conversion into usable chemical energy. For this reason, muscle cramps and pains related to physical exertion, which may be the result of the body's inability to use sugar efficiently as fuel, may signal a biotin deficiency.

### Synthesis of Fatty Acids
Many of the classic biotin deficiency symptoms involve skin-related problems, and the role of biotin in fat synthesis is often cited as a reason for this biotin-skin link. Biotin is required for the function of an enzyme in the body called *acetyl Co-A carboxylase*. This enzyme puts together the building blocks for the production of fat in the body. Fat production is critical for all cells in the body since their membranes must contain the correct fat components in order to function properly.

### Proper Skin Function
Fat production is especially critical for skin cells since they die and must be replaced very rapidly, and also because they are in contact with the outside environment and must serve as a protective barrier. When cellular fat components cannot be made properly due to biotin deficiency, skin cells are among the first cells to develop problems. In infants, the most common biotin-deficiency symptom is cradle cap—a skin condition in which crusty yellowish/whitish patches appear around the infant's scalp, head, eyebrows and the skin behind the ears. In adults, the equivalent skin condition is called seborrheic dermatitis, which is not limited to areas around the scalp but can occur in many different locations on the skin.

### Nervous System Activity Support
Because glucose and fat are used for energy within the nervous system, biotin also functions as a supportive vitamin in this area. Numerous nerve-related symptoms have been linked to biotin deficiency. These symptoms include seizures, lack of muscle coordination (ataxia), and lack of good muscle tone (hypotonia).

## WHAT ARE THE CAUSES AND SYMPTOMS OF BIOTIN DEFICIENCY?
In addition to lack of biotin-containing foods in the diet, deficient dietary intake of pantothenic acid (vitamin B5) can contribute to a functional biotin deficiency since B5 works together with biotin in many metabolic situations.

Intestinal problems should also be considered as a possible reason for biotin deficiency. Under appropriate circumstances, bacteria in the large intestine can produce biotin, but when intestinal problems create bacterial imbalance, the body is deprived of this alternative source. Consumption of raw egg whites can also contribute to a deficiency since they contain the glycoprotein avidin, which can bind to biotin, preventing its absorption.

Additionally, as many as 50% of pregnant women may be deficient in biotin, a deficiency that may increase the risk of birth defects. Preliminary research has found laboratory evidence of biotin deficiency both in the early (first trimester) and late (third trimester) stages of pregnancy.

Skin-related problems, including cradle cap in infants and seborrheic dermatitis in adults, are the most common biotin deficiency-related symptoms. Hair loss can also be symptomatic of biotin deficiency.

Nervous system-related problems, such as seizures, ataxia, and hypotonia, provide the second most common set of biotin deficiency related symptoms. Additionally, muscle cramps and pains related to physical exertion can be symptomatic of a deficiency, reflecting the body's inability to use sugar efficiently as a fuel.

## CAN YOU CONSUME TOO MUCH BIOTIN?
Reports of biotin toxicity have not surfaced in the research literature, despite the use of biotin over extended periods of time in dietary supplement doses as high as 60 milligrams (one milligram equals 1,000 micrograms) per day. For this reason, in its 1998 recommendations for intake of B-complex vitamins, the Institute of Medicine chose not to set a Tolerable Upper Intake Level (UL) for biotin.

# calcium

Best Sources of Calcium from the *World's Healthiest Foods*

| FOOD | SERVING SIZE | CALS | AMOUNT (MG) | DV (%) | DENSITY | QUALITY |
|---|---|---|---|---|---|---|
| Spinach | 1 cup | 41 | 244.8 | 24.5 | 10.6 | Excellent |
| Collard greens | 1 cup | 49 | 226.1 | 22.6 | 8.2 | Excellent |
| Basil | 2 tsp | 8 | 63.4 | 6.3 | 15.2 | Very good |
| Cinnamon | 2 tsp | 12 | 55.7 | 5.6 | 8.5 | Very good |
| Yogurt | 1 cup | 155 | 447.4 | 44.7 | 5.2 | Very good |
| Swiss chard | 1 cup | 35 | 101.5 | 10.2 | 5.2 | Very good |
| Cheese, low-fat | 1 oz-wt | 72 | 183.1 | 18.3 | 4.6 | Very good |
| Kale | 1 cup | 36 | 93.6 | 9.4 | 4.6 | Very good |
| Milk, low-fat | 1 cup | 121 | 296.7 | 29.7 | 4.4 | Very good |
| Goat's milk | 1 cup | 168 | 325.7 | 32.6 | 3.5 | Very good |
| Rosemary | 2 tsp | 7 | 28.2 | 2.8 | 7.0 | Good |
| Romaine lettuce | 2 cups | 16 | 40.3 | 4.0 | 4.6 | Good |
| Celery | 1 cup | 19 | 48.0 | 4.8 | 4.5 | Good |
| Sesame seeds | 0.25 cup | 206 | 351.0 | 35.1 | 3.1 | Good |
| Broccoli | 1 cup | 44 | 74.7 | 7.5 | 3.1 | Good |
| Cabbage | 1 cup | 33 | 46.5 | 4.7 | 2.5 | Good |
| Green beans | 1 cup | 44 | 57.5 | 5.8 | 2.4 | Good |
| Summer squash | 1 cup | 36 | 48.6 | 4.9 | 2.4 | Good |
| Garlic | 1 oz-wt | 42 | 51.3 | 5.1 | 2.2 | Good |
| Tofu | 4 oz-wt | 86 | 100.0 | 10 | 2.1 | Good |
| Mustard Seeds | 2 tsp | 7 | 38.9 | 3.9 | 2.0 | Good |
| Brussels sprouts | 1 cup | 61 | 56.2 | 5.6 | 1.7 | Good |
| Oranges | 1 each | 62 | 52.4 | 5.2 | 1.5 | Good |
| Asparagus | 1 cup | 43 | 36.0 | 3.6 | 1.5 | Good |
| Crimini mushrooms | 5 oz-wt | 31 | 25.5 | 2.6 | 1.5 | Good |

\* For more on "DV," "Density," and "Quality" Rating System, see page 805.

## FUNCTIONS

What can calcium-rich foods do for you?
- Maintain healthy, strong bones
- Support proper functioning of nerves and muscles
- Help your blood to clot

What events can indicate a need for more calcium-rich foods?
- Osteopenia (bone-thinning)
- Frequent bone fractures
- Muscle pain or spasms
- Tingling or numbness in your hands or feet
- Bone deformities and growth retardation in children

## IMPACT OF COOKING, STORAGE & PROCESSING

The amount of calcium in foods is not adversely impacted by cooking or long-term storage.

## PUBLIC HEALTH RECOMMENDATIONS

In 1998, the Institute of Medicine at the National Academy of Sciences issued new Adequate Intake (AI) levels for calcium. The recommendations are as follows:
- 0–6 months: 210 mg
- 6–12 months: 270 mg
- 1–3 years: 500 mg
- 4–8 years: 800 mg
- 9–18 years: 1,300 mg
- 14–18 years: 1,300 mg
- 19–30 years: 1,000 mg
- 31–50 years: 1,000 mg
- 51+ years: 1,200 mg
- Postmenopausal women not taking hormone replacement therapy: 1,500 mg

- Pregnant and lactating women, younger than 18 years: 1,300 mg
- Pregnant and lactating women, older than 19 years: 1,000 mg

The FDA has set the Reference Value for Nutrition Labeling for calcium at 1,000 mg. This is the recommended intake value used by the FDA to calculate the %Daily Value for calcium that may appear on food labels.

The Institute of Medicine established the Tolerable Upper Intake Level (UL) for calcium at 2,500 mg.

## WHY WE NEED CALCIUM-RICH FOODS

Minerals, like calcium, cannot be made in the body, and therefore must be attained through the foods that we eat. Calcium is one of the most abundant minerals in the human body, accounting for approximately 1.5% of total body weight. While calcium has a lot of important functions, one of its most notable is to promote bone health and prevent osteoporosis. In fact, a calcium-deficient diet is one of the factors that has been linked to the development of osteoporosis.

Other nutrients—such as magnesium, phosphorus, and the trace minerals zinc, copper and boron—also play an important role in enhancing bone density and appear in many calcium-rich foods. Therefore, gaining calcium through your diet will not only provide you with a natural source of this important nutrient, but also of others that act synergistically to promote your health. Although dairy foods have been traditionally promoted as a concentrated source of calcium, many green vegetables provide more calcium per calorie than do milk or milk products.

Getting enough calcium from your diet is specifically important in these modern times when many people's diets are filled with calcium-depleting factors. For example, sodium, caffeine, the phosphates in carbonated beverages, and excessive consumption of protein can cause an increase in calcium excretion.

## HOW DOES CALCIUM PROMOTE HEALTH?
### Promotes Bone Structure

Calcium is best known for its role in maintaining the strength and density of bones. In a process known as bone mineralization, calcium and phosphorus join to form calcium phosphate, a major component of the mineral complex hydroxyapatite that gives structure and strength to bones. If dietary calcium intake is too low to maintain normal blood levels to satisfy calcium's other important functions, the body will draw on calcium stores in the bones to maintain normal blood concentrations, which, after many years, can lead to osteoporosis.

### Other Health-Promoting Functions

Calcium also plays a role in many other physiological activities including blood clotting, nerve conduction, muscle contraction, regulation of enzyme activity, and cell membrane function.

## WHAT ARE THE CAUSES AND SYMPTOMS OF CALCIUM DEFICIENCY?

In addition to insufficient calcium intake, there are other factors that can cause calcium deficiency.

Lack of stomach acid impairs the absorption of calcium and may lead to poor calcium status. Hypochlorhydria, a condition characterized by insufficient secretion of stomach acid, affects many people and is especially common in older individuals.

Adequate intake of vitamin D is necessary for the absorption and utilization of calcium. As a result, vitamin D deficiency, or impaired conversion of the inactive to the active form of vitamin D (which takes place in the liver and kidneys), may also lead to a poor calcium status.

In children, calcium deficiency can cause improper bone mineralization, which leads to rickets, a condition characterized by bone deformities and growth retardation. In adults, calcium deficiency may result in osteomalacia, or "softening of the bone." Calcium deficiency, along with other contributing factors, can also result in osteoporosis.

Low levels of calcium in the blood (especially one particular form of calcium, called free ionized calcium) may cause a condition called tetany, in which nerve activity becomes excessive. Symptoms of tetany include muscle pain and spasms, as well as tingling and/or numbness in the hands and feet.

## CAN YOU CONSUME TOO MUCH CALCIUM?

Excessive intakes of calcium (more than 3,000 mg per day) may result in elevated blood calcium levels, a condition known as hypercalcemia. If blood levels of phosphorus are low at the same time as calcium levels are high, hypercalcemia can lead to the calcification of soft tissue. This condition involves the unwanted accumulation of calcium in cells other than bone. These negative impacts of excessively high calcium intake prompted the Institute of Medicine to establish a Tolerable Upper Intake Level (UL) of 2,500 milligrams for intake of calcium through either food and/or dietary supplements.

# carotenoids

## Best Sources of Carotenoids from the *World's Healthiest Foods*
(beta-carotene, alpha-carotene, beta-cryptoxanthin, lutein/zeaxanthin, lycopene)

| | SERVING SIZE | BETA-CAROTENE (MCG) | ALPHA-CAROTENE (MCG) | BETA-CRYPTOXANTHIN (MCG) | LUTEIN/ZEAXANTHIN (MCG) | LYCOPENE (MCG) |
|---|---|---|---|---|---|---|
| Sweet potatoes | 1 cup | 23,018 | 86 | 0 | 0 | 0 |
| Spinach | 1 cup | 11,318 | 0 | 0 | 20,354 | 0 |
| Kale | 1 cup | 10,625 | 0 | 0 | 23,720 | 0 |
| Collard greens | 1 cup | 9,147 | 171 | 38 | 14,619 | 0 |
| Carrots | 1 cup | 7,391 | 3,606 | 100 | 265 | 3 |
| Swiss chard | 1 cup | 6,391 | 79 | 0 | 19,276 | 0 |
| Winter squash | 1 cup | 5,726 | 1,398 | 0 | 2,901 | 0 |
| Romaine lettuce | 2 cup | 3,902 | 0 | 0 | 2,589 | 0 |
| Cantaloupe | 1 cup | 3,232 | 26 | 2 | 42 | 0 |
| Bell peppers | 1 cup | 2,014 | 30 | 730 | 76 | 459 |
| Broccoli | 1 cup | 1,841 | 0 | 0 | 2,367 | 0 |
| Asparagus | 1 cup | 1,087 | 0 | 0 | 1,388 | 54 |
| Papaya | 1 each | 839 | 0 | 2,390 | 228 | 0 |
| Tomatoes | 1 cup | 808 | 182 | 0 | 221 | 4,631 |
| Cayenne pepper | 2 tsp | 769 | 0 | 220 | 463 | 0 |
| Green peas | 1 cup | 752 | 35 | 0 | 4,149 | 0 |
| Brussels sprouts | 1 cup | 711 | 0 | 0 | 2,012 | 0 |
| Grapefruit | 0.5 each | 707 | 5 | 8 | 8 | 1,453 |
| Green beans | 1 cup | 525 | 0 | 0 | 886 | 0 |
| Watermelon | 1 cup | 467 | 0 | 120 | 12 | 6,979 |
| Apricots | 1 each | 383 | 7 | 36 | 31 | 0 |
| Parsley | 2 TBS | 384 | 0 | 0 | 423 | 0 |
| Celery | 1 cup | 335 | 0 | 0 | 351 | 0 |
| Olives | 1 cup | 319 | 0 | 12 | 685 | 0 |
| Summer squash | 1 cup | 229 | 0 | 0 | 4,048 | 0 |
| Figs | 8 oz-wt | 193 | 0 | 0 | 20 | 0 |

## FUNCTIONS

What can carotenoid-rich foods do for you?
- Protect your cells from the damaging effects of free radicals
- Provide a source of vitamin A
- Enhance the functioning of your immune system
- Promote eye health
- Promote lung health

What events can indicate a need for more carotenoid-rich foods?
- Low intake of fruits and vegetables
- Smoking
- Regular alcohol consumption

## IMPACT OF COOKING, STORAGE & PROCESSING

In certain cases, cooking can improve the availability of alpha- and beta-carotene in foods. Lightly steaming carrots and spinach improves your body's ability to absorb carotenoids in these foods. It is important to note, however, that in most cases, prolonged cooking of vegetables decreases the availability of these carotenoids by changing the shape of the carotenoid from its natural trans-configuration to a cis-configuration. For example, fresh carrots contain 100% all-trans beta-carotene, while canned carrots contain only 73% all-trans beta-carotene.

Lutein appears to be sensitive to cooking and storage. Prolonged cooking of green, leafy vegetables is suggested to reduce their lutein content. Additionally, the lutein content of wheat seeds has been found to decline with longer storage times.

Vine-ripened tomatoes have a higher lycopene content than tomatoes ripened off the vine. Although not all scientists agree, it is generally accepted that the availability of lycopene from tomato products is increased when these foods are processed at high temperatures or packaged with oil. If actually true, this means that your body absorbs the lycopene in canned, pasteurized tomato juice and tomato products that contain oil more easily than the lycopene found in a fresh, raw tomato.

While it appears that more research is necessary in this area, a recent study that explored the interrelationship of carotenoid (alpha-carotene, beta-carotene and lycopene) absorption with dietary fat consumption seems to be supportive of the oil-carotenoid connection. This study found that the absorption of carotenoids from salad vegetables such as spinach, romaine lettuce, cherry tomatoes, and carrots was much greater with a full-fat dressing than a reduced-fat dressing. This interrelationship makes sense since carotenoids are fat-soluble compounds.

There is minimal research specifically focusing upon the effects of cooking, storage or processing upon beta-cryptoxanthin and zeaxanthin.

## PUBLIC HEALTH RECOMMENDATIONS

In an effort to set public health recommendations, the Institute of Medicine at the National Academy of Sciences reviewed the existing scientific research on carotenoids in 2000. Despite the large body of population-based research that links high consumption of carotenoid-containing foods with a reduced risk of several chronic diseases, the Institute of Medicine concluded that this evidence was not strong enough to support a required carotenoid intake level because it is not yet known if the health benefits associated with carotenoid-containing foods are due to the carotenoids or to some other substance in the food. Therefore, to date, no recommended dietary intake levels have been established for carotenoids.

However, the National Academy of Sciences does support the recommendations of various health agencies, which encourage individuals to consume five or more servings of carotenoid-rich fruits and vegetables every day.

## WHY WE NEED CAROTENOID-RICH FOODS

Carotenoids are a phytonutrient family that represents one of the most widespread groups of naturally occurring plant pigments. Alpha-carotene, beta-carotene, beta-cryptoxanthin, lutein/zeaxanthin and lycopene are among the most abundant carotenoids in the North American diet.

Alpha-carotene, beta-carotene and beta-cryptoxanthin are considered "pro-vitamin A" compounds since they can be converted in the body into retinol, the active form of vitamin A. Among these, beta-carotene has the greatest vitamin A activity with the other two having about half that of beta-carotene.

Lutein/zeaxanthin and lycopene do share an important characteristic with these "provitamin A" carotenoids—they all have very impressive antioxidant activity. (Although separate molecules, lutein and zeaxanthin are often referred to collectively since they are usually measured together.)

Carotenoids are a great example of why whole foods (rather than dietary supplements) may be the best source of attaining nutrients for most people. While study after study shows carotenoid-rich foods to be of significant importance to preventing chronic disease, the same cannot be said of isolated carotenoid dietary supplements. This fact was brought to public attention when studies suggested that beta-carotene supplements were associated with greater risk of developing lung cancer in smokers. While it may be argued that the culprit was that the synthetic carotenoids were in a form not readily acceptable to the body, what cannot be argued is that populations who eat carotenoid-rich foods seem to enjoy better health.

Eating foods rich in carotenoids enhances your body's usage of these important nutrients since these foods naturally contain other nutrients that act in synergy with carotenoids, supporting their physiological function in your body and therefore contributing to your optimal health. Also, there are probably many other health-promoting carotenoids and phytonutrients contained in whole foods, which science has not yet identified.

## HOW DO CAROTENOIDS PROMOTE HEALTH?
### Antioxidant Activity

Carotenoids are powerful antioxidants, protecting the cells of the body from damage caused by free radicals. While they work in concert, different carotenoids have been found to have unique features. For example, lutein/zeaxanthin are especially active in the eye, protecting the retina and lens from oxidative damage, and therefore protecting against the development of cataracts and age-related macular degeneration. Lycopene is especially effective at quenching a free radical called singlet oxygen and is known for being especially effective at protecting membrane lipids from oxidation, which may be the reason that lycopene intake has been linked with reducing the risk of such health conditions as cardiovascular disease and prostate cancer.

### Prevent Vitamin A Deficiency

Alpha-carotene, beta-carotene and beta-cryptoxanthin are three of the most commonly consumed "provitamin A" carotenoids in the North American diet. Since the body can convert them into retinol, an active form of vitamin A, they can help prevent deficiency of this important nutrient. Among its other functions, vitamin A is important to maintaining a healthy immune system.

### Promote Heart Health

Lycopene is also believed to play a role in the prevention of heart disease by inhibiting free radical damage to LDL cholesterol. Before cholesterol can be deposited in the plaques that harden and narrow arteries, it must be oxidized by free radicals. With its powerful antioxidant activity, lycopene can prevent LDL cholesterol from being oxidized. Numerous research studies have also found that diets rich in carotenoid-containing foods are associated with a reduced risk of heart disease.

### Promote Eye Health

Carotenoids are found throughout the eyes, with lutein and zeaxanthin being concentrated in the retina and lens. Observational studies have noted that higher dietary intake of lutein and zeaxanthin is related to reduced risk of cataracts and age-related macular degeneration, two eye conditions for which there are minimal options when it comes to effective prevention. Researchers speculate that these carotenoids may promote eye health through their ability to protect the eyes from light-induced oxidative damage and aging through both their antioxidant actions as well as their ability to filter out UV light.

### Promote Lung Health

Research suggests that beta-cryptoxanthin may promote the health of the respiratory tract. Serum concentrations of this carotenoid have been found to be associated with improved lung function; individuals who smoke as well as those who inhale second hand smoke have been found to have lower levels of this carotenoid. In addition, the other provitamin A carotenoids—alpha-carotene and beta-carotene—may also play a role in promoting lung health since vitamin A itself is known to be necessary for proper growth and development of lung tissue.

### Promote Men's Health

Consumption of lycopene-rich foods is associated with a reduced risk of prostate cancer. Recent research has also suggested that lycopene can boost sperm concentrations in infertile men. In one study, a lycopene-supplemented diet resulted in a statistically significant improvement in sperm concentration and motility amongst the 30 infertile men being studied with six pregnancies following as a result of the trial.

### Promote Optimal Health

Increased intake of beta-cryptoxanthin has been found to be associated with reduced risk of esophageal and lung cancer while intake of lycopene is associated with reduced risk of prostate cancer. One reason that carotenoids may support optimal health is because they have the ability to stimulate cell-to-cell communication, which, if not functioning properly, may contribute to the overgrowth of cells, a condition that eventually leads to cancer.

### WHAT ARE THE CAUSES AND SYMPTOMS of CAROTENOID DEFICIENCY?

Carotenoids are fat-soluble substances, and as such require the presence of dietary fat for proper absorption through the digestive tract. Consequently, your carotenoid status may be impaired by a diet that is extremely low in fat or if you have a medical condition that causes a reduction in the ability to absorb dietary fat; these conditions include pancreatic enzyme deficiency, Crohn's disease, celiac sprue, cystic fibrosis, surgical removal of part or all of the stomach, gall bladder disease, and liver disease.

Due to low consumption of fruits and vegetables, many adolescents and young adults do not take in enough carotenoids. Smokers and drinkers have been found to eat fewer foods that contain carotenoids, while researchers also suspect that cigarette smoke destroys carotenoids.

A low dietary intake of carotenoids is not known to directly cause any diseases or health conditions, at least in the short term. However, if your intake of vitamin A is also low, a dietary deficiency of alpha-carotene, beta-carotene, beta-cryptoxanthin and/or other "provitamin A" carotenoids can cause the symptoms associated with vitamin A deficiency.

Yet, long-term inadequate intake of carotenoids is associated with chronic diseases, including heart disease and various cancers. One important mechanism for this carotenoid-disease relationship appears to be free radicals. Research indicates that diets low in carotenoids can increase the body's susceptibility to damage from free radicals. As a result, over the long term, carotenoid deficient diets may increase tissue damage from free radical activity, and increase risk of chronic diseases like heart disease and cancers.

### CAN YOU CONSUME TOO MANY CAROTENOIDS?

High intake of carotenoid-containing foods is not associated with any toxic side effects. As a result, the Institute of Medicine at the National Academy of Sciences did not establish a Tolerable Upper Intake Level (UL) for carotenoids when it reviewed these nutrients in 2000.

Excessive consumption of beta-carotene can lead to a yellowish discoloration of the skin called carotenodermia, while excessive lycopene can lead to a deep orange discoloration called lycopenodermia. Both are harmless and reversible.

While there hasn't been concern about the safety of carotenoids in foods, there has been some concern raised over the safety of carotenoid dietary supplements as reflected in studies that have shown increased risk of lung cancer in smokers taking beta-carotene supplements.

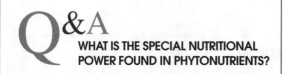

## Q&A
### WHAT IS THE SPECIAL NUTRITIONAL POWER FOUND IN PHYTONUTRIENTS?

Researchers traditionally have attributed the health-promoting effects of plant foods to their comprehensive array of vitamins, minerals and fiber. More recently, however, research studies are uncovering a new story. Plant foods contain thousands of other compounds in addition to macronutrients (carbohydrates, proteins, fats and fiber) and micronutrients (vitamins and minerals). These other compounds are collectively known as phytonutrients (phyto=plant). Simply put, phytonutrients are active compounds in plants that have been shown to provide benefit to humans when consumed.

Like us, plants are exposed to damaging radiation, toxins and pollution, and this toxic exposure results in the generation of free radicals within their cells. Free radicals are reactive molecules that can bind and damage proteins, cell membranes and DNA. Since plants can't move away from these insults, nature has provided them with a means of protection: they can make a variety of types of protective compounds—the phytonutrients. When we consume plants rich in phytonutrients, they appear to provide humans with protection as well. Investigating the ways in which phytonutrients provide this protection is one of the most exciting areas in nutrition research today, and recent findings are providing science-based explanations as to how plant foods support our health and wellness.

### Plants Contain Thousands of Phytonutrients

Most plants use sunlight as an energy source. Although to the eye sunlight appears as a single, clear, bright force, it is actually made up of many different wavelengths, some of which plants capture for the generation of energy. Others, however, are wavelengths from which plants need protection. Each plant contains literally thousands of different phytonutrients that can act as antioxidants, providing protection from potentially damaging free radicals. Many of these compounds also provide the plants with color, with their different colors each reflecting a different variety of protection they provide.

If a plant were only one color, with no shades or variations in that color, it would only be able to receive and protect against one specific wavelength of light. A plant with several different colors is like a television set with an antenna, and a plant with many different colors is like a television with a satellite dish. Most plants have a satellite dish's worth of colors—even ones that look very green to us when we eat them. Like the primer used beneath a coat of paint, these other colors are simply overshadowed by the primary color that we see.

### HOW ARE PHYTONUTRIENTS CLASSIFIED?

Some researchers estimate up to 40,000 phytonutrients will someday be fully catalogued and understood. In just the last 30 years, many hundreds of these compounds have been identified and are currently being investigated for their health-promoting qualities. At research organizations like the National Institute of Cancer, and at many universities around the world, different individual phytonutrients are being studied to identify their specific health benefits.

While phytonutrients are classified by their chemical structure, because there are so many compounds, phytonutrients are also lumped together in families depending on the similarities in their structures. Names such as terpenes are used to decribe carotenoids, some of which are precursors to vitamin A and which provide the orange, red and pink colors in foods such as carrots, tomatoes and pink shellfish; limonoids, which are found in citrus fruits and provide them with their distinctive smell; and coumarins, natural blood thinners found in parsley, licorice and citrus fruits.

The phenols, or polyphenols (poly=many), is another family of phytonutrients that has received much research attention and discussion in the scientific literature. In fact, some of the most talked about phytonutrients are in this family. They include the anthocyanidins, which give blueberries and grapes their dark blue and purple color, and the catechins, found in tea and wine, which provide the bitter taste as well as the tawny coloring in these foods. Anthocyanidins have been found to provide unique antioxidant protection from free radical damage in both water-soluble and fat-soluble environments. And, their free radical scavenging capabilities are thought to be more potent than many of the currently well-known vitamin antioxidants; anthocyanidins are estimated to have fifty times the antioxidant activity of both vitamin C and vitamin E. Flavonoids are also commonly considered phenols, although the term "flavonoids" can refer to many phytonutrients.

Lastly, the isoflavones are usually categorized as members of this phenol family. Isoflavones, which are found in soy, kudzu, red clover and rye, have been researched extensively for their ability to protect against hormone-dependent cancers, such as breast cancer.

Other phytonutrients include the organosulfur compounds, such as the glucosinolates and indoles from *Brassica* vegetables like broccoli, and the allylic sulfides from garlic and onions, all of which have been found to support our ability to detoxify noxious foreign compounds like pesticides and other environmental toxins. Organic acids are another common family of phytonutrients and include some powerful antioxidants, like ferulic acid, which are found in whole grains.

# choline

Best Sources of Choline from the *World's Healthiest Foods*

| FOOD | SERVING SIZE | CALS | AMOUNT (MG) |
|---|---|---|---|
| Eggs | 1 each | 68 | 110.4 |
| Cod | 4 oz-wt | 119 | 94.9 |
| Shrimp | 4 oz-wt | 112 | 91.7 |
| Navy beans | 1 cup | 258 | 81.5 |
| Salmon | 4 oz-wt | 261 | 74.2 |
| Brussels sprouts | 1 cup | 60 | 63.5 |
| Broccoli | 1 cup | 43 | 62.6 |
| Pinto beans | 1 cup | 234 | 60.0 |
| Kidney beans | 1 cup | 224 | 54.0 |
| Cauliflower | 1 cup | 28 | 48.5 |
| Asparagus | 1 cup | 43 | 47.0 |
| Spinach | 1 cup | 41 | 44.6 |
| Green peas | 1 cup | 134 | 44.2 |
| Milk, low-fat | 1 cup | 121 | 42.9 |
| Yogurt | 1 cup | 155 | 37.2 |
| Corn | 1 cup | 177 | 35.9 |
| Buckwheat | 1 cup | 154 | 33.6 |
| Tofu | 4 oz-wt | 86 | 31.9 |
| Cabbage | 1 cup | 33 | 30.3 |
| Crimini mushrooms | 5 oz-wt | 31 | 23.8 |
| Winter squash | 1 cup | 79 | 21.7 |
| Cashews | 0.25 cup | 196 | 20.9 |
| Avocados | 1 cup | 235 | 20.6 |
| Peanuts | 0.25 cup | 206 | 19.2 |
| Almonds | 0.25 cup | 212 | 18.5 |

\* Source:  USDA Database for the Choline Content of Common Foods (2004).

## FUNCTIONS

What can choline-rich foods do for you?
- Promote proper cell membrane function
- Assist nerve-muscle communication
- Prevent the build-up of homocysteine

What events can indicate a need for more choline-rich foods?
- Fatigue
- Insomnia
- Accumulation of fats in the blood
- Nerve-muscle problems
- Poor ability of the kidneys to concentrate urine

## IMPACT OF COOKING, STORAGE & PROCESSING

Consistent information is not available on the effects of cooking, storage, and processing on the choline content of food. Like other B complex vitamins, choline can be damaged by overexposure to heat and oxygen, and for this reason overcooking of foods high in choline is not recommended.

## PUBLIC HEALTH RECOMMENDATIONS

In 1998, the Institute of Medicine at the National Academy of Sciences issued new Adequate Intake (AI) levels for choline. The recommendations are as follows:
- 0–6 months: 125 mg
- 6–12 months: 150 mg
- 1–3 years: 200 mg
- 4–8 years: 250 mg
- 9–13 years: 375 mg

- Males 14 years and older: 550 mg
- Females 9–13 years: 375 mg
- Females 14–18 years: 400 mg
- Females 19 years and older: 425 mg
- Pregnant females: 450 mg
- Lactating females: 550 mg

The FDA has not set a Reference Value for Nutrition Labeling for choline.

Details on choline's Tolerable Upper Intake Level (UL) are provided under heading "Can You Consume Too Much Choline?"

## WHY WE NEED CHOLINE–RICH FOODS

Even though choline has only recently been officially adopted into the B family of vitamins, it has been the subject of nutritional investigations for almost 150 years. Key research discoveries about choline came in the late 1930s, when scientists discovered that tissue from the pancreas contained a substance that could help prevent fatty build-up in the liver. This substance was named choline after the Greek word *chole*, which means bile. Since the 1930s, research has shown that choline is found not only in the pancreas and liver, but is also a component of every human cell. In addition to its uniqueness as a fat-modifying substance, choline is chemically unique since it is a trimethylated molecule (a compound that has three methyl groups).

Eating foods rich in choline enhances your body's usage of this important nutrient since these foods naturally contain other nutrients that act in synergy with choline, supporting its physiological function in your body and therefore best contributing to your optimal health.

## HOW DOES CHOLINE PROMOTE HEALTH?
### Promotes Brain Health

Choline is a key component of many fat-containing structures in cell membranes. Since cell membranes are almost entirely composed of fats, the membranes' flexibility and integrity, key elements of cellular health, depend on adequate supplies of choline. Membrane structures that require choline include phosphatidylcholine and sphingomyelin, which are highly represented in the brain; choline, therefore, is particularly important for brain health.

### Support of Methyl Group Metabolism

Choline's chemical uniqueness as a trimethylated molecule makes it highly important in methyl group metabolism. Many important chemical events in the body are made possible by the transfer of methyl groups from one place to another. For example, genes in the body can be switched on or turned off in this way, and cells can use methylation to send messages

back and forth. Choline is also important in the metabolic cycle that keeps levels of homocysteine balanced.

### Support of Nervous System Activity

Choline is a key component of acetylcholine, a messenger molecule found in the nervous system that sends messages between nerves and muscles. The neurotransmitter acetylcholine is the body's primary chemical means of sending messages between nerves and muscles.

## WHAT ARE THE CAUSES AND SYMPTOMS OF CHOLINE DEFICIENCY?

In addition to poor dietary intake of choline itself, poor intake of other nutrients can result in choline deficiency. These include vitamin B3 (niacin), folic acid, and the amino acid methionine; all three nutrients are needed in order for choline to obtain the three methyl groups that compose its chemical structure. Additionally, problems including liver cirrhosis are common contributing factors to choline deficiency.

Of special importance in the relationship between choline and health is the impact of choline deficiency on the risk of coronary heart disease and other cardiovascular problems since choline deficiency can lead to homocysteine build-up. Mild choline deficiency has also been linked to fatigue, insomnia, poor ability of the kidneys to concentrate urine, problems with memory, and nerve-muscle imbalances. Choline deficiency can also cause deficiency of folic acid, another B vitamin critically important for health.

The consequences of choline deficiency are particularly visible in the liver since a lack of choline changes the way in which the liver packages and transports fat. The primary symptom of this change in fat packaging is a decrease in the blood level of VLDL (very low-density lipoprotein, a complex fat-containing molecule that the liver uses to transport fat). As part of this same unnatural pattern, levels of blood triglycerides can also become greatly increased as a result of choline deficiency.

## CAN YOU CONSUME TOO MUCH CHOLINE?

Doses of choline in the 5–10 gram/day range have been associated with reductions in blood pressure and in some subjects, feelings of faintness or dizziness. These amounts are typically much higher than the choline content of the foods in the average diet.

In 1998, the Institute of Medicine set the following Tolerable Upper Intake Level (UL) for choline: for those 1–8 years it is 1 gram; 9–13 years old, 2 grams; 14–18 years old, 3 grams; and, 19 years and older, 3.5 grams.

# chromium

Best Sources of Chromium from the *World's Healthiest Foods*

| FOOD | SERVING SIZE | CALS | AMOUNT (MCG) | DV (%) | DENSITY | QUALITY |
|------|------|------|------|------|------|------|
| Romaine Lettuce | 2 cups | 8 | 15.7 | 13.1 | 15.0 | Excellent |
| Onions | 1 cup | 61 | 24.8 | 20.7 | 6.1 | Very good |
| Tomatoes | 1 cup | 38 | 9.0 | 7.5 | 3.6 | Very good |

\* For more on "DV," "Density," and "Quality" Rating System, see page 805.

## FUNCTIONS

What can chromium-rich foods do for you?
- Help maintain normal blood sugar and insulin levels
- Support normal cholesterol levels

What events can indicate a need for more chromium-rich foods?
- Hyperinsulinemia; insulin resistance
- High blood sugar levels
- Type 2 diabetes
- High blood pressure
- High triglyceride and total cholesterol levels
- Low HDL cholesterol

## IMPACT OF COOKING, STORAGE & PROCESSING

Under most circumstances, food processing methods decrease the chromium content of foods. For example, when whole grains are milled to make flour, the chromium-containing germ and bran are removed, and consequently, most of the chromium is lost. On the other hand, acidic foods cooked in stainless steel cookware can accumulate small amounts of chromium by leaching the mineral from the cookware.

## PUBLIC HEALTH RECOMMENDATIONS

In 2001, the Institute of Medicine at the National Academy of Sciences issued new Adequate Intake (AI) levels for chromium. The recommendations are as follows:
- 0–6 months: 0.2 mcg
- 7–12 months: 5.5 mcg
- 1–3 years: 11 mcg
- 4–8 years: 15 mcg
- Males 9–13 years: 25 mcg
- Males 14–50 years: 35 mcg
- Males 51+ years: 30 mcg
- Females 9–13 years: 21 mcg
- Females 14–18 years: 24 mcg
- Females 19–50 years: 25 mcg
- Females 51+ years: 20 mcg
- Pregnant females 14–18 years: 29 mcg
- Pregnant females 19–50 years: 30 mcg
- Lactating females 14–18 years: 44 mcg
- Lactating females 19–50 years: 45 mcg

The FDA has set the Reference Value for Nutrition Labeling for chromium at 120 mcg. This is the recommended intake value used by the FDA to calculate the %Daily Value for chromium that may appear on food labels.

Details on Chromium's Tolerable Upper Intake Levels (UL) are provided under the heading "Can You Consume Too Much Chromium?"

## WHY WE NEED CHROMIUM-RICH FOODS

This essential mineral, required by the body in trace amounts, was first discovered in 1797 by a chemist in France named Louis-Nicolas Vaquelin. Many years later, a physician and research scientist in the U.S. named Walter Mertz discovered that chromium played a key role in carbohydrate metabolism, possibly by participating in formation of a special compound which he named "glucose tolerance factor," or GTF. Researchers are still not clear whether GTF is an actual chemical compound or not. But they are clear that the nutrients related to GTF—even though they may not be assembled into a single chemical structure—play an important role in blood sugar balance.

Eating foods rich in chromium enhances your body's usage of this important mineral since these foods naturally contain other nutrients that act in synergy with chromium, supporting its physiological function in your body and therefore contributing to your optimal health.

It is important to eat natural, whole foods since the refinement process strips away naturally occurring chromium. People who consume diets high in simple sugars should be especially careful about consuming enough chromium-rich foods since refined sugars rob the body of chromium by increasing its excretion. Vitamin C increases the absorption of chromium, and many chromium-rich foods come naturally packaged with this important mineral.

## HOW DOES CHROMIUM PROMOTE HEALTH?
### Controls Blood Sugar Levels

As the active component of GTF, chromium plays a fundamental role in controlling blood sugar levels. The primary function of GTF is to increase the cells' ability to regulate insulin, the hormone responsible for carrying sugar (glucose) into the cells where it can be used for energy.

After a meal, blood glucose levels begin to rise, and, in response, the pancreas secretes insulin, which lowers blood glucose levels by increasing the rate at which glucose enters the cells. To accomplish this, insulin must be able to attach to receptors on the surface of cells. GTF initiates the attachment of insulin to the insulin receptors.

### Metabolizes Cholesterol and Nucleic Acids
Chromium may also participate in cholesterol metabolism, suggesting a role for this mineral in maintaining normal blood cholesterol levels. In addition, chromium is involved in the metabolism of nucleic acids, which are the building blocks of DNA, the genetic material found in every cell.

### WHAT ARE THE CAUSES AND SYMPTOMS OF CHROMIUM DEFICIENCY?
If you have diabetes or heart disease, the amount of chromium your body needs may be increased. You may also need extra chromium if you experience physical injury, trauma or mental stress. All of these conditions increase the excretion of chromium. In addition, in the case of stress, the need for increased chromium may be also related directly to blood sugar imbalance. Under severe stress, the body increases its output of certain hormones. These hormonal changes alter blood sugar-

balance, and this altered blood sugar balance can create a need for more chromium.

Dietary deficiency of chromium is believed to be widespread in the United States since food processing methods remove most of the naturally occurring chromium from commonly consumed foods. Chromium deficiency leads to insulin resistance, a condition in which the cells of the body do not respond to the presence of insulin. Insulin resistance can lead to elevated blood levels of insulin (hyperinsulinemia) and elevated blood levels of glucose, which can ultimately cause heart disease and/or diabetes. In fact, even mild dietary deficiency of chromium is associated with Syndrome X. This medical condition features a constellation of symptoms, including hyperinsulinemia, high blood pressure, high triglyceride levels, high blood sugar levels, and low HDL cholesterol levels, all of which increase one's risk for heart disease.

### CAN YOU CONSUME TOO MUCH CHROMIUM?
Due to the limited nature of existing research studies, the Institute of Medicine at the National Academy of Sciences did not establish set a Tolerable Upper Intake Level (UL) for chromium. However, in 2001, this organization did make a recommendation that individuals with pre-existing liver or kidney disease be particularly careful to limit their chromium intake.

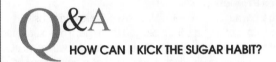

### HOW CAN I KICK THE SUGAR HABIT?

According to the *Encyclopedia of Natural Medicine* (Pizzorno and Murray, 1998), more than half of the carbohydrates consumed by people in the United States are added to foods as sweetening agents. Simply put, most of the carbohydrates we eat in this country are in the form of highly processed sugars. The typical American diet consists largely of processed foods that are loaded with refined sweeteners, with names like sucrose (table sugar), maltodextrin, fructose, lactose, and high fructose corn syrup. These sweeteners have the same amount of calories per gram as other, more healthful sources of carbohydrates such as whole grains. But, unlike whole grains, refined sweeteners are called "empty calories" because they do not contain any of the essential nutrients, such as fiber, vitamins, and minerals. Eating too much refined sugar is associated with a variety of health conditions including diabetes, hypoglycemia, obesity, poor immune function, mood fluctuations, dental caries, and premenstrual syndrome.

So, take a step towards better health and try these suggestions for eliminating refined sugar from your diet.

- **Eat more fruit:** Fruit is rich in naturally occurring sugar that can satisfy your craving for sweets. More importantly, most fruits contain fiber and several vitamins and minerals.

- **Cut out the soda:** If you are a soda drinker, you are getting too much sugar in your diet, plus a lot of other things that aren't good for you! Also, don't think you are doing yourself a favor by drinking fruit beverages. The number one ingredient in many of the fruit drinks sold in supermarkets is high fructose corn syrup. If you want to enjoy a fruit juice, choose a product that contains 100% fruit juice.

- **Leave out the spoonful of sugar:** Many of us add table sugar to hot and cold beverages. To break this habit, start by cutting the amount of sugar you add to your beverages in half, then slowly eliminate the sugar completely.

- **Bake and cook with alternatives:** If you like to make cookies and other baked goods, you probably use a lot of white and brown sugar. Try substituting a more natural sugar, such as dried organic cane juice, honey or molasses in your favorite cookie and dessert recipes. In addition, puréed fruits (such as dates, bananas and apples) or 100% fruit juice concentrate can be used in place of white and brown sugar in many recipes.

- **Use the World's Healthiest Foods as the foundation of your diet:** The foods featured in this book are whole, unprocessed, and nutrient-rich foods. By incorporating more of these foods into your diet, you will automatically reduce your consumption of refined sweeteners.

# coenzyme q

## FOOD SOURCES

Sources of Coenzyme Q include:

- Fish
- Calf's liver (and other organ meats)
- Germ portion of whole grains

Research is not currently available to classify food sources of coenzyme Q according the Quality Rating System used for other nutrients.

## FUNCTIONS

What can coenzyme Q-rich foods do for you?

- Help prevent cardiovascular disease
- Improve energy levels
- Stabilize blood sugar
- Restore the power of vitamin E

What events can indicate a need for more coenzyme Q-rich foods?

- Heart problems like angina, arrhythmia, or high blood pressure
- Problems with the gums
- Stomach ulcers
- High blood sugar
- Muscle weakness and fatigue

## IMPACT OF COOKING, STORAGE & PROCESSING

No research is currently available about the impact of cooking, storage or processing on this nutrient.

## PUBLIC HEALTH RECOMMENDATIONS

The Institute of Medicine at the National Academy of Sciences has not established a Dietary Reference Intake (DRI) nor Tolerable Upper Intake Level (UL) for coenzyme Q.

## WHY WE NEED COENZYME Q-RICH FOODS

Coenzyme Q is extremely important to our health, especially the health of our heart and blood vessels. Its chemical structure was discovered in 1957, and since that time, nearly 5,000 research studies on coenzyme Q have been published.

In many living creatures, the same chemical pathways that make vitamin E, vitamin K, and folic acid also make coenzyme Q. While the human body cannot make these other vitamins, it appears that it can make coenzyme Q.

Coenzyme Q, also called ubiquinone since it is ubiquitiously present in all our cells, is often designated as coenzyme Q10. The number "10" following its name refers to a specific part of its chemical structure.

## HOW DOES COENZYME Q PROMOTE HEALTH?
### Promotes Energy Production

Coenzyme Q lies at the heart of our cells' energy producing process. Special organelles (tiny organs) inside our cells, called mitochondria, take fat, carbohydrate and protein, and convert them into usable energy. This process always requires coenzyme Q. In some cells, like heart cells, this energy conversion process can be the difference between life and death, one of the reasons why coenzyme Q is so vital to health.

### Cell Protection

Coenzyme Q is a well-established antioxidant used by the body to protect cells from oxygen damage. The exact mechanism for this protective effect is not clear. However, in at least one study, up to 95% less damage to cell membranes has been demonstrated following supplementation with coenzyme Q.

## WHAT ARE THE CAUSES AND SYMPTOMS OF COENZYME Q DEFICIENCY?

Deficiency symptoms for coenzyme Q are not well-studied. However, deficiency of this nutrient has been clearly associated with a variety of heart problems including arrhythmia, angina, heart attack, mitral valve prolapse, high blood pressure, coronary artery disease, atherosclerosis, and congestive heart failure. Problems in regulating blood sugar have also been linked to coenzyme Q deficiency, as have problems with the gums and stomach ulcers.

Certain medications, such as statin drugs or beta blockers, can induce a deficiency of coenzyme Q.

## CAN YOU CONSUME TOO MUCH COENZYME Q?

From food sources alone, it would be impossible to obtain the hundred milligram level doses that are thought to be the starting point for toxicity. The Institute of Medicine has not established a Tolerable Upper Intake Level (UL) for coenzyme Q.

# cysteine

## FOOD SOURCES

Sources of Cysteine include:

| | | | |
|---|---|---|---|
| • Chicken | • Eggs | • Garlic | • Brussels Sprouts |
| • Turkey | • Red Bell Peppers | • Onions | • Wheat (germ) |
| • Yogurt | • Oats | • Broccoli | |

Research is not currently available to classify food sources of cysteine according the Quality Rating System used for other nutrients.

## FUNCTIONS

What can cysteine-rich foods do for you?
- Protect cells from free radical damage
- Help your body detoxify chemicals and heavy metals
- Help break down extra mucous in your lungs

What events can indicate a need for more cysteine-rich foods?
- Frequent colds
- COPD (Chronic Obstructive Pulmonary Disease)

## IMPACT OF COOKING, STORAGE & PROCESSING

No research is currently available about the impact of cooking, storage or processing on cysteine.

## PUBLIC HEALTH RECOMMENDATIONS

In 2002, the Institute of Medicine at the National Academy of Sciences set recommended protein digestibility amino acid standards for 9 amino acids or amino acid combinations. A standard of 25 milligrams per kilogram (one kilogram equals approximately 2.2 pounds) of body weight was set for intake of cysteine-plus-methionine combined. This standard applies to all individuals 1 year of age and older. For example, an individual weighing 70 pounds (31.75 kilograms) would require about 800 milligrams of cysteine-plus-methionine, whereas someone weighing 160 pounds (72.5 kilograms) would need about 1,800 milligrams.

## WHY WE NEED CYSTEINE-RICH FOODS

Cysteine is an amino acid that occurs naturally in foods and which, with the help of other nutrient cofactors, can also be manufactured in the body from the amino acid methionine. Cysteine has unique functions since it is only one of two amino acids (the other is methionione) that contains sulfur. Cysteine is an important component of the antioxidant glutathione and can also be converted into the amino acid taurine.

Eating foods rich in cysteine enhances your body's usage of this important nutrient since these foods naturally contain other nutrients that act in synergy with cysteine, supporting its physiological function in your body and therefore contributing to your optimal health.

## HOW DOES CYSTEINE PROMOTE HEALTH?
### Promotes Antioxidant Activity

As a key constituent of glutathione, cysteine has many important physiological functions. Glutathione, formed from cysteine, glutamic acid, and glycine, is found in all human tissues, with the highest concentrations found in the liver and eyes. Glutathione is a potent antioxidant, protecting fatty tissues from the damaging effects of free radicals. The antioxidant activity of glutathione is attributed specifically to the cysteine that it contains.

### Other Health-Promoting Functions

As mentioned above, cysteine is a key constituent of glutathione, a compound that also plays a vital role in the detoxification of harmful substances by the liver, which can also chelate (attach to and remove from the body) heavy metals such as lead, mercury, and cadmium. It is also believed that glutathione carries nutrients to lymphocytes and phagocytes, important immune system cells. Cysteine also has the ability to break down proteins found in mucous that settles in the lungs.

## WHAT ARE THE CAUSES AND SYMPTOMS OF CYSTEINE DEFICIENCY?

The production of cysteine in the body involves several nutrients. As a result, dietary deficiency of methionine, vitamin B-6, vitamin B12, s-adenosyl methionine or folic acid may decrease the production of cysteine.

Cysteine deficiency is relatively uncommon but may be seen in vegetarians with low intake of the plant foods containing methionine and cysteine. There is no known medical condition directly caused by cysteine deficiency, but low cysteine levels may reduce one's ability to prevent free radical damage and may result in impaired function of the immune system.

## CAN YOU CONSUME TOO MUCH CYSTEINE?

The Institute of Medicine at the National Academy of Sciences did not establish a Tolerable Upper Intake Level (UL) for cysteine or other amino acids.

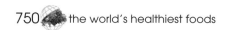

# copper

Best Sources of Copper from the *World's Healthiest Foods*

| FOOD | SERVING SIZE | CALS | AMOUNT (MG) | DV (%) | DENSITY | QUALITY |
|------|--------------|------|-------------|--------|---------|---------|
| Calf's liver | 4 oz-wt | 187 | 9.0 | 451 | 43.3 | Excellent |
| Crimini mushrooms | 5 oz-wt | 31 | 0.7 | 35.5 | 20.5 | Very good |
| Swiss chard | 1 cup | 35 | 0.3 | 14.5 | 7.5 | Very good |
| Spinach | 1 cup | 41 | .3 | 15.5 | 6.7 | Very good |
| Sesame seeds | 0.25 cup | 206 | 1.5 | 74.0 | 6.5 | Very good |
| Kale | 1 cup | 36 | 0.2 | 10.0 | 4.9 | Very good |
| Summer squash | 1 cup | 36 | 0.2 | 9.5 | 4.8 | Very good |
| Asparagus | 1 cup | 43 | 0.2 | 10.0 | 4.2 | Very good |
| Eggplant | 1 cup | 28 | 0.1 | 5.5 | 3.6 | Very good |
| Cashews | 0.25 cup | 197 | 0.8 | 38.0 | 3.5 | Very good |
| Tomatoes | 1 cup | 38 | 0.1 | 6.5 | 3.1 | Good |
| Sunflower seeds | 0.25 cup | 205 | 0.6 | 31.5 | 2.8 | Good |
| Ginger | 1 oz-wt | 20 | 0.1 | 3.0 | 2.8 | Good |
| Green beans | 1 cup | 44 | 0.1 | 6.5 | 2.7 | Good |
| Potatoes | 1 cup | 133 | 0.4 | 18.5 | 2.5 | Good |
| Sweet potatoes | 1 cup | 95 | 0.3 | 13.0 | 2.5 | Good |
| Kiwifruit | 1 each | 46 | 0.1 | 6.0 | 2.3 | Good |
| Pumpkin seeds | 0.25 cup | 187 | 0.5 | 24.0 | 2.3 | Good |
| Tofu | 4 oz-wt | 86 | 0.2 | 11.0 | 2.3 | Good |
| Walnuts | 0.25 cup | 164 | 0.4 | 20.0 | 2.2 | Good |
| Bell peppers | 1 cup | 25 | 0.1 | 3.0 | 2.2 | Good |
| Winter squash | 1 cup | 80 | 0.2 | 9.5 | 2.1 | Good |
| Soybeans | 1 cup | 298 | 0.7 | 35.0 | 2.1 | Good |
| Lentils | 1 cup | 230 | 0.5 | 25.0 | 2.0 | Good |
| Quinoa | 1 cup | 159 | 0.4 | 17.5 | 2.0 | Good |

\* For more on "DV," "Density," and "Quality" Rating System, see page 805.

## FUNCTIONS

What can copper-rich foods do for you?
- Reduce tissue damage caused by free radicals
- Maintain the health of your bones and connective tissues
- Keep your thyroid gland functioning normally
- Help your body utilize iron
- Preserve your nerves' myelin sheath

What events can indicate a need for more copper-rich foods?
- Blood vessels that rupture easily
- Bone and joint problems
- Elevated LDL and reduced HDL levels
- Frequent infections
- Iron deficiency anemia
- Loss of hair or skin color

## IMPACT OF COOKING, STORAGE & PROCESSING

Foods that require long-term cooking can have their copper content substantially reduced; for example, cooking beans may result in them losing one-half of their copper content. The processing of whole grains can also dramatically reduce copper content. In wheat, for example, the refining of the whole grain into 66% extraction wheat flour results in a drop of about 70% in the original copper that was present. Cooking with copper cookware increases the copper content of foods.

## PUBLIC HEALTH RECOMMENDATIONS

In 2000, the Institute of Medicine issued new Adequate Intake (AI) levels for copper for infants up to 1 year old and Recommended Dietary Allowances (RDAs) for all people older than 1 year old. The recommendations are as follows:

- 0–6 months: 200 mcg
- 7–12 months: 220 mcg
- 1–3 years: 340 mcg
- 4–8 years: 440 mcg
- 9–13 years: 700 mcg
- 14–18 years: 890 mcg
- 19+ years: 900 mcg
- Pregnant females 14–50 years: 1 mg
- Lactating females 14–50 years: 1.3 mg

The FDA has set the Reference Value for Nutrition Labeling for copper at 2 mg (one mg equals 1,000 mcg). This is the recommended intake value used by the FDA to calculate the %Daily Value for copper that may appear on food labels.

The Institute of Medicine established a Tolerable Upper Intake Level (UL) for copper that varies by age group: for those 1–8 years it is 1,000 mcg; 9–13 years, 5,000 mcg; 14–18 years, 8,000 mcg; and, 19 years and older, 10,000 mcg.

## WHY WE NEED COPPER-RICH FOODS
Copper is an essential trace mineral that is vitally important to health since it is involved in several important enzymatic reactions in the body. It plays such varied roles as promoting collagen maintenance, proper iron absorption and antioxidant activity. Copper is the third most abundant trace mineral in the body. Since many whole, natural foods contain ample amounts of copper, eating a diet rich in the World's Healthiest Foods can help you to fulfill your daily needs for this important nutrient.

Eating foods rich in copper enhances your body's usage of this important mineral since these foods naturally contain other nutrients that act in synergy with copper, supporting its physiological function in your body and therefore contributing to your vibrant health.

## HOW DOES COPPER PROMOTE HEALTH?
### Eliminates Free Radicals
*Superoxide dismutase* (SOD) is a copper-dependent enzyme that catalyzes the removal of superoxide radicals from the body. If not eliminated quickly, superoxide radicals cause damage to cell membranes. When copper is not present in sufficient quantities, the activity of SOD is diminished, and the damage to cell membranes caused by superoxide radicals is increased. When functioning in this enzyme, copper works together with the mineral zinc, and it is actually the ratio of copper to zinc, rather than the absolute amount of either mineral alone, that helps this enzyme to function.

### Other Health-Promoting Functions
Copper also plays a role in many other physiological activities including iron utilization, bone and connective tissue development, energy production, blood clotting, thyroid hormone production, and neurotransmitter synthesis. It also plays a role in maintaining the integrity of the myelin sheath, a covering that protects nerves.

## WHAT ARE THE CAUSES AND SYMPTOMS OF COPPER DEFICIENCY?
Certain medical conditions including chronic diarrhea, celiac sprue, and Crohn's disease result in decreased absorption of copper and may increase the risk of developing a copper deficiency. In addition, copper requires sufficient stomach acid for absorption, so if you consume antacids regularly, you may increase your risk of developing a copper deficiency. Inadequate copper status is also observed in children with low protein status and infants fed only cow's milk without supplemental copper.

Because copper is involved in many functions of the body, copper deficiency produces an extensive range of symptoms. These symptoms include iron deficiency anemia, ruptured blood vessels, osteoporosis, joint problems, brain disturbances, elevated LDL cholesterol, reduced HDL cholesterol, increased susceptibility to infection due to poor immune function, loss of pigment in the hair and skin, weakness, fatigue, breathing difficulties, skin sores, poor thyroid function, and irregular heart beat.

## CAN YOU CONSUME TOO MUCH COPPER?
In recent years, nutritionists have been more concerned about copper toxicity than copper deficiency. One partial explanation for this involves the increase in the amount of copper found in drinking water due to the switch in most areas of the country from galvanized (steel) water pipes to copper water pipes. Excessive intake of copper can cause abdominal pain and cramps, nausea, diarrhea, vomiting, and liver damage.

Postpartum depression has also been linked to high levels of copper. This is because copper concentrations increase throughout pregnancy to approximately twice the normal values, and it may take up to three months after delivery for copper concentrations to normalize.

The toxic effects of high tissue levels of copper are seen in patients with Wilson's disease, a genetic disorder characterized by copper accumulation in various organs. The treatment of Wilson's disease involves avoidance of foods and supplements rich in copper and drug treatment with chelating agents that remove the excess copper from the body.

The Tolerable Upper Intake Level (UL) for copper varies by age group: for those 1–8 years it is 1,000 mcg; 9–13 years, 5,000 mcg; 14–18 years, 8,000 mcg; and, 19 years and older, 10,000 mcg.

# dietary fiber

Best Sources of Dietary Fiber from the *World's Healthiest Foods*

| FOOD | SERVING SIZE | CALORIES | AMOUNT: TOTAL (G) | AMOUNT: SOLUBLE (G) | AMOUNT: INSOLUBLE (G) | DV (%) | DENSITY | QUALITY |
|---|---|---|---|---|---|---|---|---|
| Raspberries | 1 cup | 60 | 8.3 | 1.5 | 6.8 | 33.4 | 10 | Excellent |
| Cauliflower | 1 cup | 29 | 3.4 | 1.1 | 2.3 | 13.4 | 8.5 | Excellent |
| Collard greens | 1 cup | 49 | 5.3 | 2.4 | 2.9 | 21.3 | 7.8 | Excellent |
| Broccoli | 1 cup | 44 | 4.7 | 2.0 | 2.7 | 18.7 | 7.7 | Excellent |
| Swiss chard | 1 cup | 35 | 3.7 | n/a | n/a | 14.7 | 7.6 | Excellent |
| Spinach | 1 cup | 41 | 4.3 | 0.9 | 3.4 | 17.3 | 7.5 | Excellent |
| Celery | 1 cup | 19 | 2.0 | 0.6 | 1.5 | 8.2 | 7.7 | Very good |
| Cabbage | 1 cup | 33 | 3.5 | 1.6 | 1.9 | 13.8 | 7.5 | Very good |
| Grapefruit | 0.5 each | 60 | 2.7 | 1.7 | 1.0 | 24.0 | 7.2 | Very good |
| Green beans | 1 cup | 44 | 4.0 | 1.6 | 2.4 | 16.0 | 6.6 | Very good |
| Eggplant | 1 cup | 28 | 2.9 | 0.4 | 2.1 | 9.9 | 6.4 | Very good |
| Cranberries | 0.5 cup | 23 | 2.0 | 0.7 | 1.3 | 8.0 | 6.2 | Very good |
| Strawberries | 1 cup | 43 | 3.3 | 1.2 | 2.1 | 13.2 | 5.5 | Very good |
| Bell peppers | 1 cup | 25 | 1.8 | 0.7 | 1.1 | 7.4 | 5.3 | Very good |
| Dried peas | 1 cup | 231 | 16.3 | 5.0 | 11.2 | 65.1 | 5.1 | Very good |
| Winter squash | 1 cup | 80 | 5.7 | 0.6 | 5.1 | 23 | 5.2 | Very good |
| Kale | 1 cup | 36 | 2.6 | 1.2 | 1.4 | 10.4 | 5.1 | Very good |
| Carrots | 1 cup | 53 | 3.7 | 1.5 | 2.1 | 14.6 | 5.0 | Very good |
| Summer squash | 1 cup | 36 | 2.5 | 1.0 | 1.6 | 10.1 | 5.0 | Very good |
| Lentils | 1 cup | 230 | 15.6 | 2.6 | 13.1 | 62.6 | 4.9 | Very good |
| Brussels sprouts | 1 cup | 61 | 4.1 | 1.9 | 2.2 | 16.2 | 4.8 | Very good |
| Asparagus | 1 cup | 43 | 2.9 | 1.2 | 1.7 | 11.5 | 4.8 | Very good |
| Black beans | 1 cup | 227 | 15.0 | 4.1 | 10.8 | 59.8 | 4.7 | Very good |
| Green peas | 1 cup | 134 | 8.8 | 2.4 | 6.4 | 35.2 | 4.7 | Very good |
| Pinto beans | 1 cup | 234 | 14.7 | 5.5 | 9.2 | 58.8 | 4.5 | Very good |

* For more on "DV," "Density," and "Quality" Rating System, see page 805.

## FUNCTIONS

What can fiber-rich foods do for you?
- Support bowel regularity
- Help maintain normal cholesterol levels
- Help maintain normal blood sugar levels
- Help keep unwanted pounds off

What events can indicate a need for more fiber-rich foods?
- Constipation
- Hemorrhoids
- High blood sugar levels
- High cholesterol levels

## IMPACT OF COOKING, STORAGE & PROCESSING

Many whole foods contain five or more grams of fiber per serving, and in their whole, unprocessed form, would be highly supportive of health. When foods are processed, however, most or all of this fiber is usually lost. For example, most breads sold in the United States use an extraction process whereby the grain's germ and bran, the components that contain most of its fiber, are discarded. While fruits and vegetables in their natural state are rich in fiber, the juicing process creates a food product with virtually no fiber. Cooking does not affect the dietary fiber content of the food.

## PUBLIC HEALTH RECOMMENDATIONS

In 2002, the Institute of Medicine at the National Academy of Sciences issued Adequate Intake (AI) levels for dietary fiber. The recommendations are as follows:
- 1–3 years: 19 g
- 4–8 years: 25 g
- Males 9–13 years: 31 g

- Males 14–50 years: 38 g
- Males 51+ years: 30 g
- Females 9–13 years: 26 g
- Females 14–18 years: 26 g
- Females 19–50 years: 25 g
- Females 51+ years: 21 g
- Pregnant women: 28 g
- Lactating women: 29 g

The FDA has set the Reference Value for Nutrition Labeling for dietary fiber at 25 g. This is the recommended intake value used by the FDA to calculate the %Daily Value for dietary fiber that may appear on food labels.

The Institute of Medicine did not establish a Tolerable Upper Intake Level (UL) for dietary fiber.

## WHY WE NEED FIBER-RICH FOODS

Dietary fiber is undoubtedly one of the most talked about nutrients for health promotion and disease prevention. Promoting digestive health, keeping cholesterol levels in check, and filling you up to prevent your waistline from filling out are just some of its numerous benefits.

Processed refined foods are lacking in fiber, and therefore those who follow the average American diet receive less than the amount recommended to promote optimal health and ward off diseases. Yet, whole unrefined plant-based foods are naturally rich in fiber—yet another way eating the World's Healthiest Foods helps to keep you healthy.

Fiber has been generally classified as soluble (the type found concentrated in oat bran and barley, which is known to reduce blood cholesterol levels and reduce blood sugar) and insoluble (found in wheat, and legumes, whose function includes promoting bowel regularity). Most whole foods contain both types of fiber; however, there may be a much greater amount of one than the other. Recently, medical and nutrition experts proposed that instead of soluble and insoluble, fiber should be classified according to whether it is viscous or fermentable, as they contend that the original terms do not adequately describe the physiological effects of all the different types of fiber. Categories of fiber include: celluloses, hemicelluloses, polyfructoses, gums, mucilages, pectins, lignins and resistant starches.

## HOW DOES FIBER PROMOTE HEALTH?
### Promotes Digestive Health

Certain types of fiber are referred to as insoluble fibers because the "friendly" bacteria that live in the large intestine can ferment them. The fermentation of dietary fiber in the large intestine (colon) produces a short-chain fatty acid called butyric acid, which serves as the primary fuel for the cells of the large intestines and helps maintain the health and integrity of the colon.

In addition to producing necessary short-chain fatty acids, these bacteria play an important role in the immune system by preventing pathogenic (disease-causing) bacteria from surviving in the intestinal tract. As is the case with insoluble fiber, fibers that are not fermentable in the large intestine help maintain bowel regularity by increasing the bulk of the feces and decreasing the transit time of fecal matter through the intestines. Bowel regularity is associated with a decreased risk for colon cancer and hemorrhoids.

Two other short-chain fatty acids produced during fiber fermentation, propionic and acetic acid, are used as fuel by the cells of the liver and muscles. In addition, propionic acid may be responsible, at least in part, for the cholesterol-lowering properties of fiber.

### Reduces Cholesterol Levels

Soluble fibers lower serum cholesterol by reducing the absorption of dietary cholesterol. In addition, they combine with bile acids, which are made from cholesterol, and remove them from circulation. As a result, the liver must use additional cholesterol to manufacture new bile acids. Soluble fiber may also reduce the amount of cholesterol manufactured by the liver.

### Normalizes Blood Sugar Levels

Soluble fibers also help normalize blood glucose levels by slowing the rate at which food leaves the stomach and by delaying the absorption of glucose following a meal. They also enhance insulin sensitivity. As a result, high intake of soluble fiber plays a role in the prevention and treatment of Type 2 diabetes. In addition, by slowing the rate at which food leaves the stomach, they promote a sense of satiety, or fullness, after a meal, which can help to prevent overeating and weight gain.

## WHAT ARE THE CAUSES AND SYMPTOMS OF FIBER DEFICIENCY?

Inadequate chewing can prevent the health benefits of fiber from being realized, since insolube fibers, such as lignins, celluloses, and some hemicelluloses, require extra chewing in order to participate in biochemical processes.

There is no identifiable, isolated deficiency disease caused by lack of fiber in the diet. However, research clearly indicates that low intake of dietary fiber (less than 20 grams per day) over the course of a lifetime is associated with development of numerous health problems including constipation, hemorrhoids, colon cancer, obesity and elevated cholesterol levels.

## CAN YOU CONSUME TOO MUCH FIBER?

Intake of dietary fiber in excess of 50 grams per day may cause an intestinal obstruction in susceptible individuals. In most individuals, however, this amount of fiber will improve, rather than compromise, bowel health. Excessive intake of fiber can also cause a fluid imbalance, leading to dehydration. Individuals who decide to suddenly double or triple their fiber intake are often advised to double or triple their water intake for this reason. But an even better approach is to increase fiber intake more gradually, in the range of 50% increases over a period of time long enough for the body to naturally adjust. In addition, excessive intake of soluble fiber, typically in supplemental form, may lead to mineral deficiencies by reducing the absorption or increasing the excretion of minerals.

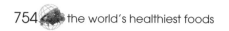

# flavonoids

Best Sources of Flavonoids from the *World's Healthiest Foods*

| ANTHOCYANINS | SERVING SIZE | CYANIDIN (MG) | DELPHINIDIN (MG) | MALVIDIN (MG) | PELARGONIDIN (MG) | PEONIDIN (MG) | PETUNIDIN (MG) |
|---|---|---|---|---|---|---|---|
| Blueberries | 1 cup | 21.9 | 42.8 | 71.4 | 4.6* | 10.2 | 17.0 |
| Raspberries | 1 cup | 52.0 | 0.6 | 1.5 | 4.6* | * | * |

| CATECHINS | SERVING SIZE | (+)-CATECHIN (MG) | (-)-EPICATECHIN (MG) |
|---|---|---|---|
| Strawberries | 1 cup | 6.4 | 0 |
| Plums | 1 each | 2.2 | 1.9 |
| Apricots | 1 each | 1.7 | 2.1 |
| Apples | 1 each | 1.3 | 11.2 |
| Raspberries | 1 cup | 1.2 | 10.2 |
| Raisins | 0.25 cup | 1.1 | 0.3 |
| Pears | 1 each | 0.4 | 5.3 |
| Cranberries | 0.5 cup | 0 | 2.0 |
| Blueberries | 1 cup | 0 | 1.6 |
| Avocados | 1 cup | 0 | 0.8 |
| Kiwifruit | 1 each | 0 | 0.3 |

| FLAVONES | SERVING SIZE | APIGENIN (MG) | LUTEOLIN (MG) |
|---|---|---|---|
| Bell peppers | 1 cup | 0 | 0.9 |
| Celery | 1 cup | 5.7 | 1.6 |
| Parsley | 2 TBS | 22.9 | 0.1 |

| FLAVONOLS | SERVING SIZE | ISORHAMNETIN (MG) | KAEMPFEROL (MG) | MYRCITIN | QUERCETIN |
|---|---|---|---|---|---|
| Apples | 1 each | * | 0 | 0 | 6.1 |
| Apricots | 1 each | * | 0 | 0 | 0.9 |
| Blueberries | 1 cup | * | * | 1.2 | 4.5 |
| Broccoli | 1 cup | * | 2.2 | * | 1.7 |
| Carrots | 1 cup | * | 0 | 0 | 0.1 |
| Celery | 1 cup | * | * | * | 4.3 |
| Cranberries | 0.5 cup | * | 0 | 2.1 | 6.7 |
| Cucumbers | 1 cup | * | 0.1 | * | 0 |
| Lemon juice | 0.25 cup | * | * | * | 0.2 |
| Onions | 1 cup | 3.1 | 0.3 | 0 | 21.2 |
| Pears | 1 each | 0.5 | 0 | 0 | 0.7 |
| Plums | 1 each | * | 0 | 0 | 0.8 |
| Raspberries | 1 cup | * | 0 | 0 | 1.0 |
| Strawberries | 1 cup | * | 1.1 | * | 0.9 |
| Tomatoes | 1 cup | * | 0.1 | 0 | 1.0 |

| FLAVONONES | SERVING SIZE | ERIODICTYOL (MG) | HESPERITIN (MG) | NARINGENIN |
|---|---|---|---|---|
| Lemon juice | 0.25 cup | 3.0 | 7.3 | 0.9 |

\* Data Unavailable

## FUNCTIONS

What can flavonoid-rich foods do for you?
- Help protect integrity of your blood vessels
- Protect cells from free radical damage
- Prevent excessive inflammation throughout your body
- Enhance the power of your vitamin C

What events can indicate a need for more flavonoid-rich foods?
- Easy bruising
- Excessive swelling after injury
- Frequent colds or infections
- Frequent nose bleeds
- Low intake of fruits and vegetables

## IMPACT OF COOKING, STORAGE & PROCESSING

Heat, degree of acidity (pH), and degree of processing can have a dramatic impact on the flavonoid content of food. Overcooking of vegetables has particularly problematic effects on this category of nutrients. For example, in fresh cut spinach, boiling extracts 50% of the total flavonoid content. With onions, boiling removes about 30% of the flavonoids.

In addition to the heat, the amount of cooking water may also play a role in flavonoid loss. A study found that zucchini, beans and carrots cooked with less water had higher polyphenolic flavonoid content than those cooked with larger volumes of water. Therefore, quick cooking methods that use little water such as steaming may be of benefit to conserving maximum amounts of flavonoids.

## PUBLIC HEALTH RECOMMENDATIONS

While flavonoids have been gaining recent attention for their health-promoting properties, currently no public health recommendations, such as Daily Reference Intakes or Daily Values, have been established for these phytonutrients.

## WHY WE NEED FLAVONOID-RICH FOODS

Flavonoids, an amazing array of over 6,000 different substances found in virtually all plants, are responsible for many of the plant colors that dazzle us with their brilliant shades of yellow, orange, and red. Classified as plant pigments, flavonoids were discovered in 1938 when a Hungarian scientist named Albert Szent-Gyorgyi used the term "vitamin P" to describe them.

Well-known flavonoids include the flavonols, quercetin, myricitin and kaempferol and the flavones, apigenin and luteolin. Flavonoids may also be named directly after the unique plant that contains them. Ginkgetin is a flavonoid from the ginkgo tree, and tangeretin is a flavonoid from the tangerine.

Flavonoid-rich foods are oftentimes foods that are also rich in vitamin C, which is important since these nutrients need each other to perform effectively. Recent findings that foods as diverse as apples, onions, berries, thyme, berries, tea and red wine had immense health-promoting activities led researchers to discover that many of their benefits may come from their flavonoids.

## HOW DO FLAVONOIDS PROMOTE HEALTH?

### Antioxidant Activity

Most flavonoids function in the human body as antioxidants. In this capacity, they help neutralize overly reactive oxygen-containing molecules and prevent them from damaging parts of cells. Particularly in traditional Chinese medicine, plant flavonoids have been used for centuries in conjunction with their antioxidant, protective properties. While flavonoids may exert their cell structure protection through a variety of mechanisms, as suggested by various research studies, one of their potent effects may be through their ability to increase levels of the powerful antioxidant glutathione.

### Inflammation Control

Inflammation—the body's natural response to danger or damage—must always be carefully regulated to prevent overactivation of the immune system and unwanted immune response. Many types of cells involved with the immune system have been shown to alter their behavior in the presence of flavonoids. Prevention of excessive inflammation appears to be a key role that many different chemical categories of flavonoids play.

### Vitamin C Support

Present-day research has clearly documented the synergistic (mutually beneficial) relationship between flavonoids and vitamin C. Many of the vitamin-related functions of vitamin C also appear to require the presence of flavonoids, as each substance improves the antioxidant activity of the other.

### Antimicrobial Activity

Test tube studies have found that several flavonoids have antimicrobial activity. For example, myricitin has been found to stop the growth of certain strains of *Staphylococcus* and *Klebsiella* bacterium while procyanin C-1 has been found to inhibit the growth of HSV-1 (herpes simplex virus).

## WHAT ARE THE CAUSES AND SYMPTOMS OF FLAVONOID DEFICIENCY?

Poor intake of fruits and vegetables—or routine intake of highly processed fruits and vegetables, whether they be overcooked or juiced—are common contributing factors to flavonoid deficiency.

Potential indicators of flavonoid deficiency include excessive bruising, nosebleeds, swelling after injury, and hemorrhoids. Generally weakened immune function, as evidenced by frequent colds or infections, can also be a sign of inadequate dietary intake of flavonoids.

## CAN YOU CONSUME TOO MANY FLAVONOIDS?

Even in very high amounts (for example, 140 grams per day), flavonoids do not appear to cause unwanted side effects. Even when raised to the level of 10% of total caloric intake, flavonoid supplementation has been shown to be non-toxic. Studies during pregnancy have also failed to show problems with high-level intake of dietary flavonoids.

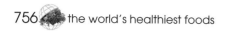

# folate

Best Sources of Folate from the *World's Healthiest Foods*

| FOOD | SERVING SIZE | CALS | AMOUNT (MCG) | DV (%) | DENSITY | QUALITY |
|------|------|------|------|------|------|------|
| Romaine lettuce | 2 cups | 16 | 152.0 | 38.0 | 43.6 | Excellent |
| Spinach | 1 cup | 41 | 262.4 | 65.6 | 28.5 | Excellent |
| Asparagus | 1 cup | 43 | 262.8 | 65.7 | 27.4 | Excellent |
| Calf's liver | 4 oz-wt | 187 | 860.7 | 215.2 | 20.7 | Excellent |
| Collard greens | 1 cup | 49 | 176.7 | 44.2 | 16.1 | Excellent |
| Broccoli | 1 cup | 44 | 93.9 | 23.5 | 9.7 | Excellent |
| Cauliflower | 1 cup | 29 | 54.6 | 13.6 | 8.6 | Excellent |
| Beets | 1 cup | 75 | 136.0 | 34.0 | 8.2 | Excellent |
| Lentils | 1 cup | 230 | 358.0 | 89.5 | 7.0 | Excellent |
| Celery | 1 cup | 19 | 33.6 | 8.4 | 7.9 | Very good |
| Brussels sprouts | 1 cup | 61 | 93.6 | 23.4 | 6.9 | Very good |
| Pinto beans | 1 cup | 234 | 294.1 | 73.5 | 5.6 | Very good |
| Black beans | 1 cup | 227 | 255.9 | 64.0 | 5.1 | Very good |
| Garbonzo beans | 1 cup | 269 | 282.1 | 70.5 | 4.7 | Very good |
| Kidney beans | 1 cup | 225 | 229.4 | 57.3 | 4.6 | Very good |
| Summer squash | 1 cup | 36 | 36.2 | 9.0 | 4.5 | Very good |
| Navy beans | 1 cup | 258 | 254.6 | 63.7 | 4.4 | Very good |
| Papaya | 1 each | 119 | 115.5 | 28.9 | 4.4 | Very good |
| Green beans | 1 cup | 44 | 41.6 | 10.4 | 4.3 | Very good |
| Cabbage | 1 cup | 33 | 30.0 | 7.5 | 4.1 | Very good |
| Bell peppers | 1 cup | 25 | 20.2 | 5.1 | 3.7 | Very good |
| Green peas | 1 cup | 134 | 101.3 | 25.3 | 3.4 | Very good |
| Lima beans | 1 cup | 216 | 156.2 | 39.1 | 3.3 | Good |
| Winter squash | 1 cup | 80 | 57.4 | 14.3 | 3.2 | Good |
| Tomatoes | 1 cup | 38 | 27.0 | 6.8 | 3.2 | Good |

\* For more on "DV," "Density," and "Quality" Rating System, see page 805.

## FUNCTIONS

What can folate-rich foods do for you?
- Support red blood cell production and help prevent anemia
- Help prevent homocysteine build-up
- Support cell production, especially skin cells
- Allow nerves to function properly

What events can indicate a need for more folate-rich foods?
- Depression; irritability
- Mental fatigue, forgetfulness, or confusion
- Insomnia
- General or muscular fatigue
- Gingivitis or periodontal disease

## IMPACT OF COOKING, STORAGE & PROCESSING

Folate contained in animal products appears to be relatively stable to cooking, unlike folate in plant products, up to 40% of which can be lost from cooking. (In general, however, animal products only tend to average about 10 micrograms of folate per 6-ounce serving. Calf's liver is an important exception, with over 1,000 micrograms in 6 ounces). Processed grains and flours may have lost up to 70% of their folate; although some manufacturers add folate back to their processed grain product, this is a voluntary procedure, and there are no standards for this process.

## PUBLIC HEALTH RECOMMENDATIONS

In 1998, the Institute of Medicine at the National Academy of Sciences issued new Recommended Dietary Allowances (RDAs) for folate. The recommendations are as follows:

- 0–6 months: 65 mcg
- 6–12 months: 80 mcg
- 1–3 years: 150 mcg
- 4–8 years: 200 mcg
- 9–13 years: 300 mcg
- 14+ years: 400 mcg
- Pregnant females: 600 mcg
- Lactating females: 500 mcg

The FDA has set the Reference Value for Nutrition Labeling for folate at 400 mcg. This is the recommended intake value used by the FDA to calculate the %Daily Value for folate that may appear on food labels.

Details of folate's Tolerable Upper Intake Levels (UL) are provided under the heading "Can You Consume Too Much Folate?"

## WHY WE NEED FOLATE-RICH FOODS

Folate is a B-complex vitamin most publicized for its importance in pregnancy and prevention of birth defects. The term "folic acid" is sometimes used interchangeably with the term "folate." Folic acid is the form of folate that is generally available in supplements and fortified foods. In food, as well as in the body, this vitamin is usually found in its folate form`. In the past few years, it has also gained recognition for the important role it plays in promoting heart health. Its name is derived from the Latin word for "foliage," reflecting its concentration in many leafy green vegetables.

Folate has a chemically complicated structure and is equally as complicated in its interaction with the human body. For example, many foods contain folate in several different forms, and some of these forms require breakdown by intestinal enzymes for their absorption. Even when the body is operating at full efficiency, only about 50% of ingested food folate is absorbed. Because of this and the popularity of folate-depleted processed foods, folate deficiency is one of the most widespread. That's one of the many reasons that it is so important to eat the World's Healthiest Foods since they are concentrated sources of this important nutrient. What's also great about these folate-rich foods is that they are also rich sources of other B-vitamins, such as B1, B2 and niacin, which are needed in adequate amounts in the body in order for folate to have optimal functioning.

## HOW DOES FOLATE PROMOTE HEALTH?
### Circulation Support

Folate helps maintain healthy circulation of the blood throughout the body by preventing build-up of homocysteine. A high serum homocysteine level is associated with increased risk of cardiovascular disease, and low intake of folate is a key risk factor for elevated homocysteine levels. Increased intake of folic acid, particularly by men, has repeatedly been suggested as a simple way to lower risk of cardiovascular disease by preventing build-up of homocysteine in the blood. Preliminary research also suggests that high homocysteine levels can lead to the deterioration of dopamine-producing brain cells and may therefore contribute to the development of Parkinson's disease. Therefore, folate deficiency may have an important relationship to neurological health.

### Cell Formation

One of folate's key functions as a vitamin is to allow for complete development of red blood cells, which help carry oxygen around the body. When folic acid is deficient, red blood cells cannot form properly and continue to grow without dividing. This condition is called macrocytic anemia, and one of its most common causes is folic acid deficiency.

Cells with very short life spans (like skin cells, intestinal cells, and most cells that line the body's exposed surfaces or cavities) are also highly dependent on folic acid for their creation. For this reason, folic acid deficiency has repeatedly been linked to problems in these types of tissue, including gingivitis, periodontal disease, seborrheic dermatitis, and vitiligo (loss of skin pigment).

### Nervous System Support

Prevention of neural tube defects in newborn infants is only one of the nervous system-related functions of folic acid. Deficiency of folate has been linked to a wide variety of nervous system problems including general mental fatigue, non-senile dementia, depression, restless leg syndrome, nerve problems in the hands and feet, irritability, forgetfulness, confusion, and insomnia. The link between folate and many of these conditions may involve the role of folate in maintaining a proper balance in the nervous system's message-carrying molecules.

## WHAT ARE THE CAUSES AND SYMPTOMS OF FOLATE DEFICIENCY?

In addition to poor dietary intake of folate, deficient intake of other B vitamins can contribute to folate deficiency. These vitamins include B1, B2, and B3, which are all involved in folate recycling. Poor protein intake can cause deficiency of folate binding protein that is needed for optimal absorption of folate from the intestines, and can also be related to an insufficient supply of certain amino acids that directly participate in metabolic recycling of folate. Excessive intake of alcohol, smoking, and heavy coffee drinking can also contribute to folate deficiency.

Because of its link with the nervous system, folate deficiency can be associated with irritability, mental fatigue, forgetfulness, confusion, depression, and insomnia. The connections between folate, circulation, and red blood cell status make folate deficiency a possible cause of general or muscular fatigue. Its role in protecting the lining of body cavities means that folate deficiency can also result in intestinal tract symptoms (like diarrhea) or mouth-related symptoms like gingivitis or periodontal disease.

## CAN YOU CONSUME TOO MUCH FOLATE?

At very high doses greater than 1,000-2,000 mcg, folate intake can trigger the same kinds of nervous system-related symptoms—insomnia, malaise, irritability, intestinal dysfunction—that it is ordinarily used to prevent. Primarily for these reasons, the Institute of Medicine set a Tolerable Upper Intake Level (UL) in 1998 of 1,000 mcg for men and women, 19 years and older. This UL was only designed to apply to "synthetic folate," defined as the forms obtained from supplements and/or fortified foods.

# glutamine

## FOOD SOURCES

Sources of Glutamine include:

| | | | |
|---|---|---|---|
| • Cabbage | • Beef | • Fish | • Dairy Products |
| • Beets | • Chicken | • Beans | |

Research is not currently available to classify food sources of glutamine according to the Quality Rating System used for other nutrients.

## FUNCTIONS

What can glutamine-rich foods do for you?
- Maintain the health of your intestinal tract
- Help your body produce glutathione, a key antioxidant nutrient
- Ensure proper acid-base balance in your body
- Help maintain your muscle mass

What events can indicate a need for more glutamine-rich foods?
- Regular high-intensity exercise
- Intestinal dysbiosis, including irritable bowel syndrome
- Frequent colds or flu
- Severe burns
- Low muscle mass or muscle wasting

## IMPACT OF COOKING, STORAGE & PROCESSING

No research shows problematic effects of cooking, storage, or processing on glutamine levels in food.

## PUBLIC HEALTH RECOMMENDATIONS

The Institute of Medicine at the National Academy of Sciences has not established a Dietary Reference Intake (DRI) or Tolerable Upper Intake Level (UL) for glutamine.

## WHY WE NEED GLUTAMINE-RICH FOODS

Glutamine is an amino acid synthesized by the body from another amino acid, called glutamic acid or glutamate. Glutamine is referred to as a conditionally essential amino acid because under certain circumstances the body is unable to produce enough glutamine to meet its needs, so it becomes "essential" during these times to obtain glutamine from the diet. Glutamine is the most abundant amino acid in the blood and muscle tissue and is especially important in maintaining the health of the gastrointestinal tract and the immune system. In recent years, glutamine has become increasingly popular among athletes, as it is believed that glutamine helps prevent infections following athletic events and speeds post-exercise recovery.

## HOW DOES GLUTAMINE PROMOTE HEALTH?
### Supports Gastrointestinal Health

Glutamine is the preferred fuel source for the cells lining the small intestine. By nourishing these cells, glutamine helps maintain the health and integrity of the gastrointestinal (GI) tract, which is vital to preserving overall well-being. Glutamine also serves as a source of fuel for muscle and immune cells.

### Other Health-Promoting Functions

Glutamine plays a role in maintaining the proper acid-base balance in the body. Glutamine also serves as precursor to the anti-oxidant glutathione, participates in glycogen synthesis (the storage form of carbohydrate), and provides nitrogen compounds for the manufacture of nucleotides that are used to make DNA and RNA.

## WHAT ARE THE CAUSES AND SYMPTOMS OF GLUTAMINE DEFICIENCY?

Because glutamine can be synthesized by the body from the amino acid glutamate, glutamine deficiency is not very common. Nevertheless, muscle and blood concentrations of glutamine are rapidly depleted when the body is confronted with any type of physical stress, such as high-intensity exercise, injury, surgery, burns, infections, and malnutrition, which cause the body to use up its stores of glutamine; during these stressful times, the body is unable to synthesize glutamine quickly enough to meet its needs for this amino acid. Consequently, people under physical stress may be at risk for glutamine deficiency.

Also, the principle site for glutamine synthesis is muscle tissue. As a result, people with low muscle mass, such as the elderly, or those with muscle wasting diseases may be at risk for glutamine deficiency.

## CAN YOU CONSUME TOO MUCH GLUTAMINE?

Consumption of glutamine from food sources alone is not known to cause any harmful effects. To date, a Tolerable Upper Intake Level (UL) has not been established for glutamine.

## HOW DOES GLUTAMINE INTERACT WITH OTHER NUTRIENTS?

One common way of making glutamine inside the body is by converting an amino acid called glutamic acid into glutamine. In order for this conversion to take place, a form of vitamin B-3 is required. Glutamic acid is itself often synthesized though a complicated conversion reaction involving three additional molecules. This complex reaction requires vitamin B-6 in order to occur. For these reasons, vitamins B-3 and B-6 can be regarded as helper nutrients when it comes to glutamine sufficiency in the body.

# lipoic acid

## FOOD SOURCES

Sources of Lipoic Acid include:

- Spinach
- Collard Greens
- Broccoli
- Beef
- Calf's Liver

Research is currently available to classify food sources of lipoic acid according to the Quality Rating System used for other nutrients.

## FUNCTIONS

What can lipoic acid-rich foods do for you?
- Maintain your antioxidant defense system
- Help regulate your blood sugar
- Help regenerate vitamin C and E supplies

What events can indicate a need for more lipoic acid-rich foods?
- High blood sugar
- Frequent colds or infections
- Eye problems like cataracts or glaucoma

## IMPACT OF COOKING, STORAGE & PROCESSING

At present, there are no studies showing the impact of cooking, storage or processing on levels of lipoic acid in foods.

## PUBLIC HEALTH RECOMMENDATIONS

The Institute of Medicine at the National Academy of Sciences has not established a Dietary Reference Intake (DRI) nor Tolerable Upper Intake Level (UL) for lipoic acid.

## WHY WE NEED LIPOIC ACID-RICH FOODS

Our bodies cannot be maximally efficient in producing energy from carbohydrates or fats without the help of lipoic acid. It is also classified as an antioxidant, and it plays a direct role in protecting our cells from oxygen damage in both water- and fat-based environments. In addition, our supplies of several different antioxidants, including vitamins E and C, cannot be successfully maintained in the absence of lipoic acid.

## HOW DOES LIPOIC ACID PROMOTE HEALTH?
### Promotes Antioxidant Protection

The antioxidant function of lipoic acid has been extensively studied, and its ability to help prevent oxygen-based damage to cells is well established. The antioxidant role of lipoic acid may be the key factor in explaining its success in preventing cataract formation in animal studies. Prevention of oxygen-based damage to nerves is also a key area of clinical research on the possible use of lipoic acid.

Because of its two-fold interactions with both water-soluble (vitamin C) and fat-soluble (vitamin E) substances, lipoic acid has been shown to prevent deficiency of both vitamins in human and animal studies. Other antioxidants seem to benefit equally from the presence of lipoic acid. These antioxidants include coenzyme Q, glutathione, and NADH (a form of niacin).

## WHAT ARE THE CAUSES AND SYMPTOMS OF LIPOIC ACID DEFICIENCY?

Since lipoic acid is found in the mitochondria (energy production units) of animal cells, individuals who eat none of the animal foods rich in lipoic acid may be at higher risk for lipoic acid deficiency than individuals who do. Similarly, vegetarians who eat no green leafy vegetables may also be at special risk, since the chloroplasts in these leaves house most of the plants' lipoic acid. Individuals with poor protein intake, and particularly those with poor intake of the amino acids methionine, cysteine, and taurine may also be at higher risk of lipoic acid deficiency.

Since lipoic acid protects proteins during aging, older individuals may be at greater risk of deficiency. Similarly, because lipoic acid is used to help regulate blood sugar, individuals with diabetes may be at special risk of deficiency. As lipoic acid is absorbed primarily through the stomach, individuals with stomach disorders such as low stomach acid may also be at increased risk of deficiency.

Because lipoic acid works so closely with many other antioxidant nutrients, deficiency symptoms for lipoic acid alone are difficult to pinpoint. Lipoic acid is required for the maintenance of vitamin C supplies, so symptoms of lipoic acid deficiency can imitate symptoms of vitamin C deficiency. These symptoms can include weakened immune function and increased susceptibility to colds and other infections.

## CAN YOU CONSUME TOO MUCH LIPOIC ACID?

Toxicity symptoms from excessive intake of lipoic acid have not been adequately studied. While there have been a few reports of adverse effects, these were from supplementation and were at dosages that are higher than can be obtained through food sources alone.

# iodine

Best Sources of Iodine from the *World's Healthiest Foods*

| FOOD | SERVING SIZE | CALS | AMOUNT (MG) | DV (%) | DENSITY | QUALITY |
|---|---|---|---|---|---|---|
| Sea vegetables | 0.25 cup | 9 | 415.0 | 276.7 | 579.1 | Excellent |
| Yogurt | 1 cup | 155 | 87.2 | 58.1 | 6.8 | Very good |
| Milk, low-fat | 1 cup | 121 | 58.6 | 39.0 | 5.8 | Very good |
| Eggs | 1 each | 68 | 23.8 | 15.8 | 4.2 | Very good |
| Strawberries | 1 cup | 43 | 13.0 | 8.6 | 3.6 | Very good |
| Cheese, low-fat | 1 oz-wt | 72 | 10.1 | 6.7 | 1.7 | Good |

\* For more on "DV," "Density," and "Quality" Rating System, see page 805.

## FUNCTIONS

What can iodine-rich foods do for you?
- Help ensure proper thyroid gland functioning

What events can indicate a need for more iodine-rich foods?
- Goiter (enlargement of the thyroid gland)
- Depression
- Fatigue
- Weakness
- Weight gain

## IMPACT OF COOKING, STORAGE & PROCESSING

Food processing practices often increase the amount of iodine in foods. For example, the addition of potassium iodide to table salt to produce "iodized" salt has dramatically increased the iodine intake of people in developed countries. In addition, iodine-based dough conditioners are commonly used in commercial bread making, which increases the iodine content of the bread.

## PUBLIC HEALTH RECOMMENDATIONS

In 2000, the Institute of Medicine at the National Academy of Sciences issued new Adequate Intake (AI) levels for iodine for infants up to 1 year old and Recommended Dietary Allowances (RDAs) for all people older than 1 year old. The recommendations are as follows:
- 0–6 months: 110 mcg
- 7–12 months: 130 mcg
- 1–8 years: 90 mcg
- 9–13 years: 120 mcg
- 14+ years: 150 mcg
- Pregnant females: 220 mcg
- Lactating females: 290 mcg

The FDA has set the Reference Value for Nutrition Labeling for iodine at 150 mcg. This is the recommended intake value used by the FDA to calculate the %Daily Value for iodine that may appear on food labels.

Details on iodine's Tolerable Upper Intake Level (UL) are provided under the heading "Can You Consume Too Much Iodine?"

## WHY WE NEED IODINE-RICH FOODS

Iodine is a trace mineral that is essential for health. We need to receive iodine from our food since this mineral has so many important functions, the most well known being its pivotal role in manufacturing the thyroid hormones, thyroxine and triiodothyronine. Thyroxine is also known as T4, as it contains four iodine atoms while triiodothyronine is known as T3 and contains three iodine atoms. Since thyroid hormones are intricately connected to so many body functions, their importance, and therefore the importance of iodine-containing foods, cannot be stressed enough.

Eating foods rich in iodine enhances your body's usage of this important mineral since these foods naturally contain other nutrients that act in synergy with iodine, supporting its physiological function in your body and therefore contributing to your optimal health.

## HOW DOES IODINE PROMOTE HEALTH?
### Regulates Thyroid Hormones

As a component of the thyroid hormones thyroxine (T4) and triiodothyronine (T3), iodine is essential to human life. Without sufficient iodine, your body is unable to synthesize these hormones, and because the thyroid hormones regulate metabolism in every cell of the body and play a role in virtually all physiological functions, an iodine deficiency can have a widespread adverse impact on your health and well-being.

### Other Health-Promoting Functions

Several other physiological functions for iodine have been suggested. Iodine may help inactivate bacteria, hence its use as a skin disinfectant and in water purification. By modulating the effect of the hormone estrogen on breast tissue, iodine may also play a role in the prevention of fibrocystic breast disease, a condition characterized by painful swelling in the breasts. Finally, researchers hypothesize that iodine deficiency impairs the function of the immune system and that adequate iodine is necessary to prevent miscarriages.

## WHAT ARE THE CAUSES AND SYMPTOMS OF IODINE DEFICIENCY?

The absorption and/or utilization of iodine are inhibited by components of certain foods. These food components, called goitrogenic compounds, are found primarily in cruciferous vegetables (for example, cabbage, broccoli and kale), soybean products, cassava root, peanuts, and millet. While overconsumption of these foods may reduce the amount of available iodine for the manufacture of thyroid hormones, cooking may partly offset this effect. For example, as much as 1/3 of the goitrogenic substances in broccoli (like isothiocyanates) may be deactivated when broccoli is simmered in water. In the early part of the 20th century, iodine deficiency was quite common in the United States and Canada. However, this problem has since been almost completely resolved by the use of iodized salt. In addition, iodine is now added to animal feed, which has increased the iodine content of commonly consumed foods, including cow's milk, which helps, but does not eliminate, the possibility of iodine deficiency.

Goiter, or enlargement of the thyroid gland, is usually the earliest symptom of iodine deficiency. Goiter is more common in certain geographical areas of the world and is attributed to lack of iodine in the diet as well as to the consumption of goitrogenic foods.

Iodine deficiency may eventually lead to hypothyroidism, which causes a variety of symptoms including fatigue, weight gain, weakness and/or depression. Interestingly, iodine deficiency can also cause hyperthyroidism, a condition characterized by weight loss, rapid heart beat, and appetite fluctuations.

## CAN YOU CONSUME TOO MUCH IODINE?

It is difficult to take in too much iodine from food sources alone. In general, even high intakes of iodine from food are well-tolerated by most people. However, in certain circumstances, excessive consumption of iodine can actually inhibit the synthesis of thyroid hormones, thereby leading to the development of goiter and hypothyroidism. Excessive iodine intake may also cause hyperthyroidism, thyroid papillary cancer, and/or iodermia (a serious skin reaction). Individuals with autoimmune thyroid disease (for example, Grave's disease or Hashimoto's disease) or those who have experienced an iodine deficiency at some point in their life may be more susceptible to the dangers of excessive iodine consumption.

In an attempt to prevent these symptoms of iodine toxicity, the Institute of Medicine established Tolerable Upper Intake Levels (UL) for iodine. They are as follows: for those 1–3 years it is 900 mcg; 4–8 years, 300 mcg; 9–13 years, 600 mcg; 14–18 years, 900 mcg; 19 years and older, 1,100 mcg; pregnant and lactating women 14–18 years, 900 mcg; and, pregnant and lactating women 19 years and older, 1,100 mcg.

## Q&A

### WHAT ARE SOME WAYS THAT I CAN INCREASE THE IODINE CONTENT OF MY DIET?

Although iodized salt has been the primary source of iodine in many meal plans for the past fifty years, excessive use of salt has also been a problem in the U.S. In many coastal communities around the world, and particularly in Asia, the primary sources of iodine in meal plans are sea vegetables. Outside of iodized salt, eggs, milk and cheese are the primary sources of iodine in the U.S. diet, and consequently, individuals who do not consume eggs or cow's milk products may especially benefit from inclusion of sea vegetables in their meal plan.

Eating sea vegetables as part of a healthy diet is nothing new. In fact, archaeological evidence suggests that Japanese cultures have been consuming sea vegetables for more than 10,000 years. While very popular in Asian cuisines, most regions and countries located by waters, including Scotland, Ireland, Norway, Iceland, New Zealand, the Pacific Islands and coastal South American countries, have been consuming sea vegetables since ancient times.

Here is some quantitative information on sea vegetables' iodine content: one gram of kelp contains between 100 and 200 mcg of iodine, one gram of wakame about 79 mcg, and one gram of dulse between 150 and 500 mcg. The variation in iodine content is related to the circumstances in which they grow.

From a nutrition perspective what's great about sea vegetables is not just that they are rich in iodine but that they also contain a host of other nutrients. Not only do they feature an array of trace minerals, but they also contain unique phytonutrients known as sulfated polysaccharides (also called fucans) that have been studied for their anti-inflammatory properties.

# iron

## Best Sources of Iron from the *World's Healthiest Foods*

| FOOD | SERVING SIZE | CALS | AMOUNT (MG) | DV (%) | DENSITY | QUALITY |
|------|------|------|------|------|------|------|
| Spinach | 1 cup | 41 | 6.4 | 35.7 | 15.5 | Excellent |
| Turmeric | 2 tsp | 16 | 1.9 | 10.4 | 11.7 | Excellent |
| Swiss chard | 1 cup | 35 | 4.0 | 22.0 | 11.3 | Excellent |
| Basil | 2 tsp | 8 | 1.3 | 7.1 | 17.0 | Very good |
| Cinnamon | 2 tsp | 12 | 1.7 | 9.6 | 14.5 | Very good |
| Romaine lettuce | 2 cups | 16 | 1.2 | 6.8 | 7.8 | Very good |
| Tofu | 4 oz-wt | 86 | 6.1 | 33.8 | 7.1 | Very good |
| Shiitake mushrooms | 8 oz-wt | 87 | 3.6 | 19.9 | 4.1 | Very good |
| Green beans | 1 cup | 44 | 1.6 | 8.9 | 3.7 | Very good |
| Parsley | 2 TBS | 3 | 0.5 | 2.6 | 17.0 | Good |
| Kale | 1 cup | 36 | 1.1 | 6.5 | 3.2 | Good |
| Shrimp | 4 oz-wt | 112 | 3.5 | 19.4 | 3.1 | Good |
| Broccoli | 1 cup | 44 | 1.4 | 7.6 | 3.1 | Good |
| Brussels sprouts | 1 cup | 61 | 1.9 | 10.4 | 3.1 | Good |
| Asparagus | 1 cup | 43 | 1.3 | 7.3 | 3.0 | Good |
| Soybeans | 1 cup | 298 | 8.8 | 49.1 | 3.0 | Good |
| Olives | 1 cup | 155 | 4.4 | 24.7 | 2.9 | Good |
| Lentils | 1 cup | 230 | 6.6 | 36.6 | 2.9 | Good |
| Venison | 4 oz-wt | 179 | 5.1 | 28.2 | 2.8 | Good |
| Pumpkin seeds | 0.25 cup | 187 | 5.2 | 28.7 | 2.8 | Good |
| Sesame seeds | 0.25 cup | 206 | 5.2 | 29.1 | 2.5 | Good |
| Celery | 1 cup | 19 | 0.5 | 2.7 | 2.5 | Good |
| Quinoa | 0.25 cup | 159 | 3.9 | 21.8 | 2.5 | Good |
| Cabbage | 1 cup | 22 | 0.5 | 2.9 | 2.4 | Good |
| Kidney beans | 1 cup | 225 | 5.2 | 28.9 | 2.3 | Good |

* For more on "DV," "Density," and "Quality" Rating System, see page 805.

## FUNCTIONS

What can iron-rich foods do for you?
- Enhance oxygen distribution in your body
- Keep your immune system healthy
- Help your body produce energy

What events can indicate a need for more iron-rich foods?
- Fatigue and weakness
- Decreased ability to concentrate
- Increased susceptibility to infections
- Depression
- Hair loss; brittle nails
- Headaches; dizziness

## IMPACT OF COOKING, STORAGE & PROCESSING

Much of the iron in whole grains is found in the bran and germ. As a result, the milling of grain, which removes the bran and germ, eliminates about 75% of the naturally occurring iron in whole grains. Refined grains are often fortified with iron, but the added iron is less absorbable than the iron that naturally occurs in the grain.

Cooking with iron cookware will add iron to food, a practice that can eventually lead to iron toxicity.

## PUBLIC HEALTH RECOMMENDATIONS

In 2000, the Institute of Medicine at the National Academy of Sciences issued new Adequate Intake (AI) levels for iron for infants up to 6 months old and Recommended Dietary Allowances (RDAs) for all people older than 6 months. The recommendations are as follows:
- 0–6 months: 0.27 mg

- 7–12 months: 11 mg
- 1–3 years: 7 mg
- 4–8 years: 10 mg
- 9–13 years: 8 mg
- Males 14–18 years: 11 mg
- Male 19+ years: 8 mg
- Females 19–50 years: 18 mg
- Females 51+ years: 8 mg
- Pregnant females 4–50 years: 27 mg
- Lactating females 14–18 years: 10 mg
- Lactating females 19–50 years: 9 mg

The FDA has set the Reference Value for Nutrition Labeling for iron at 18 mg. This is the recommended intake value used by the FDA to calculate the %Daily Value for iron that may appear on food labels.

Details on iron's Tolerable Upper Intake Level (UL) are provided under the heading "Can You Consume Too Much Iron?"

## WHY WE NEED IRON-RICH FOODS

Iron is vital to the health of the human body, and is found in every human cell, primarily linked with protein to form the oxygen-carrying molecule hemoglobin. The iron in food comes in two forms: heme iron and non-heme iron. Heme iron is found only in animal flesh, as it is derived from the hemoglobin and myoglobin in animal tissues. Non-heme iron is found in plant foods and dairy products.

It is important to eat foods that are rich in iron since several nutrients in these foods increase your body's ability to absorb iron. Mother nature is very intelligent and packaged these nutrients together in iron-rich foods. For example, iron-rich green vegetables are also concentrated sources of vitamin C, copper, and manganese, nutrients that aid iron absorption. Additionally, amino acids improve iron absorption by stimulating hydrochloric acid secretion in the stomach. Foods such as shrimp, venison, beef and calf's liver are concentrated sources of both iron and its absorption-boosting amino acids.

## HOW DOES IRON PROMOTE HEALTH?
### Oxygen Distribution

Iron serves as the core of the hemoglobin molecule, which is the oxygen-carrying component of the red blood cell. Red blood cells pick up oxygen from the lungs and distribute it to tissues throughout the body. The ability of red blood cells to carry oxygen is attributed to the presence of iron in the hemoglobin molecule.

If we lack iron, we will produce less hemoglobin, and therefore supply less oxygen to our tissues. Iron is also an important constituent of another protein called myoglobin. Myoglobin, like hemoglobin, is an oxygen-carrying molecule that distributes oxygen to muscle cells, especially to skeletal muscles and to the heart.

### Energy Production

Iron also plays a vital role in the production of energy as a constituent of several enzymes, including *iron catalase*, *iron peroxidase*, and the cytochrome enzymes. It is also involved in the production of carnitine, a nonessential amino acid important for the proper utilization of fat. The function of the immune system is also dependent on sufficient iron.

## WHAT ARE THE CAUSES AND SYMPTOMS OF IRON DEFICIENCY?

Iron absorption is decreased in people with low stomach acid (hypochlorhydria), a condition that is common in the elderly and those who use antacids frequently. In addition, iron absorption is decreased by caffeine and tannic acid found in coffee and tea and by phosphates found in carbonated soft drinks. Phytates, found in whole grains, and oxalates, found in spinach and chocolate, may also decrease iron absorption by forming complexes with the mineral, which cannot be absorbed through the digestive tract.

Although the human body conserves iron very well by reusing iron from old red blood cells to make hemoglobin for new red blood cells, iron deficiency is one of the most common nutrient deficiencies in the United States and around the world. Poor iron status may be caused by inadequate dietary intake, poor absorption, parasitic infection, and/or medical conditions that cause internal bleeding.

People who donate blood regularly, women with excessive menstrual bleeding, those who use medications (for example, antacids) that interfere with the absorption of iron, and pregnant and lactating women may be at risk for iron deficiency. In addition, the elderly, vegetarians, and children often have inadequate intake of this mineral.

Iron deficiency causes microcytic and hypochromic anemia, a condition characterized by underdeveloped red blood cells that lack hemoglobin, thereby reducing their oxygen-carrying capacity. But even before iron deficiency anemia develops, people with poor iron status may experience a variety of symptoms including fatigue, weakness, loss of stamina, decreased ability to concentrate, increased susceptibility to infections, hair loss, dizziness, headaches, brittle nails, apathy, and depression. In children, iron deficiency is associated with learning disabilities and a lower IQ.

## CAN YOU CONSUME TOO MUCH IRON?

Although iron overload is not likely to develop from food sources alone, men, because they do not experience the regular iron losses associated with the menstrual cycle in women, may be at greater risk for the problems associated with excessive iron. In recent years, excess iron intake and storage, especially in men, has been implicated as a cause of heart disease and cancer. In addition, iron has been found in increased levels in the joints of people with rheumatoid arthritis.

The Institute of Medicine set the following Tolerable Upper Intake Levels (UL) for iron: 7 months to 13 years, 40 mg; 14 years and older, 45 mg; and, pregnant or lactating women, 45 mg.

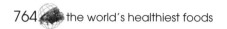

# magnesium

Best Sources of Magnesium from the *World's Healthiest Foods*

| FOOD | SERVING SIZE | CALS | AMOUNT (MG) | DV (%) | DENSITY | QUALITY |
|------|------|------|------|------|------|------|
| Swiss chard | 1 cup | 35 | 150.5 | 37.6 | 19.4 | Excellent |
| Spinach | 1 cup | 41 | 156.6 | 39.1 | 17.0 | Excellent |
| Summer squash | 1 cup | 36 | 43.2 | 10.8 | 5.4 | Very good |
| Pumpkin seeds | 0.25 cup | 187 | 184.6 | 46.1 | 4.5 | Very good |
| Broccoli | 1 cup | 44 | 39.0 | 9.8 | 4.0 | Very good |
| Basil | 2 tsp | 8 | 12.7 | 3.2 | 7.6 | Good |
| Cucumbers | 1 cup | 14 | 11.4 | 2.9 | 3.8 | Good |
| Flaxseeds | 2 TBS | 95 | 70.1 | 17.5 | 3.3 | Good |
| Green beans | 1 cup | 44 | 140.3 | 7.8 | 3.2 | Good |
| Celery | 1 cup | 19 | 13.2 | 3.3 | 3.1 | Good |
| Collard greens | 1 cup | 49 | 32.3 | 8.1 | 2.9 | Good |
| Kale | 1 cup | 36 | 23.4 | 5.8 | 2.9 | Good |
| Mustard Seeds | 2 tsp | 35 | 22.3 | 5.6 | 2.9 | Good |
| Sunflower seeds | 0.25 cup | 205 | 127.4 | 31.9 | 2.8 | Good |
| Sesame seeds | 0.25 cup | 206 | 126.4 | 31.6 | 2.8 | Good |
| Ginger | 1 oz-wt | 20 | 12.2 | 3.0 | 2.8 | Good |
| Quinoa | 1 cup | 159 | 89.3 | 22.3 | 2.5 | Good |
| Buckwheat | 1 cup | 155 | 85.7 | 21.4 | 2.5 | Good |
| Salmon | 4 oz-wt | 262 | 138.4 | 34.6 | 2.4 | Good |
| Black beans | 1 cup | 227 | 120.4 | 30.1 | 2.4 | Good |
| Beets | 1 cup | 75 | 39.1 | 9.8 | 2.4 | Good |
| Tomatoes | 1 cup | 38 | 19.8 | 5.0 | 2.4 | Good |
| Pinto beans | 1 cup | 234 | 94.1 | 23.5 | 1.8 | Good |
| Tofu | 4 oz-wt | 86 | 34.0 | 8.5 | 1.8 | Good |
| Crimini Mushrooms | 5 oz-wt | 31 | 12.8 | 3.2 | 1.8 | Good |

* For more on "DV," "Density," and "Quality" Rating System, see page 805.

## FUNCTIONS

What can magnesium-rich foods do for you?
- Relax nerves and muscles
- Build and strengthen bones
- Keep your blood circulating smoothly

What events can indicate a need for more magnesium-rich foods?
- Muscle weakness, tremor, or spasm
- Elevated blood pressure
- Imbalanced blood sugar levels
- Headaches

## IMPACT OF COOKING, STORAGE & PROCESSING

The impact of cooking and processing on magnesium can vary greatly. Since a greater percent of magnesium is found in water-soluble form, blanching, steaming, or boiling can result in a substantial loss of magnesium. For example, about one-third of the magnesium in spinach is lost after blanching, while cooking beans may result in 65% loss. In other foods, like almonds or peanuts, very little loss of magnesium results either from roasting or from processing into nut butter.

## PUBLIC HEALTH RECOMMENDATIONS

In 1997, the Institute of Medicine at the National Academy of Sciences issued Recommended Dietary Allowances (RDAs) for magnesium. The recommendations are as follows:
- 1–3 years: 80 mg
- 4–8 years: 130 mg
- 9–13 years: 240 mg
- Males 14–18 years: 410 mg
- Males 19–30 years: 400 mg

- Males 31+ years: 420 mg
- Females 14–18 years: 360 mg
- Females 19–30 years: 310 mg
- Females 31+ years: 320 mg
- Pregnant females up to 18 years: 400 mg
- Pregnant females 19–30 years: 350 mg
- Pregnant females 31–50 years: 360 mg
- Lactating females up to 18 years: 360 mg
- Lactating females 19–30 years: 310 mg
- Lactating females 31–50 years: 320 mg

The FDA has set the Reference Value for Nutrition Labeling for magnesium at 400 mg. This is the recommended intake value used by the FDA to calculate the %Daily Value for magnesium that may appear on food labels.

Details on magnesium's Tolerable Upper Intake Level (UL) are provided under the heading "Can You Consume Too Much Magnesium?"

## WHY WE NEED MAGNESIUM-RICH FOODS
Magnesium is usually referred to as a "macromineral," which means that our food must provide us with hundreds of milligrams of magnesium every day. Inside our bodies, magnesium is found mostly in our bones (60–65%), but is also concentrated in our muscles (25%), and in other cell types and body fluids. Like all minerals, magnesium cannot be made in our body and must therefore be plentiful in our diet in order for us to remain healthy. Magnesium is sometimes regarded as a "calming" mineral, since it has the ability to relax our muscles.

Eating foods rich in magnesium enhances your body's usage of this important mineral since these foods naturally contain other nutrients that act in synergy with magnesium, supporting its physiological function in your body and therefore contributing to your optimal health.

## HOW DOES MAGNESIUM PROMOTE HEALTH?
### Nerve and Muscle Relaxation
Magnesium acts together with calcium to help regulate the body's nerve and muscle tone. In many nerve cells, magnesium serves as a chemical gate blocker—as long as there is enough magnesium around, calcium can't rush into nerve cells and activate the nerve. This helps keep the nerve relaxed. If our diet provides us with too little magnesium, this gate blocking can fail, and the nerve cells can become overly activated, sending too many messages to the muscles and causing them to overcontract. This chain of events helps explain how magnesium deficiency can trigger muscle tension, soreness, spasms, cramps, and fatigue.

### Supports Bone Health
Magnesium plays a role in maintaining bone health with about two-thirds of all magnesium in our body found in our bones. The magnesium found in bone has two very different roles to play in our health. Some of it helps give bones their physical structure by being part of the bone's crystal lattice scaffolding, together with the minerals phosphorus and calcium. Bone's other reservoir of magnesium is found on its surface, and while it does not appear to be involved in the bone's structure, it does act as a storage site for magnesium that the body can draw upon in times of poor dietary supply.

### Other Health-Promoting Functions
Over 300 different enzymes, body proteins that trigger chemical reactions, require magnesium in order to function. For this reason, the functions of this mineral are especially diverse. It is involved in the metabolism of proteins, carbohydrates, and fats and also helps genes function properly. Some fuels cannot be stored in our muscle cells unless adequate supplies of magnesium are available. The metabolic roles of magnesium are so diverse that it is difficult to find a body system that is not affected by magnesium deficiency.

## WHAT ARE THE CAUSES AND SYMPTOMS OF MAGNESIUM DEFICIENCY?
In addition to poor dietary intake, problems in the digestive tract are the most common cause of magnesium deficiency. These digestive tract problems include malabsorption, diarrhea, and ulcerative colitis. Many kinds of physical stresses can contribute to magnesium deficiency, including cold, stress, physical trauma, and surgery.

Because magnesium plays such a wide variety of roles in the body, the symptoms of magnesium deficiency can also vary widely. Many symptoms involve changes in nerve and muscle function, including muscle weakness, tremor, and spasm. In the heart muscle, magnesium deficiency can result in arrhythmia, irregular contraction, and increased heart rate. Because of magnesium's role in bone structure, the softening and weakening of bone can also be a symptom of magnesium deficiency. Other symptoms can include: imbalanced blood sugar levels; headaches; elevated blood pressure; depression; and lack of appetite.

## CAN YOU CONSUME TOO MUCH MAGNESIUM?
There do not seem to be any toxicity symptoms associated with the intake of high amounts of magnesium from food, which is why the Institute of Medicine did not set a Tolerable Upper Intake Level (UL) for dietary magnesium. Alternatively, symptoms associated with high levels of magnesium from dietary supplements have been reported; the most common toxicity symptom associated with high levels of magnesium intake is diarrhea. The UL for magnesium from dietary supplements is 350 milligrams.

# manganese

Best Sources of Manganese from the *World's Healthiest Foods*

| FOOD | SERVING SIZE | CALS | AMOUNT (MG) | DV (%) | DENSITY | QUALITY |
|---|---|---|---|---|---|---|
| Cinnamon | 2 tsp | 12 | 0.8 | 38.0 | 57.8 | Excellent |
| Romaine lettuce | 2 cups | 16 | 0.7 | 35.5 | 40.8 | Excellent |
| Pineapple | 1 cup | 76 | 2.6 | 128.0 | 36.8 | Excellent |
| Spinach | 1 cup | 41 | 1.7 | 84.0 | 36.5 | Excellent |
| Turmeric | 2 tsp | 16 | 0.4 | 18.0 | 20.2 | Excellent |
| Black pepper | 2 tsp | 11 | 0.2 | 12.0 | 19.9 | Excellent |
| Collard greens | 1 cup | 49 | 1.1 | 53.5 | 19.5 | Excellent |
| Raspberries | 1 cup | 60 | 1.2 | 62.0 | 18.5 | Excellent |
| Swiss chard | 1 cup | 35 | 0.6 | 29.0 | 14.9 | Excellent |
| Kale | 1 cup | 36 | 0.5 | 27.0 | 13.4 | Excellent |
| Garlic | 1 oz-wt | 42 | 0.5 | 23.5 | 10.0 | Excellent |
| Grapes | 1 cup | 62 | 0.7 | 33.0 | 9.6 | Excellent |
| Summer squash | 1 cup | 36 | 0.4 | 19.0 | 9.5 | Excellent |
| Strawberries | 1 cup | 43 | 0.4 | 21.0 | 8.8 | Excellent |
| Oats | 1 cup | 145 | 1.4 | 68.5 | 8.5 | Excellent |
| Green beans | 1 cup | 44 | 0.4 | 18.5 | 7.6 | Excellent |
| Brown rice | 1 cup | 216 | 1.8 | 88.0 | 7.3 | Excellent |
| Garbanzo beans | 1 cup | 269 | 1.7 | 84.5 | 5.7 | Excellent |
| Tofu | 4 oz-wt | 86 | 0.7 | 34.5 | 7.2 | Very good |
| Broccoli | 1 cup | 44 | 0.3 | 17.0 | 7.0 | Very good |
| Wheat | 1 cup | 151 | 1.1 | 55.5 | 6.6 | Very good |
| Beets | 1 cup | 75 | 0.6 | 27.5 | 6.6 | Very good |
| Flaxseeds | 2 TBS | 95 | 1.3 | 64.0 | 6.0 | Very good |
| Crimini mushrooms | 5 oz-wt | 31 | 0.2 | 10.0 | 5.8 | Very good |
| Cauliflower | 1 cup | 29 | 0.2 | 8.5 | 5.4 | Very good |

* For more on "DV," "Density," and "Quality" Rating System, see page 805.

## FUNCTIONS

What can manganese-rich foods do for you?
- Protect your cells from free radical damage
- Keep your bones strong and healthy
- Maintain normal blood sugar levels
- Promote optimal function of your thyroid gland
- Maintain the health of your nerves
- Help your body synthesize cholesterol

What events can indicate a need for more manganese-rich foods?
- High blood sugar levels
- Excessive bone loss
- Low cholesterol levels
- Loss of hair color
- Skin rash
- Reproductive system difficulties

## IMPACT OF COOKING, STORAGE & PROCESSING

Significant amounts of manganese can be lost in food processing, especially in the milling of whole grains to produce flour, and in the cooking of beans. For example, three and one-half ounces of raw navy beans start out with about one milligram of manganese, which drops by 60% to 0.4 milligrams after cooking.

## PUBLIC HEALTH RECOMMENDATIONS

In 2000, the Institute of Medicine at the National Academy of Sciences issued new Adequate Intake (AI) levels for manganese. The recommendations are as follows:

- 0–6 months: 3 mcg
- 7–12 months: 600 mcg
- 1–3 years: 1.2 mg
- 4–8 years: 1.5 mg
- Males 9–13 years: 1.9 mg
- Males 14–18 years: 2.2 mg
- Males 19+ years: 2.3 mg
- Females 9–18 years: 1.6 mg
- Females 19+ years: 1.8 mg
- Pregnant or lactating females: 2 mg

The FDA has set the Reference Value for Nutrition Labeling for manganese at 2.0 mg. This is the recommended intake value used by the FDA to calculate the %Daily Value for manganese that may appear on food labels.

Details on manganese's Tolerable Upper Intake Level (UL) are provided under the heading "Can You Consume Too Much Manganese?"

## WHY WE NEED MANGANESE-RICH FOODS

Manganese, a trace mineral that participates in many enzyme systems in the body, was first considered an essential nutrient in 1931. Researchers discovered that experimental animals fed a diet deficient in manganese demonstrated poor growth and impaired reproduction. Manganese is found widely in nature, but occurs only in trace amounts in human tissues. Yet, while there may only be a relatively small amount in our bodies, manganese plays a vitally big role in maintaining our health through being a necessary cofactor of very important enzymes. Like other minerals, the body cannot make manganese, and so we must obtain this important mineral from our food.

Eating foods rich in manganese enhances your body's usage of this important mineral since these foods naturally contain other nutrients that act in synergy with manganese, supporting its physiological function in your body and therefore best contributing to your optimal health.

## HOW DOES MANGANESE PROMOTE HEALTH?
### Enzyme Activator

Manganese activates the enzymes responsible for the utilization of several key nutrients, including biotin, vitamin B1, vitamin C, and choline. It is a catalyst in the synthesis of fatty acids and cholesterol, facilitates protein and carbohydrate metabolism, and may also participate in the production of sex hormones and the maintenance of reproductive health.

In addition, manganese activates the enzymes that are important in the formation of bone. It has also been theorized that manganese is involved in the production of the thyroid hormone known as thyroxine and in maintaining the health of nerve tissue. Manganese is also a component of a variety of enzymes, playing a role in other physiological functions including blood sugar regulation.

Additionally, manganese-dependent *superoxide dismutase* (SOD) is an enzyme that has antioxidant activity and protects tissues from the damaging effects of free radicals. This enzyme is found exclusively inside the body's mitochondria (oxygen-based energy factories inside most of our cells).

## WHAT ARE THE CAUSES AND SYMPTOMS OF MANGANESE DEFICIENCY?

Poor dietary intake of manganese appears to be the most common cause of manganese deficiency. However, other factors can contribute to a need for more manganese. Like zinc, manganese is a mineral that can be excreted in significant amounts through sweat, and individuals who go through periods of excessive sweating may be at increased risk for deficiency.

Proper formation of bile in the liver and proper circulation of bile through the body are also required for manganese transport. As a result, individuals with chronic liver or gallbladder disorders may need more dietary manganese.

Because manganese plays a role in a variety of enzyme systems, dietary deficiency of manganese can impact many physiological processes. In humans, manganese deficiency is associated with poor glucose tolerance (high blood sugar levels), skin rash, loss of hair color, excessive bone loss, low cholesterol levels, and compromised function of the reproductive system. It is important to emphasize, however, that manganese deficiency is very rare in humans, and does not usually develop.

## CAN YOU CONSUME TOO MUCH MANGANESE?

Although symptoms of manganese toxicity do not typically appear even at high levels of dietary intake, in severe cases of excessive manganese consumption, individuals can develop a syndrome called "manganese madness," characterized by hallucinations, violent acts, and irritability. Overconsumption of manganese is also associated with impotency. Manganese toxicity is most likely to occur in people with chronic liver disease, as the liver plays an important role in eliminating excess manganese from the body.

The Institute of Medicine established Tolerable Upper Intake Levels (UL) for manganese. They are as follows: for those 1–3 years it is 2 mg; 4–8 years, 3 mg; 9–13 years, 6 mg; 14–18 years, including pregnant and lactating women, 9 mg; and, those older than 19 years, including pregnant and lactating women, 11 mg. It would be very unlikely for a meal plan to exceed these levels.

# niacin (vitamin b3)

Best Sources of Niacin from the *World's Healthiest Foods*

| FOOD | SERVING SIZE | CALS | AMOUNT (MG) | DV (%) | DENSITY | QUALITY |
|------|------|------|------|------|------|------|
| Crimini mushrooms | 5 oz-wt | 31 | 5.4 | 26.9 | 15.6 | Excellent |
| Tuna | 4 oz-wt | 158 | 13.5 | 67.7 | 7.7 | Excellent |
| Chicken | 4 oz-wt | 223 | 14.4 | 72.0 | 5.8 | Very good |
| Salmon | 4 oz-wt | 262 | 11.3 | 56.7 | 3.9 | Very good |
| Calf's liver | 4 oz-wt | 187 | 9.6 | 48.0 | 4.6 | Very good |
| Asparagus | 1 cup | 43 | 2.0 | 9.8 | 4.1 | Very good |
| Lamb | 4 oz-wt | 229 | 7.8 | 38.8 | 3.0 | Good |
| Turkey | 4 oz-wt | 214 | 7.2 | 36.1 | 3.0 | Good |
| Tomatoes | 1 cup | 38 | 1.1 | 5.6 | 2.7 | Good |
| Shrimp | 4 oz-wt | 112 | 2.9 | 14.7 | 2.4 | Good |
| Sardines | 4 oz-wt | 191 | 4.8 | 24.1 | 2.3 | Good |
| Summer squash | 1 cup | 36 | 0.9 | 4.6 | 2.3 | Good |
| Green peas | 1 cup | 134 | 3.2 | 16.1 | 2.2 | Good |
| Cod | 4 oz-wt | 119 | 2.8 | 14.1 | 2.1 | Good |
| Collard greens | 1 cup | 49 | 1.1 | 5.5 | 2.0 | Good |
| Peanuts | 0.25 cup | 207 | 4.4 | 22.0 | 1.9 | Good |
| Carrots | 1 cup | 53 | 1.1 | 5.6 | 1.9 | Good |
| Broccoli | 1 cup | 44 | 0.9 | 4.7 | 1.9 | Good |
| Spinach | 1 cup | 41 | 0.9 | 4.4 | 1.9 | Good |
| Eggplant | 1 cup | 28 | 0.6 | 3.0 | 1.9 | Good |
| Cauliflower | 1 cup | 25 | 0.5 | 2.6 | 1.9 | Good |
| Beef, grass-fed | 4 oz-wt | 240 | 4.4 | 22.2 | 1.7 | Good |
| Winter squash | 1 cup | 80 | 1.4 | 7.2 | 1.6 | Good |
| Raspberries | 1 cup | 60 | 1.1 | 5.5 | 1.6 | Good |
| Kale | 1. cup | 36 | 0.7 | 3.3 | 1.6 | Good |

\* For more on "DV," "Density," and "Quality" Rating System, see page 805.

## FUNCTIONS

What can niacin-rich foods do for you?
- Stabilize your blood sugar
- Support genetic processes in your cells
- Help lower cholesterol levels
- Help your body process fats

What events can indicate a need for more niacin-rich foods?
- Generalized or muscular weakness
- Digestive problems
- Skin infections
- Lack of appetite

## IMPACT OF COOKING, STORAGE & PROCESSING

Niacin is one of the more stable water-soluble vitamins and is minimally susceptible to damage by air, light, and heat.

## PUBLIC HEALTH RECOMMENDATIONS

In 1998, the Institute of Medicine at the National Academy of Sciences issued new Recommended Dietary Allowances (RDAs) for niacin. The recommendations are as follows:
- 0–6 months: 2 mg
- 6–12 months: 4 mg
- 1–3 years: 6 mg
- 4–8 years: 8 mg
- 9–13 years: 12 mg
- Males 14+ years: 16 mg
- Females 14+ years: 14 mg
- Pregnant females: 18 mg
- Lactating females: 17 mg

The FDA has set the Reference Value for Nutrition Labeling for niacin at 20 mg. This is the recommended intake value used by the FDA to calculate the %Daily Value for niacin that may appear on food labels.

Details on niacin's Tolerable Upper Intake Levels (UL) are provided under the heading "Can You Consume Too Much Niacin?"

## WHY WE NEED NIACIN-RICH FOODS

Niacin is a member of the B-complex vitamin family. The term "niacin" that is used interchangeably with vitamin B3 is actually a non-technical term that refers to several different chemical forms of the vitamin. These forms include nicotinic acid and nicotinamide (niacinamide).

Although niacin can be made in the body from the amino acid tryptophan, inadequate intake of many nutrients, including protein, iron, vitamins B1, B2, B6, and C, inhibits this conversion; therefore, it is recommended that people also ensure that they obtain adequate niacin from their diet. This is not difficult to do since many niacin-rich foods also contain the other nutrients necessary for niacin's production from tryptophan. Another reason getting your niacin from food is important is that most of these foods also contain vitamin B12, and a deficiency of this B vitamin can lead to increased excretion of niacin.

## HOW DOES NIACIN PROMOTE HEALTH?

### Energy Production

Like its fellow B-complex vitamins, niacin is important in energy production. Two unique forms of niacin (called nicotinamide adenine dinucleotide, or NAD, and nicotinamide adenine dinucleotide phosphate, or NADP) are essential for conversion of the body's proteins, fats, and carbohydrates into usable energy. Niacin is also used to synthesize starch that can be stored in the body's muscles and liver for eventual use as an energy source.

### Metabolism of Fats

Niacin plays a critical role in the chemical processing of fats in the body. The building blocks for fat-containing structures in the body (like cell membranes) typically require the presence of niacin for their synthesis, as do many fat-based steroid hormones.

### Support of Genetic Processes

Components of DNA, the primary genetic material in our cells, require niacin for their production; deficiency of niacin, like deficiency of other B-complex vitamins, has been directly linked to genetic (DNA) damage. The relationship between niacin and DNA damage appears to be particularly important in relationship to cancer and its prevention.

### Regulation of Insulin Activity

Although experts cannot agree on the precise mechanism though which niacin affects blood sugar regulation and function of the hormone insulin, the vitamin has repeatedly been shown to be involved in insulin metabolism and blood sugar regulation. Researchers continue to investigate the exact relationship between niacin, insulin, and blood sugar levels.

## WHAT ARE THE CAUSES AND SYMPTOMS of NIACIN DEFICIENCY?

Intestinal problems, including chronic diarrhea, inflammatory bowel disease, and irritable bowel disease can all trigger niacin deficiency. Because part of the body's supply comes from conversion of the amino acid tryptophan, deficiency of tryptophan can also increase risk of niacin deficiency. (Tryptophan deficiency is likely to occur in individuals with poor overall protein intake.) Physical trauma, all types of stress, long-term fever, and excessive consumption of alcohol have also been associated with increased risk of niacin deficiency.

Because of its unique relationship with energy production, niacin deficiency is often associated with general weakness, muscular weakness, and lack of appetite. Skin infections and digestive problems can also be associated with niacin deficiency.

## CAN YOU CONSUME TOO MUCH NIACIN?

In the amounts provided by food, no symptoms of toxicity have been reported in the scientific literature. The Institute of Medicine has set a Tolerable Upper Intake Level (UL) for niacin of 35 milligrams. This UL applies to men and women 19 years or older, and is limited to niacin that is obtained from supplements and/or fortified foods.

---

*Q I heard that anything fortified or enriched is bad for you. Is this true?*

A Enriched foods are not necessarily bad for you although some enriched foods are less than ideal. For example, let's look at white bread. It is made from wheat that is refined, stripped of many of its nutrients, and then has nutrients added back to it. I would much rather have bread made from whole wheat, where the nutrients you enjoy are those that are the original ones that were included in the wheat itself. Enrichment or fortification may not necessarily be bad, but philosophically I like to enjoy foods that just feature their natural compendium of nutrients, rather than those that feature nutrients that were either added back after they were removed, or added to a food but not naturally there in the first place.

# omega-3 fatty acids

Best Sources of Omega-3 Fatty Acids from the *World's Healthiest Foods*
Seafood sources (contain the omega-3 fatty acids EPA, DHA, and DPA in addition to ALA)

| FOOD | SERVING SIZE | CALS | AMOUNT (G) | DV (%) | DENSITY | QUALITY |
|------|------|------|------|------|------|------|
| Salmon | 4 oz-wt | 262 | 2.1 | 83.6 | 5.7 | Excellent |
| Scallops | 4 oz-wt | 152 | 1.1 | 44.0 | 5.2 | Very good |
| Sardines | 4 oz-wt | 191 | 1.4 | 54.4 | 5.1 | Very Good |
| Shrimp | 4 oz-wt | 112 | 0.4 | 14.8 | 2.4 | Good |
| Cod | 4 oz-wt | 119 | 0.3 | 12.8 | 1.9 | Good |
| Tuna | 4 oz-wt | 158 | 0.3 | 13.2 | 1.5 | Good |

\* For more on "DV," "Density," and "Quality" Rating System, see page 805.

Best Sources of Omega-3 Fatty Acids from the *World's Healthiest Foods*
Plant food sources (contain the omega-3 fatty acid ALA)

| FOOD | SERVING SIZE | CALS | AMOUNT (G) | DV (%) | DENSITY | QUALITY |
|------|------|------|------|------|------|------|
| Flaxseeds | 2 TBS | 95 | 3.5 | 140.4 | 26.6 | Excellent |
| Walnuts | 0.25 cup | 164 | 2.3 | 90.8 | 10.0 | Excellent |
| Cauliflower | 1 cup | 29 | 0.2 | 8.4 | 5.3 | Very good |
| Cabbage | 1 cup | 33 | 0.2 | 8.0 | 4.1 | Very good |
| Romaine lettuce | 2 cups | 16 | 0.1 | 3.2 | 3.7 | Good |
| Broccoli | 1 cup | 44 | 0.2 | 8.0 | 3.3 | Good |
| Brussels sprouts | 1 cup | 61 | 0.3 | 10.4 | 3.1 | Good |
| Winter squash | 1 cup | 80 | 0.3 | 13.6 | 3.1 | Good |
| Tofu | 4 oz-wt | 86 | 0.4 | 14.4 | 3.0 | Good |
| Summer squash | 1 cup | 36 | 0.2 | 6.0 | 3.0 | Good |
| Collard greens | 1 cup | 49 | 0.1 | 7.2 | 2.6 | Good |
| Spinach | 1 cup | 41 | 0.2 | 6.0 | 2.6 | Good |
| Kale | 1 cup | 36 | 0.1 | 5.2 | 2.6 | Good |
| Soybeans | 1 cup | 298 | 1.0 | 41.2 | 2.5 | Good |
| Strawberries | 1 cup | 43 | 0.1 | 4.4 | 1.8 | Good |
| Green beans | 1 cup | 44 | 0.1 | 4.4 | 1.8 | Good |

% DV of omega-3 fatty acids in 2 tsp of dried herbs and spices: Mustard seeds–8%

\* For more on "DV," "Density," and "Quality" Rating System, see page 805.

## FUNCTIONS

What can omega-3 fatty acid-rich foods do for you?
- Reduce inflammation throughout your body
- Keep your blood from clotting excessively
- Maintain the fluidity of your cell membranes

What events can indicate a need for more omega-3 fatty acid-rich foods?
- Depression
- Fatigue; inability to concentrate
- Dry, itchy skin; brittle hair and nails
- Joint pain

## IMPACT OF COOKING, STORAGE & PROCESSING

Omega-3 fatty acids are susceptible to damage from heat, light, and oxygen. When exposed to these elements for too long, they can become oxidized or rancid, which not only alters the flavor and smell of the oil, but also diminishes its nutritional value. In addition, the oxidation of fatty acids produces free radicals, which are believed to play a role in the development of cancer and other degenerative diseases.

## PUBLIC HEALTH RECOMMENDATIONS

In 2002, the Institute of Medicine at the National Academy of Sciences issued Adequate Intake (AI) levels for linolenic acid, the initial building block for all omega-3 fatty acids found in the body. For male teenagers and adult men, 1.6 grams per day were recommended. For female teenagers and adult women, the recommended amount was 1.1 grams per day. These guidelines do not seem as well-matched to the existing health research on omega-3 fatty acids as guidelines issued by the "Workshop on the Essentiality of and Recommended Dietary Intakes (RDI) for Omega-6 and Omega-3 Fatty Acids" in 1999 sponsored by the National Institutes of Health (NIH). This panel of experts recommended that people consume at least 1.2% of their total daily calories as omega-3 fats. To meet this recommendation, a person consuming 1,800 calories per day should eat sufficient omega-3-rich foods to provide at least 2.5 grams of omega-3 fatty acids.

## WHY WE NEED OMEGA-3-RICH FOODS

Omega-3 fatty acids are a type of polyunsaturated fat whose importance in health promotion and disease prevention cannot be overstated. The three most nutritionally important omega-3 fatty acids are alpha-linolenic acid, (ALA), eicosapentaenoic acid (EPA) and docosahexaenoic acid (DHA).

ALA is classified as "essential" because the body is unable to manufacture it on its own and because it plays a fundamental role in several physiological functions. The body can convert ALA into EPA and DHA; however, this conversion can be limited, with less than one-third of the ALA being converted into the EPA and DHA forms. For this reason vegans and vegetarians relying on ALA as their only source of omega-3 fatty acids should increase their consumption of ALA-rich foods accordingly to ensure sufficient production of its important derivatives, EPA and DHA.

EPA and DHA can also be derived directly from certain foods, most notably cold-water fish including salmon, tuna and sardines. In addition, certain types of algae contain DHA. Omega-3 fatty acids are believed to play a role in the prevention of cardiovascular disease, while DHA, in particular, is necessary for proper brain and nerve development.

By getting your omega-3 fatty acids from whole food sources, you will gain the benefit of nature's wisdom. Most omega-3 rich foods also contain vitamin E, which serves to protect the fats from oxidation, a chemical process that produces free radicals.

## HOW DO OMEGA-3 FATTY ACIDS PROMOTE HEALTH?
### Sustain Healthy Cells
Diets rich in omega-3 fats produce cell membranes with a high degree of fluidity, therefore promoting optimal functioning of the cells. In addition to their ability to receive nutrients and effectively remove wastes, a healthy membrane promotes the ability of a cell to communicate with other cells. Researchers believe that loss of cell-to-cell communication is one of the physiological events that leads to growth of cancerous tumors. Recent *in vitro* (test tube) evidence suggests that when omega-3 fatty acids are incorporated into cell membranes, they may help to protect against cancer, notably of the breast.

### Prostaglandin Production

Omega-3 fats play an important role in the production of prostaglandins, powerful hormone-like substances that regulate many important physiological functions, including blood pressure, blood clotting, nerve transmission, the inflammatory and allergic responses, the functions of the kidneys and gastrointestinal tract, and the production of other hormones.

For example, EPA and DHA serve as direct precursors for series-3 prostaglandins, which have been called "good" or "beneficial" because they reduce platelet aggregation, reduce inflammation and improve blood flow. The role of EPA and DHA in the prevention of cardiovascular disease can be explained in large part by the ability of these fats to increase the production of favorable prostaglandins.

## WHAT ARE THE CAUSES AND SYMPTOMS of OMEGA-3 FATTY ACID DEFICIENCY?

Recent statistics indicate that nearly 99% of people in the United States do not eat enough omega-3 fatty acids. In addition, in some people, the enzymes that convert ALA to EPA and DHA are underactive, so they are not able to optimally convert ALA to EPA and DHA. To increase the efficacy of this conversion, be sure that your diet includes a sufficient amounts of vitamin B6, vitamin B3, vitamin C, magnesium and zinc, cofactors of conversion enzymes. In addition, limit your intake of saturated fat and partially hydrogenated fat, as these compounds are known to decrease the activity of the conversion enzymes.

Since the symptoms of omega-3 fatty acid deficiency are very vague and can often be attributed to some other health condition or nutrient deficiencies, few people (or their physicians, for that matter) realize that they are not consuming enough omega-3 fatty acids. The symptoms of omega-3 fatty acid deficiency include fatigue, dry and/or itchy skin, brittle hair and nails, constipation, frequent colds, depression, poor concentration, lack of physical endurance, and/or joint pain.

## CAN YOU CONSUME TOO MUCH OMEGA-3 FATTY ACIDS?

In its 2002 guidelines for omega-3 fatty acid intake, the Institute of Medicine at the National Academy of Sciences declined to establish a Tolerable Upper Intake Level (UL) for omega-3s. However, research was cited showing increased risk of bleeding and hemorrhagic stroke in a few studies following supplementation with omega-3s.

Excessive consumption of omega-3 fatty acids from food sources has not known to cause any health problems.

# pantothenic acid (vitamin B5)

Best Sources of Pantothenic Acid from the *World's Healthiest Foods*

| FOOD | SERVING SIZE | CALS | AMOUNT (MG) | DV (%) | DENSITY | QUALITY |
|------|------|------|------|------|------|------|
| Crimini mushrooms | 5 oz-wt | 31 | 2.1 | 21.3 | 12.3 | Excellent |
| Cauliflower | 1 cup | 29 | 0.6 | 6.3 | 4.0 | Very good |
| Broccoli | 1 cup | 44 | 0.8 | 7.9 | 3.3 | Good |
| Calf's liver | 4 oz-wt | 187 | 2.6 | 25.9 | 2.5 | Good |
| Sunflower seeds | 0.25 cup | 205 | 2.4 | 24.3 | 2.1 | Good |
| Tomatoes | 1 cup | 38 | 0.4 | 4.4 | 2.1 | Good |
| Strawberries | 1 cup | 43 | 0.5 | 4.9 | 2.0 | Good |
| Yogurt | 1 cup | 155 | 1.5 | 14.5 | 1.7 | Good |
| Eggs | 1 each | 68 | 0.6 | 6.2 | 1.6 | Good |
| Winter squash | 1 cup | 80 | 0.7 | 7.2 | 1.6 | Good |
| Collard greens | 1 cup | 49 | 0.4 | 4.1 | 1.5 | Good |
| Swiss chard | 1 cup | 35 | 0.3 | 2.9 | 1.5 | Good |
| Corn | 1 cup | 177 | 1.4 | 14.4 | 1.5 | Good |

\* For more on "DV," "Density," and "Quality" Rating System, see page 805.

## FUNCTIONS

What can pantothenic acid-rich foods do for you?
- Help turn carbohydrates and fats into usable energy
- Improve your ability to respond to stress by supporting your adrenal glands
- Assure adequate production of healthy fats in your cells

What events can indicate a need for more pantothenic acid-rich foods?
- Fatigue, listlessness
- Sensations of weakness
- Numbness, tingling, and burning/shooting pain in the feet

## IMPACT OF COOKING, STORAGE & PROCESSING

Pantothenic acid is relatively unstable in food, and significant amounts of this vitamin can be lost through cooking, freezing, and commercial processing. For example, research on frozen foods has shown a loss of 21–70% for pantothenic acid in meats and similar losses for processed cereal grains and canned vegetables. Fruits and fruit juices lose 7–50% of their pantothenic acid during processing and packaging.

## PUBLIC HEALTH RECOMMENDATIONS

In 1998, the Institute of Medicine at the National Academy of Sciences issued new Adequate Intake (AI) levels for pantothenic acid. The recommendations are as follows:
- 0–6 months: 1.7 mg
- 6–12 months: 1.8 mg
- 1–3 years: 2 mg
- 4–8 years: 3 mg
- Males 9–13 years: 4 mg
- Males 14+ years: 5 mg
- Females 9–13 years: 4 mg
- Females 14+ years: 5 mg
- Pregnant females: 6 mg
- Lactating females: 7 mg

The FDA has set the Reference Value for Nutrition Labeling for panthothenic acid at 10 mg. This is the recommended intake value used by the FDA to calculate the %Daily Value for panthothenic acid that may appear on food labels.

Details on pantothenic acid's Tolerable Upper Intake Level (UL) are provided under the heading "Can You Consume Too Much Pantothenic Acid?"

## WHY WE NEED PANTOTHENIC ACID-RICH FOODS

Pantothenic acid, also known as vitamin B5, is a member of the B-complex family of vitamins first researched in the 1930–1940s. The name of the vitamin comes from the Greek word *pantos*, meaning "everywhere." The vitamin's name reflects its almost universal presence in nature; it is found in virtually all types of food.

Nutrients such as folate, biotin, and vitamin B12 are required for proper use of pantothenic acid in the body's metabolic pathways, while vitamin C is necessary for preventing B5 deficiency. Foods that feature pantothenic acid also feature these important vitamins as well.

In its metabolically active form, pantothenic acid gets combined with another small, sulfur-containing molecule to form coenzyme A (or simply, CoA). This conversion allows pantothenic acid to participate in a wide variety of chemical reactions.

Eating foods rich in panthothenic acid enhances your body's usage of this important vitamin since these foods naturally contain other nutrients that act in synergy with pantothenic acid, supporting its physiological function in your body and therefore contributing to your optimal health.

## HOW DOES PANTOTHENIC ACID PROMOTE HEALTH?
### Energy Production
When found in its CoA form, pantothenic acid plays a pivotal role in helping release energy from sugars, starches, and fats. Most of this energy release occurs in the energy production factories found in every cell called the mitochondria. Increased levels of pantothenic acid in the blood of marathon runners, for example, has led to interest in this vitamin as a potential aid in physical training, where sustained energy release from the mitochondria is critical.

### Production of Fats
While the CoA form of pantothenic acid is important for releasing energy stored as fat, it is equally important for the creation of important fat-containing molecules. Two basic types of fats—fatty acids and cholesterol—both require the CoA form of pantothenic acid for their synthesis. Sphingosine, a fat-like molecule that is constantly involved in the delivery of chemical messages inside our cells, also requires pantothenic acid for its synthesis.

### Changing the Shape and Function of Proteins
Sometimes it is important for the body to make small chemical changes in the shape of cell proteins. For example, if a cell does not want its proteins to be chemically broken down into other substances, it may want to modify their structure in order to prevent this chemical breakdown. One way for cells to accomplish this task is to attach acetyl chemical groups to proteins. Pantothenic acid in the form of CoA, can be used to help acetylate proteins, thereby protecting them from chemical breakdown. Additionally, sometimes this chemical process can dramatically change the function of a protein. For example, sometimes the acetylation of a protein can pave the way for its conversion into a hormone. This process is especially well researched in relationship to the body's adrenal glands, where stress-related hormone production requires participation of pantothenic acid.

## WHAT ARE THE CAUSES AND SYMPTOMS OF PANTOTHENIC ACID DEFICIENCY?
In addition to poor dietary intake, digestive problems are the most common contributing factor to pantothenic acid deficiency. The reason for this connection between poor digestion and pantothenic acid deficiency involves the CoA form of pantothenic acid which is typically found in food. Proper digestion is required to release pantothenic acid from this CoA form and allow it to be absorbed into the body from the small intestine.

Because pantothenic acid is needed to release energy from carbohydrates and fats, its deficiency is often related to low energy-related symptoms. These symptoms include fatigue, listlessness, and sensations of weakness. One rare symptom of pantothenic acid deficiency is called "burning foot syndrome." In this condition, numbness and tingling, together with burning and shooting pain, in the feet occurs.

## CAN YOU CONSUME TOO MUCH PANTOTHENIC ACID?
The amount of pantothenic acid available in food is not likely to be associated with any adverse events. In addition, because no other toxicity symptoms have been reported in the research literature, no Tolerable Upper Intake Level (UL) was established by the Institute of Medicine for pantothenic acid in its 1998 report on this vitamin.

---

## Q *Are there foods that are bad for my immune system?*

A Your immune system is not just involved in fighting invaders like bacteria, but also becomes activated when you eat foods to which you are intolerant or allergic. Reactions to allergic foods can be quick, like the anaphylactic reaction often seen with peanut or shellfish allergies, but food allergy reactions can also be delayed and cause a number of symptoms like headaches, fatigue, muscle aches, rashes and other systemic (whole body) effects. The most common allergenic foods include peanuts, shellfish, cow's milk, wheat, and soy; however, everyone is unique in their food intolerances and allergies.

Processed foods and foods produced with pesticides or not grown organically may also be problematic for your immune function. Toxic metals such as cadmium, lead and mercury are immunosuppressive. Some pesticides and preservatives can negatively affect the gastrointestinal lining. Excess sugar can also cause stress on the immune system.

# phytoestrogens

## ISOFLAVONE CONTENT OF FOODS (MG/100 GRAMS)

| | DAIDZEIN (MG) | GENISTEIN (MG) | GLYCITEIN (MG) | COUMESTEROL (MG) | FORMONONETIN (MG) | BIOCHANIN A (MG) |
|---|---|---|---|---|---|---|
| Natto (fermented soybeans) | 21.85 | 29.04 | 8.17 | n/a | n/a | n/a |
| Tempeh | 19.25 | 31.55 | 2.2 | n/a | n/a | n/a |
| Miso | 16.13 | 24.56 | 2.87 | n/a | n/a | n/a |
| Tofu | 9.44 | 13.35 | 2.08 | n/a | n/a | n/a |
| Soybeans, raw | 46.64 | 73.64 | 10.88 | 0.05 | 0.07 | 0.01 |
| Soy milk | 4.45 | 6.06 | 0.56 | n/a | n/a | n/a |
| Split peas, raw | 2.42 | 0 | n/a | 0 | 0 | 0.86 |
| Pinto beans, raw | 0.01 | 0.26 | n/a | 3.61 | trace | 0.56 |
| Peanuts | 0.03 | 0.24 | n/a | 0 | 0.01 | 0.01 |
| Navy beans, raw | 0.01 | 0.2 | n/a | 0 | 0 | 0 |
| Garbonzo beans, raw | 0.04 | 0.06 | n/a | 0 | 0 | 1.52 |
| Kidney beans, raw | 0.02 | 0.04 | n/a | 0 | 0.01 | trace |
| Green tea | 0.01 | 0.04 | n/a | 0.03 | n/a | n/a |
| Lima beans, raw | 0.02 | 0.01 | n/a | 0 | 0.01 | 0 |
| Lentils, raw | 0 | 0 | n/a | 0 | 0.01 | 0 |
| Black beans, raw | 0 | 0 | n/a | n/a | n/a | n/a |
| Green beans, cooked | 0 | 0 | n/a | 0 | trace | trace |
| Sunflower seeds | 0 | 0 | n/a | trace | 0.03 | trace |
| Flaxseeds | 0 | 0 | n/a | n/a | n/a | n/a |

U.S. Department of Agriculture, Agricultural Research Service, 2002. USDA-Iowa State University Database on the Isoflavone Content of Foods, Release 1.3–2002.
Nutrient Data Laboratory Web site: http://www.nal.usda.gov/fnic/foodcomp/Data/isoflav/isoflav.html

## INTRODUCTION

The diets of many traditional cultures throughout the world, including those of Asia and the Mediterranean region, feature plant-based foods rich in unique nutrients known as phytoestrogens. Isoflavones and lignans are the two best-studied groups of phytoestrogenic phytonutrients.

In Asia, the prominent phytoestrogens are the isoflavones found in soy foods such as soybeans, tofu, tempeh and miso as well as the lignans found in the sea vegetables. In the Mediterranean region, these isoflavone and lignan phytoestrogens are supplied by numerous foods including the legumes, seeds and vegetables that make up a significant portion of the traditional diet. Researchers suggest that phytoestrogenic nutrients help to explain part of the reason that these diets are associated with a reduced risk of certain diseases.

## WHAT ARE PHYTOESTROGENS?

The term phytoestrogen reflects the ability of these plant ("phyto") compounds to act as weak estrogenic compounds, helping to balance hormonal levels in the body.

Phytoestrogens are structurally similar to the mammalian estrogen hormone, estradiol, and can bind to estrogen receptors in the body; yet, they are thought of as having weak estrogenic activity, exhibiting only a fraction of that of estradiol. Phytoestrogens may help to balance estrogen levels, with the ability to either exert estrogenic activity if body levels of estrogen are low or anti-estrogenic activity if body levels are high.

Dietary phytoestrogen intake has been associated with reduced risk of various diseases including breast and prostate cancer. They are also suggested to be of benefit to women during times when they are experiencing fluctuating estrogen levels, such as during menopause.

## PHYTOESTROGENS IN THE DIET

Like all foods, those containing phytoestrogens are not "magic bullets" and need to be incorporated into a person's overall meal plan in a balanced and logical way. I believe that they need to be eaten in moderation like all foods.

While both isoflavones and lignans act as phytoestrogens, they each have unique properties and for most people, a healthy diet should include food sources of both. How much a person should eat would depend upon their unique health needs, but if we look at the research we can find some general recommendations.

Currently, no public health organizations in the U.S. have issued recommended daily intake levels for phytoestrogens or lignans. In Japan, a culture where the benefits of soyfoods, the most concentrated dietary source of isoflavones, have been well studied, the average intake was 50–70 total grams per day in 1995. This would translate into 2 ounces per day, an amount that is by no means daunting (the soyfoods need not be eaten every day to gain benefit as you could use 14 ounces per week as a dietary goal as well). While studies have shown therapeutic benefits of flaxseeds at ranges from 10–50 grams, most healthcare practitioners recommend 1–2 tablespoons of ground flaxseed daily for general wellness.

### Other sources of phytoestrogens

In addition to food sources of phytoestrogens, there are herbs that are concentrated in these important phytonutrients, and which are used by many women while they move through menopause. These herbs include red clover and black cohosh*.

### ISOFLAVONES

The chart on the previous page reflects the World's Healthiest Foods most concentrated in isoflavones. Daidzein and genistein are the most studied in terms of their phytoestrogenic properties. Glycetein, coumesterol, formononetin and biochanin A are also important isoflavones with health-promoting properties.

### LIGNANS

The chart on this page reflects the World's Healthiest Foods most concentrated in phytoestrogenic lignans. These lignans include secoisolariciresinol, maitiresinol and pinoresinol. They are converted in the body into the enterolignans-enterolactone and enterodiol, which act as weak estrogens to help balance the body's hormonal level (enterolignans are also known as mammalian lignans). Currently, the most thorough examination of the lignan content of foods has been to measure the amount of enterolignans into which they are converted.

## ENTEROLIGNAN PRODUCTION OF FOODS (MCG/100 GRAMS)

|  | ENTEROLACTONE/ENTERODIOL PRODUCTION (MCG) |
|---|---|
| Flaxseeds | 67,541 |
| Lentils, raw | 1,787 |
| Soybeans, raw | 1,130 |
| Sea vegetables (hijiki) | 653 |
| Kidney beans | 561 |
| Wheat | 490 |
| Navy beans | 460 |
| Garlic | 407 |
| Sunflower seeds | 396 |
| Asparagus | 374 |
| Carrots | 346 |
| Oats | 340 |
| Brown rice | 297 |
| Sweet potatoes | 295 |
| Corn | 230 |
| Broccoli | 226 |
| Pinto beans | 201 |
| Bell peppers | 195 |
| Pears | 181 |
| Peanuts | 161 |
| Rye | 160 |
| Plums | 145 |
| Cauliflower | 135 |
| Beets | 135 |
| Green peas | 122 |
| Onions | 112 |

Adapted from: Thompson LU, Robb P, Serran M, Cheung F. Mammalian Lignan Production from Various Foods. Nutr Cancer 1991;16:43-52.
Note: Food weight based upon uncooked samples.

* Standardized supplements of red clover generally contain 40 mg total isoflavones per tablet with most research studies investigating efficacy of these supplements providing approximately 80 mg isoflavones. In addition to isoflavones such as formononetin, black cohosh contains other phytonutrients such as triterpene glycosides (e.g. acetin).

# potassium

Best Sources of Potassium from the *World's Healthiest Foods*

| FOOD | SERVING SIZE | CALS | AMOUNT (MG) | DV (%) | DENSITY | QUALITY |
|---|---|---|---|---|---|---|
| Swiss chard | 1 cup | 35 | 960.8 | 27.4 | 14.1 | Excellent |
| Crimini mushrooms | 5 oz-wt | 31 | 635.0 | 18.1 | 10.5 | Excellent |
| Spinach | 1 cup | 41 | 838.8 | 24.0 | 10.4 | Excellent |
| Romaine lettuce | 2 cup | 16 | 324.8 | 9.3 | 10.7 | Very good |
| Celery | 1 cup | 19 | 344.4 | 9.8 | 9.2 | Very good |
| Broccoli | 1 cup | 44 | 505.4 | 14.4 | 6.0 | Very good |
| Winter squash | 1 cup | 80 | 895.9 | 25.6 | 5.8 | Very good |
| Tomatoes | 1 cup | 38 | 399.6 | 11.4 | 5.4 | Very good |
| Collard greens | 1 cup | 49 | 494.0 | 14.1 | 5.1 | Very good |
| Summer squash | 1 cup | 36 | 345.6 | 9.9 | 4.9 | Very good |
| Eggplant | 1 cup | 28 | 245.5 | 7.0 | 4.6 | Very good |
| Cantaloupe | 1 cup | 56 | 494.4 | 14.1 | 4.5 | Very good |
| Green beans | 1 cup | 44 | 373.8 | 10.7 | 4.4 | Very good |
| Brussels sprouts | 1 cup | 61 | 494.5 | 14.1 | 4.2 | Very good |
| Kale | 1 cup | 36 | 296.4 | 8.5 | 4.2 | Very good |
| Carrots | 1 cup | 53 | 394.1 | 11.3 | 3.9 | Very good |
| Beets | 1 cup | 75 | 518.5 | 14.8 | 3.6 | Very good |
| Papaya | 1 each | 119 | 781.3 | 22.3 | 3.4 | Very good |
| Asparagus | 1 cup | 43 | 288.0 | 8.2 | 3.4 | Very good |
| Basil | 2 tsp | 8 | 103.0 | 2.9 | 7.0 | Good |
| Cucumbers | 1 cup | 14 | 149.8 | 4.3 | 5.7 | Good |
| Turmeric | 2 tsp | 16 | 114.5 | 3.3 | 3.7 | Good |
| Bell peppers | 1 cup | 25 | 162.8 | 4.7 | 3.4 | Good |
| Cauliflower | 1 cup | 29 | 176.1 | 5.0 | 3.2 | Good |
| Apricots | 1 each | 17 | 103.6 | 3.0 | 3.2 | Good |

\* For more on "DV," "Density," and "Quality" Rating System, see page 805.

## FUNCTIONS

What can potassium-rich foods do for you?
- Help your muscles and nerves function properly
- Help lower your risk of high blood pressure
- Maintain the proper electrolyte and acid-base balance in your body
- Help maintain calcium levels

What events can indicate a need for more potassium-rich foods?
- Muscle weakness
- Confusion
- Irritability
- Fatigue
- Heart problems
- Chronic diarrhea
- Regular, intense exercise
- Use of certain diuretics

## IMPACT OF COOKING, STORAGE & PROCESSING

Potassium losses from cooking of high-potassium foods can be significant. In the case of spinach, for example, potassium levels have been shown to drop 56% after blanching for several minutes.

Sometimes this passage of potassium out of foods can be nutritionally beneficial. For example, parsley tea often contains significant amounts of potassium because this mineral is leached out of the parsley leaves and into the hot tea water.

## PUBLIC HEALTH RECOMMENDATIONS

In 2004, the Institute of Medicine at the National Academy of Sciences issued new Adequate Intake (AI) levels for potas-

sium. The recommendations are as follows:
- 0–6 months: 400 mg
- 6–12 months: 700 mg
- 1–3 years: 3,500 mg
- 4–8 years: 3,800 mg
- 9–18 years: 4,500 mg
- 14–18 years: 4,700 mg
- 19+ years: 4,700 mg
- Pregnant women: 4,700 mg
- Lactating women: 5,100 mg

The FDA has set the Reference Value for Nutrition Labeling for potassium at 3,500 mg. This is the recommended intake value used by the FDA to calculate the %Daily Value for potassium that may appear on food labels.

Details on potassium's Tolerable Upper Intake Level (UL) are provided under the heading "Can You Consume Too Much Potassium?"

## WHY WE NEED POTASSIUM-RICH FOODS

Potassium plays a critically important role in health. It is an electrolyte, which means that it conducts electricity when dissolved in water. Since the body is mostly water and many physiological functions are "sparked" by this energy potential, potassium fulfills many important roles. The balance between potassium and another electrolyte, sodium, is extremely important for maintaining cellular health. The over-consumption of sodium in our diets is just another reason supporting the need to consume potassium-rich foods, an easy recommendation to follow if your diet is rich in the World's Healthiest Foods since fruits and vegetables are very concentrated sources of potassium.

Potassium is especially important in the activity of muscles and nerves. The degree to which our muscles contract and our nerves become excitable both depend heavily on the presence of potassium in the right amount.

Potassium's ability to decrease calcium excretion is yet another reason for the importance of potassium-rich foods. Since many factors in the modern diet (including excess protein and caffeine consumption) increase calcium excretion, consuming potassium-rich fruits and vegetables may be helpful in maintaining the density and strength of your bones.

Eating foods rich in potassium enhances your body's usage of this important mineral since these foods naturally contain other nutrients that act in synergy with potassium, supporting its physiological function in your body and therefore contributing to your optimal health.

## HOW DOES POTASSIUM PROMOTE HEALTH?
### Muscle Contraction and Nerve Transmission

Potassium plays an important role in muscle contraction and nerve transmission. Many of our muscle and nerve cells have specialized channels for moving potassium in and out of the cell. Sometimes potassium moves freely in and out, and sometimes a special energy-driven pump is required. When the movement of potassium is blocked, or

when potassium is deficient in the diet, activity of both muscles and nerves can become compromised.

### Other Health-Promoting Functions

Potassium is involved in the storage of carbohydrates for use by muscles as fuel. It is also important in maintaining the body's proper electrolyte and acid-base (pH) balance. Potassium may also counteract the increased urinary calcium loss caused by the high-salt diets typical of many people, thus helping to prevent bones from thinning out at an increased rate.

## WHAT ARE THE CAUSES AND SYMPTOMS OF POTASSIUM DEFICIENCY?

In addition to poor dietary intake, overuse of muscles, as might occur in excessive physical activity, is a factor that can increase a person's need for potassium. Any events that draw excessive fluid out of the body—including excessive sweating, diarrhea, overuse of diuretics (including caffeine-containing beverages), poor water intake, or adherence to a ketogenic diet—can increase the need for potassium.

Since potassium functions in close cooperation with sodium, imbalanced intake of salt (sodium chloride) can also increase a person's need for potassium. Higher amounts of potassium are also needed by persons with high blood pressure.

Since potassium occurs naturally in a wide variety of foods, dietary deficiency of potassium is uncommon. However, if you experience excessive fluid loss through vomiting, diarrhea or sweating, or if you take certain medications, you may be at risk for potassium deficiency.

In addition, a diet that is high in sodium and low in potassium can negatively impact potassium status. The typical American diet, which is high in sodium-containing processed foods and low in fruits and vegetables, contains about two times more sodium than potassium; many health experts recommend taking in at least five times more potassium than sodium.

The symptoms of potassium deficiency include muscle weakness, confusion, irritability, fatigue, and heart disturbances. Athletes with low potassium stores may tire more easily during exercise, as potassium deficiency causes a decrease in the storage of glycogen, the fuel used by exercising muscles.

## CAN YOU CONSUME TOO MUCH POTASSIUM?

The Institute of Medicine did not establish a Tolerable Upper Intake Level (UL) for potassium. They noted that there have been no documented adverse effects of excessive consumption of potassium from food sources alone. They did note, however, that adverse effects have been documented for excess potassium from dietary supplements and salt substitutes, notably for those with kidney disease or diabetes.

# protein

Best Sources of Protein from the *World's Healthiest Foods*

| FOOD | SERVING SIZE | CALS | AMOUNT (G) | DV (%) | DENSITY | QUALITY |
|---|---|---|---|---|---|---|
| Cod | 4 oz-wt | 119 | 26.0 | 52.1 | 7.9 | Excellent |
| Tuna | 4 oz-wt | 158 | 34.0 | 68.0 | 7.8 | Excellent |
| Shrimp | 4 oz-wt | 112 | 23.7 | 47.4 | 7.6 | Excellent |
| Venison | 4 oz-wt | 179 | 34.3 | 68.5 | 6.9 | Very good |
| Turkey | 4 oz-wt | 214 | 32.6 | 65.1 | 5.5 | Very good |
| Scallops | 4 oz-wt | 152 | 23.1 | 46.2 | 5.5 | Very good |
| Chicken | 4 oz-wt | 223 | 33.8 | 67.6 | 5.4 | Very good |
| Beef, grass-fed | 4 oz-wt | 240 | 32.0 | 64.1 | 4.8 | Very good |
| Lamb | 4 oz-wt | 229 | 30.2 | 60.3 | 4.7 | Very good |
| Calf's liver | 4 oz-wt | 187 | 24.5 | 49.1 | 4.7 | Very good |
| Spinach | 1 cup | 41 | 5.4 | 10.7 | 4.7 | Very good |
| Sardines | 4 oz-wt | 191 | 22.7 | 45.3 | 4.2 | Very good |
| Crimini mushrooms | 5 oz-wt | 31 | 3.5 | 7.1 | 4.1 | Very good |
| Salmon | 4 oz-wt | 262 | 29.1 | 58.3 | 4.0 | Very good |
| Asparagus | 1 cup | 43 | 4.7 | 9.3 | 3.9 | Very good |
| Tofu | 4 oz-wt | 86 | 9.2 | 18.3 | 3.8 | Very good |
| Broccoli | 1 cup | 44 | 4.7 | 9.3 | 3.8 | Very good |
| Soybeans | 1 cup | 398 | 28.6 | 57.2 | 3.5 | Very good |
| Cheese, low-fat | 1 oz-wt | 72 | 6.9 | 13.8 | 3.4 | Very good |
| Swiss chard | 1 cup | 35 | 3.3 | 6.6 | 3.4 | Very good |
| Yogurt | 1 cup | 155 | 12.9 | 25.7 | 3.0 | Good |
| Eggs | 1 each | 68 | 5.5 | 11.1 | 2.9 | Good |
| Collard greens | 1 cup | 49 | 4.0 | 8.0 | 2.9 | Good |
| Cauliflower | 1 cup | 29 | 2.3 | 4.6 | 2.9 | Good |
| Lentils | 1 cup | 230 | 17.9 | 35.7 | 2.8 | Good |

%DVs are based on FDA's Reference Value for Nutrition Labeling for protein.

## FUNCTIONS

What can protein-rich foods do for you?
- Keep your immune system functioning properly
- Maintain healthy skin, hair and nails
- Help your body produce enzymes

What events can indicate a need for more protein-rich foods?
- Weight loss; muscle wasting
- Fatigue and weakness
- Frequent infections
- Slow growth and development in children

## IMPACT OF COOKING, STORAGE & PROCESSING

Overcooking foods containing protein can destroy heat sensitive amino acids (for example, lysine) or make the protein resistant to digestive enzymes.

## PUBLIC HEALTH RECOMMENDATION

In 2002, the Institute of Medicine at the National Academy of Sciences set Adequate Intake (AI) levels for infants 0–6 months of age and Recommended Dietary Allowances (RDAs) for protein for all age groups 7 months and older. The recommendations are as follows:
- 0–6 months: 9.1 g
- 6 months to 1 year: 13.5 g
- 1–3 years: 13 g
- 4–8 years: 19 g
- 9–13 years: 34 g
- Males 14–18 years: 52 g
- Males 19+ years: 56 g
- Females 14+ years: 46 g
- Pregnant and lactating women: 71 g

The FDA has set the Reference Value for Nutrition Labeling for protein at 50 g. This is the recommended intake value used by the FDA to calculate the %Daily Value for protein that may appear on food labels.

The Institute of Medicine did not establish a Tolerable Upper Intake Level (UL) for protein.

## WHY WE NEED PROTEIN-RICH FOODS

Protein was the first substance to be recognized as a vital part of living tissue. In fact, the word protein comes from the Greek word *proteos*, which means "primary" or "taking first place," indicating the importance of this nutrient in the function of the body. Accounting for 20 percent of our body weight, proteins perform a wide variety of functions throughout the body as vital components of body tissues, enzymes, and immune cells.

Proteins are complex molecules comprised of a combination of different amino acids, which are compounds that contain carbon, oxygen, hydrogen, nitrogen and sometimes sulfur. Amino acids link together in specific numbers and unique combinations to make each different protein. Protein is an essential component of the diet because it provides the amino acids that the body needs to synthesize its own proteins.

Proteins can carry certain nutrients (such as iron and vitamin A); therefore, inadequate protein intake may impair the function of many nutrients.

There are nine essential amino acids that we must receive from our food as our bodies cannot synthesize them on their own. Individual foods were not meant to provide us with a complete set of these essential amino acids, rather they were meant to be combined into diets and cuisines that functioned as a whole to provide all essential amino acids. Therefore, it's important to eat a wide array of protein-containing foods to ensure you meet the spectrum of your amino acid needs

## HOW DOES PROTEIN PROMOTE HEALTH?
### Provides Energy and Maintains Body Structure

Protein, providing four calories per gram, is an important source of energy for the body when carbohydrates and fats are not available. The body also uses the amino acids contained in proteins to manufacture its own proteins, including several structural proteins. Examples include myosin, actin, collagen, elastin and keratin: proteins that maintain the strength and integrity of muscles, connective tissues (ligaments and tendons), hair, skin, and nails.

### Other Health-Promoting Functions

In addition to using protein to generate energy for cellular function whenever necessary and to create structural proteins, the body uses the amino acids contained in proteins to manufacture various other protein-containing molecules that have a wide variety of important functions in the body. These include: enzymes that catalyze chemical reactions in the body; hormones involved in blood sugar regulation and thyroid hormone synthesis; transport proteins such as hemoglobin (carries oxygen) and transferrin (carries iron); lipoproteins that participate in the transportation of fat and cholesterol; antibodies, which play an important role in the immune system; and compounds that participate in the maintenance of proper fluid balance and acid-base balance.

## WHAT ARE THE CAUSES AND SYMPTOMS of PROTEIN DEFICIENCY?

Protein digestion and metabolism involves hydrochloric acid secreted by the stomach and enzymes synthesized by the pancreas. Additionally, the liver controls amino acid metabolism. Therefore any condition that compromises the function of any of these three organs can negatively impact protein status. In addition, the ability of the body to manufacture non-essential amino acids may be hampered with inadequate intake of vitamin B6.

Both adults and children can live healthfully on a low intake of protein, assuming they eat a sufficient amount of calories and all of the essential amino acids are present in the diet. For example, it would be possible to consume less than the RDA amount of protein while getting sufficient levels of amino acids if an excellent balance of high-quality, protein-containing foods was consumed. This type of balance would usually contain fish, nuts, seeds, and legumes. Protein intake as much as 25% under the RDA (in the vicinity of 40 grams per day) might be healthy if an optimal intake of amino acids was maintained and there were no existing health problems. Because affluent cultures often have protein intake above the RDAs, symptoms of protein deficiency are most often seen in impoverished people who have limited access to food. Protein-energy malnutrition, caused by low intake of both protein and calories, is especially common in children in underdeveloped nations, with symptoms including growth retardation and increased susceptibility to infections.

In developed countries, protein-energy malnutrition is most likely to affect people who have suffered severe physical trauma, which increases protein needs (for example, extensive skin burns) or those who have a medical condition or psychological problem that impacts their desire or ability to eat. The elderly are also at risk for protein-energy malnutrition.

Because meat and dairy foods are primary sources of protein in the American diet, many nutritionists caution that those following a vegetarian or vegan diet may be at risk for protein deficiency. However, vegetarians and vegans who eat a variety of vegetables, grains and legumes can easily meet or exceed current protein requirements.

## CAN YOU CONSUME TOO MUCH PROTEIN?

In the case of some chronic health problems, where protein supplies have become overtaxed and depleted, as much as 100 grams of protein per day may be needed to help restore body functions. But in general, excessive intake of protein is ill-advised. Excessive intake of protein over many years may lead to kidney problems and/or accelerated bone loss eventually leading to osteoporosis. Due to a lack of dose-response relationships at higher levels of protein intake, however, the National Academy of Sciences decided not to set a Tolerable Upper Intake Level (UL) for protein when setting protein standards in 2002.

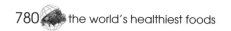

# selenium

Best Sources of Selenium from the *World's Healthiest Foods*

| FOOD | SERVING SIZE | CALS | AMOUNT (MCG) | DV (%) | DENSITY | QUALITY |
|------|------|------|------|------|------|------|
| Crimini mushrooms | 5 oz-wt | 31 | 36.9 | 52.6 | 30.4 | Excellent |
| Cod | 4 oz-wt | 119 | 53.2 | 75.8 | 11.5 | Excellent |
| Shiitake mushrooms | 8 oz-wt | 87 | 37.1 | 53.0 | 10.9 | Excellent |
| Shrimp | 4 oz-wt | 112 | 44.9 | 64.2 | 10.3 | Excellent |
| Tuna | 4 oz-wt | 158 | 53.1 | 75.8 | 8.7 | Excellent |
| Calf's liver | 4 oz-wt | 187 | 57.8 | 82.6 | 7.9 | Excellent |
| Sardines | 4 oz-wt | 191 | 48.5 | 78.1 | 7.3 | Excellent |
| Salmon | 4 oz-wt | 262 | 53.1 | 75.8 | 5.2 | Excellent |
| Mustard seeds | 2 tsp | 35 | 10.0 | 14.2 | 7.3 | Very good |
| Eggs | 1 each | 68 | 13.6 | 19.4 | 5.1 | Very good |
| Turkey | 4 oz-wt | 214 | 33.0 | 47.1 | 4.0 | Very good |
| Lamb | 4 oz-wt | 229 | 34.4 | 49.1 | 3.9 | Very good |
| Oats | 1 cup | 145 | 19.0 | 27.1 | 3.4 | Very good |
| Chicken | 4 oz-wt | 223 | 28.0 | 40.0 | 3.2 | Good |
| Tofu | 4 oz-wt | 86 | 10.1 | 14.4 | 3.0 | Good |
| Beef, grass-fed | 4 oz-wt | 240 | 27.7 | 39.5 | 3.0 | Good |
| Sunflower seeds | 0.25 cup | 205 | 21.4 | 30.6 | 2.7 | Good |
| Garlic | 1 oz-wt | 42 | 4.03 | 5.8 | 2.5 | Good |
| Broccoli | 1 cup | 20 | 2.13 | 3.0 | 2.8 | Good |
| Brown rice | 1 cup | 216 | 19.1 | 27.3 | 2.3 | Good |
| Venison | 4 oz-wt | 179 | 14.6 | 20.9 | 2.1 | Good |
| Asparagus | 1 cup | 43 | 3.1 | 4.4 | 1.8 | Good |
| Spinach | 1 cup | 41 | 2.7 | 3.9 | 1.7 | Good |
| Cheese, low-fat | 1 oz-wt | 72 | 4.1 | 5.8 | 1.5 | Good |

Brazil nuts are one of the best sources of selenium.
* For more on "DV," "Density," and "Quality" Rating System, see page 805.

## FUNCTIONS

What can selenium-rich foods do for you?
- Protect cells from free radical damage
- Enable thyroid hormone production
- Help lower your risk of joint inflammation

What events can indicate a need for more selenium-rich foods?
- Weakness or pain in the muscles
- Discoloration of the hair or skin
- Whitening of the fingernail beds

## IMPACT OF COOKING, STORAGE & PROCESSING

Like most minerals, selenium is present in many different forms in food and can vary greatly in its response to cooking and processing. High losses can occur in foods where it is found in water-soluble form and where contact with water during cooking is great. For example, when beans are cooked, 50% of the original selenium may be lost.

Additionally, in 60% extraction wheat, almost 75% of the original selenium is lost. In the case of animal foods, loss of selenium from cooking appears minimal. When a four ounce serving of beef is broiled, for example, virtually none of the selenium is lost.

## PUBLIC HEALTH RECOMMENDATIONS

In 2000, the Institute of Medicine at the National Academy of Sciences issued new Adequate Intake (AI) levels for selenium for infants up to 1 year old and Recommended Dietary Allowances (RDAs) for all people older than 1 year. The recommendations are as follows:

- 0–6 months: 15 mcg
- 6 months–3 years: 20 mcg
- 4–8 years: 30 mcg
- 9–13 years: 40 mcg
- 14+ years: 55 mcg
- Pregnant females: 60 mcg
- Lactating females: 70 mcg

The FDA has set the Reference Value for Nutrition Labeling for selenium at 70 mcg. This is the recommended intake value used by the FDA to calculate the %Daily Value for selenium that may appear on food labels.

Details on selenium's Tolerable Upper Intake Level (UL) are provided under the heading "Can You Consume Too Much Selenium?"

## WHY WE NEED SELENIUM-RICH FOODS

While selenium is considered a micromineral, meaning that it needs to be consumed daily in small amounts, its contribution to health is anything but small. Since it has been found to greatly promote the body's antioxidant potential, nutrition researchers have been suggesting strong links between this mineral and the prevention of numerous chronic diseases including cancer, heart disease, rheumatoid arthritis and asthma. Therefore, eating selenium-rich foods is an important part of a diet geared at overall wellness promotion.

Eating foods rich in selenium enhances your body's usage of this important mineral since these foods naturally contain other nutrients that act in synergy with selenium, supporting its physiological function in your body and therefore best contributing to your optimal health.

## HOW DOES SELENIUM PROMOTE HEALTH?
### Provides Antioxidant Protection

When oxygen-containing molecules in the body become too reactive, they can start damaging the cell structures around them. In chemistry, this imbalanced situation involving oxygen is called oxidative stress. Selenium helps prevent oxidative stress by working together with a group of nutrients—vitamin B3, vitamin E, vitamin C, and glutathione—to prevent oxygen molecules from becoming too reactive.

In many instances of heart disease, for example, where oxidative stress has been shown to be the source of blood vessel damage, low intake of selenium has been identified as a contributing factor to the disease. Similarly, in rheumatoid arthritis, where oxidative stress damages the area inside and around the joints, dietary deficiency of selenium has been shown to be a contributing cause.

### Thyroid Gland Support

In addition to iodine, selenium is a critical mineral for maintaining proper function of the thyroid gland. In order for the thyroid to produce the most active form of its hormone (triiodothyronine, or T3), selenium is not only essential, but also helps regulate the amount of hormone that is produced.

### Cancer Prevention

Accumulated evidence from prospective studies, intervention trials and studies on animal models of cancer has suggested a strong inverse correlation between selenium intake and cancer incidence. Several mechanisms have been suggested to explain the cancer-preventive activities of selenium. Selenium has been shown to induce DNA repair and synthesis in damaged cells, inhibit the proliferation of cancer cells, and induce their apoptosis, the self-destruct sequence the body uses to eliminate worn out or abnormal cells. In addition, selenium is incorporated at the active site of many proteins, including *glutathione peroxidase*, which is particularly important for cancer protection.

### Supports Mercury Detoxification?

Research suggests that selenium may neutralize mercury toxicity in the body. This potential benefit may be derived by two possible mechanisms: some selenium-containing compounds may directly bind with mercury while others, such as *glutathione peroxidase*, may combat the oxidative stress created by mercury.

## WHAT ARE THE CAUSES AND SYMPTOMS OF SELENIUM DEFICIENCY?

Dietary deficiency is the most common cause of selenium deficiency. Because plant content of selenium is so heavily dependent on the selenium content of the soil, researchers have been able to identify different areas of the world where selenium deficiency is particularly common. In the United States, parts of the Pacific Northwest, parts of the Great Lakes region moving eastward toward the New England states, and parts of the Atlantic Coast have been identified as selenium-deficient regions. Eating foods grown in these areas could contribute to risk of selenium deficiency.

Deficiency symptoms for selenium are difficult to determine and controversial in the research literature. Intake of selenium that is borderline or only mildly deficient has not been connected with specific symptoms in the research literature. With prolonged and severe deficiency, symptoms clearly center around two areas of the body where oxidative stress is known to take its toll: the heart and the joints.

## CAN YOU CONSUME TOO MUCH SELENIUM?

Nausea, vomiting, hair loss, skin lesions, abnormalities in the beds of the fingernail, and fingernail loss can all be symptomatic of selenium toxicity. Levels of selenium necessary to trigger these toxicity symptoms aren't usually obtained from food, since selenium-rich foods contain about 30–50 micrograms of selenium per serving. (Brazil nuts would be one exception here, since they average about 70–90 micrograms per nut.) Selenium supplementation would be a more likely cause of selenium toxicity than food ingestion.

In light of potential toxicity risks, in 2000 the National Institute of Medicine set the Tolerable Upper Intake Levels (UL) for selenium of 400 mcg per day for men and women 19 years and older.

# tryptophan

Best Sources of Tryptophan from the *World's Healthiest Foods*

| FOOD | SERVING SIZE | CALS | AMOUNT (G) | DV (%) | DENSITY | QUALITY |
|---|---|---|---|---|---|---|
| Shrimp | 4 oz-wt | 112 | 0.33 | 103.1 | 16.5 | Excellent |
| Crimini mushrooms | 5 oz-wt | 31 | 0.08 | 25.0 | 14.4 | Excellent |
| Cod | 4 oz-wt | 119 | 0.29 | 90.6 | 13.7 | Excellent |
| Tuna | 4 oz-wt | 158 | 0.38 | 118.8 | 13.6 | Excellent |
| Chicken | 4 oz-wt | 223 | 0.39 | 121.9 | 9.8 | Excellent |
| Scallops | 4 oz-wt | 152 | 0.26 | 81.3 | 9.6 | Excellent |
| Spinach | 1 cup | 41 | 0.07 | 21.9 | 9.5 | Excellent |
| Turkey | 4 oz-wt | 214 | 0.35 | 109.4 | 9.2 | Excellent |
| Tofu | 4 oz-wt | 86 | 0.14 | 43.8 | 9.1 | Excellent |
| Lamb | 4 oz-wt | 229 | 0.35 | 109.4 | 8.6 | Excellent |
| Beef, grass-fed | 4 oz-wt | 240 | 0.36 | 112.5 | 8.4 | Excellent |
| Calf's liver | 4 oz-wt | 187 | 0.25 | 78.1 | 7.5 | Excellent |
| Sardines | 4 oz-wt | 191 | 0.25 | 78.1 | 7.3 | Excellent |
| Salmon | 4 oz-wt | 262 | 0.33 | 103.1 | 7.1 | Excellent |
| Soybeans | 1 cup | 298 | 0.37 | 115.6 | 7.0 | Excellent |
| Asparagus | 1 cup | 43 | 0.05 | 15.6 | 6.5 | Very good |
| Broccoli | 1 cup | 44 | 0.05 | 15.6 | 6.4 | Very good |
| Mustard seeds | 2 tsp | 35 | 0.04 | 12.5 | 6.4 | Very good |
| Cheese, low-fat | 1 oz-wt | 72 | 0.08 | 25.0 | 6.2 | Very good |
| Cauliflower | 1 cup | 29 | 0.03 | 9.4 | 5.9 | Very good |
| Eggs | 1 each | 68 | 0.07 | 21.9 | 5.8 | Very good |
| Collard greens | 1 cup | 49 | 0.05 | 15.6 | 5.7 | Very good |
| Swiss chard | 1 cup | 35 | 0.03 | 9.4 | 4.8 | Very good |
| Cow's milk, low-fat | 1 cup | 121 | 0.10 | 31.3 | 4.6 | Very good |
| Kale | 1 cup | 36 | 0.03 | 9.4 | 4.6 | Very good |

\* For more on "DV," "Density," and "Quality" Rating System, see page 805.

## FUNCTIONS

What can tryptophan-rich foods do for you?
- Help regulate your appetite
- Elevate your mood
- Promote better sleep

What events can indicate a need for more tryptophan-rich foods?
- Depression, anxiety
- Impulsiveness
- Inability to concentrate
- Weight gain or unexpected weight loss
- Slow growth in children
- Overeating or carbohydrate cravings
- Poor dream recall
- Insomnia

## IMPACT OF COOKING, STORAGE & PROCESSING

There is no research showing problematic effects of cooking, storage, or processing on tryptophan levels in food.

## PUBLIC HEALTH RECOMMENDATIONS

In 2002, the Institute of Medicine at the National Academy of Sciences established recommended amino acid patterns for all individuals 1 year of age and older. Tryptophan was recommended at 7 milligrams per gram of protein consumed each day. Since the recommended Daily Value for protein is 50 grams per day, 350 milligrams of tryptophan would represent the current Institute of Medicine's recommendation when placed in the context of Daily Values. An alternative set of recommendations, based on milligrams of tryptophan consumed per kilogram of body weight, has been developed by the World Health Organization and is structured as follows:

- Infants up to two years: 17 mg/kg
- Children 2–10 years: 12.5 mg/kg
- Children and teens 10–18 years: 3.3 mg/kg
- Adults over 18 years of age: 3.5 mg/kg

## WHY WE NEED TRYPTOPHAN-RICH FOODS

Tryptophan is one of the essential amino acids that the body uses to synthesize the proteins it needs. An essential amino acid is one that our bodies cannot manufacture and which we must therefore get from our diets. Tryptophan works in concert with many other nutrients that are necessary for its metabolism, including vitamin B6, vitamin C, folic acid and magnesium. For this reason, it is best to get your daily supply of tryptophan from foods since tryptophan-containing foods typically include these other nutrients as well.

## HOW DOES TRYPTOPHAN PROMOTE HEALTH?
### Promotes Mood Balance

Tryptophan serves as a precursor for serotonin, a neurotransmitter that helps the body regulate appetite, sleep patterns, and mood. Because of its ability to raise serotonin levels, supplemental tryptophan has been used therapeutically in the treatment of a variety of conditions, most notably insomnia, depression, and anxiety.

### Prevention of Niacin Deficiency

A small amount of the tryptophan we get in our diet (about

3%) is converted into niacin (vitamin B3) by the liver. This conversion can help prevent the symptoms associated with niacin deficiency when dietary intake of this vitamin is low.

## WHAT ARE THE CAUSES AND SYMPTOMS OF TRYPTOPHAN DEFICIENCY?

Low dietary intake of tryptophan is the most common cause of deficiency. Dietary deficiency of tryptophan may lead to low levels of serotonin. Low serotonin levels are associated with depression, anxiety, irritability, impatience, impulsiveness, inability to concentrate, weight gain, overeating, carbohydrate cravings, poor dream recall, and insomnia. Additionally, factors such as vitamin B6 deficiency, cigarette smoking, high sugar intake, alcohol abuse, excessive protein consumption, low blood sugar, and diabetes can lead to reduced conversion of tryptophan to serotonin.

Because tryptophan is an essential amino acid, its dietary deficiency may cause the symptoms characteristic of protein deficiency, which include weight loss and impaired growth in infants and children. When accompanied by dietary niacin deficiency, lack of tryptophan in the diet may also cause pellagra, the classic niacin deficiency disease that is characterized by the "4 Ds"—dermatitis, diarrhea, dementia, and death. This condition is very rare in the United States, however, and cannot occur simply because of a tryptophan deficiency.

## CAN YOU CONSUME TOO MUCH TRYPTOPHAN?

High dietary intake of tryptophan from food sources is not known to cause any symptoms of toxicity.

---

*(Continued from Page 498)*

These differences in mercury exposure from canned tuna make it clear that light tuna (especially Pacific light tuna) is a far better choice than albacore tuna (especially Atlantic albacore tuna) when it comes to mercury exposure risk.

### How Much Total Mercury Exposure is Safe?

Safe levels of mercury exposure (including consumption of mercury-contaminated fish) are controversial because "safe" really depends on who is trying to stay safe and the specific health dangers they are facing. A very unhealthy person, perhaps in the hospital from weakness and poor nourishment, can withstand very little toxic exposure, including exposure from mercury-contaminated fish. An extremely healthy person, full of vitality, with good nutrient reserves and a robust ability to get rid of toxins would be very likely to remain fully healthy while consuming a mod-

erate amount of mercury-contaminated fish. Exactly how much could such a person eat? Here the answer would depend on the person's age, physical activity level, body size (height and weight) and other factors, including immediate performance goals. An athlete facing endurance training might not want to deplete his or her nutrient supplies at all, and might not want to ask his or her body to engage in any unnecessary detoxification of mercury. In this case, the choice might be to avoid any mercury-contaminated fish. A well-nourished, healthy person just wanting to stay generally healthy, i.e., stay safe from premature aging or premature onset of chronic disease, might choose to eat canned light tuna twice a week and simply stay with the FDA general health guidelines.

# vitamin a

Best Sources of Vitamin A from the *World's Healthiest Foods*

| FOOD | SERVING SIZE | CALS | AMOUNT (IU) | DV (%) | NUTRIENT DENSITY | QUALITY |
|------|-------------|------|-------------|--------|------------------|---------|
| Carrots | 1 cup | 53 | 34,317.4 | 686.3 | 235.5 | Excellent |
| Spinach | 1 cup | 41 | 14,742.0 | 294.8 | 128.2 | Excellent |
| Kale | 1 cup | 36 | 9,620.0 | 192.4 | 95.1 | Excellent |
| Parsley | 2 TBS | 3 | 631.8 | 12.6 | 84.2 | Excellent |
| Bell peppers | 1 cup | 25 | 5,244.0 | 104.9 | 76.0 | Excellent |
| Romaine lettuce | 2 cups | 16 | 2,912.0 | 58.2 | 66.9 | Excellent |
| Calf's liver | 4 oz-wt | 187 | 30,485.3 | 609.7 | 58.7 | Excellent |
| Swiss chard | 1 cup | 35 | 5,493.3 | 109.9 | 56.5 | Excellent |
| Sweet potatoes | 1 cup | 95 | 13,107.7 | 262.2 | 49.5 | Excellent |
| Cayenne pepper | 2 tsp | 11 | 1470.2 | 29.4 | 47.3 | Excellent |
| Collard greens | 1 cup | 49 | 5,945.1 | 118.9 | 43.3 | Excellent |
| Cantaloupe | 1 cup | 56 | 5,158.4 | 103.2 | 33.2 | Excellent |
| Winter squash | 1 cup | 80 | 7,292.9 | 145.8 | 32.8 | Excellent |
| Apricots | 1 each | 17 | 914.2 | 18.3 | 19.6 | Excellent |
| Broccoli | 1 cup | 44 | 2,280.7 | 45.6 | 18.8 | Excellent |
| Tomatoes | 1 cup | 38 | 1,121.4 | 22.4 | 10.7 | Excellent |
| Asparagus | 1 cup | 43 | 970.2 | 19.4 | 8.1 | Excellent |
| Basil | 2 tsp | 8 | 281.2 | 5.6 | 13.5 | Very good |
| Green beans | 1 cup | 44 | 833.5 | 16.6 | 6.9 | Very good |
| Brussels sprouts | 1 cup | 61 | 1,122.6 | 22.4 | 6.6 | Very good |
| Summer squash | 1 cup | 36 | 517.6 | 10.3 | 5.2 | Very good |
| Grapefruit | 0.5 each | 60 | 750.0 | 15.0 | 4.5 | Very good |
| Watermelon | 1 cup | 49 | 556.3 | 11.1 | 4.1 | Very good |
| Cucumbers | 1 cup | 14 | 223.6 | 4.5 | 6.0 | Good |
| Prunes | 0.25 cup | 102 | 844.6 | 16.9 | 3.0 | Good |

* For more on "DV," "Density," and "Quality" Rating System, see page 805.

## FUNCTIONS

What can vitamin A-rich foods do for you?
- Preserve and improve your eyesight
- Help you fight off viral infections

What events can indicate a need for more vitamin A-rich foods?
- Night blindness
- Frequent viral infections
- Goosebump-like appearance of the skin

## IMPACT OF COOKING, STORAGE & PROCESSING

Neither cooking nor storage significantly affects the amount or availability of preformed vitamin A in foods.

## PUBLIC HEALTH RECOMMENDATIONS

In 2000, the Institute of Medicine at the National Academy of Sciences issued new Adequate Intake (AI) levels for vitamin A for infants up to 1 year old, Recommended Dietary Allowances (RDAs) for people older than 1 year old and Estimated Average Requirements (EARs) for pregnant and lactating women. The recommendations are as follows and are given in both International Units (IU) and Retinol Equivalents (RE):

- 0–6 months: 1,333 IU (400 mcg RE)
- 7–12 months: 1,666 IU (500 mcg RE)
- 1–3 years: 1,000 IU (300 mcg RE)
- 4–8 years: 1,333 IU (400 mcg RE)
- 9–13 years: 2,000 IU (600 mcg RE)
- Males 14+ years: 3,000 IU (900 mcg RE)
- Females 14+ years: 2,333 IU (700 mcg RE)
- Pregnant women 18 years or younger: 2,500 IU (750 mcg RE)

- Pregnant women 19 years and older: 2,567 IU (750 mcg RE)
- Lactating women 18 years or younger: 4,000 IU (1,200 mcg RE)
- Lactating women 19 years or older: 4,333 IU (1,300 mcg RE)

The FDA has set the Reference Value for Nutrition Labeling for vitamin A at 5,000 IU. This is the recommended intake value used by the FDA to calculate the %Daily Value for vitamin A that may appear on food labels.

Details on vitamin A's Tolerable Upper Intake Level (UL) are provided under the heading "Can You Consume Too Much Vitamin A?"

## WHY WE NEED VITAMIN A-RICH FOODS

Vitamin A, identified in 1913, was the first fat-soluble vitamin to be discovered. Vitamin A is also known as retinol, a name given in reference to the participation of this compound in the functions of the retina of the eye. Vitamin A has also been called the "anti-infective" vitamin due to its role in supporting the activities of the immune system. While retinol, or pre-formed vitamin A, occurs only in foods of animal origin, some fruits and vegetables contain certain carotenoid phytonutri-ents—beta-carotene, alpha-carotene, and beta-cryptoxan-thin—that the body can convert into vitamin A. These carotenoids are sometimes referred to as "provitamin A," while retinol is called "preformed vitamin A." As nutrition researchers continue to forge the strong link between free radicals and disease development, it becomes increasingly important for people wanting to promote optimal health to ensure they consume adequate amounts of vitamin A-rich foods.

Eating foods rich in vitamin A enhances your body's usage of this important vitamin since these foods naturally contain other nutrients that act in synergy with vitamin A, supporting its physiological function in your body and therefore con-tributing to your optimal health.

## HOW DOES VITAMIN A PROMOTE HEALTH?
### Immune Function Support

Vitamin A stimulates several immune system activities, pos-sibly by promoting the growth and preventing the shrinkage of the thymus gland. It is known to enhance the function of white blood cells, increase the response of antibodies to anti-gens, and to have anti-viral activity.

In addition, retinoic acid, one of vitamin A's metabolically active forms, is needed to maintain the normal structure and function of epithelial and mucosal tissues, which are found in the lungs, trachea, skin, oral cavity, and gastrointestinal tract. These tissues, when healthy and intact, serve as the first line of defense for the immune system, providing a protective barrier that disease-causing microorganisms cannot penetrate.

### Vision Support

Vitamin A participates in the synthesis of rhodopsin, a pho-topigment found in the eye. Rhodopsin plays a fundamental role in the adaptation of the eye to low-light conditions and night vision.

### Cell Growth Support

Vitamin A is necessary for normal cell growth and develop-ment. Vitamin A is also essential for reproductive processes in both males and females and plays a role in normal bone metabolism. In addition, some of the most cutting-edge research in the field of genetics has been examining the role of vitamin A in regulating genetic events.

## WHAT ARE THE CAUSES AND SYMPTOMS OF VITAMIN A DEFICIENCY?

Since vitamin A is a fat-soluble vitamin, vitamin A deficiency may be caused by a diet that is extremely low in fat and/or the presence of certain medical conditions. In addition, chronic diarrhea caused by gastrointestinal infections and/or intestinal parasites may contribute to vitamin A deficiency. In addition, exposure to certain toxic chemicals (for example, polybrominated biphenyls and dioxin) enhances the break-down of vitamin A by the liver. Inadequate intake of protein contributes to vitamin A deficiency.

Vitamin A deficiency primarily affects the health of the skin, hair, eyes, and immune system, although loss of appetite, bone abnormalities, and growth retardation are also associ-ated with inadequate intake of this vitamin. A tell-tale sign of vitamin A deficiency is hyperkeratosis, a goosebump-like appearance of the skin caused by excessive production of keratin (a protein found in skin) that blocks hair follicles. In its initial stages, hyperkeratosis is found on the forearms and thighs, where the skin becomes dry, scaly, and rough. In its advances stages, hyperkeratosis affects the whole body, causing hair loss. Prolonged vitamin A deficiency can lead to night blindness, due to impaired production of rhodopsin, the compound in the retina responsible for detecting small amounts of light.

## CAN YOU CONSUME TOO MUCH VITAMIN A?

Toxicity can occur with excessive intakes of preformed vitamin A (not necessarily with carotenoid intake). The dosage needed to attain toxicity is such that it is difficult to attain this level from preformed vitamin A from food alone; rather, toxicity is more likely associated with prolonged intake of high levels of vitamin A supplements or accidental inges-tion of extremely high dosages. Those with poor liver func-tion are more likely to experience adverse events from excessive vitamin A intake. The Tolerable Upper Intake Level (UL) for vitamin A established by the Institute of Medicine varies by age group: for those 3 years and younger it is 2,000 IU; 4–8 years, 3,000 IU; 9–14 years, 5,666 IU; 15–18 years, 9,332 IU; 19 years and older, 10,000 IU; pregnant or lactating women 18 years or younger, 9,332 IU; and preg-nant or lactating women 19 years and older, 10,000 IU.

# vitamin B1 (thiamin)

## Best Sources of Vitamin B1 from the *World's Healthiest Foods*

| FOOD | SERVING SIZE | CALS | AMOUNT (MG) | DV (%) | DENSITY | QUALITY |
|------|------|------|------|------|------|------|
| Romaine lettuce | 2 cups | 16 | 0.1 | 7.3 | 8.4 | Very good |
| Asparagus | 1 cup | 43 | 0.2 | 14.7 | 6.1 | Very good |
| Crimini mushrooms | 5 oz-wt | 31 | 0.1 | 8.7 | 5.0 | Very good |
| Spinach | 1 cup | 41 | 0.2 | 11.3 | 4.9 | Very good |
| Sunflower seeds | 0.25 cup | 205 | 0.8 | 54.7 | 4.8 | Very good |
| Tuna | 4 oz-wt | 158 | 0.6 | 38.0 | 4.3 | Very good |
| Green peas | 1 cup | 134 | 0.4 | 27.3 | 3.7 | Very good |
| Tomatoes | 1 cup | 38 | 0.1 | 7.3 | 3.5 | Very good |
| Eggplant | 1 cup | 28 | 0.1 | 5.3 | 3.5 | Very good |
| Brussels sprouts | 1 cup | 61 | 0.2 | 11.3 | 3.4 | Very good |
| Celery | 1 cup | 19 | 0.1 | 4.0 | 3.8 | Good |
| Cabbage | 1 cup | 33 | 0.1 | 6.0 | 3.3 | Good |
| Watermelon | 1 cup | 49 | 0.1 | 8.0 | 3.0 | Good |
| Bell peppers | 1 cup | 25 | 0.1 | 4.0 | 2.9 | Good |
| Carrots | 1 cup | 53 | 0.1 | 8.0 | 2.7 | Good |
| Summer squash | 1 cup | 36 | 0.1 | 5.3 | 2.7 | Good |
| Winter squash | 1 cup | 80 | 0.2 | 11.3 | 2.6 | Good |
| Green beans | 1 cup | 44 | 0.1 | 6.0 | 2.5 | Good |
| Broccoli | 1 cup | 44 | 0.1 | 6.0 | 2.5 | Good |
| Corn | 1 cup | 177 | 0.4 | 24.0 | 2.4 | Good |
| Kale | 1 cup | 36 | 0.1 | 4.7 | 2.3 | Good |
| Black beans | 1 cup | 227 | 0.4 | 28.0 | 2.2 | Good |
| Oats | 1 cup | 145 | 0.3 | 17.3 | 2.2 | Good |
| Pineapple | 1 cup | 76 | 0.1 | 9.3 | 2.2 | Good |
| Oranges | 1 each | 62 | 0.1 | 7.3 | 2.1 | Good |

* For more on "DV," "Density," and "Quality" Rating System, see page 805.

## FUNCTIONS

What can vitamin B1-rich foods do for you?
- Maintain your energy supplies
- Coordinate the activity of nerves and muscles
- Support proper heart function

What events can indicate a need for more vitamin B1-rich foods?
- "Pins and needles" sensations
- Feeling of numbness, especially in the legs
- Muscle tenderness, particularly in the calf muscles
- Loss of appetite

## IMPACT OF COOKING, STORAGE & PROCESSING

Vitamin B1 is highly unstable and easily damaged by heat, pH, and by other chemical substances. Both sulfites and nitrites can inactivate vitamin B1. Processing of grains for use in cereals, and, in particular, heating of processed grain components, can result in the loss of more than half of the grains' vitamin B1 content.

Long-term (for example, 12 months) refrigeration of vitamin B1-containing foods can also result in substantial loss, on an average of 20-60%.

## PUBLIC HEALTH RECOMMENDATIONS

In 1998, the Institute of Medicine at the National Academy of Sciences issued new Recommended Dietary Allowances (RDAs) for vitamin B1 for all individuals 1 year and older. Adequate Intake (AI) levels were established for infants under 1 year of age. These 1998 recommendations are as follows:
- 0–6 months: 200 mcg

- 6–12 months: 300 mcg
- 1–3 years: 500 mcg
- 4–8 years: 600 mcg
- 9–13 years: 900 mcg
- Males 14+ years: 1.2 mg
- Females 14+ years: 1.1 mg
- Pregnant females: 1.4 mg
- Lactating females: 1.5 mg

The FDA has set the Reference Value for Nutrition Labeling for vitamin B1 at 1.5 mg. This is the recommended intake value used by the FDA to calculate the %Daily Value for vitamin B1 that may appear on food labels.

The Institute of Medicine did not establish a Tolerable Upper Intake Level (UL) for vitamin B1.

## WHY WE NEED VITAMIN B1-RICH FOODS

Although some vitamin B1 is stored in the body, we need to get a regular supply of it from our diet. No B-complex vitamin is more dependent on its fellow B vitamins than thiamin. Its absorption into the body requires adequate supplies of vitamins B6, B12, and folic acid, which is not a problem since many thiamin-rich foods also contain adequate amounts of these other B vitamins.

Vitamin B1 is traditionally well known for its role in the nutritional deficiency disease, beriberi. Sailing voyages were a common backdrop for the appearance of beriberi, and the addition of whole grains to ships' rations was found to prevent its occurrence. By 1926, researchers discovered that the preventive substance in whole grains that could also remedy the energy deprivation in the ships' crews was vitamin B1. Although beriberi is extremely rare in the United States, our understanding of vitamin B1 and its relationship to energy deprivation has carried over into our approach to other health problems in which vitamin B1 deficiency plays a critical role.

## HOW DOES VITAMIN B1 PROMOTE HEALTH?
### Energy Production
Most cells in the body depend on sugar as an energy source. When oxygen is used to help convert sugar into usable energy, the process of energy generation is called aerobic energy production. This process cannot take place without adequate supplies of vitamin B1 since B1 is part of an enzyme system that enables oxygen-based processing of sugar. Because vitamin B1 is so important in energy production, and because food energy is usually measured in terms of calories, vitamin B1 is often prescribed in relationship to caloric intake. For example, recommendations sometimes suggest intake of 0.5 milligrams of vitamin B1 for every 1,000 calories consumed.

### Nervous System Support
Vitamin B1 plays a key role in supporting the nervous system, where it permits healthy development of the fat-like coverings (myelin sheaths) which surround most nerves. In the absence of vitamin B1, these coverings can degenerate or become damaged.

A second type of connection between vitamin B1 and the nervous system involves its role in the production of the messenger molecule acetylcholine. This molecule, called a neurotransmitter, is used by the nervous system to relay messages between the nerves and muscles. Acetylcholine cannot be produced without adequate supplies of vitamin B1. Because acetylcholine is used by the nervous system to ensure proper muscle tone in the heart, deficiency of B1 can also result in compromised heart function.

## WHAT ARE THE CAUSES AND SYMPTOMS OF VITAMIN B1 DEFICIENCY?
The leading risk factor for vitamin B1 deficiency in the United States is alcoholism. Heavy users of coffee and tea may also have increased risk of vitamin B1 deficiency since these beverages act as diuretics and remove both water and water-soluble vitamins (like vitamin B1) from the body. Our need for vitamin B1 is also increased by chronic stress, chronic diarrhea, chronic fever, and smoking.

Because of its ability to disrupt the body's energy production, one of the first symptoms of vitamin B1 deficiency is loss of appetite that reflects the body's listlessness and malaise. Symptoms related to nerve dysfunction are commonly associated with vitamin B1 deficiency since the myelin sheaths that surround the nerves will not be formed properly without adequate supplies of this nutrient.

These nerve-related symptoms include "pins and needles" sensations or numbness, especially in the legs. Additionally, inability of the nervous system to ensure proper muscle tone in the gastrointestinal tract can lead to indigestion or constipation, and muscle tenderness, particularly in the calf muscles.

## CAN YOU CONSUME TOO MUCH VITAMIN B1?
Even at extremely high doses, vitamin B1 intake does not appear to carry a risk of toxicity. The Institute of Medicine did not establish a Tolerable Upper Intake Level (UL) for intake of vitamin B1.

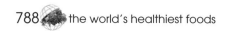

# vitamin B2 (riboflavin)

Best Sources of Vitamin B2 from the *World's Healthiest Foods*

| FOOD | SERVING SIZE | CALS | AMOUNT (MG) | DV (%) | DENSITY | QUALITY |
|---|---|---|---|---|---|---|
| Crimini mushrooms | 5 oz-wt | 31 | 0.7 | 40.6 | 23.4 | Excellent |
| Calf's liver | 4 oz-wt | 187 | 2.2 | 129.4 | 12.4 | Excellent |
| Spinach | 1 cup | 41 | 0.4 | 24.7 | 10.7 | Excellent |
| Romaine lettuce | 2 cups | 16 | 0.1 | 6.5 | 7.4 | Very good |
| Asparagus | 1 cup | 43 | 0.2 | 13.5 | 5.6 | Very good |
| Swiss chard | 1 cup | 35 | 0.2 | 8.8 | 4.5 | Very good |
| Broccoli | 1 cup | 44 | 0.2 | 10.6 | 4.4 | Very good |
| Collard greens | 1 cup | 49 | 0.2 | 11.8 | 4.3 | Very good |
| Venison | 4 oz-wt | 179 | 0.7 | 40 | 4.0 | Very good |
| Yogurt | 1 cup | 155 | 0.5 | 30.6 | 3.6 | Very good |
| Eggs | 1 each | 68 | 0.2 | 13.5 | 3.6 | Very good |
| Milk, low-fat | 1 cup | 121 | 0.4 | 23.5 | 3.5 | Very good |
| Green beans | 1 cup | 44 | 0.1 | 7.1 | 2.9 | Good |
| Celery | 1 cup | 19 | 0.1 | 2.9 | 2.8 | Good |
| Kale | 1 cup | 36 | 0.1 | 5.3 | 2.6 | Good |
| Cabbage | 1 cup | 33 | 0.1 | 4.7 | 2.6 | Good |
| Strawberries | 1 cup | 43 | 0.1 | 5.9 | 2.5 | Good |
| Tomatoes | 1 cup | 38 | 0.1 | 5.3 | 2.5 | Good |
| Cauliflower | 1 cup | 29 | 0.1 | 3.5 | 2.2 | Good |
| Goat's milk | 1 cup | 168 | 0.3 | 20 | 2.1 | Good |
| Raspberries | 1 cup | 60 | 0.1 | 7.1 | 2.1 | Good |
| Brussels sprouts | 1 cup | 61 | 0.1 | 7.1 | 2.1 | Good |
| Summer squash | 1 cup | 36 | 0.1 | 4.1 | 2.1 | Good |
| Green peas | 1 cup | 134 | 0.2 | 14.1 | 1.9 | Good |
| Plums | 1 each | 36 | 0.1 | 3.5 | 1.8 | Good |

\* For more on "DV," "Density," and "Quality" Rating System, see page 805.

## FUNCTIONS

What can vitamin B2-rich foods do for you?
- Help protect cells from oxygen damage
- Support cellular energy production
- Maintain your supply of other B vitamins

What events can indicate a need for more vitamin B2-rich foods?
- Sensitivity to light
- Tearing, burning and itching of the eyes
- Soreness around the lips, mouth, and tongue
- Cracking of the skin at the corners of the mouth

## IMPACT OF COOKING, STORAGE & PROCESSING

Heat and air do very little damage to vitamin B2, but light is a primary damaging factor for this vitamin. In studies involving the boiling of macaroni noodles, for example, prolonged exposure to light was the critical factor related to loss of vitamin B2. Due to this nutrient's sensitivity to light, high-vitamin B2-rich foods should be cooked in covered pots whenever possible and stored in opaque containers. Without prolonged exposure to light, loss of vitamin B2 from cooking and storing is typically less than 25%.

## PUBLIC HEALTH RECOMMENDATIONS

In 1998, the Institute of Medicine at the National Academy of Sciences issued new Recommended Dietary Allowances (RDAs) for vitamin B2 for all individuals 1 year of age and older. Adequate Intake (AI) levels were established for infants under 1 year of age. The recommendations are as follows:
- 0–6 months: 300 mcg
- 6–12 months: 400 mcg

- 1–3 years: 500 mcg
- 4–8 years: 600 mcg
- 9–13 years: 900 mcg
- Males 14+ years: 1.3 mg
- Females 14–18 years: 1.0 mg
- Females 19+ years: 1.1 mg
- Pregnant females: 1.4 mg
- Lactating females: 1.6 mg

The FDA has set the Reference Value for Nutrition Labeling for vitamin B2 at 1.7 mg. This is the recommended intake value used by the FDA to calculate the %Daily Value for vitamin B2 that may appear on food labels.

The Institute of Medicine did not establish a Tolerable Upper Intake Level (UL) for vitamin B2 in its 1998 recommendations.

## WHY WE NEED VITAMIN B2-RICH FOODS

Vitamin B2, also commonly called riboflavin, gets its name from its color. The root of this word is the Latin word *flavus* meaning "yellow." When a person's urine becomes bright yellow following high level supplementation with B-complex vitamins, excess riboflavin excreted in the urine is often responsible for this change in color. Because riboflavin is a component of enzymes that are necessary for everything from energy production to antioxidant status, getting enough from the foods in your diet is important for maintaining optimal health.

Eating foods rich in vitamin B2 enhances your body's usage of this important vitamin since these foods naturally contain other nutrients that act in synergy with vitamin B2, supporting its physiological function in your body and therefore best contributing to your optimal health.

### Cofactor for Homocysteine Metabolism

Vitamin B2, through its conversion to FAD, is involved in the breakdown of homocysteine. Since homocysteine excess is associated with increased risk of cardiovascular disease, maintaining adequate levels of vitamin B2 can be of benefit to heart health.

### Recycling of the Antioxidant Glutathione

Glutathione is a protein-like molecule that is responsible for preventing oxygen-based damage to cell membranes, blood vessel linings and joint tissue. Like many antioxidant molecules, glutathione must be constantly recycled. Through its role as a cofactor in the enzyme *glutathione reductase*, vitamin B2 plays an important role in recycling glutathione back into its active antioxidant form.

### Maintaining Supplies of Vitamin B2

Vitamin B2 plays an important role in maintaining supplies of its fellow B vitamins. One of the pathways used in the body to create vitamin B3 (niacin) is by conversion of the amino acid tryptophan. This conversion process is accomplished with the help of an enzyme that requires vitamin B2 to function.

## HOW DOES VITAMIN B2 PROMOTE HEALTH?
### Energy Production

Like vitamin B1, vitamin B2 plays a critical role in the body's energy production. When active in the body's energy production pathways, riboflavin typically takes the form of flavin adenine dinucleotide (FAD) or flavin mononucleotide (FMN). When riboflavin is converted into these FAD and FMN forms, it can attach to protein enzymes and allow oxygen-based energy production to occur. Proteins with FAD or FMN attached to them are often referred to as flavoproteins. Flavoproteins are found throughout the body, and particularly in locations where oxygen-based energy production is constantly needed. These locations include the heart and skeletal muscles.

## WHAT ARE THE CAUSES AND SYMPTOMS of VITAMIN B2 DEFICIENCY?

Although not as dramatic as its impact on vitamin B1, alcoholism clearly decreases the availability of vitamin B2 in the body. Heavy exercise has also been shown to increase the need for vitamin B2. Particularly in women training for athletic events, up to 10–15 times the ordinary amount of vitamin B2 may be needed to sustain optimal health. Due to the enrichment of processed grain products, wheat flour remains the primary source of vitamin B2 in the U.S. diet; individuals on specialty diets where carbohydrates like breads, grains, and pastas are avoided may be at special risk for riboflavin deficiency.

Many of the early-stage deficiency symptoms for riboflavin involve eye-related problems. These problems include excessive sensitivity to light, tearing, burning and itching in and around the eyes, and loss of clear vision. Soreness around the lips, mouth, and tongue, and cracking of the skin at the corners of the mouth are symptoms that can also be characteristic of riboflavin deficiency. Peeling of the skin, particularly around the nose, can also indicate lack of vitamin B2.

## CAN YOU CONSUME TOO MUCH VITAMIN B2?

Toxic side effects from supplemental intake of vitamin B2 (which would be at much higher doses than that found naturally in food) have not been documented in the research literature. Consequently, the Institute of Medicine did not establish a Tolerable Upper Intake Level (UL) for vitamin B2.

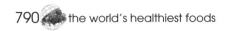

# vitamin B6

## Best Sources of Vitamin B6 from the *World's Healthiest Foods*

| FOOD | SERVING SIZE | CALS | AMOUNT (MG) | DV (%) | DENSITY | QUALITY |
|---|---|---|---|---|---|---|
| Spinach | 1 cup | 41 | 0.4 | 22.0 | 9.6 | Excellent |
| Bell peppers | 1 cup | 25 | 0.2 | 11.5 | 8.3 | Excellent |
| Garlic | 1 oz-wt | 42 | 0.4 | 17.5 | 7.5 | Very good |
| Tuna | 4 oz-wt | 158 | 1.2 | 59.0 | 6.7 | Very good |
| Cauliflower | 1 cup | 29 | 0.2 | 10.5 | 6.6 | Very good |
| Bananas | 1 each | 109 | 0.7 | 34.0 | 5.6 | Very good |
| Broccoli | 1 cup | 44 | 0.2 | 11.0 | 4.5 | Very good |
| Celery | 1 cup | 19 | 0.1 | 5.0 | 4.7 | Very good |
| Asparagus | 1 cup | 43 | 0.2 | 11.0 | 4.6 | Very good |
| Cabbage | 1 cup | 33 | 0.2 | 8.5 | 4.6 | Very good |
| Crimini mushrooms | 5 oz-wt | 31 | 0.2 | 8.0 | 4.6 | Very good |
| Kale | 1 cup | 36 | 0.2 | 9.0 | 4.5 | Very good |
| Collard greens | 1 cup | 49 | 0.2 | 12.0 | 4.4 | Very good |
| Brussels sprouts | 1 cup | 61 | 0.3 | 14.0 | 4.1 | Very good |
| Watermelon | 1 cup | 48.6 | 0.2 | 11.0 | 4.1 | Very good |
| Cod | 4 oz-wt | 119 | 0.5 | 26.0 | 3.9 | Very good |
| Swiss chard | 1 cup | 35 | 0.2 | 7.5 | 3.9 | Very good |
| Cayenne pepper | 2 tsp | 11 | 0.1 | 4.0 | 6.4 | Good |
| Turmeric | 2 tsp | 16 | 0.1 | 4.0 | 4.5 | Good |
| Tomatoes | 1 cup | 38 | 0.1 | 7.0 | 3.3 | Good |
| Carrots | 1 cup | 53 | 0.2 | 9.0 | 3.1 | Good |
| Summer squash | 1 cup | 36 | 0.1 | 6.0 | 3.0 | Good |
| Cantaloupe | 1 cup | 56 | 0.2 | 9.0 | 2.9 | Good |
| Eggplant | 1 cup | 28 | 0.1 | 4.5 | 2.9 | Good |
| Romaine lettuce | 2 cups | 16 | 0.1 | 2.5 | 2.9 | Good |

\* For more on "DV," "Density," and "Quality" Rating System, see page 805.

## FUNCTIONS

What can vitamin B6-rich foods do for you?

- Support nervous system health
- Promote proper breakdown of sugars and starches
- Help prevent homocysteine build-up in your blood

What events can indicate a need for more vitamin B6-rich foods?

- Fatigue or malaise
- Anemia
- Skin disorders including eczema and seborrheic dermatitis

## IMPACT OF COOKING, STORAGE & PROCESSING

Large amounts of vitamin B6 are lost during most forms of cooking and processing. Loss of vitamin B6 from canning of veg-etables is approximately 60–80%; from canning of fruits, about 38%; from freezing of fruits, about 15%; from conversion of grains to grain products, between 50–95%; and from conversion of fresh meat to meat by-products, 50–75%. When food is heated, the more acidic the food, the poorer the vitamin B6 retention.

## PUBLIC HEALTH RECOMMENDATIONS

In 2000, the Institute of Medicine at the National Academy of Sciences issued new Recommended Dietary Allowances (RDAs) for vitamin B6. The recommendations are as follows:

- 0–6 months: 100 mcg
- 6–12 months: 300 mcg
- 1–3 years: 500 mcg
- 4–8 years: 600 mcg
- 9–13 years: 1.0 mg

- Males 14–50 years: 1.3 mg
- Females 14–50 years: 1.2 mg
- Males 51 years and older: 1.7 mg
- Females 51 years and older: 1.5 mg
- Pregnant females: 1.9 mg
- Lactating females: 2.0 mg

The FDA has set the Reference Value for Nutrition Labeling for vitamin B6 at 2.0 mg. This is the recommended intake value used by the FDA to calculate the %Daily Value for vitamin B6 that may appear on food labels.

Details on vitamin B6's Tolerable Upper Intake Level (UL) are provided under the heading "Can You Consume Too Much Vitamin B6?"

## WHY WE NEED VITAMIN B6-RICH FOODS

Vitamin B6 is one of the best studied of all B vitamins and has one of the greatest varieties of chemical forms. The forms of this vitamin all begin with the letters "pyr," and include pyridoxine, pyridoxal, pyridoxamine, pyridoxine phosphate, pyridoxal phosphate, and pyridoxamine phosphate. The vitamin was not originally given this name, however, but was referred to as "antidermatitis factor" since skin inflammation (dermatitis) seemed to increase when foods with B6 were eliminated from the diet. Yet, the importance of vitamin B6 in the diet extends to much more than just its benefits upon the skin; it is involved in numerous physiological functions throughout the body, making it vitally important to optimal health.

Many foods that contain vitamin B6 also contain other B vitamins, which is important since vitamin B6 has key interactions with these other nutrients. For example, vitamins B2 and B3 are both needed to convert B6 into its various chemical forms. Vitamin B6 deficiency can also reduce the body's absorption of vitamin B12.

## HOW DOES VITAMIN B6 PROMOTE HEALTH?
### Support of Nervous System Activity

The role of vitamin B6 in our nervous system is very broad and involves many aspects of neurological activity. One aspect focuses on the creation of an important group of neurotransmitter messaging molecules called amines, compounds that the nervous system relies on for transmission of messages from one nerve to the next. Amines are often made from protein building blocks called amino acids, and the key nutrient for making this process occur is vitamin B6. Some of the amine-derived neurotransmitters that require vitamin B6 for their production include serotonin, melatonin, epinephrine, norepinephrine, and GABA.

### Synthesis of Essential Molecules

Nucleic acids, which are used in the creation of our DNA genetic material and many amino acids, the building blocks of proteins, require adequate supplies of vitamin B6 for their synthesis. Therefore, it is difficult to find a chemical category

of molecules in the body that does not depend in some way on vitamin B6 for its production.

### Processing of Carbohydrates

The processing of carbohydrates (sugar and starch) in our body depends on the availability of vitamin B6. This vitamin is particularly important in facilitating the breakdown of glycogen, a special form of starch stored in our muscle cells and to a lesser extent in our liver. Because carbohydrate processing plays such a key role in certain types of athletic events, researchers have looked closely at the role vitamin B6 plays in carbohydrate processing during physical performance.

### Support of Sulfur and Methyl Metabolism

Through the role it plays in the metabolism of sulfur-containing molecules, vitamin B6 is critical for maintaining hormonal balance and eliminating toxic substances through the liver. It plays a similar role with respect to methyl-containing molecules. Many important chemical events are made possible by methyl group transfer. For example, genes in the body can be switched on and turned off in this way, and cells can use the process to send messages back and forth. Through its involvement with the metabolism of chemical molecules called methyl groups, vitamin B6 also plays a role in ensuring that substances like homocysteine, which can build up excessively in the blood and increase risk of cardiovascular disease, are kept within a healthy range.

## WHAT ARE THE CAUSES AND SYMPTOMS OF VITAMIN B6 DEFICIENCY?

In addition to dietary insufficiency, smoking and the use of many prescription medications (including oral contraceptives) can contribute to vitamin B6 deficiency.

Because of its key role in the formation of new cells, vitamin B6 is especially important for healthy function of body tissue that regenerates itself quickly. The skin is exactly this type of tissue, and it is one of the first to show problems when vitamin B6 is deficient. Many skin disorders have been associated with vitamin B6 deficiency, including eczema and seborrheic dermatitis. The critical role of vitamin B6 in the formation of red blood cells means that vitamin B6 deficiency can also result in symptoms of anemia, malaise, and fatigue. The key role of vitamin B6 in the nervous system also results in many nerve-related symptoms when vitamin B6 is deficient. These symptoms can include convulsions and seizures in the case of severe deficiency.

## CAN YOU CONSUME TOO MUCH VITAMIN B6?

Imbalances in nervous system activity have been shown to result from high levels of supplemental vitamin B6 intake, but not from food intake since the dosages that have been associated with these adverse events are so much higher than can be reached with food sources alone. The Tolerable Upper Intake Level (UL) for vitamin B6 is 100 mg for adults 19 years and older.

# vitamin B12

Best Sources of Vitamin B12 from the *World's Healthiest Foods*

| FOOD | SERVING SIZE | CALS | AMOUNT (MCG) | DV (%) | DENSITY | QUALITY |
|------|------|------|------|------|------|------|
| Calf's liver | 4 oz-wt | 187 | 41.4 | 690.0 | 66.4 | Excellent |
| Sardines | 4 oz-wt | 191 | 8.2 | 137.0 | 12.9 | Excellent |
| Venison | 4 oz-wt | 179 | 3.6 | 60.0 | 6.0 | Very good |
| Shrimp | 4 oz-wt | 112 | 1.7 | 28.2 | 4.5 | Very good |
| Scallops | 4 oz-wt | 152 | 2.0 | 33.3 | 4.0 | Very good |
| Salmon | 4 oz-wt | 262 | 3.3 | 54.2 | 3.7 | Very good |
| Beef, grass-fed | 4 oz-wt | 240 | 2.9 | 48.7 | 3.6 | Very good |
| Lamb | 4 oz-wt | 229 | 2.5 | 40.8 | 3.2 | Good |
| Cod | 4 oz-wt | 119 | 1.2 | 19.7 | 3.0 | Good |
| Yogurt | 1 cup | 155 | 1.4 | 23.0 | 2.7 | Good |
| Milk, low-fat | 1 cup | 121 | 0.9 | 14.8 | 2.2 | Good |
| Eggs | 1 each | 68 | 0.5 | 8.2 | 2.2 | Good |

* For more on "DV," "Density," and "Quality" Rating System, see page 805.

## FUNCTIONS

What can vitamin B12-rich foods do for you?
- Support production of red blood cells and prevent anemia
- Allow nerve cells to develop properly
- Help your cells metabolize protein, carbohydrate, and fat

What events can indicate a need for more vitamin B-12-rich foods?
- Depression
- Nervousness
- Memory problems
- Red or sore tongue
- Tingling or numbness in feet
- Heart palpitations

## IMPACT OF COOKING, STORAGE & PROCESSING

When derived from animal foods, vitamin B12 is fairly well pre-served under most cooking conditions. For example, about 70% of the vitamin B12 present in beef is retained after broiling for 45 minutes at 350°F. Similarly, about 70% of vitamin B12 is still present after cow's milk is boiled for 2–5 minutes. Retention of vitamin B12 in plant-based foods like tempeh, a fermented food made from soy, has not been well researched.

## PUBLIC HEALTH RECOMMENDATIONS

In 1998, the Institute of Medicine at the National Academy of Sciences issued new Recommended Dietary Allowances (RDAs) for vitamin B12 for all individuals 1 year of age and older. Adequate Intake (AI) levels were set for infants under the age of 1 year. The recommendations are as follows:
- 0–6 months: 400 nanograms
- 7–12 months: 500 nanograms
- 1–3 years: 900 nanograms
- 4–8 years: 1.2 mcg
- 9–13 years: 1.8 mcg
- 14+ years: 2.4 mcg
- Pregnant females of any age: 2.6 mcg
- Lactating females of any age: 2.8 mcg

The FDA has set the Reference Value for Nutrition Labeling for vitamin B12 at 6 mcg. This is the recommended intake value used by the FDA to calculate the %Daily Value for vitamin B12 that may appear on food labels.

The Institute of Medicine did not establish a Tolerable Upper Intake Level (UL) for vitamin B12 when it set its most recent RDAs in 1998.

## WHY WE NEED VITAMIN B12-RICH FOODS

Vitamin B12 is unusual with respect to its origins. While most vitamins can be made by a wide variety of plants and spe-cific animals, no plant or animal has been shown capable of producing B12, and the exclusive source of this vitamin appears to be tiny microorganisms like bacteria, yeasts, molds, and algae. While its origins may be unusual, vitamin B12's importance is widespread since this nutrient is so vital to our health, affecting our blood, nervous system, energy level and overall feeling of wellness.

Like most vitamins, B12 can occur in a variety of forms and

can take on a variety of names. Names for vitamin B12 include cobamide, cobalamin, hydroxcobalamin, aquocobalamin, nitro-tocobalamin, and cyanocobalamin. Each of these designations contains a form of the word "cobalt," since cobalt is the mineral found in the center of the vitamin.

Eating foods rich in vitamin B12 enhances your body's usage of this important vitamin since these foods naturally contain other nutrients that act in synergy with vitamin B12, supporting its physiological function in your body and therefore best contributing to your optimal health.

## HOW DOES VITAMIN B12 PROMOTE HEALTH?
### Red Blood Cell Production
Perhaps the most well known function of vitamin B12 involves its role in the development of red blood cells. As these cells mature, they require information provided by molecules of DNA, the substance in our cells that contains genetic information. Without B12, synthesis of DNA becomes defective, and so does the information needed for red blood cell formation. The cells become oversized and poorly shaped, and begin to function ineffectively, a condition called pernicious anemia. More often than not, pernicious anemia isn't caused by a lack of vitamin B12 itself, but by a lack of intrinsic factor, a unique protein made in the stomach, upon which vitamin B12 is dependent for its absorption.

### Nerve Cell Development
A second major function of B12 involves its participation in the development of nerve cells. The myelin sheath—a coating that encloses the nerves—does not form properly whenever B12 is deficient. Additionally, protein, carbohydrates and fats all depend upon vitamin B12 for their proper cycling and movement throughout the body.

## WHAT ARE THE CAUSES AND SYMPTOMS OF VITAMIN B12 DEFICIENCY?
Stomach problems can contribute to a vitamin B12 deficiency in two ways. First, irritation and inflammation of the stomach can prevent the stomach cells from functioning properly, which may stop them from producing intrinsic factor. Lack of stomach acids can also lead to B12 deficiency since it is needed to release B12 from protein in food to which it is usually attached.

The ability of a strict vegetarian diet to supply adequate amounts of vitamin B12 remains controversial, despite increasing evidence in support of vegetarianism and its nutritional adequacy. The controversy is fueled by two somewhat divergent schools of thought. One emphasizes the fact that most animals, including humans, are capable of storing long-term supplies of B12, and therefore a daily requirement would be regarded as highly unlikely. The other school of thought, however, points to the unreliability of plants as sources of vitamin B12. Since no plant is capable of making this nutrient, the amount of B12 in plant food depends upon the relationship of the plant to soil and root-level microorganisms that make the vitamin.

Cultured and fermented bean products like tofu, tempeh, miso, and tamari (soy sauce) may or may not contain significant amounts of B12, depending upon the microorganisms used to produce them. The B12 content of sea vegetables also varies according to the distribution of microorganisms in the surrounding sea environment.

Although vitamin B12 is not the only nutrient deficiency that can contribute to occurrence of the following symptoms, its deficiency should be considered as a possible underlying factor whenever any of the symptoms listed below are present: dandruff, nervousness, decreased blood clotting, paleness, depression, fatigue, memory problems, weak pulse, and menstrual problems.

Excessive intake of folic acid can mask B12 deficiency, so individuals at risk for vitamin B12 deficiency who are also taking folic acid in supplement form should consult with their healthcare practitioner.

## CAN YOU CONSUME TOO MUCH VITAMIN B12?
No toxicity levels have been reported for vitamin B12, and no toxicity symptoms have been identified in scientific research studies. The Institute of Medicine did not establish a Tolerable Upper Intake Level (UL) for this nutrient.

Q *How can you get vitamin B12 without eating meat or other animal products?*

A It is definitely more difficult to get vitamin B12 from non-animal sources than many other nutrients. Vegans must pay attention to their intake of vitamin B12 since this vitamin occurs primarily in animal foods, and its deficiency can cause a variety of irreversible neurological problems. A study published in 1999 in the *American Journal of Clinical Nutrition* involving 245 Australian Seventh-day Adventist ministers evaluated the vitamin B12 status of lacto-ovo vegetarians and vegans who were not taking vitamin B12 supplements. Seventy three percent of the participants had low serum vitamin B12 concentrations.

Interestingly, vitamin B12 cannot be made by animals or plants, but only by microorganisms, like bacteria. When plant foods are fermented with the use of B12-producing bacteria, they end up containing B12. Otherwise, they usually don't. Sea plants are an exception to the fermented plant rule since they can contain small amounts of B12 from contact with microorganisms in the ocean. Yet, while sea vegetables, algae and fermented foods like tempeh may contain some vitamin B12, they don't necessarily contain an adequate amount. Therefore, to ensure adequate intake, many people who do not consume any animal-derived foods either look for vitamin B12-fortified foods and/or take vitamin B12 supplements.

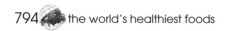
# vitamin c

Best Sources of Vitamin C from the *World's Healthiest Foods*

| FOOD | SERVING SIZE | CALS | AMOUNT (MG) | DV (%) | DENSITY | QUALITY |
|---|---|---|---|---|---|---|
| Bell peppers | 1 cup | 25 | 174.8 | 291.3 | 211.1 | Excellent |
| Parsley | 2 TBS | 3 | 10.0 | 16.6 | 110.8 | Excellent |
| Broccoli | 1 cup | 44 | 123.4 | 205.7 | 84.8 | Excellent |
| Strawberries | 1 cup | 43 | 81.7 | 136.1 | 56.7 | Excellent |
| Cauliflower | 1 cup | 29 | 54.9 | 91.5 | 57.8 | Excellent |
| Lemon juice | 0.25 cup | 15 | 28.1 | 46.8 | 55.2 | Excellent |
| Romaine lettuce | 2 cups | 16 | 26.9 | 44.8 | 51.4 | Excellent |
| Brussels sprouts | 1 cup | 61 | 96.7 | 161.2 | 47.7 | Excellent |
| Papaya | 1 each | 119 | 187.9 | 313.1 | 47.5 | Excellent |
| Kale | 1 cup | 36 | 53.3 | 88.8 | 43.9 | Excellent |
| Kiwifruit | 1 each | 46 | 57.0 | 95.0 | 36.9 | Excellent |
| Cantaloupe | 1 cup | 56 | 67.5 | 112.5 | 36.2 | Excellent |
| Oranges | 1 each | 62 | 69.7 | 116.2 | 34.0 | Excellent |
| Grapefruit | 0.5 each | 60 | 66.0 | 110.0 | 33.0 | Excellent |
| Cabbage | 1 cup | 33 | 30.2 | 50.3 | 27.4 | Excellent |
| Tomatoes | 1 cup | 38 | 34.4 | 57.3 | 27.3 | Excellent |
| Swiss chard | 1 cup | 35 | 31.5 | 52.5 | 27.0 | Excellent |
| Collard greens | 1 cup | 49 | 34.6 | 57.6 | 21.0 | Excellent |
| Raspberries | 1 cup | 60 | 30.8 | 51.3 | 15.3 | Excellent |
| Asparagus | 1 cup | 43 | 19.4 | 32.4 | 13.5 | Excellent |
| Celery | 1 cup | 19 | 8.4 | 14.0 | 13.1 | Excellent |
| Spinach | 1 cup | 41 | 17.6 | 29.4 | 12.8 | Excellent |
| Pineapple | 1 cup | 76 | 23.9 | 39.8 | 9.4 | Excellent |
| Green beans | 1 cup | 44 | 12.1 | 20.2 | 8.3 | Excellent |
| Summer squash | 1 cup | 36 | 9.9 | 16.5 | 8.3 | Excellent |

\* For more on "DV," "Density," and "Quality" Rating System, see page xxx.

## FUNCTIONS

What can vitamin C-rich foods do for you?

- Help protect cells from free radical damage
- Regenerate your vitamin E supplies
- Improve iron absorption
- Lower your cancer risk

What events can indicate a need for more vitamin C-rich foods?

- Poor wound healing
- Frequent colds or infections
- Lung-related problems

## IMPACT OF COOKING, STORAGE & PROCESSING

Vitamin C is highly sensitive to air, water, and temperature. About 25% of the vitamin C in vegetables can be lost by blanching as well as the freezing and unthawing of vegetables and fruits. Cooking of vegetables and fruits for 10–20 minutes can result in a loss of over 1/2 of the total vitamin C content. When fruits and vegetables are canned and then reheated, only 1/3 of the original vitamin C content may be left. Consumption of vitamin C-rich foods in their fresh, raw form is the best way to maximize vitamin C intake.

## PUBLIC HEALTH RECOMMENDATIONS

In 2000, the Institute of Medicine at the National Academy of Sciences issued new Adequate Intake (AI) levels for vitamin

C for infants up to 1 year old and Recommended Dietary Allowances (RDAs) for all people older than 1 year old. The recommendations are as follows:

- 0–6 months: 40 mg
- 7–12 months: 50 mg
- 1–3 years: 15 mg
- 4–8 years: 25 mg
- 9–13 years: 45 mg
- Males 14–18 years: 75 mg
- Males 19+ years: 90 mg
- Females 14–18 years: 65 mg
- Females 19+ years: 75 mg
- Pregnant females 18 years: 80 mg
- Pregnant females 19+ years: 85 mg
- Lactating females 18 years: 115 mg
- Lactating females 19+ years: 120 mg

The FDA has set the Reference Value for Nutrition Labeling for vitamin C at 60 mg. This is the recommended intake value used by the FDA to calculate the %Daily Value for vitamin C that may appear on food labels.

The Institute of Medicine established a Tolerable Upper Intake Level (UL) for vitamin C at 2,000 milligrams (2 grams) in 2000.

## WHY WE NEED VITAMIN C-RICH FOODS

Vitamin C, also called ascorbic acid, is a water-soluble essential nutrient that we must obtain from our diets. The body has a built-in vitamin C barometer, excreting any excess that is not needed. This nutrient is so critical to living creatures that almost all mammals can use their own cells to make it, although humans cannot synthesize vitamin C.

Humans vary greatly in their vitamin C requirement. It is natural for one person to need 10 times as much vitamin C as another person; and a person's age and health status can dramatically change his or her need for vitamin C.

Eating foods rich in vitamin C enhances your body's usage of this important vitamin since these foods naturally contain other nutrients that act in synergy with vitamin C, supporting its physiological function in your body and therefore best contributing to your optimal health.

Vitamin C has important interactions with several key nutrients in the body. Vitamin C can significantly enhance iron uptake and metabolism, even at food-level amounts. Absorption of calcium may be enhanced by vitamin C since calcium ascorbate forms of calcium may be better absorbed than other forms. Excessive intake of vitamin A, for example, is less toxic to the body when vitamin C is readily available. Vitamin C is involved in the regeneration of vitamin E, and these two vitamins appear to work together in their antioxidant effect.

## HOW DOES VITAMIN C PROMOTE HEALTH?
### Antioxidant Protection

Vitamin C is a primary water-soluble antioxidant in the body, disarming free radicals and preventing damage in the aqueous environment both inside and outside cells. Inside cells, a potential long-term result of excessive free radical damage to DNA is cancer. Especially in areas of the body where cellular turnover is especially rapid, such as the digestive system, preventing DNA mutations translates into preventing cancer. This may be why a good intake of vitamin C is associated with a reduced risk of colon cancer and why cardiovascular diseases, joint diseases and cataracts are all associated with vitamin C deficiency.

### Immune System Support

Vitamin C, which is also vital for the proper function of a healthy immune system, is good for preventing colds and may be helpful in preventing recurrent ear infections. The immune system relies on a wide variety of mechanisms to help protect the body from infection, including white blood cells, complement proteins, and interferons, and vitamin C is especially important in the function of these immune components.

## WHAT ARE THE CAUSES AND SYMPTOMS OF VITAMIN C DEFICIENCY?

Poor intake of vitamin C-rich vegetables and fruits is a common contributor to vitamin C deficiency. In the U.S., one third of all adults get less vitamin C from their diet than is recommended by the National Academy of Sciences, and one out of every six adults gets less than half the amount recommended. Smoking and exposure to second hand smoke also increase the risk of vitamin C deficiency.

The body's immune and detoxification systems make special use of vitamin C and overload in either of these systems can increase risk of deficiency. When the body is exposed to toxins, vitamin C is often required for the body to begin processing the toxins for elimination. Excessive toxic exposure is therefore a risk factor for vitamin C deficiency.

Full-blown symptoms of the vitamin C deficiency disease, scurvy—including bleeding gums and skin discoloration due to ruptured blood vessels—are rare in the U.S. Poor wound healing, however, is not rare, and can be a symptom of vitamin C deficiency. Weak immune function, including susceptibility to colds and other infections, can also be a telltale sign of vitamin C deficiency. Since the lining of our respiratory tract also depends heavily on vitamin C for protection, respiratory infection and other lung-related conditions can also be symptomatic of not getting enough vitamin C.

## CAN YOU CONSUME TOO MUCH VITAMIN C?

There are no documented toxicity effects for vitamin C in relation to food and diet. The Tolerable Upper Intake Level (UL) for vitamin C is 2,000 milligrams (2 grams), an amount difficult to achieve through food sources alone.

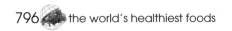

# vitamin d

Best Sources of Vitamin D from the *World's Healthiest Foods*

| FOOD | SERVING SIZE | CALS | AMOUNT (IU) | DV (%) | DENSITY | QUALITY |
|------|--------------|------|-------------|--------|---------|---------|
| Shrimp | 4 oz-wt | 112 | 162.4 | 40.6 | 6.5 | Very Good |
| Sardines | 4 oz-wt | 191 | 250.2 | 62.6 | 5.9 | Very Good |
| Milk, low-fat | 1 cup | 121 | 97.6 | 24.4 | 3.6 | Very Good |
| Cod | 4 oz-wt | 119 | 63.5 | 15.9 | 2.4 | Good |
| Eggs | 1 each | 68 | 22.88 | 5.7 | 1.5 | Good |

\* For more on "DV," "Density," and "Quality" Rating System, see page 805.

## FUNCTIONS

What can vitamin D-rich foods do for you?
- Help keep your bones and teeth strong and healthy
- Regulate the growth and activity of your cells
- Help prevent excessive inflammatory immune-related activity

What events can indicate a need for more vitamin D-rich foods?
- Thinning bones, frequent bone fractures, soft bones
- Bone deformities or growth retardation in children
- Lack of exposure to sunlight
- Being dark-skinned

## IMPACT OF COOKING, STORAGE & PROCESSING

Vitamin D is a stable compound. Neither cooking nor long-term storage significantly reduce vitamin D levels in food.

## PUBLIC HEALTH RECOMMENDATIONS

In 1997, the Institute of Medicine at the National Academy of Sciences issued new Adequate Intake (AI) levels for vitamin D. The recommendations are as follows:
- Infants and children: 5 mcg (200 IU)
- Teenagers: 5 mcg (200 IU)
- 19–50 years: 5 mcg (200 IU)
- 51–70 years: 10 mcg (400 IU)
- 70+ years: 15 mcg (600 IU)
- Pregnant and lactating women: 5 mcg (200 IU)

The FDA has set the Reference Value for Nutrition Labeling for vitamin D at 400 IU. This is the recommended intake value used by the FDA to calculate the %Daily Value for vitamin D that may appear on food labels.

Since the establishment of these vitamin D recommendations in 1997, over 3,000 research studies involving vitamin D have been published in top level science journals. Many of these studies suggest that significantly higher levels of vitamin D may be essential for certain groups of people.

These groups include persons living in more northern geographical areas, for example, residents in the Pacific Northwest or New England; obese persons; persons getting very little sunlight due to indoor jobs or personal habits, including constant use of sunscreen; and persons with naturally darker skin. Individuals in these caregories may require closer to 1000 IU than the 200–600 IU levels listed above.

Recent research suggests that the AI recommendations may be inadequate. Blood levels of no less than 30 ng/ml (nanograms per milliliter) indicate adequate supplies of vitamin D; unless able to receive sufficient sun exposure, most adults need 1,000 IU of vitamin D daily to reach and maintain these levels.

If you are concerned about your vitamin D status, ask your doctor to check your blood levels of 25(OH)D3, which is the major circulating form of vitamin D in the blood. This form of the vitamin is the true barometer of vitamin D status.

## WHY WE NEED VITAMIN D-RICH FOODS

Early in the 20th century, scientists discovered that rickets, a childhood disease characterized by improper bone development, could be prevented by a compound isolated from cod liver oil referred to as "fat-soluble factor D," now known as vitamin D. The vitamin was also called "calciferol," since it was found to boost calcium deposits in bone. We now know that without adequate vitamin D, our intestines may absorb as little as 1–15% of the calcium in the foods we eat; when our vitamin D supplies are adequate, our intestines absorb 30–80%. Because vitamin D is so important for skeletal growth and strong bones, many foods are fortified with this vitamin to ensure that children obtain adequate amounts.

There are two basic types of vitamin D. Ergosterol is the basic building block of vitamin D in plants. Cholesterol is the basic building block of vitamin D in humans. When ultraviolet light from the sun hits the leaf of a plant, ergosterol is converted into ergocalciferol, or vitamin D2. In just the same way, when ultraviolet light hits the cells of our skin, cholesterol is converted into cholecalciferol, or vitamin D3.

Vitamin D plays a role in maintaining normal blood levels of calcium. As a result, vitamin D impacts the absorption and storage of calcium. Vitamin D also stimulates the absorption of phosphorus. Vitamin D is believed to regulate the production of certain calcium-binding proteins that function in the bones and kidneys. Because these binding proteins are dependent on vitamin K, an interrelationship between vitamin D and vitamin K is also likely.

Eating foods rich in vitamin D enhances your body's usage of this important vitamin since these foods naturally contain other nutrients that act in synergy with vitamin D, supporting its physiological function in your body and therefore best contributing to your optimal health.

## HOW DOES VITAMIN D PROMOTE HEALTH?
### Maintains Proper Calcium Levels in the Blood

Although typically categorized as a fat-soluble vitamin, vitamin D actually functions more like a hormone than a vitamin. Calcitriol, the most metabolically active form of vitamin D, works with parathyroid hormone (PTH) to maintain proper levels of calcium in the blood. Calcitriol acts to increase the intestinal absorption of calcium, increase the reabsorption of calcium by the kidneys, and stimulate the release of calcium from the bone, thereby increasing blood calcium levels. Alternatively, when blood levels of calcium are high, calcitriol decreases the intestinal absorption of calcium and stimulates the bones to take up calcium, thereby decreasing blood calcium levels.

Through its relationship with calcium metabolism, vitamin D is important for maintaining not only healthy bones, but healthy teeth as well. Studies have found that in men and women over 50 years of age, lack of vitamin D increases risk of periodontal disease.

### Supports Healthy Immune Function and Prevents Excessive Inflammation

Vitamin D also helps regulate immune system activity, preventing an excessive or prolonged inflammatory response. Our immune cells, specifically our active T-cells, have receptors for vitamin D. This is important because many autoimmune diseases have a T-cell component of inflammation. Preliminary research suggests that vitamin D's anti-inflammatory effects may have benefits across a wide spectrum of health conditions including hypertension, type 1 diabetes and psoriasis.

### Regulation of Cell Activity

For many years, researchers have known that vitamin D, in the form of calcitriol, participates in the regulation of cell activity. Only recently, however, have studies confirmed the presence of a vitamin D receptor on the membrane of the cell nucleus. Signals throughout the body related to cell multiplication and natural cell death appear to depend on vitamin D. Most minerally-regulated organs, including the bone, kidney, intestine, and parathyroid glands appear to depend on vitamin D availability for their regulation. Because cell cycles play such a key role in the development of cancer, optimal vitamin D intake may turn out to play an important role in prevention and/or treatment of various cancers.

## WHAT ARE THE CAUSES AND SYMPTOMS OF VITAMIN D DEFICIENCY?

It is important for individuals with limited sun exposure to include good sources of vitamin D in their diets. Homebound individuals, people living in northern latitudes, individuals who use sunscreen and/or wear clothing that completely covers the body, and individuals working in occupations that prevent exposure to sunlight are at risk for vitamin D deficiency. Individuals with dark skin are also at risk for deficiency since their skin contains more melanin pigment, which reduces the skin's ability to produce vitamin D from sunlight. In addition, since breast milk from vitamin D-deficient mothers may not contain sufficient amounts of this nutrient, exclusively breast-fed infants may be a risk for deficiency.

Since vitamin D is a fat-soluble vitamin, a diet that is extremely low in fat and/or the presence of certain medical conditions that cause a reduction in the ability to absorb dietary fat may cause vitamin D deficiency. Under certain circumstances, the conversion of inactive forms of vitamin D to calcitriol is impaired. For example, diseases that affect the parathyroid gland, liver and/or kidney impair the synthesis of the active form of vitamin D. In addition, the production of vitamin D precursors in the skin decreases with age.

Vitamin D deficiency results in decreased absorption of calcium and phosphorus. As a result, prolonged vitamin D deficiency has a negative impact on bone mineralization. In infants and children, such a deficiency manifests itself as rickets, a condition characterized by bone deformities and growth retardation. Adults with vitamin D deficiency may experience bone thinning (osteopenia), bone pain and/or soft bones (osteomalacia).

## CAN YOU CONSUME TOO MUCH VITAMIN D?

Excessive dietary intake of vitamin D can be toxic. Toxicity of vitamin D can come from either its plant-based (D2) or animal-based (D3) form. Symptoms of toxicity include loss of appetite, nausea, vomiting, high blood pressure, kidney malfunction, and failure to thrive.

In 1997, the Institute of Medicine set Tolerable Upper Intake Levels (ULs) for vitamin D as follows: infants, 0–12 months, 25 micrograms per day; children and adults, 50 micrograms per day; and pregnant and lactating women, 50 micrograms per day.

# vitamin e

Best Sources of Vitamin E from the *World's Healthiest Foods*

| FOOD | SERVING SIZE | CALS | AMOUNT (IU) | DV (%) | DENSITY | QUALITY |
|------|------|------|------|------|------|------|
| Sunflower seeds | 1/4 cup | 205 | 40.8 | 90.5 | 7.9 | Excellent |
| Swiss chard | 1 cup | 35 | 7.5 | 16.6 | 8.5 | Excellent |
| Almonds | 1/4 cup | 205 | 20.9 | 46.4 | 4.1 | Very good |
| Spinach | 1 cup | 41 | 3.9 | 8.6 | 3.7 | Very good |
| Collard greens | 1 cup | 49 | 3.8 | 8.3 | 3.0 | Good |
| Kale | 1 cup | 36 | 2.6 | 5.6 | 2.7 | Good |
| Papaya | 1 each | 119 | 7.7 | 17.0 | 2.6 | Good |
| Olives | 1 cup | 155 | 9.0 | 20.1 | 2.3 | Good |
| Bell peppers | 1 cup | 25 | 1.5 | 3.1 | 2.3 | Good |
| Brussels sprouts | 1 cup | 61 | 3.0 | 6.7 | 2.0 | Good |
| Kiwifruit | 1 each | 46 | 2.0 | 4.3 | 1.7 | Good |
| Blueberries | 1 cup | 81 | 3.3 | 7.3 | 1.6 | Good |
| Tomatoes | 1 cup | 38 | 1.5 | 3.4 | 1.6 | Good |
| Broccoli | 1 cup | 44 | 1.7 | 3.8 | 1.5 | Good |

* For more on "DV," "Density," and "Quality" Rating System, see page 805.

## FUNCTIONS

What can vitamin E-rich foods do for you?
- Prevent cell damage from free radicals
- Protect your skin from ultraviolet light
- Allow your cells to communicate effectively

What events can indicate a need for more vitamin E-rich foods?
- Digestive system problems, especially malabsorption
- Tingling or loss of sensation in the arms, hands, legs, or feet
- Liver or gallbladder problems

## IMPACT OF COOKING, STORAGE & PROCESSING

Exposure to air and factory processing can be particularly damaging to the vitamin E content of food. In wheat, for example, where most of the vitamin E is found in the germ layer, commercial processing removes 50–90% of the food's vitamin E content. In 60% extraction wheat flour, the alpha-tocopherol content drops almost 90%, and the beta-tocopherol content drops 43%. To help protect their vitamin E content, vegetable oils like olive oil, sunflower seed oil, and peanut oil should be kept in tightly capped containers to avoid unnecessary exposure to air.

## PUBLIC HEALTH RECOMMENDATIONS

In 2000, the Institute of Medicine at the National Academy of Sciences issued new Adequate Intake (AI) levels for vitamin E for infants up to 1 year old and Recommended Dietary Allowances (RDAs) for all people older than 1 year old. The recommendations are as follows:
- 0–6 months: 4 mg (6 IU)
- 6–12 months: 6 mg (7.5 IU)
- 1–3 years: 6 mg (9 IU)
- 4–8 years: 7 mg (10.5 IU)
- 9–13 years: 11 mg (16.5 IU)
- 14+ years: 15 mg (22.5 IU)
- Pregnant females, 18+ year: 15 mg (22.5 IU)
- Lactating females, 18+ years: 19 mg (28.5 IU)

The FDA has set the Reference Value for Nutrition Labeling for vitamin E at 30mg. This is the recommended intake value used by the FDA to calculate the %Daily Value for vitamin E that may appear on food labels.

The Institute of Medicine established a Tolerable Upper Intake Level (UL) for vitamin E at 1,000 mg (1,500 IU). This daily limit applies to supplemental vitamin E only, and is intended to apply to all individuals age 19 and older.

## WHY WE NEED VITAMIN E-RICH FOODS

Even though its name makes it sound like a single substance, vitamin E is actually a family of fat-soluble vitamins that are active throughout the body. Some members of the vitamin E family are called tocopherols. These members include alpha-tocopherol, beta-tocopherol, gamma-tocopherol, and delta-tocopherol. Other members of the vitamin E family are called tocotrienols. These members include alpha-, beta-, gamma-, and delta-tocotrienol. As increasing information has become available about these forms of vitamin E, more and more of them are understood to have unique functions. Unlike most dietary supplements, which typically contain only alpha-tocopherol and often provide a strictly synthetic form of this vitamin E fraction called dl-alpha tocopherol, foods contain the full spectrum of the vitamin E family.

Eating foods rich in vitamin E enhances your body's usage of this important vitamin since these foods naturally contain other nutrients that act in synergy with vitamin E, supporting its physiological function in your body and therefore best contributing to your optimal health.

## HOW DOES VITAMIN E PROMOTE HEALTH?
### Prevention of Oxidative Stress
Although humans must breathe oxygen to stay alive, oxygen is a risky substance inside the body because it can make molecules overly reactive. When oxygen-containing molecules become too reactive, they can start damaging the cell structures around them. In chemistry, this imbalanced situation involving oxygen is called oxidative stress.

Vitamin E helps prevent oxidative stress by working together with a group of nutrients—vitamin C, vitamin B3, selenium and glutathione—to prevent oxygen molecules from becoming too reactive. Some researchers believe that vitamin E is the most important member of this oxidative stress-preventing group. Oxidative stress has been linked to a host of different chronic diseases including cardiovascular disease, arthritis, asthma, and various cancers.

### Supporting Healthy Skin
Vitamin E has sometimes been described as the "lightning rod" of the cell, allowing reactive molecules to strike the cell, like lightning, without causing damage. This "lightning rod" function of vitamin E is particularly apparent in the case of the skin, since vitamin E directly protects the skin from ultraviolet radiation (also called UV light). In numerous research studies, vitamin E applied topically to the skin has been shown to prevent UV damage. When the diet contains vitamin E-rich foods, vitamin E can travel to the skin cell membranes and exert this same protective effect.

### Promotes Cell Signaling
While most of the research on vitamin E has focused on its role in prevention of oxidative stress, a variety of new roles have recently been suggested. Most of these new roles involve the transfer of chemical information from one cell to another, or across different structures inside of a cell. This transfer of chemical information is referred to as "cell signaling," and many researchers believe that cell signaling cannot accurately take place without the help of vitamin E.

## WHAT ARE THE CAUSES AND SYMPTOMS OF VITAMIN E DEFICIENCY?
Since vitamin E is a fat-soluble vitamin, poor absorption of fat in the digestive tract can contribute to vitamin E deficiency. Some specific health conditions that can cause fat malabsorption include pancreatic disease, celiac disease, and gallbladder disease. Premature birth has also been shown to increase risk of vitamin E deficiency in infants.

Deficiency symptoms for vitamin E are difficult to pinpoint and controversial in the research literature. The area of broadest agreement involves malabsorption. In many research studies, low levels of vitamin E are associated with digestive system problems where nutrients are poorly absorbed from the digestive tract.

A second area of focus for vitamin E deficiency symptoms is called peripheral neuropathy. This area focuses on nervous system problems in the arms, hands, legs, and feet. Pain, tingling, and loss of sensation in these extremities have been associated with vitamin E deficiency. Although many healthcare practitioners report that skin problems appear closely linked to vitamin E deficiency, there are limited human research studies to support this view.

## CAN YOU CONSUME TOO MUCH VITAMIN E?
When obtained from food sources alone, vitamin E has no documented research of toxicity. The Institute of Medicine set a Tolerable Upper Intake Level (UL) for vitamin E of 1,000 mg (or 1,500 IU of vitamin E in the form of alpha-tocopherol). This daily limit applies to supplemental vitamin E only and is intended to apply to all individuals age 19 and older.

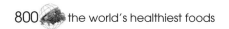

# vitamin k

Best Sources of Vitamin K from the *World's Healthiest Foods*

| FOOD | SERVING SIZE | CALS | AMOUNT (mcg) | DV (%) | DENSITY | QUALITY |
|---|---|---|---|---|---|---|
| Parsley | 2 TBS | 2.7 | 123 | 153.8 | 1025 | Excellent |
| Kale | 1 cup | 36.4 | 1062.1 | 1327.6 | 656.5 | Excellent |
| Spinach | 1 cup | 41.4 | 888.5 | 1110.6 | 482.9 | Excellent |
| Swiss chard | 1 cup | 35 | 572.8 | 716 | 368.2 | Excellent |
| Collard greens | 1 cup | 49.4 | 704 | 880 | 320.6 | Excellent |
| Romaine lettuce | 2 cup | 15.7 | 114.8 | 143.5 | 164.7 | Excellent |
| Basil | 2 tsp | 7.5 | 48.01 | 60 | 143.6 | Excellent |
| Brussel sprouts | 1 cup | 60.8 | 218.8 | 273.5 | 80.9 | Excellent |
| Broccoli | 1 cup | 43.7 | 155.2 | 194 | 79.9 | Excellent |
| Cabbage | 1 cup | 33 | 73.35 | 91.7 | 50 | Excellent |
| Asparagus | 1 cup | 43.2 | 91.8 | 114.8 | 47.8 | Excellent |
| Celery | 1 cup | 19.2 | 35.26 | 44.1 | 41.3 | Excellent |
| Sea vegetables | 0.25 cup | 8.6 | 13.2 | 16.5 | 34.5 | Excellent |
| Green beans | 1 cup | 43.8 | 20 | 25 | 10.3 | Excellent |
| Cauliflower | 1 cup | 28.5 | 11.17 | 14 | 8.8 | Excellent |
| Tomatoes | 1 cup | 37.8 | 14.22 | 17.8 | 8.5 | Excellent |
| Black pepper | 2 tsp | 10.9 | 6.88 | 8.6 | 14.2 | Very Good |
| Green peas | 1 cup | 134.4 | 41.4 | 51.8 | 6.9 | Very Good |
| Carrots | 1 cup | 52.5 | 16.1 | 20.1 | 6.9 | Very Good |
| Bell peppers | 1 cup | 24.8 | 4.51 | 5.6 | 4.1 | Very Good |
| Summer squash | 1 cup | 36 | 6.3 | 7.9 | 3.9 | Very Good |
| Cayenne pepper | 2 tsp | 11.2 | 2.89 | 3.6 | 5.8 | Good |
| Avocados | 1 cup | 235.1 | 29.2 | 36.5 | 2.8 | Good |
| Soybeans | 1 cup | 297.6 | 33.02 | 41.3 | 2.5 | Good |
| Cranberries | 0.5 cup | 23.3 | 2.42 | 3 | 2.3 | Good |

\* For more on "DV," "Density," and "Quality" Rating System, see page 805.

## FUNCTIONS

What can vitamin K-rich foods do for you?
- Allow your blood to clot normally
- Help protect against osteoporosis
- Prevent oxidative cell damage

What events can indicate a need for more vitamin K-rich foods?
- Excessive bruising and bleeding
- Digestive system problems, especially malabsorption
- Liver or gallbladder problems

## IMPACT OF COOKING, STORAGE & PROCESSING

Even though vitamin K is more resilient to processing than many vitamins, fresh foods still offer the highest amounts. Naturally occurring forms of vitamin K exist as oils and are resistant to heat and moisture, but are destroyed by acid, base, oxidizers and light; therefore, little is lost during normal cooking. Foods that are processed into low-fat versions will have less naturally occurring vitamin K, since it has been removed with the other fats. Freezing a food can decrease its vitamin K content. For example, 100 grams of raw spinach has 483 micrograms of vitamin K. One hundred grams of frozen spinach has 377 micrograms, or about 20% less.

## PUBLIC HEALTH RECOMMENDATIONS

In 2000, the Institute of Medicine at the National Academy of Sciences issued new Adequate Intake (AI) levels for vitamin K. The recommendations are as follows:
- 0–6 months: 2 mcg
- 7–12 months: 2.5 mcg

- 1–3 years: 30 mcg
- 4—8 years: 55 mcg
- 9–13 years: 60 mcg
- 14–18 years: 75 mcg
- Males 19+ years: 120 mcg
- Females 19+ years: 90 mcg
- Pregnant and lactating females up to 18 years: 75 mcg
- Pregnant and lactating females 19+ years: 90 mcg

The Institute of Medicine did not establish a Tolerable Upper Intake Level (UL) for vitamin K in its 2000 recommendations.

## WHY WE NEED VITAMIN K-RICH FOODS

There are three forms of vitamin K: vitamin K1, also called phylloquinone, is the natural, plant form of this nutrient; vitamin K2, also called menaquinone, is produced by the bacteria in animal and human intestines; and vitamin K3, also called menadione, is the synthetic version. While the three forms are about equally helpful for blood clotting, vitamin K1, the form that only occurs in green plants, is the best form for protecting against osteoporosis. Leafy green vegetables, which are rich sources of vitamin K1, also provide concentrated amounts of other bone-building nutrients, including calcium and boron.

## HOW DOES VITAMIN K PROMOTE HEALTH?

### Supports Bone Health

Vitamin K1, the form of the vitamin found in food, helps maintain bone mass because it is used to activate osteocalcin, the major noncollagen protein in bone. Activated osteocalcin anchors calcium molecules inside of the bone. Therefore, without enough vitamin K1, osteocalcin levels are inadequate, so bone mineralization is impaired. Researchers are identifying other ways in which vitamin K aids bone health. For example, vitamin K may both prevent the formation and increase the rate at which osteoclasts, the cells that break down bone, die. Low levels of blood vitamin K have been found to be associated with lower bone mineral density and higher fracture rates with dietary intake of vitamin K associated with reduced risk of hip fractures.

### Supports Healthy Blood Clotting Activity

Blood clotting is a vital function in the body that solidifies blood to prevent us from bleeding to death when a blood vessel is damaged either from an external wound or internally. Another benefit of blood clotting is that it secludes the area of an infection or injury and begins the healing process. Vitamin K is required to activate enzymes at many stages in the intricate clotting process called the clotting cascade. Without it, the amount of blood clotting proteins decreases and bleeding time increases. Vitamin K is best known as being required for blood to clot. Interestingly, it is also required to activate several proteins that decrease blood clotting. Thus, research is showing that vitamin K not only helps to initiate blood clotting, but it is also necessary for its complex regulation.

### Protects Against Oxidative Cell Damage

Although humans must breathe oxygen to stay alive, oxygen is a risky substance inside the body because its use can result in the production of free radicals. Unless quickly neutralized by antioxidants, these overly reactive, oxygen-containing molecules can damage the cell structures around them.

When vitamin K is used by an enzyme to alter proteins, it too is altered. This altered vitamin K is then regenerated and reused continuously in what is called the vitamin K cycle. During this cycle, vitamin K functions as an antioxidant, inactivating free radicals that would otherwise damage the delicate fats that are the primary constituents of our cell membranes.

## WHAT ARE THE CAUSES AND SYMPTOMS OF VITAMIN K DEFICIENCY?

Since vitamin K is a fat-soluble vitamin, poor absorption of fat in the digestive tract can contribute to vitamin K deficiency. Some specific health conditions that can cause fat malabsorption include pancreatic disease, celiac disease, and gallbladder disease. Premature birth has also been shown to increase risk of vitamin K deficiency in infants. Certain medications for heart disease block vitamin K in order to decrease blood clotting and could result in vitamin K deficiency. Anti-coagulant medications, such as Coumadin, are designed to decrease clotting by interfering with vitamin K. (Therefore, eating a diet that is high in vitamin K can make anticoagulant medications less effective. People taking anticoagulant medications, such as Coumadin, should monitor their vitamin K intake and discuss this with their physician.)

Vitamin K deficiency is rare but can cause poor blood coagulation and therefore longer bleeding time. Severe deficiency can lead to fatal anemia. When animals are deprived of vitamin K for long periods of time, they have problems crystallizing bone, and they stop growing taller.

When vitamin K deficiency does occur, it is most likely to happen in newborns, especially if they are premature, breast-fed, or their mother was taking anticoagulant medication. Babies are born with sterile intestines; therefore there are no bacteria in their intestines to produce vitamin K2, making them more susceptible to vitamin K deficiency if their diet has inadequate amounts.

## CAN YOU CONSUME TOO MUCH VITAMIN K?

Even in high doses, natural forms of vitamin K have not produced symptoms of toxicity. For this reason, the Institute of Medicine at the National Academy of Sciences chose not to set a Tolerable Upper Intake Level (UL) for vitamin K when it revised its public health recommendations for this vitamin in 2000. Consuming more than the body's needs for dietary vitamin K does not cause the blood to clot excessively in healthy people. However, this does not mean that no potential exists for adverse effects resulting from high intakes.

# zinc

Best Sources of Zinc from the *World's Healthiest Foods*

| FOOD | SERVING SIZE | CALS | AMOUNT (MG) | DV (%) | DENSITY | QUALITY |
|------|------|------|------|------|------|------|
| Calf's liver | 4 oz-wt | 187 | 10.8 | 72.0 | 6.9 | Very good |
| Crimini mushrooms | 5 oz-wt | 31 | 1.6 | 10.4 | 6.0 | Very good |
| Spinach | 1 cup | 41 | 1.4 | 9.1 | 4.0 | Very good |
| Beef, grass-fed | 4 oz-wt | 240 | 6.3 | 42.2 | 3.2 | Good |
| Lamb | 4 oz-wt | 229 | 4.6 | 30.7 | 2.4 | Good |
| Summer squash | 1 cup | 36 | 0.7 | 4.7 | 2.3 | Good |
| Asparagus | 1 cup | 43 | 0.8 | 5.1 | 2.1 | Good |
| Venison | 4 oz-wt | 179 | 3.1 | 20.8 | 2.1 | Good |
| Chard | 1 cup | 35 | 0.6 | 3.9 | 2.0 | Good |
| Shrimp | 4 oz-wt | 112 | 1.8 | 11.8 | 1.9 | Good |
| Collard greens | 1 cup | 49 | 0.8 | 5.3 | 1.9 | Good |
| Pumpkin seeds | 1/4 cup | 187 | 2.6 | 17.1 | 1.7 | Good |
| Yogurt | 1 cup | 155 | 2.2 | 14.5 | 1.7 | Good |
| Green peas | 1 cup | 134 | 1.9 | 12.7 | 1.7 | Good |
| Broccoli | 1 cup | 44 | 0.6 | 4.1 | 1.7 | Good |
| Sesame seeds | 1/4 cup | 206 | 2.8 | 18.7 | 1.6 | Good |
| Mustard seeds | 2 tsp | 35 | 0.4 | 2.9 | 1.5 | Good |

\* Oysters (not included among the World's Healthiest Foods) are one of the richest sources of Zinc with a 4 oz serving of wild Eastern Oysters containing 103 mg.

\* For more on "DV," "Density," and "Quality" Rating System, see page 805.

## FUNCTIONS

What can zinc-rich foods do for you?
- Help balance blood sugar
- Stabilize your metabolic rate
- Prevent a weakened immune system
- Support an optimal sense of smell and taste

What events can indicate a need for more zinc-rich foods?
- Frequent colds and infections
- Depression
- Impaired sense of taste or smell
- Lack of appetite
- Growth failure in children

## IMPACT OF COOKING, STORAGE & PROCESSING

Like most minerals, zinc is present in many different forms in food and can vary greatly in its response to cooking and processing. In some foods, where a greater percent of zinc is found in water-soluble form and contact with water is great, high losses of zinc can occur. For example, when navy beans are cooked, 50% of the original zinc is lost.

The processing of wheat is another example of the susceptibility of zinc to substantial loss. In 60% extraction wheat flour—the kind that is used to make over 90% of all breads, baked goods, and pastas sold in the U.S.—almost 75% of the original zinc is lost.

## PUBLIC HEALTH RECOMMENDATIONS

In 1999, the Institute of Medicine at the National Academy of Sciences issued new Recommended Dietary Allowances (RDAs) for zinc. The recommendations are as follows:

- 0–6 months: 2 mg
- 6 months–3 years: 3 mg
- 4–8 years: 5 mg
- 9–13 years: 8 mg
- Males 14+ years: 11 mg
- Females 14–18 years: 9 mg
- Females 19+ years: 8 mg
- Pregnant females 18 years or younger: 12 mg
- Pregnant females, 19+ years: 11 mg
- Lactating females under 18 years: 14 mg
- Lactating females 19+ years: 12 mg

The FDA has set the Reference Value for Nutrition Labeling for zinc at 15 mg. This is the recommended intake value used by the FDA to calculate the %Daily Value for zinc that may appear on food labels.

Details on zinc's Tolerable Upper Intake Levels (UL) are provided under the heading "Can You Consume Too Much Zinc?"

## WHY WE NEED ZINC-RICH FOODS

Eating foods rich in zinc enhances your body's usage of this important mineral since these foods naturally contain other nutrients that act in synergy with zinc, supporting its physiological function in your body and therefore best contributing to your optimal health.

Zinc is a trace mineral needed in the diet on a daily basis. The first research studies to demonstrate zinc's importance in the diet focused on the issue of growth. When foods did not supply sufficient amounts of zinc, young men were found to have impaired overall growth as well as impaired sexual maturation. These initial studies on zinc reflected some of the key functions served by this mineral, including regulation of genetic activity, and balance of carbohydrate metabolism and blood sugar.

## HOW DOES ZINC PROMOTE HEALTH?

### Supports Immune Function

Many types of immune cells appear to depend upon zinc for optimal function. Particularly in children, researchers have studied the effects of zinc deficiency (and zinc supplementation) on immune response and the number of white blood cells, including specific studies on T lymphocytes, macrophages, and B cells. In these studies, zinc deficiency has been shown to compromise white blood cell numbers and immune response, while zinc supplementation has been shown to restore conditions to normal.

### Supports Glucose Balance and Metabolic Rate

Insulin, a hormone made by the pancreas, is required to move sugar from our bloodstream into our cells. The response of our cells to insulin is called the insulin response. When the foods in our diet do not provide us with enough zinc, our insulin response decreases, and our blood sugar becomes more difficult to stabilize. Metabolic rate—the rate at which we create and use up energy—also depends on zinc for its regulation. When zinc is deficient in our diet, metabolic rate drops (along with hormonal output by our thyroid gland).

### Maintaining Smell and Taste Sensitivity

Zinc must be linked to gustin, a protein involved in our sense of taste, in order for this sense function to work properly. Because of this relationship between zinc and taste, and because taste and smell are so closely linked in human physiology, impaired sense of taste and smell are common symptoms of zinc deficiency.

### Regulates Genetic Activities

Zinc is an important regulator of many genetic activities. Zinc is essential for reading genetic instructions, and when diets do not contain foods rich in zinc, instructions can be misread, or not read at all.

## WHAT ARE THE CAUSES AND SYMPTOMS OF ZINC DEFICIENCY?

In addition to dietary deficiency, problems in the digestive tract can contribute to zinc deficiency. These problems include irritable and inflammatory bowel disorders, as well as insufficient output of digestive enzymes by the pancreas, which results in impaired digestion of food. Protein deficiency, and specifically deficiency of the amino acid cysteine, can also contribute to zinc deficiency by preventing synthesis of transport and storage molecules that are used to shuttle and store zinc in the body. Loss of zinc through chronic diarrhea or profuse sweating (as might occur with heavy physical labor or athletic training) can also contribute to deficiency of this trace mineral.

Because of the link between zinc and the taste-related protein called gustin, impaired sense of taste and/or smell are common symptoms of zinc deficiency. Depression, lack of appetite, growth failure in children, and frequent colds and infections can also be symptomatic of insufficient dietary zinc.

## CAN YOU CONSUME TOO MUCH ZINC?

Zinc toxicity has been reported in the research literature, and in 2000 the Institute of Medicine set Tolerable Upper Intake Level (UL) of 40 milligrams for daily intake of zinc for all individuals age 19 and over. This amount is difficult, but possible, to attain from food sources alone. A metallic, bitter taste in the mouth can be indicative of zinc toxicity, as can stomach pain, nausea, vomiting, and cramps.

# antioxidants

Best *World's Healthiest Food* Sources of Antioxidants

| FOOD | SERVING SIZE | BETA-CAROTENE (MCG) | SELENIUM (%DV) | VITAMIN A (%DV) | VITAMIN C (%DV) | VITAMIN E (%DV) |
|---|---|---|---|---|---|---|
| Apples | 1 each | 37.3 | 0.6 | 1.5 | 13.1 | 2.2 |
| Apricots | 1 each | 383 | 0.2 | 18.3 | 5.8 | 1.6 |
| Asparagus | 1 cup | 1,087 | 4.4 | 19.4 | 32.4 | 3.4 |
| Bell peppers | 1 cup | 2,014 | 0.4 | 104.9 | 291.3 | 3.1 |
| Blueberries | 1 cup | 46.4 | 1.3 | 2.9 | 31.4 | 7.3 |
| Broccoli | 1 cup | 1,841 | 3.0 | 45.6 | 205.7 | 3.8 |
| Brussels sprouts | 1 cup | 711 | 3.3 | 22.4 | 161.2 | 6.7 |
| Cabbage | 1 cup | 111.0 | 1.3 | 4.0 | 50.3 | 0.8 |
| Cantaloupe | 1 cup | 3,232 | 0.9 | 103.2 | 112.5 | 1.2 |
| Carrots | 1 cup | 7,391 | 1.9 | 686.3 | 18.9 | 2.8 |
| Cauliflower | 1 cup | 8.7 | 0.9 | 0.4 | 91.5 | 0.3 |
| Cayenne pepper | 2 tsp | 786 | 0.5 | 29.4 | 4.5 | 0.8 |
| Collard greens | 1 cup | 9,147 | 3.0 | 118.9 | 57.6 | 8.3 |
| Cranberries | 0.5 cup | 17.1 | 0.4 | 0.4 | 10.7 | 0.3 |
| Figs | 8 oz-wt | 193 | 1.9 | 6.47 | 7.6 | 10.1 |
| Grapefruit | 0.5 each | 707 | 1.5 | 15.0 | 110.0 | 1.6 |
| Green beans | 1 cup | 525 | 0.7 | 16.6 | 20.2 | 0.9 |
| Green peas | 1 cup | 752 | 4.3 | 19.1 | 37.9 | 3.1 |
| Kale | 1 cup | 10,625 | 1.7 | 192.4 | 88.8 | 5.6 |
| Olives | 1 cup | 319 | 1.7 | 10.8 | 2.0 | 20.1 |
| Oranges | 1 each | 93.0 | 0.9 | 5.4 | 116.2 | 1.6 |
| Papaya | 1 each | 839 | 2.6 | 17.3 | 313.1 | 17.0 |
| Parsley | 2 TBS | 384 | 0.0 | 12.6 | 16.6 | 0.3 |
| Raspberries | 1 cup | 14.8 | 1.1 | 3.2 | 51.3 | 2.8 |
| Romaine lettuce | 2 cup | 3,902 | 0.3 | 58.2 | 44.8 | 2.5 |
| Shiitake mushrooms | 8 oz-wt | - | 53.0 | - | 10.0 | - |
| Spinach | 1 cup | 11,318 | 3.9 | 294.8 | 29.4 | 8.6 |
| Strawberries | 1 cup | 10.1 | 1.4 | 0.8 | 136.1 | 1.0 |
| Sunflower seeds | 0.25 cup | - | 30.6 | 0.4 | 0.8 | 90.5 |
| Sweet potatoes | 1 cup | 23,018 | 0.8 | 262.2 | 28.4 | 0.9 |
| Swiss chard | 1 cup | 6,391 | 2.3 | 109.9 | 52.5 | 16.6 |
| Tomatoes | 1 cup | 808 | 1.0 | 22.4 | 57.3 | 3.4 |
| Watermelon | 1 cup | 467 | 0.2 | 11.1 | 24.3 | 1.2 |
| Winter squash | 1 cup | 5,726 | 1.2 | 145.8 | 32.8 | 1.3 |

For more information on other nutrients with antioxidant functions, see carotenoids (page 740), flavonoids (page 754), niacin (page 768), zinc (page 802) and cysteine (page 749).

(Note: "-" indicates data is unavailable. For more information, please see page 805)

# the world's healthiest foods' quality rating system methodology

In order to quantify the nutrient richness of each of the World's Healthiest Foods in both this book and the www.whfood.org website, a team of top nutritionists and I designed the World's Healthiest Foods Quality Rating System ("Rating System").

This Rating System qualifies foods as "excellent," "very good" and "good" sources of nutrients, providing you with a simple, yet reliable, way to determine the nutritional attributes of a food. These quality descriptions don't just take a food's nutrient contribution into consideration; rather, they evaluate this nutrient contribution in relationship to the amount of calories a food contains. This way you can evaluate foods in terms of their ability to maximize your intake of important nutrients without having to exceed your individual caloric intake goals. (For more on the importance of nutrient richness, see page 24.)

To help you better understand the categorization of foods as "excellent," "very good" or "good" sources of a particular nutrient, I want to provide you with some background as to how these quality ratings were derived.

## Rating System Categories

We began with a computerized analysis of the nutritional contents of the World's Healthiest Foods using the nutritional analysis software, Food Processor for Windows (ESHA

| EXCELLENT | DENSITY>=7.6 | AND | DV>=10% | OR | DV>=75% |
|-----------|--------------|-----|---------|-----|---------|
| VERY GOOD | DENSITY>=3.4 | AND | DV>=5% | OR | DV>=50% |
| GOOD | DENSITY>=1.5 | AND | DV>=2.5% | OR | DV>=25% |

## Quality Rating System: Spinach Example

To further illustrate, let's look at an example. The example for spinach below shows how the two-part formula using the %DV and Density values for folic acid, dietary fiber and omega-3 fatty acids determines that spinach is an excellent source of folic acid, a very good source of dietary fiber and a good source of omega-3 fatty acids.

**EXCELLENT: Folic acid**
One cup of spinach contains 262 mcg of folic acid, which is 66% of this nutrient's DV. This cup of spinach contains 41 calories, or 2.3% of the DV for daily caloric intake. To get the Density rating, we compare (divide) the %DV for folic acid (66%) by the %DV for calories (2.3%) and get 28.5. This is its Density. Reflecting on the chart above, since its Density is greater than 7.6 AND it has a %DV greater than 10%, it qualifies as an "excellent" source of folic acid.

**VERY GOOD: Dietary fiber**
One cup of spinach contains 4.3 mg of dietary fiber, which is 17% of this nutrient's DV. Comparing that to its 2.3% DV for calories, we find that its Density rating for dietary fiber is 7.5. While spinach does not provide greater than the 50% DV for dietary fiber required to qualify it as a "very good" source of this nutrient based upon that specific criterion, it does have a Density greater than 3.4 AND has a DV greater than 5%; this combination qualifies it as a "very good" source according to the criterion in the chart above.

**GOOD: Omega-3 fatty acids**
One cup of spinach contains 0.15 g of omega-3 fatty acids, which is 6% of this nutrient's DV. Comparing that to the 2.3% DV for calories, we find that its Density rating for omega-3 fatty acids is 2.6. While spinach does not provide greater than the 25% DV for omega-3s to qualify it as a "good" source of this nutrient based upon that specific criterion, it does have a Density greater than 1.5 AND has a DV greater than 2.5%; this combination qualifies it as a "good" source according to the criterion in the chart above.

Research, Salem, Oregon, USA). In other words, we started with a food like spinach, and we analyzed how much vitamin C, vitamin A, zinc, protein, etc. that food contained in one commonly eaten serving.

For each food we found the %Daily Value (DV) contribution of each nutrient, as well as the food serving's %DV contribution of calories (for more on DV, see below); the comparison of the two became the Density, and is the first (and most important) part of the formula to determine the food's quality rating. We then picked a simple, three-category system for rating all foods: "excellent," "very good" and "good." The definitions of these rating qualifications are shown in the chart on the previous page.

## Daily Values (DVs)

In reality, the goal that each individual should strive for in terms of daily nutrient and caloric intake varies depending upon his or her personal needs. Yet, to help individuals meet their nutritional needs, government agencies have created standard recommendations for intake. The most up-to-date ones in the U.S. are those created by the Institute of Medicine and are known as the Dietary Reference Intakes (DRIs). Yet, since these DRIs can have many values for each nutrient (varying by age, gender and whether a woman is pregnant or lactating), we chose not to use these as our Daily Value (DV) standard. Rather, for most nutrients we chose to use the U.S. Food and Drug Administration's "Reference Values for Nutrition Labeling" as our standard for DVs. These are the values used by food manufacturers in the "Food Facts" portion of their product's label.

For other nutrients, for example for those where there were no "Reference Values," we derived a DV based upon the latest research or opinion of nutrition science experts. For example, we chose 2.5 grams as the Daily Value for omega-3 fatty acids; this was derived from recommendations of a panel of experts at a workshop sponsored by the National Institutes of Health in 1999, including Artemis Simopoulos, MD, Alexander Leaf, MD, and Norman Salem, Jr., Ph.D., who concluded that at least 1.2% of total calories should consist of omega-3 fatty acids. Since we used 1,800 calories as the reference diet for the Rating System, this translated into the 2.5 grams per day of omega-3 fatty acids that we chose for this nutrient's DV. The 1,800 calories chosen as the reference diet is based upon the Institute of Medicine's recommendation for sedentary women, age 31-50.

## Total Nutrient Richness Chart

Once the density ratings for each food were calculated, I wanted to create a quantitative way that each food's density could be compared. This was the number that was to become the Total Nutrient Richness, featured in each of the Nutrient Richness Charts as well as the Total Nutrient Richness Chart on page 21. The number is a reflection of how many "excellent," "very good" and "good" ratings a food had. Each "excellent" was assigned a value of 4, each "very good" a value of "2" and each "good" a value of 1. These were added together to arrive at the Total Nutrient Richness score.

## Nutritional Analysis Charts

In addition to the Nutrient Richness Chart featured for each food, each food chapter also includes a nutritional analysis that contains information on the amounts of over 60 nutrients that may be featured in that food. In addition to providing the amount of the nutrient, it also provides the %DV for many nutrients (some nutrients do not yet have established DVs).

As noted above, the nutrient profiles are derived from Food Processor for Windows software by ESHA Research. Of the 21,629 food records contained in the ESHA foods database, most of them—including those of the World's Healthiest Foods—lacked information for specific nutrients. In the nutritional analysis chart for each food, the designation "—" was chosen to represent those nutrients for which there was no measurement included in the ESHA foods database.

Data on phytonutrient values in an individual food's Nutrient Richness Chart were derived from the USDA National Nutrient Database for Standard Reference, Release 17 (2004) (http://www.nal.usda.gov/fnic/foodcomp/search) and the USDA Nutrient Data Laboratory, Agricultural Research Ser-vice. USDA Database for the Flavonoid Content of Selected Foods–2003 (http://www.nal.usda.gov/fnic/foodcomp/Data/Flav/flav.html). Oftentimes, information on phytonutrients may be cited in the text of individual food chapters without values appearing in the Nutrient Richness Chart; that is because there were either no measurements or no appreciable measurements for these phytonutrients featured in these databases.

# healing with the world's healthiest foods

*The focus in the past was on curing disease. The future belongs to its prevention.*
— George Mateljan

The World's Healthiest Foods can help promote vibrant health and energy. Research studies continue to confirm that eating a diet concentrated in nutrient-rich foods is one of the best things that you can do to enjoy optimal health and reduce the risk of disease. These studies have focused on both the overall dietary pattern of eating more whole foods as well as the benefits that individual foods provide. For example, studies show that the calcium in collard greens builds healthy bones and the omega-3 fatty acids in fish and flaxseeds support skin health while lycopene-rich tomatoes promote men's health and garlic helps maintain healthy cholesterol levels.

Yet, it's not just the research study results that are confirming the benefits of nutrient-rich foods. Speak with anyone who has changed their diet and began eating more whole foods, like the World's Healthiest Foods, and they'll attest to the improvement in health, energy and vitality that they have experienced.

In this section of the book, you'll find an overview of 21 health-related topics and what to eat, and what to avoid, if you are trying to enhance your health in these areas. These topics range from diseases such as rheumatoid arthritis to lifestyle concerns such as achieving more restful sleep.

*(Continued on Page 810)*

# anti-inflammatory foods

**Eat more of these World's Healthiest Foods:**

### Essential

- Foods rich in omega-3 fatty acids including fish such as salmon, tuna, sardines and cod, as well as flaxseeds and walnuts (page 770)

  The omega-3 fatty acids EPA and DHA found in fish serve as direct precursors for series-3 prostaglandins and resolvins, which reduce inflammation. Flaxseeds and walnuts are rich in the omega-3 fatty acid ALA, whose dietary intake is associated with reduced production of inflammatory compounds such as cRP, vCAM and IL-6.

- Herbs and spices such as turmeric, rosemary and ginger (page 691)

  Volatile oils and other phytonutrients contained in numerous herbs and spices are being studied for their potent anti-inflammatory properties.

### Avoid:

- Foods rich in omega-6 fatty acids such as sunflower oil, corn oil and other vegetable oils

  Excessive consumption of omega-6 fatty acids, notably with low intake of omega-3 fatty acids, can trigger the synthesis of pro-inflammatory compounds.

### Supportive

- Garlic (page 258) and onions (page 268)

  Contain compounds that inhibit *lipoxygenase* and *cyclooxygenase* enzymes, thus markedly reducing inflammation.

- Extra virgin olive oil (page 328)

  Rich in both antioxidant polyphenols and monounsaturated fats that inhibit production of inflammatory compounds.

- Conventionally grown produce with high pesticide residues (page 171)

  In animal studies, certain pesticides have been shown to overstimulate enzymes involved in chemical signaling, causing imbalance that has been linked to inflammation.

# asthma

**Eat more of these World's Healthiest Foods:**

### Essential

- Foods rich in omega-3 fatty acids including fish such as salmon, tuna, sardines and cod, as well as flaxseeds and walnuts (page 770)

  Studies have shown a strong link between eating fish, intake of omega-3 fatty acids and lower rates of asthma.

- Organically grown fruits and vegetables (page 113)

  Concentrated in vitamin C, vitamin E, selenium, beta-carotene and flavonoids, nutrients that promote lung health.

### Avoid:

- Milk and other dairy products

  Commonly cited as increasing the severity of asthmatic symptoms.

- Rosemary, sage, oregano and peppermint

  Contain rosmarinic acid, an antioxidant that encourages cells to make compounds that keep airways open for easy breathing.

- Turmeric and ginger

  Feature phytonutrients that interrupt the activation of a biological compound linked with inflammatory diseases such as asthma.

### Supportive

- Extra virgin olive oil (page 328)

  Consumption of olive oil is linked to reduced risk of developing asthma.

# colds and flu

## Eat more of these World's Healthiest Foods:

### Essential

- Fish rich in omega-3 fatty acids including salmon, tuna, sardines and cod (page 453)

    Omega-3 fatty acids are the precursors for series-3 prostaglandins, compounds that are involved in the regulation of the immune system.

- Organically grown fruits and vegetables

    Rich in vitamins C, E and A (through their concentration of carotenoids), which are all vital to a well functioning immune system.

- Onions (page 268)

    Onions contain compounds that have antibiotic properties and serve as anti-inflammatory agents, helpful in reducing the severity of respiratory congestion associated with the common cold.

### Avoid:

- Cooking oils exposed to high heat (page 52)

    Can produce immune system damaging substances.

- Excessive consumption of calories and fat

    Can weaken immune system strength.

- Garlic (page 258)

    Contains sulfur-containing compounds, such as allicin, that have been shown to be effective against common infections like colds and flu.

- Shiitake mushrooms (page 316)

    Contain the phytonutrient lentinan, which has been found to power up the immune system and strengthen its ability to fight infection.

### Supportive

- Nuts and seeds (page 501)

    Rich in the minerals selenium and zinc, which are important for immune system support. Walnuts and flaxseeds provide ALA, an omega-3 fatty acid that produces compounds necessary for the immune system to function properly.

- Refined grain products, white sugar and processed foods (page 658)

    Deplete the body of vitamins and minerals necessary for promoting immunity.

- Refined sugar

    Reduces the responsiveness of your immune cells and lowers your immune defenses.

# diabetes mellitus, type 2

## Eat more of these World's Healthiest Foods:

### Essential

- Fish rich in omega-3 fatty acids including salmon, tuna, sardines and cod

    Omega-3 fatty acids have been shown to be helpful for cardiovascular health and several studies have shown that type 2 diabetes occurs much less frequently in populations that eat fish regularly compared to populations that don't eat much fish.

- Legumes (page 587)

    Concentrated in fiber, protein and other nutrients that have a beneficial effect on blood sugar regulation.

- Organically grown vegetables, especially green leafy vegetables (such as Swiss chard, mustard greens and kale) and sweet potatoes (page 85)

    Rich in antioxidant nutrients such as vitamin C, vitamin E, carotenoids and flavonoids. Sweet potatoes contain special compounds thought to be beneficial for glucose balance.

- Garlic (page 258)

    May provide protection against cardiovascular disease, a well-known complication of type 2 diabetes.

- Onions (page 268)

    Rich in chromium, an important mineral for helping to regulate blood sugar.

- Tomatoes (page 164)

    Tomatoes are a good source of chromium and

antioxidant nutrients, and tomato juice can reduce the tendency toward blood clotting in persons with type 2 diabetes.

- Cinnamon (page 702)

    Both test tube and animal studies have shown that compounds in cinnamon not only stimulate insulin receptors but also significantly increase cells' ability to use glucose.

- Organically grown fruit (page 335)

    Rich in antioxidant nutrients, fresh fruits have been shown to have stabilizing effects on blood sugar levels when consumed in small amounts at a time.

- Red and purple fruits

    Anthocyanins, plant pigment phytonutrients found in cranberries, cherries, blueberries and other red and purple fruits, may help lower blood sugar levels in people with diabetes.

## Avoid:

- Concentrated sugars

    Cause elevations in blood glucose levels.

- Dried fruit (page 338)

    When watery portion is removed to make dried fruit, the sugar concentration becomes too high.

- Excessive iron-containing foods, particularly red meat

    Some individuals with diabetes, particularly men, may have too high levels of iron in their bodies, which may contribute to their risk of complication from blood sugar problems.

- Fruit juices (page 338)

    Too much whole food fiber, water, vitamins and phytonutrients are usually removed in the processing of whole fruit into fruit juice, and it's

## Supportive

- Walnuts (page 528)

    A great source of the omega-3 fatty acid ALA, walnuts may help lower a diabetic's heart disease risk.

- Whole grains, especially buckwheat (page 657)

    Whole grains contain beneficial dietary fiber and buckwheat contains a substance called chiro-inositol that may play an important role in the regulation of blood sugar.

- Soyfoods (page 594)

    Rich in protein and fiber, soyfoods can be generally supportive of blood sugar balance and may also help individuals with diabetes by improving kidney function.

- Extra virgin olive oil (page 328)

    Studies have shown that meals containing olive oil can have beneficial effects on blood sugar balance.

much easier to consume excessive amounts of sugar from fruit juice.

- Excessive total fats

    High-fat diets are associated with an increased risk for diabetes as well as an increase risk in heart disease, a concern for diabetics.

- Saturated fats

    Meals high in saturated fats have been shown to trigger insulin resistance and raise blood insulin levels more than desired.

- Foods that contain trans fats

    Trans fats are directly linked to an increased risk for insulin resistance as well as to an increased risk for blood clots, which can lead to heart attack or stroke.

*(Continued from Page 807)*

Please remember that this information is for educational purposes only. Causes of a health condition may vary owing to people's biochemical individuality; the details of the correct dietary approach for one person experiencing a certain health condition may not be the same for another person since the underlying factors causing the manifestation of symptoms may vary. As such, treatment of any health condition should be done with the guidance of a licensed health-care practitioner. If you'd like more details on dietary strategies to support health, please visit www.whfoods.org.

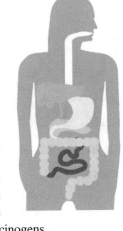

# digestive health

## Eat more of these World's Healthiest Foods:

### Essential

- Cruciferous vegetables including broccoli, kale, cauliflower and Brussels sprouts (page 153)

  Some studies show that eating just two or more servings of these vegetables a week can decrease colon cancer risk by 20–40%.

- Onions, garlic and leeks (page 258 and 268)

  These *Allium* family vegetables are rich sources of substances called organosulfur compounds, which have been found to increase the body's ability to break down harmful chemicals that can damage intestinal cells.

- Organically grown fruits, especially apples, grapefruit, cranberries and blueberries

  Fruits are rich in nutrients such as fiber, which supports healthy elimination and the growth of beneficial intestinal bacteria, as well as phytonutrients that that can help support circulation to the digestive tract, and may lower the risk of certain cancers, including breast and colon cancer.

- Whole grains (page 657)

  An excellent source of fiber and B-vitamins, nutrients known for the ability to promote digestive health or the metabolism of food components like carbohydrates.

- Yogurt (page 644)

  Fermented dairy products are rich in certain types of beneficial bacteria, which normally live in the human intestines. These bacteria have been shown to help protect colon cells from the damaging effects of carcinogens.

### Supportive

- Foods rich in omega-3 fatty acids including fish such as salmon, tuna, sardines and cod (page 453)

  Several studies have shown that populations that consume a good amount of fish have lower rates of colon cancer.

- Turmeric (page 700)

  Turmeric is a seasoning rich in curcumin, a substance that has been shown in numerous research studies to have very strong antioxidant and anti-inflammatory actions in the body.

- Ginger (page 708)

  Research suggests that ginger may lower the risk for certain cancers, including colon cancer. It has also been found to be helpful for nausea, notably from motion sickness and pregnancy.

- Soyfoods (page 594)

  Soyfoods contains compounds called sphingolipids that have been found to reduce the development of colon cancer in experimental animals.

## Avoid:

- Alcohol

  Many studies have shown an association between overconsumption of alcoholic beverages and an increased risk of colorectal cancer. The negative effects of alcohol are greatest in people who also have a low intake of the B-vitamin, folate.

- Red meat

  Several studies have shown that high intakes of meats, particularly fattier red meats and processed meats, are associated with an increased risk of colon cancer.

- Refined sugar

  Highly processed, refined sugar does not provide the digestive tract with any supportive vitamins or minereals, and it may reduce the activity of immune cells that must function within the digestive tract.

- Saturated and omega-6 fatty acids

  Those who consume large amounts of fat in their diets may have twice the risk of developing colon cancer compared to those who consume low-fat diets. The types of fats that seem to present the greatest problems when consumed in excessive amounts are long-chain saturated fats and the longer-chain omega-6 fatty acids, especially arachidonic acid.

# fatigue reduction and enhanced energy

**Eat more of these World's Healthiest Foods:**

**Essential**

- Low-glycemic index carbohydrates, particularly during the first half of the day (page 342)

    Examples include vegetables, certain fruits, nuts and seeds.

- Organically grown fruits and vegetables

    Rich in B vitamins, magnesium, chromium and other nutrients essential for optimal energy production.

- High-quality sources of protein (page 778)

    Eat these foods with each meal, especially during the first half of the day. Examples include legumes, nuts, fish, lean meat and poultry.

- Foods containing essential fatty acid and monounsaturated fats (page 770)

    Eat small amounts of these types of foods with each meal. Examples include extra virgin olive oil, almonds, walnuts, pecans, flaxseeds, pumpkin seeds, salmon, sardines, cod and tuna.

- Herbs and spices such as ginger, black pepper, cinnamon, rosemary, garlic, turmeric, chili pepper and fennel (page 691)

    Help support digestion.

**Follow these dietary strategies:**

- Eat frequently, if necessary, and keep healthy snacks close at hand.

- Eat lightly, only until you begin to feel satisfied. Because light eating places less of a burden on your digestion, you will feel lighter and more energetic.

- Eat slowly, deliberately and thankfully.

- Eat real food in which you can identify the actual source of the ingredients. Is it from whole or processed grains? Is it from fresh fruits and vegetables? Was it overcooked? Does it actually appear wholesome to you?

- Consider establishing your own "happy hour"—a relaxing and enjoyable hour before dinner that primes your mood and digestion. The origin of "happy hour" was simply a social hour spent enjoying bitter herbal (and not necessarily alcoholic!) beverages that warmed digestive fires.

- Consider a gentle after-dinner walk, respecting your own limits.

**Avoid:**

- Avoid foods or drinks to which you are sensitive (page 719).

- Avoid the temptations of stimulants and sweet snacks, especially soft drinks, coffee and candy.

- Limit your alcohol intake to low levels enjoyed not too regularly. If your fatigue is related to carbohydrate metabolism, avoid alcohol completely.

- Limit foods or drinks having a high-glycemic index since they can upset blood sugar balance (page 342).

# hair and nail health

**Eat more of these World's Healthiest Foods:**

**Essential**

- Biotin-containing foods such as Swiss chard, cooked eggs, almonds and walnuts (page 736)

  Biotin deficiency has been associated with hair loss, seborrheic dermatitis and brittle nails.

- Foods that provide adequate amounts of protein throughout the day (page 778)

  Since hair is made up primarily of protein, adequate protein is a very important factor for healthy hair.

- Foods rich in omega-3 fatty acids including fish such as salmon, tuna, sardines and cod as well as flaxseeds and walnuts (page 770)

  Symptoms of omega-3 fatty acid deficiency include brittle hair.

- Spinach, kale and other dark leafy greens

  Rich in both beta-carotene, which is converted to hair-healthy vitamin A, as well as lutein, which is a powerful antioxidant.

# heart disease (including atherosclerosis)

**Eat more of these World's Healthiest Foods:**

**Essential**

- Fish rich in omega-3 fatty acids including salmon, tuna, sardines and cod (page 453)

  Fish and omega-3 intake reduce triglycerides and are associated with reduced risk of stroke and heart attack.

- Organically grown fruits and vegetables

  Rich in nutrients that promote heart health such as vitamin B6, vitamin C, magnesium and antioxidant flavonoids and carotenoids.

- Garlic and Onions (page 258 and 268)

  Contain compounds that have been shown to lower cholesterol levels, lower blood pressure in cases of hypertension and slow the rate of arterial plaque growth.

- Tomatoes (page 164)

  A great source of lycopene, a carotenoid antioxidant whose dietary intake is associated with reduced risk of heart disease.

- Cranberries (page 410)

  Rich in polyphenolic antioxidants, intake of cranberries has been associated with improved blood vessel function.

- Oats (page 664)

  Contain beta-glucan, which reduces cholesterol levels, and avenathramides, antioxidants that prevent free-radical damage to LDL.

- Whole grains (page 657)

  Intake of whole grains is associated with reduced progression of atherosclerosis and reduced risk of heart disease.

- Walnuts (page 528)

  Have been found to reduce total and LDL cholesterol and increase the elasticity of arteries.

- Flaxseeds (page 512)

  Found to reduce total and LDL cholesterol levels.

- Almonds (page 534)

  Found to reduce total cholesterol and LDL levels, almonds are rich in heart-healthy vitamin E.

- Soyfoods (page 594)

  Soyfoods have been found to significantly decrease the risk of heart disease and lower LDL and total cholesterol, triglyceride levels and risk of blood clots.

- Extra virgin olive oil

  Protects against LDL oxidation, one of the first steps in atherosclerosis development.

- Green Tea (page 716)

  Contains flavonoids, whose intake has been associated with a significant decrease in risk of cardiovascular disease mortality.

## Avoid:

- Foods high in cholesterol and saturated fats

  As much as 80% of all elevated cholesterol levels may be due to excessive amounts of cholesterol and saturated fat in the diet.

- Foods that contain trans fats

  Trans fats cause elevations in LDL levels and increase the risk and progression of atherosclerosis.

# high cholesterol

### Eat more of these World's Healthiest Foods:

### Essential

- Organically grown vegetables (page 85)

  Rich in nutrients such as vitamin E, vitamin C, beta-carotene and niacin that help to reduce cholesterol oxidation and reduce LDL levels.

- Garlic and Onions (page 258 and 268)

  These *Allium* family vegetables contain sulfur-containing phytonutrients that inhibit cholesterol synthesis with dietary consumption found to reduce total and LDL cholesterol levels.

- Organically grown fruits, including cranberries, grapes and blueberries (page 335)

  Contain polyphenol phytonutrients, including pterostilbene, which can help prevent the oxidation of cholesterol and increase levels of HDL cholesterol.

- Cranberries (page 410)

  Preliminary research suggests that cranberries may increase HDL levels.

- Fish rich in omega-3 fatty acids including salmon, tuna, sardines and cod (page 453)

  These fish are rich in omega-3 fatty acids, which have been found to reduce VLDL cholesterol, as well as the amino acid taurine, which may decrease cholesterol absorption in the intestines.

- Legumes (page 587)

  In addition to a diet rich in fruits and vegetables and low in saturated fats, the soluble fiber concentrated in legumes has been found to lower elevated levels of LDL and improve the ratio of LDL to HDL.

- Oats (page 664)

  Oats are rich in beta-glucan that reduces cholesterol levels as well as unique antioxidant compounds called avenanthramides that can help prevent free radicals from damaging LDL cholesterol.

- Barley (page 660)

  Rich in beta-glucan, barley may significantly lower total and LDL cholesterol.

- Nuts (page 501)

  Rich in heart-healthy monounsaturated fats as well as phytosterols, plant compounds that help to reduce total and LDL cholesterol as well as LDL oxidation.

- Flaxseeds (page 512)

  Intake of flaxseeds has been found to reduce total and LDL cholesterol.

- Brown rice (page 676)

  Rich in nutrients that can help maintain healthy cholesterol levels, brown rice's bran oil has been found to also lower LDL cholesterol.

- Soyfoods (page 594)

  Consumption of soy protein decreases total and LDL cholesterol and increases HDL cholesterol.

### Avoid:

- Foods high in cholesterol and saturated fats

  Can lead to elevated cholesterol levels with excessive dietary intake of foods rich in saturated fat and cholesterol strongly associated with increased risk of atherosclerosis and heart disease.

- Foods that contain trans fats

  Increase LDL cholesterol levels.

# hypertension (high blood pressure)

**Eat more of these World's Healthiest Foods:**

### Essential

- Organically grown fruits and vegetables, especially leafy greens and cruciferous vegetables such as broccoli, cauliflower and cabbage (page 85)

  > Concentrated in nutrients, such as calcium, magnesium and potassium, which have beneficial effects on blood pressure.

- Fish rich in omega-3 fatty acids including salmon, tuna, sardines and cod (page 453)

  > Omega-3 fatty acids have been associated with improvements in mean arterial pressure and systolic and diastolic blood pressure.

- Legumes (page 587)

  > Rich in nutrients including folic acid, whose intake has been associated with reduced risk of hypertension.

- Whole grains, including oats (page 657)

  > Rich in vitamins and minerals associated with improved blood pressure control.

### Supportive

- Garlic and Onions (page 258 and 268)

  > Sulfur-containing compounds in garlic and onions may help to lower blood pressure.

- Celery (page 202)

  > A compound found in celery, 3-n-butyl phthalide, has been shown to lower blood pressure in experimental animals.

- Potatoes (page 292)

  > Contain blood pressure-lowering compounds called kukoamines.

### Avoid:

- Foods high in saturated fat

  > Saturated fats decrease the elasticity, integrity and healing capacity of blood vessels.

- Alcohol

  > In susceptible individuals, even moderate alcohol consumption can damage arteries and contribute to chronically elevated blood pressure.

- Caffeine

  > Can promote the body's stress response, releasing hormones that rapidly elevate blood pressure.

- Sodium

  > Excessive consumption of dietary sodium, coupled with diminished dietary potassium, is a common cause of high blood pressure.

- Refined sugar

  > Excessive intake of highly processed, refined sugar can deplete the body of vitamins and minerals necessary for controlling lipid levels as well as for protecting the blood vessels.

# memory, concentration and mood

**Eat more of these World's Healthiest Foods:**

### Essential

- Foods rich in omega-3 fatty acids including fish such as salmon, tuna, sardines and cod, as well as flaxseeds and walnuts (page 770)

  > – Several research studies have found dietary intake of fish as well as the ALA that is found in flaxseeds and walnuts to be associated with a reduced incidence of depression.

– Adequate levels of omega-3 fatty acids, particularly DHA, are necessary for optimal learning abilities.

– Individuals with ADHD have been found to have reduced levels of essential fatty acids, such as DHA, EPA and DGLA.

### Supportive

- Organically grown fruits and vegetables

### Avoid:

- Highly processed foods

  These food do not provide the nutrients needed for the central nervous system to function optimally.

- High sugar foods

  Excessive intake of sugar can cause problematic peaks and then drops in blood sugar that have

Deeply colored fruits and vegetables are rich in not only vitamins and minerals but also phytonutrients that have great antioxidant activity.

- Extra virgin olive oil and avocados
  (page 328 and 298)

  These foods are rich in monounsaturated fats that support the integrity of your blood vessels and nerve wrappings.

been associated with mood disturbances and reduced concentration.

- Unwanted food additives

  These may cause hypersensitivity reactions in some individuals. For example, the yellow dye tartrazine has been found to be associated with irritability and sleep disturbances in some children.

# menopausal symptoms

**Eat more of these World's Healthiest Foods:**

### Essential

- Fish rich in omega-3 fatty acids including salmon, tuna, sardines and cod (page 453)

  Omega-3 fatty acids have been found to reduce risk of heart disease and may help regulate hormone levels.

- Soyfoods (page 594)

  A diet rich in soyfoods can be cardioprotective and is often recommended to reduce some symptoms associated with menopause, such as hot flashes.

- Flaxseeds (page 512)

  The richest source of a type of lignan that acts

like estrogen and helps to balance hormone levels.

- Legumes (page 587)

  Also contain phytoestrogenic compounds that act like weak estrogens.

### Supportive

- Whole grains (page 657)

  Concentrated sources of fiber that also contain phytoestrogens.

- Sea vegetables (page 310)

  Contain lignans that may be helpful with hot flashes.

### Avoid:

- Spicy foods
  - Some women report that spicy foods trigger hot flashes.

# migraines

**Eat more of these World's Healthiest Foods:**

### Essential

- Fish rich in omega-3 fatty acids including salmon, tuna, sardines and cod (page 453)

- Omega-3 fatty acids have anti-inflammatory actions and the ability to prevent blood vessels from squeezing shut when they shouldn't.

**Avoid:**

- Foods that cause allergic reactions (page 719)

    Many reports indicate that around 40% of migraine patients improve significantly when they remove certain foods they react to from their diet.

- Salt

    For some migraine sufferers, large amounts of salt can act as migraine triggers.

- Excessive saturated fat

    Individuals following diets low in saturated fats have found a significant reduction in their migraine attacks.

- Vasoactive amines contained in such foods as chocolate, aged cheese, fermented sausage, red wine, sour cream and pickled herring

    If not well metabolized, they can cause the blood vessels near the brain to squeeze shut, triggering a migraine attack.

# osteoarthritis

**Eat more of these World's Healthiest Foods:**

**Essential**

- Organically grown fruits and vegetables

    Rich in nutrients important for healthy joints including vitamin C and beta-carotene.

- Fish rich in omega-3 fatty acids including salmon, tuna, sardines and cod (page 453)

    The omega-3 fatty acids EPA and DHA have anti-inflammatory effects while the protein and vitamin D in fish help to support joint health.

- Nuts and seeds (page 501)

    Contain anti-inflammatory monounsaturated fats and the omega-3 fatty acid ALA.

- Ginger (page 708)

    Contains active components that lower the body's production of substances that can cause joint inflammation.

**Supportive**

- Whole grains (page 657)

    Often concentrated in folic acid, selenium, copper and other nutrients important for joint health.

**Avoid:**

- A diet low in essential nutrients since it has been shown to contribute to the development or progression of osteoarthritis. This translates into a diet centered around:

    - Highly refined products such as white rice, white bread and white pasta.
    - Excessive saturated fats.
    - Foods that contain trans fats.

# osteoporosis

**Eat more of these World's Healthiest Foods:**

**Essential**

- Organically grown fruits and green leafy vegetables

    Contain nutrients such as calcium, magnesium, potassium and B vitamins that are integral to bone health.

- Dairy products (if you don't have sensitivity to milk) (page 629)

    Rich in bone-building calcium and vitamin D.

- Fish rich in omega-3 fatty acids including salmon, tuna, sardines and cod (page 453)

    New research provides evidence that omega-3 fatty acids can decrease bone turnover rates.

**Avoid:**

- Coffee

    Caffeine increases calcium excretion.

- Excess salt

    Salty foods cause kidneys to remove additional calcium from the body.

- Refined sugar

    Eating too much refined sugar increases urinary calcium loss.

- Soft drinks

    If soft drinks provide the body with an excessive amount of phosphorus, the body may leach calcium from the bones, which would then become lost in the urine.

# prostate health

## Eat more of these World's Healthiest Foods:

### Supportive

- Tomatoes (page 164)

    Tomatoes are rich in lycopene as well as other nutrients that seem to act synergistically to help promote prostate health. A meta-analysis (grouping of studies) found that men who ate the highest amounts of raw tomatoes had an 11% reduction in risk for prostate cancer.

- Soyfoods (page 594)

    Men who eat soyfoods have been found to have a lower risk of prostate cancer. The phytoestrogens in soy, such as genistein and daidzein, inhibit *5-alpha-reductase*, the enzyme that converts testosterone to dihydrotestosterone.

- Pumpkin seeds (page 522)

    Pumpkin seeds are not only rich in prostate-health-promoting zinc, but also contain chemical substances called cucurbitacins that may prevent the body from converting testosterone into a much more potent form of this hormone called dihydrotestosterone. Without dihydrotestosterone, it is more difficult for the body to produce more prostate cells and therefore more difficult for the prostate to keep enlarging.

# restful sleep

## Eat more of these World's Healthiest Foods:

### Supportive

- Evening meal should be geared towards relaxation and good digestion:
    - Emphasis should be on low-to-medium glycemic index carbohydrates, such as whole grains, a mixed green salad or lightly sautéed vegetables rather than high-glycemic-index, blood-sugar-elevating carbohydrates (page 342).
    - Include a small portion of a healthy fat-containing food, such as olive oil, avocado, nuts or seeds.
    - Include herb tea (especially chamomile or peppermint) or other non-stimulating water-based beverage.
    - Include only moderate amounts of fresh or dried fruit for dessert, if dessert is desired.
    - Should be eaten about four hours before bedtime so that the main digestive effort is finished before sleep and so the energy from these foods can be released gradually throughout the night.
    - If it is necessary for you to eat a snack at bedtime, choose one or two of the following:
        - small cup of herb tea or warm milk (soy, nut, or dairy)—not so much that you must wake up to use the restroom in the middle of the night.
        - small serving of fresh or dried fruit.
        - small handful of raw nuts or seeds.
    - Should be light. For example: steamed vegetables served with beans, grains, or nuts and seeds.

# rheumatoid arthritis

## Eat more of these World's Healthiest Foods:

### Essential

- Fish rich in omega-3 fatty acids including salmon, tuna, sardines and cod (page 453)

    Populations who enjoy a good amount of fish in their diets also enjoy fairly low rates of rheumatoid arthritis.

- Organically grown fruits and vegetables

    Rich in nutrients such as vitamin C, beta-carotene, copper and calcium that are supportive of rheumatic health.

### Avoid:

- Foods that cause allergic reactions (page 719)

    Some individuals with rheumatoid arthritis have found that their symptoms are worse after they eat certain foods.

- Dairy Products

    Some individuals with rheumatoid arthritis have antibodies against milk proteins, which can lead to inflammation.

- Gluten (primarily found in wheat) (page 720)

    Many individuals with rheumatoid arthritis have been found to have antibodies against gluten, which can lead to inflammation.

- Omega-6 fatty acids

    Excess intake of omega-6 fatty acids can make

- Extra virgin olive oil (page 320)

    Research studies have shown that rheumatoid arthritis patients who increase their intake of olive oil, which has anti-inflammatory properties, experience a dramatic reduction in symptoms.

### Supportive

- Yogurt (page 644)

    Contains active cultures of "friendly" bacteria that can reduce toxin-producing intestinal bacteria that contribute to rheumatoid arthritis.

rheumatoid arthritis worse because too many of these substances will be converted into messaging substances that increase inflammation.

- Meat

    A high intake of meat may worsen the symptoms of rheumatoid arthritis and many individuals with rheumatoid arthritis experience improvement in their condition when they switch to a vegetarian or vegan diet.

- Saturated fat

    Many saturated fats that are commonly overconsumed in the U.S. diet are also associated with increased production of pro-inflammatory substances in the body.

# skin health

## Eat more of these World's Healthiest Foods:

### Essential

- Organically grown fruits and vegetables

    Rich in antioxidant nutrients such as vitamin C, vitamin E, carotenoids and flavonoids.

- Foods rich in omega-3 fatty acids including fish such as salmon, tuna, sardines and cod as well as flaxseeds and walnuts (page 770)

    Omega-3 fatty acids inhibit the production of

### Avoid:

- Foods that cause allergic reactions (page 719)

inflammatory compounds involved in the progression of skin conditions. Walnuts and flaxseeds contain ALA, which can help reduce inflammatory responses in the skin and can help keep the skin cell membranes functioning properly.

- Water, filtered

    Good hydration with high-quality water is essential for skin health.

Many individuals find that certain foods trigger skin symptoms such as dermatitis and breakouts.

# vision health

**Eat More of These World's Healthiest Foods:**

**Essential**

- Organically grown vegetables, including cruciferous vegetables such as broccoli, cabbage, kale and mustard greens (page 153)

    Many vegetables are rich in beta-carotene and lutein/zeaxanthin, important for vision health. Cruciferous vegetables contain sulforaphane, an antioxidant phytonutrient found to protect retinal cells from free-radical damage.

- Fish rich in omega-3 fatty acids including salmon, tuna, sardines and cod (page 453)

    The omega-3 fatty acid DHA is highly concentrated in cell membranes of the retina. Consumption of fish has been found to be associated with a lower likelihood of age-related macular degeneration (ARMD).

- Organically grown fruit (page 335)

    Dietary intake of fruit has been found to inversely related to risk of ARMD. Many fruits, including berries, also contain antioxidant flavonoids, which may play an important role in protecting eye health.

# for vital health and energy

Many scientists now agree that only nutrient-rich foods deliver all the vitamins, minerals and anti-oxidants that our bodies need because our bodies work as a whole and not as isolated parts. As convenient as it is to talk about foods that support the nervous system, or foods that support the cardiovascular system, the more lasting way to support health is by supporting all body systems through a meal plan that takes into account not only the nervous system but the way that the nervous system interacts with the endocrine system and immune system and other body tissues. A balanced and varied foods diet such as the "Healthiest Way of Eating Plan" is the best way we know of to accomplish this.

Here are some daily dietary guidelines that you can find in the 4-Week Healthiest Way of Eating Plan:

- Enjoy a wide range of nutrient-rich foods, like the World's Healthiest Foods, each day.
- Eat fresh fruits with every meal and/or as snacks.
- Enjoy a large salad with your lunch.
- Have at least two vegetable side dishes with your dinner.
- Eat foods rich in omega-3 fatty acids—such as fish, nuts, seeds, and leafy greens—each day.
- Limit saturated fats and omega-6 fatty acids and avoid trans fats.
- Buy local and organically grown foods, rather than conventionally grown foods, whenever possible.
- Choose whole grains over refined grains.
- Eat protein-containing or fat-containing foods when you eat carbohydrate-containing foods so as to minimize elevations in blood sugar.
- Use natural sweeteners—such as honey, cane juice, maple syrup, blackstrap molasses, agave syrup and stevia—in place of refined sugar and artificial sweeteners.
- Drink adequate amounts of filtered water each day.
- Avoid refined and processed foods and those with chemical additives, preservatives, flavors and colors.
- Refrain from excessive caffeine and alcohol.

# food sensitivity elimination plan

Did you know that if you have symptoms such as

| | |
|---|---|
| **Fatigue** | **Depression** |
| **Migraines** | **Indigestion** |
| **Poor memory** | **Sinus congestion** |
| **Dark circles or puffiness under the eyes** | **Chronic ear infection** |
| | **Joint inflammation** |
| **Mood swings** | **Attention deficit disorder** |
| **Bloating** | **Eating disorders** |
| **Fluid retention** | |

you may be experiencing a sensitivity (or intolerance) to particular foods in your diet? Sensitivities to food can take many different forms and affect 60–70% of the population. Unlike food allergies (see page 719) food sensitivities do not involve the immune system and cannot be clinically tested. This can make it very difficult for people to make the connection between their symptoms and the food they eat.

Do not confuse food sensitivities with food allergies. For example, it is possible to be sensitive to milk and yet not have an actual allergic reaction to milk. Lactose intolerance is one way that a sensitivity to milk may manifest; lactose intolerance is caused by a deficiency of the enzyme (lactase) that digests the sugars found in milk. In the United States, approximately 15–30% of all adults are lactose intolerant. Others forms of food sensitivities can be caused by poor functioning of the digestive tract (gluten intolerance), reactions to natural or synthetic chemicals (food additives such as MSG or sulfites) or even to some naturally occurring substances in food (salicylates or amines).

In the United States, the foods listed below are those most commonly associated with food sensitivities:

| | |
|---|---|
| • **Beef** | • **Chicken** |
| • **Corn** | • **Cow's milk** |
| • **Eggs** | • **Kiwi fruit** |
| • **Oranges** | • **Peanuts** |
| • **Pork** | • **Shellfish** |
| • **Soy** | • **Spinach** |
| • **Strawberries** | • **Tomatoes** |
| • **Tree Nuts\*** | • **Wheat** |

*\* Primarily walnuts, but also potentially including other tree nuts such as hazelnuts, pecans, almonds, or cashews.*

Other foods and additives likely to cause food sensitivities include:

| | |
|---|---|
| • **Alcohol** | • **Caffeine-containing beverages** |
| • **Chocolate** | • **Fermented (hard) cheese** |
| • **MSG** | • **Refined sugar** |
| • **Smoked meats** | • **Sulfites** |
| • **Vinegar** | • **Red wines** |

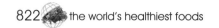

# elimination plan

To identify which foods might be problematic for you and determine if you have undiagnosed sensitivities to food, you might try following the Elimination Plan. It is composed of two easy phases. In the 1st phase you eat a variety of foods not likely to be associated with food sensitivities for 1 week (see list below). In 2nd phase, you reintroduce others foods to see if you are sensitive to them. In addition, any foods that you eat frequently and crave should be highly suspect as foods to which you are sensitive and included among those you eliminate for this trial period.

## What Are the Best Foods to Eat?

### PHASE 1

While it is best to avoid specific foods during the Elimination Plan, there are also some foods that are preferable to include as part of your meals because as a group they are less likely to be associated with food sensitivities than the group of foods you will be eliminating. Eat the foods below for at least 1 week. I recommend that the meals you enjoy during the Elimination Plan consist of approximately 8 parts of fruits and vegetables and 2 parts of protein-rich foods. It is also especially important to select organically grown foods whenever possible. Chew your food well to increase saliva production to help digestion.

| | |
|---|---|
| • Cabbage | • Apples |
| • Carrots | • Grapes |
| • Celery | • Lemons |
| • Collard greens | • Pears |
| • Garlic | |
| • Green beans | • Brown Rice |
| • Green peas | • Black beans |
| • Kale | • Garbanzo beans |
| • Olive oil | • Lentils |
| • Onion | • Pumpkin Seeds |
| • Lettuce | • Sesame Seeds |
| • Sea vegetables | • Sunflower Seeds |
| • Summer squash | |
|    (zucchini) | • Cod |
| • Sweet potatoes | • Salmon |
| • Swiss chard | • Lamb |
| • Winter squash | |

As you will notice, an integral part of helping you to identify sensitivities to foods during the Elimination Plan is to enjoy meals primarily comprised of vegetables, fruits, beans and fish. These are the health-promoting foods that study after study has shown to be of immeasurable benefit to health.

*\* It is best to consult with your healthcare professional when undertaking an elimination approach to determine food sensitivities.*

## Phase 1 Elimination Menu:

(sample menu based on an average 1800 calories per day\*):

### BREAKFAST:

1 cup of green tea with lemon juice. A bowl of fruit or vegetables served with 1 cup of brown rice topped with ground sunflower seeds.

### LUNCH:

1 cup of green tea with lemon juice.

A large salad made from 4 cups romaine lettuce topped with ground pumpkin seeds tossed with Mediterranean Dressing (page 143). Serve with "Quick Broiled" Lamb (page 573) or garbanzo or black beans.

**Dessert:** Apple

### DINNER:

1 cup of green tea with lemon juice.

2 cups mixed green salad topped with sesame seeds. Serve with "Quick Broiled" salmon or cod (page 481) and 2 servings of vegetables, such as the Mediterranean Feast (See page 277)

**Dessert:** Grapes

**Snack:** Fruit, nuts, seeds or crudités

### PHASE 2

After following the above diet for 1 week, you then begin to reintroduce avoided foods one at a time, one per day. The first list from which to reintroduce includes asparagus avocados, beets, bell peppers, broccoli, Brussels sprouts, cauliflower, cucumbers, blueberries, watermelon, flaxseeds and quinoa. These are foods that are not associated with sensitivity reactions in many people. After that, you reintroduce another avoided food, one food per day. When you reintroduce the foods you avoided notice any adverse reactions that you may have. If you develop any symptoms that compromise your feelings of wellness when reintroducing a food, that food may be problematic to you. (For more on Food Sensitivity see page 719.)

# references

## SELECTED REFERENCES

### Part 1: What are the World's Healthiest Foods? and Part 2: The Healthiest Way of Eating Plan

Ames BN. Micronutrients prevent cancer and delay aging. Toxicol Lett 1998;103:5–18.

Baker BP, Benbrook CM, Groth E 3rd, et al. Pesticide residues in conventional, integrated pest management (IPM)-grown and organic foods: insights from three US data sets. Food Addit Contam 2002;19(5):427–46.

Bazzano LA, He J, Ogden LG, et al. Dietary fiber intake and reduced risk of coronary heart disease in US men and women: the National Health and Nutrition Examination Survey I Epidemiologic Follow-up Study. Arch Intern Med 2003;163(16):1897–904.

Bruce B, Spiller GA, Klevay LM, et al. A diet high in whole and unrefined foods favorably alters lipids, antioxidant defenses, and colon function. J Am Coll Nutr 2000;19(1):61–7.

Clydesdale FM. Optimizing the diet with whole grains. Crit Rev Food Sci Nutr 1994;34(5–6):453–71.

Craig WJ. Phytonutrients: guardians of our health. J Am Diet Assoc 1997;97(10 Suppl 2):S199–204.

Foster-Powell K, Holt SH, Brand-Miller JC. International table of glycemic index and glycemic load value: 2002. AJCN 2002;76(1):5–56.

Giovannucci E, Rimm EB, Liu Y, et al. A prospective study of tomato products, lycopene, and prostate cancer risk. J Natl Cancer Inst 2002;94(5):391–8.

Grinder-Pedersen L, Rasmussen SE, Bugel S, et al. Effect of diets based on foods from conventional versus organic production on intake and excretion of flavonoids and markers of antioxidative defense in humans. J Agric Food Chem 2003;51(19):5671–6.

Hu FB, Stampfer MJ, Manson JE, et al. Frequent nut consumption and risk of coronary heart disease in women: prospective cohort study. BMJ 1998;317(7169):1341–5.

Jacobs DR, Pereira MA, Meyer KA, et al. Fiber from whole grains, but not refined grains, is inversely associated with all-cause mortality in older women: the Iowa women's health study. J Am Coll Nutr 2000;19(3 Suppl):326S–330S.

Joshipura KJ, Hu FB, Manson JE, et al. The effect of fruit and vegetable intake on risk for coronary heart disease. Ann Intern Med 2001;134(12):1106–14.

Kushi LH, Folsom AR, Prineas RJ, et al. Dietary antioxidant vitamins and death from coronary heart disease in postmenopausal women. N Engl J Med 1996;334(18):1156–62.

Liu Rui H. Potential synergy of phytochemicals in cancer prevention: mechanism of action. J Nutr. 2004;134(12): 3479S–85S.

Liu S, Stampfer MJ, Hu FB, et al. Whole-grain consumption and risk of coronary heart disease: results from the Nurses' Health Study. Am J Clin Nutr 1999;70(3):412–9.

Lu C, Toepel K, Irish R, et al. Organic diets significantly lower children's dietary exposure to organophosphorus pesticides. Environ Health Perspect 2006;114(2):260–3.

O'Dea K. Cardiovascular disease risk factors in Australian aborigines. Clin Exp Pharmacol Physiol 1991;18(2):85–8.

Omenn GS, Goodman GE, Thornquist MD, et al. Effects of a combination of beta carotene and vitamin A on lung cancer and cardiovascular disease. N Engl J Med 1996;334:1150–5.

Quattrucci E, Masci V. Nutritional aspects of food preservatives. Food Addit Contam 1992;9(5):515–25.

Reddy MB, Love M. The impact of food processing on the nutritional quality of vitamins and minerals. Adv Exp Med Biol 1999;459:99–106.

Sacks FM, Svetkey LP, Vollmer WM, et al. DASH-Sodium Collaborative Research Group. Effects on blood pressure of reduced dietary sodium and the Dietary Approaches to Stop Hypertension (DASH) diet. DASH-Sodium Collaborative Research Group. N Engl J Med 2001;344(1):3–10.

Slavin JL, Jacobs D, Marquart L. Grain processing and nutrition. Crit Rev Biotechnol 2001;21(1):49–66.

United States Congress. Organic Foods Production Act of 1990. Public Law 701–624: 1990; Title 21, U.S. 1990 Farm Bill.

Willett W, Stampfer MJ. Total energy intake: implications for epidemiologic analyses. Am J Epidemiol 1986;124(1):17–27.

Worthington V. Nutritional quality of organic versus conventional fruits, vegetables, and grains. J Altern Complement Med 2001;7(2):161–73.

## Part 3: Healthiest Way of Cooking

Balogh Z, Gray JI, Gomaa EA, et al. Formation and inhibition of heterocyclic aromatic amines in fried ground beef patties. Food Chem Toxicol 2000;38(5):395–401.

Becalski A, Lau BP, Lewis D, et al. Acrylamide in foods: occurrence, sources, and modeling. J Agric Food Chem 2003;51:802–8.

Bugianesi R, Salucci M, Leonardi C, et al. Effect of domestic cooking on human bioavailability of naringenin, chlorogenic acid, lycopene and beta-carotene in cherry tomatoes. Eur J Nutr 2004;43(6):360–6.

Esterbauer H. Cytotoxicity and genotoxicity of lipid-oxidation products. Am J Clin Nutr 1993;57(5 Suppl): 779S–785S; discussion 785S–786S.

Kikugawa K, Hiramoto K, Kato T. Prevention of the formation of mutagenic and/or carcinogenic heterocyclic amines by food factors. Biofactors 2000;12(1–4):123–7.

Kimura M, Itokawa Y. Cooking losses of minerals in foods and its nutritional significance. J Nutr Sci Vitaminol (Tokyo) 1990;36 Suppl 1:S25–32.

Larsson BK. Formation of polycyclic aromatic hydrocarbons during the smoking and grilling of food. Prog Clin Biol Res 1986;206:169–80.

Livny O, Reifen R, Levy I, et al. Beta-carotene bioavailability from differently processed carrot meals in human ileostomy volunteers. Eur J Nutr 2003;42(6):338–45.

Mosha TC, Gaga HE, Pace RD, et al. Effect of blanching on the content of antinutritional factors in selected vegetables. Plant Foods Hum Nutr 1995;47(4):361–7.

Muller JP, Steinegger A, Schlatter C. Contribution of aluminum from packaging materials and cooking utensils to the daily aluminum intake. Z Lebensm Unters Forsch 1993 Oct;197(4):332–41.

Nursal B, Yucecan S. Vitamin C losses in some frozen vegetables due to various cooking methods. Nahrung 2000;44(6):451–3.

Prochaska LJ, Nguyen XT, Donat N, et al. Effects of food processing on the thermodynamic and nutritive value of foods: literature and database survey. Med Hypotheses 2000 Feb;54(2):254–62.

Reddy MB, Love M. The impact of food processing on the nutritional quality of vitamins and minerals. Adv Exp Med Biol 1999;459:99–106.

Thorkelsson G. The effect of processing on the content of polycyclic aromatic hydrocarbons and volatile N-nitrosamines in cured and smoked lamb meat. Bibl Nutr Dieta 1989;188–98.

Vallejo F, Tomás-Barberán FA, García-Viguera C. Phenolic compounds content in edible parts of broccoli inflorescences after domestic cooking. J Sci Food Agric 2003;83(14):1151–6.

## Part 4: The World's Healthiest Foods Support Healthy Cells

Ames, BN. Micronutrient deficiencies. A major cause of DNA damage. Ann N Y Acad Sci 1999;889:152–6.

Bland J. *Genetic Nutritioneering*. Lincolnwood, IL: Keats, a division of NTC/Contemporary Publishing Group, Inc.; 1999.

Groff JL, Gropper SS, Hunt SM. *Advanced Nutrition and Human Metabolism*. New York: West Publishing Company; 1995.

Levin B. *Environmental nutrition: understanding the link between environment, food quality, and disease*. Vashon Island, Washington: HingePin Publishing; 1999.

Mascio PD, Murphy ME, Sies H. Antioxidant defense systems: the role of Carotenoids, tocopherols, and thiols. Am J Clin Nutr 1991;53:194S–200S.

Moore D. *Dependent Gene: The Fallacy of Nature vs, Nurture*. New York: Henry Holt & Company; 2003.

Orzechowski A, Ostaszewski P, Jank M, et al. Bioactive substances of plant origin in food-impact on genomics. Reprod Nutr Dev 2002;42(5):461–77.

Pedersen B, Eggum BO. The influence of milling on the nutritive value of flour from cereal grains. Part 2. Wheat. Qual Plant Plant Fds Hum Nutr 1983;33:51–61.

Simopolous AP. Diet and Gene Interactions. Food Technology 1997;51(3):66–69.

Smith, J.D. Apolipoprotein E4: an allele associated with many diseases. Annals of Medicine 2000;32:118–27.

Toborek M, Hennig B. The role of linoleic acid in endothelial cell gene expression. Relationship to atherosclerosis. Subcell Biochem 1998;30:415–36

## Part 5: 100 World's Healthiest Foods

*For more references on specific foods, please see the bottom of the individual food's article on the whfoods.org website (http://whfoods.org/foodstoc.php)*

### FOOD CHAPTERS–GENERAL

Adel A. *Kader. Postharvest Technology of Horticultural Crops, Second Edition*. 1992. University of California Division of Agriculture and Natural Resources Publication 3311.

Delahaut KA, Newenhouse AC. *Growing Vegetable Crops in Wisconsin, A Guide for Fresh Market Growers*. 1997, 1998 University of Wisconsin Extension Publication Series:A3684–A3688.

Ensminger AH, Ensminger, ME, Kondale JE, et al. *Foods & Nutrition Encyclopedia*. Clovis, California: Pegus Press; 1986.

Fortin, Francois, Editorial Director. *The Visual Foods Encyclopedia*. New York, NY: Macmillan; 1996.

Grieve M. *A Modern Herbal*. New York, NY: Dover Publications; 1973.

Kitinoja L, Kader AA. 1995. *Small-scale postharvest handling practices: A manual for horticultural crops (3rd edition)*. Univ. Calif. Postharvest Horticulture Series No. 8.

Mendosa, R. Revised International Table of Glycemic Index (GI) and Glycemic Load (GL) Values—2002. www.mendosa.com/gilists.htm

Pizzorno Jr. JE, Murray MT. Textbook of Natural Medicine (2nd edition). New York, NY: Churchill Livingstone; 1999.

USDA Nutrient Data Laboratory, Agricultural Research Service. USDA Database for the Flavonoid Content of Selected Food-2003. http://www.nal.usda.gov/fnic/food-comp/Data/Flav/flav.html

USDA Nutrient Data Laboratory, Agricultural Research Service. USDA National Nutrient Database for Standard Reference, Release 17 (2004). http://www.nal.usda.gov/fnic/foodcomp/

Wood, Rebecca. *The Whole Foods Encyclopedia*. New York, NY: Prentice-Hall;1998.

## VEGETABLE CHAPTERS

Ali M, Bordia T, Mustafa T. Effect of raw versus boiled aqueous extract of garlic and onion on platelet aggregation. Biofactors 2000;13(1–4):257–63.

Andorfer JH, Tchaikovskaya T, Listowsky I. Selective expression of glutathione S-transferase genes in the murine gastrointestinal tract in response to dietary organosulfur compounds. Carcinogenesis 2004;25(3):359–67.

Beecher C. Cancer preventive properties of varieties of Brassica oleracea: a review. Am J Clin Nutr 1994;59(Suppl):166S–70S.

Blondin C, Chaubet F, Nardella A, et al. Relationships between chemical characteristics and anticomplementary activity of fucans. Biomaterials 1996 Mar;17(6):597–603.

Brown MJ, Ferruzzi MG, Nguyen ML, et al. Carotenoid bioavailability is higher from salads ingested with full-fat than with fat-reduced salad dressings as measured with electrochemical detection. Am J Clin Nutr. 2004 Aug;80(2):396–403.

Cheney G. Rapid healing of peptic ulcers in patients receiving fresh cabbage juice. Cal Med 70 (1949):10–14.

Edenharder R, Keller G, Platt KL, et al. Isolation and characterization of structurally novel antimutagenic flavonoids from spinach (Spinacia oleracea). J Agric Food Chem 2001;49(6):2767–73.

Etminan M, Takkouche B, Caamano-Isorna F. The role of tomato products and lycopene in the prevention of prostate cancer: a meta-analysis of observational studies. Cancer Epidemiol Biomarkers Prev. 2004;13(3):340–5.

Fahey JW, Haristoy X, Dolan PM et al. Sulforaphane inhibits extracellular, intracellular, and antibiotic-resistant strains of Helicobacter pylori and prevents benzopyrene-induced stomach tumors. Proc Natl Acad Sci USA 2002;99(11):7610–5.

Fowke JH, Chung FL, Jin F, et al. Urinary isothiocyanate levels, brassica, and human breast cancer. Cancer Res 2003;63(14):3980–6.

Grube BJ, Eng ET, Kao YC, et al. White Button Mushroom Phytochemicals Inhibit Aromatase Activity and Breast Cancer Cell Proliferation. J Nutr 2001;131(12):3288–93.

Hirano R, Sasamoto W, Matsumoto A, et al. Antioxidant ability of various flavonoids against DPPH radicals and LDL oxidation. J Nutr Sci Vitaminol (Tokyo). 2001;47(5):357–62.

Hou WC, Chen YC, Chen HJ, et al. Antioxidant activities of trypsin inhibitor, a 33 KDa root storage protein of sweet potato (Ipomoea batatas (L.) Lam cv. Tainong 57). J Agric Food Chem 2001;49(6):2978–81.

Huxley RR, Neil HAW. The relation between dietary flavonol intake and coronary heart disease mortality: a meta-analysis of prospective cohort studies. Eur J Clin Nutr 2003;57:904–908.

Ioku K, Aoyama Y, Tokuno A, et al. Various cooking methods and the flavonoid content in onion. J Nutr Sci Vitaminol (Tokyo). 2001;47(1):78–83.

Johnson IT. Glucosinolates: bioavailability and importance to health. Int J Vitam Nutr Res 2002 Jan;72(1):26–31.

Jong SC, Birmingham JM. Medicinal and therapeutic value of the shiitake mushroom. Adv Appl Microbiol 1993;39:153–84.

Jorge PA, Neyra LC, Osaki RM, et al. Effect of eggplant on plasma lipid levels, lipidic peroxidation and reversion of endothelial dysfunction in experimental hypercholesterolemia. Arq Bras Cardiol 1998;70(2):87–91.

Keys A, Menotti A, Karvonen MJ, et al. The diet and 15-year death rate in the seven countries study. Am J Epidemiol 1986;124(6):903–15.

Kusano S, Abe H. Antidiabetic activity of white skinned sweet potato (Ipomoea batatas L.) in obese Zucker fatty rats. Biol Pharm Bull 2000;23(1):23–6.

Longnecker MP, Newcomb PA, Mittendorf R, et al. Intake of carrots, spinach, and supplements containing vitamin A in relation to risk of breast cancer. Cancer Epidemiol Biomarkers Prev 1997;6(11):887–92.

Lopez Ledesma R, Frati Munari AC, Hernandez Dominguez BC, et al. Monounsaturated fatty acid (avocado) rich diet for mild hypercholesterolemia. Arch Med Res 1996;27(4):519–23.

Ludikhuyze L, Rodrigo L, Hendrickx M. The activity of myrosinase from broccoli (Brassica oleracea L. cv. Italica): influence of intrinsic and extrinsic factors. J Food Prot. 2000;63(3):400–3.

Martinez-Dominguez E, de la Puerta R, Ruiz-Gutierrez V. Protective effects upon experimental inflammation models of a polyphenol-supplemented virgin olive oil diet. Inflamm Res 2001;50(2):102–6.

McKillop DJ, Pentieva K, Daly D. The effect of different cooking methods on folate retention in various foods that are amongst the major contributors to folate intake in the UK diet. Br J Nutr. 2002;88(6):681–8.

Michnovicz JJ, Bradlow HL. Altered estrogen metabolism and excretion in humans following consumption of indole-3-carbinol. Nutr Cancer 1991;16(1):59–66.

Nanba H, Mori K, Toyomasu T, et al. Antitumor action of shiitake (Lentinus edodes) fruit bodies orally administered to mice. Chem Pharm Bull (Tokyo) 1987;35(6):2453–8.

Nishimura H, Takahashi T, Wijaya CH, et al. Thermochemical transformation of sulfur compounds in Japanese domestic Allium, Allium victorialis L. J Agric Food Chem 2002;50(26):7684–90.

Noda Y, Kneyuki T, Igarashi K, et al. Antioxidant activity of nasunin, an anthocyanin in eggplant peels. Toxicology 2000;148(2–3):119–23.

Sesso HD, Liu S, Gaziano JM, et al. Dietary lycopene, tomato-based food products and cardiovascular disease in women. J Nutr;133(7):2336–41.

Sheela CG, Kumud K, Augusti KT. Anti-diabetic effects of onion and garlic sulfoxide amino acids in rats. Planta Med. 1995;61(4):356–7.

Skoldstam L, Hagfors L, Johansson G. An experimental study of a Mediterranean diet intervention for patients with rheumatoid arthritis. Ann Rheum Dis. 2003;62(3):208–14.

Song K, Milner JA. The influence of heating on the anti-cancer properties of garlic. American Society for Nutritional Sciences. 2001 [Supplement]:1054S–1057S.

Stintzing FC, Schieber A, Carle R. Identification of beta-lains from yellow beet (Beta vulgaris L.) and cactus pear [Opuntia ficus-indica (L.) Mill.] by high-performance liquid chromatography-electrospray ionization mass spectrometry. J Agric Food Chem. 2002;50(8):2302–7.

Tavani A, Negri E, La Vecchia C. Food and nutrient intake and risk of cataract. Ann Epidemiol 1996;6(1):41–46.

Terahara N, Konczak-Islam I, Nakatani M, et al. Anthocyanins in callus induced from purple storage root of Ipomoea batatas L. Phytochemistry 2000;54(8):919–22.

Tesoriere L, Butera D, D'Arpa D, et al. Increased resistance to oxidation of betalain-enriched human low density lipoproteins. Free Radic Res. 2003;37(6):689–96.

Tsi D, Tan BK. The mechanism underlying the hypocholesterolaemic activity of aqueous celery extract, its butanol and aqueous fractions in genetically hypercholesterolaemic RICO rats. Life Sci 2000;66(8):755–67.

Unlu NZ, Bohn T, Clinton SK, et al. Carotenoid absorption from salad and salsa by humans is enhanced by the addition of avocado or avocado oil. J Nutr 2005;135(3):431–6.

Verhagen H, Poulsen HE, Loft S, et al. Reduction of oxidative DNA-damage in humans by Brussels sprouts. Carcinogenesis 1995;16(4):969–70.

Visioli F, Bellomo G, Galli C. Free radical-scavenging properties of olive oil polyphenols. Biochem Biophys Res Commun 1998;247(1):60–4.

Willcox JK, Catignani GL, Lazarus S. Tomatoes and cadio-vascular health. Crit Rev Food Sci Nutr 2003;43(1):1–18.

## FRUIT CHAPTERS

Avorn J, Monane M, Gurwitz JH, et al. Reduction of bacteriuria and pyruia after using cranberry juice. JAMA 1994;272:590.

Boyer J, Liu RH. Apple phytochemicals and their health benefits. Nutr J 2004;3(1):5.

Cho E, Seddon JM, Rosner B, et al. Prospective study of intake of fruits, vegetables, vitamins, and carotenoids and risk of age-related maculopathy. Arch Ophthalmol. 2004;122(6):883–92.

Committee on Safety of Medicines. Interactions between warfarin and cranberry juice: new advice. Curr Prob Pharmacovigil 2004;30:9.

Dahan A, Altman H. Food-drug interaction: grapefruit juice augments drug bioavailability—mechanism, extent and relevance. Eur J Clin Nutr. 2004;58(1):1–9.

Dunjic BS, Svensson I, Axelson J, et al. Green banana protection of gastric mucosa against experimentally induced injuries in rats. A multicomponent mechanism. Scand J Gastroenterol 1993;28(10):894–8.

Forastiere F, Pistelli R, Sestini P, et al. Consumption of fresh fruit rich in vitamin C and wheezing symptoms in children. SIDRIA Collaborative Group, Italy (Italian Studies on Respiratory Disorders in Children and the Environment). Thorax. 2000;55(4):283–8.

Freedman JE, Parker C 3rd, Li L, et al. Select flavonoids and whole juice from purple grapes inhibit platelet function and enhance nitric oxide release. Circulation 2001;103(23):2792–8.

Hills BA, Kirwood CA. Surfactant approach to the gastric mucosal barrier: Protection of rats by banana even when acidified. Gastroenterology 1989;97:294–303.

Honow R, Laube N, Schneider A, et al. Influence of grapefruit-, orange- and apple-juice consumption on urinary variables and risk of crystallization. Br J Nutr Aug;90(2):295–300.

Kahkonen MP, Hopia AI, Heinonen M. Berry phenolics and their antioxidant activity. J Agric Food Chem 2001;49(8):4076–82.

Kalt W, Forney CF, Martin A, et al. Antioxidant capacity, vitamin C, phenolics, and anthocyanins after fresh storage of small fruits. J Agric Food Chem 1999;47(11):4638–44.

Karakaya S, El SN, Tas AA. Antioxidant activity of some foods containing phenolic compounds. Int J Food Sci Nutr 2001;52(6):501–8.

Kurowska EM, Manthey JA. Hypolipidemic effects and absorption of citrus polymethoxylated flavones in hamsters with diet-induced hypercholesterolemia. Agric Food Chem. 2004;52(10):2879–86.

Liu M, Li XQ, Weber C, et al. Antioxidant and antiproliferative activities of raspberries. J Agric Food Chem 2002;50(10):2926–30.

Miyagi Y, Miwa K, Inoue H. Inhibition of human low-density lipoprotein oxidation by flavonoids in red wine and grape juice. Am J Cardiol 1997;80(12):1627–31.

Pearson DA, Tan CH, German JB, et al. Apple juice inhibits low density lipoprotein oxidation. Life Sci 1999;64(21):1913–20.

Rakhimov MR. Pharmacological study of papain from the papaya plant cultivated in Uzbekistan (Article in Russian). Eksp Klin Farmakol 2000;63(3):55–7.

Rimando AM, Kalt W, Magee JB, et al. Resveratrol, pterostilbene, and piceatannol in vaccinium berries. J Agric Food Chem. 2004;52(15):4713–9.

Rodrigues A, Sandstrom A, Ca T, et al. Protection from cholera by adding lime juice to food—results from community and laboratory studies in Guinea-Bissau, West Africa. Trop Med Int Health 2000;5(6):418–22.

Sable-Amplis R, Sicart R, Agid R. Further studies on the cholesterol-lowering effect of apple in humans. Biochemical mechanisms involved. Nutr Res 1983;3:325–8.

Serraclara A, Hawkins F, Perez C, et al. Hypoglycemic action of an oral fig-leaf decoction in type-I diabetic patients. Diabetes Res Clin Pract 1998;39(1):19–22.

Simon JA, Hudes ES, Perez-Perez GI. Relation of serum ascorbic acid to Helicobacter pylori serology in US adults: the Third National Health and Nutrition Examination Survey. J Am Coll Nutr;22(4):283–9.

Sun J, Chu YF, Wu X, et al. Antioxidant and antiproliferative activities of common fruits. J Agric Food Chem 2002 Dec 4;50(25):7449–54.

Tona L, Kambu K, Ngimbi N, et al. Antiamoebic and phytochemical screening of some Congolese medicinal plants. J Ethnopharmacol. 1998;61(1):57–65.

Tsao R, Yang R, Young JC, et al. Polyphenolic profiles in eight apple cultivars using high-performance liquid chromatography (HPLC). J Agric Food Chem 2003;51(21):6347–53.

Walker AF, Bundy R, Hicks SM, et al. Bromelain reduces mild acute knee pain and improves well-being in a dose-dependent fashion in an open study of otherwise healthy adults. Phytomedicine 2002;9(8):681–6.

Wills RB, Scriven FM, Greenfield H. Nutrient composition of stone fruit (Prunus spp.) cultivars: apricot, cherry, nectarine, peach and plum. J Sci Food Agric 1983;34(12):1383–9.

## FISH & SHELLFISH CHAPTERS

Bernard-Gallon DJ, Vissac-Sabatier C, Antoine-Vincent D et al. Differential effects of n-3 and n-6 polyunsaturated fatty acids on BRCA1 and BRCA2 gene expression in breast cell lines. Br J Nutr 2002;87(4):281–9.

Cho E, Hung S, Willett WC, et al. Prospective study of dietary fat and the risk of age-related macular degeneration. Am J Clin Nutr. 2001;73(2):209–18.

Environmental Working Group. Analysis of polychlorinated biphenyls (PCBs) in farmed versus wild salmon sold in the United States (http://www.ewg.org/reports/farmedPCBs). July 30, 2003.

Erkkila A, Lichtenstein A, Mozaffarian D, et al. Fish intake is associated with a reduced progression of coronary artery atherosclerosis in postmenopausal women with coronary artery disease. Am J Clin Nutr 2004; 80(3):626–32.

Fernandez E, Chatenoud L, La Vecchia C, et al. Fish consumption and cancer risk. Am J Clin Nutr 1999;70(1):85–90.

Foran JA, Carpenter DO, Hamilton MC, et al. Risk-based consumption advice for farmed Atlantic and wild Pacific salmon contaminated with dioxins and dioxin-like compounds. Environ Health Perspect. 2005;113(5):552–6.

He K, Song Y, Daviglus ML, et al. Fish consumption and incidence of stroke: a meta-analysis of cohort studies. Stroke. 2004;35(7):1538–42.

Iribarren C, Markovitz JH, Jacobs DR, et al. Dietary intake of n-3, n-6 fatty acids and fish: Relationship with hostility in young adults—the CARDIA study. Eur J Clin Nutr. 2004;58(1):24–31.

Kalmijn S, van Boxtel MP, Ocke M, et al. Dietary intake of fatty aids and fish in relation to cognitive performance at middle age. Neurology. 2004;62(2):275–80.

Noaghiul S, Hibbeln JR. Cross-national comparisons of seafood consumption and rates of bipolar disorders. Am J Psychiatry. 2003;160(12):2222–7.

Rose DP, Connolly JM. Omega-3 fatty acids as cancer chemopreventive agents. Pharmacol Ther 1999;83(3):217–44.

Storey A, McArdle F, Friedmann PS, et al. Eicosapentaenoic acid and docosahexaenoic acid reduce UVB- and TNF-alpha-induced IL-8 secretion in keratinocytes and UVB-induced IL-8 in fibroblasts. J Invest Dermatol. 2005;124(1):248–55.

## NUTS & SEEDS CHAPTERS

Bradamante S, Barenghi L, Villa A. Cardiovascular protective effects of resveratrol. Cardiovasc Drug Rev 2004;22(3):169–88.

Brooks JD, Ward WE, Lewis JE, et al. Supplementation with flaxseed alters estrogen metabolism in postmenopausal women to a greater extent than does supplementation with an equal amount of soy. Am J Clin Nutr 2004;79(2):318–25.

Chen CY, Milbury PE, Lapsley K, et al. Flavonoids from almond skins are bioavailable and act synergistically with vitamins C and E to enhance hamster and human LDL resistance to oxidation. J Nutr 2005;135(6):1366–73.

Fraser GE. Nut consumption, lipids, and risk of a coronary event. Clin Cardiol 1999;22(7 Suppl):III11–5.

Fukuda T, Ito H, Yoshida T. Antioxidative polyphenols from walnuts (Juglans regia L.). Phytochemistry; 63(7):795–801.

Hirata F, Fujita K, Ishikura Y, et al. Hypocholesterolemic effect of sesame lignan in humans. Atherosclerosis 1996;122(1):135–36.

Hu FB, Stampfer MJ. Nut consumption and risk of coronary heart disease: a review of epidemiologic evidence. Curr Atheroscler Rep 1999;1(3):204–9.

Lucas EA, Wild RD, Hammond LJ, et al. Flaxseed improves lipid profile without altering biomarkers of bone metabolism in postmenopausal women. J Clin Endocrinol Metab 2002;87(4):1527–32.

Nesbitt PD, Thompson LU. Lignans in homemade and commercial products containing flaxseed. Nutr Cancer 1997;29(3):222–7.

Ros E, Nunez I, Perez-Heras A, et al. A walnut diet improves endothelial function in hypercholesterolemic subjects: a randomized crossover trial. Circulation 2004;109(13):1609–14.

Tapsell LC, Gillen LJ, Patch CS, et al. Including Walnuts in a Low-Fat/Modified-Fat Diet Improves HDL Cholesterol-to-Total Cholesterol Ratios in Patients With Type 2 Diabetes. Diabetes Care 2004;27(12):2777–83.

Tsai CJ, Leitzmann MF, Hu FB, et al. Frequent nut consumption and decreased risk of cholecystectomy in women. Am J Clin Nutr 2004;80(1):76–81.

Wien MA, Sabate JM, Ikle DN, et al. Almonds vs complex carbohydrates in a weight reduction program. Int J Obes Relat Metab Disord 2003;27(11):1365–72.

Yamashita K, Nohara Y, Katayama K, et al. Sesame seed lignans and gamma-tocopherol act synergistically to produce vitamin E activity in rats. J Nutr 1992;122(12):2440–6.

Zhao G, Etherton TD, Martin KR, et al. Dietary {alpha}–Linolenic Acid Reduces Inflammatory and Lipid Cardiovascular Risk Factors in Hypercholesterolemic Men and Women. J Nutr 2004;134(11):2991–2997.

### POULTRY & LEAN MEATS CHAPTERS

Dhonukshe-Rutten RA, Lips M, de Jong N et al. Vitamin B-12 status is associated with bone mineral content and bone mineral density in frail elderly women but not in men. J Nutr. 2003;133(3):801–7.

Hyun T, Barrett-Connor E, Milne D. Zinc intakes and plasma concentrations in men with osteoporosis: the Rancho Bernardo Study. Am J Clin Nutr 2004:80(3):715–721.

Kiatoko M, McDowell LR, Bertrand JE, et al. Evaluating the nutritional status of beef cattle herds from four soil order regions of Florida. I. Macroelements, protein, carotene, vitamins A and E, hemoglobin and hematocrit. J Anim Sci 1982;55(1):28–37.

Neale RJ, Obanu ZA, Biggin RJ, et al. Protein quality and iron availability of intermediate moisture beef stored at 38 degrees C. Ann Nutr Aliment 1978;32(2–3):587–96.

### BEANS & LEGUMES CHAPTERS

Azevedo L, Gomes JC, Stringheta PC, et al. Black bean (Phaseolus vulgaris L.) as a protective agent against DNA damage in mice. Food Chem Toxicol 2003;41(12):1671–6.

Chen YM, Ho SC, Lam SS, et al. Soy isoflavones have a favorable effect on bone loss in Chinese postmenopausal women with lower bone mass: a double-blind, randomized, controlled trial. J Clin Endocrinol Metab 2003;88(10):4740–7.

Desroches S, Mauger JF, Ausman LM, et al. Soy protein favorably affects LDL size independently of isoflavones in hypercholesterolemic men and women. J Nutr 2004;134(3):574–9.

Kritz-Silverstein D, Goodman-Gruen DL. Usual dietary isoflavone intake, bone mineral density, and bone metabolism in postmenopausal women. J Womens Health Gend Based Med 2002;11(1):69–78.

Lee MM, Gomez SL, Chang JS, et al. Soy and isoflavone consumption in relation to prostate cancer risk in China. Cancer Epidemiol Biomarkers;12(7):665–8.

Menotti A, Kromhout D, Blackburn H, et al. Food intake patterns and 25-year mortality from coronary heart disease: cross-cultural correlations in the Seven Countries Study. The Seven Countries Study Research Group. Eur J Epidemiol 1999;15(6):507–15.

Queiroz Kda S, de Oliveira AC, Helbig E et al. Soaking the common bean in a domestic preparation reduced the contents of raffinose-type oligosaccharides but did not interfere with nutritive value. J Nutr Sci Vitaminol (Tokyo) 2002 ;48(4):283–9.

Wagner JD, Schwenke DC, Greaves KA, et al. Soy protein with isoflavones, but not an isoflavone-rich supplement, improves arterial low-density lipoprotein metabolism and atherogenesis. Arterioscler Thromb Vasc Biol 2003;23(12):2241–6.

### DAIRY & EGGS CHAPTERS

Blumberg J, Johnson E. Lutein and disease prevention. Papers presented at the annual American Dietetic Association Conference, San Antonio, TX, October 26, 2003 and at the First International Scientific Symposium On Eggs and Human Health: The Transition from Restrictions to Recommendations, USDA, Washington, DC, September 23.

Cho HJ, Ham HS, Lee DS, et al. Effects of proteins from

hen egg yolk on human platelet aggregation and blood coagulation. Biol Pharm Bull 2003;26(10):1388–92.

Chung HY, Rasmussen HM, Johnson EJ. Lutein bioavailability is higher from lutein-enriched eggs than from supplements and spinach in men. J Nutr 2004;134(8):1887–93.

Cornish J, Callon KE, Naot D, et al. Lactoferrin is a potent regulator of bone cell activity and increases bone formation in vivo. Endocrinology 2004;145(9):4366–74.

Meydani SN, Ha WK. Immunologic effects of yogurt. Am J Clin Nutr 2000;71(4):861–72.

Wang K, Li S, Liu C, et al. Effect of ingesting Lactobacillus- and Bifidobacterium-containing yogurt in subjects with colonized Helicobacter pylori. Am J Clin Nutr 2004;80(3):737–41.

## WHOLE GRAINS CHAPTERS

Anderson JW, Hanna TJ, Peng X, et al. Whole grain foods and heart disease risk. J Am Coll Nutr 2000;19(3 Suppl):291S–9S.

Bach Knudsen KE, Serena A, Kjaer AK et al. Rye bread in the diet of pigs enhances the formation of enterolactone and increases its levels in plasma, urine and feces. J Nutr 2003; 133(5):1368–75.

Chen CY, Milbury PE, Kwak HK, et al. Avenanthramides phenolic acids from oats are bioavailable and act synergistically with vitamin C to enhance hamster and human LDL resistance to oxidation. J Nutr 2004;134(6):1459–66.

Delaney B, Nicolosi RJ, Wilson TA, et al. Beta-glucan fractions from barley and oats are similarly antiatherogenic in hypercholesterolemic Syrian golden hamsters. J Nutr 2003;133(2):468–75.

Hogberg L, Laurin P, Falth-Magnusson K, et al. Oats to children with newly diagnosed coeliac disease: a randomised double blind study. Gut 2004;53(5):649–654.

Jacobs DR, Pereira MA, Meyer KA, et al. Fiber from whole grains, but not refined grains, is inversely associated with all-cause mortality in older women: the Iowa women's health study. J Am Coll Nutr 2000;19 (3 Suppl):326S–330S.

Jenkins AL, Jenkins DJ, Zdravkovic U, et al. Depression of the glycemic index by high levels of beta-glucan fiber in two functional foods tested in type 2 diabetes. Eur J Clin Nutr;56(7):622–8.

Johnsen NF, Hausner H, Olsen A, et al. Intake of whole grains and vegetables determines the plasma enterolactone concentration of Danish women. J Nutr. 2004; 134(10):2691–7.

Juntunen KS, Laaksonen DE, Autio K, et al. Structural differences between rye and wheat breads but not total fiber content may explain the lower postprandial insulin response to rye bread. Am J Clin Nutr 2003;78(5):957–64.

McKeown NM, Meigs JB, Liu S, et al. Carbohydrate Nutrition, Insulin Resistance, and the Prevalence of the Metabolic Syndrome in the Framingham Offspring Cohort. Diabetes Care 2004;27(2):538–546.

## HERBS & SPICES CHAPTERS

al-Sereiti MR, Abu-Amer KM, Sen P. Pharmacology of rosemary (Rosmarinus officinalis Linn.) and its therapeutic potentials. Indian J Exp Biol 1999;37(2):124–30.

Borrelli F, Capasso R, Aviello G, et al. Effectiveness and safety of ginger in the treatment of pregnancy-induced nausea and vomiting. Obstet Gynecol. 2005;105(4):849–56.

Calucci L, Pinzino C, Zandomeneghi M et al. Effects of gamma-irradiation on the free radical and antioxidant contents in nine aromatic herbs and spices. J Agric Food Chem 2003; 51(4):927–34.

Chithra V, Leelamma S. Coriandrum sativum changes the levels of lipid peroxides and activity of antioxidant enzymes in experimental animals. Indian J Biochem Biophys 1999;36(1):59–61.

Deshpande UR, Gadre SG, Raste AS, et al. Protective effect of turmeric (Curcuma longa L.) extract on carbon tetrachloride-induced liver damage in rats. Indian J Exp Biol 1998;36(6):573–7.

Dorman HJ, Deans SG. Antimicrobial agents from plants: antibacterial activity of plant volatile oils. J Appl Microbiol 2000 Feb;88(2):308–16.

Gonzalez R, Dunkel R, Koletzko B, et al. Effect of capsaicin-containing red pepper sauce suspension on upper gastrointestinal motility in healthy volunteers. Dig Dis Sci 1998;43(6):1165–71.

Hautkappe M, Roizen MF, Toledano A, et al. Review of the effectiveness of capsaicin for painful cutaneous disorders and neural dysfunction. Clin J Pain 1998;14:97–106.

Khan A, Safdar M, Ali Khan MM, et al. Cinnamon improves glucose and lipids of people with type 2 diabetes. Diabetes Care. 2003;26(12):3215–8.

Kiuchi F, Iwakami S, Shibuya M, et al. Inhibition of prostaglandin and leukotriene biosynthesis by gingerols and diarylheptanoids. Chem Pharm Bull 1992;40(2):387–91.

Kubo I, Fujita K, Kubo A, et al. Antibacterial Activity of Coriander Volatile Compounds against Salmonella choleraesuis. J Agric Food Chem. 2004;52(11):3329–32.

Mujumdar AM, Dhuley JN, Deshmukh VK, et al. Antiinflammatory activity of piperine. Jpn J Med Sci Biol 1990;43(3):95–100.

Nagabhushan M, Bhide SV. Curcumin as an inhibitor of cancer. J Am Coll Nutr. 1992;11(2):192–8.

Ouattara B, Simard RE, Holley RA, et al. Antibacterial activity of selected fatty acids and essential oils against six meat spoilage organisms. Int J Food Microbiol 1997;37(2–3):155–62.

Srivastava KC, Mustafa T. Ginger (Zingiber officinale) in rheumatism and musculoskeletal disorders. Med Hypothesis 1992;39:342–8.

Zheng GQ, Kenney PM, Lam LK. Anethofuran, carvone, and limonene: potential cancer chemopreventive agents from dill weed oil and caraway oil. Planta Med 1992;58(4):338–41.

## Part 6: Biochemical Individuality

Assimos DG, Holmes RP. Role of diet in the therapy of urolithiasis. Urol Clin North Am. 2000;27(2):255–68.

Blanco C. Latex-fruit syndrome. Curr Allergy Asthma Rep 2003;3(1):47–53.

Conaway CC, Getahun SM, Liebes LL, et al. Disposition of glucosinolates and sulforaphane in humans after ingestion of steamed and fresh broccoli. Nutr Cancer 2000;38(2):168–78.

Crittenden RG, Bennett LE. Cow's milk allergy: a complex disorder. J Am Coll Nutr. 2005;24(6 Suppl): 582S–91S.

Curhan GC. Epidemiologic evidence for the role of oxalate in idiopathic nephrolithiasis. J Endourol 1999; 13(9):629–31.

Dalvi RR, Bowie WC. Toxicology of solanine: an overview. Vet Hum Toxicol 1983;25(1):13–5.

Environmental Working Group. Report card: pesticides in produce. http://www.foodnews.org/reportcard.php

Gunnison AF, Jacobsen DW. Sulfite hypersensitivity. A critical review. CRC Crit Rev Toxicol 1987;17(3):185–214.

Palosuo K, Varjonen E, Kekki OM, et al. Wheat omega-5 gliadin is a major allergen in children with immediate allergy to ingested wheat. J Allergy Clin Immunol 2001;108(4):634–8.

Sarwar G, Brule D. Assessment of the uricogenic potential of processed foods based on the nature and quantity of dietary purines. Prog Food Nutr Sci 1991;15(3):159–81.

Sheen SJ. Detection of nicotine in foods and plant materials. J Food Sci 1988;53(5):1572–3.

Urbano G, Lopez-Jurado M, Aranda P, et al. The role of phytic acid in legumes: antinutrient or beneficial function? Physiol Biochem 2000;56(3):283–94.

Varjonen E, Vainio E, Kalimo K Antigliadin IgE— indicator of wheat allergy in atopic dermatitis. Allergy 2000;55(4):386–91.

Vatn MH, Grimstad IA, Thorsen L, et al. Adverse reaction to food: assessment by double-blind placebo-controlled food challenge and clinical, psychosomatic and immunologic analysis. Digestion 1995;56(5):421–8.

## Part 7: Health-Promoting Nutrients from the World's Healthiest Foods

*For more references on specific nutrients, please see the bottom of the individual nutrients articles on the whfoods.org website (http://whfoods.org/nutrientstoc.php)*

Adlercreutz H, Mazur W. Phyto-oestrogens and Western diseases. Ann Med 1997;29(2):95–120.

Agarwal S, Rao AV. Carotenoids and chronic diseases. Drug Metabol Drug Interact 2000;17(1–4):189–210.

Chandra RK. Micronutrients and immune functions. Ann NY Acad Sci 1990;587:9–16.

Institute of Medicine. *Dietary Reference Intakes for Calcium, Phosphorus, Magnesium, Vitamin D, and Fluoride.* Washington, DC: National Academy Press; 1997.

Institute of Medicine. *Dietary Reference Intakes for Energy, Carbohydrate, Fiber, Fat, Fatty Acids, Cholesterol, Protein, and Amino Acids (Macronutrients).* Washington, DC: National Academy Press; 2005.

Institute of Medicine. *Dietary Reference Intakes for Thiamin, Riboflavin, Niacin, Vitamin B6, Folate, Vitamin B12, Pantothenic Acid, Biotin, and Choline.* Washington, DC: National Academy Press; 1998.

Institute of Medicine. *Dietary Reference Intakes for Vitamin A, Vitamin K, Arsenic, Boron, Chromium, Copper, Iodine, Iron, Manganese, Molybdenum, Nickel, Silicon, Vanadium, and Zinc.* Washington, DC: National Academy Press; 2001.

Institute of Medicine. *Dietary Reference Intakes for Vitamin C, Vitamin E, Selenium, and Carotenoids.* Washington, DC: National Academy Press; 2000.

Institute of Medicine. *Dietary Reference Intakes for Water, Potassium, Sodium, Chloride, and Sulfate.* Washington, DC: National Academy Press; 2004.

Institute of Medicine. *Dietary Reference Intakes: Proposed Definition of Dietary Fiber.* Washington DC: National Academy Press; 2001.

Institute of Medicine. *The Role of Protein and Amino Acids in Sustaining and Enhancing Performance.* Washington, DC: National Academy Press; 1999.

Middleton E, Kandaswami C. Effects of flavonoids on immune and inflammatory cell function. Biochem Pharmacol 1992;43(6):1167–1179.

# index

## A

# the author

George Mateljan has had a lifelong interest in food. From the time he was five years old, his favorite room in the house was the kitchen, where he watched as his mother lovingly spent hours preparing meals for the family. He still vividly remembers seeing a bowl full of ingredients transformed into dough that rose as if by magic. Then, after the dough went into the oven, he was tantalized by the fragrant aroma of it baking. He loved the wonderful look and taste of golden loaves of warm bread fresh from the oven.

By watching food being prepared for many years, George learned to appreciate the way each season brought forth its own special foods, including fresh fruits and vegetables. In the spring and summer, there were sweet, juicy strawberries, raspberries, apricots and many types of melons. In the fall, there were apples, oranges and sweet potatoes. And in the winter, there were hearty root vegetables such as beets, carrots and potatoes. George's favorite times were the holidays when he helped prepare special festive dishes.

George's continued passion for food sent him to the ends of the earth to learn about it. He has spent over 30 years traveling to over 80 countries around the world. He experienced cuisines from many cultures renowned for their health and longevity and appreciated the different foods and ways of preparing them that were unique to each.

George's education in biochemistry helped his understanding of what he learned through observing, tasting and formal training to create this better and healthier way of cooking. George earned a certificate studying French cuisine at the renowned La Varenne cooking school near Paris. He studied Italian cooking at the Guiliano Bugialli's cooking school in Florence. He refined his skills at the Gourmet's Oxford in England.

George was disappointed that he couldn't find nutritious, tasty and convenient foods for himself and his family, so in 1970 he founded Health Valley Foods, the first company to produce healthy prepared foods in the United States. As time went on, Health Valley produced thousands of convenient, enjoyable products that were packed with nutrition and flavor yet completely free from the white flour, refined sugar, hydrogenated fats, excess salt, chemical preservatives and artificial colors that are standard in highly processed foods.

George not only focused on the preparation of healthy foods, he also led the way in using safe, truthful, environmentally-friendly packaging and encouraged and supported organic farming. Health Valley Foods has since became the gold standard for healthy, tasty, conveniently-prepared foods.

In 1996, George sold Health Valley Foods. He felt that after 26 years he had inspired a number of others to establish companies to produce nutritious, conveniently-prepared foods, and it was time to turn his energies and resources toward the next phase of helping people enjoy eating healthier. Today, he shares, free of charge, his passion to help others, and his experiences and knowledge with everyone who wants to know about the "Healthiest Way of Eating" through the not-for-profit George Mateljan Foundation.

Over the years, George had come to identify which foods were among the World's Healthiest. And he also knew that in order to eat them on a regular basis the preparation of these foods had to fit the individual tastes and lifestyles of people in today's busy world. So, George worked to create and develop preparation methods and recipes that allow people to enjoy delicious and exciting flavors in easy and affordable ways. His Foundation supports an extensive website and the publication of books to share this information with you.

George has published five books that have been read and used by millions of people. This book is a culmination of his travels and personal experiences. It contains in-depth information on the techniques, recipes and menus that help make the "Healthiest Way of Eating" enjoyable, practical and personalized. It's the most recent example of how George's lifelong love of food can help people enjoy the World's Healthiest Foods to achieve vibrant health and energy and to live a longer and healthier life.

Thank YOU for walking your talk! Thank YOU for giving back! YOUR efforts to educate and inspire your fellow humans are appreciated. Very few people share their insights, wealth and success with others, so when I see someone like yourself who does,I wanted to take the time to say THANKS! — Mike

# The George Mateljan Foundation

*"Dedicated to help make a healthier world"*

The George Mateljan Foundation was established by George Mateljan to discover, develop and share scientifically proven information about the benefits of healthy eating through the World's Healthiest Foods website (whfoods.org) and to offer this information to you free of charge. The Foundation is also committed to the publication of books, such as the World's Healthiest Foods Essential Guide for the Healthiest Way of Eating, which are designed to complement the information on the website and provide easy, practical ways to integrate the "Healthiest Way of Eating" into your lifestyle.

## The Independent Perspective

The Foundation is not-for-profit so it can offer an independent perspective that is not influenced by commercial interests or advertising. Its only purpose is to help you discover the many joys and benefits of healthy eating. The Foundation's independent perspective can help provide clear and easy-to-understand knowledge on how people of all ages and backgrounds can achieve vibrant health and energy.

## Beliefs

The Foundation believes that true good health is more than just the absence of disease; it is a state where you enjoy all the energy and benefits life has to offer. One of the keys to achieving good health is to use the power of nutrient-rich foods to positively affect how you feel, how much energy you have, and the length and quality of your life. There is clear and definitive scientific evidence that nutrient-rich foods play an important and significant role in reducing the risk of degenerative diseases, and in providing long-term health and longevity.

The Foundation also believes that nutrient-rich foods not only have the power to provide good health, they also have the power to provide the pure joy of eating, and the joy of sharing with others. Each individual is unique, so everyone is not fit into the same "food formula." Biochemical individuality is respected and a wide variety of nutrient-rich food options are provided. That way each individual can discover the personalized information, recipes, cooking methods and menu plans to meet his or her needs.

## Our Mission

The George Mateljan Foundation's mission is to offer the latest scientific information about the benefits of the World's Healthiest Foods and the specific nutrients they provide. Equally important, the Foundation offers practical, simple and affordable ways to enjoy them that fit your individual lifestyle.

## Focus: Helping Everyone Learn How to Eat Healthier for Free

The George Mateljan Foundation is focused on using the power of nutrient-rich foods to achieve and maintain good health and the prevention of disease. George has devoted his life to discovering and understanding the benefits of the "Healthiest Way of Eating," and because of his passion for helping people, he believes that information on how to achieve vibrant health and energy should be accessible to everyone. So he has made the Foundation's website, www.whfoods.org, available free of charge, to anyone interested in learning about the "Healthiest Way of Eating."

The profits from the sale of this book go to the George Mateljan Foundation, a not-for-profit organization, which provides funding for research and education to promote the "Healthiest Way of Eating" and the "Healthiest Way of Cooking." The Foundation is dedicated to help make a healthier world.

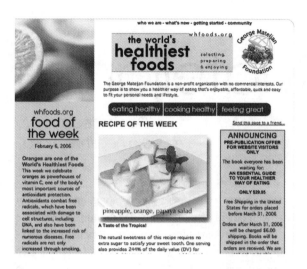

# the world's healthiest foods website

In addition to The World's Healthiest Foods: Essential Guide to the Healthiest Way of Eating, the George Mateljan Foundation has created the World's Healthiest Foods website (www.whfoods.org). This online resource, launched in 2001, provides extensive information on enjoyable and convenient ways to eat healthier. The George Mateljan Foundation is a non-profit organization with no commercial interests. Our purpose is to show you the healthiest way of eating that's enjoyable, affordable and easy and will fit your personal needs and lifestyle.

The book and the website are designed to complement each other, helping you to better understand the benefits of the "Healthiest Way of Eating." While the book provides many features not included on the website, whfoods.org utilizes the inherent technology of the Internet and is designed to offer extensive up-to-date information, interactivity, colorful pictures, animated graphics and video capability.

## #1 Website

For the last two years the whfoods.org website has come up #1 when doing a Google search for "healthiest foods." It has also recently been recognized as an extraordinarily good website and awarded as:

*#1 'Best of the Best' in Healthy Eating in 'The Web's Greatest Hits for 2005'*

*by Lynie Arden*

## We Keep the Website Current

Each week the website highlights one of the World's Healthiest Foods that is currently in season and provides the latest information about that food and a "Recipe of the Week" featuring that food. We also provide a "Food Tip of the Week" and "Breakthrough Scientific Information," which reports on the latest findings from recent scientific papers. "Ask George," provides in-depth information on a new topic each week. Additionally, the website offers a free Weekly Bulletin for which you can sign up; it contains information about the website's "Food of the Week" as well as an editorial about what is current in the world of nutrition and the "Healthiest Way of Eating." The website is updated each week with the latest scientific findings having to do with the World's Healthiest Foods.

## What the Website Has to Offer

### IN-DEPTH INFORMATION

Whfoods.org is a veritable encyclopedia, providing information on important topics concerning food, nutrition and preparation. The information combines scientific research and the expertise of nutrition and cooking professionals, presented in a style that is both intelligent and easy-to-understand. As the website is supported by the George Mateljan Foundation and not by any advertising interests, it provides education in a thorough and unbiased way, entirely free of charge.

One of the most frequent comments that we hear from website users is their appreciation of just how much information is provided. The website features detailed information on the World's Healthiest Foods and over 100 recipes. It shows you how to prepare foods, enhance flavor and nutritional value, and enjoy healthy meals, many of which can be prepared in as little as 15 minutes. We also provide information on nutrients, popular diets, nutrition through the lifestages… the list goes on and on. And with an easy-to-use search feature, you can find all of the information on any topic you are researching in a matter of a few seconds.

On the whfoods.org website you will find extensive and comprehensive information about organically grown foods. It will help you to decipher the U.S. government's organic regulations as well as understand how to read organic food labels. Additionally, it provides a research-based investigation into why organic foods are not only better for your health but for the health of the planet as well.

The website also provides an in-depth look into other topics including digestion, food sensitivities, and cellular nutrition. Not only does this information provide intelligent insights into subjects that lie at the essence of nutrition and healthy living, but it includes animated graphics designed to create a visual context that relays the information in a more educational and enjoyable way.

# What Can the World's Healthiest Foods Website Do for You?

### ASK THE FOOD ADVISOR

Whfoods.org makes great use of the available technology offered by the Internet. You will find interactive features such as the "Food Advisor," a unique program developed to help you assess and improve your diet. By spending no more than five minutes completing the questionnaire, you can receive valuable information that highlights nutrients that may be deficient in your diet, as well as food and recipe recommendations that will help you fulfill your individual nutritional needs. Since the results are based upon your diet and targeted for your specific requirements, you will receive recommendations that are tailored just for you.

### ASK GEORGE AND THE Q & A LIBRARY

Although the whfoods.org website is a comprehensive resource, we realize that there still may be individual questions that remain unanswered. Therefore "Ask George" is a feature that enables you to ask a team of professional nutritionists your personal questions about the nutritional benefits of a particular food, how to prepare it or generally how to eat healthier. The Q & A Library is also a great place to find answers to questions about food, nutrition, the latest news, organic foods and a host of other topics.

### 5-MINUTE IN-HOME COOKING SCHOOL

To help you to better experience how nutrient-rich foods can benefit your health, the website provides the In-Home Cooking School that shows you how to easily prepare these foods. It features over 100 preparation tips with text and animated photographs that visually show you how to easily prepare foods.

### WHFOODS KITCHEN

The WHFoods Kitchen provides information about preparing some of your favorite foods, how to cook healthy foods with the seasons, and healthy meal planning.

### RECIPES AND RECIPE ASSISTANT

There are over 100 quick and easy recipes that have been created especially for the website. Each recipe features both a Nutrient Richness Chart as well as a complete nutritional profile. Additionally, the website features the Recipe Assistant that can perform a search on the website's database of recipes, looking for ones that highlight either a particular food or nutrient in which you are interested.

### SEND US A FAVORITE RECIPE

Another interactive feature on the website is "Send Us a Favorite Recipe" where you can post your own original healthy recipe and enjoy those of other website users.

### FEELING GREAT MENU

The Feeling Great Menu is a great way to start you on your path to the "Healthiest Way of Eating." It provides you with 7 days of recipes and snacks that are highly nutritious and easy to prepare. A nutrient analysis is presented for each day's menu so you know precisely the nutritional benefits you will be deriving from any one day. And it is flexible as well. You can interchange the recipes with other favorites you find on the list of recipes created specifically for the website and enjoy!

### LOG ON...

While The World's Healthiest Food Essential Guide to the Healthiest Way of Eating serves as a timeless reference for cooking and health, whfoods.org provides you with additional information that can help you enjoy the World's Healthiest Foods. So continue your journey of healthier eating and log on to www.whfoods.org.

### LETTERS FROM OUR READERS

As the testimonials featured on the website profess, whfoods.org is a unique site that can help to enrich your life by assisting you in the journey of healthier eating. Here are some examples:

*"I was totally amazed when I first saw your site. It was like… er… look, strange, no annoying ads trying to sell you something… hey, no paying for access to "really useful information" section. Is this for real? Let me click on every link on the left just to be sure there isn't a login trap somewhere. No, seriously; top-notch layout, enormous quantity of excellent info, very well organized, overall "no nonsense, no mystique" attitude… That's what a good website should be all about and that's something you rarely see around. Thanks for putting this up. Thank you!"—Nenad*

*Your site is priceless! I rely on your site for so much information. Thanks for all you do.—Peg*

*I would like to say thank you to the creator and those who contribute to www.whfoods.org. This is a clear and informative website that allows the viewer to make sensible decisions based on credible scientific research. —Nushien*

*First let me start off by saying how great this site is, how amazing the recipes are and how much it has helped me to maintain a healthy lifestyle and make better food choices.—Janis*

*This site is excellent! This is a very informative, educative and interesting site which every health conscious person must visit. A great and easy way to learn about the goodness of food and healthy living.—Jay*

*Thanks for such a comprehensive and informative site. This site empowers me to find out for myself what foods are going to serve my body best and those which serve no purpose. So, in short, thanks! I am now a regular visitor.—Phoebe*

*Thank you for your work... Wow! This is such a great site. It's so refreshing to see a non-biased site on nutrition. I have never come across a site so complete, informative and helpful.—Darden*

*Really enjoy your site—helps keep me healthy—James*

*This is the most reliable site where we can be sure of getting right, unbiased information!!—Richa*

*Wonderful site! I came across this site a year or two ago and was quite impressed and continue to be. I appreciate so much the variety and quality of content and that all is well referenced and regularly updated (and that you tell us what has been updated). Thank you for the great resource.—Rebecca*

*I am so happy to have stumbled upon this site! I have been referencing it for some time; whenever I am curious about what I am eating. I just look it up! I love the history, the addition of updated studies, and the description of the functions each highlighted nutrient has on our bodies. Overall, this is a terrific source of info for health-conscious people who are serious about feeding themselves and their families nutritious foods.—Erika*

*I love your site. It is informative, thoughtful and a tremendous contribution to society.—Anestine*

*Incredible webpage. I can't believe the amount of work you have put into this site. Everything you say is advice and information. This site is a wealth of important info and I thank you for putting it together. It truly is making a difference so all your hard work is worth it!—Holmes*

*I wish to thank you very much for your wonderful website! I tell everyone I can about your website and how educational and informative it is. You provide a wealth of knowledge, and I feel your site is the very best on the entire internet. Thank you again for providing such excellent information about health and nutrition. You do make a difference in people's lives by the wealth of knowledge you provide.—Valerie*

*Thank you! Just a note to congratulate and to thank you for a most informative and health-inspiring site. I have been consulting your web pages for the past 2 months, and am applying the basic good food know-how to my whole family.—Lisa*

*Firstly, let me compliment you on a superb web site, informative, colorful and educational. Excellent in fact... I know I trawled through hundreds of sites looking for the food information you have on your site. Thank you again for a great service and a great site. I have received more information from your site than anywhere else (including Oxford University Medical Dept)!! Thank you again for a great service and a great site.—Barry*

*My doctor turned me on to your website. I have to say that this is the BEST website of its kind that I have ever seen! The amount of useful info is amazing! Although I am now eating many of the foods you list, I have plans to add more. I also understand HOW these foods keep me healthy. Thanks for a GREAT job and keep it up!! I'm also sending your web address to friends and family members.—Deb*

*Finally, an honest answer about food and everything you should know about it in an easy to use and easy to ready way.—AR*

*From one nonprofit to another, I seriously applaud you in your work. When other nonprofits stand up and applaud you, it does mean something. Fantastic website! Fantastic information!—LeAnn*

## HEALTHCARE PROFESSIONALS

*I am ecstatic to have found your website. I'm a board certified family physician. It is very refreshing to see this site which offers untainted, vital information which hopefully will empower people to understand and make better nutritional choices. I'm placing it on top of my favorites list.—James*

*LET ALL MY PATIENTS FOLLOW YOUR ADVICE. I am really impressed, and I want to promote your site and advice to all my patients. I would love to be a part of your mission.—Dr. Chary*

*As a nutritionist I provide your site to my patients.—Lada*